AIIMS-MAMC-PGI IMAGING SERIES

DIAGNOSTIC RADIOLOGY

Musculoskeletal and Breast Imaging

PIONEERS OF AIIMS-MAMC-PGI IMAGING SERIES

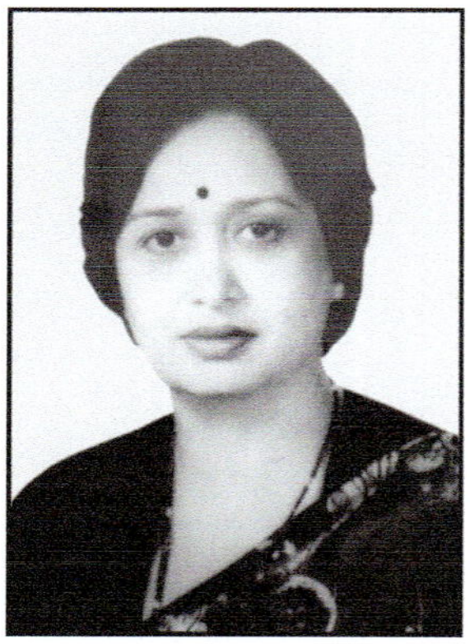

Manorama Berry

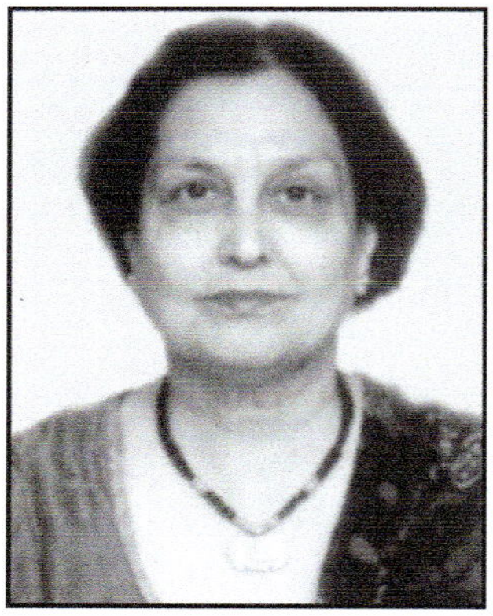

Sudha Suri

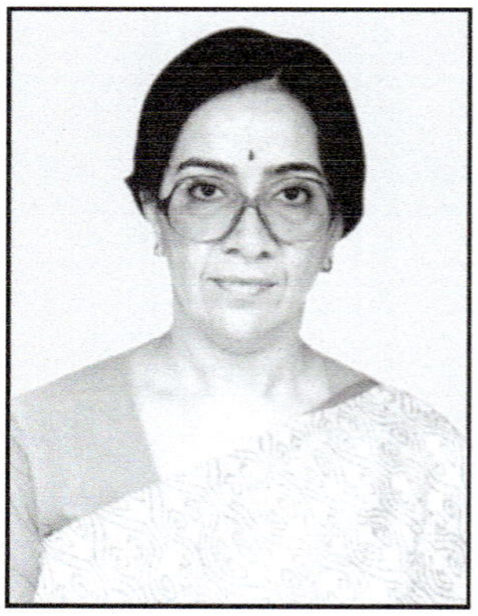

Veena Chowdhury

PAST EDITORS

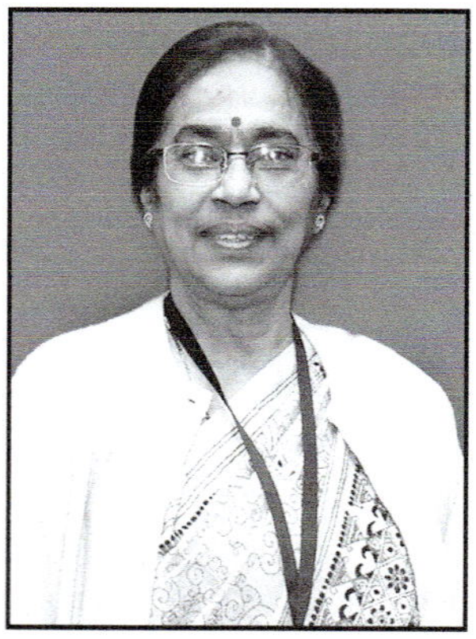

Sima Mukhopadhyay

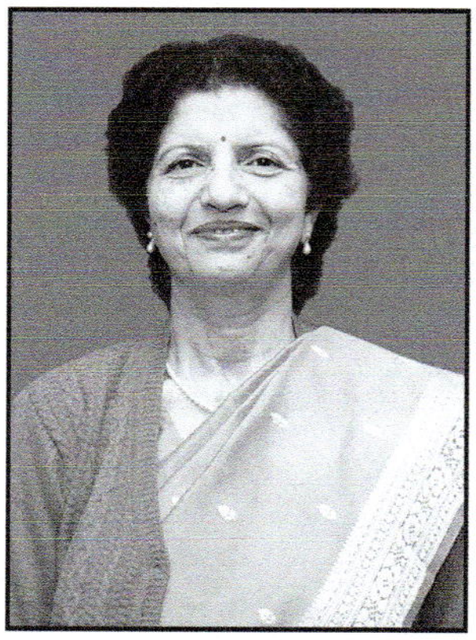

Sushma Vashisht

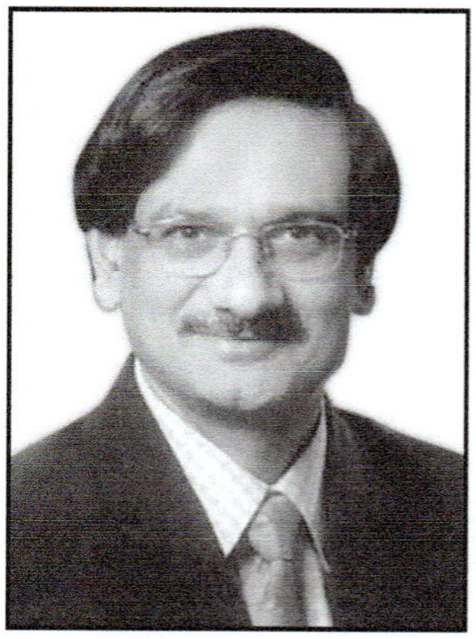

Niranjan Khandelwal

AIIMS-MAMC-PGI IMAGING SERIES

DIAGNOSTIC RADIOLOGY

Musculoskeletal and Breast Imaging

Fourth Edition

Editors

Manavjit Singh Sandhu
MD FICR
Professor and Head
Department of Radiodiagnosis
Postgraduate Institute of Medical Education and Research
Chandigarh, India

Arun Kumar Gupta
MD FAMS
Professor and Head
Department of Radiodiagnosis
All India Institute of Medical Sciences
New Delhi, India

Anju Garg
MD
Director-Professor and Head
Department of Radiodiagnosis
Maulana Azad Medical College
New Delhi, India

Associate Editors

Mahesh Prakash
MD MAMS FIACM FICR
Professor
Department of Radiodiagnosis
Postgraduate Institute of Medical
Education and Research
Chandigarh, India

Anindita Sinha
MD MAMS
Additional Professor
Department of Radiodiagnosis
Postgraduate Institute of Medical
Education and Research
Chandigarh, India

JAYPEE

JAYPEE BROTHERS MEDICAL PUBLISHERS

The Health Sciences Publisher

New Delhi | London

Jaypee Brothers Medical Publishers (P) Ltd

Headquarters
EMCA House
23/23-B, Ansari Road, Daryaganj
New Delhi 110 002, India
Landline: +91-11-23272143, +91-11-23272703
+91-11-23282021, +91-11-23245672
E-mail: jaypee@jaypeebrothers.com

Corporate Office
4838/24, Ansari Road, Daryaganj
New Delhi 110 002, India
Phone: +91-11-43574357
Fax: +91-11-43574314
E-mail: jaypee@jaypeebrothers.com

Overseas Office
J.P. Medical Ltd
83 Victoria Street, London
SW1H 0HW (UK)
Phone: +44 20 3170 8910
E-mail: info@jpmedpub.com

EU GPSR Authorised Representative
Logos Europe, 9 rue Nicolas Poussin
17000, La Rochelle, France
Phone: +33 (0) 6 67 93 73 78
E-mail: contact@logoseurope.eu

Website: www.jaypeebrothers.com
Website: www.jaypeedigital.com

Diagnostic Radiology: Musculoskeletal and Breast Imaging

First Edition: 1998
Second Edition: 2005
Reprint Edition: 2011
Third Edition: 2012
Fourth Edition: 2021
Reprint: **2026**

ISBN: 978-93-90020-55-3

Printed in India

Contributors

Ajay Kumar MD
Professor
Department of Radiodiagnosis
Postgraduate Institute of Medical Education and Research
Chandigarh, India

Akshay Saxena MD DNB FICR
Professor
Department of Radiodiagnosis
Postgraduate Institute of Medical Education and Research
Chandigarh, India

Alpana Manchanda MD
Director-Professor
Department of Radiodiagnosis
Maulana Azad Medical College
New Delhi, India

Anindita Sinha MD MAMS
Additional Professor
Department of Radiodiagnosis
Postgraduate Institute of Medical Education and Research
Chandigarh, India

Anjali Prakash DMRD DNB MNAMS
Director-Professor
Department of Radiodiagnosis
Maulana Azad Medical College
New Delhi, India

Anju Garg MD
Director-Professor and Head
Department of Radiodiagnosis
Maulana Azad Medical College
New Delhi, India

Ankur Goyal MD DNB MNAMS
Associate Professor
Department of Radiodiagnosis
All India Institute of Medical Sciences
New Delhi, India

Arun Kumar Gupta MD FAMS
Professor and Head
Department of Radiodiagnosis
All India Institute of Medical Sciences
New Delhi, India

Ashu Seith Bhalla MD MAMS FICR
Professor
Department of Radiodiagnosis
All India Institute of Medical Sciences
New Delhi, India

Atin Kumar MD DNB MNAMS FICR
Professor
Department of Radiodiagnosis
(Trauma Center Division)
All India Institute of Medical Sciences
New Delhi, India

Chirag Kamal Ahuja MD DM
Associate Professor
Department of Radiodiagnosis
Postgraduate Institute of Medical Education and Research
Chandigarh, India

Deep Narayan Srivastava
MD MBA FAMS FICR
Professor
Department of Radiodiagnosis
All India Institute of Medical Sciences
New Delhi, India

Devasenathipathy Kandasamy
MD DNB FRCR
Additional Professor
Department of Radiodiagnosis
All India Institute of Medical Sciences
New Delhi, India

Ekta Dhamija MD
Associate Professor
Department of Radiodiagnosis
(BRA IRCH Division)
All India Institute of Medical Sciences
New Delhi, India

Gaurav Shanker Pradhan
MBBS DMRD DNB
Director-Professor
Department of Radiodiagnosis
Maulana Azad Medical College
New Delhi, India

Gita Devi MD DNB
Assistant Professor
Department of Radiodiagnosis
Postgraduate Institute of Medical Education and Research
Chandigarh, India

Harish Bhujade
MD Fellowship (Interventional Radiology)
Assistant Professor
Department of Radiodiagnosis
Postgraduate Institute of Medical Education and Research
Chandigarh, India

Jyoti Kumar MD DNB MNAMS FICR
Professor
Department of Radiodiagnosis
Maulana Azad Medical College
New Delhi, India

Kushaljit Singh Sodhi
MD PhD MAMS FICR
Professor
Department of Radiodiagnosis
Postgraduate Institute of Medical Education and Research
Chandigarh, India

Madhavi Tripathi
MD DNB (Nuclear Medicine)
Additional Professor
Department of Nuclear Medicine and PET
All India Institute of Medical Sciences
New Delhi, India

Madhusudhan KS MD MAMS FRCR
Additional Professor
Department of Radiodiagnosis
All India Institute of Medical Sciences
New Delhi, India

Mahesh Prakash MD MAMS FIACM FICR
Professor
Department of Radiodiagnosis
Postgraduate Institute of Medical Education and Research
Chandigarh, India

Manavjit Singh Sandhu MD FICR
Professor and Head
Department of Radiodiagnosis
Postgraduate Institute of Medical Education and Research
Chandigarh, India

Mandeep Kang MD MAMS FICR
Professor
Department of Radiodiagnosis
Postgraduate Institute of Medical Education and Research
Chandigarh, India

Manisha Jana MD DNB FRCR
Additional Professor
Department of Radiodiagnosis
All India Institute of Medical Sciences
New Delhi, India

Manphool Singhal MD DNB MAMS
Additional Professor
Department of Radiodiagnosis
Postgraduate Institute of Medical Education and Research
Chandigarh, India

Mukesh Kumar Yadav
(MD Radiodiagnosis)
Formerly Associate Professor
PGIMER, Chandigarh
Associate Professor
Department of Radiodiagnosis
All India Institute of Medical Sciences (IRCH)
New Delhi, India

Nidhi Prabhakar MD DNB
Senior Research Associate
Department of Radiodiagnosis
Postgraduate Institute of Medical Education and Research
Chandigarh, India

Paramjeet Singh MD
Professor
Department of Radiodiagnosis
Postgraduate Institute of Medical Education and Research
Chandigarh, India

Priyanka Naranje MD DNB MNAMS
Associate Professor
Department of Radiodiagnosis
All India Institute of Medical Sciences
New Delhi, India

Radhika Batra MD DNB
Assistant Professor
Department of Radiodiagnosis
Maulana Azad Medical College
New Delhi, India

Raju Sharma MD MAMS FICR
Professor
Department of Radiodiagnosis
All India Institute of Medical Sciences
New Delhi, India

Rakesh Kumar DRM DNB PhD
Professor and Head
Diagnostic Nuclear Medicine Division
Department of Nuclear Medicine and PET
All India Institute of Medical Sciences
New Delhi, India

Rashmi Dixit MD
Director-Professor
Department of Radiodiagnosis
Maulana Azad Medical College
New Delhi, India

Sameer Vyas MD DM
Additional Professor
Department of Radiodiagnosis
Postgraduate Institute of Medical Education and Research
Chandigarh, India

Sapna Singh MD DNB MNAMS
Professor
Department of Radiodiagnosis
Maulana Azad Medical College
New Delhi, India

Shamim Ahmed Shamim
MD (Nuclear Medicine)
Associate Professor
Department of Nuclear Medicine
All India Institute of Medical Sciences
New Delhi, India

Shivanand Gamanagatti
MD MAMS FICR
Professor
Department of Radiodiagnosis
(Trauma Center Division)
All India Institute of Medical Sciences
New Delhi, India

Smita Manchanda MD DNB
Associate Professor
Department of Radiodiagnosis
All India Institute of Medical Sciences
New Delhi, India

Smriti Hari MD MAMS
Professor
Department of Radiodiagnosis
All India Institute of Medical Sciences
New Delhi, India

Surabhi Vyas MD DNB MNAMS
Additional Professor
Department of Radiodiagnosis
All India Institute of Medical Sciences
New Delhi, India

Swati Gupta MD DNB FRCR
Assistant Professor
Department of Radiodiagnosis
Maulana Azad Medical College
New Delhi, India

Tulika Singh MD
Additional Professor
Department of Radiodiagnosis
Postgraduate Institute of Medical Education and Research
Chandigarh, India

Ujjwal Gorsi (MD Radiodiagnosis)
Associate Professor
Department of Radiodiagnosis
Postgraduate Institute of Medical Education and Research
Chandigarh, India

Uma Debi MD
Associate Professor
Department of Radiodiagnosis
Postgraduate Institute of Medical Education and Research
Chandigarh, India

Veenu Singla MD
Professor
Department of Radiodiagnosis
Postgraduate Institute of Medical Education and Research
Chandigarh, India

Vikas Bhatia MD DM
Assistant Professor
Department of Radiodiagnosis
Postgraduate Institute of Medical Education and Research
Chandigarh, India

Preface to the Fourth Edition

The scope and use of various imaging modalities in musculoskeletal radiology and breast imaging has increased manifold since the publication of the third edition of this book. While radiographs remain the cornerstone of diagnosis of musculoskeletal lesions, this edition also highlights the basics and advances in cross-sectional imaging with special emphasis and coverage of imaging with MRI.

The first edition of *Musculoskeletal and Breast Imaging* was published in 1998; the second edition in 2005; followed by the third edition in 2012.

The present edition has incorporated 4 new chapters in the musculoskeletal subsections and 2 new chapters in the breast subsection. The content has been divided into 7 different subsections, beginning with current concepts and interventions. The first section deals with all imaging modalities in musculoskeletal imaging. There is an updated section on MR imaging, including new additions of imaging of wrist and ankle; peripheral nerve imaging and imaging of prosthetic joints. All chapters have been thoroughly revised.

The second part of the book contains updated chapters on Breast imaging and interventions and includes two new chapters on *Male Breast Imaging* and *Advances in Breast Imaging*.

We hope this edition will serve as a concise yet comprehensive guide for students and practitioners of radiodiagnosis as well as a ready reckoner to clinicians in understanding the basics as well as current advances in imaging and interventions.

The editors take this opportunity to thank the faculty of the three institutions who have put their collective experience and effort in this book. We would also like to express our appreciation to Shri Jitendar P Vij (Group Chairman), Mr Ankit Vij (Managing Director), Ms Chetna Malhotra Vohra (Associate Director–Content Strategy), Ms Nedup Denka Bhutia (Development Editor) and the other staff of M/s Jaypee Brothers Medical Publishers (P) Ltd, New Delhi, India, for their professionalism and dedication towards publication of this book.

Manavjit Singh Sandhu
Arun Kumar Gupta
Anju Garg

Preface to the First Edition

There has been a significant increase in the awareness as well as in the actual incidence of detection of disorders related to the musculoskeletal system and the breast over the years. At the same time, a continuous revolution, occurring in the field of imaging over these years, has given a new insight in the proper diagnosis, management and follow-up of these disorders. With the availability of a large number of imaging techniques today, including conventional radiology, computed tomography (CT), magnetic resonance imaging (MRI), ultrasonography (USG), interventional procedures and radioisotope studies, each having its own merits and limitations, it has become essential on the part of the present day radiologist to be able to advise and use the most cost-effective methodology in a given clinical situation. Such a need assumes even a greater importance in the limited resources situation of a developing country. It is necessary for a radiologist of today to learn the basic aspects and the role of various imaging modalities in a given clinical situation for taking the fullest advantage of these modalities. The need for a closer cooperation and understanding of each other's role between the radiologist and a clinician had never been felt greater before.

The present book on *Musculoskeletal and Breast Imaging*, the fifth in the series of AIIMS-MAMC-PGI imaging courses, is a further attempt in this direction. The book has been broadly divided into two sections, i.e., the musculoskeletal disorders and the breast disorders, each section dealing at length with the relevant imaging techniques and their interpretations in various disease processes. There are 19 chapters, dealing with all important aspects of these systems.

The multimodality imaging approach to bone, soft tissue and joint diseases is presented while retaining the major emphasis on conventional radiological findings. There are separate sections devoted to imaging modalities for infections and inflammations, metabolic bone disorders and tumors. The text is intended to assist in the interpretation of imaging studies of patients with these disorders and in suggesting the appropriate imaging technique to the clinicians involved in their care.

The role of mammography in early diagnosis of breast cancer and in helping in breast conservation need not be overemphasized. The section on breast imaging deals in detail with the role of screening mammography, its relevance as it pertains to our country, the current status of various other imaging modalities and future directions in the imaging of breast. The purpose of this book is to provide the reader with essential information in all important aspects of the subspecialty of musculoskeletal and breast imaging, and we hope that it serves as a compliment to the AIIMS-MAMC-PGI course, through its concise, comprehensive and current survey on the subject.

We are grateful to all our faculty staff and other eminent teachers for contributing their experiences through their excellent write-ups in all these volumes providing a balanced view on the modern day practice of Radiology in various clinical situations. We also thank the series publishers M/s Jaypee Brothers Medical Publishers (P) Ltd, New Delhi, India, Shri Jitendar P Vij (Chairman and Managing Director) and other staff, for timely publication of all these volumes in an excellent form. But for their active and persistent involvement, such a gigantic task would not have been a reality. We do sincerely hope that all these volumes, including the present one published under the AIIMS-MAMC-PGI imaging course series, shall be able to fulfill the desired aims and shall continue to guide the readers in their daily office practice of radiology. Readers response shall always remain the ultimate guiding spirit in this direction.

Manorama Berry
Veena Chowdhury
Sudha Suri
Sima Mukhopadhyay

Contents

Section 5: MRI of Joints

Section 6: Miscellaneous MSK-trauma/Soft Tissue/Nerve/Prosthetics Imaging

Section 7: Breast Imaging and Interventions

SECTION

1

Current Concepts and Intervention

CHAPTER

1

Current Concepts in Cross-sectional Imaging of Musculoskeletal Diseases

Shivanand Gamanagatti, Ankur Goyal, Raju Sharma

INTRODUCTION

Imaging of musculoskeletal diseases has seen a paradigm shift with increased emphasis on cross-sectional modalities including high-resolution ultrasound (HRUS), computed tomography (CT), and magnetic resonance imaging (MRI). HRUS is fast becoming the modality of choice for evaluation of soft tissue structures while CT serves to accurately assess bone pathology. MRI provides excellent contrast resolution of both marrow disorders as well as soft tissue diseases. This chapter provides an insight into the role of ultrasound (US) and CT and focuses on MRI assessment of musculoskeletal diseases.

Cross-sectional imaging of the musculoskeletal system has made immense progress in the last two decades. The pace of innovation has been maximum in MRI and it has become a versatile and virtually indispensable imaging modality for many musculoskeletal applications. Developments such as high-performance magnetic resonance (MR) systems and optimized coil technology have led to improvements in spatial resolution and signal-to-noise and better cost-effectiveness of MR studies.[1] This in turn has led to improved diagnosis in shorter period of time and better understanding of complex orthopedic disorders. This chapter aims to briefly outline the basic principles of musculoskeletal MRI and highlights the recent advances in this exciting and ever-changing specialty.

ULTRASONOGRAPHY

Musculoskeletal US is currently gaining popularity by leaps and bounds. Not only radiologists, but other specialties are also increasingly using US for both diagnostic and therapeutic purposes. US is a multiplanar cross-sectional imaging modality which provides high-resolution information regarding soft tissue structures. Low cost, dynamic evaluation, and unrestricted field-of-view (FOV) work in its favor along with the opportunity to combine with comprehensive clinical examination. There are no contraindications, radiation exposure or risks involved and US can be repeated any number of times. Portability of the US equipment has enabled its use in the operation theaters as well as in the sports field.

Ultrasound probe frequencies ranging from 5 to 18 MHz are optimal for musculoskeletal imaging. US waves travel through different soft tissues at different speeds based on the propagation speed of that tissue. The propagation speed depends not only on the density of the tissue, but also on the number of internal reflective structures, for example, tendon fibers, which absorb or reflect the sound wave energy. The transducer also acts as a receiver for the reflected sound waves. In brief, less dense structures such as fluid that lack tissue interfaces will appear as dark or hypoechoic, whereas more dense structures with multiple interfaces such as tendon will appear brighter or hyperechoic. The tissue interfaces also produce typical features of a tissue, such as the regular parallel lines of a tendon or ligament, which aid in their identification. US is an operator dependent technique; hence it is important for the radiologist to be well trained for performing musculoskeletal studies.

Ultrasound provides excellent spatial contrast for evaluation of tendons, ligaments, and nerves. The ligaments can be seen as fibrillar structures and any tears can be easily seen **(Fig. 1)**. Stress maneuvers can be applied while doing US so as to diagnose nonretracted tears as well. US is used to evaluate a wide spectrum of tendon diseases such as degenerative/traumatic tears of the rotator cuff, ankle tendons, as well as tenosynovitis, tendinosis, and masses **(Figs. 2 and 3)**. Nerves can be easily scanned throughout their course and comparison with the contralateral side can also be done in equivocal cases **(Figs. 4A and B)**. Panoramic view (extended FOV) function helps to demonstrate longitudinal structures (which are longer than the probe length) by moving the probe along the same. Joint effusions, synovial thickening, and bony erosions are also easily discernible and Doppler signal aids in assessment of active synovitis **(Figs. 5A to D)**. US has become a valuable tool in diagnosis and follow-up of patients with inflammatory arthritis to demonstrate early inflammatory changes such as synovitis, tenosynovitis, enthesitis, and also helps in identification of early bone erosions with added advantage of color Doppler to visualize the vascularity. Tumor and tumor-like masses (including vascular malformations) can also be comprehensively evaluated using US and Doppler.

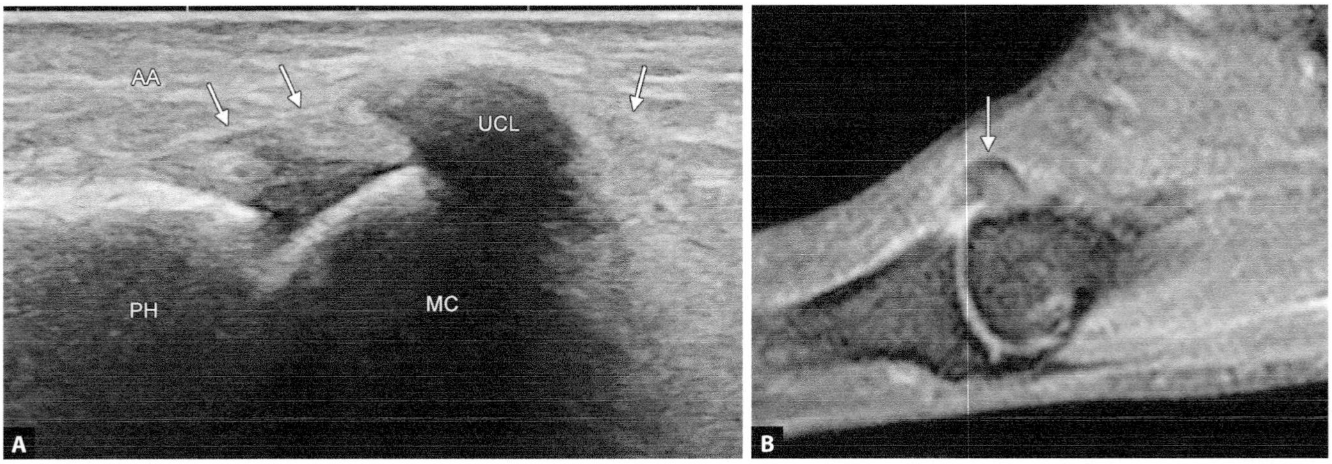

Figs. 1A and B: (A) Ultrasound image along the ulnar collateral ligament (UCL) of the thumb shows retracted ligament with adductor aponeurosis (AA) interposed between the ligament and its distal insertion, suggesting Stener lesion; (B) Coronal proton density (PD) fat suppression magnetic resonance image shows the same findings (arrow shows retracted UCL in B). (MC: metacarpal; PH: phalanx)

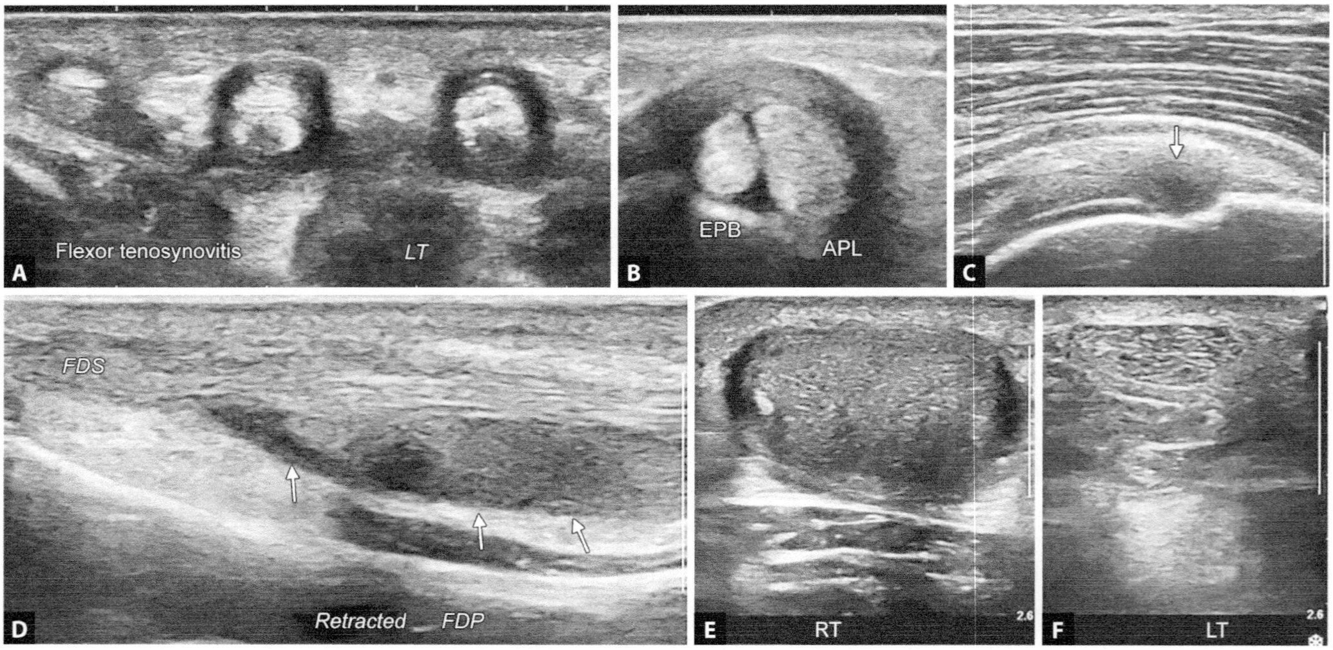

Figs. 2A to F: Ultrasound spectrum of tendon disorders. (A) Axial ultrasound image shows presence of hypoechoic tenosynovitis around the flexor tendons of the left hand; (B) Ultrasound image shows de Quervain's tenosynovitis around the first extensor compartment tendons; (C) Ultrasound image in oblique coronal plane along the long axis of supraspinatus shows hypoechogenicity at insertion site (arrow), suggesting tendinosis; (D) Oblique sagittal image shows retracted tendon of flexor digitorum profundus after glass-cut injury of the hand; (E) Axial ultrasound image shows bulky hypoechoic degenerated Achilles tendon in contrast to small echogenic contralateral tendon (F). (APL: abductor pollicis longus; EPB: extensor pollicis brevis; FDP: flexor digitorum profundus; FDS: flexor digitorum superficialis; LT: left; RT: right)

US permits real time imaging, which allows for provocative maneuvers to detect entities which are not well shown on static imaging such as elbow flexion maneuver to elicit ulnar nerve subluxation at cubital tunnel, hip flexion to elicit snapping of iliopsoas tendon, and real-time muscle contraction in diagnosis of myofascial herniation.

Ultrasound elastography may serve to distinguish benign from malignant soft tissue masses. Also, elastography may detect tendon degeneration before it becomes apparent on gray-scale US. *Contrast-enhanced US (CEUS)* employing gas microbubbles is another addition to US armamentarium, which enables accurate detection of solid viable components in a soft tissue mass. This contrast media is exhaled via lungs and thus can be safely used even in the presence of renal dysfunction. CEUS provides real-time dynamic assessment of perfusion

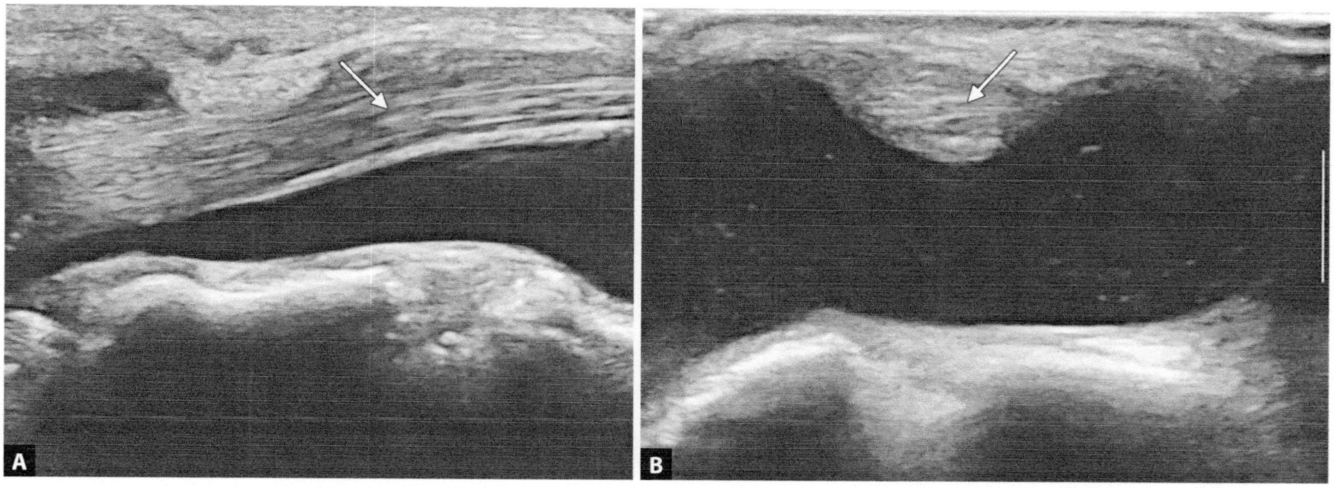

Figs. 3A and B: Longitudinal and transverse ultrasound images of ankle showing large fluid collection along the intact tibialis anterior tendon (arrows) suggestive of tenosynovitis.

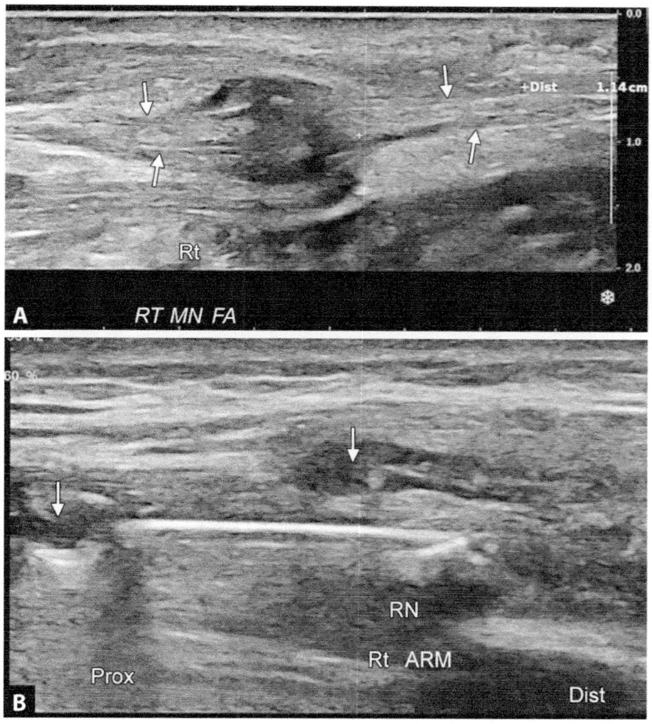

Figs. 4A and B: Ultrasound images showing nerve diseases. (A) Long-axis ultrasound image along the median nerve shows complete transection with discontinuity of epineurium and neuroma in continuity; (B) Another patient with radial nerve transection shows separation and retraction of the nerve ends, forming neuromas (arrows).

and thus aids in distinguishing high-flow and low-flow lesions. Contrast-enhancement may also serve to assess disease activity in synovial inflammation.

Ultrasound is widely used to guide musculoskeletal interventional procedures such as joint fluid aspiration, drainage of fluid collections, tissue biopsy, injection of tendon sheaths, joints, bursae, and peritendinous soft tissues (e.g., common extensor tendon at lateral epicondyle for tennis elbow) **(Figs. 5A to D)**. Also, US provides a viable imaging method in the presence of metallic prosthesis, to evaluate periprosthetic collections, hematoma, and ligaments, since prosthesis produce artifacts on MRI.

It may be noted however, that US may not be a standalone modality and correlation with radiographs or other cross-sectional modalities may be required to clinch the diagnosis.

COMPUTED TOMOGRAPHY

Computed tomography is the investigation of choice for evaluation of bony structures. With the introduction of MRI, role of CT in musculoskeletal imaging has somewhat declined, particularly for soft tissue imaging. Nonetheless, CT has certain inherent advantages that make it a robust tool for some musculoskeletal pathology. CT is most commonly used to evaluate bone trauma, for acute fractures of spine, to detect subtle fractures when the radiograph is normal, fractures of complex anatomical areas such as pelvis, maxillofacial area, and scapula, evaluation of intra-articular fractures, to plan operative reduction of complex fractures, and to diagnose osseous nonunion of fractures. In trauma setting, CT is the workhorse, serving as the gold standard to diagnose complex and multiple fractures. Many classification systems of traumatic fractures are also based on CT and help in deciding the management. CT has obviated the need of taking radiographs at different angulations and projections in sick patients. CT is also used to evaluate various measurements such as after joint replacement, angle of femoral neck anteversion prior to rotation osteotomy, tibial tuberosity-trochlear groove (TT-TG) distance in case of recurrent patellar dislocation, and measurements in evaluation of scoliosis and femoroacetabular impingement. More recently,

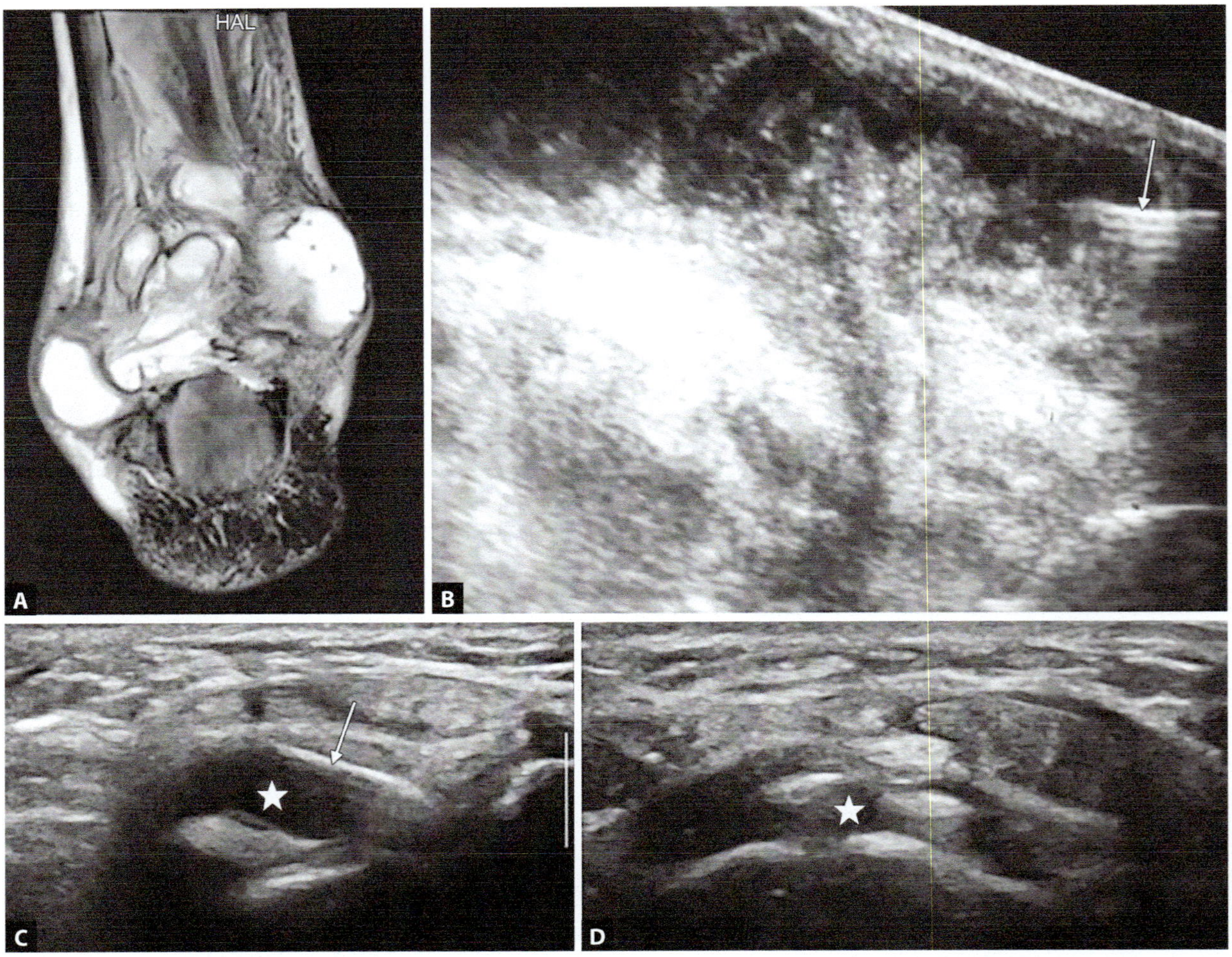

Figs. 5A to D: Ultrasound-guided interventions. (A) Coronal short tau inversion recovery (STIR) image shows multiple collections in the ankle joint; (B) Ultrasound image shows severe synovial thickening with effusion with aspiration needle in situ (arrow); (C) Ultrasound image in a different patient of dorsal wrist ganglion (star) shows needle in situ (arrow) for fenestration of the wall; (D) Development of echogenicity within the ganglion cyst (star) after steroid injection.

dual-energy CT has become available and has the capability to provide added information regarding tissue composition, artifact reduction, and image optimization. These advantages of dual-energy CT are used to evaluate crystal deposition disorders like gout, orthopedic implant imaging by reducing metal artifacts (high kV images), trabecular acute bone marrow edema through the use of material decomposition protocol, i.e., virtual noncalcium (VNCa) application **(Figs. 6A to C)**.

Computed tomography is very sensitive for identification of calcium especially to detect matrix mineralization in osseous tumors, chondroid tumors **(Figs. 7A to D)** and to detect calcified nidus in osteoid osteoma **(Figs. 8A to C)**. The other niche indications of CT include suspected partial/stress fractures, bony avulsion fractures, osteoid osteoma, hemangioma, etc. Other applications include, contrast-enhanced CT for evaluation of soft tissue abscess, CT arthrography to evaluate various intra-articular pathology, and CT angiography for vascular encasement **(Figs. 9A and B)** whenever MR is contraindicated or MRI is unavailable or when osteochondral disease is to be evaluated. Low-dose CT is now emerging as a new promising tool to detect early sacroiliitis.

MAGNETIC RESONANCE IMAGING

Magnetic resonance imaging is currently considered the gold standard imaging investigation for the evaluation of bone marrow and soft tissue structures.

Hardware Issues

The basic prerequisites for optimized MRI of the musculoskeletal system are high spatial and contrast resolution and high sensitivity for the visualization of free water. The high-field systems (3 Tesla) are now widely available and provide very high-quality images of the musculoskeletal system. Faster gradients, improvements

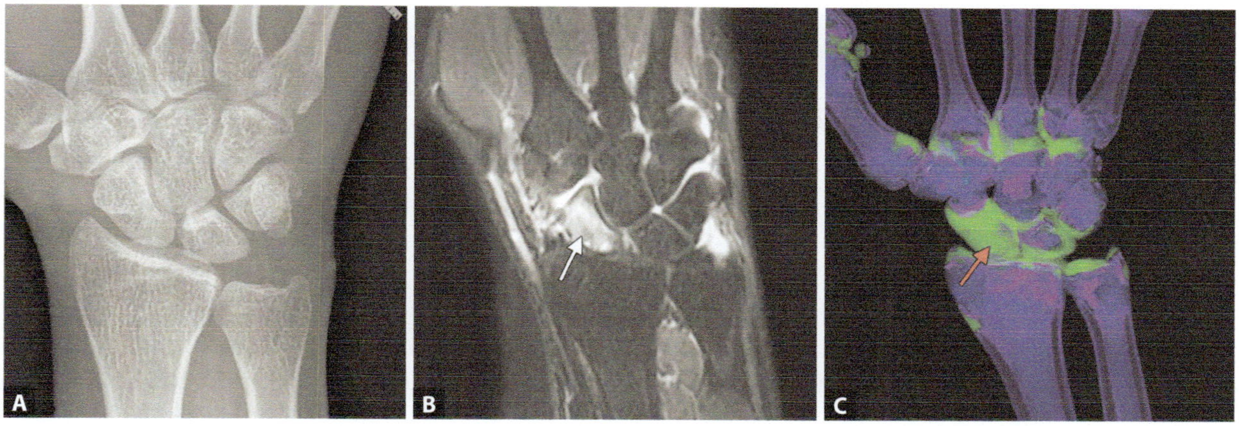

Figs. 6A to C: Posteroanterior (PA) radiograph of wrist (A), coronal short tau inversion recovery (STIR) magnetic resonance image (B), and coronal virtual noncalcium (VNCa) image (C) generated from the dual-energy acquisition, show no obvious abnormality on radiograph (A), nonspecific marrow edema involving scaphoid bone (arrow) without any fracture line in magnetic resonance imagining (B) and trabecular acute bone marrow edema (green color) (red arrow) through the use of material decomposition protocol (VNCa).

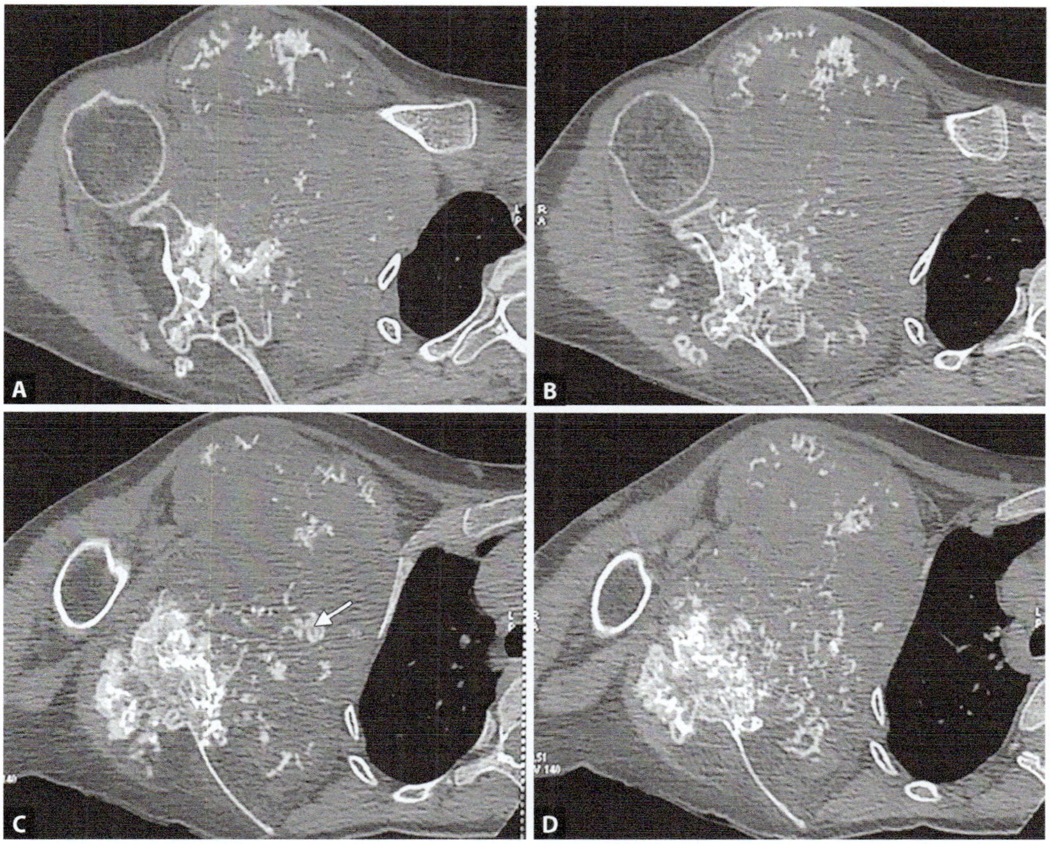

Figs. 7A to D: Axial CT images of right shoulder showing large destructive lesion involving body of right scapula associated with large soft tissue component having chondroid type of calcification (arrow) suggestive of chondrosarcoma arising from exostosis.

in surface coil design, and development of new and faster sequences have all contributed to the fact that MRI has become the modality of choice for evaluation of the musculoskeletal system.[1,2] The use of parallel imaging and motion reduction techniques like periodically rotated overlapping parallel lines with enhanced reconstruction (PROPELLER) and BLADE have further enhanced the image quality of MR images.[2] Scanners are now available which allow imaging in the weight bearing, upright position, and also in flexion and extension (kinematic MRI). This allows evaluation of dynamic postural and functional changes in degenerated discs,[3] as well as

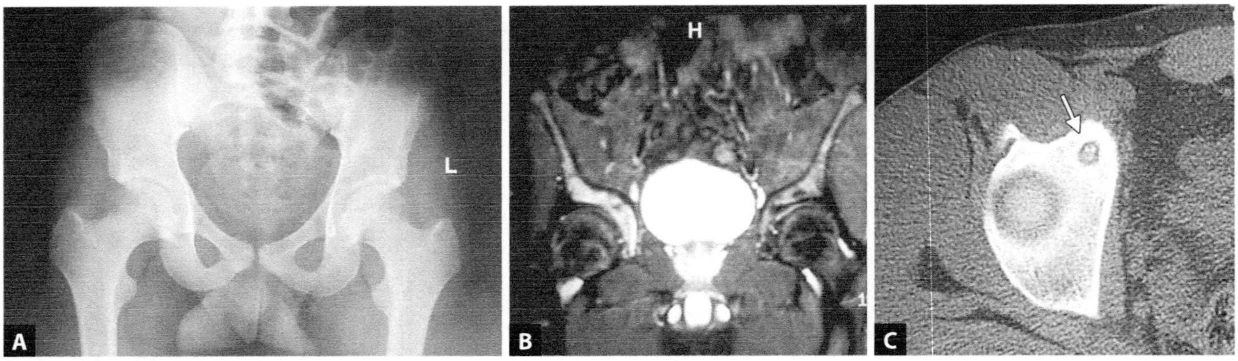

Figs. 8A to C: Anteroposterior (AP) radiograph of pelvis (A), coronal short tau inversion recovery (STIR) magnetic resonance image (B) and axial computed tomography section of acetabulum show no obvious abnormality on radiograph (A), nonspecific marrow edema involving acetabulum and right iliac blade (B) and partially calcified nidus within anterior column of acetabulum (arrow) on computed tomography (C).

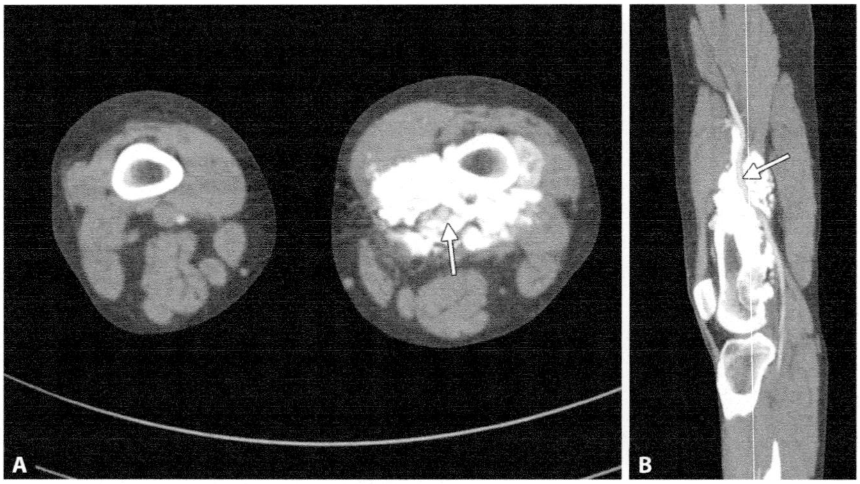

Figs. 9A and B: Axial and sagittal CT angiography images showing juxtacortical ossified lesion arising from posterior cortex of left femur which is encasing the superficial femoral artery (arrows).

dynamic evaluation of joints. Upright and kinematic MRI may detect minor neural foraminal compromise related to posture. However, these scanners are open configuration with low magnetic field strength, which may compromise resolution and are therefore suitable for few niche indications.

Choosing the appropriate coil is important to obtain high-quality images. The smallest coil possible, that allows the required anatomical coverage, should be used to get the maximum signal. Surface coils that can be placed on or close to the region of interest should be used. Most new coils are made with a phased array design. These are made of several smaller coils placed in a series and provide the combined advantage of high-resolution images and a wide FOV. 16-channel coils are now available for musculoskeletal applications.

3T Imaging

The 3T imaging has many advantages in the musculoskeletal system. Imaging at higher field strengths gives better signal-to-noise ratio (SNR), resulting in higher resolution images and shorter scan times. The SNR at 3T is about twice that at 1.5T and 3T scanners are being widely used for musculoskeletal imaging **(Fig. 10)**. Research studies are being conducted at 7T systems also. Not only SNR but also spatial resolution and the contrast to noise ratio can be enhanced on 3T scanners. The collective benefit gives rise to better delineation of the small intrinsic structures of joints. Many studies have documented higher accuracy and greater degree of confidence using 3T imaging, in the diagnosis of meniscal tears, defects in articular cartilage, triangular fibrocartilage pathology, etc. However, 3T imaging is unlikely to replace the need for MR arthrography in lesions like labral tears.[2,4]

The sequences and protocols need to be modified for optimum imaging at 3T. Improved sequence design and widespread use of parallel imaging are likely to improve the image quality at 3T even further.

Sequences

Many different options are available to image the musculoskeletal system. The aim is to get all the diagnostic

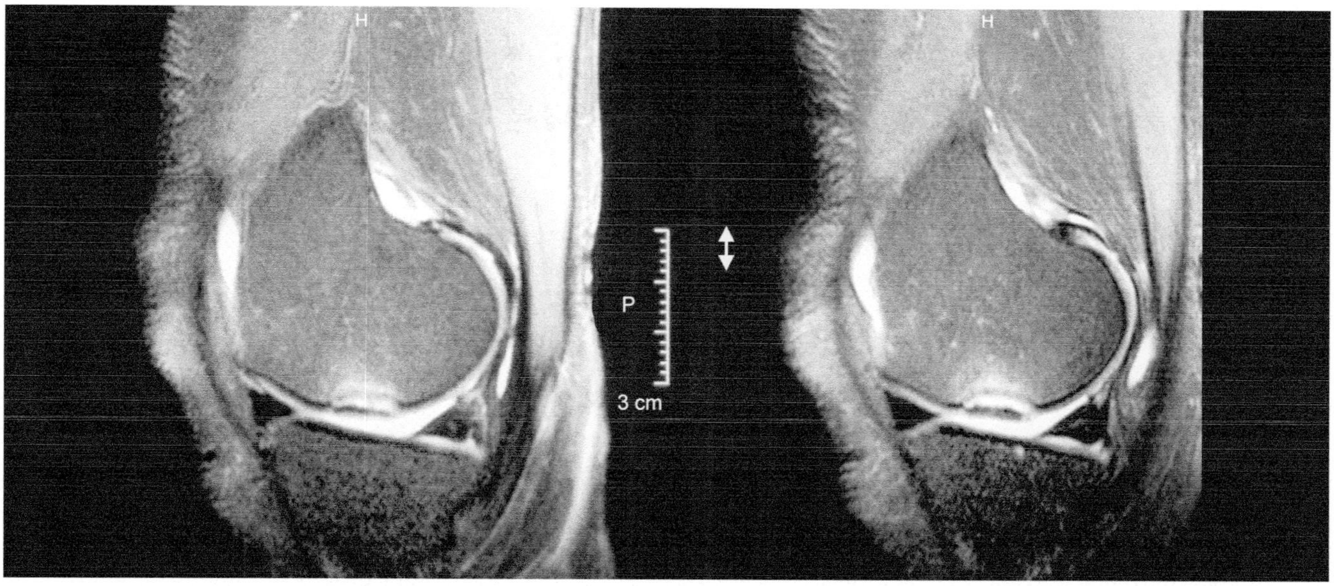

Fig. 10: Sagittal fat suppressed T2-weighted (T2W) image acquired on a 3 Tesla scanner shows a small detached ossific fragment in the articular surface of medial femoral condyle with fluid signal intensity between the fragment and the underlying bone, suggesting osteochondritis dissecans. The image has a high signal-to-noise ratio with excellent delineation of anatomy.

information necessary in as short a time as possible. This can only be done by adopting a judicious protocol for which it is important to know the merits and demerits of the different types of sequences. It is a good practice to have a standard protocol tailored to a specific clinical indication for a given MR scanner. T1-weighted (T1W) sequence is good for delineation of anatomy and marrow pathology, proton density sequence for meniscal tears, articular cartilage **(Fig. 11)**, and ligament pathology and T2-weighted (T2W) sequence for detecting soft tissue component of tumors **(Figs. 12A and B)**, edema, etc. For most musculoskeletal applications, proton density and T2W sequences are coupled with fat suppression (FS).

Fast Spin-echo Sequences

This group of sequences allows for much more rapid acquisition of images than the conventional spin-echo (SE) method. This is done by acquiring several samples in the time in which one sample is obtained in the conventional SE technique. The time saved is directly proportional to the number of samples also known as the echo train length.[1] This decreases overall imaging time thereby decreasing the motion artifacts and increasing the throughput. Alternatively, the time saved can be used for obtaining additional signal averages and increasing the matrix size to improve the signal and resolution, respectively.

However, the fast spin-echo (FSE) technique has some disadvantages. Firstly the signal intensity of fat remains quite bright on these T2W images. As a result, pathology in subcutaneous fat or marrow may be obscured, due to the similarity in the signal intensity of fat and fluid. This problem can be resolved by combining this technique with fat saturation **(Figs. 12A and B)**, which is now routinely employed.[1,2] Secondly the FSE technique can result in blurring along tissue margins when long echo train lengths are used. This may result in missing subtle pathology such as meniscal tears in the knee.

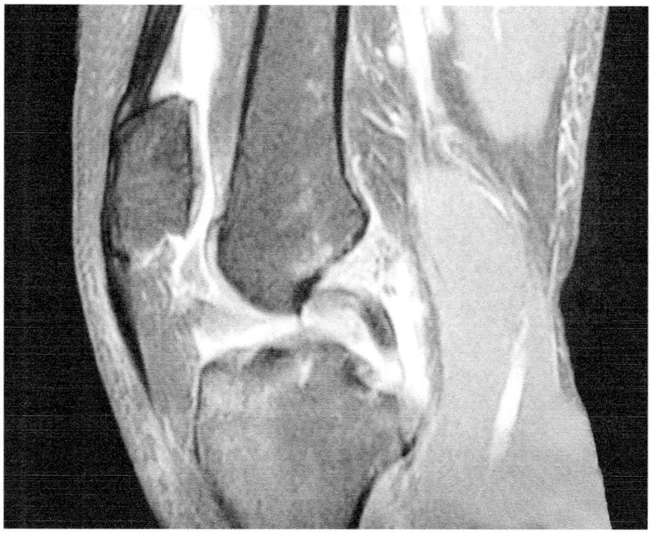

Fig. 11: Sagittal fat suppression proton density (PD) image shows good delineation of hyaline articular cartilage (gray signal intensity along posterior aspect of patella) and cruciate ligaments in the knee. Anterior cruciate ligament is disrupted with no normal fibers identified, and there is buckling of posterior cruciate ligament (PCL), suggesting complete anterior cruciate ligament (ACL) tear.

Gradient-recalled Echo Sequences

These sequences were originally developed to produce T2W images in less time than was possible with

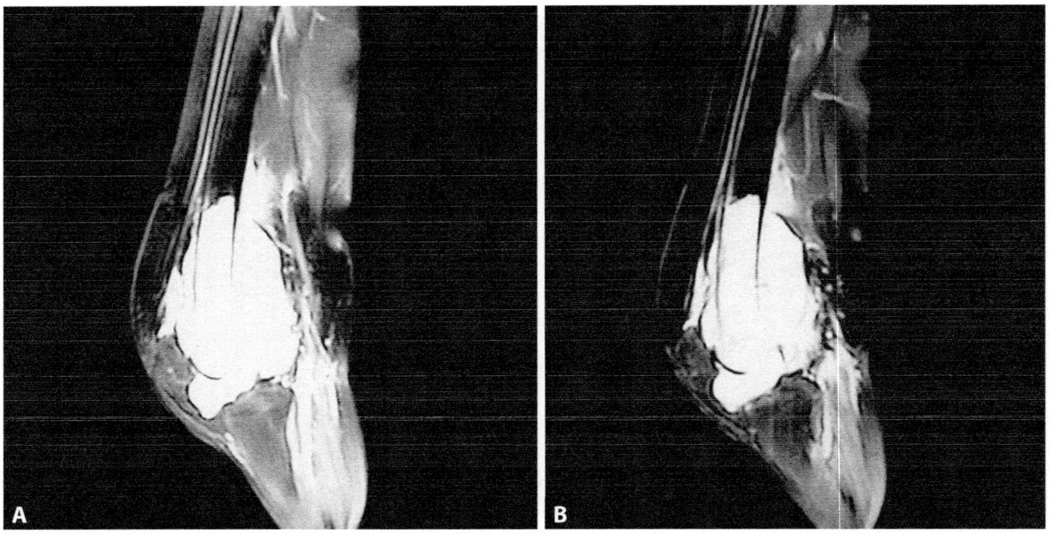

Figs. 12A and B: Sagittal fat suppression T2-weighted image of the knee gives excellent depiction of the extraosseous and intraosseous extent of the tumor in a case of osteosarcoma of the distal femoral end. Also note the intra-articular extension of the tumor.

conventional SE techniques. They can be performed either with a two-dimensional (2D) or three-dimensional (3D) volume technique. In 3D imaging, the signal from an entire volume of tissue is obtained at one time and this data can be partitioned into extremely thin slices such that the voxel dimensions are nearly isotropic.[2] This allows for high-resolution imaging and is especially useful when evaluating extremely small structures such as ligaments in the wrist. These 3D sequences also provide the ability to create reformatted images in virtually any plane. Ligaments and articular cartilage are particularly well demonstrated with these sequences. Dual-echo steady state (DESS) is a 3D steady state gradient-recalled echo (GRE) sequence with a good SNR and strong T2 contrast. It is useful for the differentiation of synovial fluid and cartilaginous structures. Multiecho data image combination (MEDIC) is a multiecho GRE sequence that provides good T2W images and has been found useful in joint imaging **(Fig. 13)**.

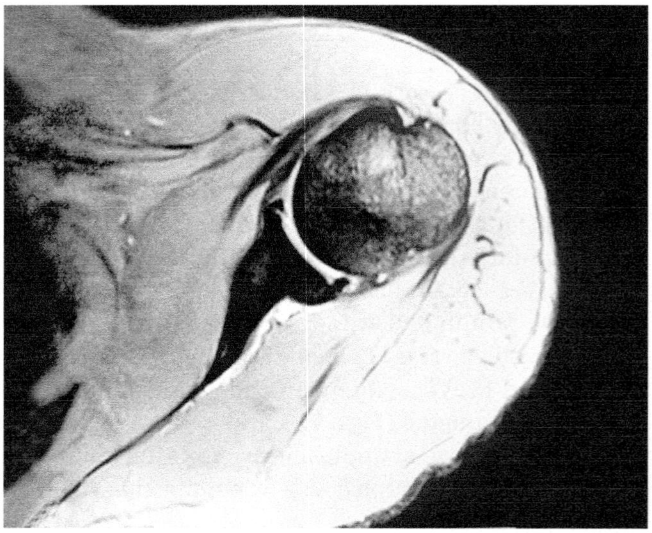

Fig. 13: Axial fat suppression gradient-echo image [multiecho data image combination (MEDIC)] of the shoulder. Anterior and posterior glenoid labrums are well seen as hypointense triangular structures.

Gradient-recalled echo sequences are extremely sensitive to susceptibility effects. This is advantageous when searching for subtle areas of hemorrhage, detecting loose bodies and soft tissue gas. Conversely drawbacks of this effect include overestimating the size of osteophytes in spine imaging and gross artifacts when imaging patients with metallic hardware.

Fat Suppressed Sequences

Detection of a pathological process is often hindered by the presence of strong signal from neighboring adipose tissue. In such cases, suppression of the fat signal offers improved conspicuity and sensitivity.[1] FS is commonly employed with FSE T2W sequences on which fat is very bright. It is also frequently coupled with gadolinium enhanced images where the hyperintense signal from enhancing abnormalities may be masked by hyperintense fat. Fat saturated T1W images are also used with gadolinium arthrography. Diffusion-weighted imaging (DWI) also employs FS.

Two main techniques used to accomplish FS are frequency selective (chemical fat saturation) and short tau inversion recovery (STIR) imaging. A problem with the frequency selective fat saturation is the potential for inhomogeneous suppression of fat signal. It relies on adequate separation of fat and water peaks, which occurs only at high-field strength (greater than 1 T), and hence it is not available on low-field scanners.[1] The STIR technique relies on the relaxation properties of fat protons rather than their resonant frequency. It produces more homogeneous FS, because it is not as sensitive to field inhomogeneity as the frequency selective technique **(Fig. 14)**. However, STIR sequence should not be used with intravenous or intra-articular gadolinium because the contrast agent has similar relaxation properties to fat protons and therefore its signal intensity may be saturated along with fat on the STIR images.

A third method of FS is the Dixon technique or fat-water separation technique. This is also based on the difference in the precessional frequency of protons in fat and water. However, unlike chemical fat sat it uses a spectrally nonselective radiofrequency (RF) pulse, with echo times (TEs) that capture the phase difference between fat and water protons. When fat and water are in-phase, the signal is maximal and when they are out-of-phase there is destructive interference between fat and water magnetization vectors. At 1.5 T, the TE for the in-phase image is 4.6 ms or a multiple of 4.6 and the TE for the opposed-phase image is 2.3 ms or a multiple of 2.3. The fat and water in-phase and out-phase images can be added or subtracted to produce water only or fat only images. This two-point Dixon technique is sensitive to magnetic field inhomogeneity and to overcome this, a three-point Dixon method has been developed where one in-phase and two opposed-phase images (one at 2.3 ms shorter and another sequence with TE 2.3 longer than the nominal TE) are acquired. The three images are analyzed and a phase map is generated from which fat only, water only, and combined images can be created. This technique is called iterative decomposition of fat and water with echo asymmetric and least-square estimation (IDEAL). The Dixon technique can be applied to regions of complex anatomy and can be used with SE, FSE, as well as GRE sequences. Its disadvantages include sensitivity to magnetic field inhomogeneity and potential blurring with FSE sequences.[2]

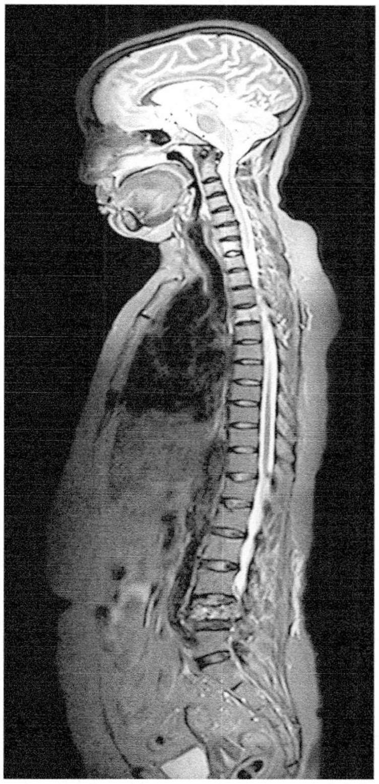

Fig. 14: Sagittal short tau inversion recovery (STIR) image of the whole spine shows hyperintensity and decreased vertebral height involving multiple vertebrae, suggesting multiple metastases in a known case of malignancy. There is homogeneous suppression of fat.

Role of Contrast

Gadolinium-diethylenetriaminepentaacetic acid (Gd-DTPA) is a paramagnetic compound and is a T1 contrast agent. For musculoskeletal applications it can be administered by the intravenous and intra-articular route. Its major application in musculoskeletal MRI is in the setting of infections **(Fig. 15)**, where it can help to distinguish cellulitis from abscess. It is used in evaluating bone and soft tissue tumors to differentiate cystic from solid lesions for perfusion studies and for directing biopsy to the enhancing viable tumor rather than nonenhancing necrotic component.[1] Time-resolved MR angiography enables rapid acquisition at multiple time points so that scrolling the maximal intensity projection slabs provides images similar to digital subtraction angiography (DSA). This is especially useful in the evaluation of vascular tumors and malformations. Gadolinium is also useful in

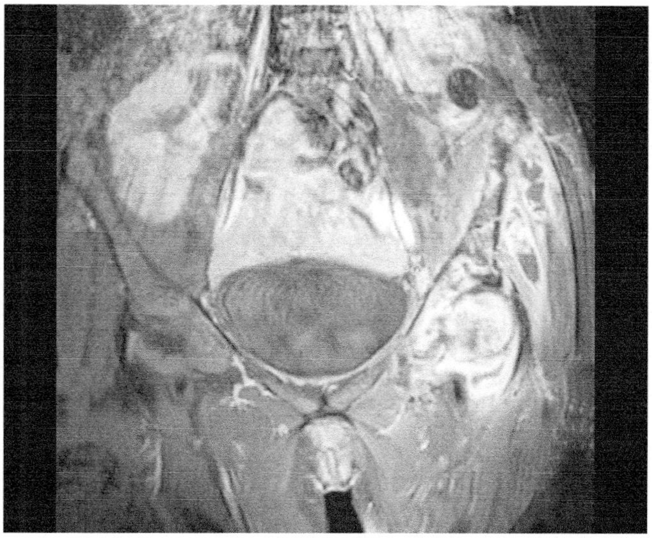

Fig. 15: Utility of contrast administration. Coronal fat suppression postgadolinium T1-weighted image shows abnormal synovial enhancement in a case of tuberculosis (TB) of left hip with multiple rim-enhancing abscesses within the joint cavity and in the surrounding soft tissues.

imaging postoperative spine to differentiate scar tissue from nonenhancing disc material.[2] MR arthrography is useful for the diagnosis of subtle pathology like labral tears.

Reduction of Metallic Artifact from Orthopedic Hardware

Patients with metallic implants and orthopedic hardware frequently need to be imaged. Although they are mostly MR compatible, they can give rise to significant artifact and image distortion. Radiologists should be aware of the steps that can be taken to reduce these artifacts. If there is any doubt of the MR compatibility of the prosthesis, an alternative imaging modality like US should be used.

The degree of metal artifact is related to field strength and imaging at lower field magnets will decrease the metallic artifact. The long axis of the prosthesis should be positioned parallel to the external magnetic field (B0) to minimize artifacts. Other steps that can be taken to reduce in-plane metal artifacts are aligning the frequency encoding direction along the long axis of the implant, increasing the receiver bandwidth, increasing matrix size, and reducing the FOV. FSE sequences with long echo train length are least susceptible to metal artifacts and should be preferred over gradient-echo sequences.[2] STIR and Dixon-based FS work better than chemical-shift in reducing artifacts. Metal artifact reduction sequences (MARS) refer to SE sequences with high bandwidths, increased echo-train length, increased matrix, and decreased echo spacing. MARS may refer to a proprietary sequence but may be better used to refer to an optimized protocol to reduce in-plane distortions. A typical MARS protocol includes STIR coronal, T1 and T2 spin-echo axial and proton-density coronal images. WARP is a proprietary sequence which includes multidirectional view-angle tilting (VAT) to further optimize MARS.

Artifacts due to metal in the adjacent plane (through-plane artifacts) can be reduced by using special multispectral sequences like multiacquisition variable-resonance image combination (MAVRIC) or slice encoding for metal artifact correction (SEMAC). The former uses multiple overlapping acquisitions at different frequencies while the latter uses an additional slice-encoding gradient to FSE. MAVRIC uses multiple frequency-selective excitations, multidirectional VAT, computational postprocessing, and reduces in-plane artifacts as well. Sterile fluid collections are a common complication of metallic prosthesis, especially with metal-on-metal implants **(Figs. 16A to D)**.

Normal Appearance of Musculoskeletal Tissues

It is useful to know the normal appearance of various tissues on different MR sequences and the optimal sequence for each, as this can be applied to any anatomical region. Cortical bone is dark on all sequences whereas the medullary cavity shows a variable signal depending on whether the marrow is hematopoietic or fatty. The distribution of red and yellow marrow changes with age. STIR, fat suppressed FSE T2, and T1W sequences are ideal for imaging marrow pathology, whereas GRE sequences are not useful for bony evaluation. MRI is very sensitive to evaluation of occult osseous trauma **(Figs. 17A and B)** when radiographs are normal and for early diagnosis of marrow infiltrative disorders and for this purpose STIR sequence is the most sensitive.[2]

Articular cartilage is dark gray on STIR and FSE T2W sequences, and is bright on GRE sequences. Fibrocartilage like the menisci and glenoid labrum are dark on all sequences. Meniscal tears are best demonstrated on short TE sequences like T1 and proton density images.

Tendons are generally dark on all pulse sequences. Useful sequences are GRE T2*, T1, and FSE T2. Tendons are usually best imaged in the axial plane. Tears and tendonitis are seen as hyperintense areas but it is important to know some pitfalls for this finding. Tendons may show slightly increased signal intensity close to the site of osseous insertion. This is due to nontendinous fatty material getting interposed between tendon fibers. Another important cause is the magic angle phenomenon, which can give rise to a hyperintense signal in the tendons that are oriented at 55° to the main magnetic field B0. However, this bright signal is seen only on the short TE images (T1W and proton density) and not on T2W images.[1] Common sites where this artifactual hyperintensity may be seen are the posterior tibial tendon in the ankle, rotator cuff in the shoulder, and posterior cruciate ligament in the knee. Changing the position for instance imaging the ankle in 20° plantar flexion can help to overcome this artifact by changing the angle of the tendon with respect to the main magnetic field vector. In addition to hyperintense signal within the tendon, attention should also be paid to any thickening or fluid around the tendon as is seen in tenosynovitis.

Normal synovium is not usually visualized unless it is pathologically thickened. Postgadolinium T1W fat saturated images are useful for delineation of thickened synovium. It may be difficult to distinguish hypertrophied synovium from synovial fluid on T2W and STIR images. Hypertrophied synovium is commonly seen in tubercular and rheumatoid arthritis (RA).

Muscle is of intermediate signal intensity on all sequences. T1W sequences are good to show the anatomy and detect subacute hemorrhage and fatty atrophy. T2W or STIR sequences are sensitive for the diagnosis of muscle strain, myositis, and intramuscular tumors. These sequences are sensitive but unfortunately nonspecific for muscle pathology.

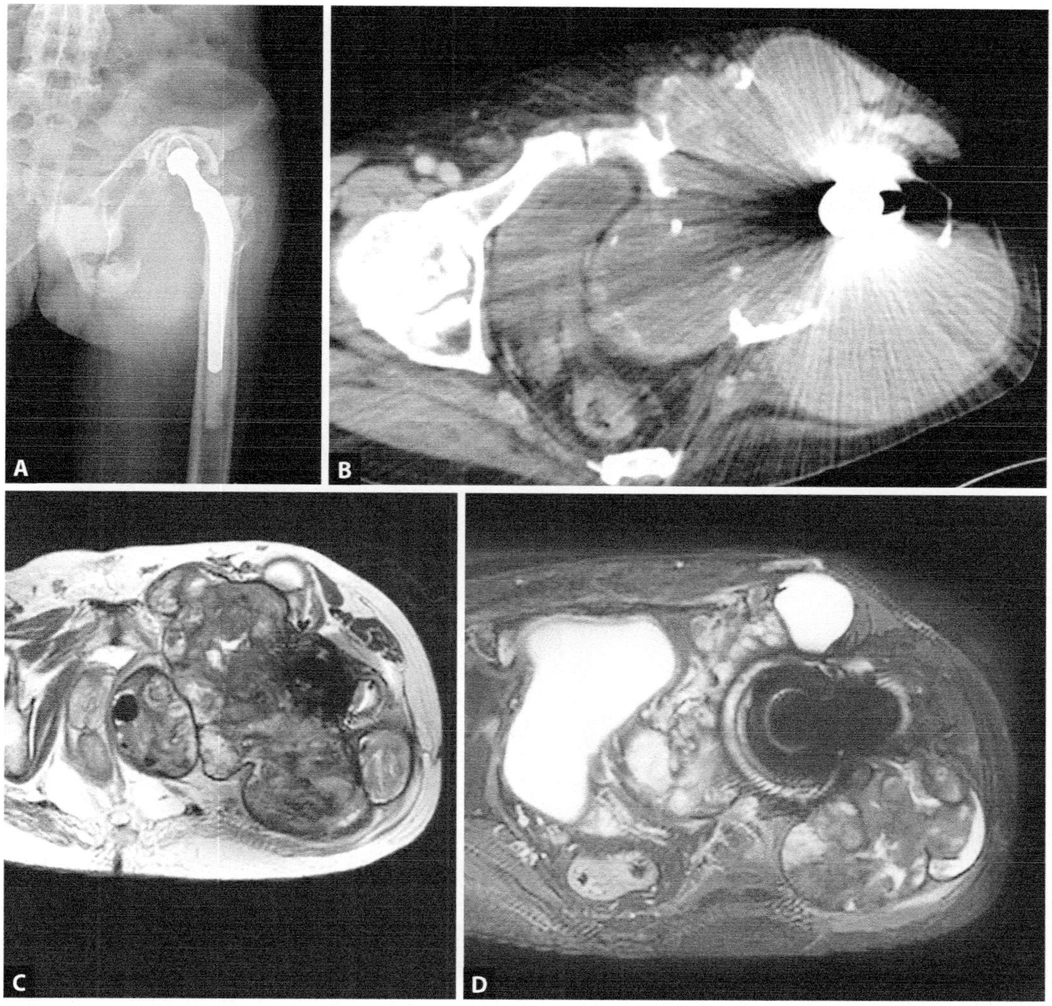

Figs. 16A to D: Anteroposterior (AP) radiograph of left hip (A), axial CT section (B), axial T1-weighted (T1W) and T2-weighted (T2W) fat-saturated magnetic resonance images (C and D) of left hip replacement showing lytic destructive lesion involving left ischium, acetabulum, and medial cortex of left femur (A) associated with large soft tissue component (B), which is showing hypointense signal intensity on both T1W and T2W magnetic resonance images suggestive of metallosis.

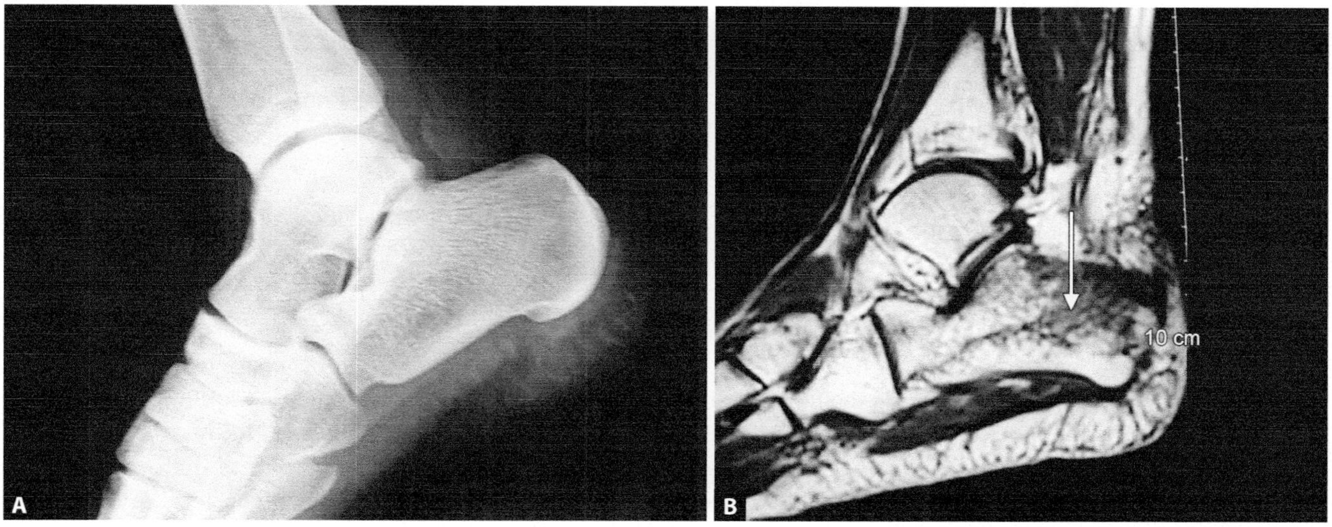

Figs. 17A and B: Lateral radiograph (A) and sagittal T1-weighted magnetic resonance image (B) of young adult, who had history of fall from height, showing normal appearing calcaneum without any obvious fracture on radiograph (A) and hypointense fracture line involving calcaneum (B) (arrow) suggesting occult fracture.

Imaging of Articular Cartilage

Articular cartilage imaging has become increasingly important in the setting of aging population where osteoarthritis is a leading cause of chronic disability. Accurate assessment of abnormalities has become essential with advanced surgical and pharmacological treatments proving to be useful in the management of cartilage pathology.

There are two types of cartilage assessment sequences based on their usefulness for morphological or compositional evaluation. To assess the morphology, standard SE and gradient echo sequences, FSE and 3D spin-echo and gradient sequences are available.[5,6] These sequences allow the detection of morphological defects in cartilage and are also used for semiquantitative analysis.

To assess the collagen and proteoglycan content of cartilage matrix, compositional assessment techniques like T2 mapping, delayed gadolinium-enhanced MRI of cartilage (d-GEMRIC), T1ρ (rho) mapping, sodium imaging, and diffusion-weighted techniques are available, but are mostly used at the research level.[2,7]

Morphological Assessment of Cartilage

On SE T1W, proton density **(Fig. 11)** and T2W sequences, articular cartilage is of intermediate signal intensity.[8] With both conventional and advanced MR techniques several investigators have reported a bilaminar, and occasionally, a trilaminar appearance of articular cartilage on MRI. However, the laminar signals may not correspond to the histologic zones. Many MR artifacts like truncation, partial volume, chemical shift, and magic angle can contribute to or obscure the laminated appearance. Routine MR evaluation of a joint includes conventional SE, FSE, and GRE technique.[9] FS methods improve the contrast between the cartilage and fatty marrow. The cartilage appears bright due to an increase in the dynamic range. This technique is easily combined with the routine sequences to provide high contrast images of the cartilage. The use of 3D imaging methods in conjunction with FSE and GRE sequences allows for less than 1 mm slice thickness and greatly improved spatial resolution. 3D spoiled gradient in the steady state (3D SPGR) or 3D fast low-angle shot (FLASH) has been suggested to be one of the most useful techniques for assessment of cartilage lesions. Due to the availability of high-speed gradient MRI systems, interest has recently been renewed in steady-state free precession (SSFP), a rapid GRE imaging technique using a balanced gradient. This is known as balanced turbo field echo (BTFE) or true fast imaging with steady precession (FISP) imaging. SSFP has superior SNR compared with other GRE techniques and has excellent contrast behavior with varying dependence on T1 and T2. Synovial fluid appears bright due to its long T2. The limitation of this sequence is image degradation due to local magnetic field inhomogeneities at a long repetition time (TR). 3D DESS images have been generated by combining images from first and second echoes in a steady state. These images show a high contrast between cartilage and joint fluid.[6,10] Similarly, 3D-water-selective cartilage scan (WATS) (water excitation) shows bright signal in cartilage and fatty bone marrow appears dark, increasing the contrast.

Chondromalacia, osteoarthritic degeneration, osteochondral defects or inflammatory erosions are the common cartilage abnormalities seen on MRI.[8] Cartilage degeneration may be superficial or basal. The MR grading is mainly based on the depth of the abnormality (partial or full-thickness) which is seen as a focal signal alteration. Conventional MR techniques show 52–95% accuracy for lesion detection, which is higher for severe lesions. However, use of FSE 3D SPGR and delayed MR arthrography techniques have increased the sensitivity for early and surface lesions.[10]

Direct (joint injection) or indirect (intravenous injection with delayed imaging) MR arthrography is another cartilage imaging method and is especially useful for detecting superficial lesions. Indirect arthrography with intravenous administration of diluted gadolinium may be performed when direct arthrography is inconvenient or not logistically feasible. It is based on the concept that intravenous contrast over time will diffuse into the joint space, so that semiarthrographic T1W images can be obtained. MR contrast agents do not produce signal themselves but affect the relaxivity of the surrounding structures; consequently a very low concentration can affect numerous surrounding molecules. The advantages are it does not involve a joint injection or fluoroscopic guidance. In addition, vascularized or inflamed tissue will enhance with this method. It works best in joints like the wrist, ankle, and shoulder but not in large joints like the knee.[2]

Compositional Analysis of Cartilage

The macromolecular network of articular cartilage consists of collagen and proteoglycans. The collagen provides the framework for the tissue and is the main source for tensile and shear strength, whereas glycosaminoglycans provide compressive strength.

T2 mapping: T2 of hyaline cartilage is highly sensitive to alterations of cartilage matrix. A multiecho sequence is used to measure T2 values and a quantitative color coded map can be generated representing variations in T2 relaxation time within articular cartilage. Areas of early degeneration are seen as areas of higher T2 as compared to normal cartilage. T2 maps can be used to monitor the effectiveness of cartilage repair.[7,11]

d-GEMRIC: In this technique, the joint is exercised for 10 minutes after the injection of Gd-DTPA and T1 mapping is done 90 minutes after the injection of Gd. The delay is required to allow gadolinium to penetrate the full thickness of the articular cartilage. It is based on the fact that ions in the interstitial fluid of cartilage are distributed on the basis of the concentration of negatively charged glycosaminoglycan molecules. When anionic molecules like Gd-DTPA enter cartilage, they are distributed in areas where the concentration of glycosaminoglycans is low. The concentration of Gd-DTPA can be estimated by measuring T1, T1 mapping of cartilage after administration of Gd-DTPA allows quantitative assessment of glycosamine content. This technique may become the noninvasive method of assessing glycosaminoglycan content in cartilage after various methods of repair.[2,7,11]

T1 rho mapping: This technique assesses both collagen and glycosaminoglycan content and can detect early degenerative changes. However, an additional RF pulse has to be applied after the magnetization has been tipped in the transverse plane. It is a more time-consuming technique and no large trials have been done using this method.[7,11]

Musculoskeletal Tumors

MRI has a vital role in the detection, confirmation, and preoperative evaluation of malignant and aggressive benign musculoskeletal tumors. Though plain radiographs are the initial modality for the diagnosis of bone tumors, MRI is indispensable for elucidation of the intra- and extraosseous extent of the tumor, its categorization as intra- or extracompartmental, assessment of the neurovascular structures and the adjacent joint **(Figs. 18 to 21)**.[1] MRI is also the best technique to detect skip lesions, which are often missed by other imaging means. The plain radiograph is the modality most likely to yield a specific diagnosis **(Fig. 18A)**, whereas MRI is crucial for accurate local staging of a malignant tumor.

In general, musculoskeletal tumors have a nonspecific appearance on MRI and this modality is not reliable in determining the histology of bone tumors in most cases. Occasionally, it may enable a specific diagnosis on account of pathognomonic signal characteristics, for example, vertebral hemangioma, soft tissue lipoma **(Figs. 19A and B)**, etc. Therefore, one should be wary of interpreting the MR scan in a suspected tumor without reviewing the radiographs.

Magnetic resonance imaging may detect bone tumors, which are easy to overlook or are not visible on plain radiographs **(Figs. 21A and B)**. This is particularly true in the pelvis and sacrum and in patients with hematological malignancies. In patients with bone pain and a negative plain radiograph, MRI is more sensitive and specific than nuclear scan.[1]

All preoperative imaging of musculoskeletal tumors should be done before a biopsy is performed as it may aid in biopsy planning. Hemorrhage and edema resulting from a biopsy may alter the MR appearance and create difficulty in evaluating the lesion. The tumor should be imaged in at least two planes usually parallel and perpendicular to the long axis of the involved bone.

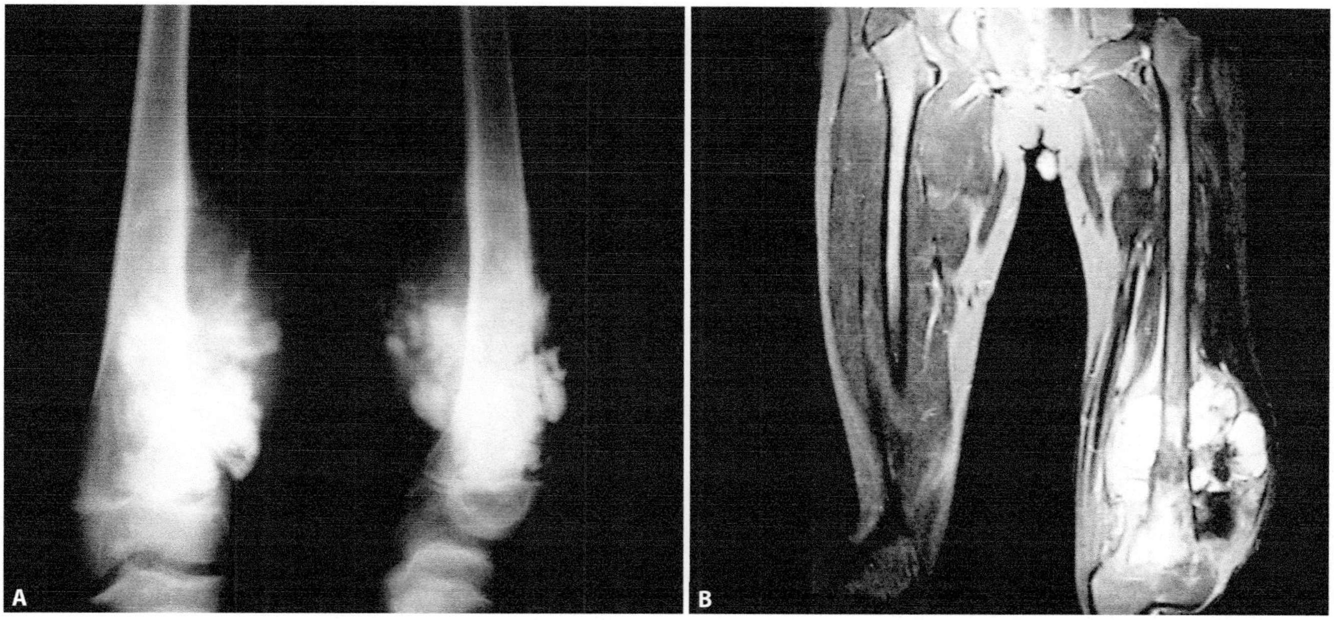

Figs. 18A and B: Frontal and lateral radiographs of the knee (A), show osteosarcoma of the distal femoral metaphysis with permeative involvement and osteoid pattern of matrix mineralization extending into the soft tissues. Coronal short tau inversion recovery (STIR) image (B), using body coil shows the complete extent of the tumor, which facilitates optimal surgical management.

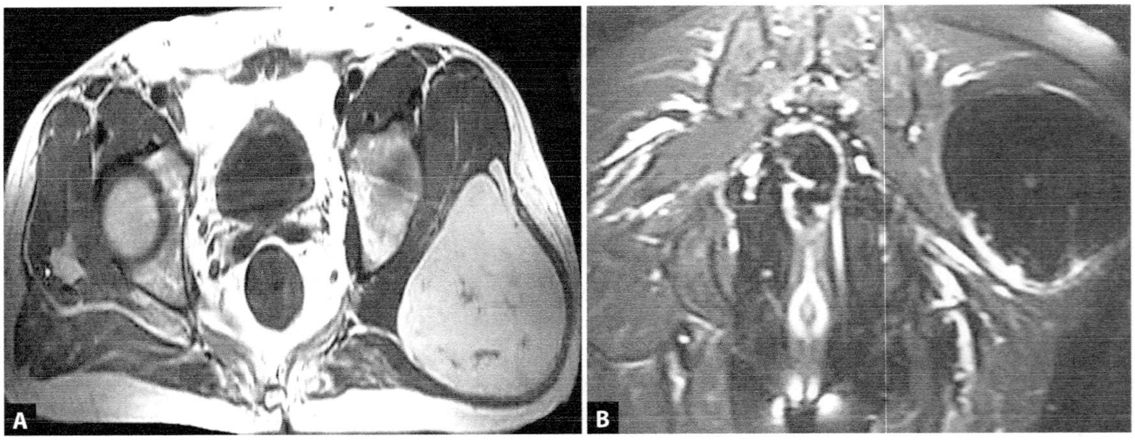

Figs. 19A and B: Axial T1-weighted image (A) shows a well-defined hyperintense mass lesion in the left gluteal region which completely loses signal on coronal fat suppressed image; (B) Indicative of fat within, suggesting the diagnosis of soft tissue lipoma. Also note that the signal intensity of the lesion parallels that of subcutaneous fat.

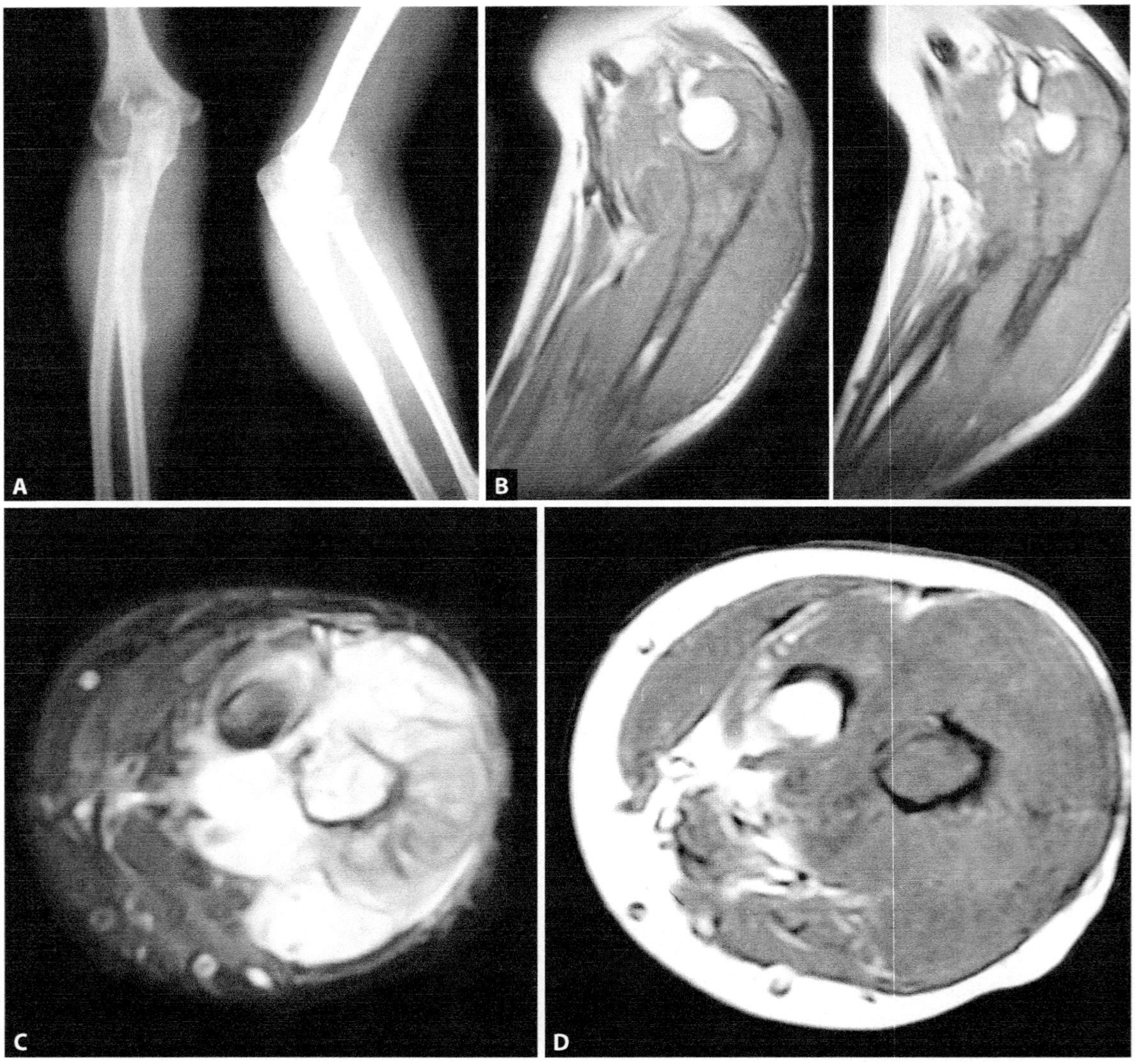

Figs. 20A to D: Frontal and lateral radiographs of the elbow (A) show permeative lytic bone destruction with ill-defined margins involving proximal ulna with Codman's triangle, cortical breech, soft tissue extension and osseous mineralization, suggesting osteosarcoma. Sagittal T1-weighted (T1W) image (B), clearly demonstrates the intraosseous extent and extension into surrounding soft tissues. Axial T2-weighted (T2W) (C) and T1W (D) images depict the extent of tumor, cortical disruption, and soft tissue extension with sparing of the neurovascular bundle.

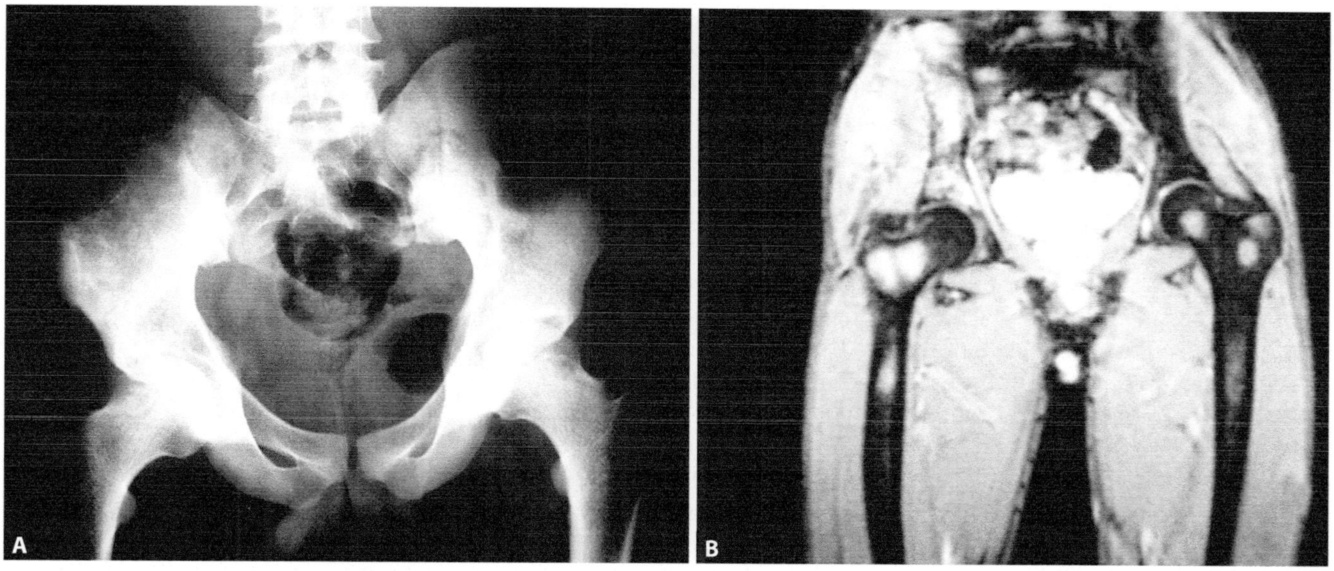

Figs. 21A and B: Frontal radiograph of the pelvis (A) shows an ill-defined permeative lytic lesion in the right iliac wing. Short tau inversion recovery (STIR) coronal image (B) clearly shows that there are multiple well-defined hyperintense lesions in bilateral femoral necks also, indicative of bony metastases. These lesions were not apparent on radiographs. The primary tumor was proven to be Ewing's sarcoma.

The imaging protocol includes an initial large FOV T1W or STIR study using the body coil **(Fig. 18B)**. This is useful in detection of skip lesions and for planning subsequent sequences. Surface coil images are then obtained in the coronal or sagittal planes to display the extent of the lesion in all three dimensions. The accurate assessment of the craniocaudal extent and exact distance of the proximal and distal margins from a nearby landmark, such as a joint line is crucial for planning a limb-salvage procedure and selection of a suitable prosthesis.[1] Axial images best demonstrate the relationship of the tumor to the neurovascular bundle **(Figs. 19A and B)**. The elucidation of the intraosseous tumor extent as well as the skip lesions needs inclusion of a T1W or STIR sequence **(Figs. 18, 20, and 21)**. However, overestimation of the tumor extent may occur on STIR images due to peritumoral edema. The extraosseous extent is exquisitely demonstrated on a T2W sequence **(Figs. 12A and B)** due to the contrast provided by the low-signal muscles. Adjacent bright fat is best suppressed by a fat saturation technique to further increase the contrast on T2W images. MRI has a high negative predictive value for neurovascular or joint involvement by the tumor, though joint involvement tends to get overdiagnosed based on MRI. A GRE sequence is helpful in clear identification of the neurovascular bundle and contrast administration is not required for extent delineation of bone tumors.[12]

Use of Advanced Magnetic Resonance Techniques

Diffusion-weighted Imaging

Diffusion can be assessed both qualitatively and quantitatively and is a measure of tumor cellularity and cell membrane integrity. It can be used for detection and characterization of bone tumors as well as assess the response to chemotherapy. DWI sequences are done at different b values ranging from 0 to 1,000. Typically, benign lesions lose their signal intensity as b value increases whereas cellular tumors retain their signal intensity. The apparent diffusion coefficient (ADC) can be used for quantitative assessment. Low ADC values are seen in cellular tumors because of restricted diffusion.

Diffusion-weighted imaging can also be used to assess response to chemoradiotherapy. Tumor necrosis caused by these modalities increases the ADC value which can be used as a surrogate marker for response.[13]

Magnetic Resonance Neurography

An MRI of the nerves employs high-resolution thin T1W and T2W SE, 3D isotropic T2 sampling perfection with application optimized contrast (SPACE) or VISTA or CUBE, 3D STIR and volume diffusion-weighted images. 3D diffusion-weighted reverse FISP (3D DW PSIF) has also been advocated especially to evaluate small nerves and differentiate them from vascular signals. Diffusion tensor imaging and color tractography can be done to look for any loss of anisotropy indirectly suggesting the functional status of the nerve fibers.

Whole Body Magnetic Resonance Imaging

Whole body MRI (WB-MRI) provides a radiation-free alternative to positron-emission tomography (PET)/CT for evaluation of multifocal and multisystem diseases. Common musculoskeletal indications include detection of lesions, evaluation of tumor load (staging), and follow-up (assessment of treatment response) in case of lymphoma, multiple myeloma, and metastases **(Fig. 22)**.[14] It is also useful in detection of occult primary neoplastic lesion in diseases like oncogenic osteomalacia or identifying the focus of infection in chronic fever of unknown origin. The sequences which are done as part of whole body imaging include STIR, diffusion-weighted imaging with background suppression (DWIBS), and postcontrast T1W imaging. WB-MRI has been found to be more sensitive than bone scan and choline PET/CT for identifying bone metastases from prostatic carcinoma.[14] WB-MRI can aid in evaluating multiple lesions in case of neurofibromatosis and vascular malformations. Quantification techniques have been described for WB-DWI and include calculation of total diffusion volume (TDV) and global ADC. TDV is based on aggregated volume of segmented high signal intensity areas (corresponding to high cellularity tumor) on high b-value DWI image and gives estimate of total disease burden.[15] Corresponding ADC value of the entire volume is known as global ADC and various histogram parameters can be calculated.

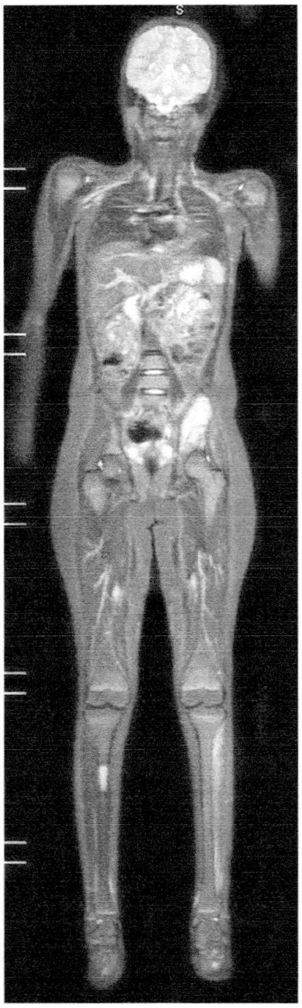

Fig. 22: Whole body short tau inversion recovery (STIR) image shows a large lesion in the left iliac blade and another lesion in the right tibia in a case of multiple metastases.

Zero Echo Time Magnetic Resonance Imaging

Zero echo time (ZTE) MRI demonstrates increased contrast resolution of the osseous outline and thus may exclude the need to do CT in evaluation of cases like bony Bankart.[16] Ultrashort echo time (UTE) MRI is used in better visualization of tendons, menisci, and calcified zone of hyaline cartilage. ZTE is a further extension of the same concept to evaluate structures with short TE and acquisition is done immediately after the application of RF pulse (TE ~8 ms).[16] ZTE MR allows simultaneous evaluation of marrow edema, bone outline, and subchondral cysts.[15]

New Rapid Acquisition Sequences

Compressed sensing serves to accelerate the MR acquisition by acquiring less data via undersampling of the k-space. This is usually combined with parallel imaging to enable high acceleration factors but the role is still investigational in musculoskeletal diseases. Limitations include image blurring and poor visibility of low-contrast structures. Machine-learning reconstructions are also being explored to speed up acquisition. Multislice/multiband imaging employs simultaneous acquisition of information from multiple slices, rather than doing so sequentially [simultaneous multislice (SMS)]. However the problems for musculoskeletal application include altered contrast between the soft tissue structures and loss of image quality.

Conventional MR is unable to provide a specific histologic diagnosis and is unreliable for differentiating benign from malignant neoplasms. Neoadjuvant chemotherapy is used in many bone tumors like osteosarcoma and Ewing's sarcoma. The evaluation of response to chemotherapy on routine MR is based on size reduction, which is unreliable and may take time. These problems can be addressed by using techniques like dynamic contrast-enhanced perfusion imaging, proton spectroscopy, diffusion imaging, intravoxel incoherent motion (IVIM), in-phase/opposed-phase MRI, and texture analysis.[13,17]

Dynamic Perfusion Imaging

T1W gradient echo sequence is repeated rapidly a number of times after an injection of gadolinium bolus (0.1 mmol/kg) followed by a saline chase. Time signal intensity curves are generated in much the same way as is done in breast imaging. In general, malignant tumors show greater enhancement at a faster rate **(Figs. 23A to D)** and a rapid wash out as compared to benign tumors.[17] This technique coupled with conventional MR, spectroscopy and DWI may help in narrowing the list of differential diagnosis, better assess the extent of disease, distinguish responders to chemotherapy from nonresponders, and differentiate residual/recurrent tumor from radiation necrosis.

The former enhance early and more rapidly whereas post-therapy changes enhance later and more slowly.[13] Time-resolved 4D MR angiography is another method of dynamic postcontrast imaging which is useful for characterizing vascular malformations. The principle behind this sequence is that center of the k-space is repeatedly sampled while periphery is sampled only once during acquisition, thus reducing scan time. Commercially this is available as time-resolved angiography with interleaved stochastic trajectories (TWIST) or time-resolved angiography with keyhole method (TRAK) or time-resolved imaging of contrast kinetics (TRICKS). Multiple fast 3D acquisitions of the region of interest are obtained sequentially and almost a real-time effect is perceived.

Proton Spectroscopy

It can be performed using a single voxel technique with a point resolved spectroscopy sequence (PRESS) and TE of 135 ms. The choline peak and choline/creatine ratio has been shown to distinguish benign from malignant bone and soft tissue tumors **(Figs. 23A to D)**. The voxel should be placed on areas showing early and intense enhancement. The caveat is that some metabolically active tumors like giant cell tumor may also show choline peak.[17]

Positron-emission Tomography–Magnetic Resonance Imaging

Hybrid PET-MRI systems offer high-contrast resolution of MRI along with metabolic information from PET. They

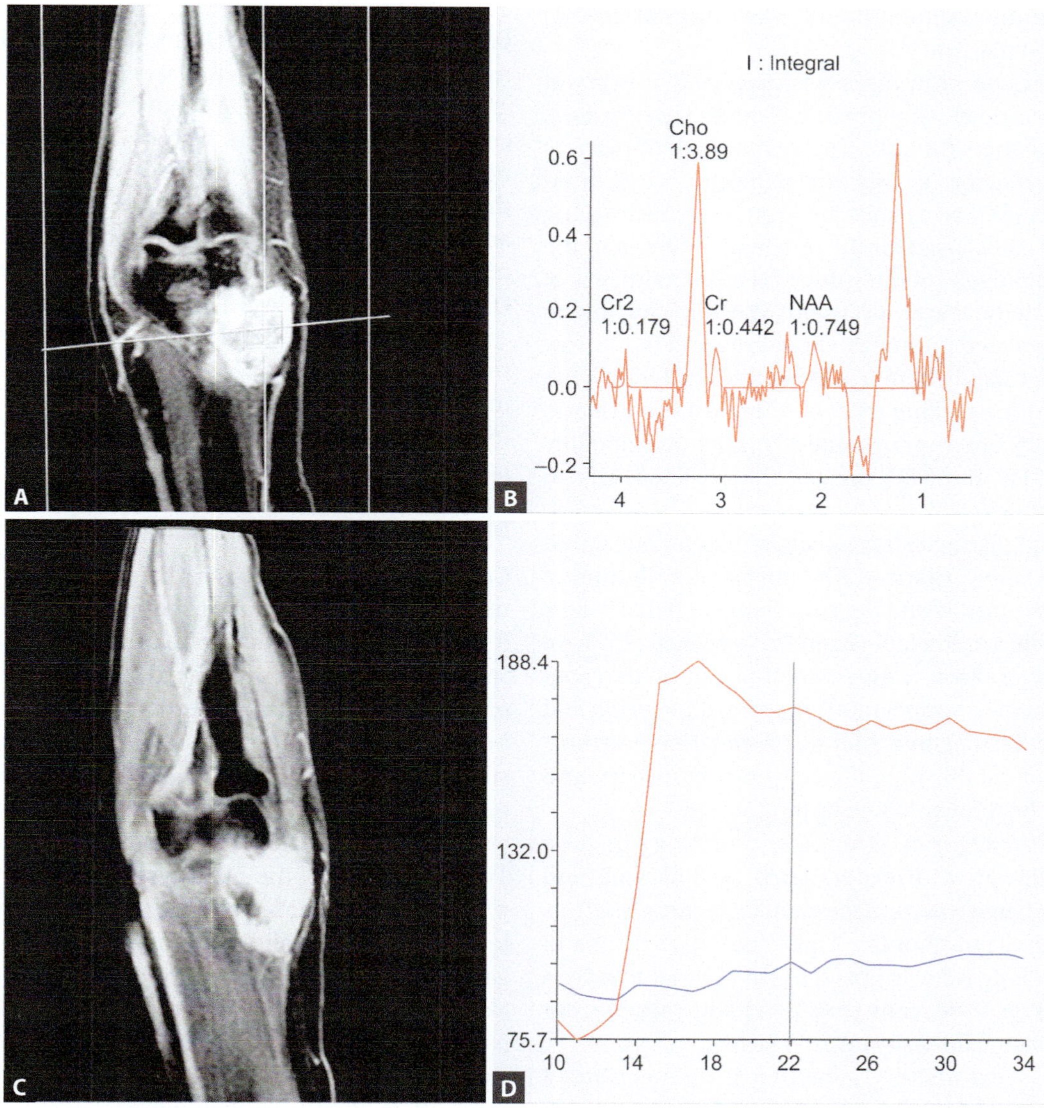

Figs. 23A to D: Coronal fat suppression (FS) postgadolinium image (A) of the elbow showing the placement of voxel for single voxel magnetic resonance spectroscopy in enhancing lesion seen in distal humeral metaphysis. There is elevated choline peak (B), suggesting malignant bone tumor. Coronal postgadolinium FS T1-weighted image (C) of the elbow showing the placement of region of interest (ROI) for generation of perfusion map of the lesion to show contrast kinetics. Time signal intensity curve (D) of the same lesion shows rapid uptake and washout of the contrast, indicating malignant neoplasm.

have been found useful in the T-staging, follow-up, and therapeutic response assessment of musculoskeletal sarcomas.[18] This may also prove useful in multiple myeloma and diffuse metastases. Potential nononcological applications include stress fractures and evaluation of arthritides.

Marrow Imaging

Conventional radiographic techniques are very insensitive to marrow infiltration and tumors. CT may detect gross metastatic disease of the spine but is of limited use in imaging primary and metastatic neoplasms in the rest of the skeleton. Radionuclide bone scanning is insensitive to certain marrow neoplasms such as lymphoma and multiple myeloma. MRI has the major advantage of imaging the bone marrow directly and its excellent contrast resolution allows the differentiation of normal from infiltrated marrow.[1,2]

When diffuse marrow disease is suspected a survey of the entire spine, pelvis, and proximal femora is performed, because this is where the bulk of the hematopoietic marrow exists. For a marrow survey the patient is positioned supine. The phased array coils are used for spine imaging and the body coil is used for the proximal femora and the pelvis. Sagittal images of the spine and coronal images of the pelvis and femora are most useful. WB-MRI can now be routinely performed for metastatic survey and in marrow infiltrative diseases. There is a technique called DWIBS which is ideal for picking up foci of metastatic disease, lymphoma, etc., and may become a competitive modality for PET-CT. T1W and STIR images are most sensitive to marrow pathology.[1]

An MRI can distinguish between hematopoietic or red marrow from yellow marrow. The normal distribution of red and yellow marrow and the conversion of red to yellow marrow occur in a predictable manner based on age.[2] There is a vast array of marrow disorders that can be detected on MRI although the appearance may be nonspecific and only a differential diagnosis may be offered. However, MRI is excellent for establishing the presence of disease and also for directing biopsy to an appropriate site.

Important categories of marrow pathology include marrow proliferative disorders such as leukemia and myeloma and marrow replacement disorders such as metastases and lymphoma.[1] The usual appearance of marrow pathology is low signal intensity (equal to or less than muscle) on T1W scans **(Fig. 24A)** and variable, but usually high-signal intensity on T2W scans.

An MRI is exquisitely sensitive for detection of metastatic disease and surpasses all other imaging techniques in this regard. A common clinical problem is the distinction between metastatic deposits from an acute osteoporotic collapse, especially in a patient with a known primary tumor. Both may show a fractured vertebral body with replacement of normal marrow by low signal intensity on T1W scans. Features that suggest tumor are abnormal signal intensity extending into the pedicles and other posterior elements, involvement of the entire vertebral body by the abnormal signal intensity, associated soft tissue mass, and multiple bone lesions. In osteoporotic fractures, the abnormal signal intensity does not involve the entire vertebral body, but has a horizontal line or band separating the abnormal signal intensity from the normal fatty marrow signal.[1] It has been reported that GRE opposed-phase sequence may be helpful based on the fact that some fat is still present in benign lesions such as osteoporotic fractures. Hence, osteoporotic fractures are supposed to show lower signal intensity than the metastatic lesions. Diffusion-weighted images have also been successfully used for the purpose of this differentiation.[1] The vertebral lesions due to marrow infiltration by tumor become hyperintense on DWI **(Figs. 24B and C)** whereas osteoporotic collapsed vertebra remains hypointense. In- and opposed-phase images have also been used in this context. Collapse due to osteoporosis will retain some normal fatty marrow which will show loss of signal on the opposed-phase image. On the other hand, metastatic and marrow infiltrative disease replaces the fatty marrow completely and hence does not show this signal loss **(Figs. 24D and E)**.

Magnetic resonance can also be used to monitor the response of marrow pathology such as leukemia and metastases to treatment. Serial MRI has been shown to be useful in confirming remission and detecting relapse in patients with leukemia.

Musculoskeletal Infections

Conventional radiographs remain the initial imaging modality of choice for suspected osteomyelitis. However, it is insensitive to the detection of early osteomyelitis. MRI scores over radiography, CT, and scintigraphy in detection of early osteomyelitis. However, the MR appearance is nonspecific and similar to infiltrating neoplasms and stress fractures and the clinical context is important in reaching the correct diagnosis.[19] MR is also superior to other modalities in delineating the soft tissue involvement. The elucidation of the full extent facilitates preoperative planning of the maximal degree of debridement or the level of the amputation. FS techniques combined with gadolinium administration further increase the sensitivity for detection of involved areas. Contrast administration is also helpful in distinguishing abscess **(Fig. 15)** from surrounding cellulitis, increasing the conspicuity of the sinus tracts by causing their walls to enhance and clearly demonstrating the nonenhancing sequestra within enhancing granulation tissue.[20]

In infants and children, involvement of the unossified physis and epiphysis is best shown by MRI.

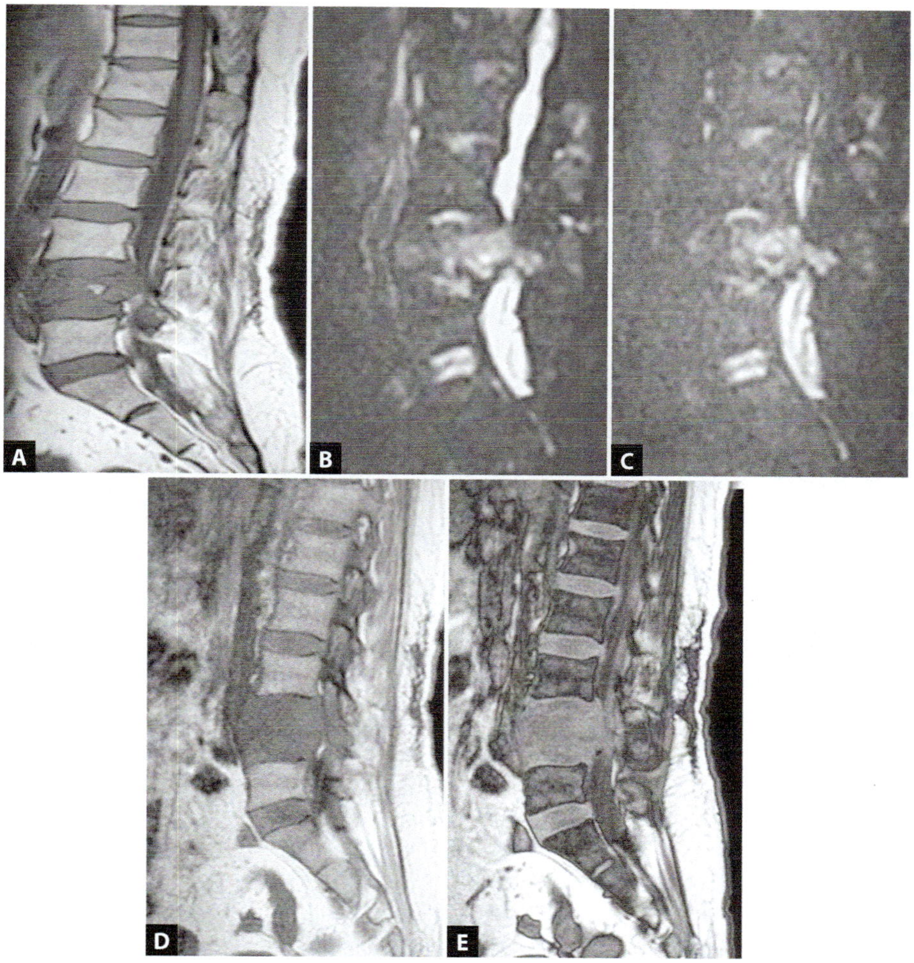

Figs. 24A to E: Sagittal T1-weighted (T1W) image (A) of lumbosacral spine shows altered signal intensity with partial collapse of L4 vertebra. Diffusion-weighted images at b 0 s/mm^2 (B) and b 400 s/mm^2 (C) show retention of signal at higher b value, suggesting restricted diffusion. Sagittal T1W in-phase (D) and opposed-phase (E) images show suppression of marrow signal in the normal vertebrae. However, L4 vertebra shows no loss of signal. Diffusion restriction and absence of signal suppression on opposed-phase images are markers of malignant vertebral involvement. This was proven to be metastatic vertebral collapse.

Inflammatory Arthritis

Radiography has been the imaging modality of choice in RA, primarily because of its reproducibility and feasibility. Currently MRI is being used widely for recruiting patients into clinical trials as well as monitoring disease progression over time, because of its advantage of simultaneous imaging of key structures other than bone (synovium and surrounding soft tissues) that are important in inflammatory arthritis. MRI is also a useful tool in evaluating patients with early RA. It can detect pre-erosive synovitis and can also identify early bone damage before it becomes apparent on radiography. In early RA, wrist and hand involvement is usually bilateral. Some authors perform bilateral MRI of the wrists or hands. However, it is preferred to study the dominant or more painful wrist in order to reduce the study time. The technical recommendations of the OMERACT (Outcome Measures in Rheumatoid Arthritis Clinical Trials) group for MRI studies of RA patients should include at least the following sequences:

- Imaging in two planes (coronal and axial)
- T1-weighted imaging before and after the administration of gadolinium, fat saturated imaging is preferable after administration
- A fat saturated T2W sequence or a STIR sequence.[21]

Interventional Magnetic Resonance Imaging

Due to restricted patient access on conventional high and midfield MR machines and unacceptable speed on the older low-field systems, MRI was not considered as a guidance tool for interventional procedures earlier. Since the introduction of open magnet designs offering a nearly free patient access, interest has now focused on interventional MR. In addition, short bore high-field systems presently allow satisfactory patient access combined with high-performance imaging capabilities.

A simultaneous creation of an adequate array of MR compatible instruments has made MR interventions viable.[22] Percutaneous biopsies and drainage procedures are currently the easiest procedures to be performed under MR control. These do not require dedicated hard or software modifications and are thus attractive and clinically useful.

Three types of magnets are clinically used for percutaneous biopsies: (1) open low-field magnets (0.2–0.35 T), (2) open midfield system (0.5 T), and (3) closed short bore magnets (1–1.5 T). Improved patient access with open magnet allows interventions in any desired plane and patient position. To begin with, horizontally open magnets were used. Recently, experience with vertically open units has also been reported. Vertically open units permit unrestricted vertical and side access to the patient at the most homogeneous portion of the magnetic field. The other advantage is a horizontally directed main magnetic field along the long axis of the bore, which ensures that the needle trajectory is never parallel to the field.[23] In closed systems, instrument manipulation can only be performed with the patient outside the magnet. However, due to higher field strength, image quality as well as the imaging speed is better.

For instrument visualization, the susceptibility artifact provided by the nonferromagnetic alloys of MR compatible needles is used. The size of the artifact is inversely proportional to the size of the instrument and directly proportional to the field strength and to the angle the instrument makes with the main magnetic field. Typically, biopsy needles are displayed as dark areas surrounded by a brighter rim.[24] Several vendors on the market offer MR compatible needles at present. Fine needles of 20–24G with different tip configurations and cutting needles of 14–18G are commercially available. The overall performance of a MR compatible needle is inferior to a stainless steel needle due to relatively blunt surfaces and softer alloys. For drainage procedures MR compatible sets consisting of MR compatible guidewires, dilators, and drainage catheters are available.

Imaging protocol consists of fast localizers in three planes followed by a fast multislice T2W SE sequence. A postcontrast GRE sequence may be used to select the appropriate biopsy site. In the closed magnet, needle tracking is done by following a procedure similar to that used in CT-guided interventions. After defining the target region, a T1W or T2W compatible grid is fixed to the skin of the patient to aid in selecting needle entry site. The angle and distance from skin to the lesion can be obtained by using standard scanner software. The needle track can be controlled step-by-step during advancement of the needle. In the open magnet, a palpating finger may be used instead of a grid for entry site. The instrument can be tracked by continuous repetition of a fast imaging sequence.[22]

Primary and secondary bone and soft tissue lesions can be accessed by MR-guided interventional procedures. Due to its multiplanar capability, MR allows visualization of the entire planned biopsy pathway including orthogonal and oblique scans. Lack of ionizing radiation is an obvious advantage.[24] The unique advantage of MR interventions is in transcutaneous biopsy of bone marrow lesions of unknown origin, as their display and localization is possible exclusively on MR. However, the available armamentarium to perform MR-guided transcortical bone biopsy is limited, though a MR compatible coaxial bone biopsy system has recently been developed.[22] Although lesion access by MR is good for appendicular skeleton, CT is preferred for biopsy of the axial skeleton due to superior spatial resolution.

CONCLUSION

The scope of musculoskeletal radiology has widened over the last few years and to a large extent this has been possible because of the exquisite detail provided by the versatile technique of MRI. There has been a resurgence of interest in US as a noninvasive simple tool for dynamic evaluation of musculoskeletal pathology. The advent of dual-energy CT has led to some new applications like evaluation of gout and marrow imaging based on the VNCa images. High-field MRI, DWI, dynamic contrast-enhanced imaging, MR spectroscopy, and other advances have further enhanced the utility of this modality. However, elegant display of pathology alone does not suffice, as diagnosis based on images alone, especially MR images, is nonspecific. For the optimal use of this technology the radiologist must couple these images with an in depth knowledge of pathophysiology and clinical perspective so that he can guide the referring clinician appropriately. "Seeing better" should be coupled with "knowing more" to make the optimum use of the high tech modality of MRI.[25]

REFERENCES

1. Helms CA, Anderson MW, Major NM, Kaplan P, Dussault R. Musculoskeletal MRI, 2nd edition. Philadelphia: WB Saunders Co; 2009.
2. Stoller DW. Magnetic Resonance Imaging in Orthopaedics and Sports Medicine, 3rd edition. Philadelphia: Lippincott Williams & Wilkins; 2007.
3. Zou J, Yang H, Miyazaki M, Morishita Y, Wei F, McGovern S, et al. Dynamic bulging of intervertebral discs in the degenerative lumbar spine. Spine. 2009;34(23):2545-50.
4. Ramnath RR. 3T MR imaging of the musculoskeletal system (Part II): clinical applications. Magn Reson Imaging Clin N Am. 2006;14(1):41-62.
5. Koff MF, Potter HG. Noncontrast MR techniques and imaging of cartilage. Radiol Clin N Am. 2009;47(3):495-504.
6. Strickland CD, Kijowski R. Morphologic imaging of articular cartilage. Magn Reson Imaging Clin N Am. 2011;19(2):229-48.

7. Choi JA, Gold GE. MR imaging of articular cartilage physiology. Magn Reson Imaging Clin N Am. 2011;19(2):249-82.
8. Suh JS, Lee SH, Jeong EK, Kim DJ. Magnetic resonance imaging of articular cartilage. Eur Radiol. 2001;11(10):2015-25.
9. Sonin AH, Pensy RA, Mulligan ME, Hatem S. Grading articular cartilage of the knee using fast spinecho proton density-weighted MR imaging without fat suppression. Am J Roentgenol. 2002;179(5):1159-66.
10. Reeder SB, Pelc NJ, Alley MT, Gold GE. Rapid MR imaging of articular cartilage with steady-state free precession and multipoint fat-water separation. Am J Roentgenol. 2003;180(2):357-62.
11. Crema MD, Roemer FW, Marra MD, Burstein D, Gold GE, Eckstein F, et al. Articular cartilage in the knee: current MR imaging techniques and applications in clinical practice and research. Radiographics. 2011;31(1):37-61.
12. Peabody TD, Gibbs CP, Simon MA. Current concepts review—evaluation and staging of musculoskeletal neoplasms. J Bone Joint Surg Am. 1998;80(8):1204-18.
13. Garner HW, Kransdorf MJ, Peterson JJ. Posttherapy imaging of musculoskeletal neoplasms. Radiol Clin North Am. 2011;49(6):1307-23.
14. Petralia G, Padhani AR. Whole-body magnetic resonance imaging in oncology: uses and indications. Magn Reson Imaging Clin N Am. 2018;26(4):495-507.
15. Donners R, Blackledge M, Tunariu N, Messiou C, Merkle EM, Koh DM. Quantitative whole-body diffusion-weighted MR imaging. Magn Reson Imaging Clin N Am. 2018;26(4):479-94.
16. Breighner RE, Endo Y, Konin GP, Gulotta LV, Koff MF, Potter HG. Technical developments: zero echo time imaging of the shoulder: enhanced osseous detail by using MR imaging. Radiology. 2018;286(3):960-6.
17. Costa FM, Canella C, Gasparetto E. Advanced magnetic resonance imaging techniques in the evaluation of musculoskeletal tumors. Radiol Clin North Am. 2011;49(6):1325-58.
18. Kogan F, Broski SM, Yoon D, Gold GE. Applications of PET-MRI in musculoskeletal disease. J Magn Reson Imaging. 2018;48(1):27-47.
19. Boutin RD, Brossmann J, Sartoris DJ, Reilly D, Resnick D. Update on imaging of orthopedic infections. Orthop Clin North Am. 1998;29(1):41-66.
20. D Towers J. The use of intravenous contrast in MRI of extremity infection. Semin Ultrasound CT MR. 1997;18:269-75.
21. Narváez JA, Narváez J, De Lama E, De Albert M. MR imaging of early rheumatoid arthritis. Radiographics. 2010;30(1):143-63.
22. Adam G, Bücker A, Nolte-Ernsting C, Tacke J, Günther R. Interventional MR imaging: percutaneous abdominal and skeletal biopsies and drainages of the abdomen. Eur Radiol. 1999;9(8):1471-8.
23. Genant JW, Vandevenne JE, Bergman AG, Beaulieu CF, Kee ST, Norbash AM, et al. Interventional musculoskeletal procedures performed by using MR imaging guidance with a vertically open MR unit: assessment of techniques and applicability. Radiology. 2002;223(1):127-36.
24. Ghelman B. Biopsies of the musculoskeletal system. Radiol Clinics North Am. 1998;36(3):567-80.
25. Feldman F. Musculoskeletal radiology: then and now. Radiology. 2000;216(2):309-16.

CHAPTER 2

Nuclear Medicine Imaging for Musculoskeletal Disorders

Rakesh Kumar, Madhavi Tripathi, Shamim Ahmed Shamim

INTRODUCTION

Musculoskeletal system is a dynamic organ system, which responds to systemic as well as to localized stress and, hence, apart from anatomical visualization, it requires physiological evaluation. Nuclear medicine techniques provide the physician with physiologically detailed images that can give insight, which cannot always be accomplished, from plain radiograph or even with computed tomography (CT) and magnetic resonance imaging (MRI). The major advantage of nuclear medicine imaging stems from the fact that functional changes appear much before anatomical changes. Hence, nuclear medicine imaging allows early detection of diseases affecting musculoskeletal system. The present chapter summarizes the nuclear medicine techniques used for musculoskeletal imaging and their utility in various benign and malignant pathologies involving the musculoskeletal system.

Table 1: Radiotracers used for skeletal scintigraphy.

Tracers for skeletal imaging	*Nonspecific*	*Tumor-specific*
Planar and SPECT	^{99m}Tc MDP	
	^{99m}Tc HEDP	
PET	18F-Fluoride	*Ga-68 DOTANOC-NET
	*18F FDG	*!Ga-68 PSMA-prostate cancer

*Localizes in bone marrow and bone metastases.
!This tracer localizes to prostate-specific membrane antigen (PSMA) expression on prostate cancer cells and also in neovascularization, thus has been found to localize to bone metastases in breast, anaplastic thyroid cancer, adrenocortical cancer (ACC), etc.
(FDG: fluorodeoxyglucose; HEDP: hydroxyethylidene diphosphonic acid; MDP: methylene diphosphonate; NET: neuroendocrine tumor; PET: positron emission tomography; SPECT: single photon emission computed tomography)

BONE SCINTIGRAPHY

In spite of newer developments in the field of nuclear medicine, bone scintigraphy (BS) remains the most commonly employed method for musculoskeletal imaging. It is performed following the intravenous administration of bone-seeking radiopharmaceuticals. These compounds are usually phosphonates labeled with ^{99m}Technetium (^{99m}Tc). The most widely used is ^{99m}Tc-methylene diphosphonate (MDP) **(Table 1)**. Others are ^{99m}Tc-ethylene hydroxy-diphosphonate (EHDP) and ^{99m}Tc-hydroxymethylene diphosphonate (HDP). The presence of P-C-P bonds makes these compounds resistant to hydrolysis by bone phosphatases, thereby increasing the biological half-life. 3–4 hours after intravenous injection about 25–35% of radiotracer is retained in the normal adult skeleton, the rest is excreted in the urine via the kidney. These phosphorus-containing complexes attach themselves to the hydroxyapatite crystal on the bone surface by chemisorption.[1] Thus, they localize at the site of direct and indirect osteoblastic activation. Autoradiographic studies revealed that the ^{99m}Tc-labeled phosphonates are mainly taken up in the mineral phase of skeletal bone at the site of reactive bone formation. This osteoblastic activation can be seen because of wide array of pathologies, thereby decreasing the specificity. The routine BS employs whole body anterior and posterior sweep images. In addition, dynamic flow and pool images are acquired in selected cases.

SPECT AND SPECT/CT

Given the lack of anatomical information provided by planar BS, especially in the regions of complex anatomy, additional methods are employed. Single photon emission tomography (SPECT) is being routinely used in such a scenario. It gives three-dimensional pictures and is beneficial in patients with normal planar images despite symptoms and in those with equivocal findings.[2] SPECT imaging is most useful for the evaluation of the thoracolumbar spine, skull, and pelvis. These areas have extensive surrounding soft tissue and/or complicated body contours, and thus superior image contrast provided by SPECT improves lesion detection. The decision to perform single field-of-view SPECT studies has been guided by suspicious findings on planar imaging or localized clinical symptoms. However, even with plain

SPECT, correlation with anatomical imaging is usually needed. SPECT/CT imaging with hybrid cameras has been introduced to overcome this shortcoming and to provide both anatomical and functional information in a single setting.

PET AND PET/CT

In contrast to routine gamma camera imaging, positron emission tomography (PET) imaging is based on the detection of high energy (511 KeV) annihilation photons emitted by positron-emitting radionuclides. The inherent physics of positron decay allows tomographic imaging without the need for collimators, thereby improving the sensitivity and resolution. The lack of anatomical information on PET alone has been overcome with introduction of hybrid PET/CT. In fact, the availability of hybrid PET/CT systems has made PET alone redundant. Although, PET and PET/CT had greatest impact in the field of cancer imaging, its application for other areas including musculoskeletal disorders is being actively investigated. In clinical practice, most PET studies are performed with 2-[^{18}F] fluoro-2-deoxy-D-glucose (FDG), a glucose analog. It is actively taken up by cells with increased glucose metabolic rate via specific glucose transporters (GLUT-1 and GLUT-4) and is phosphorylated by hexokinases to FDG-6-phosphate, which is retained.[3] Nowadays, FDG-PET is being increasingly used for imaging primary and secondary musculoskeletal tumors as well as infections. Another important tracer in the context of skeletal imaging is ^{18}F-fluoride **(Table 1)**. It can also be used for quantitative studies of skeletal kinetics.[4] Although there are differences between ^{18}F-fluoride and ^{99m}Tc-diphosphonate, it is probable that the mechanism of uptake in bone is the same, i.e., adsorption onto bony surfaces with predilection for sites of active bone formation.[5] The uptake of ^{18}F-fluoride is approximately twofold higher and its blood clearance is significantly faster compared with the ^{99m}Tc-diphosphonates, resulting in an increased bone-to-background ratio. Ga-68 prostate-specific membrane antigen (PSMA) PET-CT is a new addition, is used for prostate cancer staging, particularly for bone metastasis, and shows high sensitivity and specificity for bone metastasis. In addition, PET offers high sensitivity and high resolution, and therefore enables to perform highly accurate whole-body screening for metastases.[6]

MUSCULOSKELETAL TUMOR IMAGING

Metastasis

Skeletal metastasis is the most common bone malignancy. It affects approximately two-thirds of cancer patients, with breast cancer being the leading cause in women, prostate cancer in men, followed by lung cancer in both genders. Accurate assessment of skeletal involvement is essential for optimal management of these patients.[7] Many patients with bone metastases are identified during initial staging, routine follow-up, or on investigation for rising tumor markers. For the past few decades, planar BS has been the most frequently performed imaging study in the evaluation of metastatic bone disease. Although scintigraphic findings alone are often nonspecific for skeletal pathologies, this technique reportedly has an exquisite sensitivity. Radiographs are found to be negative in 30–50% of patients with positive bone scan. The most common pattern of bone metastasis is multiple "hot" spots distributed randomly throughout the skeleton.[8] A lytic metastasis usually presents as a photopenic area with increased activity at the margin of the lesion. False negative results in BS are seen in avascular lesions, in the presence of rapidly growing pure osteolytic metastases with no reactive increased osteoblastic activity, or in lesions with low bone turnover (multiple myeloma and hepatocellular cancer). Specificity of BS is generally lower, due to a known increased blood flow and bone remodeling in response to a variety of disease processes, including trauma, infection, inflammation, and osteoarthritis. Therefore, further assessment with other imaging modalities, mainly CT and MRI, and in some cases, histologic confirmation may be required for precise diagnosis.[9]

Addition of SPECT has been reported to detect 20–50% more lesions in the spine compared with planar scintigraphy.[10] It increases both the sensitivity and specificity of bone scans.[11] The use of SPECT for the assessment of suspicious vertebral lesions on planar BS had a negative predictive value of 98%. The sensitivity and specificity of bone SPECT for diagnosis of bone metastases are 87–92 and 91–93%, respectively.[12] The decision to perform single field-of-view SPECT studies has been guided by suspicious findings on planar imaging or localized clinical symptoms. Newly developed half-time whole body SPECT protocols provide tomographic assessment of the entire skeleton within an acceptable image acquisition time, with subsequent improvement in sensitivity and an increased detection rate of asymptomatic small skeletal metastases.[13] However, even with SPECT correlation with high-quality anatomic images, CT or MRI may still be needed for diagnosis. Hybrid SPECT/CT devices equipped with multislice CT scanners further improve the sensitivity and specificity of BS. It has been shown to be superior to planar BS and SPECT for skeletal metastasis of breast and lung cancers.[14,15] Foci of increased tracer activity on BS, suspicious of representing malignant bone lesions, may not show any morphologic abnormality on CT as functional changes precede anatomical changes, and therefore cannot be confirmed as such. The present consensus is to do SPECT/CT of suspicious planar BS lesions only if the lesion remains equivocal even after SPECT **(Figs. 1A to E)**.

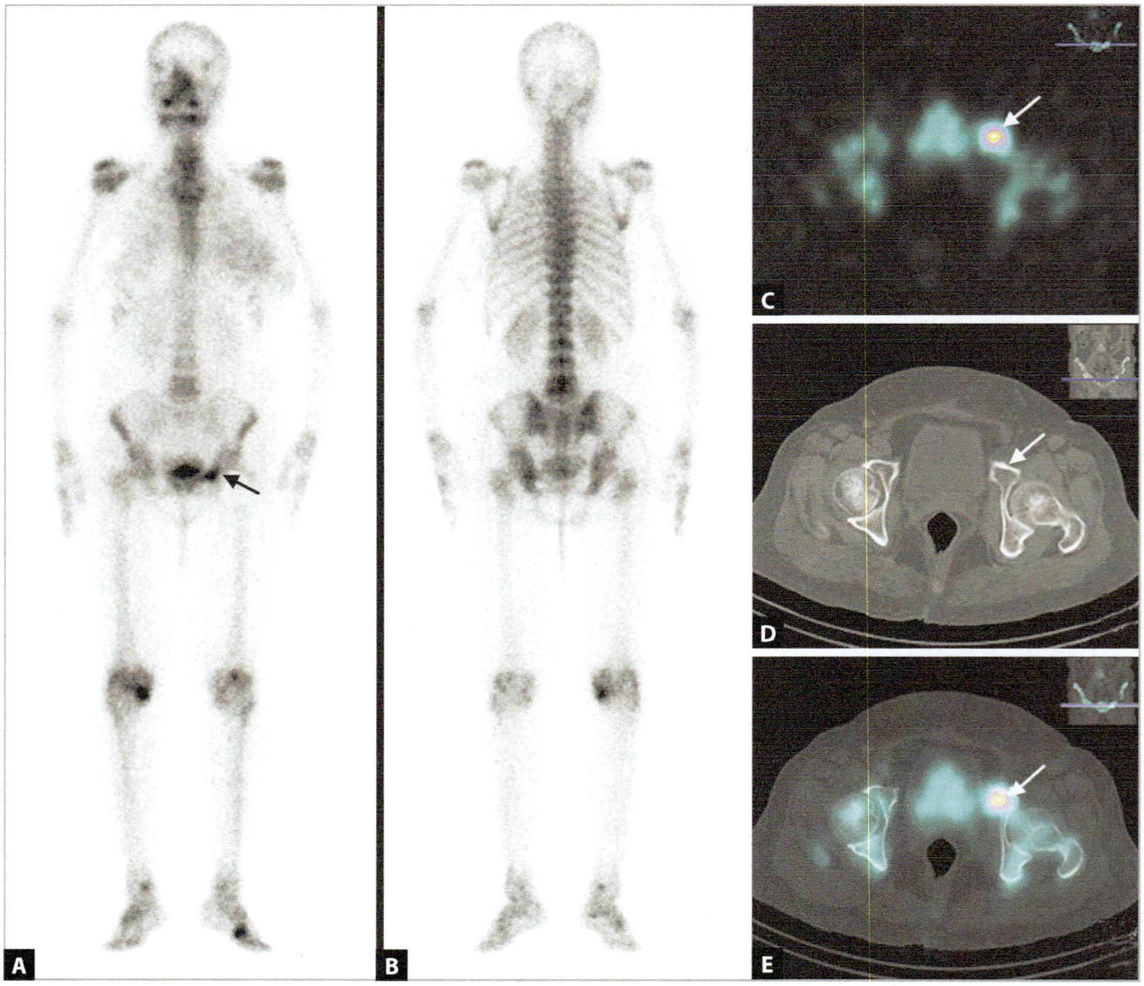

Figs. 1A to E: A 37-year-old carcinoma of breast patient for staging. (A and B) Planar bone scintigraphy showed a suspicious focal uptake in left superior pubic rami (arrow). SPECT (C), CT (D), and SPECT (E) images showed lytic lesion with increased tracer uptake (arrows) suggesting metastasis.

Several studies have shown the superiority of the ^{18}F-fluoride PET over BS for the diagnosis of skeletal metastases; the former demonstrated a higher number of the lesions and a higher contrast between normal and abnormal bone.[16] Although the superb resolution and high abnormal-to-normal bone ratio of ^{18}F-fluoride PET can potentially lower the specificity, hybrid PET-CT imaging should help differentiate benign versus malignant lesions **(Figs. 2A to C)**.[17] ^{18}F-fluoride has shown to be highly sensitive for detecting lytic and sclerotic bone metastasis in breast cancer,[18] prostate cancer,[19] and lung cancer.[20] There has been the suggestion that ^{18}F-fluoride could be more cost effective than the bone scan and that a case can be made for it replacing the bone scan.[21] Increased FDG activity at the sites of skeletal lesions represents active tumor itself, whereas increased ^{99m}Tc-MDP or ^{18}F-fluoride activity represents a blastic activity/reparative process in response to tumor and destroyed bone. Compared with BS or ^{18}F-fluoride, FDG-PET is reported to be more sensitive for lytic lesions and bone marrow disease but less sensitive for blastic lesions.[22] It has an additional advantage: the ability to assess extraskeletal metastatic disease, including muscle metastasis.[23] Recent data almost invariably have shown that BS is more sensitive than FDG-PET for detection of blastic/sclerotic lesion, whereas FDG-PET is more sensitive for lytic lesions and bone marrow involvement **(Figs. 3A to D)**.[24] The lower sensitivity of FDG-PET for detecting sclerotic lesions can be complemented by CT, which may obviate the need for BS.[2] For prostatic bone metastasis, Ga-68 PSMA can be used in addition to BS **(Figs. 4A to E)**. It is generally agreed that the overall sensitivity of FDG-PET and BS for all lesions is comparable, but PET has a higher specificity, resulting in an overall higher accuracy. The utility of FDG-PET-CT for bone metastasis has already been shown in breast cancer, lung cancer, lymphoma, multiple myeloma, and neuroblastoma.[25-27] Another very important advantage of FDG-PET-CT is its ability to assess response to therapy in bone metastasis. Although BS has been used to assess the efficacy of treatment and to follow breast cancer patients,

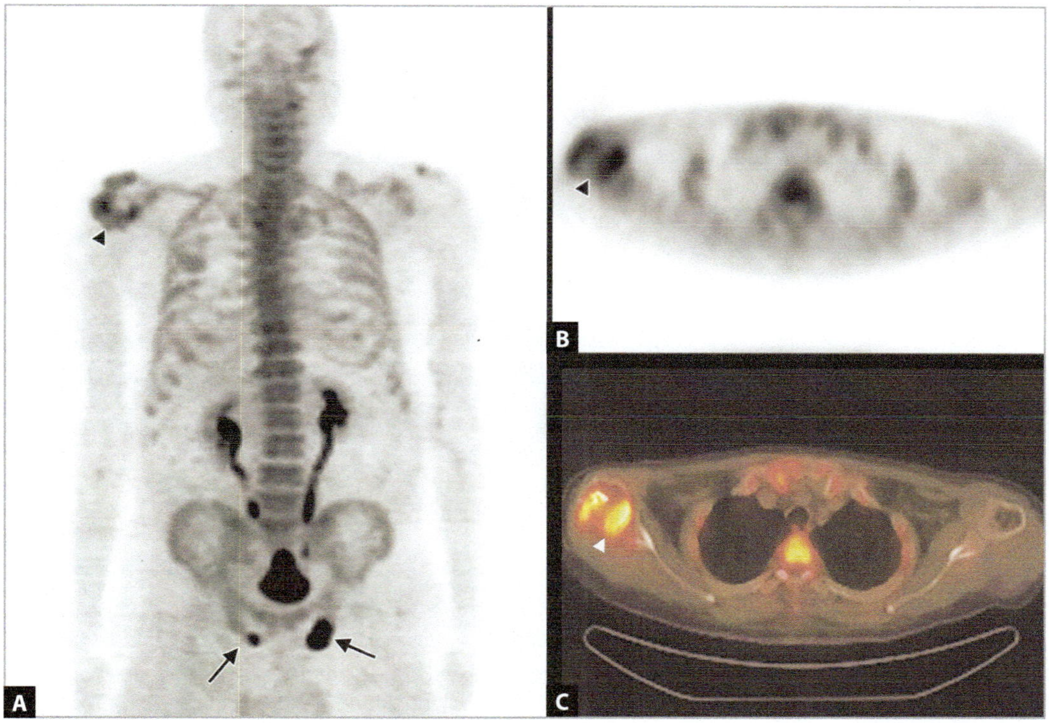

Figs. 2A to C: A 60-year-old male with carcinoma of prostate and rising prostate-specific antigen (PSA). (A and B) ^{18}F-fluoride PET maximum intensity projection (MIP) images show focal tracer uptake in bilateral pubic rami (arrows) suggestive of metastasis. Also, noted was tracer uptake in right shoulder (arrowhead); (C) On PET-CT images, this uptake was diagnosed to be degenerative change (arrowhead).

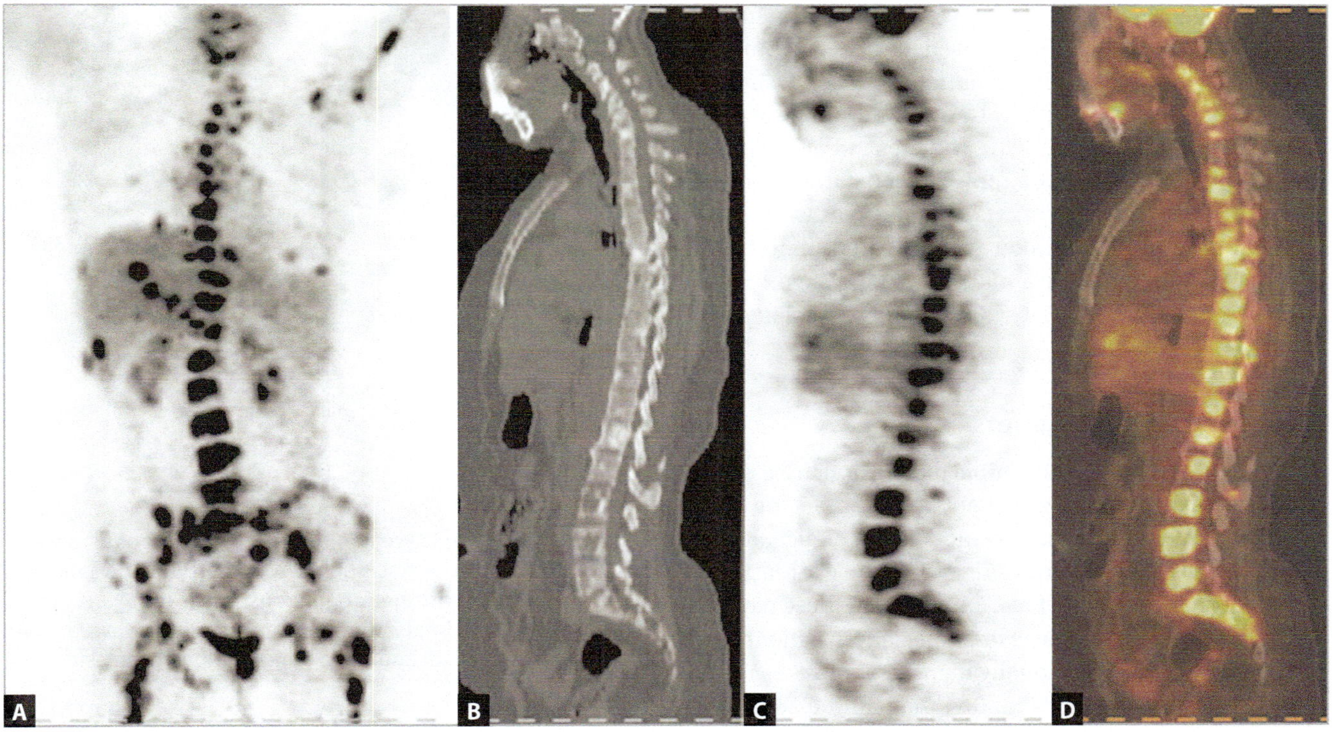

Figs. 3A to D: A 35-year-old female with known breast cancer underwent PET-CT scan for staging. ^{18}F-FDG whole body projection image (A) shows focal areas of increased radiotracer uptake suggestive of metastases. Lytic sclerotic bone lesions and FDG uptake in multiple vertebrae in CT, PET, and PET-CT sagittal sections (B to D). There are many lesions showing focal FDG uptake no sclerosis on CT suggestive of marrow metastases.

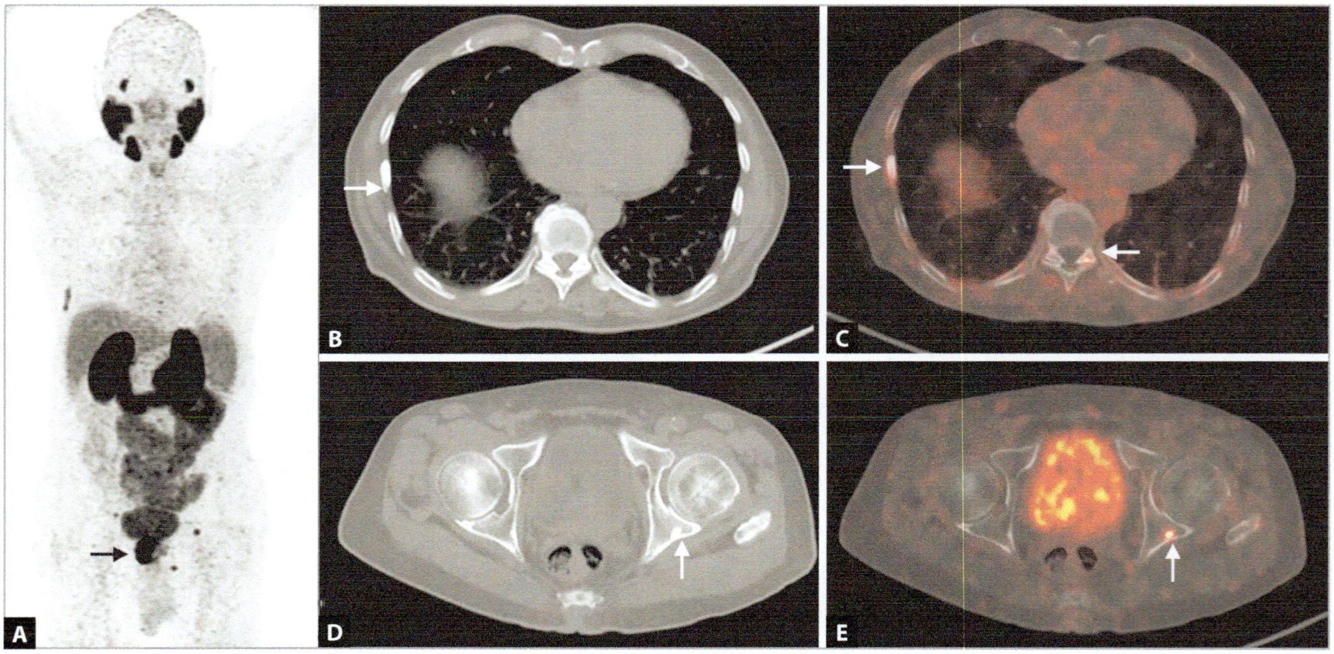

Figs. 4A to E: (A) ^{68}Ga-PSMA PET/CT maximum intensity projection image showing heterogeneous increased uptake in prostatic bed with focal uptake in left hip region and physiological uptake in salivary gland, kidney, and bowel loops; (B) Axial CT image showing sclerotic lesion in the rib and left pedicle of vertebra, (C) corresponding fused PET/CT image showing focal uptake (arrows)—consistent with metastases; (D) Axial CT image showing sclerotic lesion in the left acetabulum, corresponding fused PET/CT image (E) showing focal uptake—consistent with metastasis.

the early response to any treatment cannot be assessed by BS. Moreover, BS may show persistent increased activity even in treated lesions for several weeks to months. In most malignancies, FDG-PET has proved an effective modality for early assessment of therapeutic response by showing rapid reduction in FDG uptake by the tumors in responders following chemotherapy.[28] The changes in FDG standard uptake value (SUV) with therapy showed correlation with the overall clinical assessment of response as well as with the change in tumor marker value. Flare phenomenon which is considered to be a marker of response on BS has also been described on FDG-PET but only associated with antiestrogen therapy.[29]

Primary Malignant Tumors

Bone scan has no role in the initial diagnosis or assessment of the extent of primary malignant bone tumors for which MRI is considered the imaging modality of choice. Rather, whole-body BS is generally reserved for evaluation of metastatic bone disease **(Figs. 5A and B)** in these patients. Calcified pulmonary metastases, especially in patients with osteosarcoma, are occasionally identified on BS as focally increased tracer uptake **(Fig. 5A)** that can be accurately localized using SPECT/CT. High-resolution CT is the mainstay for the evaluation of pulmonary metastases.

Functional imaging with FDG-PET provides unique information with regard to the metabolic activity of bone and soft tissue tumors **(Figs. 6A to G)**. This may help characterize indeterminate lesions and guide targeted biopsy of the most metabolically active area within larger tumors. This aspect is particularly important in many soft

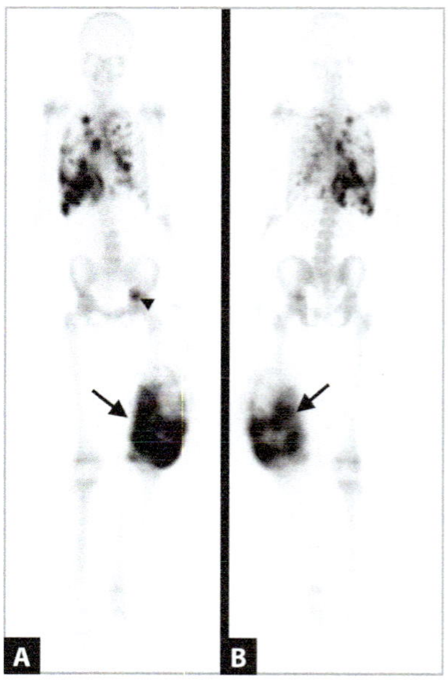

Figs. 5A and B: A 16-year-old male with osteosarcoma of left femur. Planar bone scintigraphy (A and B) shows mass in left femoral shaft with heterogeneous tracer uptake (arrows), consistent with primary tumor. In addition, it showed bone metastasis (arrowhead) and osteogenic pulmonary metastasis.

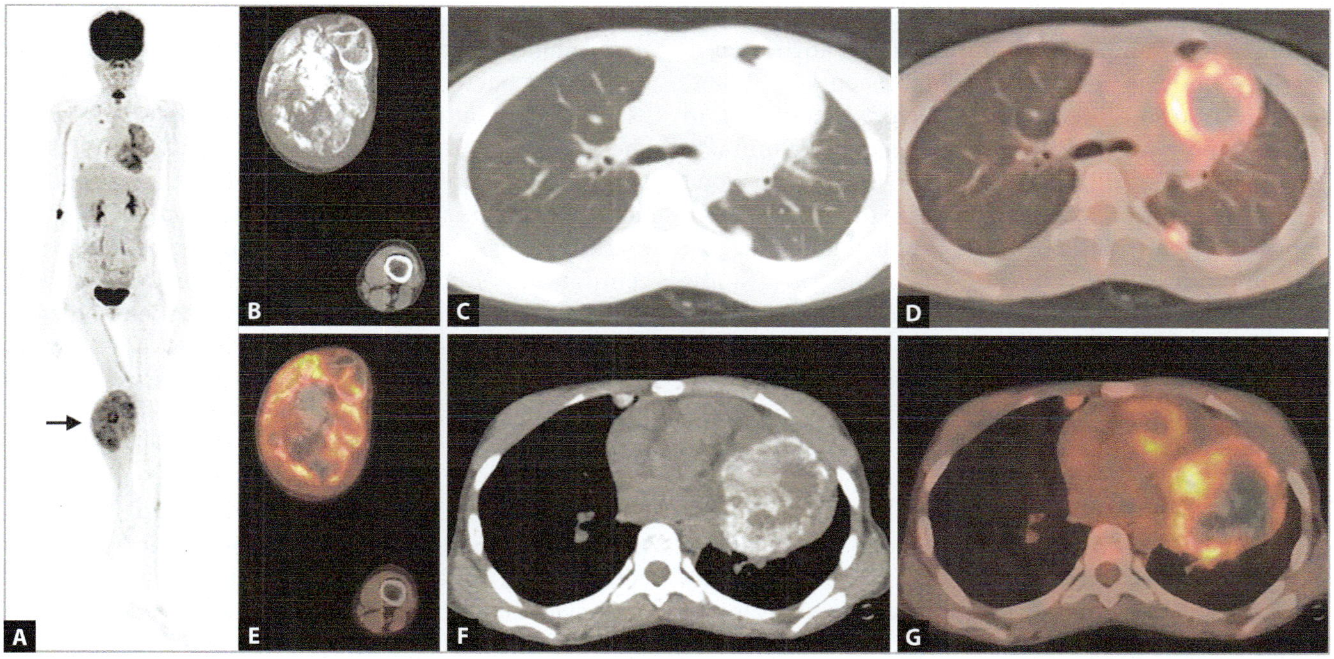

Figs. 6A to G: (A) ^{18}F-FDG PET/CT maximum intensity projection images of patient with osteosarcoma of right tibia showing expansile heterogeneous FDG uptake the right knee region (arrow), axial CT and fused PET/CT images at the proximal shaft of right tibia showing FDG avid expansile primary (B and E). Axial CT (C and F) and fused PET/CT (D and G) images at the thoracic level showing multiple calcified masses and nodules (consistent with metastases).

tissue and bone tumors which are of mixed grade and/or cell type. In one study of soft tissue tumors, there was a statistically significant difference in SUV between benign and malignant lesions, although there was considerable overlap between the two groups and only lipomas and hemangiomas were consistently non-FDG avid.[30] Dual-time point PET imaging can be utilized to increase the accuracy of differentiating benign from malignant soft tissue lesions.[31] FDG-PET may also be used for more accurate staging of histologically confirmed tumors, in therapy response assessment to detect progression or response of disease ahead of morphological changes in the tumor and in the early detection of recurrent disease. The degree of FDG uptake by tumors pre- and post-therapy correlates well with histological response, often prior to demonstrable changes on anatomical imaging.[32] FDG-PET is also useful for the detection of tumor recurrence and has been found to be more sensitive than magnetic resonance (MR), especially when MR findings are equivocal.[33] SUV on FDG-PET is an important prognostic factor in most musculoskeletal tumors and has been shown to be a reliable independent prognostic indicator.[34,35]

Benign Tumors

Bone scan is a highly sensitive investigation for the diagnosis of osteoid osteoma. A negative bone scan virtually rules out the diagnosis of osteoid osteoma. A three-phase bone scan shows increased blood flow and blood pool and a "focal" area of intense uptake on delayed images.[36] Some surgeons have used intraoperative scintigraphic probes to localize osteoid osteoma. In addition, BS has been used for detecting recurrence after radiofrequency ablation of osteoid osteoma. Other benign lesions, which can show increased uptake, are aneurysmal bone cyst, chondroblastoma, enchondroma, etc. However, there is no specific pattern pertaining to these lesions on BS alone. With the availability of hybrid SPECT/CT, these lesions can be characterized with greater certainty by employing their CT characteristics.

INFECTION IMAGING

Acute and Chronic Osteomyelitis

Bone scintigraphy is used as a complementary imaging procedure in the evaluation of infection. The classic findings are increased regional blood flow and blood pool with a corresponding increased uptake on delayed images. This is different from cellulitis where only increase in blood flow and blood pool in the soft tissue with no increased radiotracer uptake on delayed image is seen. ^{99m}Tc MDP has a high sensitivity (82–95%) and accuracy (90%) for detecting acute, uncomplicated osteomyelitis, becoming positive within 28–48 hours after the onset of symptoms. Compared with anatomic modalities, the radionuclide bone scan has the further advantage of detecting multiple foci of disease which can be seen especially in children. However, other conditions (e.g., fractures, neuropathic joints, and arthritis) may mimic osteomyelitis on bone scanning alone, decreasing its specificity.[37] Although adding a fourth phase (24-hour image) is advocated to increase the specificity, with a high accuracy of 85%, the clinical results are not impressive.[38] In addition, in pediatric population, BS can show reduced radiotracer uptake, which is attributed to increased pressure on blood vessels, stripping away of periosteum via the accumulation of pus and interruption of blood supply due to plugging and thrombosis. This can lead to a false negative study. About 30% of patients with acute osteomyelitis will progress to have subacute or chronic osteomyelitis **(Figs. 7A to E)**. Bone scan remains positive for months even after successful treatment of acute osteomyelitis. It is difficult to differentiate healing from chronic active disease.[39]

Other radiotracer, such as ^{67}Ga-citrate and ^{111}In-oxine/^{99m}Tc-hexamethyl-propylene amine oxime (HMPAO)-labeled leukocyte imaging, has been extensively used in musculoskeletal infection, either alone or in combination with BS. ^{67}Ga-citrate localize to the site of infection via several pathway including increased vascular permeability at the site of infection, binding to lactoferrin and direct bacterial uptake.[40] Reported sensitivity for ^{67}Ga-citrate scintigraphy ranges from 25 to 80%, with a specificity of 67%.[41] It has proven to be extremely useful in detecting infection in the immunocompromised population. It is usually done in combination with BS for musculoskeletal infection. However, ^{67}Ga-citrate scintigraphy suffers from poor image quality, long scanning time, and significantly higher patient radiation dose leading to decline in its use with advent of better tracers. Labeled leukocytes can overcome some of the disadvantages of BS. Its uptake is dependent on the chemotaxis of labeled leukocytes at the site of infection. ^{111}In-oxine/^{99m}Tc HMPAO-labeled leukocyte imaging have shown increased specificity—upto 80–90%—compared to BS for detecting infection, particularly when complicating conditions are present. As the majority of leukocytes labeled are neutrophils, the procedure is most useful for identifying neutrophil-mediated inflammatory

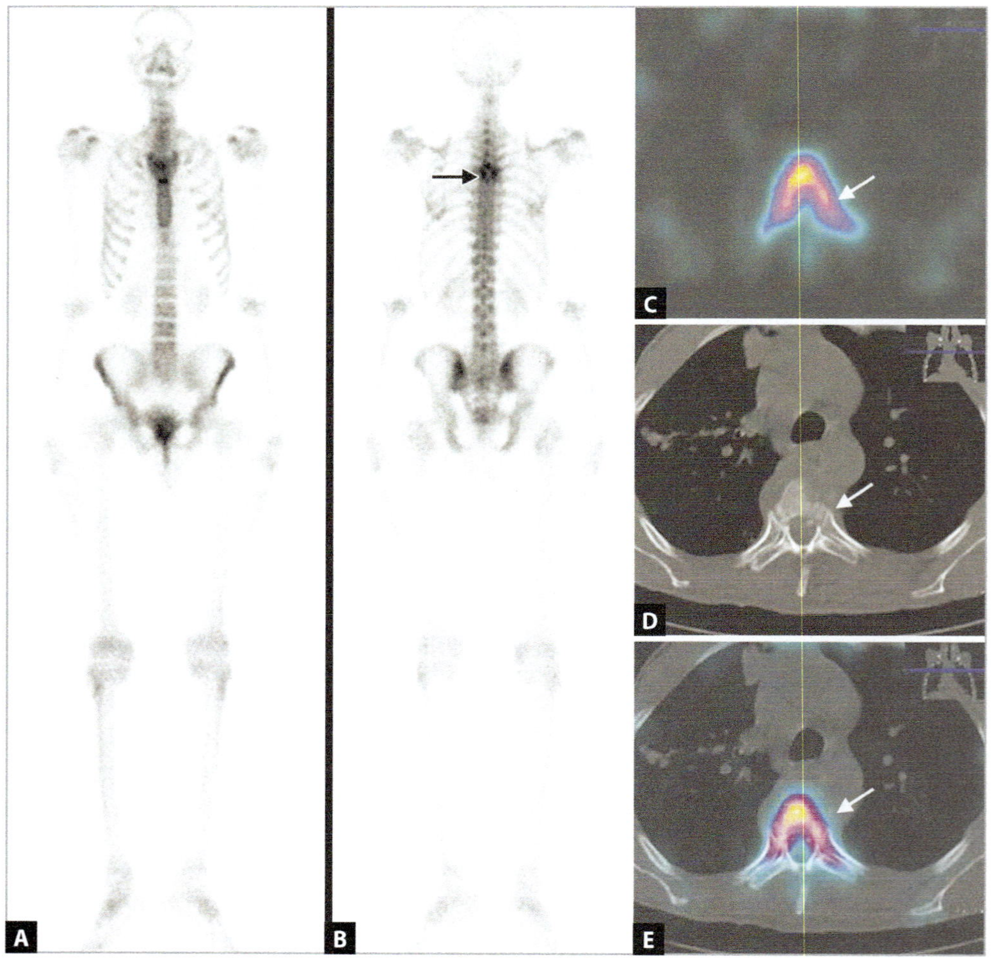

Figs. 7A to E: A 35-year-old male with backache. (A and B) Planar bone scintigraphy showed increased irregular tracer uptake in D6 vertebra (arrow). SPECT (C), CT (D), and SPECT-CT (E) images showed destructive changes in D6 vertebra with increased tracer uptake along with paravertebral fluid collection (arrows). The findings were highly suspicious for tuberculosis and confirmed at histopathology.

processes, such as bacterial infections. It is less useful for those illnesses in which the predominant cellular response is other than neutrophilic, such as tuberculosis.[42] Additionally, in contrast to other locations in the skeleton, labeled leukocyte imaging is of limited value for detecting spinal osteomyelitis.[43] Also, their performance requires the withdrawal of a large amount of blood (50 cc); it is also costly, is labor intensive, and has the inherent limitations related to personnel safety, including the risks of infection and cross-contamination from handling blood products. All these factors limit their routine use. Additional use of SPECT/CT with BS, ^{67}Ga-citrate and ^{111}In-oxine/^{99m}Tc HMPAO-labeled leukocyte improves the specificity of these studies for detecting osteomyelitis.[44]

PET-CT-based radiotracers such as ^{18}F-FDG-labeled white blood cell (WBC) and plain ^{18}F-FDG are also being explored for infection imaging. These agents have shown better sensitivity and specificity than SPECT agents and are currently in use for infection imaging **(Figs. 8A to I)**.

Diabetic Foot

Pedal ulcers with or without osteomyelitis is a very common complication in patients with long-standing diabetes. Foot osteomyelitis frequently presents without systemic illness and with no obvious clinical symptoms or signs, besides the ulcer, and imaging studies are often needed to confirm the diagnosis. Although routinely performed, the accuracy of three-phase BS for pedal osteomyelitis is modest with large prospective study demonstrating a sensitivity of 67% and specificity of 43%.[45] With the presence of associated Charcot arthropathy, the diagnosis becomes more difficult. Addition of SPECT-CT in this scenario appears promising.[46] It can show focal bone destruction versus arthropathic changes, thereby clinching the diagnosis **(Figs. 9A to D)**. Labeled leukocyte imaging may be more sensitive for detecting clinically unsuspected pedal osteomyelitis and is useful for monitoring response to medical therapy.[47] But a major drawback is the fact that even neuropathic joints may accumulate labeled leukocyte; hence, it is not useful when both infection and Charcot joint coexist.[48]

Prosthetic Infection

With improving surgical techniques and availability of better prosthetics, the number of patients opting for the same is increasing. Although the clinical results of joint replacement surgery are usually excellent, these implants do fail. Aseptic loosening due to mechanical factors and inflammatory reaction to prosthetic components is the most common cause for implant failure followed by infection. Infection is perhaps the most serious complication of joint arthroplasty, ranging in frequency from ~1–2% for primary implants to ~3–5% for revision implants.[49] Because their treatments are so different, the importance of distinguishing infection from aseptic loosening of prosthesis cannot be overemphasized. Although BS is sensitive for detecting complications of prosthetic surgery, it cannot reliably distinguish among the causes for failure. Although routinely advocated, periprosthetic uptake patterns are not too useful for differentiating infection from aseptic loosening.[50] Addition of ^{67}Ga-citrate scintigraphy to BS only provides

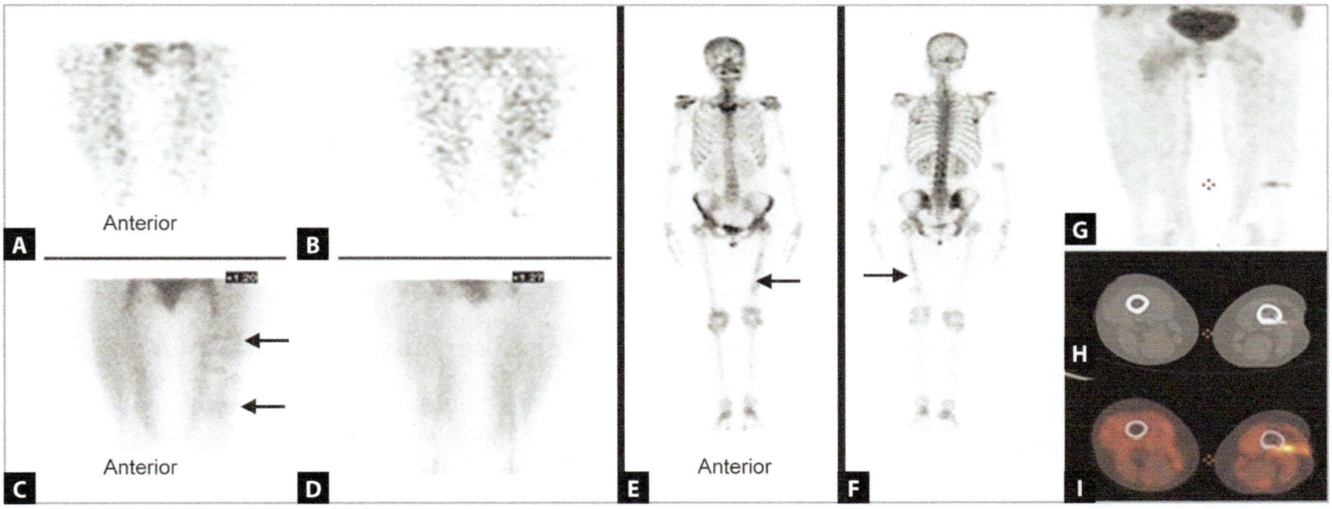

Figs. 8A to I: ^{99m}Tc MDP three-phase bone scintigraphy images (Flow A and B, soft tissue/blood pool phase—C and D, delayed phase E and F) and ^{18}F-FDG-PET/CT images (images G to I) of a 37-year-old female with chronic osteomyelitis of left femur. The flow phase images were within normal limits; however, pool showed mild increased radiotracer accumulation in the mid and distal thigh region and delayed phase images showed mild tracer uptake in the mid and distal shaft of femur. FDG-PET/CT was done to rule out infection which showed small area of increased radiotracer uptake in the cortex of distal shaft of femur with calcific changes and increased uptake in the adjacent bone suggestive of residual infection which was confirmed by biopsy culture.

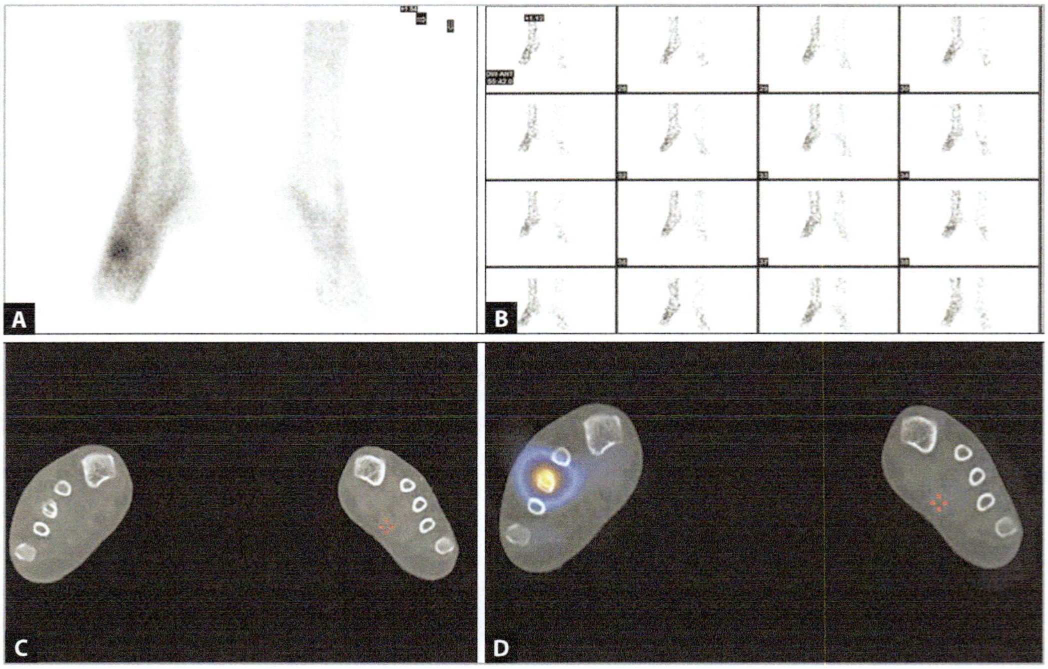

Figs. 9A to D: 35-year-old male, known case of diabetic mellitus, having foot ulcer, referred for bone scan to differentiate between cellulitis and osteomyelitis. Blood pool (A) and blood flow (B) images show focal area of increased radiotracer uptake in distal foot region. Axial CT (C) and fused SPECT-CT (D) images showing involvement of right third metatarsal bone—consistent with osteomyelitis.

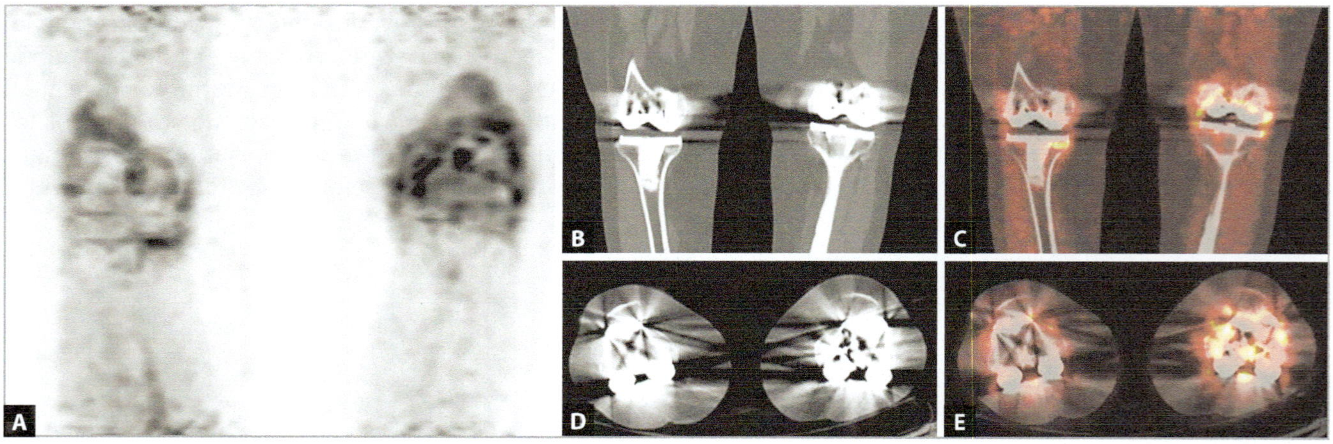

Figs. 10A to E: ^{18}F-FDG WBC PET/CT maximum intensity projection image of both knee joint showing increased FDG-labeled WBC accumulation around the prosthesis of left knee joint. Corresponding coronal (A) and axial images of CT (B and D) and fused PET/CT (C and E) show periprosthetic accumulation of labeled WBCs consistent with culture positive prosthetic infection.

moderate improvement in accuracy.[51] Labeled leukocyte scintigraphy though theoretically presents the advantage of differentiating aseptic loosening from infection, the actual results has been variable.[52,53] Poor sensitivity is ascribed to the chronicity of the process, whereas poor specificity is ascribed to nonspecific inflammation. Addition of BS or marrow scintigraphy might improve the specificity of this test, though there is no general consensus.[54] ^{18}F-FDG-labeled WBC scan and F-18 FDG-PET-CT are also used in these days for distinguishing aseptic and septic loosening **(Figs. 10A to E)**.

FDG-PET-CT for Musculoskeletal Infection

Experimental studies have shown that mononuclear cells and neutrophilic granulocytes have increased FDG uptake when activated during the so-called respiratory burst, which they experience while fighting an infection.[55] This forms the basis for its use in musculoskeletal infections. It provides better resolution and shorter test duration compared to conventional radionuclide procedures, albeit with higher cost and radiation exposure. It should also be remembered that FDG is not specific for infection, and increased FDG uptake also is observed in inflammatory arthritis, osteoarthritis, fractures, normally healing bone, and degenerative changes.[56] For acute and subacute bone and soft tissue infections, sensitivities of 98% and specificities from 75 to 99% have been reported with FDG-PET.[57] It is especially useful in cases of chronic infections where BS has major limitations. It has been shown to be superior to labeled leukocyte imaging for chronic musculoskeletal infections.[58] Its specificity is higher, if recently (<4 months) traumatized or operated bone is excluded. Though initial results were excellent, FDG-PET-CT appears to be less useful for diabetic foot infection.[59] It is inferior to labeled leukocyte imaging for this purpose. Moreover, altered glucose and insulin dynamics in these patients makes FDG technically challenging. Regarding FDG-PET in patients with suspicion of joint prosthesis infection; initial studies showed promising results and reported sensitivities of 90% and specificities of 89% in the diagnosis of infected lower limb prostheses.[60] Accuracy of FDG-PET was 96% for hip prostheses, 81% for knee prostheses, and 100% for other orthopedic devices. However, when associated with loosening, FDG-PET cannot differentiate between septic and aseptic loosening, as both conditions can cause increased FDG uptake.[61] The reason for the increased FDG uptake around the prosthesis in aseptic loosening is likely an inflammatory immune reaction to the prosthetic material. In a large series, the accuracy of FDG-PET for diagnosing infection of the failed prosthetic joint was low, and varied between 47 and 71% depending on different criteria used to evaluate the images.[62] In fact, it was inferior to combined labeled leukocyte/marrow imaging in this series. It should be remembered that image interpretation in patients with prosthetic devices can be affected by attenuation-correction-induced artifacts. Therefore, it is necessary to examine the nonattenuation corrected scans because they show less prominent reconstruction artifacts.[63]

MUSCULOSKELETAL TRAUMA

Stress Fractures

Stress fractures are two types: (1) Fatigue fractures, which are caused by repeated abnormal stress on normal bones, bone scan shows fusiform increased radiotracer uptake involving the posterior tibial cortex and (2) insufficiency fractures resulting from normal stress on abnormal bone. The latter is seen in patients with underlying bone disease such as osteoporosis, osteomalacia, Paget's disease, and fibrous dysplasia. Because clinical assessment usually is not definitive in these injuries, diagnostic imaging is often required. Plain-film radiography is usually the first examination performed when a stress fracture is suspected. Unfortunately, sensitivity of this method for stress fracture may be as low as 15%.[64] BS, however, is extremely sensitive in detecting stress fractures because it assesses bone metabolism rather than bone anatomy **(Figs. 11A to C)**. In fact for stress fracture at certain sites such as metatarsal bones, it is considered to be the reference method. Sacral insufficiency fractures have a classic appearance on BS, highly specific pattern of horizontal uptake in the body of the sacrum and vertical uptake in the alae, resulting in the "Honda" or "H" sign.[36] Addition of SPECT/CT is likely to improve the accuracy of BS, especially by improving the anatomical localization.

Shin Splints

The clinical entity shin splints is characterized by exercise-induced pain and tenderness on palpation along the posteromedial border of tibia. It results generally from unaccustomed biomechanical stress on the tibia. Shin splints are not fractures and can be distinguished from stress fractures by their linear activity rather than round or fusiform activity.[65] In addition, blood flow and blood pool images are almost always normal. Delayed images of BS demonstrate involvement of the posterior tibial cortex, longitudinally oriented uptake involving one-third of the length of the bone **(Figs. 12A to G)**.

Fractures in Childhood

Very young children may present with failure to move a limb or joint. A history may not be available, especially in preschool children. Bone scans can identify unsuspected sites of fractures in such children. In addition, it can be useful to identify child abuse in children at risk. Radiological skeletal survey and whole-body scintigraphy does offer complementary information that is not available from either study alone.[66] More than 50% of such cases demonstrate diaphyseal injuries.[67] Rarely, fracture of the first rib may be the sole manifestation of abuse. Of course, knowledge of normal BS appearance for the age of child is essential for interpreting such a study.

Sport Injuries

The blood pool phase of BS is very important in detection of soft tissue injuries. Hyperemia is evident in the affected structure with delayed uptake apparent only if there is necrosis/calcification or close apposition of adjacent bony structures, as with tendonitis of the extensor and abductor pollicis tendons and the adjacent radius or tibialis posterior tendonitis and the medial malleolus. SPECT/CT adds by anatomically localizing the site of involvement. It can in addition guide the site of injection, when required.

METABOLIC BONE DISEASE IMAGING

Metabolic bone disorders represent a heterogeneous group of skeletal pathologies that can lead to global or focal

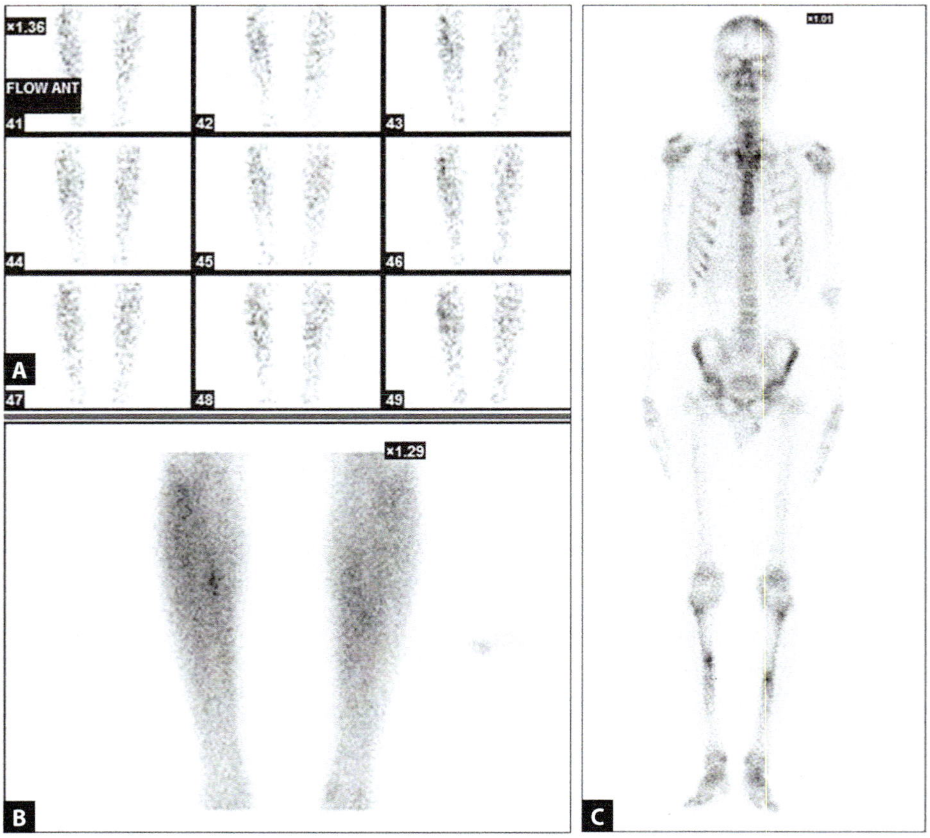

Figs. 11A to C: A 25-year-old active male complain of pain in bilateral leg, bone scan showed focal area of increased radiotracer in bilateral tibial region in flow (A), pool (B), and delayed static (C) images suggestive of bilateral stress fractures.

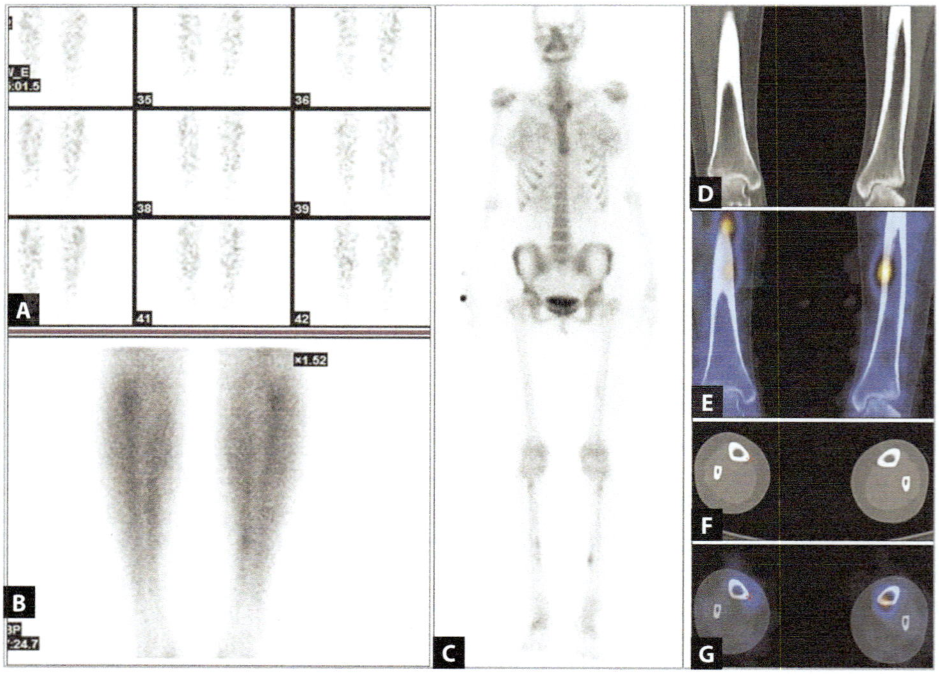

Figs. 12A to G: An 18-year-old sports female complains of pain in both legs. Flow (A) and pool (B) images show mild increased radiotracer uptake along the posterolateral border, also noted increased radiotracer along the posterolateral border in delayed static images (C) in addition to focal uptake. CT (D) and fused (E) coronal images, no changes noted on CT images; however, linear uptake noted in the right tibia and focal uptake in mid shaft of the left tibia. Transaxial CT (F) and fused (G) images, on CT, there is no change noted; however, focal uptake noted along the medial boarder of both tibia.

changes in bone metabolism. The superior sensitivity of BS can be valuable for diagnosis, detection of complications, and monitoring of treatment response **(Figs. 13A and B)**. The continuous improvement in gamma camera hardware and software with the addition of SPECT, and more recently, hybrid SPECT/CT, has maintained a role for nuclear medicine methods in bone disease despite the improvements seen in morphologic imaging techniques.

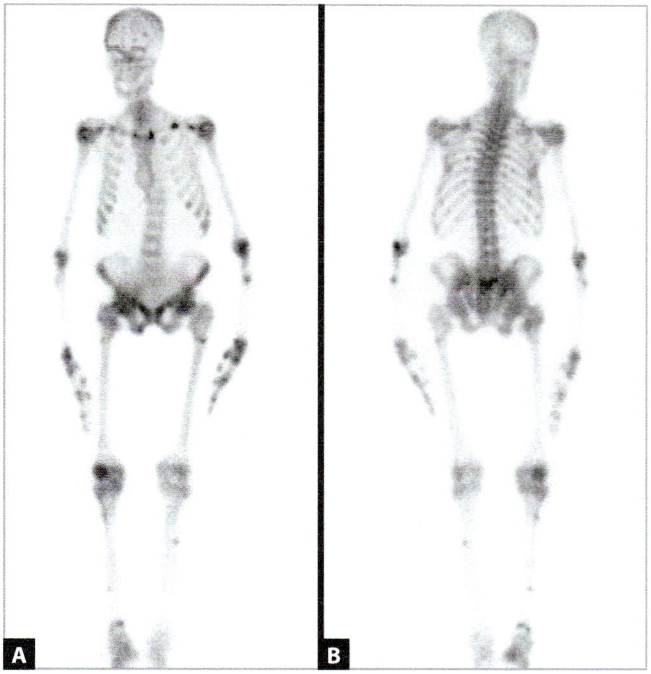

Figs. 13A and B: A 29-year-old female presented with multifocal body ache. Biochemical evaluation showed decreased serum calcium. (A and B) Planar bone scintigraphy images showed classical features of metabolic bone disease-increased bone to soft tissue activity, hot calvarium, tie sternum, nonvisualization of kidneys, and multiple pseudofractures classical for osteomalacia.

Paget's Disease

The initial step in Paget's disease is increased osteoclastic resorption, followed by compensatory osteoblastic activity and increased bone formation. Most patients with Paget's disease have polyostotic disease. Bone scans are a convenient way to evaluate the whole skeleton and has shown a greater sensitivity for detecting affected sites in symptomatic patients in comparison with radiographic skeletal surveys.[68] Characteristically, affected bones show intensely increased activity, extending from the end of a bone and spreading either proximally or distally, often showing a "V"-shaped leading edge **(Figs. 14A to D)**. Many different patterns describing vertebral uptake have been reported as being specific for pagetic involvement, including clover, heart, and Mickey Mouse signs.[69] Apart from localizing the sites of multifocal involvement, another important use of BS is monitoring response to therapy (bisphosphonates). For this purpose, BS is better than measurement of serum alkaline phosphatase alone. The bone scan appearances can be unusual after successful bisphosphonate treatment, resultant heterogeneous uptake sometimes mimicking metastatic disease. As ^{18}F-fluoride PET is better suited to assess bone mineral kinetics, it has also been used to monitor response to bisphosphonate therapy.[70]

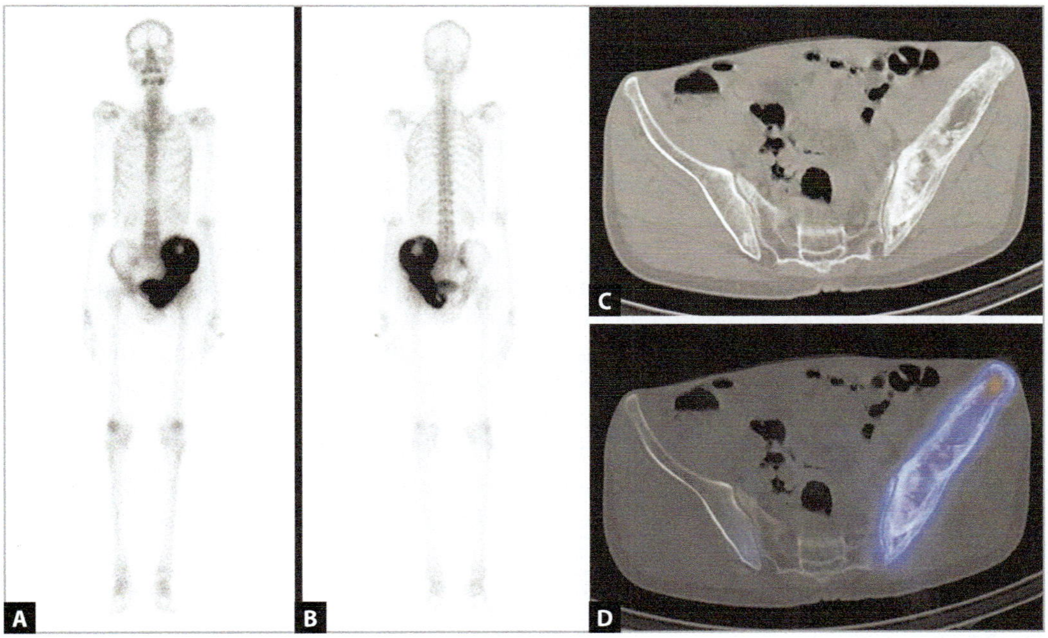

Figs. 14A to D: A 57-year-old female complains of pain in the left hip. Anterior (A) and posterior (B) images show intense radiotracer uptake in the left iliac bone in delayed static images. Transaxial CT (C) and fused (D) images, on CT, there is lytic and sclerotic changes in left iliac bone noted. There is no other lesion in the rest of whole body bone scan.

Hyperparathyroidism

The diagnosis of hyperparathyroidism is biochemical and BS has no routine role in diagnosis. Bone scans are often used to help differentiate the causes of hypercalcemia, in particular, hyperparathyroidism versus malignancy, so that typical features of metabolic bone disorders may be recognized. The most common bone scan appearance is similar to a superscan from other metabolic bone disorders, and uptake of diphosphonate in areas of ectopic calcification also may be seen. Multiple focal areas of abnormal radiotracer uptake in bone scan are suggestive of brown tumors in such patients, which can be well characterized on SPECT/CT.[36]

Renal Osteodystrophy

Renal osteodystrophy is due to a combination of bone disorders as a consequence of chronic renal dysfunction, and often demonstrates the most severe cases of metabolic bone disease. It may comprise osteoporosis, osteomalacia, adynamic bone, and secondary hyperparathyroidism in varying degrees. The most common bone scan appearance is similar to a superscan from other metabolic bone disorders. A clue in differentiating this type of scintigraphic pattern from others is that there may be a lack of bladder activity in view of renal failure. Quantitative measurements of bone metabolism in renal osteodystrophy using ^{18}F-fluoride have been compared with bone histomorphometry and have shown a close relationship.[71]

Osteoporosis and Osteomalacia

Bone scans have no routine clinical role in the diagnosis of osteoporosis *per se* but is most often used in established osteoporosis to diagnose fractures, particularly at sites that are difficult to image with plain film radiography (e.g., sacrum and ribs), and may be particularly useful in the diagnosis of vertebral fractures and in distinguishing malignancy-related vertebral fractures from osteoporotic ones. The characteristic appearance of this type of fracture is of intense, linearly increased tracer uptake at the affected vertebral level which in metastatic collapse extends into the posterior elements and is limited to the body only in osteoporotic collapse. In addition, bone scan is extremely helpful in assessing the age of the fracture. Also, other causes of bone pain can be reliably excluded in osteoporotic patients on BS. Osteomalacia on the other hand shows features similar to other metabolic bone disease. This is probably because of increased osteoid formation. The detection of pseudofractures with this technique is more sensitive than that with radiography.[72]

Bone Dysplasias

Fibrous dysplasia is characterized by a slow, progressive, replacement of the medullary cavity by fibrocollagenous tissue. There is usually intense hyperemia and intense uptake with well-delineated margins on BS. Failure of preservation of the bony outline differentiates fibrous dysplasia from Paget's disease. Identification of polyostotic involvement, which is often asymptomatic, is the main indication for BS.[73] In addition, secondary complications in fibrous dysplasia can be demonstrated on BS. In several other uncommon congenital dysplasias, skeletal abnormalities are usually obvious radiologically. BS can occasionally provide images that are of interest but, more importantly, reflect current physiological activity. The BS findings are variable depending on the type and the site of dysplasia. Additionally, BS might be used for monitoring therapy response.

Avascular Necrosis

Avascular necrosis (AVN) is a common condition affecting up to 30% of individuals with underlying medical conditions requiring steroids. Although the hip is most commonly involved, AVN may affect many other bones, such as lunate (Kienböck's disease), navicular (Kohler's disease), scaphoid (post-fracture), and jaw (post-bisphosphonate therapy). Although MRI is the investigation of choice, a three-phase BS provides useful information to diagnose AVN. A unique advantage of BS is its ability to identify AVN earlier than MRI (72 hours vs. 6 days).[74] Up to 85%, BS may be normal for first 48 hours, the femoral head then shows decreased activity ("cold") for a variable period followed by increased activity due to reparative process. BS is highly sensitive (98%) and specific (95%) for the diagnosis of AVN.[75] SPECT images improve sensitivity to detect AVN. SPECT/CT images are very useful, especially when evaluating small bones.

Complex Regional Pain Syndrome (Reflex Sympathetic Dystrophy)

The complex regional pain syndrome (CRPS) comprises a spectrum of sensory, autonomic, and motor features that predominantly affect the extremities. CRPS I occurs in the absence of definable neurological abnormality. Radiological changes of bone resorption are late findings and hence three-phase BS has been widely utilized in both the diagnosis and the monitoring of treatment. The BS pattern of reflex sympathetic dystrophy (RSD) varies significantly, depending upon the stage of the disease. In early stages, there is increased blood flow and blood pool with increased bone uptake on delayed images **(Figs. 15A to E)**. A characteristic feature is periarticular uptake of radiotracer. In later stages of RSD, bone scan shows normal or even decreased blood flow and blood pool but increased uptake on delayed images on the affected side.[76] In addition, patients with BS abnormalities have higher response rate (90%) to systemic steroid therapy as compared to those without BS findings (36%).[77]

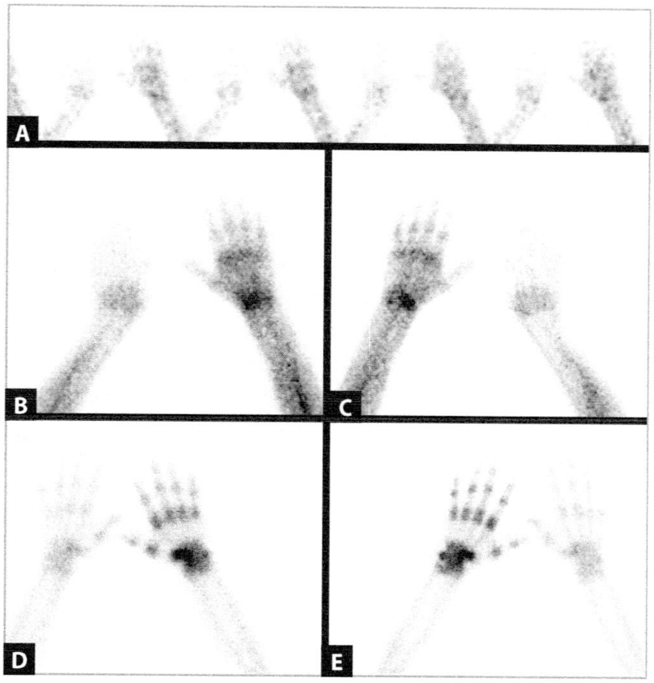

Figs. 15A to E: A 42-year-old male presented with swelling and pain in the left hand 3 months after a minor surgery. Three-phase bone scintigraphy showed increased blood flow (A) and pool (B and C) in the left hand along with classical periarticular uptake in small joints (D and E in delayed images, suggestive of CRPS (reflex sympathetic dystrophy).

JOINT IMAGING

The role of BS is usually complementary to anatomical imaging for joint disease. The major role of BS is in the early detection of subclinical synovitis and monitoring its response to treatment. Scintigraphy is sensitive for the early detection of sacroiliitis, although MRI is used routinely. Three-phase bone scans are as sensitive as MRI for identifying early rheumatoid arthritis. Bone scans are very sensitive for the diagnosis of septic arthritis and become abnormal much earlier than radiographs. Multiphase BS shows increased flow and blood pool in soft tissue and joint and diffuses increased uptake in bones around joints on delayed images. This is especially useful in pediatric population.

FUTURE DIRECTION AND THERANOSTICS

Further improvement in imaging technology and development of newer radiopharmaceuticals will keep on strengthening and redefining the role of nuclear medicine imaging. Routine use of SPECT/CT and PET/CT on one hand will improve the accuracy and on the other hand will broaden the range of indications with respect to musculoskeletal imaging. Another exiting development is hybrid PET/MRI, which when clinically available, might revolutionize musculoskeletal imaging providing high quality images (anatomical and functional) with less radiation burden. PET tracers such as ^{18}F-fluoroestradiol, ^{18}F-fluorothymidine, and ^{18}F-fluorocholine will improve the utilization of PET/CT for diagnosis, response monitoring, and prognostication of musculoskeletal tumors. In addition, FDG as well as FDG-labeled leukocyte PET/CT might gain more and more ground for infection imaging.

CONCLUSION

Despite challenges from morphological imaging, nuclear medicine imaging techniques continue to have a major role in a range of neoplastic, infective, inflammatory, metabolic, and traumatic musculoskeletal diseases. In future, with widespread availability of hybrid modalities, its role in musculoskeletal imaging will continue to expand.

REFERENCES

1. Fogelman I. Skeletal uptake of diphosphonates: a review. Eur J Nucl Med. 1980;5(6):473-6.
2. Even-Sapir E. Imaging of malignant bone involvement by morphologic, scintigraphic and hybrid modalities. J Nucl Med. 2005;46(8):1356-67.
3. Kubota R, Yamada S, Kubota K, Ishiwata K, Tamahashi N, Ido T. Intratumoral distribution of uorine-18-uorodeoxyglucose in vivo: high accumulation in macrophages and granulation tissues studied by microautoradiography. J Nucl Med. 1992;33(11):1972-80.
4. Blake GM, Park-Holohan SJ, Cook GJ, Fogelman I. Quantitative studies of bone with the use of 18F-fluoride and ^{99m}Tc-methylene diphosphonate. Semin Nucl Med. 2001;31:28-49.
5. Schirrmeister H, Guhlmann A, Elsner K, Kotzerke J, Glatting G, Rentschler M, et al. Sensitivity in detecting osseous lesions depends on anatomic localization: planar bone scintigraphy versus 18F PET. J Nucl Med. 1999;40(10):1623-9.
6. Schirrmeister H. Detection of bone metastases in breast cancer by positron emission tomography. Radiol Clin North Am. 2007;45(4):669-76.
7. Van der Wall H, Clarke S. The evaluation of malignancy: metastatic bone disease. In: Ell PJ, Gambhir SS, (Eds). Nuclear Medicine in Clinical Diagnosis and Treatment. Edinburgh: Churchill Livingstone; 2004. pp. 641-55.
8. Krasnow AZ, Hellman RS, Timins ME, Collier BD, Anderson T, Isitman AT. Diagnostic bone scanning in oncology. Semin Nucl Med. 1997;27(2):107-41.
9. Tryciecky EW, Gottschalk A, Ludema K. Oncologic imaging: interactions of nuclear medicine with CT and MRI using the one scan as the model. Semin Nucl Med. 1997;27(2): 142-51.
10. Gates GF. SPECT bone scanning of the spine. Semin Nucl Med. 1998;28(1):78-94.
11. Savelli G, Mafoli L, Maccauro M, De Deckere E, Bombardieri E. Bone scintigraphy and the added value of SPECT (single photon emission tomography) in detecting skeletal lesions. Q J Nucl Med. 2001;45(1):27-37.

12. Kosuda S, Kaji T, Yokohama H, Yokokawa T, Katayama M, Iriye T, et al. Does bone SPECT actually have lower sensitivity for detecting vertebral metastasis than MRI? J Nucl Med. 1996;37(6):975-8.
13. Even-Sapir E, Flusser G, Lerman H, Lievshitz G, Metser U, et al. SPECT/multislice low-dose CT: a clinically relevant constituent in the imaging algorithm of nononcologic patients referred for bone scintigraphy. J Nucl Med. 2007;48(2):319-24.
14. Sharma P, Singh H, Kumar R, Bal C, Thulkar S, Seenu V, et al. XBone scintigraphy in breast cancer: added value of hybrid SPECT-CT and its impact on patient management. Nucl Med Commun. 2012;33(2):139-47.
15. Sharma P, Kumar R, Singh H, Bal C, Julka PK, Thulkar S, et al. Indeterminate lesions on planar bone scintigraphy in lung cancer patients: SPECT, CT or SPECT-CT? Skeletal Radiol. 2012;41(7):843-50.
16. Petrén-Mallmin M, Andréasson I, Ljunggren O, Ahlström H, Bergh J, Antoni G, et al. Skeletal metastases from breast cancer: uptake of 18F-fluoride measured with positron emission tomography in correlation with CT. Skeletal Radiol. 1998;27(2):72-6.
17. Even-Sapir E, Metser U, Mishani E, Lievshitz G, Lerman H, Leibovitch I. The detection of bone metastases in patients with high-risk prostate cancer: 99mTc-MDP planar bone scintigraphy, single- and multi-field-of-view SPECT, 18F-Fluoride PET, and 18F-Fluoride PET/CT. J Nucl Med. 2006;47(2):287-97.
18. Schirrmeister H, Guhlmann A, Kotzerke J, Santjohanser C, Kühn T, Kreienberg R, et al. Early detection and accurate description of extent of metastatic bone disease in breast cancer with fluoride ion and positron emission tomography. J Clin Oncol. 1999;17(8):2381-9.
19. Langsteger W, Heinisch M, Fogelman I. The role of fluorodeoxyglucose, 18F-dihydroxyphenylalanine, 18F-choline, and 18F-Fluoride in bone imaging with emphasis on prostate and breast. Semin Nucl Med. 2006;36(1):73-92.
20. Schirrmeister H, Glatting G, Hetzel J, Nüssle K, Arslandemir C, Buck AK, et al. Prospective evaluation of clinical value of planar bone scan, SPECT and 18F-labeled NaF PET in newly diagnosed lung cancer. J Nucl Med. 2001;42(12):1800-4.
21. Hetzel M, Arslandemir C, Konig HH, Buck AK, Nüssle K, Glatting G, et al. F-18 NaF PET for detection of bone metastases in lung cancer: accuracy, cost-effectiveness, and impact on patient management. J Bone Miner Res. 2003;18(12):2206-14.
22. Cook GJ, Houston S, Rubens R, Maisey MN, Fogelman I. Detection of bone metastases in breast cancer by 18FDG PET: differing metabolic activity in osteoblastic and osteolytic lesions. J Clin Oncol. 1998;16(10):3375-9.
23. Yilmaz M, Elboga U, Celen Z, Isik F, Tutar E. Multiple muscle metastases from lung cancer detected by FDG PET/CT. Clin Nucl Med. 2011;36(3):245-7.
24. Yang SN, Liang JA, Lin FJ, Kao CH, Lin CC, Lee CC. Comparing whole body (18)F-2-deoxyglucose positron emission tomography and technetium-99m methylene diphosphonate bone scan to detect bone metastases in patients with breast cancer. J Cancer Res Clin Oncol. 2002;128(6):325-8.
25. Cheran SK, Herndon JE 2nd, Patz EF Jr. Comparison of whole-body FDG-PET to bone scan for detection of bone metastases in patients with a new diagnosis of lung cancer. Lung Cancer. 2004;44(3):317-25.
26. Antoch G, Vogt FM, Freudenberg LS, Nazaradeh F, Goehde SC, Barkhausen J, et al. Whole-body dual-modality PET/CT and whole-body MRI for tumor staging in oncology. JAMA. 2003;290(24):3199-206.
27. Kushner BH. Neuroblastoma: a disease requiring a multitude of imaging studies. J Nucl Med. 2004;45(7):1172-88.
28. Stafford SE, Gralow JR, Schubert EK, Rinn KJ, Dunnwald LK, Livingston RB, et al. Use of serial FDG PET to measure the response of bone-dominant breast cancer to therapy. Acad Radiol. 2002;9(8):913-21.
29. Mortimer JE, Dehdashti F, Siegel BA, Trinkaus K, Katzenellenbogen JA, Welch MJ. Metabolic flare: indicator of hormone responsiveness in advanced breast cancer. J Clin Oncol. 2001;19(11):2797-803.
30. Aoki J, Watanabe H, Shinozaki T, Takagishi K, Tokunaga M, Koyama Y, et al. FDG-PET for pre- operative differential diagnosis between benign and malignant soft tissue masses. Skeletal Radiol. 2003;32(3):133-8.
31. Chen YM, Huang G, Sun XG, Liu JJ, Chen T, Shi YP, et al. Optimizing delayed scan time for FDG PET: comparison of the early and late delayed scan. Nucl Med Commun. 2008;29(5):425-30.
32. Evilevitch V, Weber WA, Tap WD, Allen-Auerbach M, Chow K, Nelson SD, et al. Reduction of glucose metabolic activity is more accurate than change in size at predicting histopathologic response to neoadjuvant therapy in high-grade soft-tissue sarcomas. Clin Cancer Res. 2008;14(3):715-20.
33. Dimitrakopoulou-Strauss A, Strauss LG, Schwarzbach MH, Burger C, Heichel T, Willeke F, et al. Dynamic PET 18F-FDG studies in patients with primary and recurrent soft-tissue sarcomas: impact on diagnosis and correlation with grading. J Nucl Med. 2001;42(5):713-20.
34. Adler LP, Blair HF, Makley JT, Williams RP, Joyce MJ, Leisure G, et al. Noninvasive grading of musculoskeletal tumors using PET. J Nucl Med. 1991;32(8):1508-12.
35. Ioannidis JP, Lau J. 18F-FDG PET for the diagnosis and grading of soft tissue sarcoma: a meta-analysis. J Nucl Med. 2003;44(5):717-24.
36. Sartoris DJ. Skeletal System: The Requisites. St Louis: Mosby; 2001. pp. 110-44.
37. Palestro CJ, Torres MA. Radionuclide imaging in orthopedic infections. Semin Nucl Med. 1997;27(4):334-45.
38. Israel O, Gips S, Jerushalmi J, Frenkel A, Front D. Osteomyelitis and soft-tissue infection: differential diagnosis with 24 hour/ 4 hour ratio of Tc-99m MDP uptake. Radiology. 1987;163(3):725-6.

39. Anderson SE, Heini P, Sauvain MJ, Stauffer E, Geiger L, Johnston JO, et al. Imaging of chronic recurrent multifocal osteomyelitis of childhood first presenting with isolated primary spinal involvement. Skeletal Radiol. 2003;32(6):328-36.
40. Palestro CJ. The current role of gallium imaging in infection. Semin Nucl Med. 1994;24(2):128-41.
41. Pineda C, Vargas A, Rodriguez AV. Imaging of osteomyelitis: current concepts. Infect Dis Clin N Am. 2006;20(4): 789-825.
42. Fineman DS, Palestro CJ, Kim CK, Needle LB, Vallabhajosula S, Solomon RW, et al. Detection of abnormalities in febrile AIDS patients with In-111-labeled leukocyte and GA-67 scintigraphy. Radiology. 1989;170(3):677-80.
43. Whalen JL, Brown ML, McLeod R, Fitzgerald RH Jr. Limitations of indium leukocyte imaging for the diagnosis of spine infections. Spine. 1991;16(2):193-7.
44. Linke R, Kuwert T, Uder M, Forst R, Wuest W. Skeletal SPECT/CT of the peripheral extremities. AJR Am J Roentgenol. 2010;194(4):W329-35.
45. Shults DW, Hunter GC, McIntyre KE, Parent FN, Piotrowski JJ, Bernhard VM. Value of radiographs and bone scans in determining the need for therapy in diabetic patients with foot ulcers. Am J Surg. 1989;158(6):525-30.
46. Heiba SI, Kolker D, Mocherla B, Kapoor K, Jiang M, Son H, et al. The optimized evaluation of diabetic foot infection by dual isotope SPECT/CT imaging protocol. J Foot Ankle Surg. 2010;49(6):529-36.
47. Newman LG, Waller J, Palestro CJ, Hermann G, Klein MJ, Schwartz M, et al. Leukocyte scanning with 111In is superior to magnetic resonance imaging in the diagnosis of clinically unsuspected osteomyelitis in diabetic foot ulcers. Diabetes Care. 1992;15(11):1527-30.
48. Hayashida K, Ochi T, Fujimoto M, Owaki H, Shimaoka Y, Ono K, et al. Bone marrow changes in adjuvant-induced and collagen-induced arthritis. Interleukin-1 and interleukin-6 activity and abnormal myelopoiesis. Arthritis Rheum. 1992;35(2):241-5.
49. Hanssen AD, Rand JA. Evaluation and treatment of infection at the site of a total hip or knee arthroplasty. Instr Course Lect. 1999;48:111-22.
50. Aliabadi P, Tumeh SS, Weissman BN, McNeil BJ. Cemented total hip prosthesis: radiographic and scintigraphic evaluation. Radiology. 1989;173(1):203-6.
51. Love C, Tronco GG, Yu AK, Marwin S, Nichols K, Palestro C. Diagnosing the infected prosthetic hip: an intraindividual comparison of three- phase bone, bone, gallium, bone/gallium, leukocyte, leukocyte/bone, and leukocyte/marrow imaging. Eur J Nucl Med Mol Imaging. 2007;34(Suppl 2):(P) S384.
52. Pring DJ, Henderson RG, Rivett AG, Krausz T, Coombs RR, Lavender JP. Autologous granulocyte scanning of painful prosthetic joints. J Bone Joint Surg Br. 1986;68(4):647-52.
53. Wukich DK, Abreu SH, Callaghan JJ, Van Nostrand D, Savory CG, Eggli DF, et al. Diagnosis of infection by preoperative scintigraphy with indium labeled white blood cells. J Bone Joint Surg Am. 1987;69(9):1353-60.
54. Love C, Tronco GG, Yu AK, Marwin S, Nichols K, Palestro C, et al. Diagnosing lower extremity prosthetic joint infection: intraindividual comparison of leukocyte/marrow and leukocyte/bone imaging. J Nucl Med. 2007;48(Suppl):62.
55. Mochizuki T, Tsukamoto E, Kuge Y, Kanegae K, Zhao S, Hikosaka K, et al. FDG uptake and glucose transporter subtype expressions in experimental tumor and inflammation models. J Nucl Med. 2001;42(10):1551-5.
56. Beckers C, Jeukens X, Ribbens C, André B, Marcelis S, Leclercq P, et al. (18)F-FDG PET imaging of rheumatoid knee synovitis correlates with dynamic magnetic resonance and sonographic assessments as well as with the serum level of metalloproteinase-3. Eur J Nucl Med Mol Imaging. 2006;33(3):275-80.
57. Stumpe KD, Dazzi H, Schaffner A, von Schulthess GK. Infection imaging using wholebody FDG-PET. Eur J Nucl Med. 2000;27(7):822-32.
58. de Winter F, van de Wiele C, Vogelaers D, de Smet K, Verdonk R, Dierckx RA. Fluorine-18 fluorodeoxyglucose positron emission tomography: a highly accurate imaging modality for the diagnosis of chronic musculoskeletal infections. J Bone Joint Surg Am. 2001;83(5):651-60.
59. Familiari D, Glaudemans AW, Vitale V, Prosperi D, Bagni O, Lenza A, et al. Can sequential 18F-FDG PET/CT replace WBC imaging in the diabetic foot? J Nucl Med. 2011;52(7):1012-9.
60. Zhuang H, Duarte PS, Pourdehnad M, Maes A, Van Acker F, Shnier D, et al. The promising role of 18F-FDG PET in detecting infected lower limb prosthesis implants. J Nucl Med. 2001;42(1):44-8.
61. Reinartz P, Mumme T, Hermanns B, Cremerius U, Wirtz DC, Schaefer WM, et al. Radionuclide imaging of the painful hip arthroplasty: positronemission tomography versus triple-phase bone scanning. J Bone Joint Surg Br. 2005;87(4):465-70.
62. Love C, Scott EM, Tomas MB, Krauss ES, Tronco GG, Bhargava KK, et al. Diagnosing infection in the failed joint replacement: a comparison of coincidence detection 18F-FDG and 111In-labeled leucocyte/99mTc-sulfur colloid marrow imaging. J Nucl Med. 2004;45(11):1864-71.
63. Goerres GW, Ziegler SI, Burger C, Berthold T, Von Schulthess GK, Buck A. Artifacts at PET and PET/CT caused by metallic hip prosthetic material. Radiology. 2003;226(2): 577-84.
64. Donohoe KJ. Selected topics in orthopedic nuclear medicine. Orthop Clin North Am. 1998;29(1):85-101.
65. Barai S, Kumar R, Dhanpati H, Malhotra R, Dasan JB, Bandopadhyaya GB, et al. Bone scintigraphy in sports injuries. Ortho Today. 2003;5:29-32.
66. Mandelstam SA, Cook D, Fitzgerald M, Ditchfield M, Carty H. Complementary use of radiological skeletal survey and bone scintigraphy in detection of bony injuries in suspected child abuse. Arch Dis Child. 2003;88(5):387-90.

67. Kleinman PK. Shaken babies. Lancet. 1998;352(9130):815-6.
68. Fogelman I, Carr D. A comparison of bone scanning and radiology in the assessment of patients with symptomatic Paget's disease. Eur J Nucl Med. 1980;5(5):417-21.
69. Rotés-Sala D, Monfort J, Solano A, Miralles E, Vila J, Carbonell J. The clover and heart signs in vertebral scintigraphic images are highly specific of Paget's disease of bone. Bone. 2004;34(4):605-8.
70. Installé J, Nzeusseu A, Bol A, Depresseux G, Devogelaer J-P, Lonneux M. 18F-Fluoride PET for monitoring therapeutic response in Paget's disease of bone. J Nucl Med. 2005;46(10):1650-58.
71. Messa C, Goodman WG, Hoh CK, Choi Y, Nissenson AR, Salusky IB, et al. Bone metabolic activity measured with positron emission tomography and 18F-Fluoride ion in renal osteodystrophy: correlation with bone histomorphometry. J Clin Endocrinol Metab. 1993;77(4):949-55.
72. Fogelman I, McKillop JH, Greig WR, Boyle IT. Pseudofractures of the ribs detected by bone scanning. J Nucl Med. 1977;18(12):1236-7.
73. Fukumitsu N, Dohi M, Midda K, Nakada N, Sunagawa Y, Harada J, et al. Bone scintigraphy in polyostotic fibrous dysplasia. Clin Nucl Med. 1999;24(6):446-7.
74. Conway WF, Totty WG, McEnery KW. CT and MRI imaging of the hip. Radiology. 1996;198(2):297-307.
75. Collier BD, Carrera GF, Johnson RP, Isitman AT, Hellman RS, Knobel J, et al. Detection of femoral head avascular necrosis in adults by SPECT. J Nucl Med. 1985;26(9):979-87.
76. Ruffin D. Natural history of reflex sympathetic dystrophy syndrome. J Nucl Med. 1984;25:423-9.
77. Kozin F, Genant HK, Bekerman C, McCarty DJ. The reflex sympathetic dystrophy syndrome. II. Roentgenographic and scintigraphic evidence of bilaterality and of periarticular accentuation. Am J Med. 1976;60(3):332-8.

CHAPTER 3

Angiography and Interventions in Musculoskeletal Lesions

Deep Narayan Srivastava, Madhusudhan KS

INTRODUCTION

With increasing use of computed tomography (CT) and magnetic resonance imaging (MRI) in the diagnosis of bone and soft tissue lesions, angiography is not being used as commonly as before, however, if the procedure is used properly in conjunction with other diagnostic studies, it can play a valuable role in the diagnosis and treatment of bone and soft tissue lesions. The role of angiointerventions and nonvascular musculoskeletal interventions is increasing and will be discussed.

TECHNIQUE

Diagnostic Angiography

The common femoral artery is the commonly used entry site for percutaneous approach because of its accessibility, the ease of compression against the femoral head for hemostasis, and the low rate of complications when punctured. The left or right femoral artery is punctured by Seldinger technique and an arterial sheath is placed. Usually the contralateral femoral artery is used to approach the lesion in lower limb region. Through this, arterial sheath angiographic catheter is advanced into the arteries supplying the lesion. A wide variety of preshaped 4/5 F angiographic catheters are available for selective and superselective catheterization. The catheter is placed selectively in the major vessel supplying the tumor and angiographic runs are taken with contrast medium injection. Various selective injections are taken depending upon the tumor supply.

Visualization of both the arterial and venous circulations is desirable in all cases. The radiographs/frames are obtained initially at two frames/second for 3–4 seconds followed by every 2 seconds for a total of 25–30 seconds. The amount of contrast injection depends on the size and location of the lesion.

Digital subtraction angiograms (DSAs) are superior to conventional angiograms since the superimposed bones, calcifications and also other limb supports in trauma patients can be subtracted resulting in better image quality because of which reliable evaluation of vascular supply of the lesion is possible.

Magnification angiograms are sometimes required for visualization of tiny vessels.

Angioembolization

The term embolization refers to the introduction of an embolic agent into a vessel through a selectively placed catheter to achieve therapeutic vascular occlusion. The advent of catheters with hydrophilic coating, microcatheters, torque control guidewires and various embolic materials has allowed precise and safe delivery of occluding agents to anywhere in the body using the blood vessels as a roadway. In certain situations, these embolizing materials are also injected into the lesion directly under image guidance without angiographic route.

The embolization is usually performed using the access used for diagnostic angiography. After the initial diagnostic angiography, the angiographic catheter is advanced into the artery supplying the tumor before introduction of embolic material. The selective and superselective embolization is a safe interventional procedure for any vascular lesion. Sometimes small caliber catheters like microcatheters (2–3 F) are also used for this. It is also important to weigh the risks of the procedure against those of noninterventional and surgical therapies. The embolization should preferably be performed in angiography suite equipped with C-arm mounted image intensifier with DSA of high-quality resolution. A portable ultrasound scanner is always useful in the assessment of nonpalpable arteries, veins and also for direct percutaneous puncture of lesion.

ANGIOGRAPHY IN BONE TUMORS

The role of angiography in bone tumors is limited because of the following reasons:

- If the definitive angiographic features of malignancy are present, it can be assumed that the lesion is malignant, but a normal arteriogram does not entirely rule out a malignancy.[1]
- It is often not possible to distinguish between various types of bone tumors from the angiographic features alone.

The angiographic features of malignancy include neovascularity, pooling or laking of contrast material, tumor stain or blush, encasement and occlusion of vessels, extension of the tumor vascularity outside the bone, displacement of vessels, arteriovenous shunts, abnormal draining veins, tumor invasion of veins, etc.

Neovascularity and pooling of contrast are important features of malignancy; however, these may also be present in some benign lesions like giant cell tumor, aneurysmal bone cyst, osteoblastoma, Paget's disease, benign nerve sheath tumor and certain hemangiomas **(Figs. 1 to 3)**. These lesions can easily be differentiated by their clinical and plain radiographic features.

The presence of a tumor blush does not indicate malignancy but may suggest the size and extent of the tumor. Angiography, however, does not always define the complete intraosseous extent of the tumor and skip metastases within the bone are not always seen.[2]

The angiographic information about the displacement or encasement of vessel is important if a radical local resection is planned in limb salvage surgeries.

Early arteriovenous shunting is not a reliable sign of malignancy, however, the identification of large abnormal draining veins is important to facilitate early ligation and prevent tumor embolization during surgery.[2]

Some bone tumors in which diagnostic angiography is sometimes indicated are discussed here.

Osteochondroma

These bone tumors because of their size and location may cause vascular complications in the form of thrombosis and pseudoaneurysms[3,4] as well as displacement of vessels. Angiography can show all these complications **(Figs. 4A and B)**. The tumor usually does not show hypervascularity or abnormal vessels.

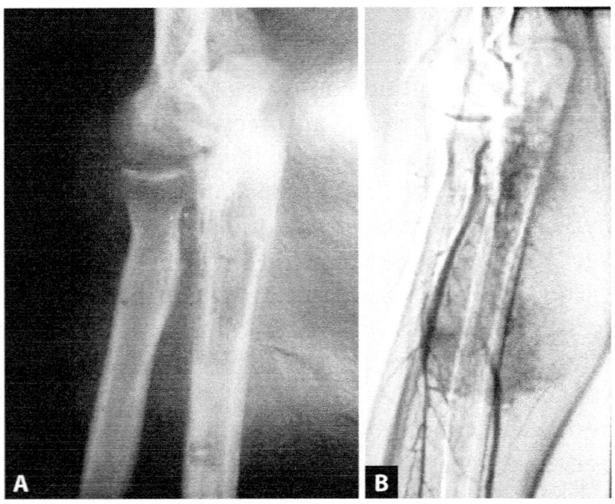

Figs. 1A and B: Ewing's tumor. (A) Lytic lesion with periosteal reaction and soft tissue mass of ulna; (B) Pooling of contrast material is seen on digital subtraction angiography (DSA).

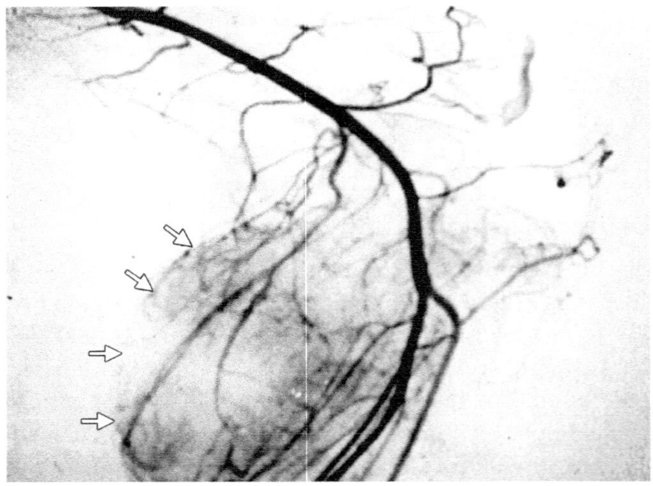

Fig. 2: Benign nerve sheath tumor. The digital subtraction angiography (DSA) showing blush of contrast (arrows).

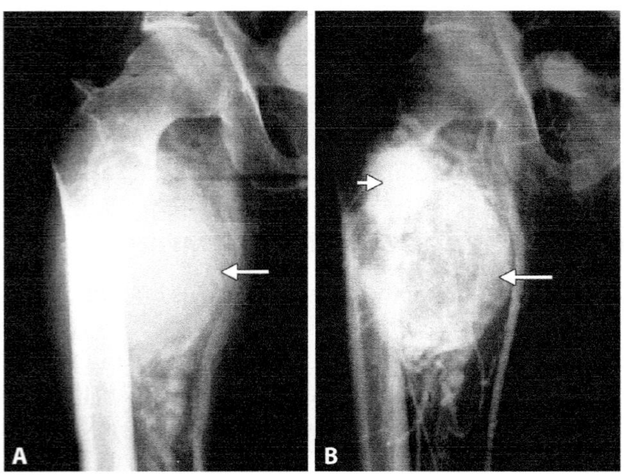

Figs. 3A and B: Angiography shows highly vascular mass with pooling of contrast in a case of hemangioma of femur (small arrow) with extraosseous component (large arrows).

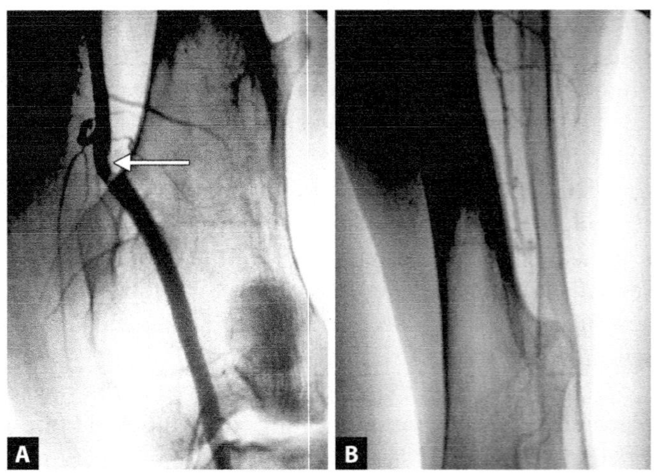

Figs. 4A and B: Multiple osteochondroma. (A) Displacement and narrowing (arrow) of femoral artery; (B) Thrombosis of leg vessels.

Osteoid Osteoma

In the absence of classical roentgenographic findings, angiography can be helpful when the diagnosis is in doubt.[5] The angiographic feature is dense, circumscribed blush in the early arterial phase which persists in late venous phase. This feature differentiates it from osteomyelitis, Brodie's abscess and stress fractures that do not have the feature of dense vascular blush.

Osteosarcoma

Angiography can demonstrate that the tumor is malignant, and accurately define the degree of soft tissue extension; however, skip areas within the medullary canal are not always detected.[2] MRI is useful in defining the intraosseous and extraosseous extent of the tumor and its anatomic relationship to nearby structures.

Giant Cell Tumor

Angiography can accurately define the intraosseous as well as extraosseous extent of the tumor because the tumors are usually hypervascular and show neovascularity, intense blush and early venous filling. This is of particular importance in view of the high recurrence rate of the tumor and its ability to become malignant after treatment. The MRI is useful in the limb salvage surgeries in the assessment of extent of tumor and the anatomic relationship to nearby structures and joint.

Aneurysmal Bone Cyst

Angiography can differentiate aneurysmal bone cyst from giant cell tumor. On angiography, it is poorly vascularized tumor, devoid of arteriovenous fistulae and soft tissue invasion.[6] The clinical course and plain radiographic findings are very useful for the diagnosis of this lesion.

ANGIOGRAPHY IN BONE AND SOFT TISSUE LESIONS OF VASCULAR ORIGIN

Hemangioma

Hemangiomas can be grouped into four categories: (1) capillary, (2) cavernous, (3) venous hemangiomas and (4) arteriovenous malformations (AVMs). Hemangiomas usually involve the soft tissues (most commonly skeletal muscles) but can also involve bones.[7] Arteriography can define the extent, degree of vascularity, source of vascular supply, local recurrence in follow-up case and differentiate from AVMs.[8] Angiography may show mild to marked vascularity with coarse, irregular, enlarged arteries and pooling of contrast material **(Figs. 3 and 5)**. Arteriovenous shunting may be seen. The osseous hemangiomas may have dilated vascular spaces **(Figs. 3A and B)**. Venous hemangioma is rarely seen on arteriography but is usually seen on venography[9] **(Figs. 6A to D)**. Sometimes it is difficult to ascertain the entire lesion on angiography.[10] The MRI is useful in depicting the full extent of the lesion and the relationship to surrounding structures **(Figs. 6A to D)**. Angiography sometimes cannot differentiate a benign hemangioma from a malignant vascular tumor.[8]

In cavernous hemangioma, arteriography demonstrates normal sized arteries that may show late venous staining on delayed films. They do not require treatment as they do not change with time and rarely bleed, but a common problem is local pain due to distention of the lesion or superimposed thrombosis. The embolization of regional arterial branches is not always useful, but injection of sclerosing agent by direct puncture technique has shown good results **(Fig. 5)**.

Klippel-Trenaunay syndrome (KTS) is a congenital vascular abnormality consisting of a cutaneous nevus, varicose veins and bone and soft tissue hypertrophy affecting one or more limbs. Venography is very useful in demonstrating the characteristic venous anomaly [Klippel-Trenaunay (KT) vein], which is a large lateral superficial venous channel that often communicates with profunda femoris or iliac veins **(Figs. 7A to C)**. MRI with its multiplanar imaging abilities has the advantage of demonstrating the full extent of venous malformation and the status of muscle and soft tissues.[9]

Arteriovenous malformations tend to grow at the same rate as the individual, unlike the pattern of rapid growth and involution seen in hemangioma. The angiographic findings include enlarged, tortuous feeding arteries, a dense nidus of malformations and early opacification of draining veins. The AVMs are refractory to treatment.

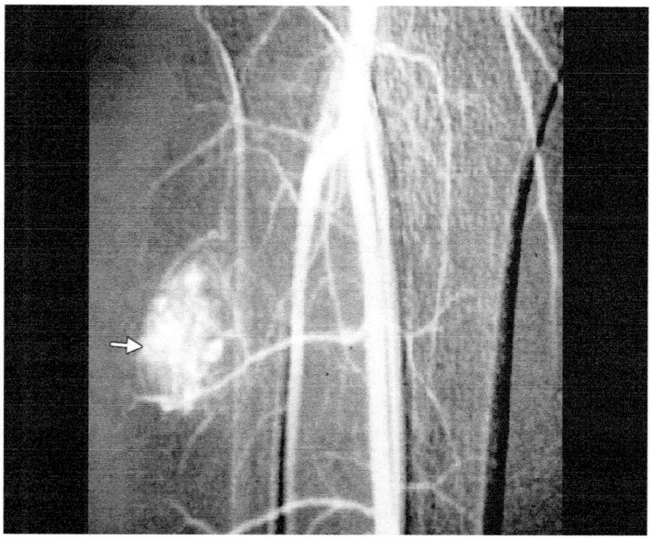

Fig. 5: Soft tissue hemangioma leg. Digital subtraction angiography shows fine vessels with some pooling of contrast (arrow). This painful lesion was successfully treated by percutaneous injection of sclerosing agent.

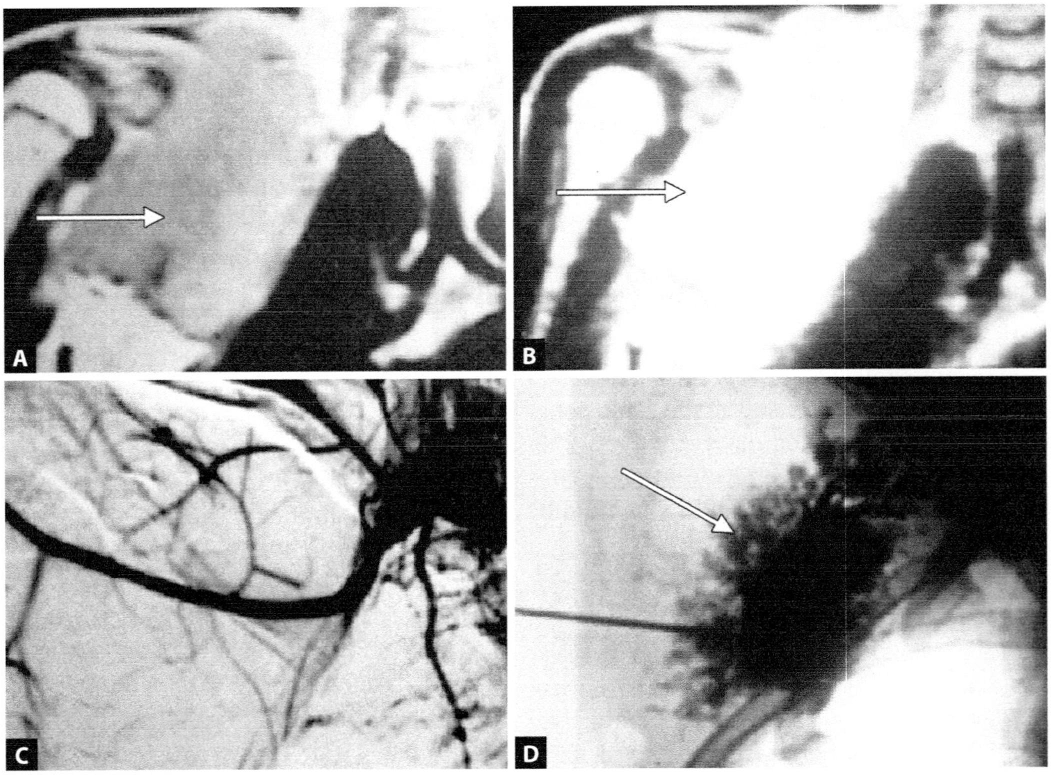

Figs. 6A to D: Venous hemangioma (arrows) of axilla with supraclavicular extension. The mass is mildly hyperintense to muscles on T1-weighted image (T1WI) (A) Hyperintense on T2WI; (B) On digital subtraction angiography (DSA), the mass is not vascular with mass effect over axillary artery with splaying of its lateral thoracic and subscapular branches; (C) No early venous filling seen. Percutaneous aspiration and injection of contrast shows multiple dilated vascular spaces; (D) The pain disappeared and the size was reduced after injection of sclerosing agent through the same needle.

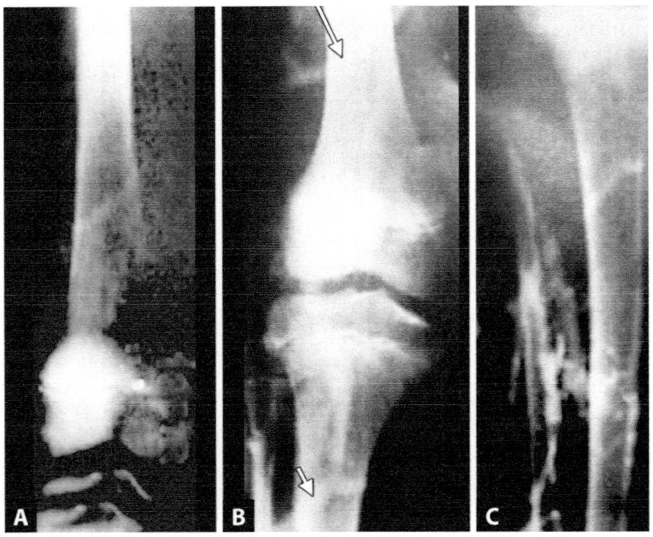

Figs. 7A to C: Ascending phlebogram showing two Klippel–Trenaunay veins, one communicating with the popliteal vein (small arrow), and the other with the superficial femoral vein (large arrow).

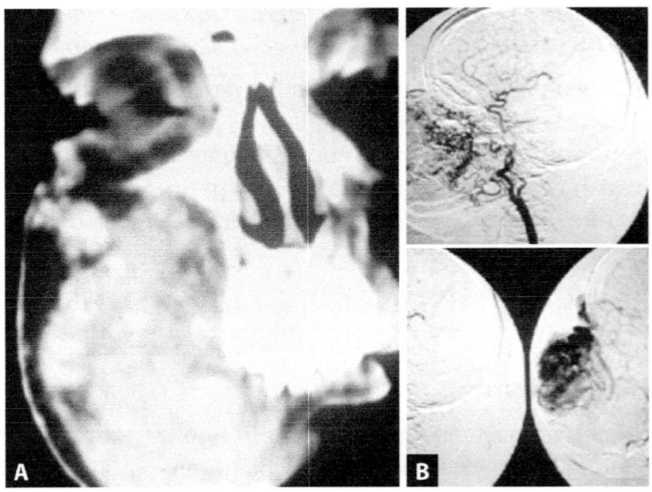

Figs. 8A and B: Arteriovenous malformations of cheek. (A) Computed tomography (CT) shows soft tissue vascular mass overlying maxilla, mandible, and inferior orbital margin; (B) On digital subtraction angiography (DSA), the mass is supplied by branches of left external carotid artery with early venous filling.

Mechanically disturbing a stable lesion (after surgical ligation or proximal embolization of feeding arteries) can result in significant worsening due to development of new collaterals. Transcatheter embolization close to nidus of the lesion has now attained a primary role in the management of AVMs, but proximal occlusion of feeding vessels by an endovascular embolic agent or surgical ligation will provide poor clinical result with recurrence **(Figs. 8A and B).**[11,12] The angiography can tell about the size, number and location of these lesions **(Figs. 9A and B).**

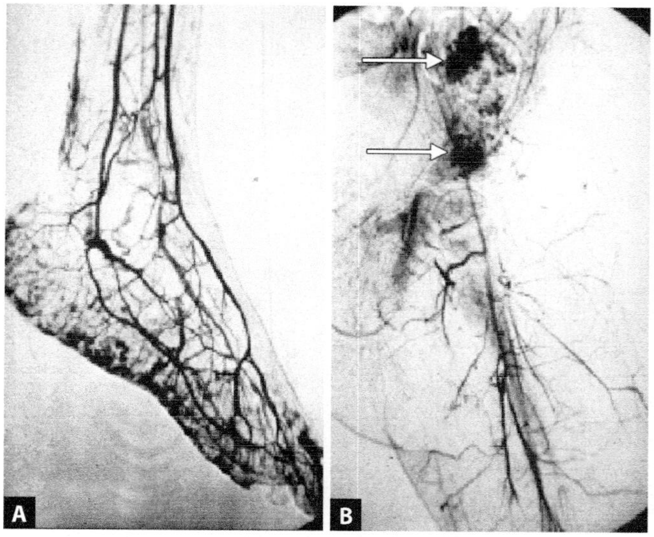

Figs. 9A and B: Multiple hemangiomas involving (A) left foot and (B) gluteal muscles (arrows).

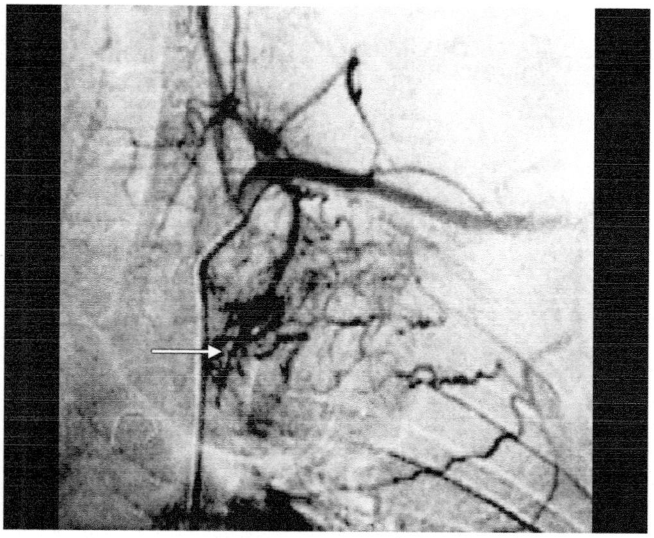

Fig. 10: Hemangiopericytoma. A well-demarcated hypervascular mass (arrow) with homogeneous blush seen on delayed images.

In lesions of extremities, injection of sclerosing agent or alcohol by direct puncture technique is safe and useful.

Hemangiopericytoma

These are hypervascular tumors and are seen as a prolonged dense stain on angiogram.[13] There may be displacement of the major arteries **(Fig. 10)**.

Angiosarcoma

The angiographic features include highly irregular, tortuous arteries with pooling of contrast,[14] arteriovenous shunts and encasement of vessels.

ANGIOGRAPHY IN METASTATIC TUMORS IN BONE AND SOFT TISSUES

Most metastatic lesions have the same vascular characteristics that are exhibited by their primary tumors.[15] Angiography cannot distinguish between different types of metastases. It also cannot distinguish a primary osseous or soft tissue tumor from a secondary growth.

ANGIOGRAPHY IN PERIPHERAL TRAUMA

Angiography has an important role in the management of patients with suspected vascular injury both for diagnosis and treatment. Angiography is both sensitive and specific for the diagnosis of vascular injury (active bleeding, pseudoaneurysms and arteriovenous fistula) **(Figs. 11 and 12)**. Transcatheter embolization is effective, safe and can be a definitive therapy for suitable arterial injuries. In arteriovenous fistula, early intervention is very useful. Early intervention in hemodynamically unstable patients with pelvic fractures is essential to reduce the morbidity of the injury.[16] In pelvic fractures, percutaneous embolization of uncontrolled pelvic hemorrhage is a lifesaving technique **(Figs. 12A and B)**. Small aneurysms can be treated by sonoguided manual compression or coil embolization **(Figs. 13 and 14)**. The intra-arterial thrombolytic therapy can also be used in arterial thrombosis **(Figs. 15A and B)**.

IMAGE-GUIDED INTERVENTIONS IN BONE AND SOFT TISSUE LESIONS

The commonly used image-guided interventions are fine needle aspiration cytology and Trucut biopsies, embolizations, intra-arterial chemotherapies, vertebroplasties, radiofrequency and laser ablation of benign bone lesions.

Aspiration Cytology and Biopsy

The role of aspiration cytology is limited since most lesions require biopsy. Percutaneous biopsy is less invasive, requires smaller dose of anesthetics and analgesics, causes minimal bleeding and biopsy tract contamination, and is a cost-effective method. However, it is less reliable in obtaining an adequate representative specimen for grading and further special studies. For heterogeneous tumors, very myxoid or cystic lesions and bone tumors without soft tissue component, a needle core may not give a high diagnostic yield. The hemangioma and AVMs usually do not require histological confirmation because of characteristic imaging features. For biopsy, various size Trucut needles (11–18G) are used. For bone biopsy, thick needles (11G) with diamond tip are preferred. Ultrasound guidance is always preferred though CT and fluoroscopy is required for vertebral and other bone lesions.

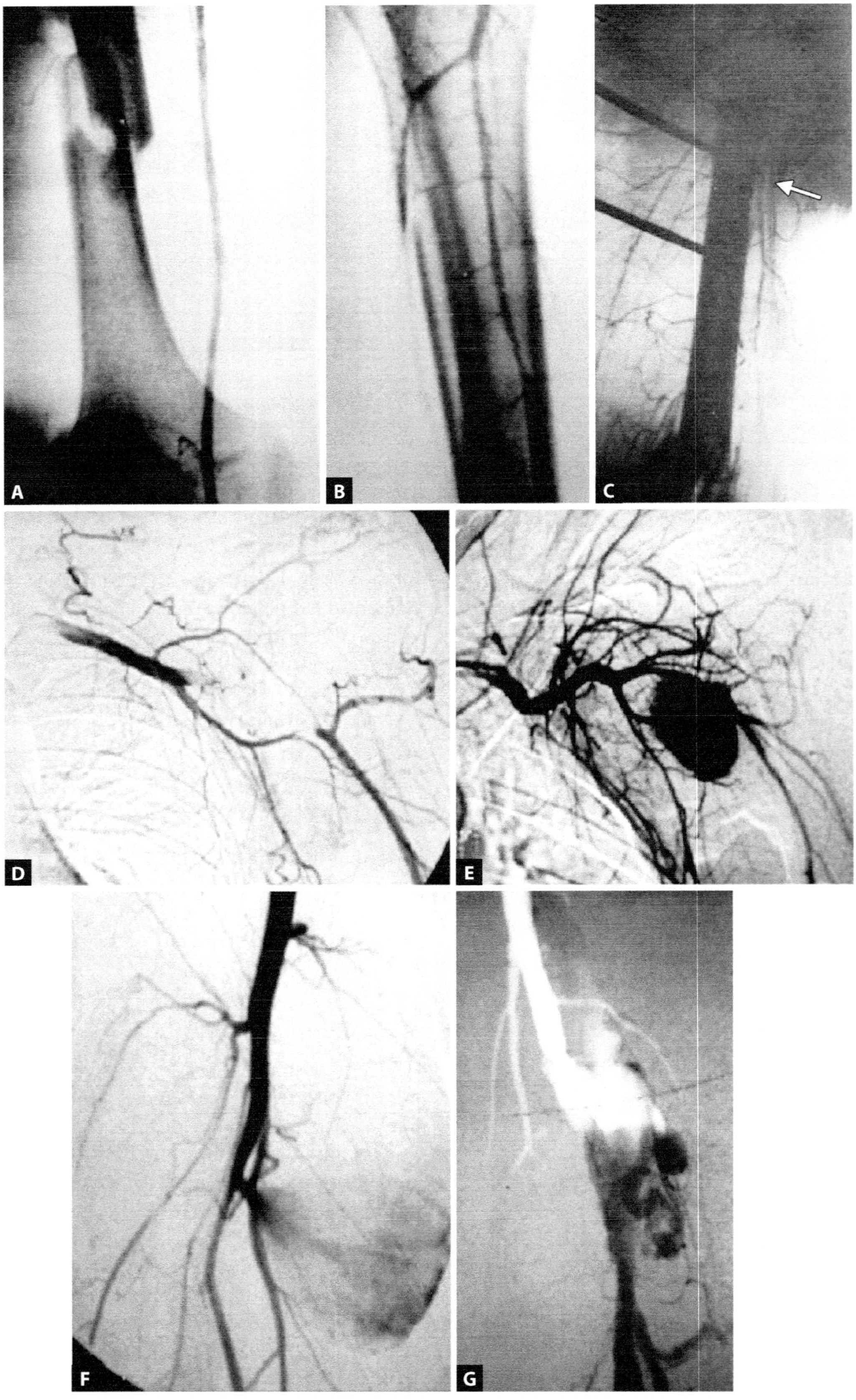

Figs. 11A to G: The digital subtraction angiography (DSA) in different patients of trauma. (A and B) Fracture femur and fibula with patent arteries; (C) Fracture femur with thrombosed superficial femoral artery (arrow) with collaterals; (D) Soft tissue injury left shoulder with thrombosed axillary artery-brachial artery is filling from collaterals; (E) Large pseudoaneurysm from axillary artery; (F) Large pseudoaneurysm from right superficial femoral artery; (G) Arteriovenous fistula between popliteal artery and vein.

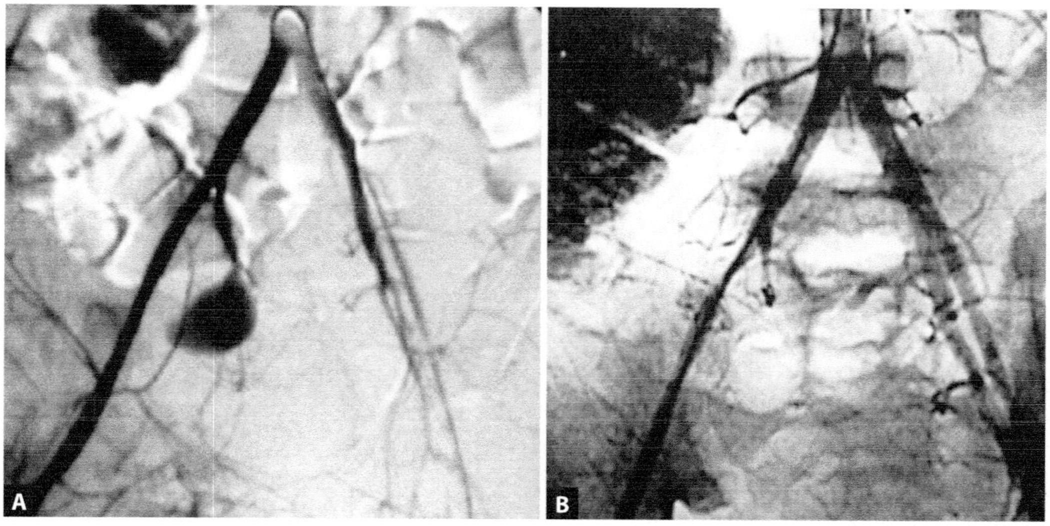

Figs. 12A and B: Post-traumatic pelvic bleeding. (A) Digital subtraction angiography (DSA) showing bleeding from right internal iliac artery trunk; (B) Which stopped after steel coil embolization.

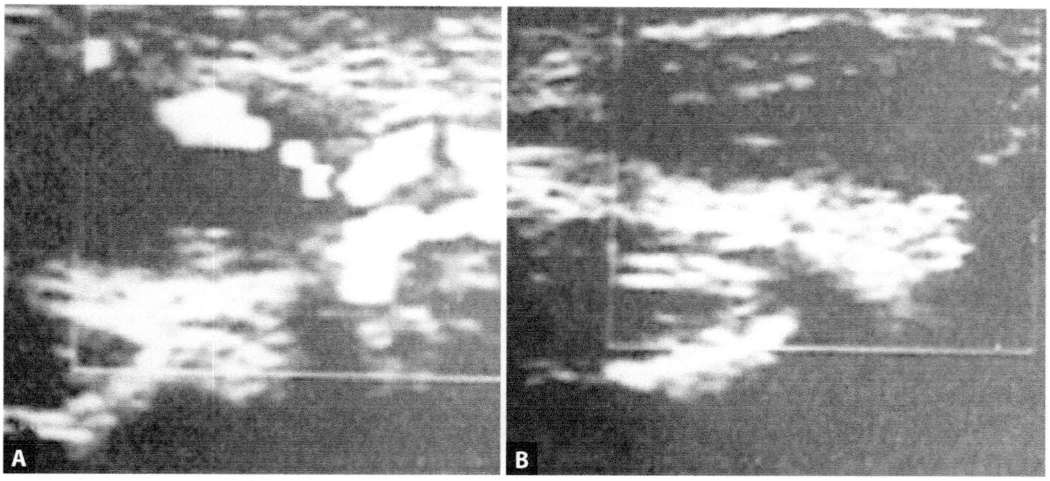

Figs. 13A and B: (A) Ultrasound showing pseudoaneurysm of femoral artery; (B) Developed after transfemoral arteriography, treated by manual compression.

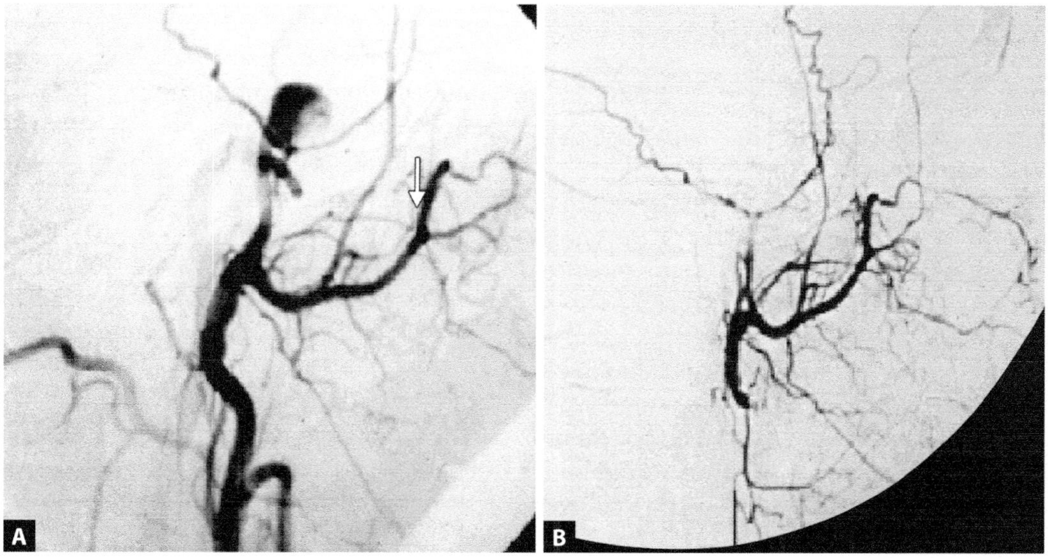

Figs. 14A and B: (A) Post-traumatic pseudoaneurysm from superficial temporal artery (arrow). This was treated by ultrasound-guided percutaneous coil embolization; (B) Post-treatment digital subtraction angiography (DSA) is not showing aneurysm.

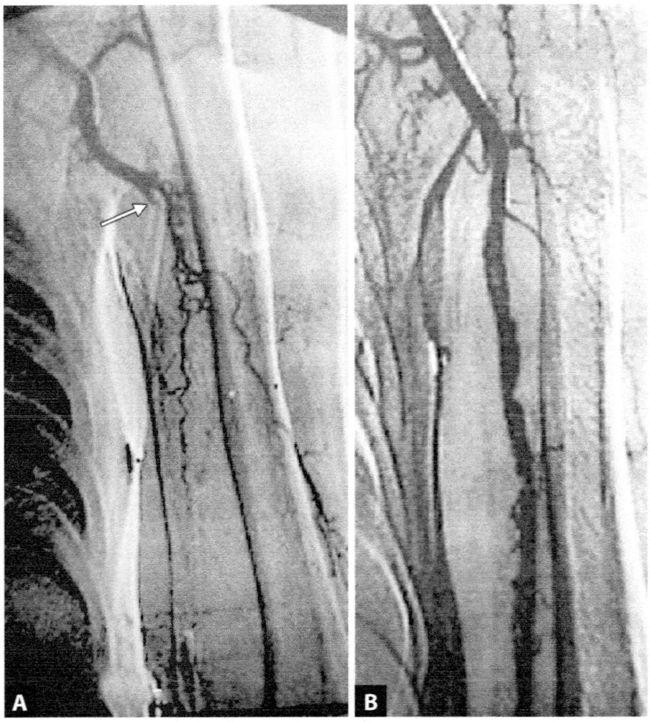

Figs. 15A and B: (A) Post-traumatic acute thrombosis (arrow) of brachial artery; (B) Recanalized after intra-arterial thrombolytic infusion.

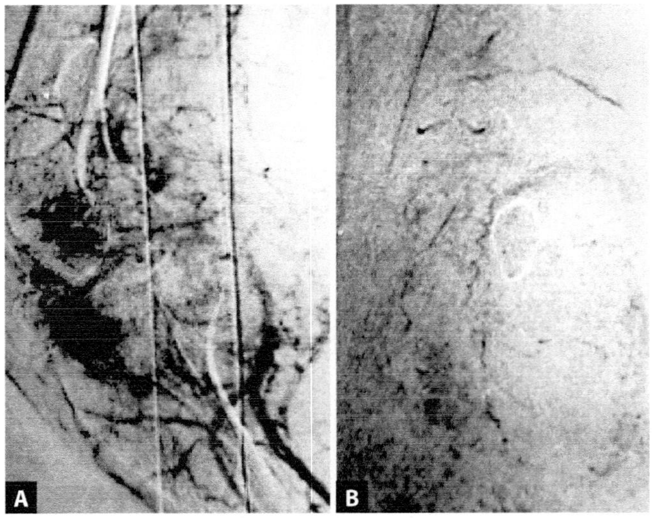

Figs. 16A and B: Preoperative embolization of a very large hemangioma around knee for reconstructive surgery. (A) Pre-embolization angiogram; (B) Postembolization angiogram.

Embolization

Preprocedural Preparations

The patient must be informed about the procedure, benefits, alternative procedures and potential complications. The patient should be well hydrated and standby general anesthesia may be needed for uncooperative patients and children. Severe coagulopathy should be corrected and sometimes antibiotics are also given. The sedation is given during the procedure depending upon the type and duration of the procedure.

Indications

The indications of embolization in bone and soft tissue tumors are as follows:

1. *To control hemorrhage*: If there is internal or external bleeding from the tumor, angioembolization is sometimes done as an emergency procedure.
2. *To reduce peroperative bleeding*: It has been used in various soft tissue and bone tumors and hemangiomas to decrease intraoperative blood loss, which improves surgical vision and allows safer and faster surgery.[16,17] Voigt et al. reported the use of Gelfoam embolization in patients with deforming vascular malformations in the craniofacial area.[18] The procedure allows reconstructive surgery to be carried out with decreased blood loss with good cosmetic results **(Figs. 16A and B)**.
3. *As palliative treatment*: In previously treated (surgery and/or embolization) cases of recurrent or residual AVMs if intravascular access is difficult, direct puncture of the symptomatic lesion can be performed[18] by Chiba needle and alcohol or sclerosing agent can be injected directly in tumor bed (nidus) until flow is occluded. The embolization of the soft tissue tumors may result in severe, prolonged muscle pain if acute muscle ischemia takes place. Therefore, for palliation of pain in patients with inoperable tumors, embolization should be cautiously used.
4. *To relieve from chronic pain due to tumors*: It has been reported that therapeutic arterial occlusion in pelvic tumors[19] and in metastatic deposits[16] gives symptomatic relief of pain. The major vessels of supply are embolized with Gelfoam followed by steel coils to occlude the vessels permanently **(Figs. 17A and B)**. Embolization with particles (transcatheter) or percutaneous instillation of sclerosing agent has been used to control pain associated with a peripheral hemangioma **(Fig. 5)**.[20]
5. *As a part of treatment*: In hemangiomas, angioembolization decreases the chance of recurrence **(Figs. 18A to C)**.[21] A study has shown that this not only decreases the size but also controls a persistent left-to-right shunt.[22]

Transarterial embolization should be considered in the treatment algorithm of primary or secondary bone tumors. Specific benefit is present where there is a high risk of bleeding at surgery, where there is spinal involvement and neural encroachment, where active bleeding is present or in awkward surgical locations where prolonged surgery is anticipated.[23]

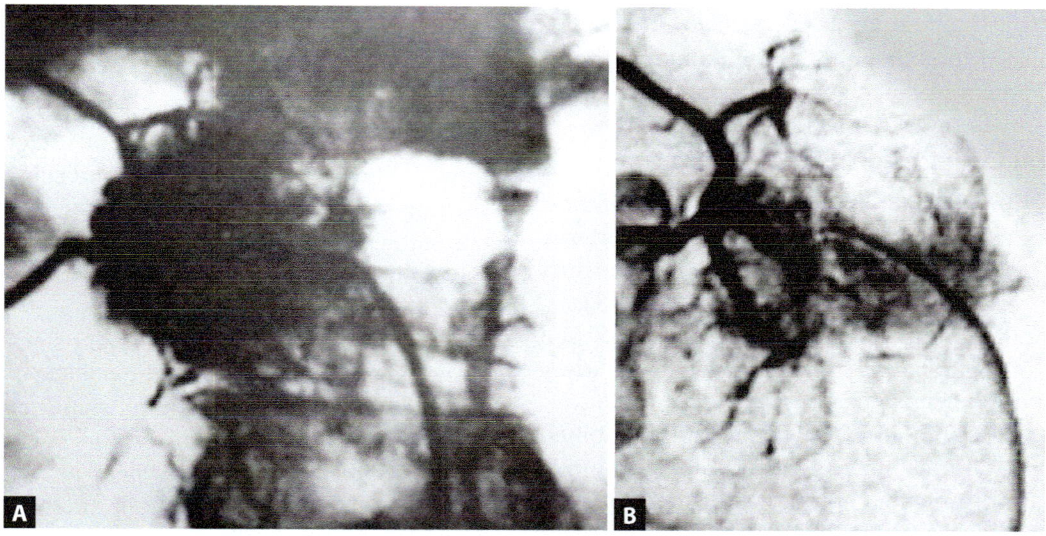

Figs. 17A and B: Painful metastatic deposit in the spine treated by therapeutic arterial occlusion. (A) Pre-embolization; (B) Postembolization angiograms.

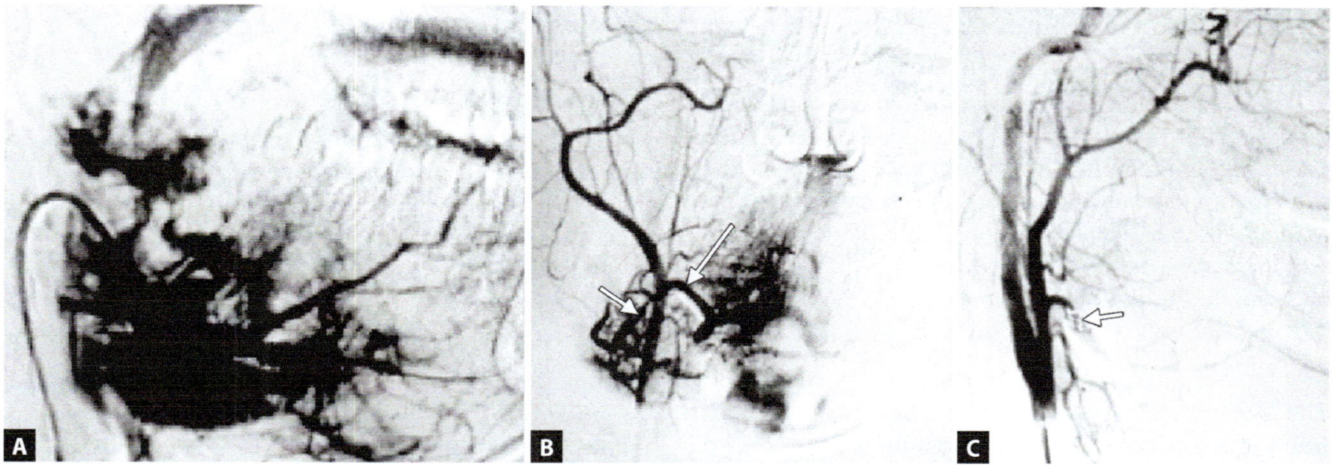

Figs. 18A to C: (A) Hemangioma submandibular region; (B) Supplied by right facial and lingual arteries (arrows); (C) The common origin of which embolized by steel coils (arrow).

Embolizing Materials

There are various types of embolizing materials available. The selection of the material depends upon the duration, extent and level of occlusion. The materials can be categorized as short, intermediate and long-acting or as particulate or liquid agents depending upon the physical properties. The commonly used embolizing materials have been listed in **Table 1**.

Table 1: Commonly used embolizing materials.

Type of embolizing agent	*Examples and duration*
Particulate agents	Absorbable (Temporary) • Autologous blood clot • Gelfoam Nonabsorbable (Permanent) • Polyvinyl alcohol particles • Microspheres
Mechanical agents	Nonabsorbable (Permanent) • Steel coils • Detachable balloons
Liquid agents	Nonabsorbable (Permanent) • Isobutyl 2-cyanoacrylate • Ethanol • Sodium tetradecyl sulfate

Complications

The common complication is postembolization syndrome in the form of nausea, vomiting, fever and pain due to tissue ischemia. The uncommon complications reported are inadvertent embolization, misplaced or migrated steel coils, abscess formation, spinal cord injury, aneurysm formation or vessel rupture.

Contraindications

The contraindications are patients with hemorrhagic diathesis and puncture site infection.

Intra-arterial Chemotherapy

Patients with sarcomas not amenable to cure by surgical resection alone can benefit from preoperative intra-arterial chemotherapy. Intra-arterial chemotherapy permits limb-sparing resection with less morbidity **(Fig. 19)**.[23,24] In this, chemotherapeutic drug is injected in tumor bed with the help of angiographic catheter placed in the artery supplying the tumor.

Neoadjuvant chemotherapy protocols using combined intra-arterial and intravenous agents to treat high-grade osteosarcoma and malignant fibrous histiocytoma of bone in an attempt to improve survival have also been tried with good results.[25]

Percutaneous Vertebral Body Augmentation Procedures

Percutaneous vertebroplasty is a well-accepted interventional procedure for the treatment of painful vertebral lesions. The technique first introduced in 1984[26] for a vertebral hemangioma, has been subsequently used for the treatment of numerous lesions causing back pain associated with vertebral involvement like osteoporotic vertebral collapse, metastatic disease, multiple myeloma and symptomatic vertebral hemangiomas.

Technique

The procedure consists of instilling acrylic bone cement into the affected vertebra through a bone biopsy needle by a percutaneous approach. The cement consists of polymethyl methacrylate (PMMA) (obtained by mixing liquid monomer to the powdered polymer), which is mixed just before the injection. The cement is injected into the lesion after needle placement, under fluoroscopic control.[27] The cement polymerizes and subsequently sets, affording support to the vertebra **(Figs. 20A to C)**. The steps of the procedure are:

1. Patient is placed in prone position on angiography/fluoroscopy table.
2. The procedure is performed under sterile conditions. The skin over the center of the pedicle is anesthetized with local anesthesia. A small skin incision is made and bone biopsy needle is positioned with its tip in the center of the midpoint of the pedicle.
3. The needle is advanced under anteroposterior (AP) and lateral fluoroscopy till the junction of the anterior and middle third of the vertebral body. Approximately 6 mL of PMMA cement is injected.
4. Patient is placed in supine position for 3 hours after the procedure and is discharged after 6 hours.

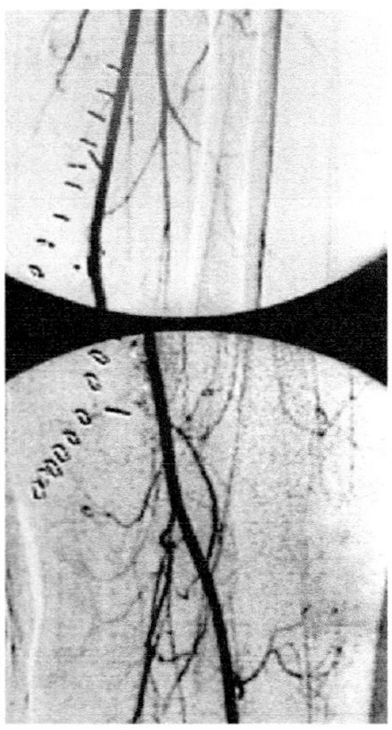

Fig. 19: Soft tissue sarcoma thigh. Postoperative angiogram was done to look for residual mass and intra-arterial chemotherapy.

Results

Vertebroplasty results in relief of pain with decrease in analgesic use. It provides strength so prevents further collapse and pain relief by coagulating the tissue. The relief is obtained irrespective of the cause of pain, and is long-lasting.[27]

Complications

The incidence of complications is less though various complications associated with the procedure are as follows:

- Cement leaks outside the vertebra are mostly inconsequential, but can cause local or radicular pain, neurological damage and pulmonary embolism.
- Inaccurate needle placement can injure nerve root or spinal cord.
- Pain exacerbation may occur due to substantial cement leaks.
- Rarely puncture site infection and bleeding may occur.

Future Directions

Although vertebroplasty can give considerable pain relief, it is not very useful in vertebral body height restoration. A new technique called kyphoplasty[28] involves the inflation of a bone tamp within the vertebral body to restore the height of the vertebra, and subsequently placing bone cement for augmentation of strength.

Another new technique is vesselplasty, alternative to vertebroplasty and kyphoplasty. It was devised to prevent the leakage of bone cement and restore vertebral body height. In this procedure, cement is injected into a

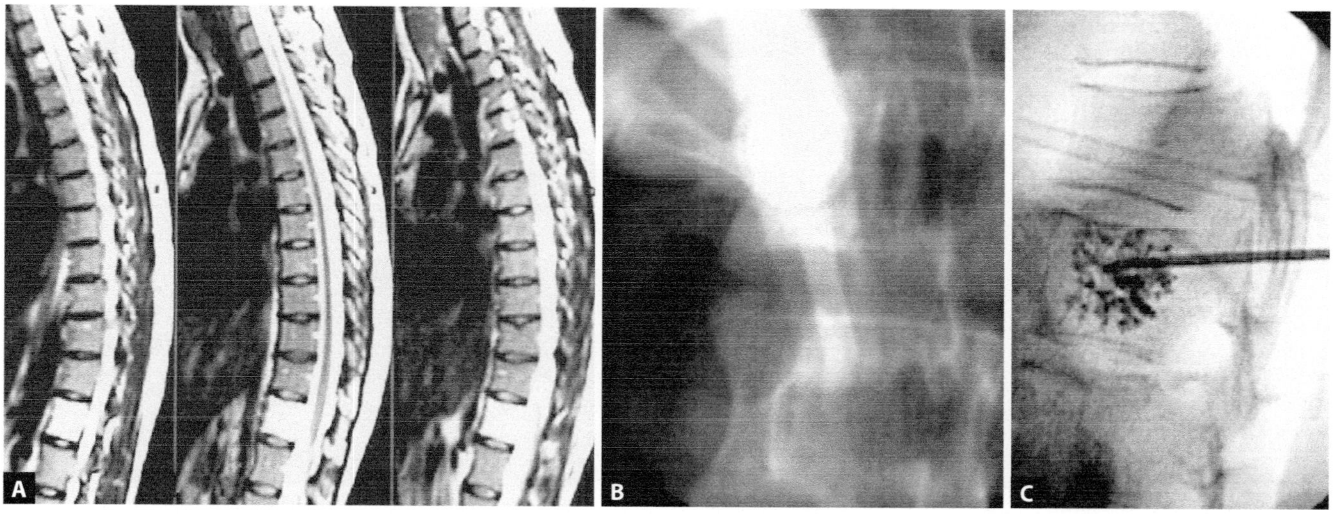

Figs. 20A to C: (A) A 30-year-old female with symptomatic D12 vertebral hemangioma, successfully treated with percutaneous vertebroplasty using polymethyl methacrylate bone cement. T2-weighted (T2W) pretreatment magnetic resonance (MR) shows D12 vertebral body hemangioma; (B) The vertebroplasty needle is seen in position with (C) injected bone cement.

balloon positioned in the vertebral body, thus reducing the incidence of leak. Vesselplasty has shown statistically significant benefits in patients with symptomatic vertebral compression fractures.[29] Recently in the treatment of burst fractures with posterior wall retropulsion and no neurologic deficit, armed kyphoplasty using intravertebral distraction devices, such as vertebral body stents and SpineJack, could be effective in fracture reduction, internal fixation, and indirect central canal decompression. In selected cases, it might represent a suitable minimally invasive treatment option, stand alone or in combination with posterior stabilization.[30]

Vertebroplasty is becoming a well-established modality in the management of the aforementioned conditions, and is relatively safe.[31]

Percutaneous Treatment of Disc Herniation

Low backache is one of the major causes of chronic pain and morbidity. Treatment of herniated disc has evolved from open surgical techniques to minimally invasive or microtherapeutic procedures under local anesthesia. These include percutaneous laser disc decompression (PLDD), percutaneous ozone therapy and percutaneous/endoscopic nucleotomy.

In PLDD, laser energy is delivered into nucleus pulposus by laser fiber, through a needle. The aim of PLDD is to vaporize a small portion of the nucleus pulposus. The ablation of this small volume results in reduction of intradiscal pressure, thus reducing the disc herniation[32] **(Figs. 21A to D)**. This technology has been improved further to deliver proper energy without damaging the nerve.[33]

In percutaneous ozone treatment, mixture of ozone-oxygen gas is administered into nucleus pulposus through the needle. This mixture has a direct effect on the proteoglycans of the nucleus pulposus, resulting in release of water molecules and subsequent degeneration of matrix and reduction of volume[34] **(Figs. 22A to C)**.

Both PLDD and percutaneous ozone therapy are not used for uncontained herniations or sequestered disc. In both the procedures, patient is positioned prone and using either fluoroscopy or CT guidance a lumbar puncture needle (18–21G) is inserted into the center of the disc. After proper position of the needle, for PLDD, an optical fiber is advanced through the needle and proper laser energy is given. For ozone treatment, approximated 4 mL ozone-oxygen mixture is injected with an ozone concentration of 27 μg/mL.[35]

PERCUTANEOUS ABLATION OF BONE TUMORS

Percutaneous image-guided tumor ablation with thermal energy source such as radiofrequency, laser or microwave energy is used in the treatment of both benign (osteoid osteoma, osteoblastoma, enchondroma, etc.) and malignant (metastatic) lesions in place of surgery due to potential benefits such as minimal invasiveness, reduced cost and morbidity.[36]

The procedure is performed with CT guidance either under general anesthesia or conscious sedation. A proper bone biopsy needle is placed into the lesion with the help of a hammer or a drill. Radiofrequency probe or laser fiber is introduced through the cannula and proper

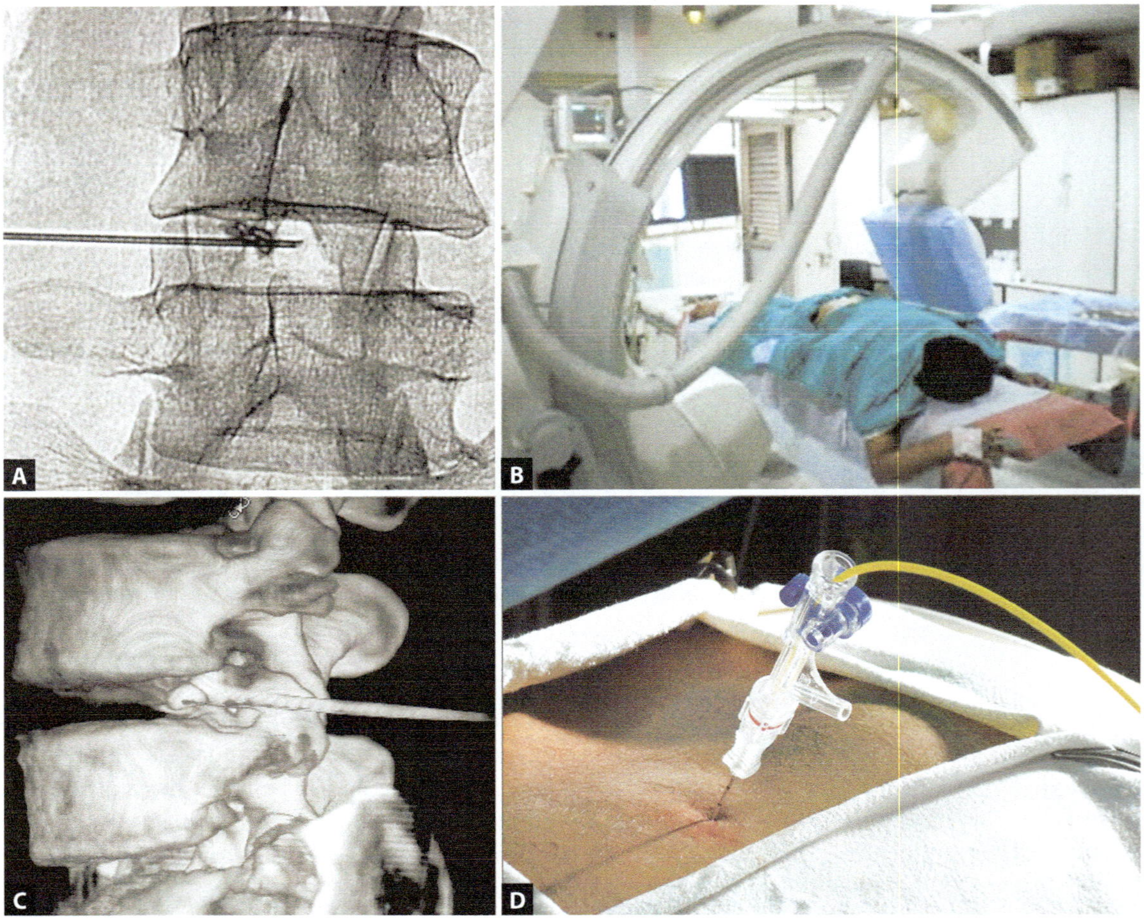

Figs. 21A to D: Percutaneous laser treatment of herniated disc. (A) A lumbar puncture needle is placed into the disc under fluoroscopy; (B and C) Needle position can be checked by doing rotation angiogram and three-dimensional (3D) reconstruction image; (D) After proper position of needle, optical fiber is advanced through the needle and laser energy is deposited.

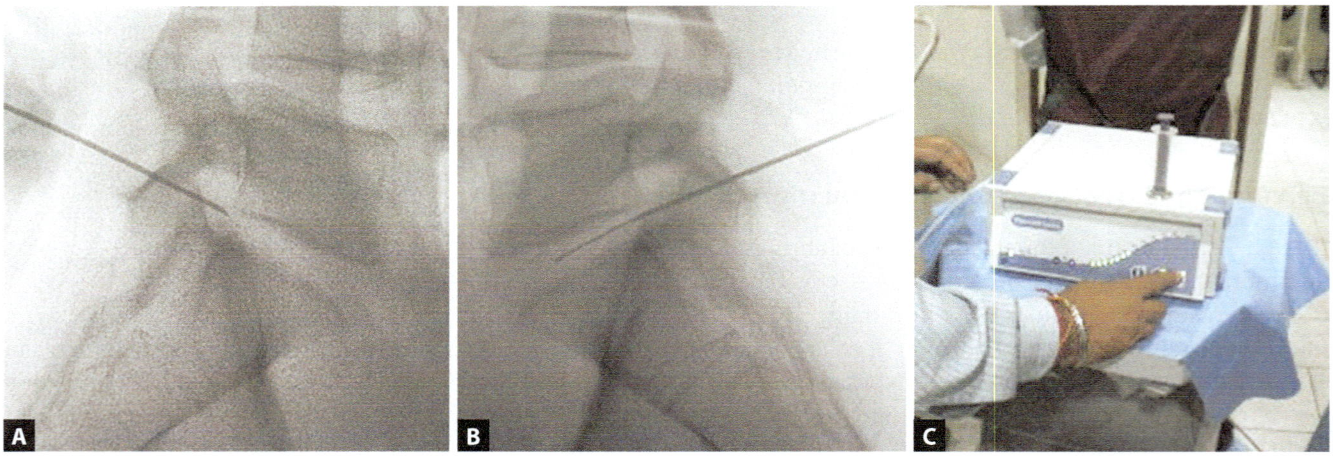

Figs. 22A to C: Percutaneous ozone treatment of herniated disc. (A and B) A lumbar puncture needle is placed into the disc under fluoroscopy; (C) Ozone gas is injected after preparing it from ozone generator machine.

energy is delivered for ablation **(Figs. 23A to F)**. CT-guided radiofrequency ablation (RFA) is proven to be a safe and effective procedure for the treatment of osteoid osteomas. When compared to surgical excision, it shows a significant reduction in hospitalization cost and duration. With its almost negligible postprocedural complications and a low rate of recurrence, RFA is at the moment is the treatment of choice for these bone tumors.[37]

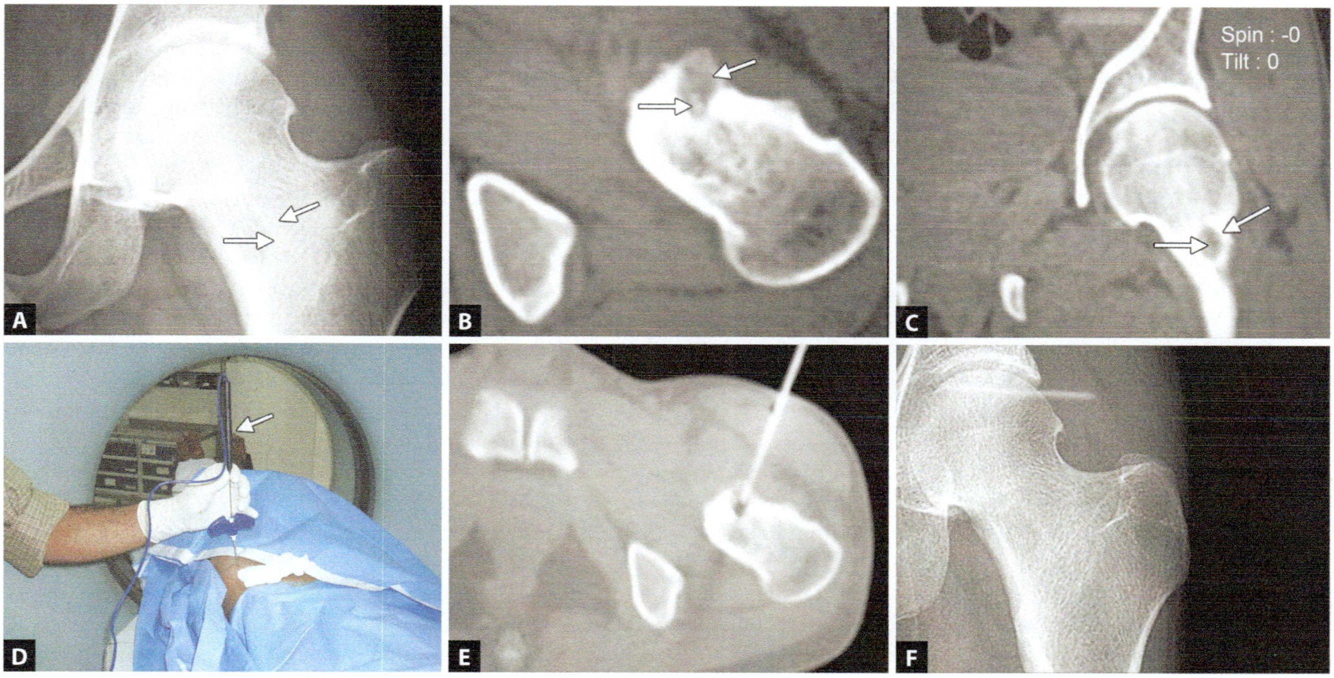

Figs. 23A to F: Percutaneous radiofrequency (RF) ablation of osteoid osteoma. Radiograph of left hip anteroposterior (AP) view (A), unenhanced axial (B) and coronal (C) computed tomography (CT) images showing a small calcified nidus (small arrow) with surrounding sclerosis (long arrow). After placement of bone biopsy needle (small arrow) into the lesion under CT guidance, the stylet was withdrawn and the RF probe (long arrow) was introduced (D). Axial CT image at the time of procedure (E) showing tip of the biopsy needle in the lesion. Post-treatment (1 week) AP radiograph (F) does not show nidus and patient is asymptomatic.

REFERENCES

1. Voegeli E, Uehlinger E. Arteriography in bone tumors. Skeletal Radiol. 1976;1:3-14.
2. Hudson TM, Haas G, Enneking WF, Hawkins IF Jr. Angiography in the management of musculoskeletal tumors. Surg Gynecol Obstet. 1975;141:11-21.
3. Han SK, Henein MH, Novin N, Giargiana FA. An unusual arterial complication seen with a solitary osteochondroma. Am Surg. 1977;43:471-2.
4. Gomez-Reino JH, Radin A, Gorevic PD. Pseudoaneurysm of the popliteal artery as a complication of an osteochondroma. Skeletal Radiol. 1979;4:26-8.
5. Lateur L, Baert AL. Localisation and diagnosis of osteoid osteoma of the carpal area by angiography. Skeletal Radiol. 1977;2:75-9.
6. deSantos LA, Murray JA. The value of arteriography in the management of aneurysmal bone cyst. Skeletal Radiol. 1978;2:137-41.
7. Bliznak J, Staple TW. Radiology of angiodysplasias of the limb. Radiology. 1974;110:35-44.
8. Levin DC, Grodon DH, McSweeney J. Arteriography of peripheral haemangiomas. Radiology. 1976;121:625.
9. Srivastava DN, Gulati M, Thulkar S, Berry M. Klippel-Trenaunay syndrome: unusual magnetic resonance features. Australas Radiol. 1998;42:88-9.
10. Bartlely O, Wickbom I. Angiography in soft tissue hemangiomas. Acta Radiol. 1959;51:81-94.
11. Bjarnason H. Vascular embolotherapy. In: Ferral H, Bjarnason H, Qian Z (Eds). Synopsis of Castaneda's Interventional Radiology, 1st edition. Philadelphia: Lippincott Williams and Wilkins; 2001. pp. 27-45.
12. Rosen RJ, Riles TS. Arteriovenous malformations. In: Strandness D, van Breda A (Eds). Vascular Diseases: Surgical and Interventional Therapy. New York: Churchill Livingstone; 1994. p. 1126.
13. Yaghmai I. Angiographic manifestations of soft tissue and osseous hemangiopericytomas. Radiology. 1978;126: 653-9.
14. Unni KK, Ivins JC, Beabout JW, Dahlin DC. Hemangioma, hemangiopericytoma, and hemangioendothelioma (angiosarcoma) of bone. Cancer. 1971;27:1403-14.
15. Yaghmai I. Angiography of Bone and Soft Tissue Lesions. New York: Springer; 1979.
16. Hoffer EK, Borsa JJ, Bloch RD, Fontaine AB. Endovascular techniques in the damage control setting. Radiographics. 1999;19:1340-8.
17. Feldman F, Casarella WJ, Dick HM, Hollander BA. Selective intra-arterial embolization of bone tumors: a useful adjunct in the management of selected lesions. Am J Roentgenol Radium Ther Nucl Med. 1975;123:130-9.
18. Voigt K, Schwenzer N, Stoeter P. Angiographic, operative, and histologic findings after embolization of craniofacial angiomas. Neuroradiology. 1978;16:424-7.
19. Doppman JL, Pevsner P. Embolization of arteriovenous malformations by direct percutaneous puncture. AJR Am J Roentgenol. 1983;140:773-8.

20. Wallace S, Granmayeh M, deSantos LA, Murray JA, Romsdahl MM, Bracken RB, et al. Arterial occlusion of pelvic bone tumor. Cancer. 1979;43:322-8.
21. Hemmy DC, McGee DM, Armbrust FH, Larson SJ. Resection of a vertebral hemangioma after preoperative embolization: a case report. J Neurosurg. 1977;47:282-5.
22. Mitty HA, Kleiger B. Partial embolization of large peripheral hemangioma for pain control. Radiology. 1978;127:671-2.
23. Owen RJ. Embolization of musculoskeletal tumors. Radiol Clin North Am. 2008;46(3):535-43.
24. Keus RB, Rutgers EJ, Ho GH, Gortzak E, Albus-Lutter CE, Hart AA. Limb-sparing therapy of extremity sarcomas: treatment outcome and long-term functional results. Eur J Cancer. 1994;30A:1459-63.
25. Hugate RR, Wilkins RM, Kelly CM, Madsen W, Hinshaw I, Camozzi AB. Intra-arterial chemotherapy for extremity osteosarcoma and MFH in adults. Clin Orthop Relat Res. 2008;466(6):1292-301.
26. Galibert P, Deramond H, Rosat P, Le Gars D. Preliminary note on the treatment of vertebral angioma by percutaneous acrylic vertebroplasty. Neurochirurgie. 1987;33:166-8.
27. Barr JD, Barr MS, Lemley TJ, McCann RM. Percutaneous vertebroplasty for pain relief and spinal stabilization. Spine (Phila Pa 1976). 2000;25:923-8.
28. Ledlie JT, Renfro M. Balloon kyphoplasty: one-year outcomes in vertebral body height restoration, chronic pain, and activity levels. J Neurosurg. 2003;98:36-42.
29. Flors L, Lonjedo E, Leiva-Salinas C, Martí-Bonmatí L, Martínez-Rodrigo JJ, López-Pérez E, et al. Vesselplasty: a new technical approach to treat symptomatic vertebral compression fractures. AJR Am J Roentgenol. 2009;193:218-26.
30. Venier A, Roccatagliata L, Isalberti M, Scarone P, Kuhlen DE, Reinert M, et al. Armed kyphoplasty: an indirect central canal decompression technique in burst fractures. AJNR Am J Neuroradiol. 2019;40(11):1965-72.
31. Gangi A, Guth S, Imbert JP, Marin H, Dietemann JL. Percutaneous vertebroplasty: indications, technique, and results. Radiographics. 2003;23:e10.
32. Gupta AK, Bodhey NK, Jayasree RS, Kapilamoorthy TR, Kesavadas C, Krishnamoorthy T, et al. Percutaneous laser disc decompression: clinical experience at SCTIMST and long-term follow-up. Neurol India. 2006;54:164-7.
33. Meng C, Li Y, Wang S, Yu J, Kou D, Liu C. Application of a modified optical fiber in targeted percutaneous laser disc decompression of lumbar disc herniation: a retrospective study. Exp Ther Med. 2019;18(5):3552-62.
34. Baabor MG, Vazquez PF, Sanchez JA. Automated nucleotomy and nucleolysis with ozone. Acta Neurochir Suppl. 2011;108:97-101.
35. Andreula CF, Simonetti L, De Santis F, Agati R, Ricci R, Leonardi M. Minimally invasive oxygen-ozone therapy lumber disc herniation. AJNR Am J Neuroradiol. 2003;24:996-1000.
36. Ruiz Santiago F, Garcia MD, Alvarez LG, Montes JL, García MR, Fernández JM. Percutaneous treatment of bone tumors by radiofrequency thermal ablation. Eur J Radiol. 2011;77(1):156-63.
37. Filippo MD, Russo U, Papapietro VR, Ceccarelli F, Pogliacomi F, Vaienti E, et al. Radiofrequency ablation of osteoid osteoma. Acta Biomed. 2018;89(1):175-85.

SECTION

2

Infections of Bones and Joints

CHAPTER

4

Tuberculosis of Bones and Joints

Gaurav Shanker Pradhan, Rashmi Dixit, Jyoti Kumar

INTRODUCTION

Tuberculosis (TB) is endemic throughout the Indian subcontinent.[1] This is of concern, as with the advent of drug-resistant cases and increase in number of immunocompromised patients, the disease prevalence will only increase and management becomes problematic. The causative etiological agent for tubercular affliction of bone is *Mycobacterium tuberculosis.*[2-4]

ETIOPATHOGENESIS

Osteoarticular TB begins in the synovium or in the metaphyseal spongiosa. Synovial infection can occur by contiguous spread or due to hematogenous spread.

Hematogenous spread can occur from lung primary or postprimary focus, or from any other visceral, lymph nodal source of infection. Simultaneous involvement of viscera, lymph nodes, and parts of skeletal system suggest spread of infection through arterial blood supply. The bacillus usually lodges in the spongiosa of the metaphysis. Lesion is usually destructive and accompanied by pus formation. The metaphyseal lesion may infect the joint through subperiosteal space, through capsule or through destruction of the epiphyseal plate. In contrast to pyogenic infections, sequestration and periostitis are not very common. Ischemic necrosis and endarteritis may result in very small sequestrum formation which is usually not radiologically visible. It may become visible as a result of calcification. Marked exudative reaction is, however, a common feature. Granulation tissue spreads onto the free surface of cartilage eroding it in patches, insinuating between cartilage and subchondral bone, advancing from periphery to the center causing loosening and separation of cartilaginous tissue, causing necrosis of cartilage with erosion of exposed bone. Marginal erosions are characteristics of TB in weight-bearing joints such as hip, knee, and ankle. Wedge-shaped necrotic foci may become evident on either side of joint leading to the appearance of "kissing sequestra". Necrosed cartilage, fibrinous material form "rice bodies" in synovial joints, tendon sheaths, and bursae.[5,6] Abscesses that form may track along fascial planes and result in sinus formation. Plaques of irregular bone, if present in walls of chronic abscess or sinus suggest diagnosis of long-standing tubercular infection.

Bacille Calmette-Guérin (BCG) osteitis that can occur following BCG vaccination runs a benign course with localization of the *Bacillus* in epiphysis and metaphysis with extension across growth plate. It resembles chronic osteomyelitis radiologically, but responds to antitubercular therapy (ATT).

Synovial sheath infections are common with nontypical *Mycobacterium* (other than *M. tuberculosis* and *M. bovis*), with history of trauma (puncture wounds), surgery, immunocompromised status, and exposure to contaminated marine life.

Tuberculosis has been seen as a late complication of implant surgery (6–12 months postoperation). This has been attributed to extensive surgery, use of implants, and favorable conditions for circulating mycobacteria such as diabetes mellitus, corticosteroids, and immunocompromised status.[6,7]

CLINICAL FEATURES

Clinical features include insidious onset, low-grade fever, anorexia, weight loss, and night sweats. The patient may present with night pains, painful limitation of movement, muscle wasting, regional lymph node involvement, and neurologic symptoms.

Weight-bearing joints such as hip, knee, and ankle are commonly involved, though any part of the skeleton can get involved by the disease process.[8,9]

RADIOLOGICAL FEATURES

Pathologic affliction of the disease can be categorized as under:

- Inflammatory edema and exudates (predestructive stage)
- Necrosis and cavitation
- Destruction and deformation
- Healing and repair.

Tubercular infection in bones is said to develop 2–3 years after primary focus, so the diagnosis is usually delayed, in contrast to pyogenic infections which are seen

2–3 weeks after clinical presentation. Further changes in bone on plain radiograph, are usually appreciable 2–4 months after onset of disease in the bone. The infection originates in the metaphysis and it can cross the growth plate. There is usually no sclerosis and small sequestra are absorbed. Diaphysial lesions are rare and multiple cystic lucencies are rarer still.

Investigations include anteroposterior and lateral radiographs of the involved region and a radiograph of the chest.

Stage of synovitis: In early synovial disease there is soft tissue swelling and joint widening due to effusion and synovial hypertrophy. The first radiological sign may be juxta-articular osteoporosis. Patchy areas of trabecular or bony destruction may be evident. In the center of osteolytic lesion or cavity, there may be sequestrum or calcification of the caseous tissue, giving appearance of an irregular soft, feathery, coke-like sequestrum **(Fig. 1)**. If there is secondary superadded infection, subperiosteal reaction may result. As a result of localized hyperemia, growth plate may show overgrowth, especially in childhood.

Stage of arthritis: Later in the disease, the articular margin and bony cortices may be hazy (blurring and fuzzy) giving rise to "washed-out appearance". With involvement of articular cartilage there is narrowing and reduction of joint space. Juxta-articular osteopenia, peripherally located osseous lesions, and gradual narrowing of joint space are considered pathognomonic of tubercular osteoarthritis and are referred to as "Phemister triad" **(Fig. 2)**.

Early loss of articular joint space is more typically seen in rheumatoid arthritis and thus helps in differentiating from TB.

Stage of advanced arthritis: In advanced cases, there is collapse of bone, subluxation or dislocation, migration of bone and resultant deformity of joint.[10,11]

With healing, there is remineralization and cortical and articular margins become distinct. Fibrous ankylosis may occur during healing phase. In contrast to pyogenic arthritis, the development of bone ankylosis is uncommon in tuberculous arthritis.

Ultrasonography is helpful in the evaluation of large joints, like hip joint, to demonstrate joint effusion, synovitis, and capsular thickening. Synovial thickening can be seen as hypoechoic intra-articular soft tissue. Fluid in joint space and bursal fluid can be anechoic or hypoechoic (thick exudates). In tenosynovitis, the synovial sheath along tendons is thick and heterogeneous with minimal fluid suggestive of chronic tenosynovitis. It can, in addition, indicate presence of associated soft tissue abscess such as psoas abscess. It can also demonstrate cortical disruption, irregularity of articular margins, and associated soft tissue swelling. Calcification in abscess, if any, can also be seen. Further, evaluation of tendon sheaths and bursal spaces and smaller joints such as wrist, hand, foot, and ankle is also possible. Guided joint fluid aspiration or synovial biopsy is possible under ultrasound guidance.

Computed tomography (CT) is helpful in demonstrating lytic areas and marginal erosions much before plain radiographs.[12]

Swelling in soft tissues, granulation, exudations, abscess, and early calcification can also be demonstrated much earlier. Joint space can also be better evaluated by CT scan.

The predestructive stage can be visualized by magnetic resonance imaging (MRI) and also probably by bone scans. The plain radiographs and CT scan are not likely to detect the stage of inflammatory edema and exudates.

Isotope bone scan or MRI may reveal subclinical active lesion in 40% of patients, in addition to the presenting lesion. Out of technetium-99m, gallium-67,

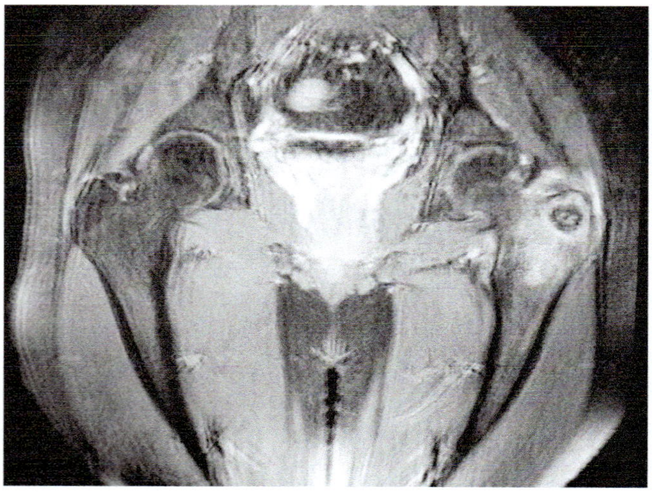

Fig. 1: In the center of osteolytic lesion in left femur, there is a small irregular sequestrum picked up on MRI [image en Grelot].

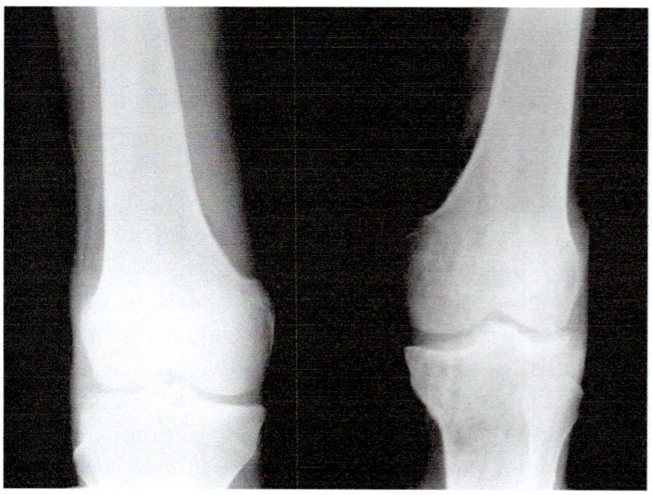

Fig. 2: Diffuse osteopenia with lytic lesion seen at the lateral articular margin of tibia with relative preservation of joint spaces in a case of tuberculosis of left knee.

and indium-111 isotopes used in skeletal scintigraphy, technetium-99m is the most sensitive, though not specific. So a positive scan helps in localizing the suspicious region and is also helpful for follow-up.

Fluorine fluorodeoxyglucose positron emission tomography (^{18}F-FDG-PET) has also been found useful in localizing tubercular disease and in differentiating soft tissue infection from osseous infection.[4,5,13]

Synovial hypertrophy is most commonly seen in osteoarticular TB on MRI. Hypointense areas on T2-weighted images (T2WI) suggesting hemosiderin deposition, rim of synovial lesions on pregadolinium T1-weighted images (T1WI) and fluid loculations with enhancing synovial rims and erosions on post-gadolinium images may be helpful in characterizing the lesion as tubercular when the radiographs are normal **(Fig. 3)**.

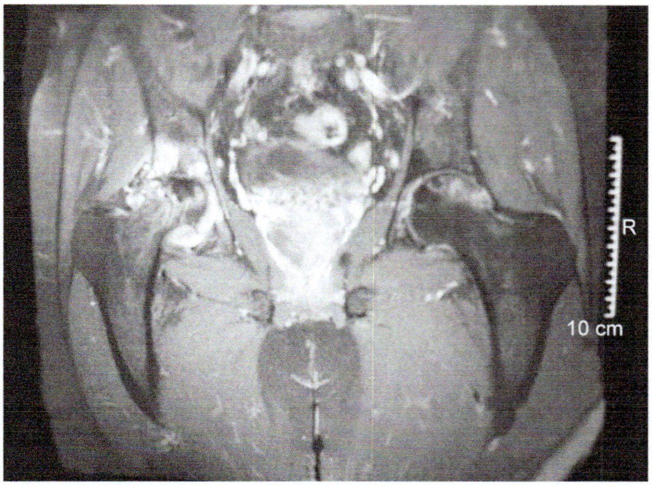

Fig. 3: Fluid loculations with enhancing synovial rims and erosions on postgadolinium images in a case of tuberculosis of right hip.

Magnetic resonance imaging can be helpful in diagnostic evaluation:

- *Short-tau inversion recovery (STIR) imaging, inversion recovery [repetition time (TR) >2,000 ms; echo time (TE) >30 ms; inversion-time (TI) = 120–150 ms)]*: Fat-saturation technique that results in markedly decreased signal intensity from fat and strikingly increased signal from fluid and edema. Inversion recovery is an extremely sensitive tool for detecting tissue and marrow pathology. Fast spin echo (FSE)-STIR sequence is used with most of our musculoskeletal protocols.
- T2-weighted sequences are sensitive in picking up high signal of joint fluid and make it a sensitive method to detect joint effusion.
- T2-weighted images depict synovial proliferation as hypointense, while contrast-enhanced MR shows marked enhancement after gadolinium injection.
- Caseating granulomas with solid centers give a characteristic hypointense signal to the synovium on T2WI.
- Chondral lesions and subchondral bone erosions may be visible at a stage, when the joint space is still well preserved.
- *Penumbra sign* may be present. A thin intermediate signal intensity rim along the periphery of a bone or soft tissue abscess on unenhanced T1WI may be seen, due to layer of granulation tissue along its wall. It is useful in identifying soft tissue abscesses.
- In the pelvis and extremities, routine protocols should include T1, STIR, and postgadolinium T1WI. Section thickness used in the pelvis is 7 mm and in the extremities, 4 mm.
- MRI can be helpful in detecting bone marrow inflammation, intraosseous abscess, sequestrum, cortical destruction, cloaca, and sinus tract formation **(Figs. 4A to C)**.

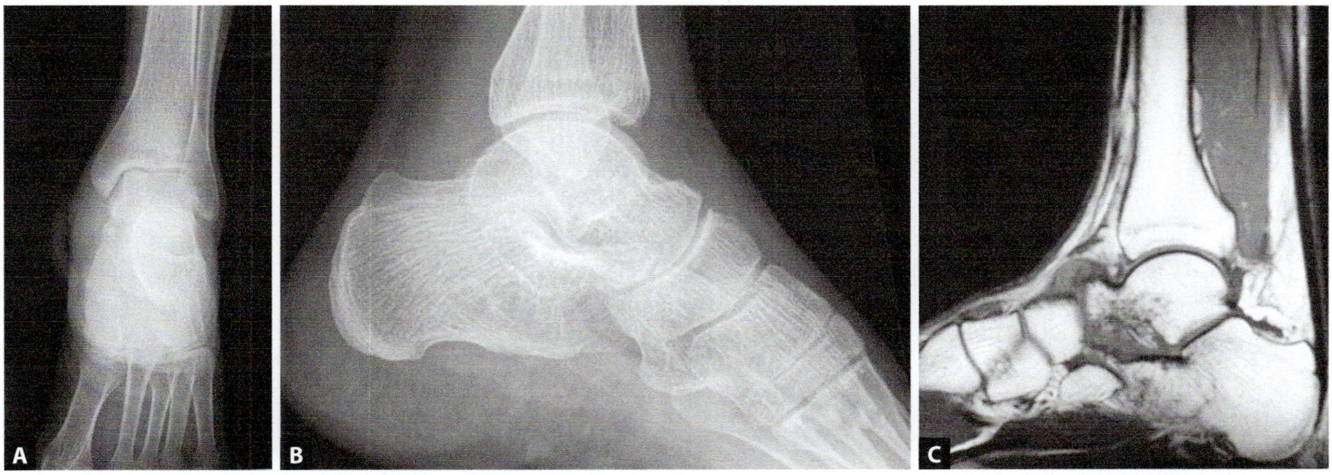

Figs. 4A to C: (A and B) Plain X-rays of ankle showing subtle osteolytic lesion in anterior aspect of talus on right side; (C) MRI showing markedly destructive lesion in anterior aspect of talus with associated soft tissue abnormality.

- Tenosynovitis may be seen in active (hygromatous) and chronic (serofibrinous) phase and bursitis may be seen as distended bursa or multiple small abscesses.[4,9,14]

Skeletal TB involving parts of body other than spine can be classified according to region of involvement:

- *Tuberculosis of joints*: Tubercular arthritis
- *Tuberculosis of long and flat bones*: Tubercular osteomyelitis
- *Tuberculosis of short tubular bones*: Tubular dactylitis.

TUBERCULOSIS OF JOINTS (ARTHRITIS)

Hip Joint

Lesion can arise in acetabulum, synovium, femoral epiphysis or metaphysis (Babcock's triangle) or spread to the hip from foci in the greater trochanter or ischium. If there is tubercular involvement of the upper end of femur (being entirely intracapsular), the joint is involved early in disease and there is destruction of articular margins of femoral head and acetabulum. Hip involvement is seen in about 15% of cases of osteoarticular TB.[15]

Tubercular lesion may start in the greater trochanter or the overlying bursa. There may be surface erosion or lytic lesion may be present in greater trochanter. TB of the greater trochanter may involve the overlying trochanteric bursa without involving the hip joint for a fairly long period of time.

Stage of Synovitis

The patient may present with irritable hip with plain radiograph being normal **(Fig. 5)**. Soft tissue swelling, marked deossification with radiologically significant osteoporosis appearing 12–18 weeks after symptoms may be present. Displacement of fat planes and positive obturator sign occur due to flexion deformity (reduced obturator foramina size).

Ultrasound, CT, and MRI are more sensitive in this stage to detect increased joint space and accumulation of fluid. Investigations may be repeated, at 3–6 weeks' interval, to help in establishing the diagnosis.

Differential diagnosis includes traumatic or nonspecific transient synovitis, Perthes' disease, slipped capital femoral epiphysis, and low-grade pyogenic infections.

Stage of Arthritis

There is deformity of the hip joint. In addition to osteoporosis, localized erosions may be seen in periarticular region **(Fig. 6)**. The destruction of articular cartilage leads to erosion of acetabular margin and femoral head with reduction of joint space. Lesions can usually be picked up on CT, before they are apparent on plain radiographs.[7,9]

Stage of Advanced Arthritis

With progression of disease, there is destruction of articular cartilage, acetabulum, femoral head, capsule, and ligaments. The capsule may also get thickened and contracted **(Figs. 7A to C)**. The upper end of femur may displace upward, dorsally breaking the Shenton's line and leaving the lower part of acetabulum empty (wandering acetabulum; **Fig. 8**). Bone loss can lead to bird-beak appearance with intrapelvic protrusion. If femoral head, neck are grossly destroyed and collapsed in an enlarged acetabulum, this appearance is called "mortar and pestle" appearance **(Fig. 9)**.

Radiological classification for TB of hip (Shanmugasundaram's classification) is useful in assessing relationship between various radiological types and functional outcome in which various radiological types have been described such as traveling acetabulum, dislocated hip, Perthes' type, protrusio acetabuli, atrophic type, and mortar and pestle type **(Figs. 10A to C)**.[16]

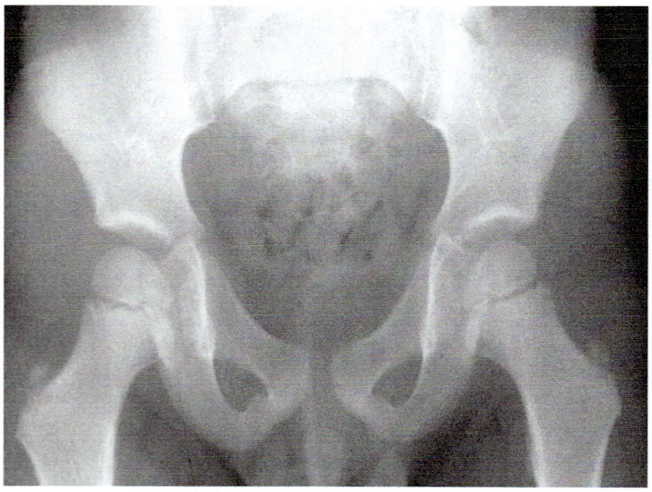

Fig. 5: Plain X-ray of pelvis showing relatively well-maintained hip joint on left side in an early case of tuberculosis of left hip with hip joint effusion on ultrasound.

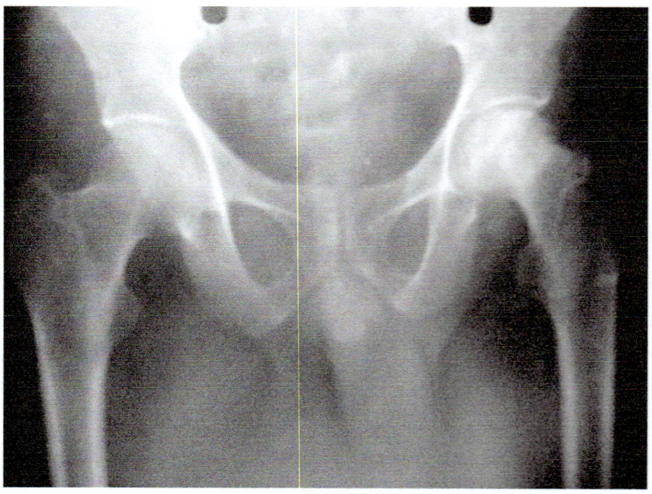

Fig. 6: Tubercular arthritis of left hip showing periarticular osteopenia, indistinct articular surfaces and erosions of femoral head and neck with relative preservation of joint space.

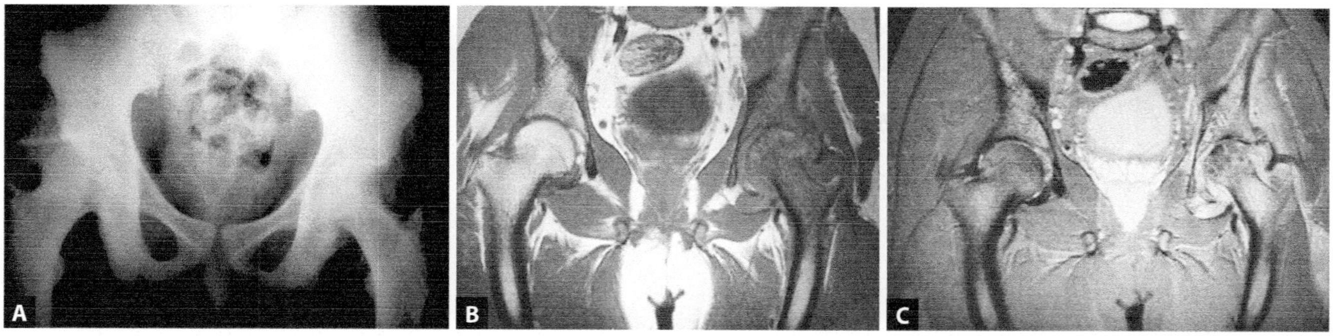

Figs. 7A to C: (A) Plain X-ray of pelvis showing erosion of the lateral aspect of femur head and neck with markedly reduced joint space on left side; (B and C) Altered marrow signal intensity in the left femoral head and neck appearing hypointense on T1 and hyperintense on short-tau inversion recovery (STIR) magnetic resonance images.

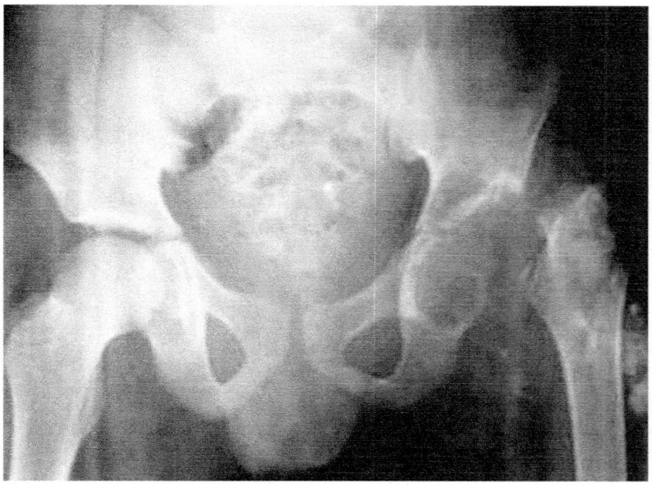

Fig. 8: Plain X-ray of pelvis showing destruction and subluxation of upper end of left femur, being displaced upwards and dorsally resulting in "wandering acetabulum".

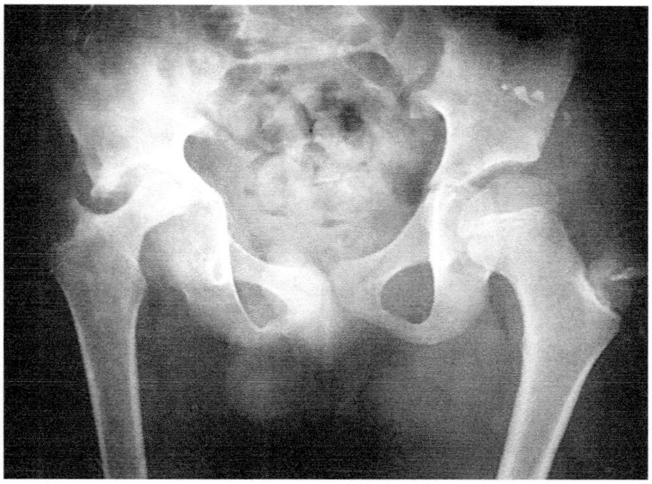

Fig. 9: Plain X-ray of pelvis showing gross destruction of right femoral head and neck with collapse contained within the enlarged acetabulum giving "mortar and pestle appearance".

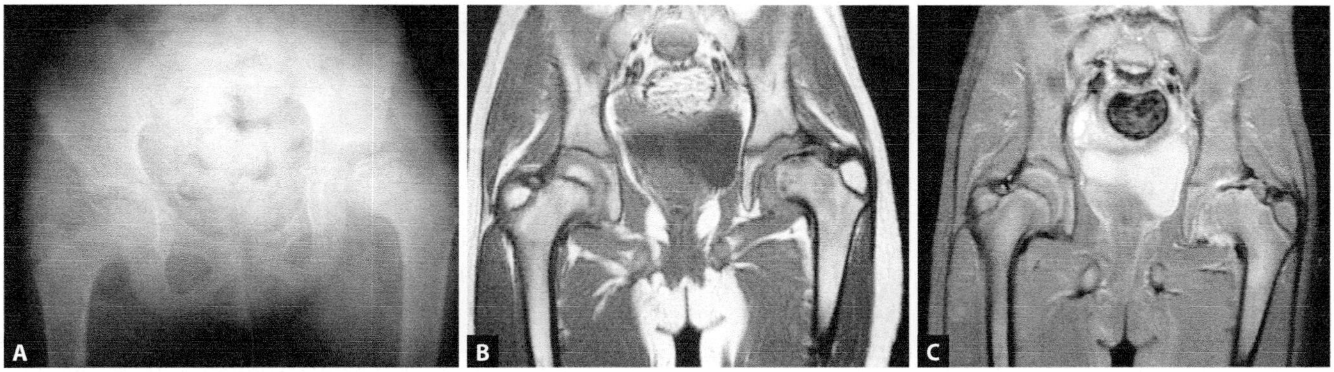

Figs. 10A to C: (A) There is evidence of irregularity, partial collapse and sclerosis of epiphysis of left femoral head suggestive of Perthes' type appearance in a case of tuberculosis of left hip joint; (B and C) Flattening of the left femur capital epiphysis in the same case, which appears diffusely hypointense on T1 and short-tau inversion recovery suggestive of sclerosis with marrow signal alteration noted in the left femoral neck.

Knee Joint

Patients with tubercular involvement of knee can present with pain, limitation of movement or swelling, in addition to general clinical features of TB.

The knee joint has the largest intra-articular space and is involved in about 10% cases of osteoarticular TB. The initial focus may be in synovium or subchondral bone of distal femur, proximal tibia, or patella.[17]

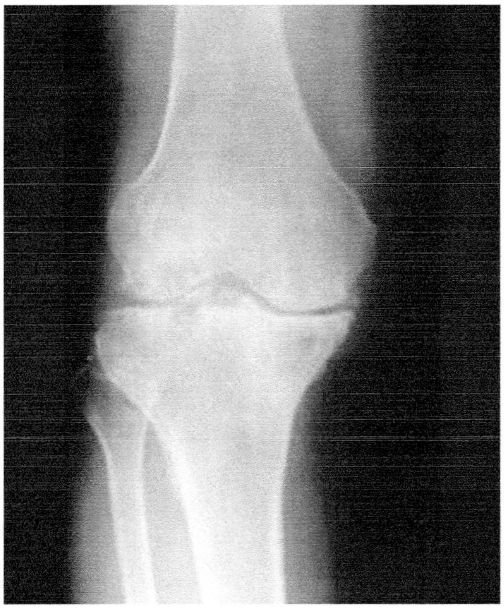

Fig. 11: Plain X-ray of knee joint showing juxta-articular osteopenia with fuzziness of articular margins numerous marginal erosions and loss of joint space.

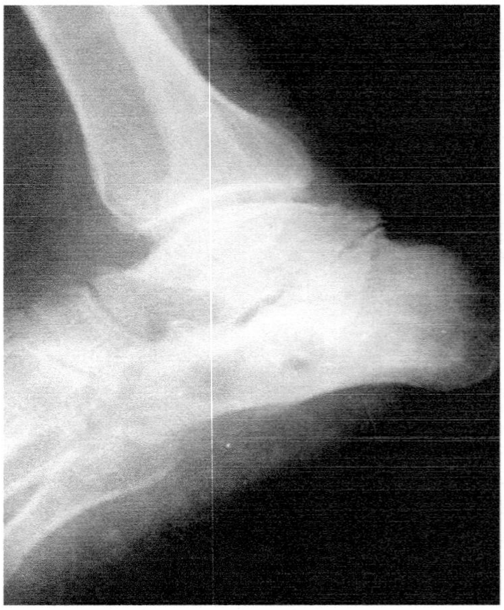

Fig. 12: Plain X-ray of ankle joint showing marginal erosions at subtalar joint with indistinct articular surfaces and loss of joint space.

In the synovial stage, there is osteoporosis, soft tissue swelling due to synovial effusion, thickened synovium and capsule. Synovial infection in childhood can lead to effusion, osteoporosis, accelerated growth, and maturation resulting in big bulbous squared epiphysis.[18] Synovitis can also cause widening of the intercondylar notch. Synovial inflammation with cartilage destruction leads to bony involvement in subarticular region and pus formation in joint.

As arthritis sets in, there is loss of definition of articular surfaces, marginal erosions, decreased joint space, and destruction of bones **(Fig. 11)**.

In advanced arthritis, there is bony destruction with joint space reduction and deformity. Translocation of tibia can occur with respect to femur posteriorly, laterally, or superiorly.

The differential diagnosis includes juvenile rheumatoid arthritis, villonodular synovitis, osteochondritis dissecans, and hemophilia.

Diagnosis can be aided by clinical sign and symptoms, radiologically by noting regional osteopenia, bony destructive lesions, and joint involvement with pathologic confirmation by fluid analysis or synovial biopsy.

Ankle and Foot

Swelling, limp, and pain may be the early presenting features in TB of ankle joint. The swelling is evident in front of the joint, around the malleoli, and tendoachilles insertion. Marked osteoporosis with or without erosions and osteolytic lesions may be present in active stage of disease. There may be unsharpness of articular surfaces along with reduction of joint space **(Fig. 12)**.

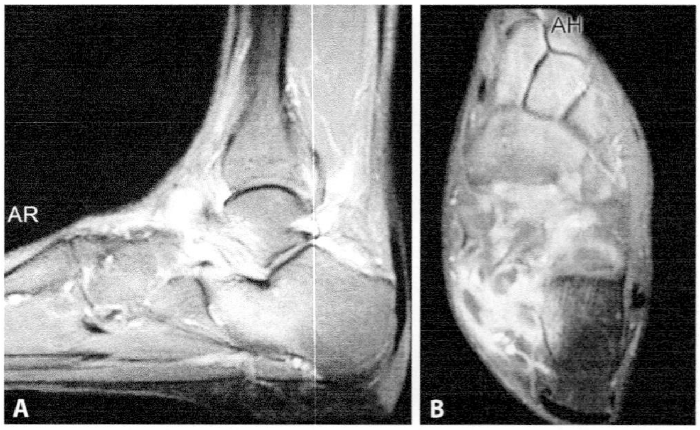

Figs. 13A and B: MRI of ankle joint in a case of talocalcaneal tuberculosis showing bony destruction involving talus, multiple collections along with rim enhancement in the subtalar region with cloaca and sinus tract formation.

In long-standing cases, gross destruction of bones and sinus formation can result. The ankle joint can show pathological anterior dislocation. Rarely, periosteal reaction may occur.

In tubercular affliction of foot, common involvement is seen of calcaneum, subtalar and midtarsal joints, anterior two-thirds of calcaneum being commonly affected.

Talus, metatarsal bones, navicular, cuneiform, cuboid can all get involved.[19] Radiographs can reveal presence of osteolyic lesion with or without coke-like sequestrum. Tubercular infection rapidly spreads across the intercommunicating synovial channels, so multiple bones are commonly involved **(Figs. 13A and B)**.

Differential diagnosis of tubercular affliction includes maduramycosis and neuropathic foot due to various causes, osteochondritis dissecans of talus.

Shoulder

Tubercular disease involving the shoulder joint is rare. It is more frequent in adults and the incidence of coexisting pulmonary TB is high. The sites of involvement include humeral head, scapula (glenoid, coracoid process, and spine of scapula), and acromioclavicular joint.

In the shoulder joint, the initial tubercular destruction is typically widespread because of the small surface contact area of articular cartilage. There is painful restriction of movement of shoulder in abduction and internal rotation with wasting of associated muscles, as the disease becomes chronic.[20]

Radiologically, there is osteoporosis with erosion of articular margins (fuzzy) with osteolytic lesion involving head of humerus, glenoid or both **(Fig. 14)**. The lesion may mimic giant cell tumor. Sinus formation can also occur. In advanced cases, inferior subluxation of the humeral head and fibrous ankylosis may result **(Fig. 15)**. In atrophic variety of tubercular affliction of shoulder, the disease runs a benign course without pus formation called *caries sicca* and small pitted erosions on the humeral head may be seen. The classical dry type is more common in adults while the fulminating variety with cold abscess or sinus formation is more common in children.[21]

Since the joint space is small, multiple and large osseous destructive lesions are commonly seen. MRI can show synovial lesions as well as the osseous lesions.

Differential diagnosis includes periarthritis, post-traumatic stiff shoulder. Aspiration of joint fluid or biopsy may be required to arrive at the diagnosis.

Elbow

Tubercular involvement is seen in about 2–5% cases.

Humeral condyles, radial head, and olecranon are frequently involved **(Fig. 16)**. Rarely the disease is synovial in origin.

Radiographic features in articular type include involvement of humerus and ulna, osteoporosis, blurring of articular cortex, and early compromise of joint space, while in extra-articular type ulna is more frequently involved with destructive lesions seen in olecranon or coronoid process.[9,21] Periostitis may also be seen.

Radiographs may depict blurring of articular margins due to synovial involvement. Osteolytic lesions may be seen around the elbow joint. In advanced case, there is decreased joint space and subchondral bone destruction.[20,21] Periostitis commonly affects the ulna.

Osteoid osteoma involving lateral condyle which is intra-articular and osteochondritis dissecans can cause diagnostic dilemma.

Wrist and Carpus

It is a rare site, usually affecting adults. Sites of involvement include distal radius, scaphoid, capitate, and lunate, with or without involvement of adjacent tendon sheaths **(Fig. 17)**.

Radiographic features include intense osteoporosis, soft tissue swelling, erosions of articular margins and cartilage destructions, periosteal reaction, and early appearance of ossification centers.

All carpal bones tend to get involved in adults while more localized lesions are seen in children. This is thought to be due to thicker articular cartilage in children.[22] With cartilage destruction, the carpal bones become crowded and adjacent bones tend to get involved. Intense demineralization is present in carpus, distal radius and ulna, metacarpals being usually spared. This serves as a differentiating feature from rheumatoid arthritis.

Sacroiliac Joints

These are affected more often in young adults than children and the involvement is usually unilateral. Sacroiliac joint infection is usually associated with TB of spine.

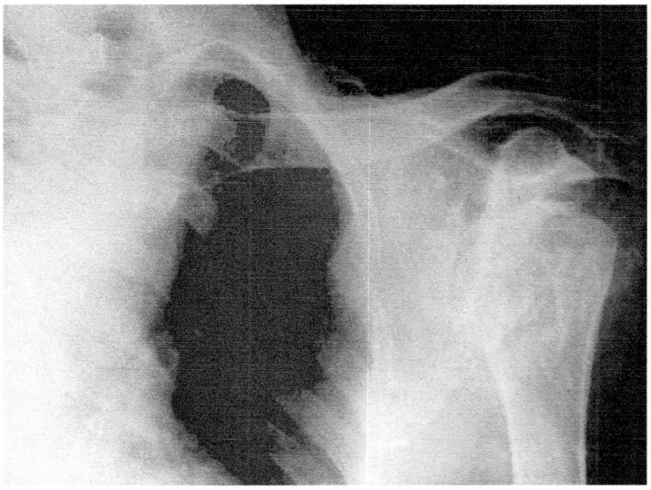

Fig. 14: Plain X-ray of left shoulder joint showing erosions and deformity of humeral head and acetabular margin with osteopenia and periarticular calcification.

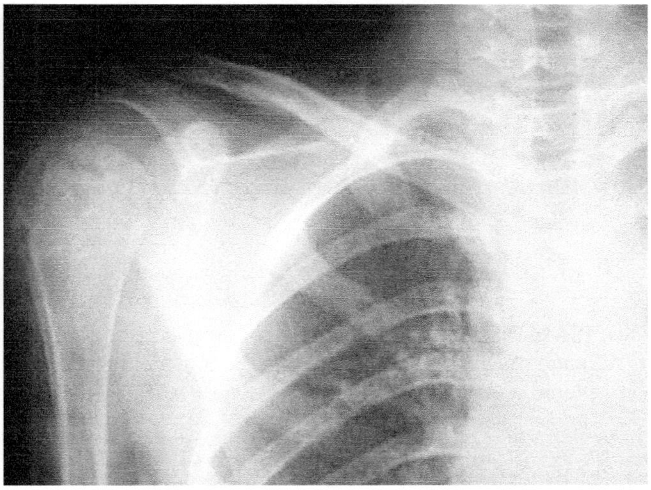

Fig. 15: Plain X-ray of right shoulder joint showing fuzzy articular margins and osteolytic lesions in proximal part of right humerus with pathological subluxation of head of humerus.

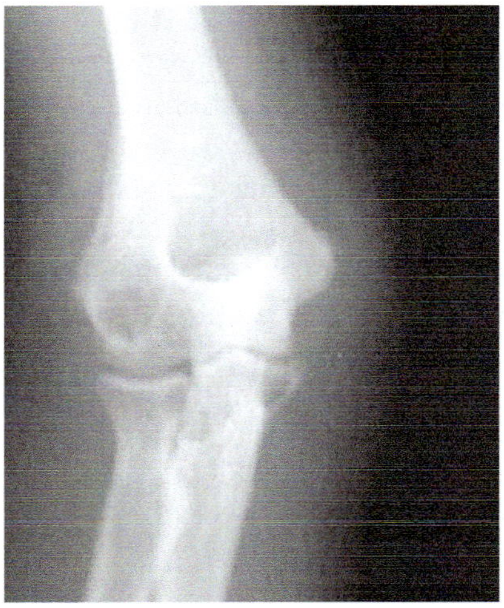

Fig. 16: Plain X-ray of right elbow joint showing multiple osteolytic lesions within the radius, ulna, and capitulum.

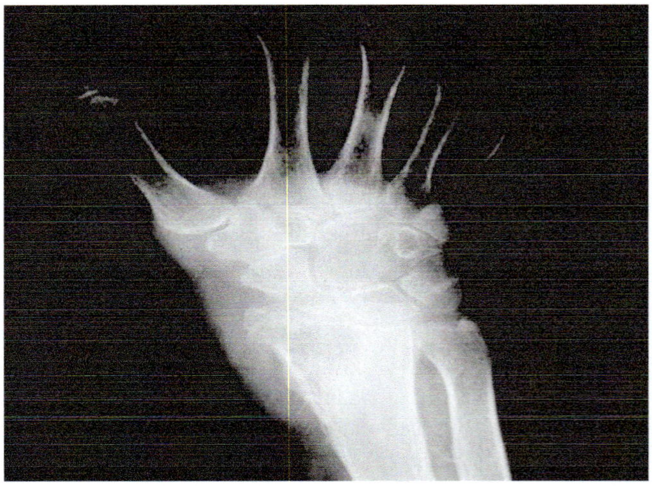

Fig. 17: Plain X-ray of right wrist joint showing irregular area of lytic destruction seen in distal metaphysis of radius with osteoporosis and soft tissue swelling.

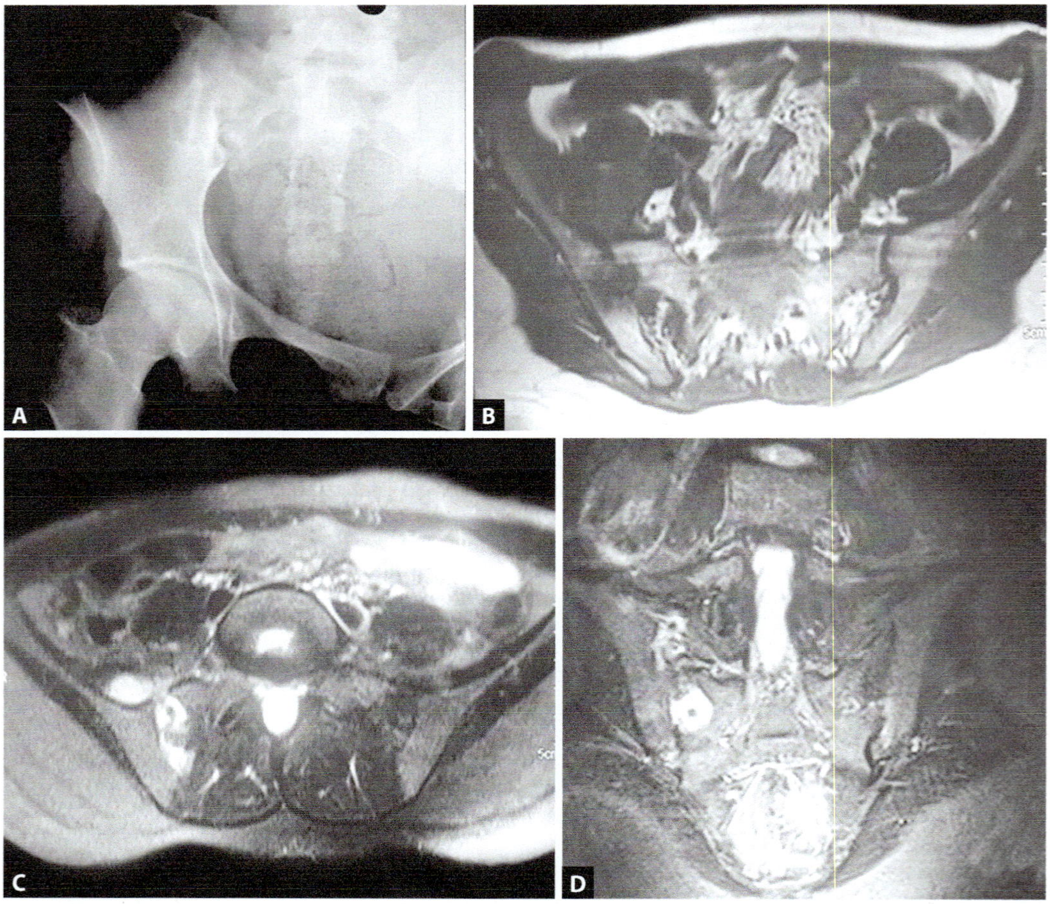

Figs. 18A to D: (A) Plain X-ray of pelvis showing large erosions with surrounding sclerosis at right sacroiliac joint; (B and C) Axial T1W and T2W image shows hypointensity along iliac blade with hyperintense signal on T2 likely to be marrow edema with synovial proliferation with altered signal intensity in iliacus muscle; (D) STIR MR image showing hyperintense synovium in right sacroiliac joint.

Radiographic features include irregularity and fuzziness of articular surfaces starting at the inferior surface. Subarticular erosions may be present causing widening of joint space. Both the sclerosis and erosions predominate on the iliac side while punched out lesions may be seen in ilium or sacrum **(Figs. 18A to D)**.

Articular erosions cause widening of the joint space and infection is associated with abscess formation over the back of the joint which may later calcify. Articular erosion cause widening of the joint space and tubercular infection is associated with abscess formation. This abscess may remain intrapelvic or extend under the glutei muscles.[23]

Magnetic resonance imaging is the ideal means of evaluating the complex anatomy of sacroiliac joints. Coronal imaging of the sacroiliac joints, parallel to the plane of the sacrum allows direct comparison of one sacroiliac joint to the other.[23,24]

BCG OSTEITIS

Bacille Calmette-Guérin is a vaccine of an attenuated bovine tubercular *Bacillus*. Although complications are unusual, generalized BCG infection and bone and joint infection can occur after BCG vaccination. Due to hematogenous spread of BCG infection to the skeleton, it is not usually associated with immunologic disorder and has a favorable prognosis.

Radiologically, BCG osteomyelitis affects children between 6 months and 6 year. It usually affects epiphysis and metaphysis of tubular bone especially around the knee, ribs, the sternum, the small bones of hand and feet. Lesions are more common on same side of the body as the vaccine was injected. Solitary lesions predominate and are seen as well-defined lytic foci.

Foucard and Helmstedt had suggested parameters to establish diagnosis of BCG-induced osteitis as follows:[23]

- BCG vaccination in the neonatal period.
- A period of less than 4 years between vaccination and symptom onset.
- No contact between the child and any adults with TB.
- A consistent clinical profile.
- Histopathology suggestive of TB

TUBERCULOSIS OF LONG AND FLAT BONES

Tubercular osteomyelitis occurs in roughly 3% of patients suffering from bone or joint TB, with multifocal involvement in about 7% cases. Flat bones are commonly involved and include sternum, scapula, ischium, and rarely skull. The lesions tend to be simultaneous in onset and progression and generally affect persons with low immune resistance. Symmetric well round, oval cystic lesions, with little or no periosteal reaction initially, may be present **(Fig. 19)**. In untreated cases, laminated periosteal reaction may be seen **(Figs. 20A to D)**. Sequestra formation is uncommon in adults, though in children large sequestra may be seen as the intraosseous vasculature is more prone to thrombosis. Joint involvement is rare as the lesions are diaphyseal or metphyseal.[24,25] There is no sclerosis, abscess or sinus formation, so it is also called as closed cystic TB.

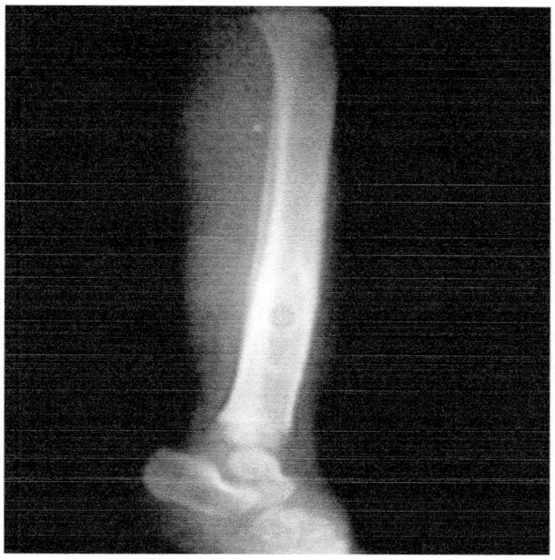

Fig. 19: Plain X-ray of right leg with ankle lateral view showing well- defined round osteolytic area seen in the shaft of tibia, in a case of diaphyseal tuberculosis.

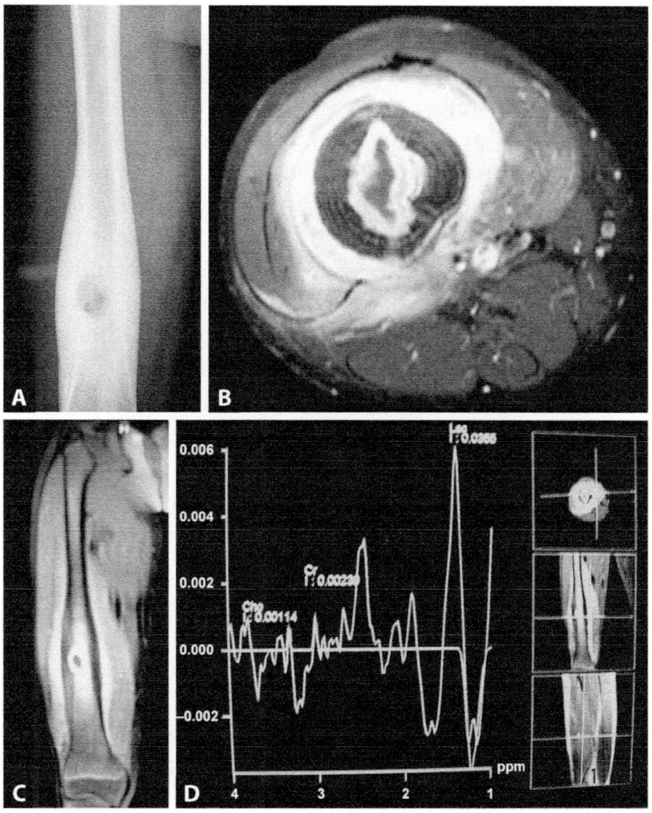

Figs. 20A to D: (A) Plain X-ray of right thigh showing well-defined round osteolytic area in the shaft of right femur, along with marked laminated periosteal reaction; (B and C) Magnetic resonance axial and coronal images showing intraosseous abscess in right femur, along with marked laminated periosteal reaction; (D) Magnetic resonance spectroscopic image showing prominent lactate peak in a case of diaphyseal tuberculosis.

Differential diagnosis includes polyostotic fibrous dysplasia, eosinophilic granuloma of the bone, and enchondromatosis. Isolated tubercular involvement of bone is rare (2–3% of all cases).

Pathology

Bones are involved as a result of hematogenous spread from a primary focus, usually in the lung or the lymphatic system. Granulomatous lesion develops within the bone at the site of deposition of the *Mycobacterium*, usually metaphysis, which is the site of infection. Earliest lesion appears as eccentric osteolytic lesion in the shaft near the epiphysis or metaphysis. Epiphyseal growth plate offers little resistance resulting in transphyseal spread of infections.

Two types of lesions are described. *Caseous exudative type*, in which there is destruction of bony trabeculae, softening and caseation necrosis followed by formation of tuberculous pus or cold abscess and *granular type caries sicca*, where predominantly granulation tissue is formed with minimal caseation.

Tuberculosis of Long Bones

Two varieties of long bone TB occur:

1. Metaphyseal type, in which oval or round focus in metaphysis ultimately crosses into the epiphysis and further to involve the joint. Femur and tibia being the most commonly affected bones.
2. Cystic (diaphyseal type) generally affecting children and young adults. There is presence of well-defined round or oval lytic areas involving and expanding the diaphysis. Large sequestra may be seen in diaphysis, due to thrombosis of intraosseous vasculature in children. Tibia is the most common bone involved. Joint involvement is infrequent. Solitary involvement is predominant although multifocal involvement can occur. Multiple cystic diaphyseal lesions can occur rarely. The condition is symmetrical in distribution, with simultaneous onset, progression, and regression. Multifocal tuberculous osteomyelitis also known as *osteitis cystica tuberculosa multiplex.*[25]

Multiple sites of involvement are seen in children, while in adults, involvement is more often confined to a single bone. The earliest lesion appears as an eccentric area of osteolysis in the metaphysis. Little or no surrounding reactive bone and local osteopenia are salient features.

The radiographic appearance may be somewhat different in children as compared to adults. In young patients, the lesions may be symmetrical and favor metaphyseal region. They are usually osteolytic and well-defined, without sclerosis, and may show variable size while in adults, the lesions are smaller, located in the long axis of bone, and may show well-defined sclerotic margins.

On MRI, early focus of altered marrow signal with irregular margins and cortical invasion with ill-defined soft tissue may be seen. Eccentric lesion with cortical breach may show irregular breach or hyperintensity within the cortical black line while small communicating abscesses are better appreciated on postcontrast T1WI as enhancing rings of juxtacortical inflammatory tissue and are a strong predictor of TB.

Flat Bones

Ribs

Rib involvement is seen in about 2% cases of bone TB, adults being generally affected. Nearly one-third of patients will have pulmonary TB or TB at other sites. Patient may present with pain, tenderness, and fluctuant chest wall swelling. There is bony rib expansion with punched out lesions and destruction which may be poorly marginated, posterior half of ribs being most commonly affected **(Fig. 21)**. Associated extrapleural soft tissue abscesses presenting as cold abscesses are commonly seen. The abscess may present as chest wall discharging sinus.[5,7]

Scapula

Scapula is a rare site for tubercular infection. The infective focus may be present in acromion, spine, neck, superior or inferior angle of scapula. The patient can present with pain and swelling around scapula. CT and MRI are helpful in early detection of lesions.[23,24]

Sternum

Sternum is involved in about one and a half percent of cases. An irregular destructive lesion along with presence of retrosternal and presternal soft tissue mass may be seen. There is paucity of sclerosis or periostitis.[24]

Skull

Frontal bone is the most common site to be involved in bones of cranial vault. Ill-defined lytic lesion may be the only radiological feature seen, with overlying cold abscess

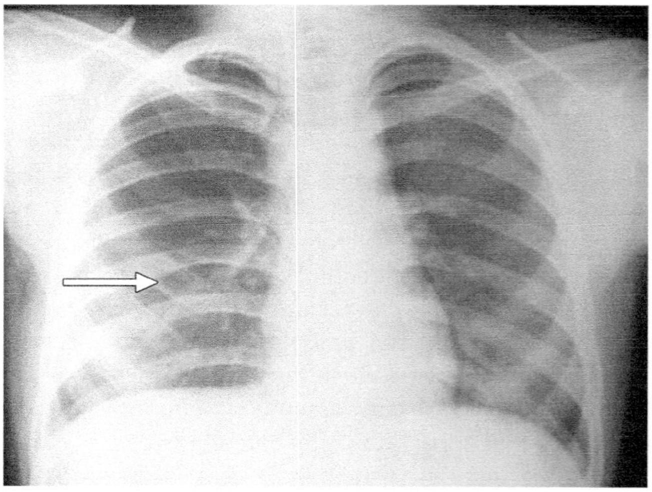

Fig. 21: Plain X-ray of chest showing lytic lesion involving anterior end of right 3rd rib in a case of rib tuberculosis.

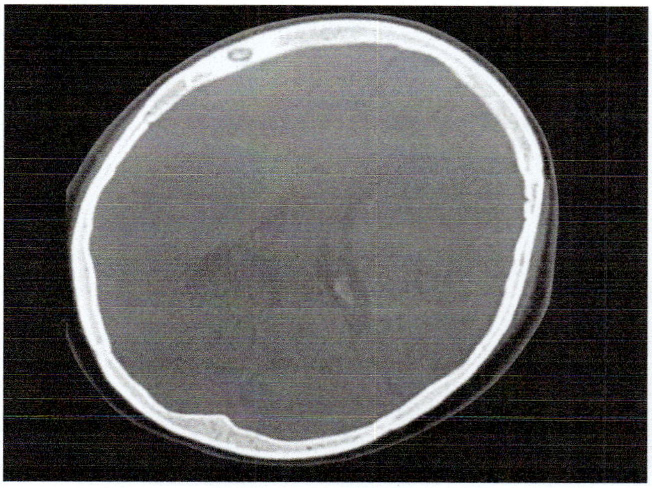

Fig. 22: Plain CT scan of cranium showing button sequestrum in the right parietal bone.

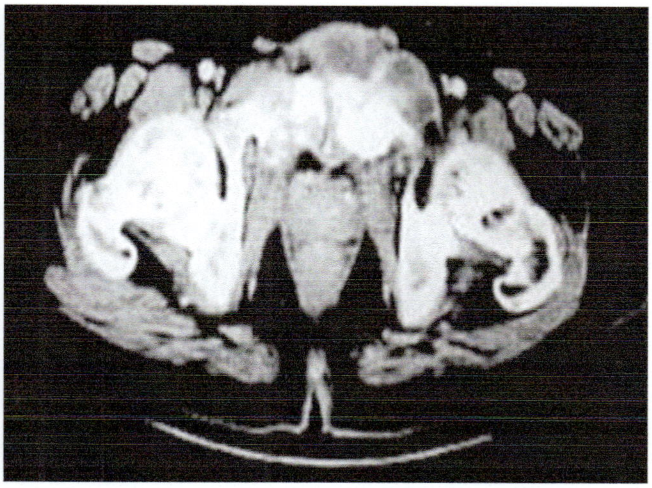

Fig. 23: Axial CT scan showing bilateral pubic bone erosions with subcutaneous small cold abscess.

(Pott's puffy tumor). Button sequestrum can also be sometimes seen **(Fig. 22)**. Facial bones and mandibular involvement is extremely rare.[8,9]

Pelvis

Isolated tubercular lesion may occur in iliac bone, ischial tuberosity, and ischiopubic ramus. Radiologically, lytic lesions without surrounding sclerosis or periosteal reaction may be seen. Infection may extend to involve pubic symphysis **(Fig. 23)**.

Sternoclavicular Joint

Tuberculosis of the sternoclavicular joint is rare. It is usually seen in the region of medial end and presents with a painful swelling. Cold abscess and sinus can result as a complication. MRI can be a useful modality to detect early erosions and associated soft tissue swelling. Biopsy may be necessary in doubtful cases. Differential diagnosis includes rheumatoid arthritis, multiple myeloma, metastasis, and low-grade pyogenic infections.[11,14,24]

Acromioclavicular Joint

Tuberculosis of the acromioclavicular joint is also rare. It is usually seen in the region of lateral end of clavicle and presents with a painful swelling.[24] Clavicle may rarely be involved without involvement of adjoining joints. There may be diffuse thickening and honeycombing, multiple cystic cavities, and sequestra formation such as pyogenic infections. Biopsy may be necessary to confirm the diagnosis.

TUBERCULOSIS OF SHORT BONES

Tuberculosis of short tubular bones is referred to as tubercular dactylitis. It is primarily a disease of childhood. The disease primarily affects short tubular bones of hands and feet.

Hand bones are more commonly affected than bones of feet. Proximal phalanges of 2nd and 3rd fingers and metacarpals of 3rd and 4th fingers are frequently involved in tubercular dactylitis.

Clinical features include soft tissue swelling, which may be followed by pain and numbness. Swelling due to abscess formation may occur. There is usually no fever or other signs of inflammation. Boyer and Nelaton first described tubercular dactylitis. The short tubular bones show cystic expansion as if with air and the condition has been characteristically described as "spina ventosa", spina meaning short bone and ventosa meaning expanded with air.[23]

Initial bony lesion is in the marrow. The disease is characterized by bone destruction and fusiform expansion of the bone, often accompanied by soft tissue swelling. It is more marked in diaphysis of metacarpals and metatarsals in children. Periosteal reaction and sequestra are uncommon. Healing is gradual by sclerosis.[24]

Magnetic resonance imaging may demonstrate intraosseous involvement earlier than with other imaging modalities **(Figs. 24A and B)**.

This condition needs to be differentiated from syphilitic dactylitis, in which there is bilateral and symmetric involvement, more periostitis, less soft tissue swelling and less sequestrations and from pyogenic osteomyelitis in which there is marked periostitis. The differential diagnosis also includes sarcoidosis, hemoglobinopathies, and hyperparathyroidism.[24]

Tuberculosis of Tendon Sheaths and Bursae

While TB can involve any bursa or tendon sheath, the tendon sheaths of hand and wrist and trochanteric bursa are commonly involved.[25]

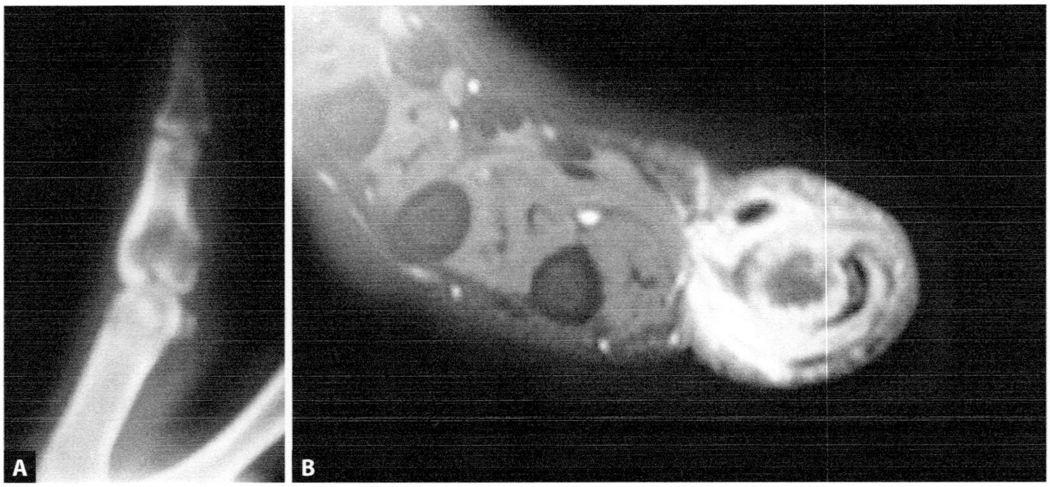

Figs. 24A and B: (A) Plain X-ray of right thumb showing cystic expansile lesion of the proximal shaft of proximal phalanx of right thumb with pathological fracture; (B) MRI of the same patient showing bone marrow inflammation along with marked enhancing synovium on postgadolinium images, in a biopsy proven case of tuberculosis.

Primary investigation to confirm the diagnosis of tenosynovitis and to reveal the degree and extent of tendon and tendon sheath involvement is ultrasonography. Sonograms can be quickly obtained along virtually any orientation and very high-frequency transducers provide exquisite spatial and contrast resolution.

In chronic tenosynovitis, tendon and synovial thickening predominate with relatively little synovial sheath effusion, while in acute suppurative tenosynovitis, synovial sheath effusion is the predominant feature.[25]

Magnetic resonance imaging helps in delineating the precise extent of soft tissue involvement and any associated osseous or joint involvement. Three stages of tuberculous tenosynovitis have been described:

1. The *hygromatous stage* is characterized by the presence of fluid inside the tendon sheath without associated sheath thickening.
2. The *serofibrinous stage* is characterized by thickening of the flexor tendons and synovium, with multiple tiny hypointense nodules within the hyperintense synovial fluid on T2WI. These tiny nodules correspond to the *rice* bodies.
3. The *fungoid stage* is characterized by a soft tissue mass involving the tendon and tendon sheath. Among bursal infections, the most commonly affected locations are trochanteric, subacromial, subgluteal, and radioulnar wrist bursa. Plain radiography may demonstrate local osteopenia due to hyperemia in long-standing bursitis or focal osteolytic bone destruction (e.g., greater trochanter or the humeral head) due to local pressure of the enlarged bursa. The wall of the distended bursa may contain calcifications, which may be visible on radiographs.[8,25] On MRI, two patterns of involvement have been reported. A uniform distension of the bursa or multiple small abscesses in the bursa may be seen or low-signal intensity material within the fluid-filled bursa on T2WI may be seen due to the presence of caseous necrosis and fibrotic material.

Atypical Mycobacterial Infection

Infections due to atypical mycobacteria are also seen in specific clinical setting. Skin and pulmonary disease are most frequent, however, skeletal changes may also be noted. The infection may be seen in immunocompromised patients, those with renal transplants or those receiving corticosteroids. Infection can lead to osteomyelitis, septic arthritis, tenosynovitis, and bursitis.[20,23,25]

Radiologically, multiple lesions may be seen, metaphysis and diaphysis of long bones being usually affected. Discrete lesions may be present with sclerotic margins but osteoporosis is not marked. Abscesses and sinus tract can also be seen.

Tubercular Infection of Prosthetic Joint

Prosthetic joint infection may develop, due to reactivation of tubercular arthritis for which the operation had been performed.[26] Arthrocentesis and specimens are required for establishing the diagnosis.

CONCLUSION

It is difficult to diagnose the disease in its earliest stage as the clinical and radiologic findings are nonspecific in initial stages. We should have a high level of clinical suspicion, as the disease is endemic in our country. At this stage, cross-sectional imaging and histological examination can lead to correct diagnosis. In advanced cases, diagnosis is not much of a problem and imaging helps in supplementing and guiding therapeutic procedures.

REFERENCES

1. Yochum TR, Row LJ. Infection: non-suppurative osteomyelitis (tuberculosis). Essentials of Skeletal Radiology, 2nd edition. Philadelphia: Lippincott Williams and Wilkins; 1996.
2. Moore SL, Rafii M. Imaging of musculoskeletal and spinal tuberculosis. Radiol Clin North Am. 2001;39(2):329-42.
3. Bhan S, Nag HL. Skeletal tuberculosis. In: Sharma SK (Ed). Tuberculosis, 2nd edition. New Delhi: Jaypee Brothers Medical Publishers (P) Ltd; 2009. pp. 342-72.
4. Sawlani V, Chandra T, Mishra RN, Aggarwal A, Jain UK, Gujral RB. MRI features of tuberculosis of peripheral joints. Clin Radiol. 2003;58(10):755-62.
5. Grainger and Allison's Diagnostic Radiology: A Textbook of Medical Imaging, 4th edition. UK: Churchill Livingstone; 2005. pp. 2069-70.
6. Greenspan A. Orthopedic Imaging: A Practical Approach, 4th edition. Philadelphia: Lippincott Williams and Wilkins; 2004. pp. 798-9.
7. Tuli SM. Tuberculosis of the Skeletal System. New Delhi: Jaypee Brothers Medical Publishers (P) Ltd; 1997.
8. Sutton D. Textbook of Radiology and Imaging, 7th edition. UK: Churchill Livingstone; 2003. pp. 1166-71.
9. Resnik D, Kransdorf MJ. Bone and Joint Imaging, 3rd edition. Philadelphia: Elsevier Saunders; 2005. pp. 758-65.
10. Riddley N, Shaikh MI, Remedios D, Mitchell R. Radiology of skeletal tuberculosis. Orthopedics. 1998;21(11):1213-20.
11. Ebnezar J. Textbook of Orthopedics, 3rd edition. New Delhi: Jaypee Brothers Medical Publishers (P) Ltd; 2006. pp. 499-519.
12. Morris BS, Varma R, Garg A, Awasthi M, Maheshwari M. Multifocal musculoskeletal tuberculosis in children: appearances on computed tomography. Skeletal Radiol. 2002;31(1):1-8.
13. Yago Y, Yukihiro M, Kuroki H, Katsuragawa Y, Kubota K. Cold tubercular abscess identified by FDG PET. Ann Nucl Med. 2005;19(6):515-8.
14. Griffth JF, Kumta SM, Leung PC, Cheng JC, Chow LT, Metrewell C. Imaging of musculoskeletal tuberculosis: a new look at old disease. Clin Orthop Relat Res. 2002;398:32-9.
15. Babhulkar SS, Pande S. Tuberculosis of the hip. Clin Orthop Relat Res. 2002;398:93-9.
16. Shanmugasundaram TK. A clinicoradiological classification of tuberculosis of hip. Current Concepts in Bone Joint Tuberculosis. Madras: International Bone and Joint Club; 1983.
17. Hoffman EB, Allin J, Campbell JA, Leisegang FM. Tuberculosis of the knee. Clin Orthop Relat Res. 2002;398: 100-6.
18. Lee AS, Campbell JA, Hoffman EB. Tuberculosis of the knee in children. J Bone Joint Surg Br. 1995;77(2):313-8.
19. Dhillon MS, Nagi ON. Tuberculosis of the foot and ankle. Clin Orthop Relat Res. 2002;398:107-13.
20. Singh NV. Fundamental of Orthopedics, 1st edition. New Delhi: New Age International (P) Ltd; 2011. pp. 236-44.
21. Malaviya AN, Kotwal PP. Arthritis associated with tuberculosis. Best Pract Res Clin Rheumatol. 2003;17(2): 319-43.
22. Gardam M, Lim S. Mycobacterial osteomyelitis and arthritis. Infect Dis Clin North Am. 2005;19(4):819-30.
23. Harisinghani GM, McLoud TC, Shepard JO, Ko JP, Shroff MM, Mueller PR. Tuberculosis from head to toe. Radiographics. 2000;20(2):449-70.
24. Babhulkar SS, Pande SK. Unusual manifestations of osteoarticular tuberculosis. Clin Orthop Relat Res. 2002;398:114-20.
25. Boutin RD, Brossmann J, Sartoris DJ, Reilly D, Resnick D. Update on imaging of orthopedic infections. Orthop Clin North Am. 1998;29(1):41-65.
26. Kaya M, Nagoya S, Yamashita, Niiro N, Fujita M. Periprosthetic infection of the hip in a patient with no previous history of tuberculosis. J Bone Joint Surg Br. 2006;88(3):394-5.

CHAPTER 5

Nontubercular Bone and Joint Infections

Anindita Sinha, Manphool Singhal, Kushaljit Singh Sodhi

INTRODUCTION

Osteomyelitis refers to the infection of cortical bone and its marrow space. It is classified into three forms: (1) acute, (2) subacute, and (3) chronic. Subacute osteomyelitis is insidious in presentation as compared to the acute form. Chronic osteomyelitis is a continuous low-grade recurring infection. The pathogens causing osteomyelitis can be bacteria, viruses, mycobacteria or treponemes (syphilis). Pyogenic osteomyelitis is the most common.[1,2] Plain radiographs, scintigraphy, ultrasonography (USG), computed tomography (CT), and magnetic resonance imaging (MRI), all play an important role in the diagnosis of osteomyelitis, but overall diagnostic accuracy does not exceed more than 80–90%.[3] Presence of previous or chronic osteomyelitis, adjoining soft tissue infection, fracture, surgery, and prosthesis are the factors which make the diagnosis difficult.

IMAGING MODALITIES

Plain radiographs are the first imaging study asked for in the workup of osteomyelitis. If cortical irregularity, periosteal reaction, deep soft tissue swelling, and demineralization are detected, additional imaging may not be required to diagnose osteomyelitis.[3] However, only 5% of radiographs are positive in the early course of disease. Less than one-third reveal abnormality by 1 week while 90% are positive only by 3–4 weeks.[4] This delay constrains the utility of plain radiographs in the early diagnosis of osteomyelitis.

Computed tomography offers advantages over conventional radiographs in terms of early detection of bony changes, better visualization of axial skeletal involvement (e.g., spine, pelvis, sternum) and better delineation of overlapping bony abnormalities like thick periosteal reaction or sequestra in chronic osteomyelitis.

Radionuclide scintigraphy is the most sensitive investigation available for diagnosing acute osteomyelitis though the specificity is not as good.[3] 99mTc-labeled methylene diphosphonate (99mTc-MDP), 99mTc-hydroxymethylene diphosphonate (99mTc-HMDP), and gallium-67 (^{67}Ga) citrate are the most commonly used radionuclide agents. The sensitivity and specificity for combined 99mTc ^{67}Ga scanning are 50% and 78%, respectively.[5] Indium-111-labeled white blood cell (leukocyte) scanning (^{111}In WBC) has a higher sensitivity and specificity of 83% and 94%, respectively. Recently introduced Indium-111-labeled polyclonal immunoglobulin (IgG) has the highest sensitivity and specificity of 92% and 95–100%, respectively.[6,7] False negatives occur due to ischemic bone with no isotope uptake.[8] High-resolution USG is being increasingly used for diagnosis of acute osteomyelitis. Positive findings can be detected much earlier than on plain radiographs. Deep soft tissue swelling is the earliest sign which can be detected within 2–3 days of onset. The other changes include periosteal elevation seen as a hyperechoic line and subperiosteal fluid collection **(Fig. 1)**. Cortical breach is seen as a focal defect in the cortex.[9] In a prospective study of 25 patients done to assess the role of ultrasound in acute osteomyelitis, the authors found the presence of deep soft tissue swelling, periosseous fluid **(Fig. 2)**, and periosteal elevation has positive predictive value of 100% in first 3 days after the onset of symptoms.[10]

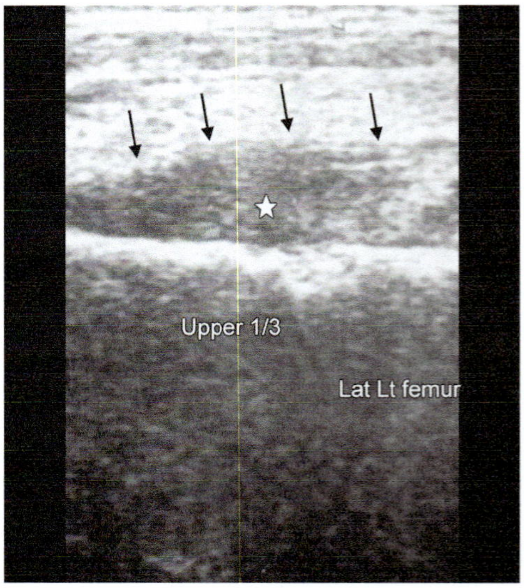

Fig. 1: Acute osteomyelitis. High-resolution ultrasonography (USG) of femur shows periosteal elevation (arrows) (hyperechoic line) with subperiosteal fluid collection (star).

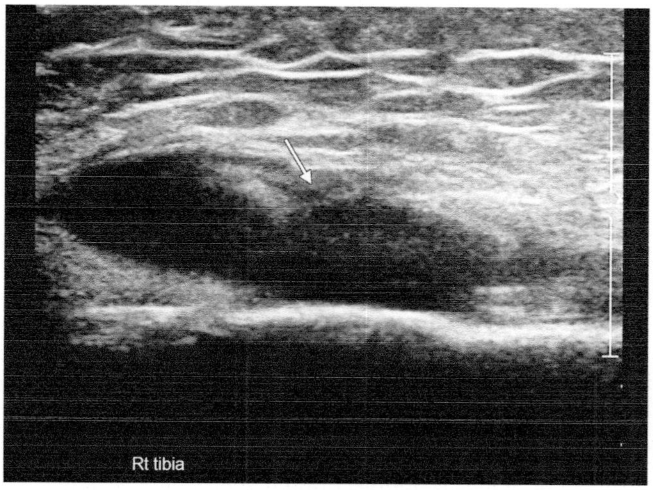

Fig. 2: High-resolution ultrasonography (USG) of tibia shows extraosseous fluid collection in a boy with acute osteomyelitis (arrow).

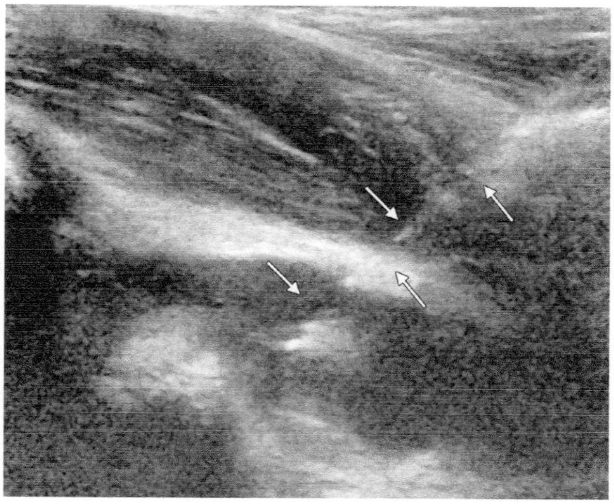

Fig. 3: USG-guided percutaneous aspiration of periosteal fluid. Note the needle in situ (arrows).

Ultrasonography is also an excellent method to detect presence of fluid in the joint which may be an indirect sign to suggest osteomyelitis especially of femur and humerus in an infant. In reactivation of chronic osteomyelitis, USG can demonstrate abscess or sinus tract formation in soft tissues which are characteristic of acute osteomyelitis. USG guidance can also be used for percutaneous aspiration of fluid from the joint or periosteal collection for diagnostic purposes **(Fig. 3)**.

Magnetic resonance imaging due to its multiplanar imaging capability, excellent tissue characterization and high-resolution is now the imaging modality of choice for the early diagnosis of osteomyelitis and overlying soft tissue involvement.[11] It has a sensitivity and specificity of 92–100% and 89–100%, respectively.[12] MRI is better than scintigraphy in evaluation of axial skeletal osteomyelitis because of better anatomical delineation.[13] In addition, MRI can distinguish soft tissue infection with periostitis from osteomyelitis.[14] Moreover, the complications of osteomyelitis like soft tissue and bone abscesses, physeal involvement, and septic arthritis can also be diagnosed which can help in further management such as determining the need for percutaneous or surgical drainage in addition to antibiotic therapy.[15-17]

ACUTE OSTEOMYELITIS

Acute osteomyelitis is usually hematogenous in origin and generally follows skin infection. *Staphylococcus aureus* is the most common offending pathogen. Common age of presentation is 2–16 years with a male preponderance, the latter being attributed to greater exposure to trauma.

Clinical Features

Patients present with local or systemic symptoms with local tenderness, swelling, restriction of motion, fever, irritability, and poor feeding (in infants).

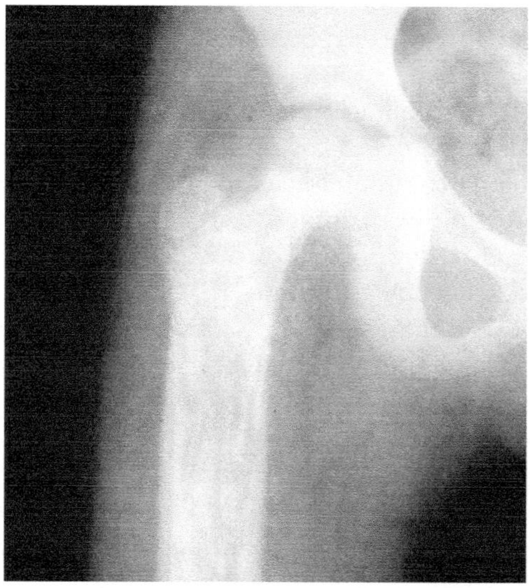

Fig. 4: Chronic osteomyelitis in a child. Radiograph of the right hip showing diffuse ill-defined lytic areas affecting the entire upper shaft of femur with cortical thickening. Note the sparing of epiphysis and the joint.

Pathophysiology of osteomyelitis varies in infants, children and adults, being related to the structural and vascular differences of bone at these ages. The blood-borne microbial emboli lodge in the metaphysis because of sluggish blood flow in this region. In children older than 1 year, the epiphyseal plate blocks extension of the infection **(Fig. 4)**, so the infection spreads laterally into the subperiosteal space or to the joint in which synovial reflections extend beyond the epiphysis to metaphysis, such as the shoulder and hip joints. In infants, small capillaries cross the epiphyseal growth plate and thus permit extension of infection to the epiphysis and the joint. In adults, the epiphyseal plate is fused and no longer forms a barrier to the spread of infection from metaphysis to the adjacent joint. Thus, acute pyogenic arthritis is a frequent complication of osteomyelitis in infants and adults **(Fig. 5)**.

The infarcted bone is reabsorbed by formation of granulation tissue and the dead cortex usually forms sequestrum. Reparative new bone formation starts roughly 10 days after the onset of infection and new bone is generally laid down along both periosteal and endosteal surfaces resulting in formation of involucrum. Cloacae appear at the site of dead periosteum.

Neonatal osteomyelitis presents with few clinical signs despite multiple sites of involvement, and hence, a complete skeletal survey is warranted in such cases.[18] Premature infants requiring umbilical catheterization are at higher risk for osteomyelitis.[19] Radionuclide bone scintigraphy is advocated in all patients with suspected neonatal osteomyelitis, following initial radiographs.[20]

A soft tissue component, subperiosteal abscess and dense involucrum are more striking in infants than in adults and children. This has been attributed to less rigid bone of infants and easy penetration of periosteum by the abscess.

In adults, direct inoculation from penetrating injury, surgery or adjacent soft tissue infection and periprosthetic infections are common causes of osteomyelitis.[21]

Immunocompromised patients with diabetes mellitus, human immunodeficiency virus/acquired immunodeficiency syndrome (HIV/AIDS), malnutrition, renal or liver failure are prone to developing osteomyelitis. Local factors like lymphedema, vascular stasis, and radiation also predispose to developing osteomyelitis.

Organisms: Bacterial—*Staphylococcus aureus* is the most common organism involved in hematogenous infection or direct inoculation, with methicillin-resistant *S. aureus* being a common pathogen, which is hard to treat. *Pseudomonas*, *Klebsiella* osteomyelitis occur in intravenous (IV) drug users.[22] Fungal osteomyelitis is common in immunocompromised patients.

Radiologic Features

Radiographs

The earliest radiographic changes are seen 7–14 days after onset of infection in the form of soft tissue swelling and small single or multiple osteolytic areas affecting the metaphysis **(Fig. 6)**. Extrusion of infected contents from the medullary cavity due to increased intramedullary pressure, through cortical bone into the subperiosteal space, which is loose in children causes a subperiosteal abscess formation and elevation of the periosteum.[22]

The periosteal reaction is typically lamellar and nodular and layered new bone formation after 3–6 weeks.[2] The dead bone (sequestrum) also forms at 3–8 weeks. It appears dense since it does not participate in normal bone mineral metabolism because of loss of its vascular supply. Osteopenia in the surrounding bone due to hyperemia enhances the density of the sequestrum. Once the acute phase has subsided, remodeling reverts the appearance of bone to normal in infants and children but in adults the sclerosis and cortical irregularity persist.

Patients with sickle cell disease have an unusual propensity for *Salmonella* osteomyelitis. This infection is diaphyseal and difficult to differentiate from a bone infarct. Localized cortical fissuring or tunneling is a characteristic and early feature of this entity.[23]

Despite its low sensitivity in detecting early osteomyelitis, radiographs should be the primary modality of investigation. MRI with or without contrast is the next appropriate investigation. Ultrasound may also be done, especially in cases of foreign body-induced osteomyelitis.[24]

Bone Scintigraphy

The bone scintigraphy shows positive findings much earlier than plain radiographs, usually within 3 days and sometimes within 24 hours of onset of infection.

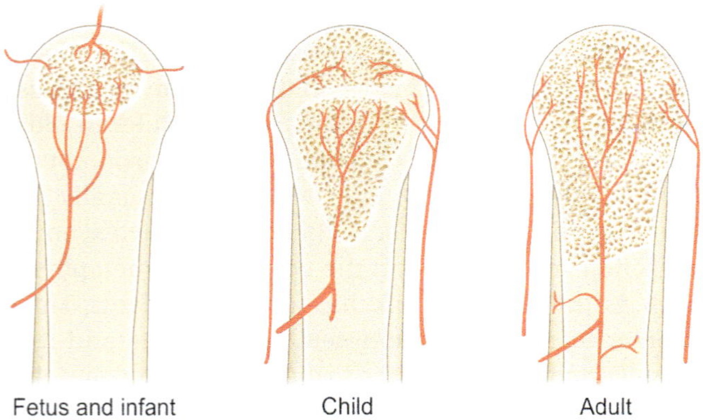

Fig. 5: Schematic diagram of vascular supply of the epimetaphyseal region in the infant, child, and adult.

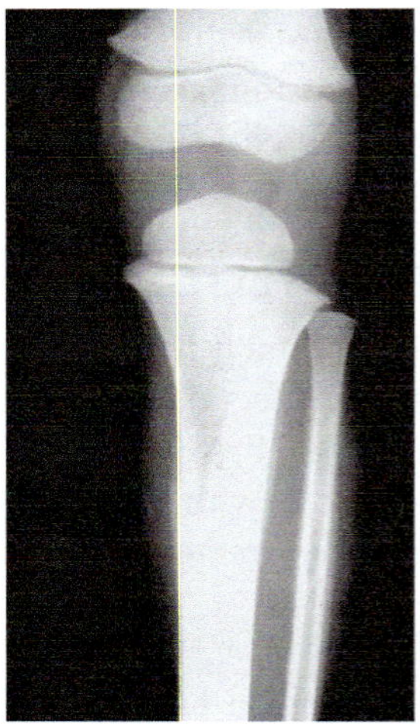

Fig. 6: Acute osteomyelitis of tibia. Radiograph of leg shows small lucencies in the metaphysis along with thin periosteal reaction.

Traditionally, "triple phase" bone scanning is done, using technetium 99mTc agents. The first phase shows the "blood flow", the second phase shows the "blood pool" of the inflamed region and the third phase, which is acquired after 2–4 hours, shows the uptake by bone. Osteomyelitis is "hot" on all phases. However, in patients presenting within 48 hours, the isotope bone scan may reveal a "cold" spot on account of vasospasm. A false-positive result can occur in degenerative disease, healing fracture, inflammatory arthritis, and loose prosthesis. But these conditions do not show increased activity in early (I and II) phases, unlike osteomyelitis. Deep soft tissue infection with periostitis and diabetic osteopathy also cannot be differentiated from osteomyelitis on the basis of bone scanning alone.[3] MRI is considered superior to bone scan in distinguishing these two entities.

Magnetic Resonance Imaging

Magnetic resonance imaging is the modality of choice for early diagnosis of osteomyelitis. Early diagnosis is essential to prevent chronic changes in bone with bone destruction or deformity which are irreversible. MRI shows intramedullary signal change due to bone marrow edema as early as 1 or 2 days after infection.[25]

Magnetic resonance imaging features of acute osteomyelitis include low signal intensity due to pus or edema partially or fully replacing marrow signal on T1-weighted (T1W) image and high-signal intensity on T2-weighted (T2W) and fluid-sensitive images [fat-suppressed T2W and short tau inversion recovery (STIR) sequences] with postcontrast enhancement **(Figs. 7A to C)**. Intraosseous, subperiosteal, and soft tissue abscesses if present appear as well-circumscribed areas of focally decreased signal intensity on T1W images with increased signal intensity equal to that of fluid on fluid-sensitive sequences and rim enhancement on contrast T1W images.[15,26,27]

Rim enhancement of the abscess is useful in differentiating phlegmonous tissue from abscess which needs urgent surgical or image-guided intervention.[28]

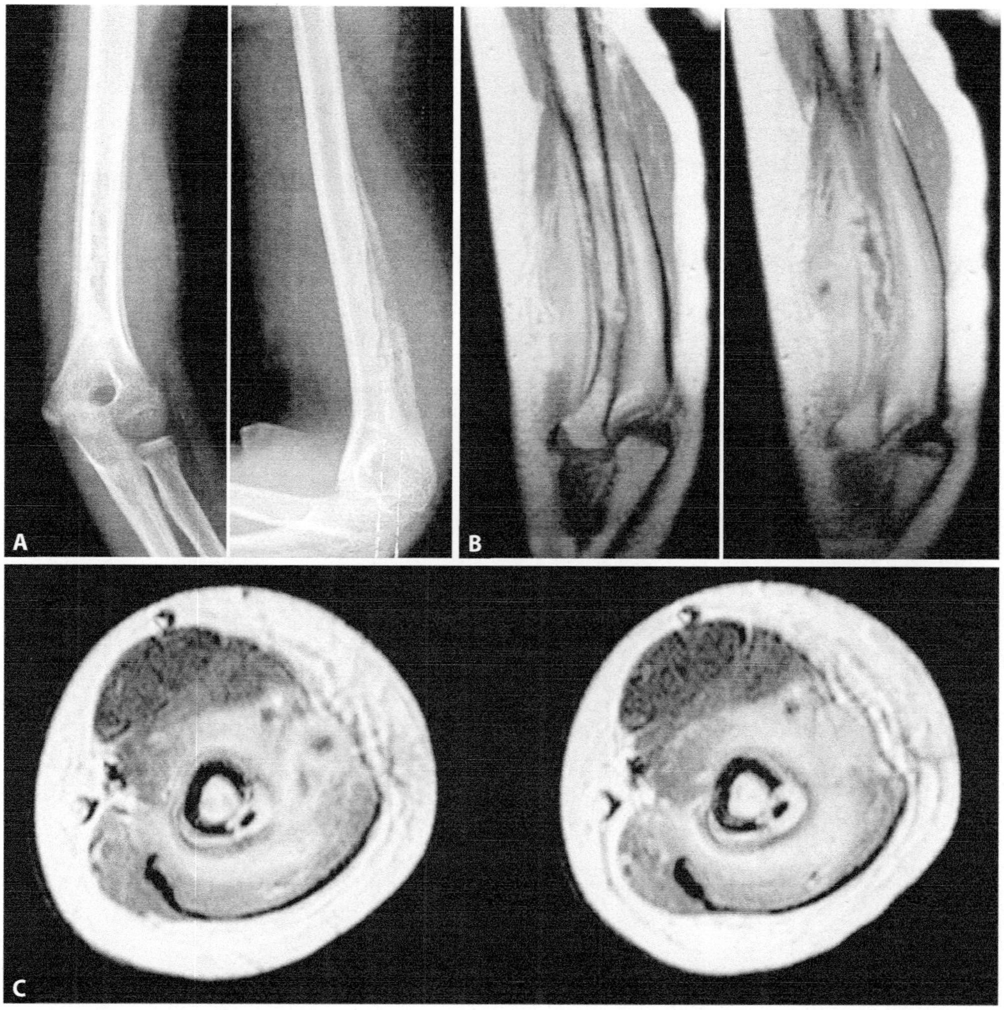

Figs. 7A to C: Acute osteomyelitis. (A) Plain X-rays show smooth periosteal reaction with cortical irregularity in the lower third of humerus; Postcontrast sagittal (B) and axial (C) MR images show cortical irregularity with break in the outline and periosseous fluid collection with increased signal in the adjacent soft tissues.

Magnetic resonance imaging has also been shown to be more sensitive and specific than isotope bone scanning in the detection, localization, and differentiation of osteomyelitis, cellulitis, and abscess. Cellulitis and osteomyelitis may have similar soft tissue changes. However, in cellulitis, the bone is normal.[29]

Differential diagnosis of osteomyelitis:[22] Tumors such as Ewing's sarcoma, leukemia, Langerhans cell histiocytosis may mimic acute osteomyelitis even on MRI. Presence of intervening interspersed intramedullary fat within the lesion, peripherally enhancing rim of soft tissue (abscess) rather than heterogeneous enhancement of tumor-associated soft tissue go in favor of osteomyelitis. Osteomyelitis also causes more rapid progressive bone destruction.

Stress fractures and osteoid osteoma can also mimic osteomyelitis. Osteoid osteoma enhances rapidly on MRI and has a rounded configuration—whereas intraosseous abscesses are irregular or oblong.

LOCALIZED OSTEOMYELITIS (BRODIE'S ABSCESS)

Localized osteomyelitis or Brodie's abscess is a limited osteomyelitis caused either by organisms of low virulence or high resistance in the host. Presentation with insidious pain is most common, which may exacerbate at night and be relieved by nonsteroidal anti-inflammatory drugs (NSAIDs) (like osteoid osteoma). It occurs most frequently at one end of the bone, but it may also occur in the diaphysis. Tibia is most commonly involved bone, followed by femur, although any bone can be affected.[30]

It is seen as a well-circumscribed osteolytic focus surrounded by a sclerotic margin **(Figs. 8A to C)**. Occasionally, a metaphyseal serpiginous channel with sclerotic border marks the tract of infection. This feature is considered characteristic of nontubercular etiology like *Staphylococcus, Streptococcus* or *Haemophilus.*[2] When the lesion is small, it may be difficult to identify on plain radiographs and CT/MRI may be required. The close differential diagnosis of Brodie's abscess is an osteoid osteoma as on imaging both these conditions closely simulate each other (T2 hyperintense nidus, sclerotic rim, and bone edema); however, on T1W MRI scans, a "penumbra sign" has been described as a central intermediate or hypointense zone of pus, a discrete rim of the abscess wall of marginally higher signal intensity than the abscess cavity, sclerosis which is hypointense, and surrounding marrow edema of lower signal intensity than fatty bone marrow, which often enhances after contrast. This has been postulated to be due to the presence of active, vascular, inflammatory granulation tissue around the abscess.[31]

Epiphyseal lesions can be mistaken for aneurysmal bone cyst or chondroblastoma.

CHRONIC OSTEOMYELITIS

Chronic bone infections usually result from inadequately treated acute osteomyelitis or from infection following compound bone fractures. Pain, local swelling, discharge

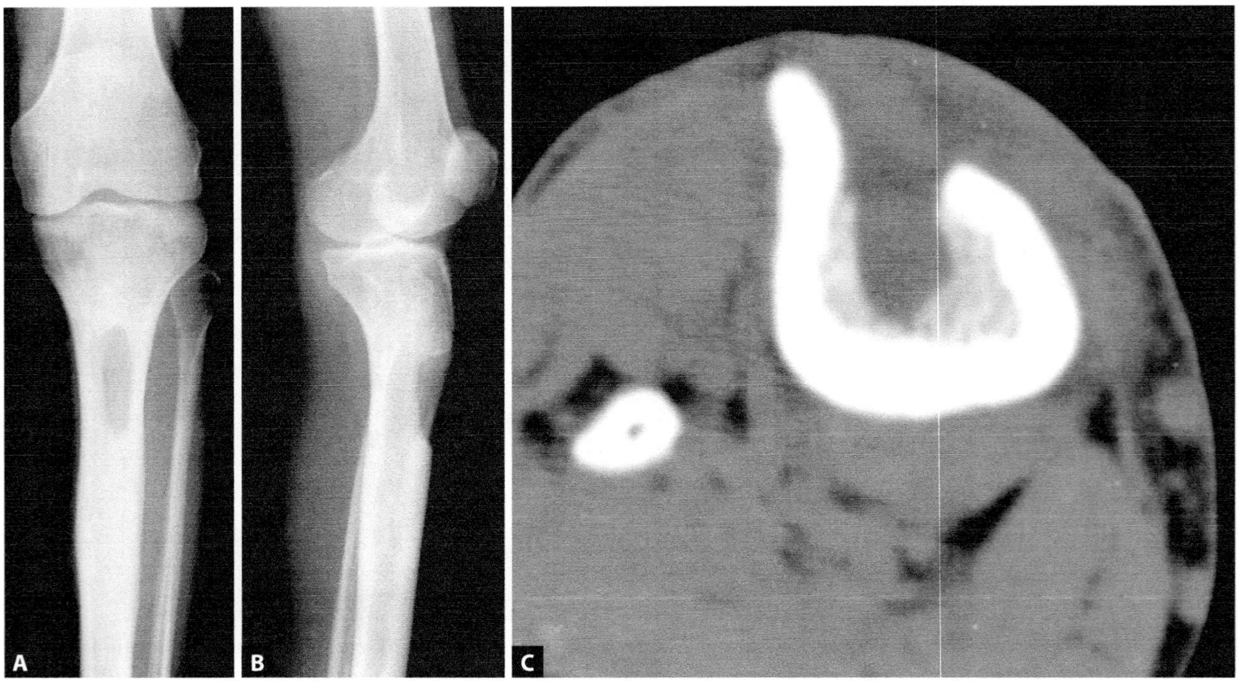

Figs. 8A to C: (A and B) Plain X-ray; and (C) Axial CT images showing Brodie's abscess in the upper end of tibia.

from wound, sinus formation, and systemic signs and symptoms (fever, malaise, nausea, and vomiting) may be present.

Conventional radiographs show cloacae, involucrum or sequestrum **(Figs. 9 and 10)**. There are sclerotic and lucent areas admixed with cortical thickening and deformities. The radiographic impression regarding the activity of infectious process is often equivocal, and one relies heavily on clinical findings such as the presence of a sinus tract.[25] At times, it is imperative to review previous films as it may be difficult to differentiate inactive and active chronic osteomyelitis. In osteomyelitis of the skull, typically no sclerosis is seen **(Figs. 11A and B)**.

Scintigraphy is more useful in determining activity. Routine 99mTc-MDP scanning shows increased uptake, but is often nondiagnostic, since even after 1–2 years following successful treatment, a positive isotope bone scan is not uncommon.[3] ^{67}Ga has been recommended as the optimal agent. Following successful treatment, ^{67}Ga uptake should decrease to a normal level.

Magnetic resonance imaging findings correspond to the pathologic features. On MR images, the involucrum

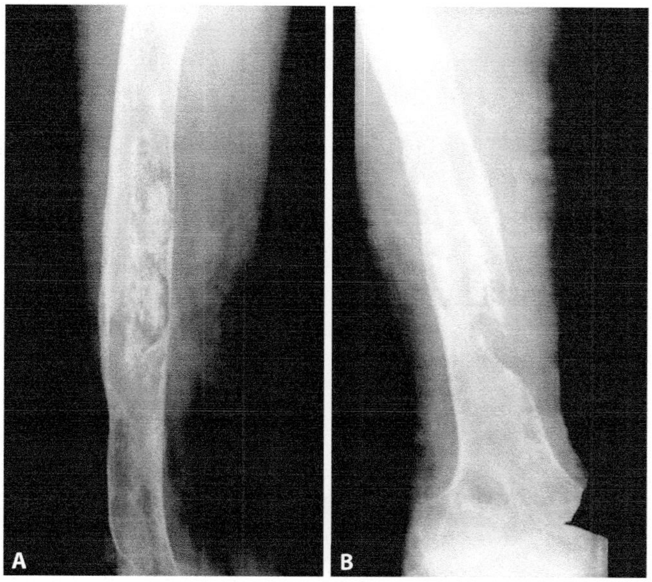

Figs. 9A and B: Chronic osteomyelitis of the femoral bone. Diaphyseal lucent areas represent cloacae formation with sequestrum seen as radiodense opacities.

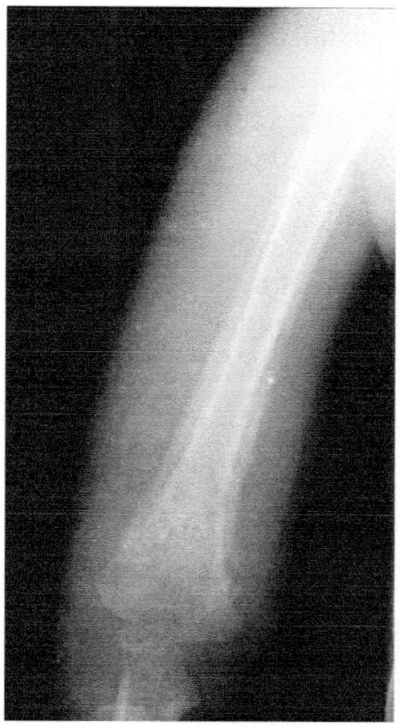

Fig. 10: Chronic osteomyelitis. Radiograph of right arm showing involucrum surrounding distal two-thirds of humerus.

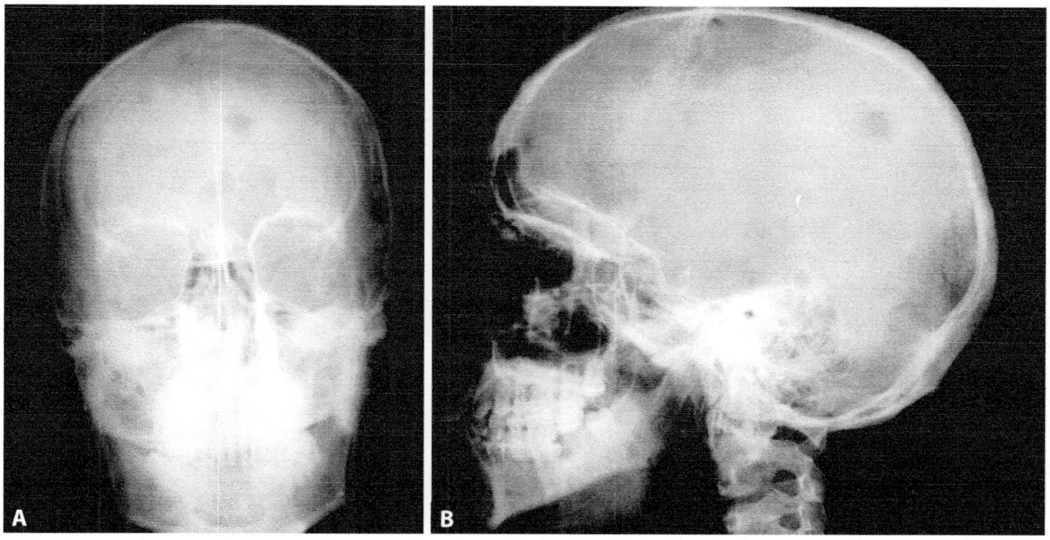

Figs. 11A and B: Chronic osteomyelitis of skull vault. Anteroposterior and lateral skull radiographs showing multiple lytic areas with no surrounding sclerosis.

manifests as a well-defined rim of low-signal intensity on all sequences surrounding the infected bone marrow.

Granulation tissue surrounding the infection appears as hypointense on T1W images, hyperintense on T2W and STIR images, and shows enhancement after gadolinium-diethylenetriamine pentaacetic acid (Gd-DTPA).

Magnetic resonance imaging has been advocated as the imaging modality to distinguish regions of active infection from uninvolved marrow or fibrotic regions representing scars from previous infection or trauma.[25] Active foci of infection tend to have a low-to-intermediate signal intensity on T1W and high-signal intensity on T2W and fluid-sensitive images which is in marked contrast to the low-signal of thickened, surrounding bone.[32,33]

However, persistent hyperintensity on T2W images may also be seen in postsurgical granulation tissue and does not necessarily imply persistent infection. Comparison with previous imaging is essential as persistent infection leads to progressive increase in intramedullary hyperintensity.[34]

Sequestrum is an isolated fragment of devitalized bone within an area of active infection shows low-signal intensity on all sequences, and does not enhance.

Sinus tract is identified as a linear or curvilinear area of low-signal on T1W and high-signal on T2W and STIR images extending in contiguity from the medullary cavity, with disruption of the cortex, to the skin.

Soft tissue inflammation is seen as bright signal on T2W and STIR images, enhancing after contrast. Sometimes soft tissue abscess may also develop **(Figs. 12A to D)**.[32,33]

SCLEROSING OSTEOMYELITIS OF GARRE

Sclerosing osteomyelitis of Garre is a rare type of chronic osteomyelitis occurring in children and young adults, presenting with insidious onset of local pain. Symptoms recur at intervals for several years and then subside gradually. There is a predilection for involvement of mandible and shafts of long bones. Radiological appearance is of intense sclerosis resulting in thickened bone **(Fig. 13)**. Areas of frank bony destruction are rare. It is distinguished from Ewing's tumor by the absence of lamellations of periosteal reaction and permeative bone destruction.

SYPHILIS OF BONE

Syphilis is caused by *Treponema pallidum* and is of three types:

1. Congenital syphilis, present at birth or in early infancy
2. Late congenital syphilis
3. Acquired syphilis

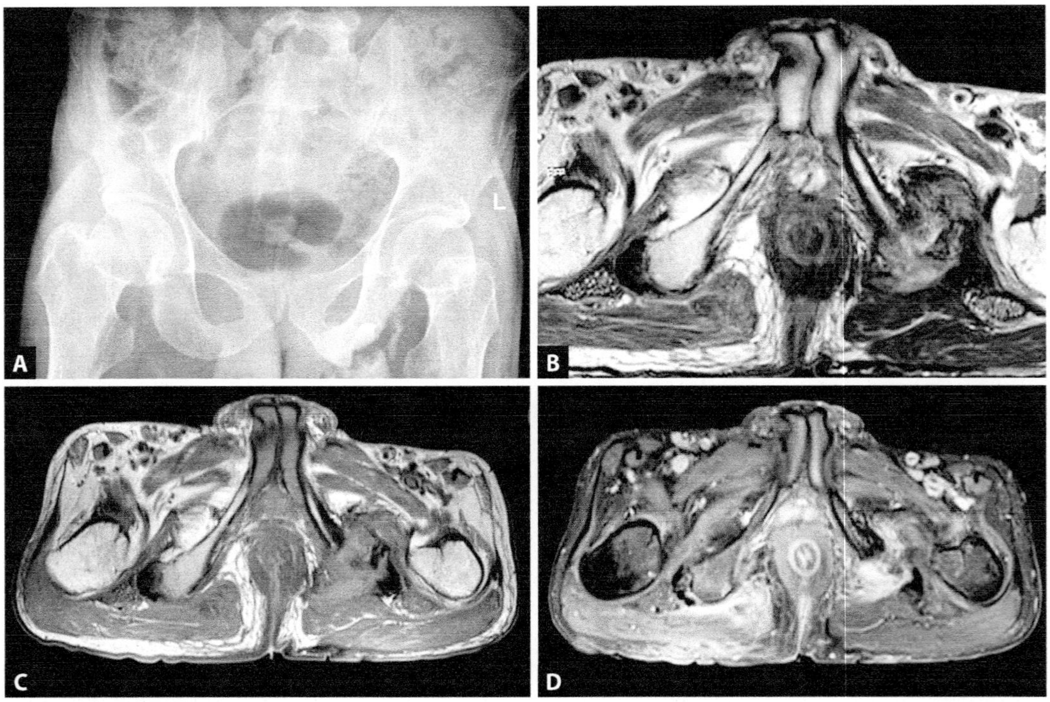

Figs. 12A to D: (A) Plain X-ray of hip joints reveals erosions along the inferior border of left ischium with sclerosis; (B) Axial T2-weighted; (C) T1-weighted; and (D) Postcontrast T1 fat-saturated MR images show a large area of lytic destruction involving the left ischium associated with a large inflammatory tissue which is of high signal on T2W and hypointense on T1W images involving the gluteal muscles. The marrow of the left ischium also shows increased signal consistent with marrow edema. Few small peripherally enhancing collections are also seen representing abscesses. The gluteal muscles on the right side also show inflammatory changes.

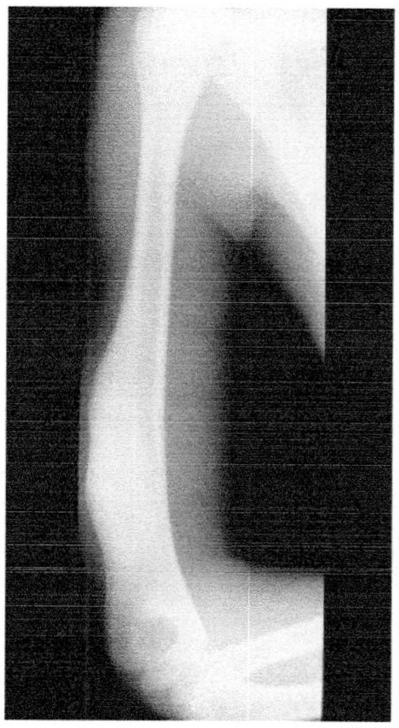

Fig. 13: Chronic sclerosing osteomyelitis of Garre. Long-standing osteomyelitis with endosteal thickening of cortex with obliteration of medullary cavity.

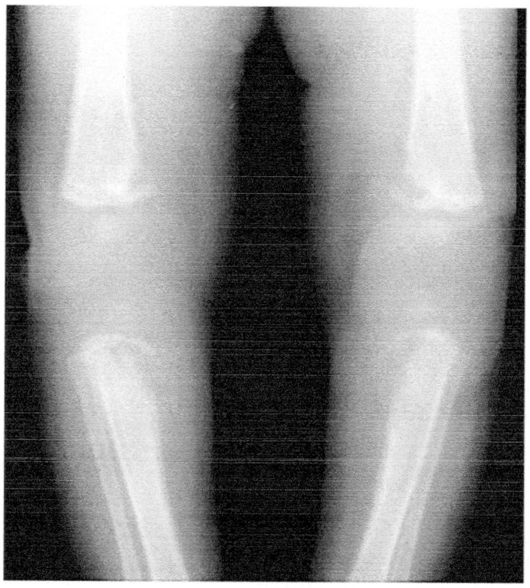

Fig. 14: Congenital syphilis. Radiograph of both knees of an infant showing symmetrical marginal destruction of medial aspect of tibia and femur in juxtaepiphyseal area and metaphyseal bands.

Congenital (Infantile) Syphilis

Congenital (infantile) syphilis is a systemic disease due to transplacental transmission of the spirochetes. Clinical features include, fever, failure to thrive, saddle nose, Hutchinson's teeth, and pseudoparalysis due to painful bone lesions, etc. Serologic diagnostic tests include the Venereal Disease Research Laboratory (VDRL), fluorescent treponemal antibody absorption (FTA-ABS) tests. Osseous abnormalities include luetic metaphysitis, diaphysitis and periostitis. Radiologically, the earliest change is in the metaphysis, with widening of the zone of provisional calcification. The epiphyseal plate appears wide and dense. The outstanding feature is symmetrical involvement of multiple bones especially at the upper end of tibia and lower end of femur. Symmetrical destruction of medial portion of the proximal tibial metaphysis (Wimberger's sign) is common and pathognomonic of syphilis. It should not be confused with Wimberger's ring sign (around an osteoporotic epiphysis in scurvy) **(Fig. 14)**.

The earliest diaphyseal change is focal cortical destruction. Later there may be extensive destruction of bone. Periosteal reaction can be solid or lamellated. In the skull, irregular, osteolytic lesions are seen.

Late Congenital Syphilis

In this condition, syphilitic bony lesions do not become evident until childhood or early adult life. The lesions are due to gumma or syphilitic endarteritis. There is minimal bone destruction which is overshadowed by extensive new bone proliferation. This results in diffuse thickening of cortical bone and lamellated periosteal reaction. This lesion causes typical thickening of the upper half of tibial cortex anteriorly and is called "Saber Tibia" **(Fig. 15)**.

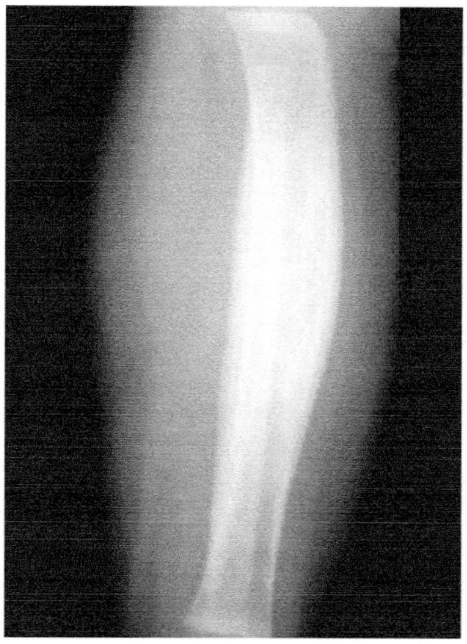

Fig. 15: Saber tibia. Extensive cortical thickening affecting the shaft of tibia which is widened.

Acquired Syphilis

Osseous changes in acquired syphilis manifest as periostitis and osteomyelitis with dense osteosclerosis. Long bones and skull are most frequently involved. The earliest change is periosteal reaction. The affected bone shows thickened cortex with narrowing of medullary canal. Gummas cause osteolytic lesion of variable size and shape. The skull shows predominantly osteolytic lesions, and outer table is more often involved.

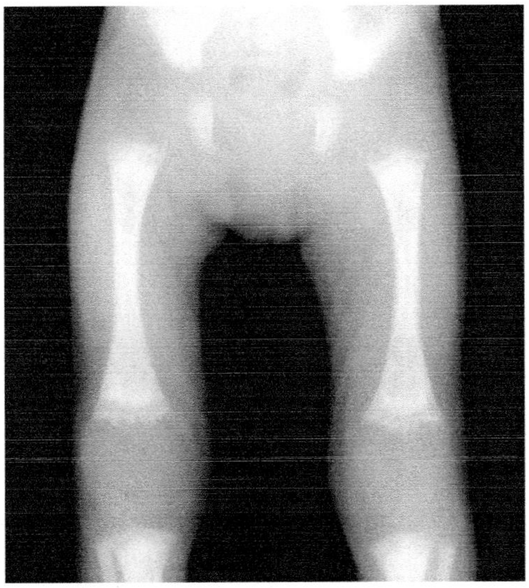

Fig. 16: Rubella. Radiograph of both lower limbs shows the typical metaphyseal bands and trabecular irregularity in metaphysis extending longitudinally. Note absence of periosteal reaction.

RUBELLA OSTEOMYELITIS

Congenital rubella infection occurs following maternal rubella in the early months of pregnancy. The characteristic radiological feature is metaphyseal lucent bands and trabecular irregularity, extending longitudinally from the epiphysis. It is seen in the upper and lower extremities, predominantly in the distal end of femur and proximal end of the tibia (celery stalk appearance) **(Fig. 16)**. Bone changes can be confused with syphilis. Absence of periosteal reaction in congenital rubella helps in differentiating from congenital syphilis.

ACTINOMYCOSIS OF BONE

It is a chronic osteomyelitis caused by gram-positive organism, *Actinomyces israelii*, which grows in colonies and appears as yellow (sulfur) granules in pus. They are common saprophytes in the gastrointestinal tract and infection occurs after a dental procedure or trauma to mouth and jaw. The most common bones involved are vertebrae/mandible, symphysis pubis, tibia, and foot bones. *Actinomyces* is also being isolated increasingly from periprosthetic joint infections.[35]

Radiologically, there is bone destruction without new bone formation. Vertebral osteomyelitis resembles tuberculosis, although discs are usually spared.[2] Ribs respond to actinomycosis by periosteal reaction and thickening, a feature which is most suggestive though, not diagnostic.

MADUROMYCOSIS

Maduromycosis is a form of chronic osteomyelitis due to granulomatous inflammation caused by a wide variety of pathogens including fungi or *Actinomyces*. The infection occurs by entry of organism through minor trauma to skin, usually foot (Madura foot). The disease is painless and presents as swelling, sinus formation and marked deformity **(Figs. 17 and 18)**.

Radiologically, periosteal reaction is the most common lesion and is usually lamellated. The disease arises primarily in soft tissues and secondarily erodes the adjoining cortex and medulla. There is little, if any, osteopenia. The disease is painless, and characteristically, the sequestrum is absent.

LEPROSY OF BONE

Leprosy is a chronic granulomatous infection caused by *Mycobacterium leprae*. In lepromatous leprosy, the disease predominantly affects the skin, mucous membranes, and the viscera. Bone involvement can rarely occur by direct lepromatous granulation tissue or by endarteritis causing bone infarcts. In tuberculoid (neural) type, there is predominant involvement of nerves which become thickened and nodular. The bone changes are secondary to neurotrophic disturbances causing recurrent trauma and infection which go unnoticed.

Radiographically, there is diffuse osteopenia and ill-defined small osteolytic areas with soft tissue swelling are seen. Periosteal reaction is rare. In later stages, erosions or resorption of phalangeal tufts are seen along with soft tissue atrophy **(Figs. 19A and B)**. Nonspecific changes including soft tissue swelling and contractures are also seen. Calcification of nerves, if observed, is classical of leprosy. Nasal septal irregularity, thinning and perforation are not well appreciated on plain radiography, but these abnormalities are very well demonstrated on CT.

DIABETIC FOOT

Infection is the primary problem requiring hospitalization of diabetic patient with foot problems often necessitating amputation. Foot problems account for as much as one-fourth of hospital admissions among diabetic patients.[36] The pathological changes are often a combination of neuropathy, vasculopathy or infection.

Conventional radiographs show osteomyelitis or neuropathic changes in the foot bones (sensitivity and specificity 75% each) **(Fig. 20)**.[37]

Scintigraphy can identify early osteopathy at a time when the conventional radiograph is normal, but its specificity is very low.[37] [111]In WBC scanning is more specific than 99mTc bone scan since it is not affected by increased bone turnover from neuropathy or fracture.[38]

Magnetic resonance imaging can visualize marrow directly and is found to have the lowest false-positive rate compared to both scintigraphy as well as plain radiography.[37]

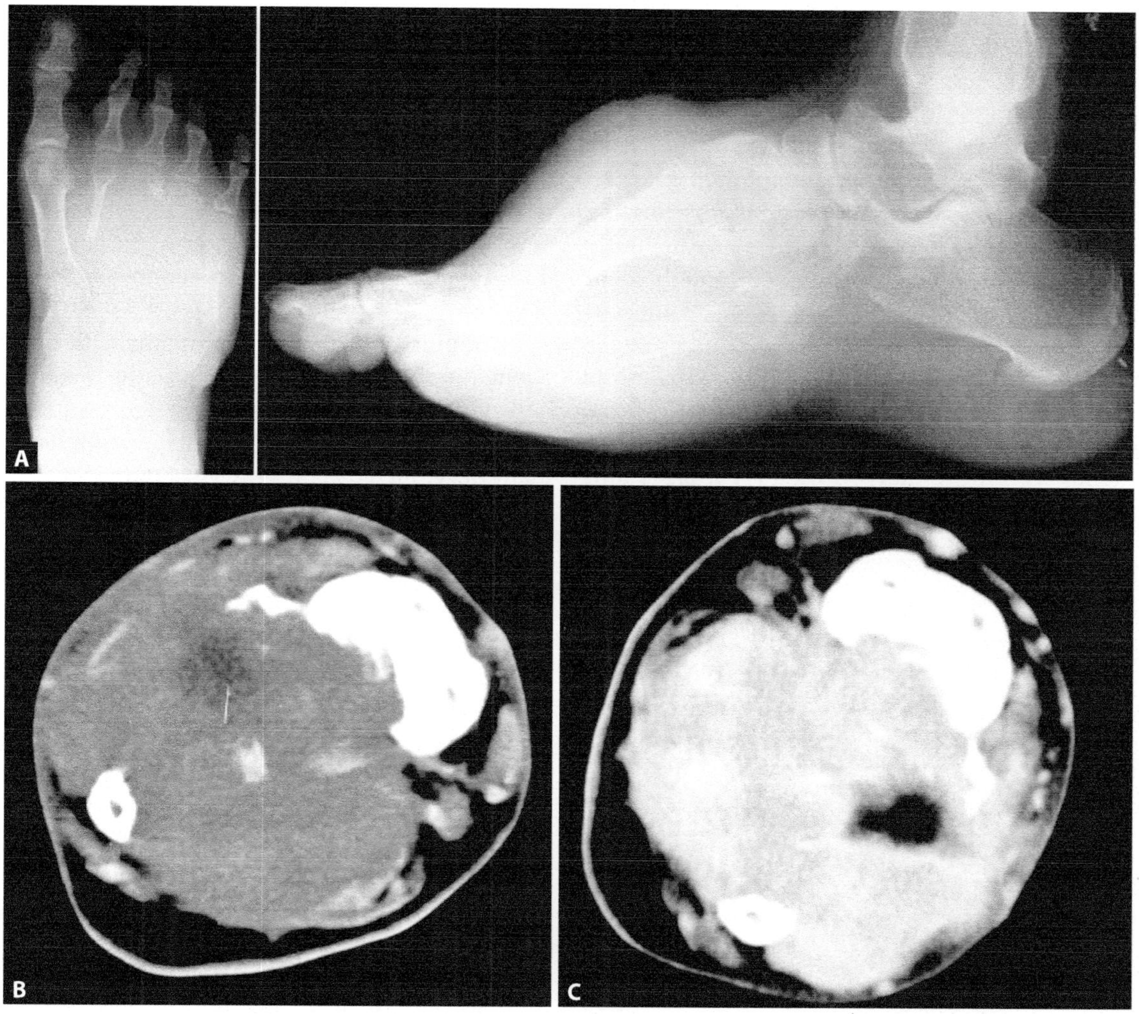

Figs. 17A to C: Maduromycosis. (A) Plain X-rays; and (B and C) Axial CT pre- and postcontrast images. There is a large soft tissue swelling in the foot with destruction of 2–4th metatarsals. On CT, an enhancing soft tissue lesion with secondary destruction of metatarsal shafts is seen.

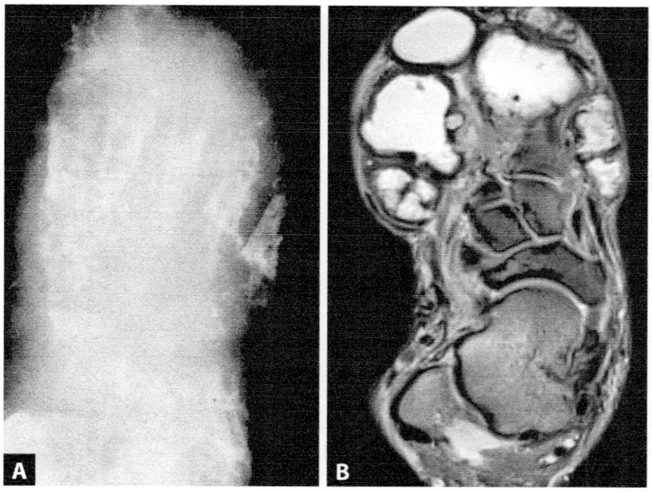

Figs. 18A and B: Maduromycosis. (A) Infiltrative destruction of the tarsal and metatarsal bones with large soft tissue component; (B) Axial proton density-weighted fat-saturated image of the foot of another patient with eumycetoma shows multiple hyperintense nodules with hypointense rim in subcutaneous tissue with a central dot-in-circle sign.

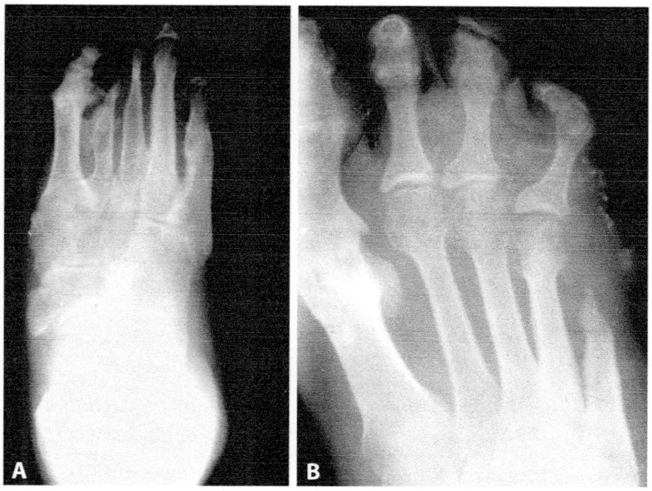

Figs. 19A and B: Leprosy. (A and B) Osteopenia with "licked candy appearance" of the metatarsals. Note the absence of the phalanges of the 5th toe (B) due to bony resorption.

Early stages of neuroarthropathy may mimic foot osteomyelitis both clinically and on imaging **(Table 1)**. In the early stages where radiography is usually normal, MRI may show soft tissue edema, fluid collections, effusions, and bone marrow abnormalities. Neuropathic changes are primarily periarticular, differentiating it from osteomyelitis which almost occurs secondary to overlying ulcer at predictable sites. Neuroarthropathy usually involves the tarsometatarsal and metatarsophalangeal joints, while calcaneum, cuboid, and malleoli are affected by osteomyelitis. However, both neuropathic changes and osteomyelitis can coexist, making imaging diagnosis difficult.

In neuroarthropathy, MRI typically shows a preserved marrow signal within the marrow on T1W images and subarticular T2 hyperintensity while rest of the bone is normal. Midfoot involvement, periarticular, subchondral or polyarticular involvement favors a neuroarthropathy over osteomyelitis.[39]

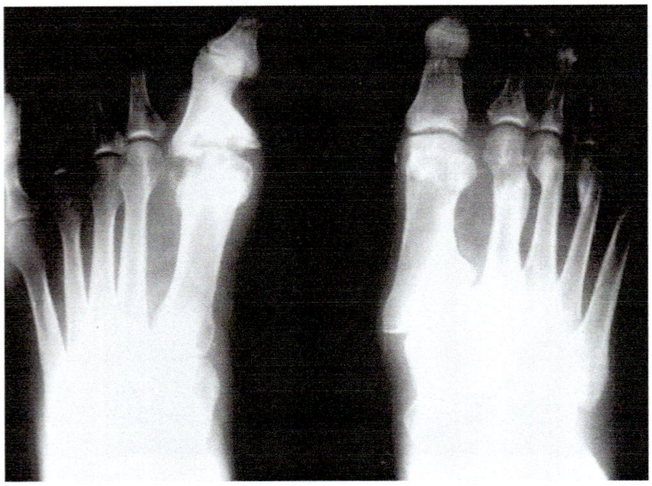

Fig. 20: Diabetic foot. There is narrowing of first metatarsophalangeal joint (right) and tarsometatarsal joint (left) with articular erosion and marked sclerosis of adjacent bone. Lucencies in soft tissues are due to air.

This finding is consistently different from early osteomyelitis where a high signal within the nonperiarticular marrow on T2W images is seen with or without changes in T1W images. Abscess, overlying ulcer, and sinus tract are diagnostic of infection; however, imaging goal is to diagnose infections early before these develop.

A trophic ulcer due to neuropathy with bone marrow edema in adjacent bone may cause diagnostic confusion between neuroarthropathy and osteomyelitis. However, 61% of such patients with marrow edema have or eventually developed osteomyelitis in a retrospective study.[40]

Concurrent infection in the adjacent soft tissues, synovium (infectious arthritis), muscles and tendons (tenosynovitis) may reveal increased signal on T2W and STIR images which may enhance on postgadolinium scans, and contrast enhancement is important to differentiate infectious myositis from changes in muscles due to ischemia or neuropathy associated denervation edema since extensive soft tissue and muscle inflammation also occur in acute Charcot neuro-osteoarthropathy (CNO)[41] **(Figs. 21A to F)**.

A sign known as the ghost sign has been described in osteomyelitis where the bones become hypointense and difficult to differentiate from surrounding muscle and inflammation on T1W images, but become prominent after contrast administration due to enhancement.[42]

Contrast should be judiciously administered since many patients have renal dysfunction and is not mandatory for diagnosis. Recent studies on dynamic postcontrast imaging have demonstrated that it can differentiate between neuroarthropathy and osteomyelitis.

Table 1: Differentiating features between osteomyelitis and neuropathic arthropathy in diabetic foot.

	Osteomyelitis	*Neuropathic arthropathy*
Distribution	Usually focal involvement	Multiple bones and joints are involved
Location	Peripheral location at weight-bearing areas, e.g., toes, metatarsal heads, calcaneus	Midfoot is predominantly involved
Associated deformity	Usually not seen. Can be ± if associated neuropathic joint	Commonly + along with destruction and debris
Soft tissue changes	Commonly overlying ulcer and draining sinus can be demonstrated	Overlying skin usually intact, edema +
Bone marrow involvement	Hyperintense on T2/STIR, hypointense on T1W image associated with postgadolinium enhancement	Acute stage—mimics osteomyelitis Chronic stage—decreased T1/T2 signal or normal marrow signal
Pattern of bone marrow edema	Usually single bone is affected with diffuse bone marrow edema	Usually periarticular and subchondral in location
Ghost sign	+	–

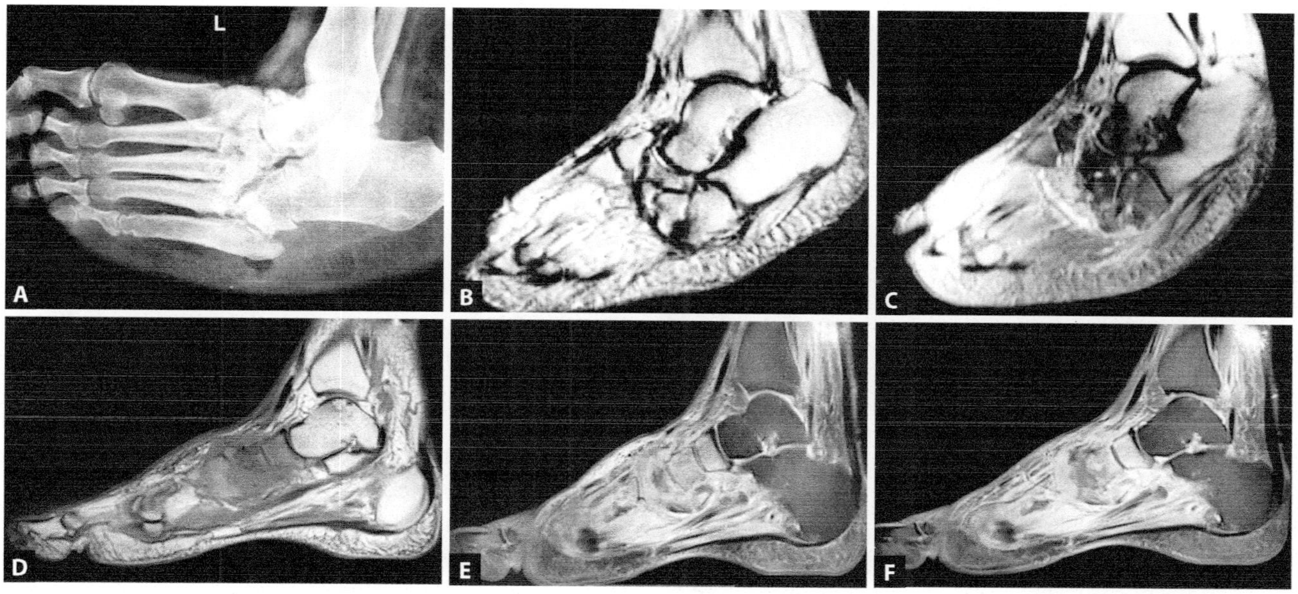

Figs. 21A to F: (A to C) Diabetic foot (Charcot's neuroarthropathy). (A) Plain radiograph of foot shows dislocation of joints of midfoot and tarsometatarsal joints and with reduced joint spaces and erosions. The bones show mixed lytic and sclerotic areas; (B) T1-weighted (T1W) MR image shows dislocated-disorganized joints of foot with markedly hypointense areas of bony sclerosis; however, marrow signal is maintained; (C) Postcontrast T1W image shows thickened enhancing synovium at tarsometatarsal joints with enhancing muscles of plantar surface; (D to F) Diabetic foot with osteomyelitis. Sagittal T1W image (D) shows hypointense tarsal bones which show osteitis (E) and intense postcontrast enhancement of bones and adjacent muscles (F).

Values of K^{trans} (volume transfer constant), K_{ep} (volume of contrast that returns to vascular compartment), and V_e (extracellular volume) are significantly higher in osteomyelitis.[43] Time-intensity curves also may be helpful in differentiating infection from neuropathic changes with rapid wash in and a steep curve in osteomyelitis.[44]

Soft tissue infection of foot occurs especially over pressure points such as metatarsals where organisms enter via superficial ulceration. Gas may be noted in infective tissues, because of gas-producing organisms such as *Escherichia coli*, without implying the presence of gangrene.

HYDATID DISEASE

Bone involvement is rare accounting for 0.5–2% cases. The most commonly involved bones are the spine, pelvis, femur, tibia, ribs, skull, scapula, humerus, and fibula.[45,46] The hydatid disease in the bone and joint begins in childhood and grows at a very slow rate and hence is seldom diagnosed in childhood. The bone offers mechanical resistance; hence cyst cannot assume its typical spherical shape and enlarges along the path of least resistance. Over the time, the trabeculae are absorbed and cortex is breached, resulting in fracture. Then, the disease spreads to surrounding structures and becomes symptomatic.

Hydatid disease should be suspected whenever cystic lesions are seen in the bone especially in the endemic areas.

The bone shows expanded medullary cavity with thinned out cortex with cortical breach or complete fracture. Typically, there is no periosteal reaction or new bone formation. On MRI, the infested bone reveals multiple cysts which exhibit medium-to-low signal on T1W images and high signal on T2W images **(Figs. 22A to D)**.[45,46]

SEPTIC ARTHRITIS

Septic arthritis is usually hematogenous in origin but may follow local trauma, joint aspiration, soft tissue infection or periarticular osteomyelitis. Arthroscopic procedures are complicated by septic arthritis in 0.04–3.4% of patients.[8] *S. aureus* is the most common invader followed by *Neisseria gonorrhoeae*, *Streptococcus*, *Haemophilus*, and anaerobic organisms.[30]

Onset of bacterial arthritis is usually abrupt with high fever, chills, and one or more severely tender swollen joints. Knee joint is most frequently affected (40–50%) followed by hip (20–25%), shoulder, wrist, elbow and ankle. Sternoclavicular, sacroiliac, and manubriosternal joints are more often involved in IV drug abusers.

Bone scan is the investigation of choice for early diagnosis of septic arthritis. Although not specific, bone scanning is very sensitive and when negative can rule out the possibility of infected joint.[9] CT demonstrates bone changes much earlier than plain films and is superior in demonstrating the extent of infection. MRI is extremely

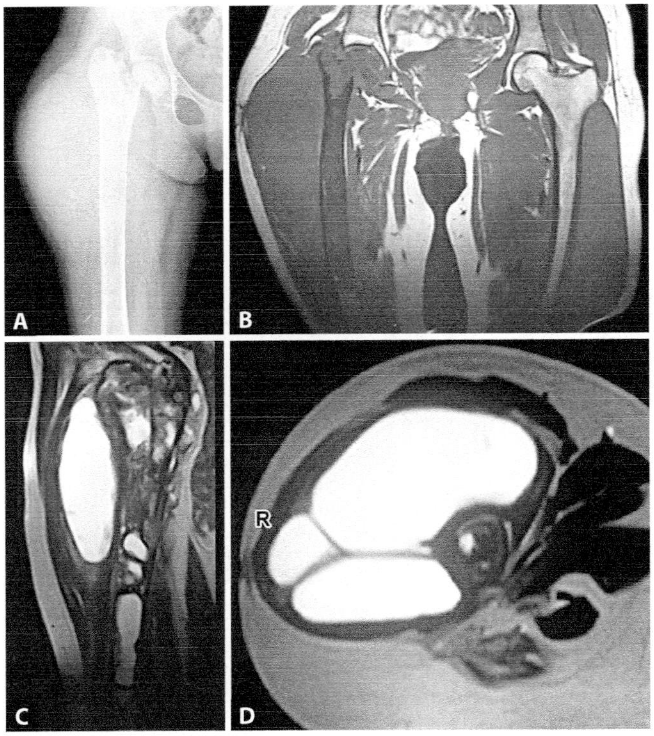

Figs. 22A to D: (A) Plain radiograph demonstrates expanded medullary cavity with endosteal scalloping in right femur and thinned out cortex. There is pathological fracture neck of femur with proximal migration of greater trochanter. A large soft tissue shadow is also seen along the lateral aspect with foci of calcifications; (B) Coronal T1W MR image showing altered marrow signal of medullary cavity (hypointense when compared to left femur) with a large hypointense lesion along lateral aspect of upper thigh. Note pathological fracture neck of right femur; (C) Sagittal T2W MR image showing multiple cysts in the medullary cavity of right femur with small cysts in adductor group of muscles and large cysts along lateral aspect of thigh; (D) Axial T2W MR image showing a multiseptated cystic lesion along lateral aspect of femur. Note a small cyst in the medullary cavity.

sensitive in the depiction of joint fluid, cartilage damage, marrow changes, and medullary bone destruction, but cannot differentiate infectious from noninfectious joint effusions.[47]

Radiological patterns are different in adults and infants. Plain radiographs are usually normal in early course of disease. Soft tissue swelling is the first radiographic sign of acute pyogenic arthritis. Hyperemia associated with pyogenic arthritis causes rapid, juxta-articular osteoporosis with disappearance of subchondral white line. Periarticular edema obliterates the adjacent fat planes. At this stage, effusion is identifiable. Earliest bone change occurs 8–10 days after the onset of infection.[48] There is loss of definition of the margins due to osteoporosis with small focal articular erosions followed by progressive destruction of cartilage leading to reduction in joint space. Untreated infection can lead to extensive bone destruction and loss of cortical outline. In later stages, subluxation or even dislocation can occur. With healing, sclerotic bone reaction occurs resulting in irregular articular surface. If the entire cartilage is destroyed, then bony ankylosis follows **(Figs. 23A and B)**.[49]

In infants and children, distention of joint capsule due to fluid can cause joint space widening and even subluxation, especially of the hip and shoulder. In neonates, physiological ossification of femoral head is absent, thus plain radiographs are of limited value. USG in such cases may reveal joint effusion with/without internal echoes **(Fig. 24)**. Thickened synovial membrane is seen as irregular echogenic membrane surrounding the fluid. Joint effusion can also occur as sympathetic response to adjacent focus of osteomyelitis. Arthrocentesis with bacterial cultures is therefore essential in such cases to document joint infection.

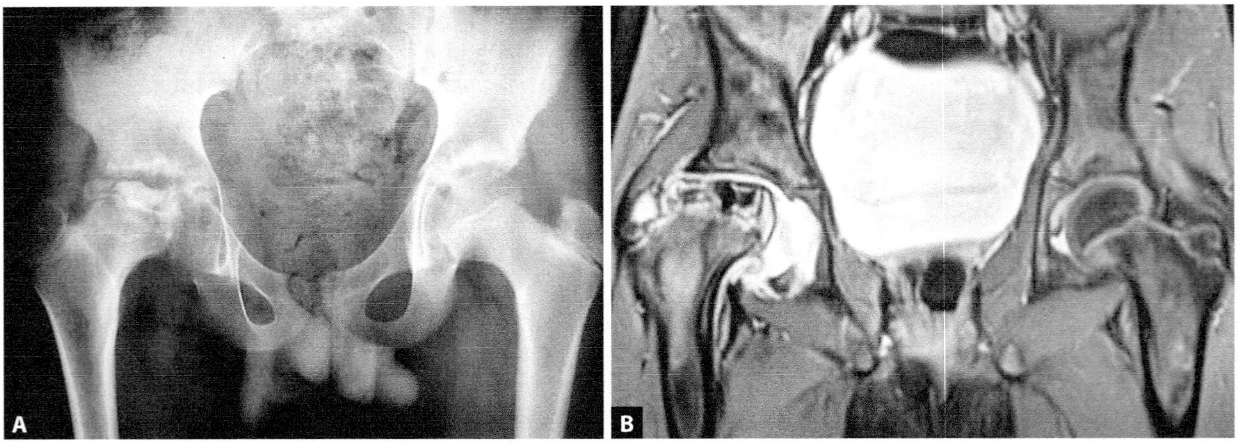

Figs. 23A and B: (A) Plain X-ray of hip joints reveals irregular articular margins of right femoral joint with sclerosis. The femoral epiphysis is fragmented, flattened and irregular with superimposed changes of avascular necrosis secondary to infection with increased teardrop distance due to effusion; (B) Postcontrast T1W MR image demonstrates thickened enhancing synovium with intraosseous abscesses in the femoral epiphysis and bone destruction. Also the metadiaphyseal marrow shows enhancement.

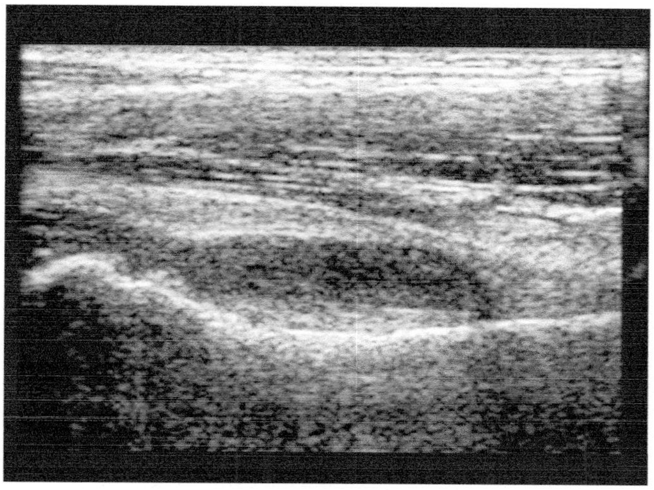

Fig. 24: Ultrasonography image in an infant shows joint effusion in hip joint with dependent debris.

In pediatric population, distinguishing transient synovitis from septic arthritis is extremely important and in such cases the USG may not differentiate as both the conditions manifest as synovial thickening, joint effusions, and alteration in surrounding soft tissues. MRI can differentiate these two conditions as in transient synovitis, there are minimal to almost nil marrow changes (high signal changes in T2W and STIR images which show postcontrast enhancement).[50]

Bone changes in gonococcal arthritis are indistinguishable from tuberculosis. Destruction is more rapid and serial films are helpful in distinguishing the two. Similarly, brucellar arthritic changes are also indistinguishable from tubercular joint; however, *Brucella* involves most commonly sacroiliac joints and usually unilaterally.[49] Fungal arthritis is most commonly due to *Candida*, coccidiosis, and blastomycosis. Radiologically, there is soft tissue swelling, periarticular osteopenia, relative joint space preservation and bony erosions but differentiation from tuberculosis is difficult.

TRANSIENT SYNOVITIS

Transient synovitis is a common self-limiting cause of acute hip pain in children which generally subsides within 2 weeks. Children between 4 and 10 years of age are prone to transient synovitis and the condition is more common in male children.

Clinical features: Acute hip or groin pain, limp, restriction of motion, refusal to bear weight and systemic symptoms of fever are common. A prior history of upper respiratory tract infection is often present. Erythrocyte sedimentation rate (ESR), C-reactive protein (CRP), and WBC counts may be raised. Although no infectious agent has been isolated, elevated viral titers have been found. Though the disease is self-limiting, recurrence rates range between 0 and 26%.[51] Among the recurrent and persistent cases, a significant proportion progress to Legg-Calvé-Perthes disease.

Common cause of acute hip pain in pediatric age group includes septic arthritis, transient synovitis, and Legg-Calvé-Perthes disease. It is important to differentiate between infectious and noninfectious causes. Dynamic contrast-enhanced MRI shows early decreased enhancement of femoral head epiphysis on time-intensity curves in patients with septic arthritis.[52]

CHRONIC RECURRENT MULTIFOCAL OSTEOMYELITIS

Chronic recurrent multifocal osteomyelitis (CRMO) is an idiopathic autoinflammatory bone disorder of children and adolescents characterized by recurrent episodic osseous pain at one or multiple sites over several years.[53]

It is usually a diagnosis of exclusion once underlying infection and neoplasia has been ruled out. Median age of presentation is of 10 years with a range of 9–14 years, with youngest age at presentation being 6 months.[53] Biopsy of the osseous lesions shows an inflammatory reaction. No organisms are demonstrated.

The combination of synovitis, acne, pustulosis, hyperostosis, and osteitis is designated as SAPHO and is seen as the adult counterpart of CRMO. CRMO is associated with a number of dermatological (psoriasis, palmoplantar pustulosis, etc.), gastrointestinal (Crohn's and ulcerative colitis), genetic (Majeed syndrome), and autoimmune conditions such as Wegener's granulomatosis and Takayasu's arteritis.[53]

The most common sites of disease are the metaphyses or metaphyseal equivalents of the tubular bones, most frequently in the lower limb bones followed by clavicle, spine, ribs, sternum, pelvis, mandible.[53,54] Clavicle involvement is a characteristic finding as this is an uncommon location for hematogenous osteomyelitis. Symmetric involvement is common. In early stages, osteolytic lesion is noted which shows progressive sclerosis during late stages. Lesions can be purely osteolytic, osteolytic with a sclerotic rim, mixed lytic and sclerotic, and purely sclerotic. Characteristically, there is no sequestration.[54] Mild periosteal reaction may be noted. MRI findings include bone marrow edema with heterogeneous contrast enhancement within the affected bone. Abscess formation and soft tissue changes are usually not seen in CRMO **(Fig. 25)** differentiating CRMO from the other types of multifocal osteomyelitis **(Figs. 26A and B)**.

Clinical course of the disease lasts for 7–10 years. Treatment usually includes anti-inflammatory drugs for symptomatic relief.

Major differentials that should be considered are (acute and subacute) osteomyelitis, Langerhans cell osteomyelitis, and Ewing's sarcoma.

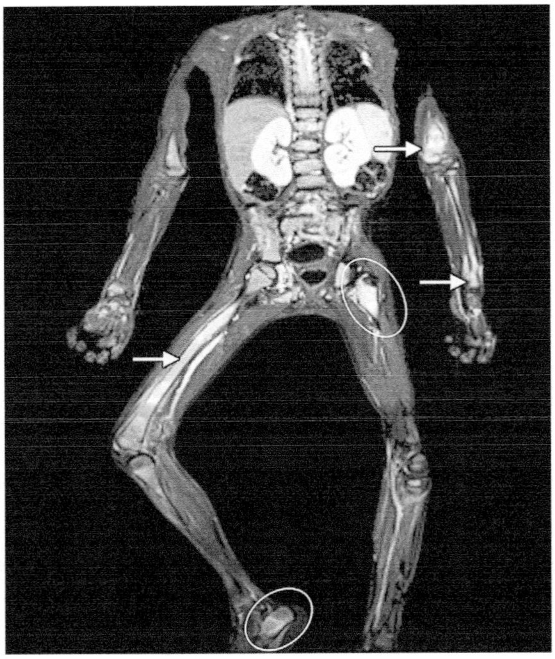

Fig. 25: Whole-body coronal short tau inversion recovery (STIR) sequence in a patient with chronic recurrent multifocal osteomyelitis (CRMO) shows multifocal areas of intramedullary hyperintensity in metaphysis of humerus radii, proximal femur, and calcaneum. Bone marrow edema is seen in diaphysis of right femur.

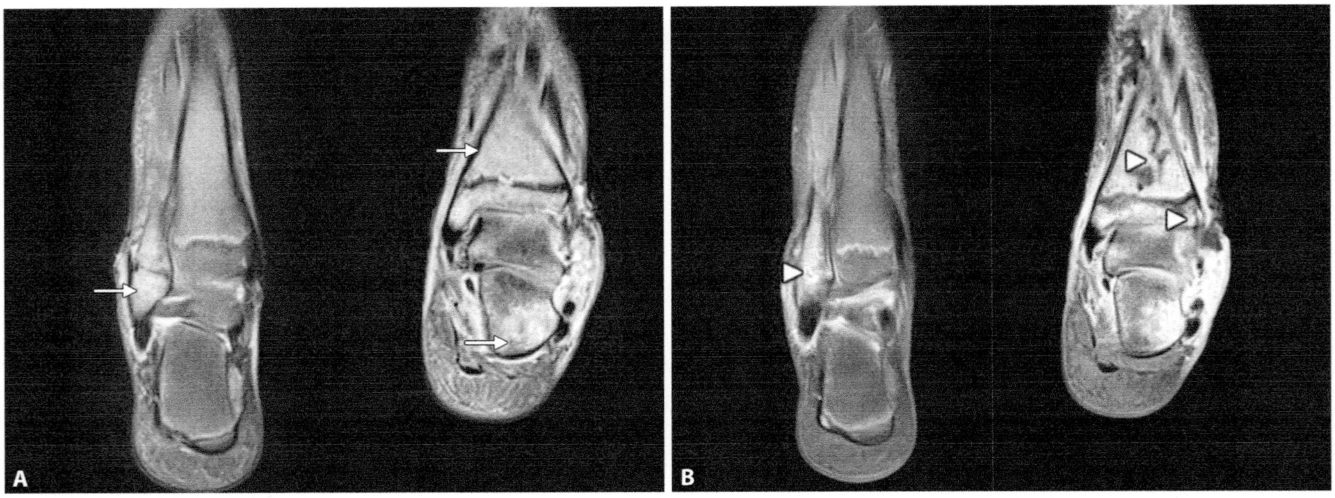

Figs. 26A and B: (A) Coronal T2-weighted; and (B) Postcontrast T1-weighted fat-saturated images show multifocal areas of osteitis in right lower fibula, tibia, and calcaneus (arrows in A), with areas of intraosseous and extraosseous abscesses (arrowheads in B) evident after contrast enhancement with surrounding tenosynovitis and soft tissue inflammation.

FUNGAL OSTEOMYELITIS

The incidence of fungal bone and joint infections has increased in solid organ transplant, chemotherapy, long-term corticosteroid, and HIV-positive individuals. Although pyogenic organisms are the most common type of infection in the immunocompromised patient, but fungal infections have also increased in number in this population. Infection either directly extends from the overlying skin or is hematogenous in origin. In the setting of an indolent infection with associated marked osseous deformity, fungal infection should be considered. Clinical features include pain in the involved region along with signs of systemic illness. No specific imaging features are known till date and it is difficult to differentiate from other infective/inflammatory causes of arthritis.

PERIPROSTHETIC INFECTIONS

Periprosthetic joint infections are a major complication of joint arthroplasties and incidence ranges between 1 and 2.5% in primary arthroplasties to 4% in revision arthroplasties.[55]

Infections can present early within 4 weeks of surgery and are typically caused by highly virulent bacteria (*S. aureus*, streptococci, and enterococci).[55] Clinically, there is evidence of local inflammation, swelling, and pain. Delayed wound healing, wound dehiscence, persistent discharge or a sinus tract can develop.

Delayed infections most commonly occur after the first month but within the first year, though delayed infection can occur at any time, especially in first 3 years. Delayed infections present with insidious clinical symptom of chronic pain, stiffness, and fistula formation.

Imaging: Serial radiographs showing a rapidly developing periprosthetic lucency of >2 mm or a focal osteolysis at the metal-bone or bone-cement interface. Similar findings of lucency can be found in aseptic loosening, which however, does not progress as rapidly as loosening due to infection. Conventional radiographs have a low sensitivity and specificity for periprosthetic infections but should be the first imaging modality. Serial radiographs are essential to evaluate the loosening.

Computed tomography scan evidence of periosteitis and joint distension are indicative of infection.

Magnetic resonance imaging is challenging with metallic artifacts from prosthetic devices and implants. Imaging techniques for metal artifact reduction include increasing bandwidth, decreasing slice thickness, view angle tilting (using a slice selection gradient during read out of the signal) or slice-encoding for metal artifact correction (SEMAC) or multiacquisition variable-resonance image combination (MAVRIC) technique on a 1.5 T MR scanner.[56]

Imaging findings of soft tissue edema, soft tissue mass, fluid around the prosthesis, bone marrow edema, and bone destruction are indicative of infection. Soft tissue mass and bone destruction are indicative of tumor recurrence in patients after tumor resection.[56]

White blood cell labeled with ^{111}In has a high degree of sensitivity, specificity, and accuracy (96–97%) in diagnosing periprosthetic joint infections and is the preferred modality of choice, although fluorodeoxyglucose-positron emission tomography (FDG-PET) also has similar sensitivity and specificity. These modalities remain constrained due to lack of widespread availability.[57,58]

REFERENCES

1. Greenfield GB. Cardinal roentgen features. In: Greenfield GB (Ed). Radiology of Bone Diseases, 5th edition. Philadelphia: JB Lippincott; 1990.
2. Edeiken J. Edeiken's Roentgen Diagnosis of Diseases of Bone, 4th edition. Baltimore: Williams and Wilkins; 1990. pp. 973-1084.
3. Wegener WA, Alavi A. Diagnostic imaging of musculoskeletal infection. Roentgenography; gallium, indium-labeled white blood cell, gammaglobulin, bone scintigraphy. Orthop Clin North Am. 1991;22:401-18.
4. Wheat J. Diagnostic strategies in osteomyelitis. Am J Med. 1985;78:218-24.
5. Markel KD, Brown ML, Dewanjee MK, Fitzgerald RH. Comparison of indium-labeled leukocyte imaging with sequential technetium-gallium scanning in the diagnosis of low grade musculoskeletal sepsis. A prospective study. J Bone Joint Surg Am. 1985;67:465-76.
6. Rubin RH, Fischman AJ, Callahan RJ, Khaw BA, Keech F, Ahmad M, et al. 111In-labelled nonspecific immunoglobulin scanning in the detection of focal infection. N Eng J Med. 1989;321:935-40.
7. D'Angelo GL, Ogilive-Harris DJ. Septic arthritis following arthroscopy with cost benefit analysis of antibiotic prophylaxis. Arthroscopy. 1988;4:10-4.
8. Mujoomdar M, Russell E, Dionne F, Moulton K, Murray C, McGill S. Appendix 2.5 Diagnosis of acute osteomyelitis. In: Mujoomdar M, Russell E, Dionne F, Moulton K, Murray C, McGill S (Eds). Optimal Use Report: Optimizing Health System Use of Medical Isotopes and Other Imaging Modalities [Internet]. Ottawa (ON): Canadian Agency for Drugs and Technologies in Health; 2012.
9. Esterhai JL Jr, Gelb I. Adult septic arthritis. Orthop Clin North Am. 1991;22:503-14.
10. Desai RV, Khandelwal N, Gupta S, Suri S, Gill SS, Suri S. Role of ultrasound in acute Osteomyelitis. Asian Oceanian J Radiol. 2001;6:159-65.
11. Modic MT, Pflanze W, Feiglin DH, Belhobek G. Magnetic resonance imaging of musculoskeletal infections. Radiol Clin North Am. 1986;24:247-58.
12. Schanwecker DS, Braunstein EM, Wheat LJ. Diagnostic imaging of osteomyelitis. Infect Dis Clin North Am. 1990;4:441-63.
13. Modic MT, Feiglin DH, Piraino DW, Boumphrey F, Weinstein MA, Duchesneau PM, et al. Vertebral osteomyelitis: assessment using MR. Radiology. 1985;157:157-66.
14. Unger E, Moldfsky P, Gatenby R, Hartz W, Broder G. Diagnosis of osteomyelitis by MR imaging. Am J Roentgenol. 1988;150:605-10.
15. Morrison WB, Schweitzer ME, Batte WG, Radack DP, Russel KM. Osteomyelitis of the foot: relative importance of primary and secondary MR imaging signs. Radiology. 1998;207:625-32.
16. Jaramillo D, Treves ST, Kasser JR, Harper M, Sundel R, Laor T. Osteomyelitis and septic arthritis in children: appropriate use of imaging to guide treatment. Am J Roentgenol. 1995;165:399-403.
17. Beltran J, Noto AM, McGhee RB, Freedy RM, McCalla MS. Infections of the musculoskeletal system: high-field-strength MR imaging. Radiology. 1987;164:449-54.
18. Brill PW, Winchester P, Krause AN, Symchych P. Osteomyelitis in a neonatal intensive care unit. Radiology. 1979;131:83-8.
19. Mok M, Reilly RJ, Ash JM. Osteomyelitis in the neonate. Radiology. 1982;145:677-82.
20. Bressler EL, Conway JJ, Weiss SC. Neonatal osteomyelitis examined by bone scintigraphy. Radiology. 1984;152:685-8.
21. Cierny G, Mader JT, Pennick JJ. A clinical staging system for adult osteomyelitis. Contemp Orthop. 1985;10:17-37.
22. Lee YJ, Sadigh S, Mankad K, Kapse N, Rajeswaran G. The imaging of osteomyelitis. Quant Imaging Med Surg. 2016;6(2):184-98.
23. Rosen Ra, Morehouse HT, Karp JH, Yu GS. Intracortical fissuring in osteomyelitis. Radiology. 1981;141:17-20.

24. Beaman FD, von Herrmann PF, Kransdorf MJ, Adler RS, Amini B, Appel M, et al. ACR Appropriateness Criteria® suspected osteomyelitis, septic arthritis, or soft tissue infection (excluding spine and diabetic foot). J Am Coll Radiol. 2017;14(5S):S326-37.
25. Jaramillo D. Infection: musculoskeletal. Pediatr Radiol. 2011;41(Suppl 1):S127-34.
26. Connolly SA, Connolly LP, Drubach LA, Zurakowski D, Jaramillo D. MRI for detection of abscess in acute osteomyelitis of the pelvis in children. Am J Roentgenol. 2007;189:867-72.
27. Karchevsky M, Schweitzer ME, Morrison WB, Parellada JA. MRI findings of septic arthritis and associated osteomyelitis in adults. Am J Roentgenol. 2004;182:119-22.
28. Collins MS, Schaar MM, Wenger DE, Mandrekar JN. T1-weighted MRI characteristics of pedal osteomyelitis. Am J Roentgenol. 2005;185:386-93.
29. Cooper C, Cawley MI. Bacterial arthritis in an English Health district. A 10-year-review. Ann Rheum Dis. 1986;45:458-63.
30. Olasinde AA, Oluwadiya KS, Adegbehingbe OO. Treatment of Brodie's abscess: excellent results from curettage, bone grafting and antibiotics. Singapore Med J. 2011;52(6):436-9.
31. Gulati Y, Maheshwari AV. Brodie's abscess of the femoral neck simulating osteoid osteoma. Acta Orthop Belg. 2007;73:648-52.
32. Quinn SF, Murray W, Clerk RA, Cochran C. MR imaging of chronic osteomyelitis. J Comput Assist Tomogr. 1988;12:113-7.
33. Mason MD, Zlatkin MB, Esterhai JL, Dalinka MK, Velchik MG, Kressel HY. Chronic complicated osteomyelitis of the lower extremity evaluation with MR imaging. Radiology. 1989;173:355-9.
34. Pineda C, Espinosa R, Pena A. Radiographic imaging in osteomyelitis: the role of plain radiography, computed tomography, ultrasonography, magnetic resonance imaging, and scintigraphy. Semin Plast Surg. 2009;23:80-9.
35. Könönen E, Wade WG. Actinomyces and related organisms in human infections. Clin Microbiol Rev. 2015;28:419-42.
36. Brodsky JW, Schneidler C. Diabetic foot infections. Orthop Clin North Am. 1991;22:473-89.
37. Yuh WT, Corson JD, Baraniewski HM, Rezai K, Shamma AR, Kathol MH, et al. Osteomyelitis of the foot in diabetic patients: evaluation with plain film, 99mTc-MDP bone scintigraphy and MR imaging. Am J Roentgenol. 1989;152:795-800.
38. Keenam AM, Tindel NL, Alavi A. Diagnosis of pedal osteomyelitis in diabetic patients using current scintigraphy techniques. Arch Intern Med. 1989;149:2262-6.
39. Toledano TR, Fatone EA, Weis A, Cotten A, Beltran J. MRI evaluation of bone marrow changes in the diabetic foot: a practical approach. Semin Musculoskelet Radiol. 2011;15(3):257-68.
40. Duryea D, Bernard S, Flemming D, Walker E, French C. Outcomes in diabetic foot ulcer patients with isolated T2 marrow signal abnormality in the underlying bone: should the diagnosis of "osteitis" be changed to "early osteomyelitis"? Skeletal Radiol. 2017;46(10):1327-33.
41. Leone A, Vitiello C, Gullì C, Sikora AK, MacagninoS, Colosimo C. Bone and soft tissue infections in patients with diabetic foot. Radiol Med. 2020;125(2):177-87.
42. Donovan A, Schweitzer ME. Use of MR imaging in diagnosing diabetes-related pedal osteomyelitis. Radiographics. 2010;30:723-36.
43. Liao D, Xie L, Han Y, Du S, Wang H, Zeng C, et al. Dynamic contrast-enhanced magnetic resonance imaging for differentiating osteomyelitis from acute neuropathic arthropathy in the complicated diabetic foot. Skeletal Radiol. 2018;47(10):1337-47.
44. Noguerol TM, Luna Alcalá A, Beltrán LS, Gómez Cabrera M, Broncano Cabrero J, Vilanova JC. Advanced MR imaging techniques for differentiation of neuropathic arthropathy and osteomyelitis in the diabetic foot. Radiographics. 2017;37(4):1161-80.
45. Pedrosa I, Saiz A, Arrazola J, Ferreirós J, Pedrosa CS. Hydatid cyst: radiologic and pathologic features and complications. Radiographics. 2000;20:795-817.
46. Dhatt S, Singhal M, Tripathy SK, Tahasildar N, Sen R. Primary hydatidosis of femur: a case report and review of the literature. Eur J Orthop Surg Traumatol. 2010;20:401-5.
47. Tang JS, Gold RH, Bessett LW, Seeger LL. Musculoskeletal infection of the extremities: evaluation with MR Imaging. Radiology. 1988;166:205-9.
48. Manaster BJ. Adult chronic hip pain: radiographic evaluation. Radiographics. 2000;20:S3-25.
49. Edeiken J. Edeiken's Roentgen Diagnosis of Diseases of Bone, 4th edition. Baltimore: Williams and Wilkins; 1990. pp. 593-601.
50. Yang WJ, Im SA, Lim GY, Chun HJ, Jung NY, Sung MS, et al. MR imaging of transient synovitis: differentiation from septic arthritis. Pediatr Radiol. 2006;36:1154-8.
51. Asche SS, van Rijn RM, Bessems JH, Krul M, Bierma-Zeinstra SM. What is the clinical course of transient synovitis in children: a systematic review of the literature. Chiropr Man Therap. 2013;21(1):39.
52. Kim EY, Kwack KS, Cho JH, Lee DH, Yoon SH. Usefulness of dynamic contrast-enhanced MRI in differentiating between septic arthritis and transient synovitis in the hip joint. Am J Roentgenol. 2012;198:428-33.
53. Khanna G, Sato TS, Ferguson P. Imaging of chronic recurrent multifocal osteomyelitis. Radiographics. 2009;29(4):1159-77.
54. Iyer RS, Thapa MM, Chew FS. Chronic recurrent multifocal osteomyelitis: review. Am J Roentgenol. 2011;196:S87-91.
55. Izakovicova P, Borens O, Trampuz A. Periprosthetic joint infection: current concepts and outlook. EFORT Open Rev. 2019;4(7):482-94.
56. Jiang M, He C, Feng JM, Li ZH, Chen Z, Yan FH, et al. Magnetic resonance imaging parameter optimizations for diagnosis of periprosthetic infection and tumor recurrence in artificial joint replacement patients. Sci Rep. 2016;6:36995.
57. Palestro CJ, Kim CK, Swyer AJ, Capozzi JD, Solomon RW, Goldsmith SJ. Total-hip arthroplasty: periprosthetic indium-111-labled leukocyte activity and complementary technetium-99mm-sulfur colloid imaging in suspected infection. J Nucl Med. 1990;31:1950-5.
58. Chryssikos T, Parvizi J, Ghanem E, Newberg A, Zhuang H, Alavi A. FDG-PET imaging can diagnose periprosthetic infection of the hip. Clin Orthop Relat Res. 2008;466:1338-42.

CHAPTER

6

Tuberculosis of the Spine

Rashmi Dixit, Gaurav Shanker Pradhan, Radhika Batra

INTRODUCTION

The spine is the most frequent site of osseous involvement by tuberculosis accounting for about 50% of cases.[1,2] The disease was first described by Sir Percival Pott in 1779, hence, the name Pott's disease.[3] There has been a resurgence of the disease even in developed countries following the human immunodeficiency virus (HIV) pandemic.

Tubercular spondylitis is defined as an infection by *Mycobacterium tuberculosis* of one or more of the extradural components of the spine namely the vertebrae, intervertebral discs, paraspinal soft tissues, and epidural space.[4,5] It is associated with disproportionate amount of morbidity due to its tendency to produce significant deformity and neurologic complications therefore prompt diagnosis and treatment are of utmost importance.

PATHOPHYSIOLOGY

The spread of tuberculosis to the spine is usually by hematogenous route.[2] Hematogenous seeding may arise from a primary focus in the lung or other extraosseous foci such as lymph nodes, gastrointestinal tract (GIT), or any other viscera which may be active or quiescent.[6]

Lower dorsal and lumbar vertebrae are most frequently involved followed by midthoracic and cervical region.[7] The C2-C7 region is reportedly involved in 3–5% of cases[8,9] and the atlantoaxial articulation in less than 1% of cases.[10-12] Usually, two continuous vertebrae are involved but several vertebrae may be affected, skip lesions, and solitary vertebral involvement may also be seen.[7] The so-called skip lesion or a second lesion not contiguous with the more obvious lesion is seen in 4–10% of cases.[4,13]

The infection usually begins in the cancellous, paradiscal area of the vertebral body and less often in the central portion or anterior surface. There is softening of the vertebral body which gets easily compressed to produce either wedging or total collapse. The normal kyphotic curve in the thoracic spine accentuates the pressure on the anterior portion of the vertebral body, producing anterior wedging resulting in kyphus with a gibbus deformity.[6,7]

As infection spreads to the adjacent disc, the disc space narrows. The intervertebral disc is avascular in adults and spread of infection to the disc can occur by extension through the subchondral bone via cartilaginous end plate or beneath the anterior or posterior longitudinal ligament to involve the peripheral disc. Disc space narrowing can also occur due to disc herniation into the weakened vertebral body with subsequent infection of the herniated disc.[6] The intervertebral disc, however, is relatively resistant to infection by *M. tuberculosis*. This is thought to be due to a lack of proteolytic enzymes in the *Mycobacterium* as compared with pyogenic bacteria.[14] The avascularity of the disc may also prevent it from serving as an initial site of infection. Hence it has been suggested that disc involvement occurs only when the disc has lost its nutritional support due to involvement of adjacent vertebral bodies.[2] Disc space narrowing thus occurs later and is less pronounced in tubercular infection than in pyogenic infection.[14-16] Although the vertebral body is involved more often than the posterior elements, these latter structures may be affected initially or predominantly in some persons.[17,18]

A marked exudative lesion due to hypersensitivity reaction to *Mycobacterium* results in formation of thick pus containing serum, leukocytes, caseous material, tubercle bacilli, and bone fragments, which tracks through the pre- and paravertebral soft tissues forming pre- and paravertebral abscesses. The exudate penetrates ligaments and follows the path of least resistance along fascial planes, blood vessels, and nerves to distant sites from the original bony lesion as cold abscess. The abscesses may further extend into the spinal canal producing an epidural abscess and cord compression.[7] Spread of infection can occur beneath the anterior longitudinal ligament, involving adjacent vertebral bodies.

CLINICAL FEATURES

Tuberculous spondylitis can occur in any age group, but, majority of the patients are under 30 years of age at the time of diagnosis. The disease is rare in the first year of life but when it occurs, it tends to be more severe with greater bone destruction and multiple vertebral involvement.[7,8] Symptoms and signs are variable.[4] Some patients may be afebrile and free of systemic symptoms until late stage of the disease, others may present with constitutional symptoms before symptoms related to the spine manifest. The usual presentation is with persistent spinal pain, local tenderness, and limitation of spinal mobility.[4,7]

Paraparesis may be apparent in about 20–30% of all patients with spinal tuberculosis.[4,7] In the cervical region, the incidence is much higher and over 40% cases may be associated with quadriparesis.[4,8] Paraplegia may be *early onset*, which develops during the active phase of the disease or *late onset* which may appear many years after the disease has become quiescent, even without any evidence of reactivation. Early-onset paraplegia is usually due to cord compression by epidural abscess or granulation tissue, pathological subluxation or dislocation, sequestered bone, or disc fragments. Nonmechanical causes include inflammatory cord edema which could be a result of vascular stasis, bacterial toxins, or granulation tissue due extension of tuberculous inflammation through the meninges to the cord. Rarely endarteritis may cause cord infarction. Late-onset paraplegia can occur due to dural fibrosis, severe kyphoscoliotic deformity, spinal canal stenosis, gliosis of cord, or sequestra from vertebral body. Late-onset paraplegia has a less favorable prognosis as compared to early onset paraplegia.[7]

LABORATORY INVESTIGATIONS[19-24]

Blood investigations reveal relative lymphocytosis, low hemoglobin and elevated ESR in active disease. The mantoux test is nondiagnostic in an endemic region and may be negative in immunodeficient individuals. The sensitivity of staining for acid-fast bacilli may vary from 25 to 75%. A long incubation period of 4–6 weeks is required for culture, although BACTEC radiometric culture is faster and takes around 2 weeks. Polymerase chain reaction (PCR) can distinguish between typical and atypical mycobacteria and is an efficient and rapid method of diagnosis. A positive PCR, however, cannot substitute culture and does not indicate disease activity, as it does not distinguish between live and dead microorganisms.

IMAGING MODALITIES

Conventional Radiographs

Radiographs are the usual initial investigation, but they are often negative in early disease **(Figs. 1A to D)**.[25] More than 30–50% of mineral has to be lost before a radiolucent lesion becomes apparent on plain films and 2–5 months are needed for this.[2,7] Plain films are also limited in the

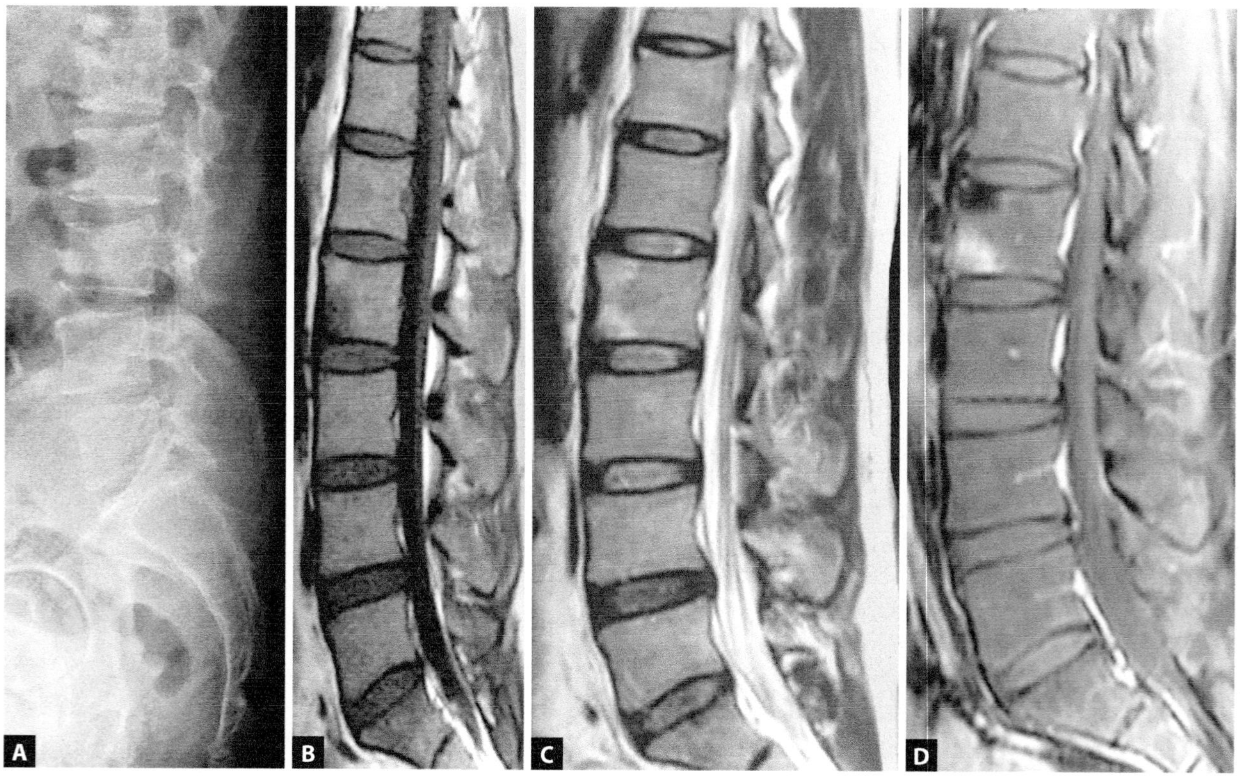

Figs. 1A to D: (A) Lateral radiograph L-S spine of a 25-year-old male presenting with low backache and fever reveals normal vertebrae and disc spaces; (B) T1W, (C) T2W, and (D) postcontrast T1W fat suppressed sagittal images of the same patient show an area of signal alteration in the anteroinferior part of L2 vertebral body appearing hypointense on T1W, hyperintense on T2W images and showing patchy enhancement on the postcontrast images.

evaluation of areas such as craniovertebral junction, cervicodorsal junction, posterior neural arches, and sacrum.

Computed Tomography

Advantages of computed tomography (CT) evaluation in cases of tubercular spondylitis include early detection of bone and soft tissue changes when plain films are normal, better anatomic localization and characterization of lesions, evaluation of areas difficult to evaluate on plain films such as craniovertebral junction, cervicodorsal junction, and sacrum, and providing guidance for biopsy and surgical approach. It is also an excellent technique for detection of bone fragments, soft tissue calcification, and to demonstrate the exact extent of deformity in chronic cases.[13,26,27] However, a routine CT examination may overlook lesions outside the chosen scan volume.[4] With the use of multirow detector scanners, the entire spine can be covered though with an increased radiation burden **(Figs. 2A and B)**. Furthermore CT is less useful than magnetic resonance for early diagnosis of spondylitis as inflammatory marrow changes in the vertebral body, an early sign of infection, are not well depicted on CT scanning.[28] In addition, soft tissue structures within the bony spinal canal are poorly delineated.[4,28] In the cervicothoracic region, epidural involvement may be missed even on contrast-enhanced CT (CECT), without intrathecal contrast enhancement because of beam hardening artifacts. For this reason, the effect of extradural disease on the thecal sac, spinal cord and neural elements is difficult to evaluate properly.[28]

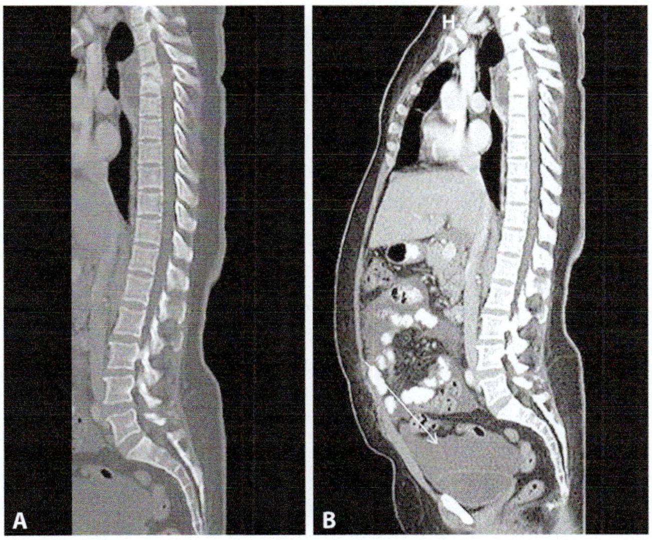

Figs. 2A and B: Sagittal reconstructions at bone (A) and soft tissue (B) settings from a multislice CT acquisition for disseminated tuberculosis reveal reduction of disc space between D4 and D5, destruction of endplates and a peripherally enhancing prevertebral abscess due to tubercular involvement. Note the extended coverage and presence of free fluid in the abdomen (arrow).

Magnetic Resonance Imaging

The superiority of magnetic resonance imaging (MRI) in the detection and staging of inflammatory and infective disorders of the spine is generally accepted making MR the imaging modality of choice in these conditions.[15,28,29] MRI is useful to detect disease in areas difficult to evaluate on plain films such as the CV junction. It demonstrates of early bone marrow involvement or edema and allows unparalleled evaluation of the spinal canal and cord. Soft tissue and intraosseous abscesses are also well demonstrated on MRI.[28] It has higher sensitivity for early disease than bone scan and plain films.[2] MRI also scores over CT in the detection of early disease due to its sensitivity to detect bone marrow edema which is best depicted on short tau inversion recovery (STIR) and T1W images.[28] The changes at this stage, however, are nonspecific.

In addition, skip lesions are more easily and more often detected by MRI as compared to CT. Incidence of multilevel noncontiguous vertebral tuberculosis is generally reported to be between 1.1 and 16%, but an incidence as high as 71.4% has been reported when using whole spine MRI **(Figs. 3A to D)**.[30] MR is also superior to CT for detection of epidural, meningeal, and cord involvement.[31,32] Planning the surgical approach can be facilitated by MRI because of the clear display of the extent of the active infection and its complications including involvement of neural arch.

While tuberculosis can be confidently diagnosed when the characteristic imaging features are present, at times it may be difficult to distinguish this from other causes of bone marrow edema in early stages and from other conditions such as metastases and myeloma in atypical cases. Diffusion-weighted (DW)-MRI and apparent diffusion coefficient (ADC) values have been used to help in the differentiation of spinal tuberculosis from other lesions of similar appearance. However, an overlap of ADC values was noted with metastatic disease, hence, these must be interpreted in association with clinical history and routine MR findings.[33,34] MRI does have disadvantages. Calcification, the hallmark of tubercular infection and small bone fragments are not readily detectable by MRI. Small bone fragments in an epidural abscess are important to detect when surgical management is being considered so that they can be accurately removed. Gradient echo (T2*W) images demonstrate calcification better than spin-echo images. The low signal of calcification or bone fragments is more prominent on these images and closely matches calcification seen on CT. Demonstration of bone fragmentation on T2*W images is also considered characteristic of tuberculosis even in the absence of abscess formation.[35] The other disadvantage is that interventional procedures are difficult to perform with MRI.

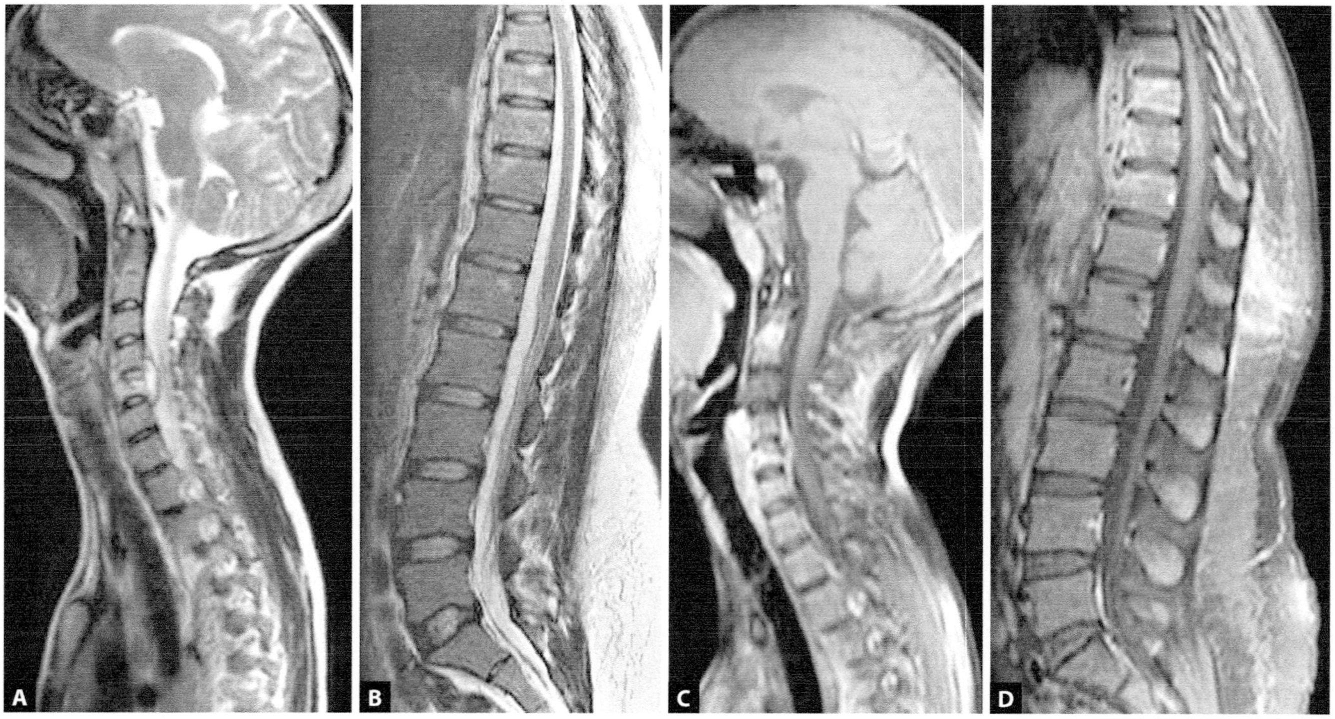

Figs. 3A to D: Sagittal T2-weighted images of the cervical (A) and lumbosacral spine (B) in a case of multifocal caries spine reveal hyperintense marrow signal in C5 and D8 to D11 vertebrae. A T2 hyperintense epidural soft tissue is noted at C5 and in the prevertebral region in the lower dorsal spine; (C and D) Postcontrast images reveal abnormal enhancement in the above vertebrae, and soft tissues. Additional foci of enhancement in C2 and posterior to spinous processes in the lumbar region are also seen. Note the relative preservation of the intervertebral discs.

Nuclear Medicine Scintigraphy[30,32-40]

Bone scintigraphy using technetium diphosphonate is economical but nonspecific for early detection of tuberculous spondylitis. Reported sensitivities vary from 87.5 to 95%. Uptake is usually increased and multiple sites in disseminated disease may be seen which may mimic metastases. However, Lifeso and Weaver reported false-negative bone scan findings in 35% of plain film positive lesions. The authors noted a high incidence of negative Gallium scans as well. This may be explained by a purely lytic and avascular early phase of the disease. False-negative bone scans are seen with disseminated tuberculosis, cervical spine lesions, and isolated neural arch lesions. Posterior neural arch lesions are more readily detectable when cross-sectional nuclear medicine imaging is performed. The pitfalls of limited anatomic resolution, nonspecificity, and false-negative examinations limit the use of scintigraphy in tuberculous spondylodiscitis. These techniques also cannot distinguish between the different causes of infection, but they are useful to identify the area of interest which can then be evaluated further to establish the diagnosis.

Fluorodeoxyglucose-positron emission tomography (FDG-PET) and PET-CT have high sensitivity for detection of chronic osteomyelitis.[41,42] Tubercular lesions are found to have increased FDG uptake in regions of active granulomatous inflammation with cold areas that represent necrosed tissue containing pus. PET-CT can also delineate the sinus tracks without the need for contrast instillation which is an added advantage of PET-CT. If CECT is incorporated along with the PET-CT, the complete extent of osseous, marrow and soft tissue involvement can be delineated. Moreover, it is useful to distinguish active disease from residual fibrotic tissue, detect multiple occult foci, for monitoring response to treatment and providing information on disease spread. It is also a useful tool to guide the site of biopsy or other interventional procedures.

Tuberculosis can be a common cancer mimic on PET/CT, producing uptake patterns that are indistinguishable from that of malignant processes. Though high standardized uptake values (SUVs) >2.5 have been attributed to malignant lesions, high values (up to 21) have been seen in tuberculosis as well. Several groups have attempted to improve the specificity of an ^{18}F-FDG-PET by imaging the abnormal sites at dual time points after its administration including additional delayed imaging at 90–120 minutes.[43,44] At malignant sites, the FDG uptake continues to increase for several hours, which can be demonstrated by the increase in SUVs. On the other hand, in inflammatory lesions, uptake peaks at approximately 60 minutes after administration and the SUVs either stabilize or decline thereafter. Hence, Alavi et al.[35] concluded that imaging at two time points after FDG administration may help distinguish between malignant and inflammatory disorders. However, other authors have found equivocal results with dual point time imaging (45 and 120 minutes post-FDG injection). Another approach to increase the diagnostic accuracy of PET is the combined use of ^{18}F-FDG and C-11 acetate as the latter accumulates in tumors and not in inflammatory lesions.

The exact role of FDG-PET and PET-CT in tuberculosis and other inflammatory diseases is evolving. With the development of newer and more specific radiotracers like positron emitter-labeled antituberculous drug molecules such as isoniazid (INH) and rifampicin in the future, PET/CT may play a significant role in establishing an early diagnosis and effective monitoring of therapeutic response.

IMAGING APPEARANCES

Imaging features in tubercular spondylitis consist of the vertebral, disc space, and the soft tissue changes. Paravertebral abscesses are an important early feature of Pott's spine. Extension of tubercular spondylodiscitis to the adjacent soft tissues is common, incidence varying from 55 to 96%[1,4,45] and rarely may precede any visible vertebral lesion.[6] This extension usually occurs anterolaterally and is less often observed directly posteriorly in the peridural space.[6,45]

Associated changes in the spinal cord and rare variants of disease such as extraosseous extradural granuloma may be detected by modern imaging techniques.

CONVENTIONAL RADIOGRAPHS

The radiographic appearances vary depending on the initial focus of infection within the vertebra. There are mainly four sites of infection in the vertebra, i.e., paradiscal, anterior subperiosteal, central, and appendiceal.

Paradiscal

This is the most common type of lesion, also called marginal, intervertebral, subarticular, or metaphyseal lesion. The disease process most often begins in the anterior vertebral body adjacent to the superior or inferior endplate.[1,15] Two contiguous vertebral bodies are involved in about 50% of cases of tubercular osteomyelitis. Demineralization and loss of definition of the endplates is seen. There is minimal or no periosteal reaction or reactive sclerosis in the remaining part of the vertebra.[1,2,18] Eventually, the adjacent intervertebral disc is narrowed **(Fig. 4)**. Rarely, the disc space may remain intact for a long time. This causes difficulty in diagnosis, as disc space narrowing is an important diagnostic feature It helps to differentiate tuberculosis from traumatic collapse, metastases, solitary myeloma, and porotic collapse where disc space narrowing is absent.[18]

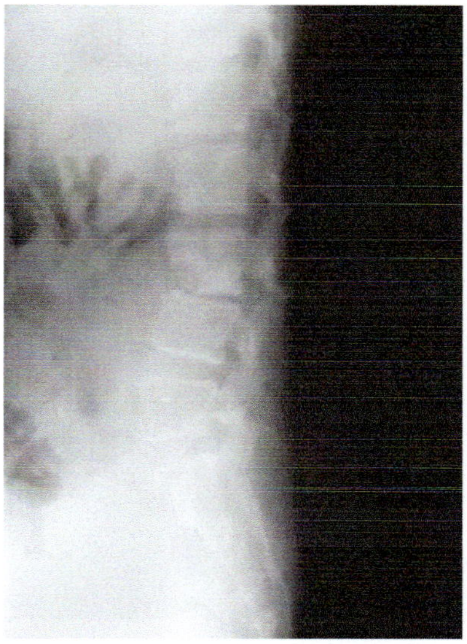

Fig. 4: Lateral radiograph L-S spine showing reduction of L3-L4 disc space with erosion of the anteroinferior aspect of L3 vertebral body—marginal variety of caries.

With progressive destruction anterior wedging or collapse occur resulting in varying degrees of kyphosis. The morbidity is greater when three or more vertebral bodies are involved, the angle of kyphosis is more than 25°, and when the vertebrae have lost more than 20% anterior height. Scoliosis may occasionally be seen with asymmetric or unilateral destruction of vertebral bodies and discs and is virtually confined to the lower thoracic and lumbar vertebrae. This is not as frequent as kyphosis.[6]

Central

The central type of lesion starts in the center of the vertebral body. A lytic area with absence of normal trabeculae is seen in the central part of the vertebral body away from the disc margin **(Fig. 5)**.

This gradually enlarges and the vertebral body may expand or balloon out like a tumor. In later stages concentric collapse occurs, almost resembling a vertebra plana. Paravertebral abscesses may be absent or minimal. The disc space is either not affected or only minimally affected.[6,7,18]

Anterior Subperiosteal

This type of infection begins at the anterior vertebral margin underneath the periosteum and spreads beneath the anterior longitudinal ligament producing subtle anterior erosions of multiple vertebrae. The clinical symptoms are out of proportion to the minor radiographic abnormalities **(Figs. 6A and B)**. Disc destruction may be late and anterior erosions may not be apparent on plain radiographs.

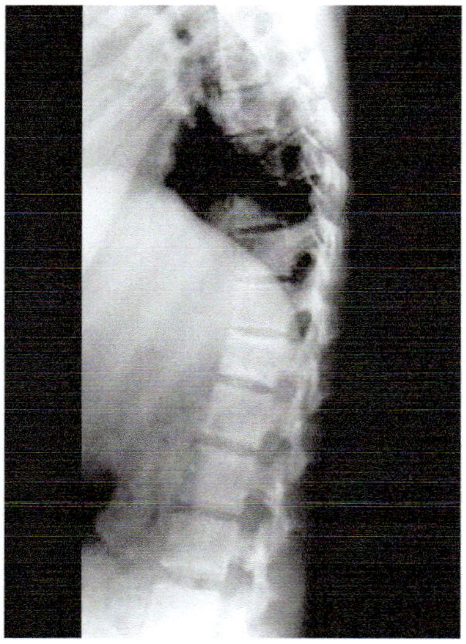

Fig. 5: Lateral radiograph D-L spine showing a lytic area with lack of normal trabeculae in the center of D12 vertebral body. There is mild reduction of vertebral height and minimal sclerosis, adjacent disc spaces are, however, normal—central caries.

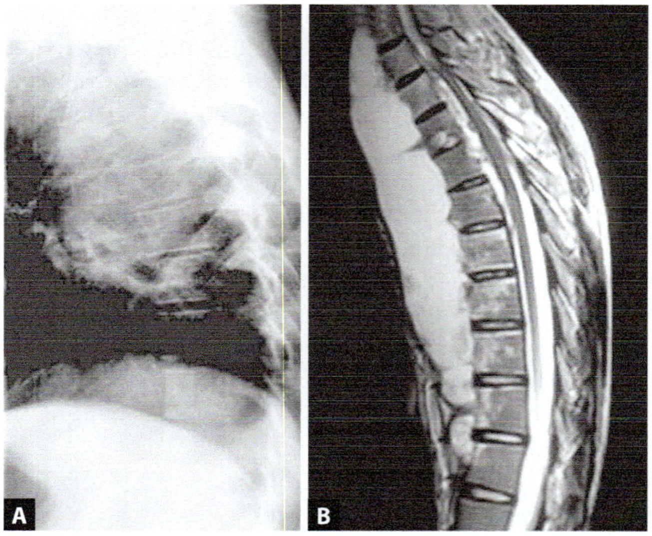

Figs. 6A and B: (A) X-ray dorsal spine lateral view in a patient with anterior subperiosteal caries shows indistinct the anterior cortices of multiple dorsal vertebrae; (B) Sagittal T2W MR image of the same reveals the entire extent of pathology with patchy hyperintense signal in multiple dorsal vertebrae, erosions of the anterior cortices and a large prevertebral abscess. A small ventral epidural collection with dorsal displacement of the upper thoracic cord is also noted.

Appendiceal or Neural Arch Tuberculosis

The neural arch or vertebral arch includes the spinous process, the laminae, the transverse processes and the pedicle as well as the lateral masses of the atlas, as embryologically, they are equivalent to the neural arch. Overall, the neural arch involvement is reported to range from 2 to 30% of cases usually along with vertebral body involvement.[4,13] Isolated involvement of the neural arch with complete sparing of vertebral bodies and intervertebral discs is rare, constituting less than 2% of all the cases of spinal tuberculosis in nonendemic areas and 5–10% in endemic areas.[4,46] Neural arch tuberculosis (NAT) is being increasingly recognized with the use of cross-sectional imaging **(Figs. 7A to C)**. It is reported NAT usually affects the cervical and upper dorsal spine while the classical variety is the most common at the lumbodorsal region.[47] Radiographic findings in NAT include erosion of pedicles, laminae, the posterior cortex of the vertebra, the adjacent ribs in the dorsal spine with relative sparing of the disc and a large paraspinal mass.[6] Involvement of pedicles (usually unilateral) and laminae is most common in tubercular spondylitis whereas pyogenic spondylitis more often involves the facet joints.[47-49] When there is bilateral involvement of the posterior elements associated with body involvement, gross instability can lead to cord compression and paralysis.

Identification of coexisting posterior and anterior involvement is essential for presurgical planning. Since anterior stabilization depends on posterior stability, anterior, and posterior stabilization must be performed.[2] Simple decompression and debridement with chemotherapy work well for isolated NAT.[50] Paraplegia associated with NAT reportedly has a better prognosis than that with typical spinal tuberculosis.[46]

Occasionally, unilateral large bridging osteophytes may occur due to irritation of the bone by inflammatory process with periosteal new bone formation or due to ossification in ligaments. They are more common in the lumbar spine as it bears most of the body weight.

Abscess formation associated with tubercular spondylitis can produce soft tissue opacity on radiographs that appear out of proportion to the bone destruction. The opacity is usually bilateral. It may be globular, which implies pus under tension or fusiform in shape. Involvement of three or more vertebral levels is common paravertebral abscess may be absent or minimal in central caries. A cervical abscess produces widening of the prevertebral soft tissues **(Fig. 8)**. In the thoracic region, the posteromedial pleural line is displaced outward resulting in a characteristic fusiform shape called the "birds nest" appearance.[7] An anterior paravertebral or subligamentous abscess between T4 and T10 vertebrae may produce the so called aneurysmal effect, i.e., erosions or gouge defects on the anterior and lateral surfaces of the vertebral bodies probably due to transmitted aortic pulsations. The intervertebral discs are resistant to pressure atrophy, hence are spared.[6,7,18,51] An abscess at the dorsolumbar junction has a poorly defined lower border and is called a "petering abscess" **(Fig. 9)**. In the lumbar region, tracking of the abscess along the psoas produces bulge of the psoas

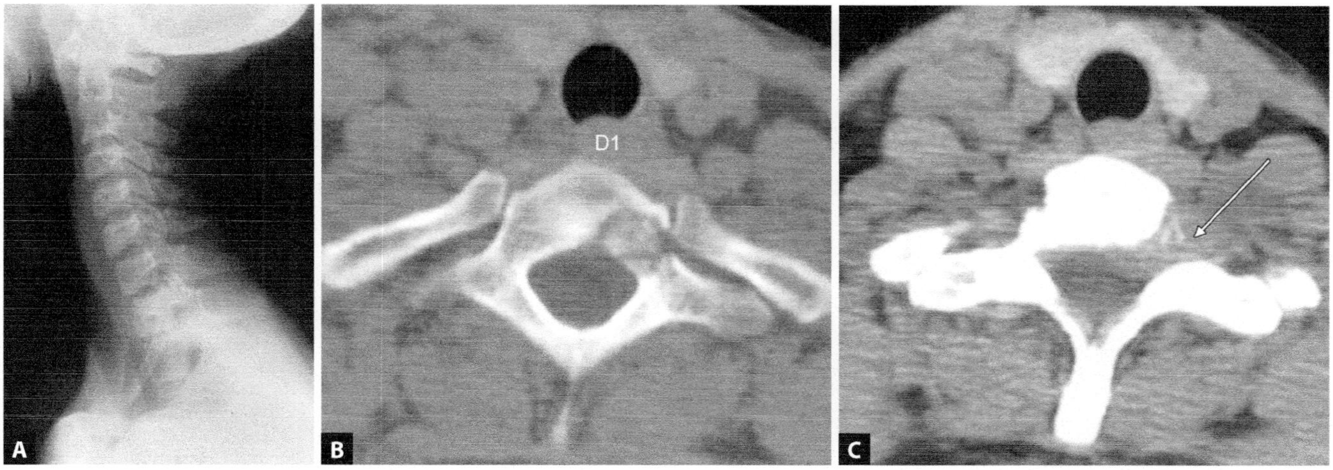

Figs. 7A to C: X-ray cervical spine lateral view with the shoulders pulled down reveals no abnormality; (A) Axial CT sections bone (B) and soft tissue (C) windows showing lytic lesions involving the left pedicle and posterior body of D1 vertebra. Associated soft tissue extending into the spinal canal is also seen (arrow)—neural arch tuberculosis.

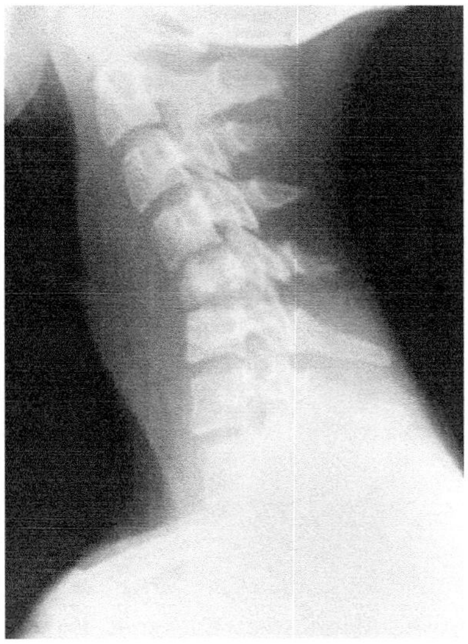

Fig. 8: Lateral radiograph cervical spine in a patient with caries C5 vertebra showing reversal of the cervical lordosis, widening of the prevertebral soft tissues and anterior displacement of the airway due to an associated abscess.

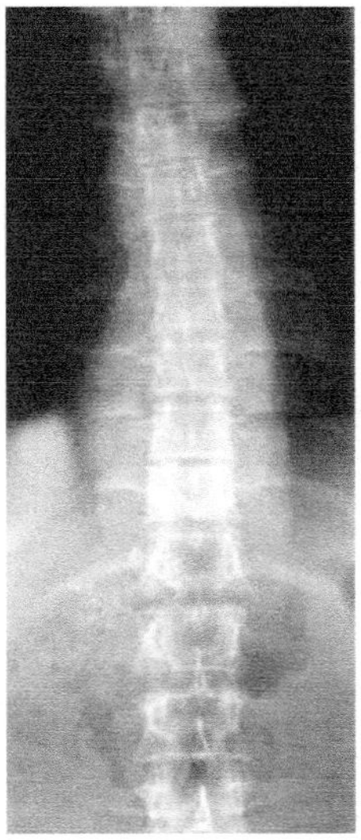

Fig. 9: X-ray D-L spine anteroposterior view of a patient with tuberculosis D10-D11 vertebrae showing a characteristic "petering abscess" with indistinct inferior margins. Subtle amorphous calcification is seen on the right side.

outline.[6,7,51] Abscesses may calcify which is thought to be characteristic for tuberculosis, since calcification in nontubercular abscesses is uncommon. Psoas abscesses show two patterns of calcification—faint amorphous deposits and tear drop-shaped calcification.[6] Calcification generally becomes more dense as healing occurs, rarely it may decrease or disappear on serial X-rays.[6]

Unusually, sclerotic changes and periosteal reaction mimicking nontubercular infection may be seen. Cystic and multilocular patterns of involvement may be seen probably due to malnourishment and poor immunological status. However, in general, marked sclerosis, less destruction and collapse, small or no paravertebral abscess more rapid clinical course should suggest a nontubercular etiology on conventional radiographs.[52]

Computed Tomography

Four patterns of bone destruction have been described:[13] on CT, i.e., fragmentary—47% **(Fig. 10)**, osteolytic—33% **(Fig. 11)**, subperiosteal—10% **(Figs. 12A and B)**, and well-defined lytic with sclerotic margins—10%. The fragmentary type is the most common and most typical. In this type numerous residual, small bone fragments are seen embedded in a soft tissue mass. Similar appearance has also been described in involved areas of vertebral appendages.[46] The appearance has been attributed to the absence of proteolytic enzymes required to lyse

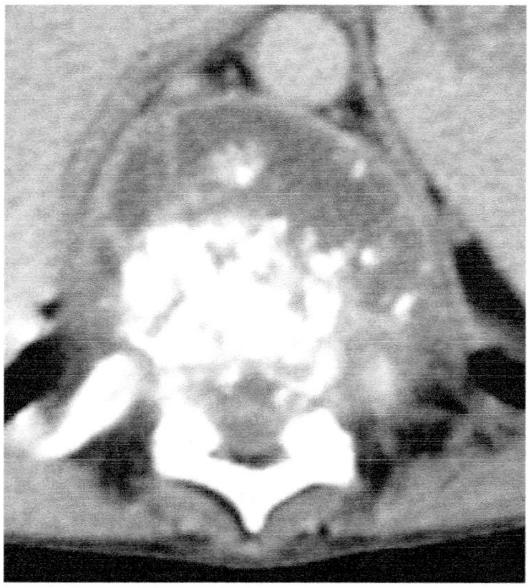

Fig. 10: Postcontrast axial CT scan showing characteristic fragmentary destruction of the vertebral body with an associated multiloculated pre- and paravertebral abscess.

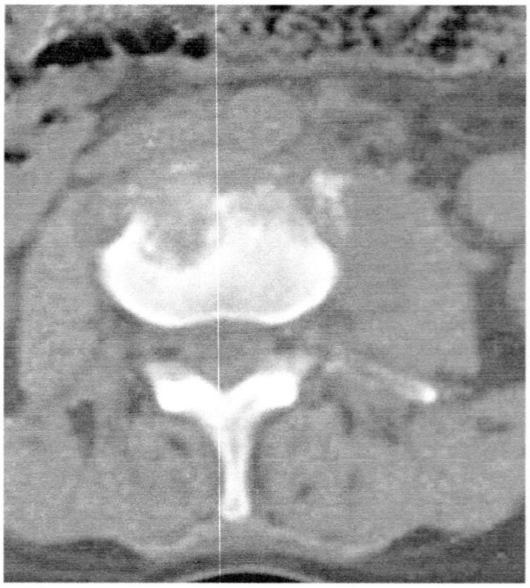

Fig. 11: Axial CT scan showing an osteolytic lesion in the anterior vertebral body in a case of caries spine.

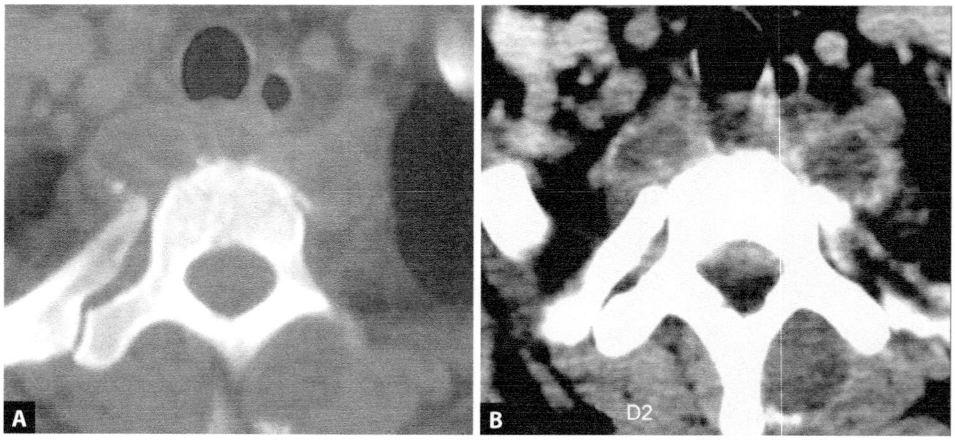

Figs. 12A and B: Axial CT scans—bone (A) and soft tissue (B) window settings in a case of subperiosteal caries showing subtle erosions of the anterior cortex of the D2 vertebra. Associated collections are noted in the pre- and paravertebral soft tissues anteriorly. Note another collection in the left posterior paraspinal region.

bone in tuberculosis .[13] Bone fragments may move to the surrounding structures—the spinal canal, paravertebral soft tissues, and psoas muscles. It is especially important to localize such fragments prior to surgical removal which is easily done on CT.[13] Some authors describe that the vertebral bodies appear to have "exploded" with peripheral bony fragments. This is unlike pyogenic spondylitis which shows multiple small erosions like a "pepper pot" and no calcification. Disc space narrowing, multilevel involvement, and kyphosis are also demonstrated and are particularly well seen on multiplanar reconstructions.[4,26]

Computed tomography can also show small amount of calcification not visible on plain radiographs **(Fig. 13)**.[28]

Fat planes around the vertebral body are obliterated early in the course of abscess formation.[4] Soft tissue abscesses are well-demonstrated on axial scans and multi-planar reconstructions.[4,13] These have been characterized by their CT attenuation values with granulation tissue showing high attenuation while abscesses appear as low density lesions with thick a hyperdense rim representing the wall of the inflammatory cavity. Rim enhancement surrounding the low attenuation collection is seen. This is also called the "*rind sign*".[6] Granulation tissue shows a more homogeneous enhancement **(Figs. 14A and B)**. CT can also demonstrate epidural extension of these soft tissue masses with cord compression but these changes are best delineated on MR.

The combination of a multilocular and calcified paraspinal abscess with thick enhancing rim along with vertebral body fragmentation strongly favors tuberculous rather than pyogenic infection or neoplasm. CT though not always pathognomonic, facilitates CT-guided FNA/biopsy so that histo/cytopathological, or microbiological diagnosis can be established.[4,21,53-55]

Magnetic Resonance Imaging

The involved vertebrae show marrow signal alteration appearing hypointense on T1W and relatively hyperintense on T2W images. Loss of cortical definition of the affected vertebrae may also be seen.[4,50] Intervertebral disc is involved in 46–72% of cases though relatively later than pyogenic spondylitis. The internuclear cleft within the disc is a normal finding in patients older than 30 years, and its loss on imaging, in combination with a high-signal intensity, is sign of discitis **(Figs. 15A and B)**.[4,45] In children, the hydrated discs do not form a good barrier to infection and are involved in most patients imaged.[26] Occasionally, the disc space is preserved despite extensive bone destruction, the so-called *floating disc sign*. Involvement of the neural arch is also detected well by MRI **(Fig. 16)**. Enhanced MR studies may demonstrate inhomogeneous enhancement in the region of marrow infiltration.

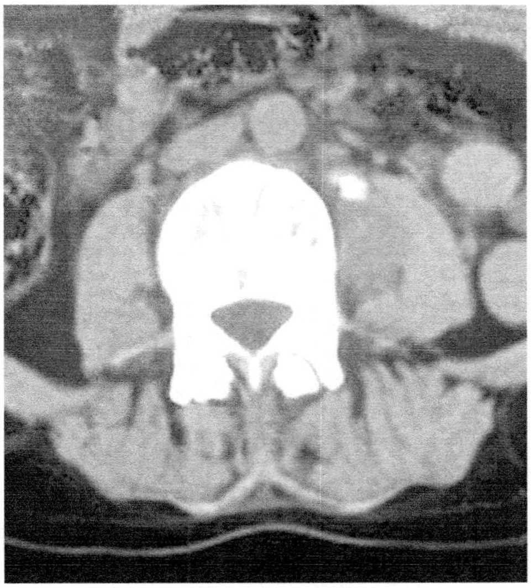

Fig. 13: Axial CT section showing a left psoas abscess with a small speck of calcification.

Paraspinal soft tissue masses are seen in approximately 71% of cases on MRI.[56] On T1W images loss of the uniform psoas muscle signal intensity and enlargement of the affected muscle is seen while on T2W images there is an increase in signal intensity **(Fig. 17)**. Postcontrast studies reveal thick rim enhancement around intraosseous and paraspinal soft tissue abscesses **(Fig. 18)**. More uniform enhancement is seen with granulation tissue or phlegmon.[4,44,56,57] MR is useful in delineating the communication between vertebral and paravertebral components of abscesses with epidural extension being seen 61% of involved vertebrae[45,56] The soft tissue masses displace the thecal sac and the spinal cord is distorted. Postcontrast fat suppressed T1W sequences are the best to demonstrate meningeal and epidural inflammatory soft tissues, with improved definition of cord and nerve root compromise **(Figs. 19A and B)**.[15] Heavily T2W fast spin-echo sequences can also be applied to generate myelographic images showing thecal sac compression.[56]

Disruption of the endplate reportedly has high sensitivity and specificity for diagnosis of spinal tuberculosis,[58] i.e., 100% and 81.4%, respectively. Other features with high sensitivity and specificity include paravertebral soft tissue shadow (96.8% and 85.3%) and a high-signal intensity of the intervertebral disc on the T2W image (80.6% and 82.4%). The overall sensitivity and specificity for diagnosis are 100% and 88.2%, respectively.

Cord Changes

Conventional radiographs provide little information if any, on the status of the cord which is inadequately assessed on

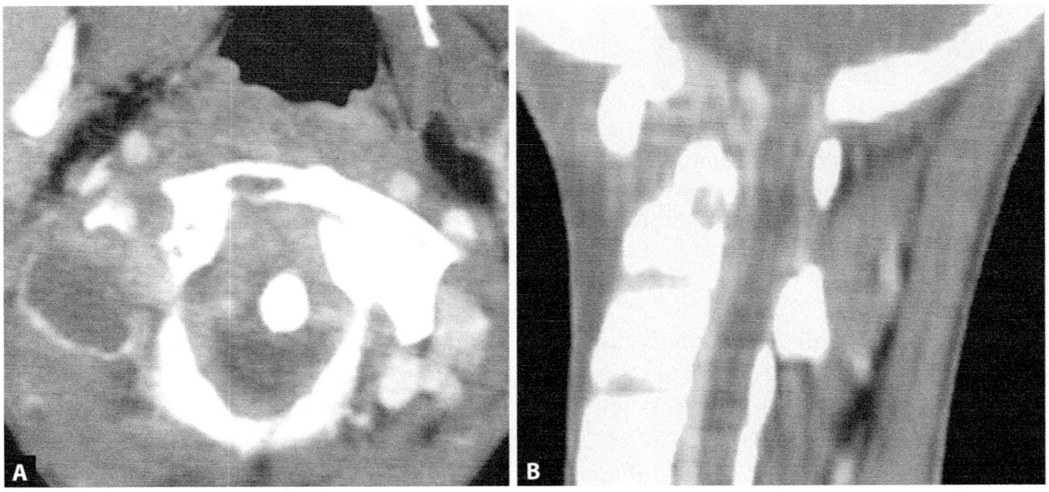

Figs. 14A and B: Axial postcontrast CT myelogram (A) with sagittal multiplanar reconstruction (B) in a patient with caries C1-C2 showing atlantoaxial dislocation with erosions of the right lateral mass of C1 and the dens. A peripherally enhancing abscess is noted on the right side while homogeneously enhancing granulation tissue is seen in the predental space.

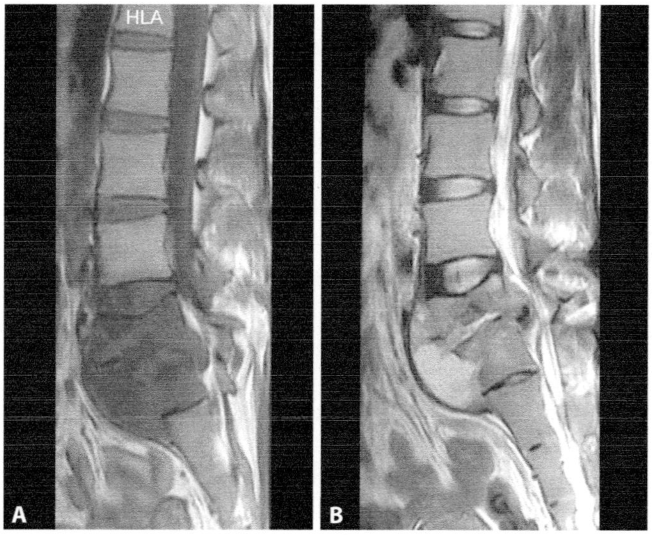

Figs. 15A and B: Sagittal T1W (A) and T2W (B) MR scans of a patient with tuberculosis L5-S1 show collapse of L5 vertebral body, hypointense marrow signal of L5-S1 and loss of cortical definition on the T1W image. The intervening disc space is reduced with hyperintense signal on the T2W image suggesting discitis. A prevertebral abscess lifting up the anterior longitudinal ligament and a small ventral epidural collection are also seen.

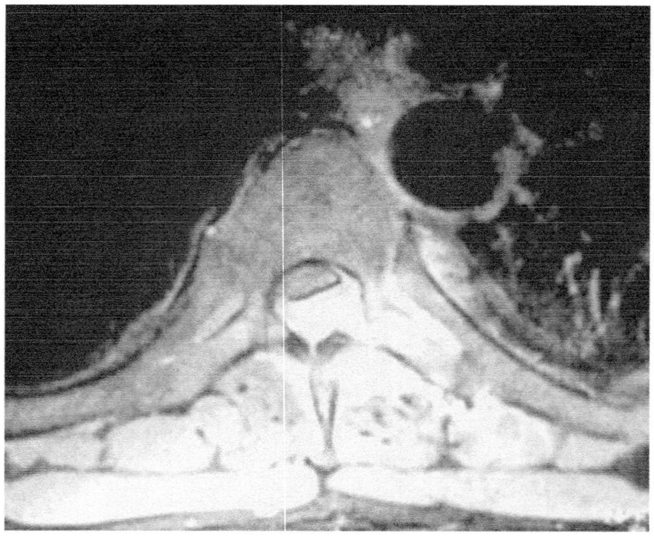

Fig. 16: Postcontrast T1W fat suppressed axial MR section through a thoracic vertebra showing patchy enhancement in the left pedicle, lamina, transverse process, and the adjacent rib. Homogeneously enhancing granulation tissue is noted in the left paraspinal region and dorsal epidural space displacing the cord anteriorly—neural arch tuberculosis.

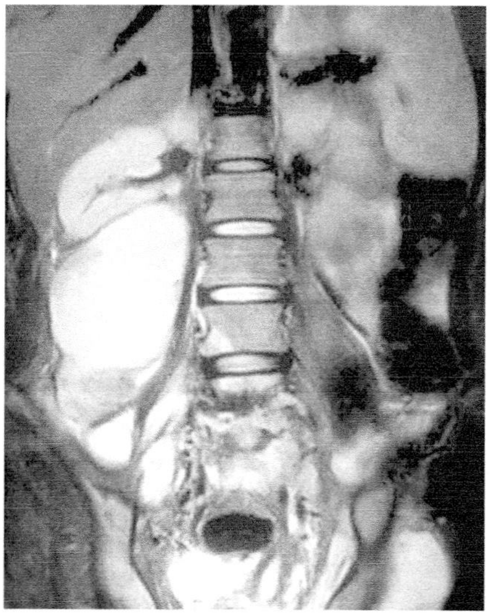

Fig. 17: STIR coronal scan in a patient with lumbosacral caries depicts partial collapse and hyperintense signal involving L4-L5 vertebrae. There is a disproportionately large psoas abscess on the right side lifting up the inferior pole of right kidney.

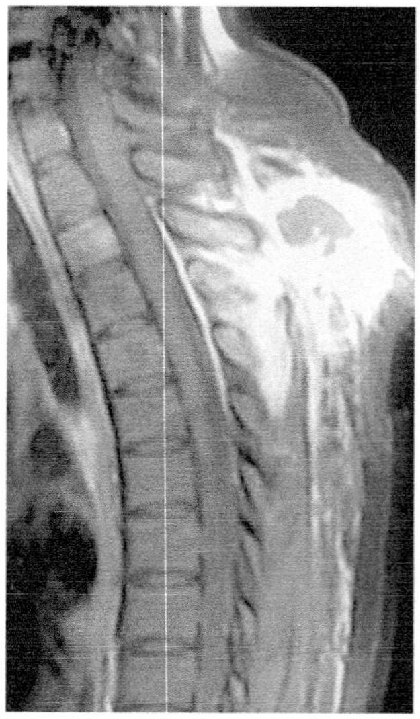

Fig. 18: Postcontrast T1W sagittal MR image of a patient with caries spine showing erosion of the spinous process of D3 vertebra with a large abscess showing thick peripheral rim enhancement.

CT as well. MRI, on the other hand because of its superior soft tissue contrast is the technique of choice to assess the cord. Cord changes may result in neurological deficit or paraplegia.

Paraplegia in patients with *active disease*—tubercular abscesses, granulation tissue, debris, internal gibbus, or subluxation may cause cord compression due to *mechanical pressure*. The spinal cord may be able with stand some degree of pressure, especially when it develops slowly as in tuberculosis. It is reported that good cord function may be seen even with 40–50% decrease in cord diameter. The midsagittal cord diameter and presence of cerebrospinal fluid (CSF) signal anterior to cord at the apex of the deformity at presentation have been shown to correlate with neurological deficit. Ambulatory patients had greater cord dimensions and CSF signal persisting

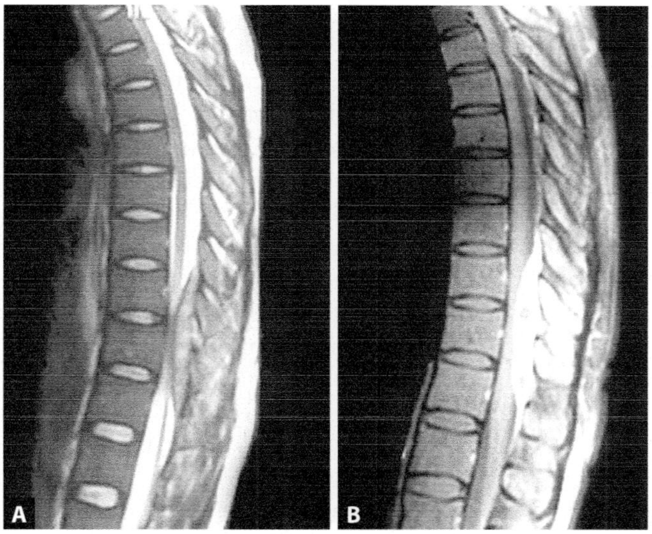

Figs. 19A and B: Sagittal T2W (A) and postcontrast fat suppressed T1W (B) MR images in a patient with neural arch tuberculosis D-L spine show nearly homogeneously enhancing dorsal epidural granulation tissue with resultant cord compression. Note the abnormal enhancement in the adjacent spinous processes and interspinous region.

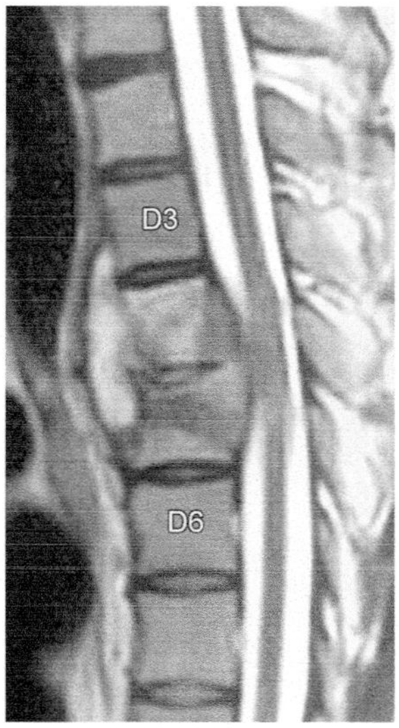

Fig. 20: Sagittal T2W MR image of the cervicodorsal spine in a patient of caries D4-D5 shows reduction in disc space with altered marrow signal in the involved vertebrae and associated prevertebral and ventral epidural collections. The cord is mildly expanded at this level with T2 hyperintense signal due to cord edema.

anterior to cord at the apex of the deformity in this study.[59] Unrelieved compression of the spinal cord results in loss of neurons, gliosis, and demyelination of cord substance in the damaged segment.

Intrinsic changes in the spinal cord may also lead to paraplegia. Spinal cord may show edema, myelomalacia, or syringomyelia **(Fig. 20)**. Edema is seen as hyperintense signal on T2W images but no signal alteration on T1 while myelomalacia shows a T1 hypointense signal (higher than that of CSF) as well and may be associated with thinning of the cord. A syrinx is a tubular, well-defined fluid-filled region within the spinal cord with tapered ends and may be septated. The signal characteristics of a syrinx are typically those of CSF. Edema of the cord is associated with good recovery of neurological function following treatment, while a poor outcome is likely when there is syrinx or myelomalacia. Rarely a small tuberculoma of the cord may be responsible for neurological deficits presenting as spinal tumor syndrome **(Figs. 21A and B)**.[60] Mild atrophy of the cord may persist following treatment even with good neurological outcome.[26,60]

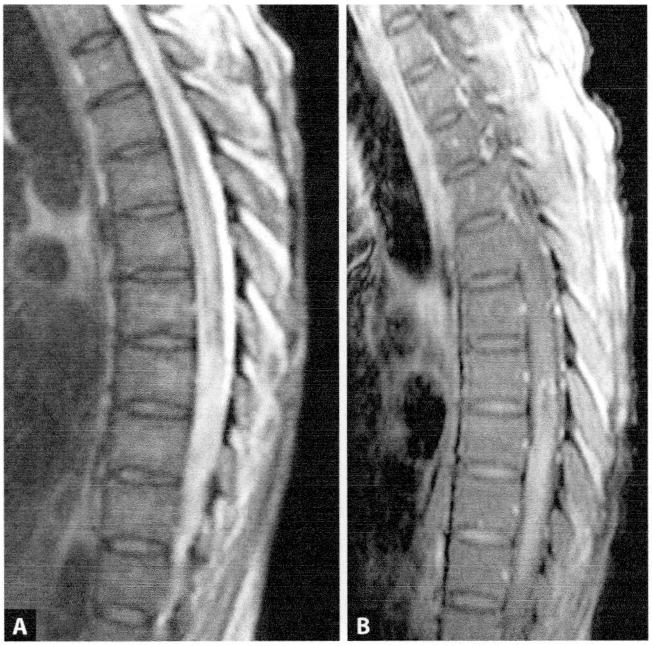

Figs. 21A and B: T2W (A) and postcontrast T1W (B) sagittal images of a patient with tubercular myelitis reveal cord swelling and edema appearing hyperintense on the T2W image with patchy enhancement on the postcontrast image.

According to some authors, MR findings may also be a useful guide to treatment strategy. When MR shows a predominantly fluid collection in the extradural space, compressing the cord with evidence of myelitis or edema only, a good response to conservative treatment is seen. If the extradural compression is due to granulation tissue with little fluid, early surgical decompression may be beneficial.[21] *Paraplegia* with *healed disease*[21] may occur when the initial lesion has healed with a residual severe deformity, even after a gap of 10–20 years. It is produced by stretching of the spinal cord over an internal anterior bony projection, producing gliosis. MRI shows severe atrophy of the cord and/or syringohydromyelia, or constricting scarring of and around the dura **(Figs. 22A and B)**. Symptomatic severe stenosis of the lumbar canal and ossification of the ligamentum flavum adjacent to severe

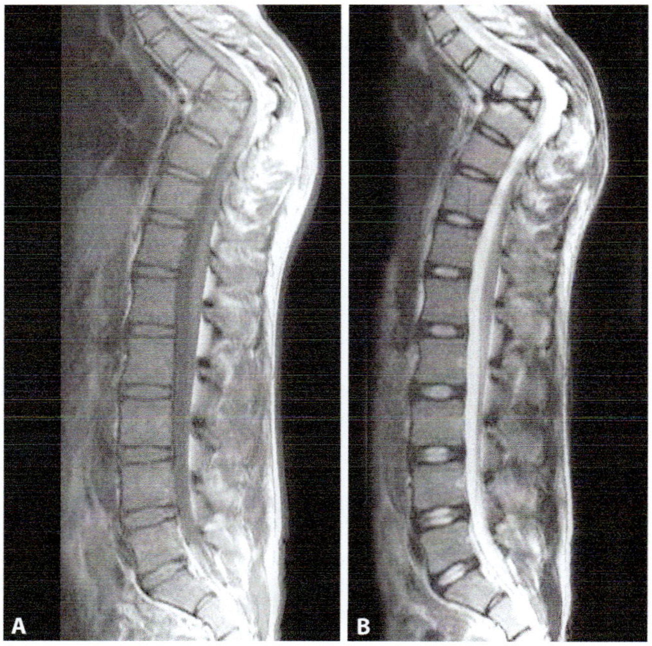

Figs. 22A and B: T1W (A) and T2W (B) images of the dorsolumbar spine in an old treated case of tuberculosis spine reveal near complete destruction of D8 vertebra and partial destruction of the adjacent D7 and D9 with fatty marrow signal and gross kyphotic deformity. There is resultant stretching and thinning of the cord but no signal change suggestive of cord atrophy. Note the fibrofatty proliferation along the dorsal epidural space appearing hyperintense on both T1W and T2W images.

kyphosis may produce an incomplete neurological deficit. Reactivation of the disease is found in 30–40% of old cases on exploration.

ATYPICAL SPINAL TUBERCULOSIS[21]

The classical paradiscal tubercular lesion is easily recognized and treated. Atypical spinal tuberculosis is defined as compressive myelopathy with no visible or palpable spinal deformity and without the radiological appearance of a typical vertebral lesion. Such lesions are not only infrequent, but also difficult to diagnose in the early stages with more chance of neurological complications. Atypical lesions may present as an intraspinal tubercular granuloma, involvement of the neural arch, compressive myelopathy in single vertebral disease, a concertina collapse of a vertebra, or a sclerotic vertebra. Granulomatous lesions of the epidural, intradural, or intramedullary spaces present as a compressive myelopathy, the *spinal tumor syndrome*, without obvious radiological signs. Tubercular granuloma should be considered in the differential diagnosis of spinal tumor syndrome in zones endemic for tuberculosis.

Extraosseous extradural granuloma is a rare variant that leads to an extradural granulomatous lesion in the absence of bone involvement. The route of infection is most likely hematogenous. It is more common in men than women, and usually involves the dorsal epidural space in the thoracic region. Clinically, there are features of compressive radiculomyelopathy. On pathologic examination, a granulomatous membrane is found ensheathing and compressing the spinal cord or cauda equina.[6] MR shows the pathology well. The lesion is T1 isointense and shows mixed signal on T2W images. Uniform enhancement is seen, if the inflammatory tissue is phlegmonous while rim enhancement is seen, if abscess formation or caseation has occurred **(Figs. 23A to C)**.[5] Epidural tuberculous abscess may also be seen in along with arachnoiditis, myelitis, intramedullary tuberculoma, etc.[61]

Post-treatment Follow-up

Conventional Radiographs

While on treatment, sequential radiographs can be repeated to assess the degree of healing. However, radiological evidence of healing is evident late on radiographs. It lags behind by about 3 months.[21] Evidence of bone destruction or loss of vertebral height may progress up to 14 months after treatment initiation and should not necessarily be considered a poor response.[62] Soft tissue paravertebral masses may also progress while on treatment reaching a maximum size within 1.5 months, and may take up to 15 months to resolve. Although MRC trials (multicenter randomized controlled trials of Medical Research Council, UK) have shown persistent changes in plain radiological appearances of the vertebral column up to 3 years after completion of treatment, these changes were attributed to new bone formation and ankylosis.[63] Signs of healing include the lesion remaining static or regressing on serial radiographs, better definition of lesion margin, and sclerosis **(Fig. 24)**. Increased density of the vertebral body with healing can lead to the appearance of an ivory vertebra. The phenomenon is usually seen in the lumbar region **(Fig. 25)**.[6] Calcific debris which progresses to fusion on serial films may be seen in 3 weeks, although it can take up to 27 months for any evidence of fusion to appear.[62] Fusion of contiguous vertebrae is generally regarded as the surest sign of healing tuberculosis although there is no actual proof of this **(Fig. 26)**.[62]

The healed status of disease or end point of treatment is not clearly defined for tuberculosis. Clinical and radiological evidence of healing with no recurrence after 2 years is generally referred to as "healed status."[21] It is, however, well known that reactivation of disease may occur years later.

Computed Tomography

Features of resolution such as increase in vertebral bone density, with reduction in the size of paraspinal soft tissue

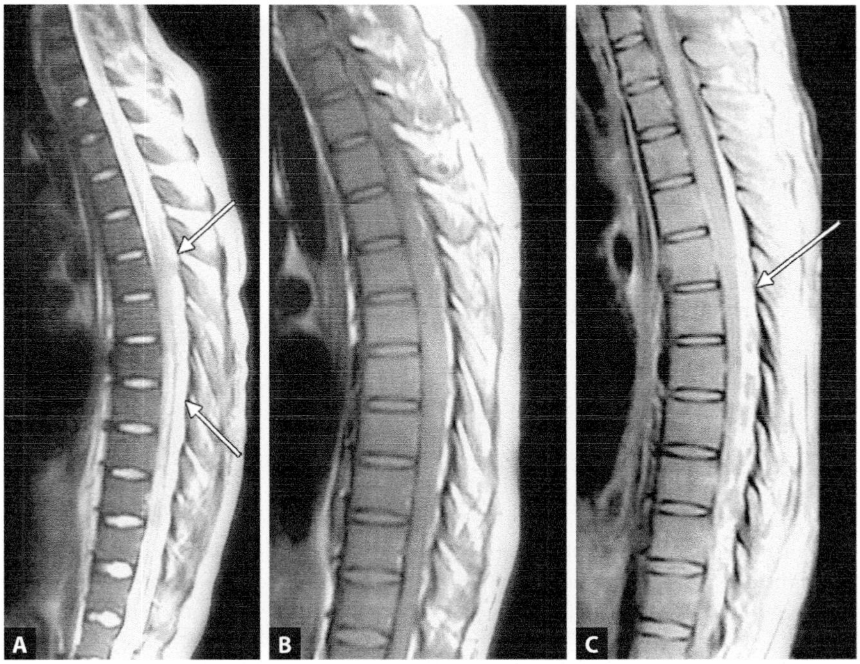

Figs. 23A to C: Extraosseous extradural granuloma: Sagittal T2W (A), T1W (B), and postcontrast (C) MR images show normal vertebral and intervertebral disc morphology and signal intensity pattern. A long segment, crescentic dorsal epidural abscess showing heterogeneous signal on T1W and T2W images with irregular peripheral contrast enhancement (arrows) causing anterior displacement of thecal sac is seen.

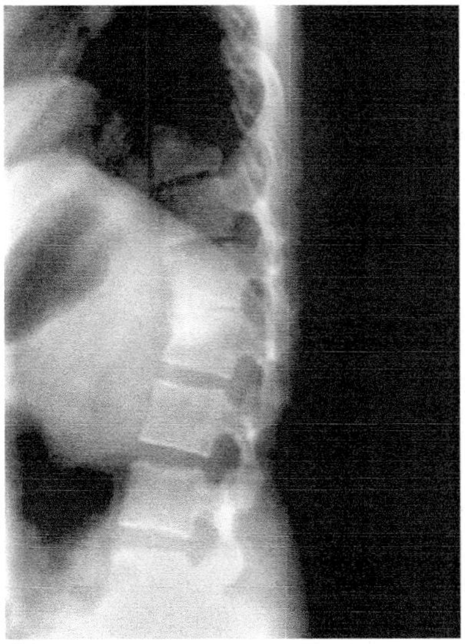

Fig. 24: Lateral radiograph D-L spine in a case of healing tuberculosis shows reduced disc space between D12 and L1 vertebrae with sclerosis adjacent to the vertebral end plates.

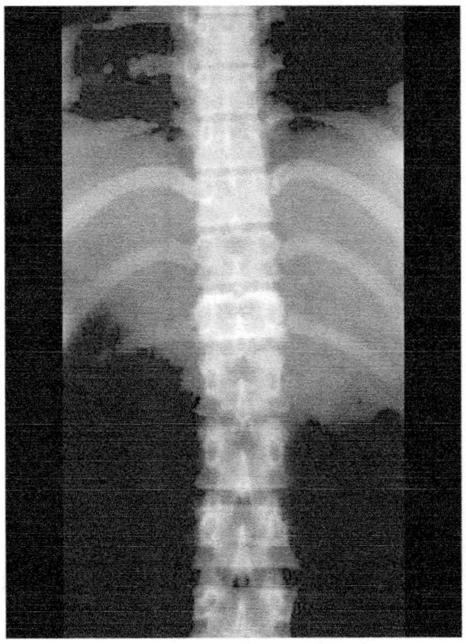

Fig. 25: X-ray D-L spine AP view showing sclerosis of D12 vertebra giving the appearance of ivory vertebra in a patient with healing caries.

masses as edema and inflammatory exudate subside are readily apparent on sequential CT examinations.[4] The inflammatory reaction in the bone marrow, however, is not well depicted **(Figs. 27A and B)**.[28]

Magnetic Resonance Imaging[40,47,56,64,65]

Post-therapy follow-up can also be done with MR. The earliest sign of healing is a reduction in the amount of soft tissue masses or collections. However, enlargement of the soft tissue mass or bone destruction does not indicate failed treatment. A high-signal intensity rim on the T1W sequences at the edge of the osseous lesion represents healing **(Fig. 28)**. A progressive sequential increase in signal intensity on T1W image is apparent with resolution **(Fig. 29)**. Reduction in gadolinium enhancement and eventual loss of enhancement are useful signs of healing.

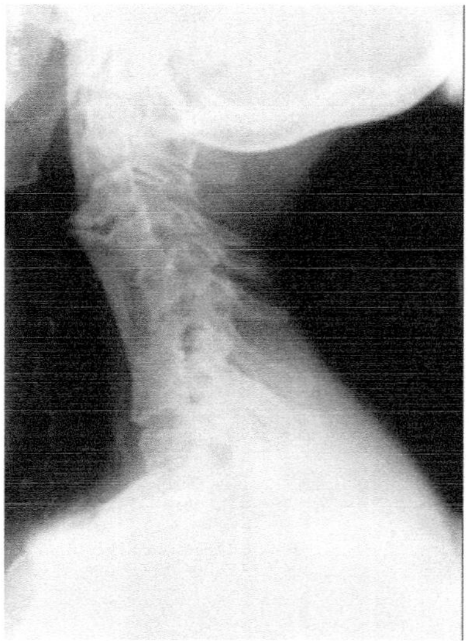

Fig. 26: Lateral radiograph of the cervical spine shows fusion of multiple cervical vertebral forming a large osseous block in a patient with healed tuberculosis of the cervical spine.

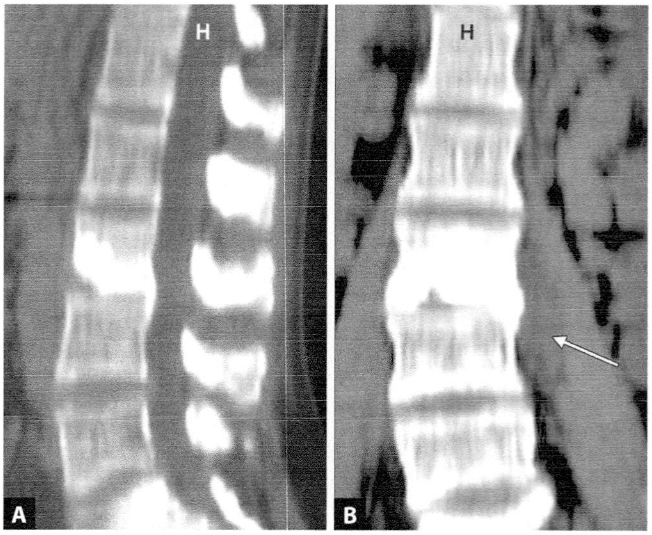

Figs. 27A and B: Sagittal and coronal CT reconstructions of the lumbar spine of a patient on anti-tubercular treatment (ATT) showing sclerosis of the inferior body and end plate of L1 vertebra with reduced L1-L2 disc space suggestive of healing disease.

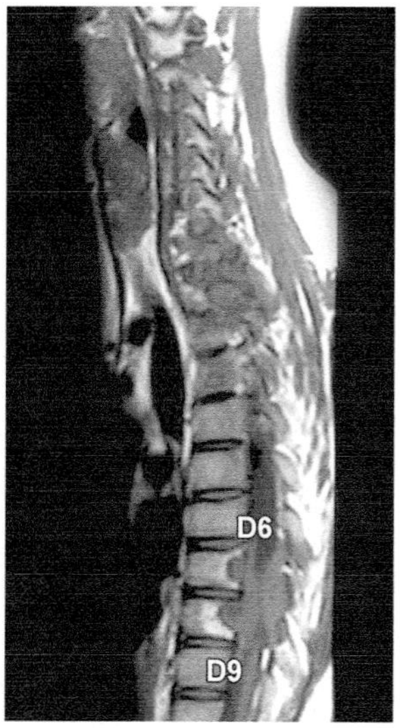

Fig. 28: Sagittal T1W MR image of the cervicodorsal spine of a patient after 3 months of ATT shows erosions of the posterior cortex of D7-D8 vertebrae. These lesions show marginal hyperintense signal signifying healing lesions.

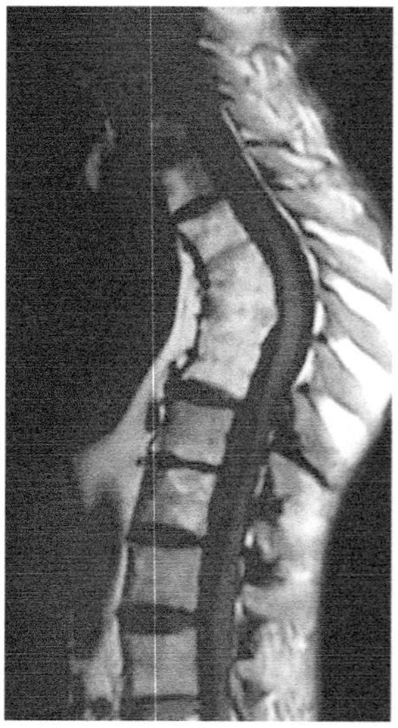

Fig. 29: Sagittal T1W MR image of the dorsal spine in a patient with healed caries spine shows kyphosis with complete absence of disc space between multiple dorsal vertebrae which appear hyperintense on the T1W image due to fatty replacement.

However, persistent or even increasing enhancement does not necessarily indicate worsening or treatment failure. MRI is also useful in the detection of reactivation of old tubercular spondylitis. The change of signal from low signal in healed tuberculosis to high signal on T2W images suggests active disease. Reactivation may present with an isolated psoas abscess without evidence of bony lesions.

The question whether treatment end point should be determined based on MR findings remains controversial. A significant proportion of patients may have radiological evidence of persistent disease activity in the form of discitis, vertebral body abscess, marrow edema, or multifocal intraosseous abscess with persistent cord compression after 6 months of treatment. Both the British and American Thoracic Societies, based on the evidence of the MRC trials, advocate short course chemotherapy (6 months) for adult uncomplicated fully sensitive spinal tuberculosis. However, the authors felt that in a significant proportion of patients, longer durations of treatment (more than 6 months) may be required as their MR scans were abnormal even though there was apparent disease resolution clinically. Other authors have suggested that the persistence of MRI abnormalities after 12 months of treatment does not require further treatment in patients with good clinical and laboratory outcome. MRI alone should not determine when treatment should be stopped. Repeat MRI is probably not necessary in patients who have a clinical and laboratory improvement during treatment.

Although these studies have evaluated only a limited number of patients they highlight the fact that there are currently no universally accepted guidelines, more studies need to be performed to achieve consensus on the interpretation and use of this powerful modality in the follow-up of spinal tuberculosis patients.

Positron Emission Tomography/ Computed Tomography[66-68]

^{18}F-fluorodeoxyglucose-PET may be useful for discriminating residual and nonresidual spinal infection after treatment healed disease demonstrates absence of uptake. In a recent study, both contrast-enhanced MR and FDG-PET were used for follow-up, with treatment being continued till contrast enhancement or FDG uptake was negative suggestive of healed status. ^{18}F-FDG-PET was considered to be better at demonstrating healed status than MRI.

DIFFERENTIAL DIAGNOSIS

The differential diagnosis of tubercular spondylodiscitis includes pyogenic and fungal infections, degenerative disc disease, brucellosis, neoplasms, etc.

Clinically patients of *degenerative spondylosis* present with radicular pain and no systemic symptoms, but vertebral infection with radicular pain may be misdiagnosed as degenerative disease, if the patient is afebrile. With degenerative disease, the disc space is usually not markedly narrowed, bone density and end plate definition are preserved. On MR disc desiccation produces a low signal on T2W images unlike discitis which is bright. After intravenous contrast infected discs enhance strongly whereas degenerated discs only occasionally minimally.[17]

When infection is considered, a history of chronicity and insidious progression suggests tubercular rather than *pyogenic infection*. In tuberculosis, osteoporosis with absence of sclerosis is seen on plain films. Involvement of multiple contiguous vertebrae, the entire vertebral body, loss of cortical definition, more frequent involvement of posterior elements, disproportionally large paraspinal masses, especially with calcification or a thick rim of enhancement, subligamentous spread to three or more vertebral levels, and presence of skip lesions favor a tubercular etiology. Disc involvement is said to occur later in tuberculosis as compared to pyogenic infections. However, differentiation from pyogenic infection can at times be difficult.[1,17]

Brucellosis is an indolent infection such as tuberculosis. Typically brucellar spondylitis is common in the lower lumbar spine, with minimal paraspinal soft tissue masses, no gibbus deformity, and presence of gas within the disc. On MR images, vertebral body morphology and cortical margins are maintained despite evidence of osteomyelitis.

Sarcoidosis can produce findings identical to those of tuberculosis including multifocal vertebral lesions with paraspinal masses.[1]

When a solitary vertebra is involved, differentiation from *metastatic disease* in adults and from *eosinophilic granuloma* in children may be difficult. Spinal lesions, such as *lymphoma,* that affect consecutive vertebrae or neoplasms, such as *multiple myeloma* and *chordoma,* that involve contiguous vertebrae and discs can add to the diagnostic difficulty.[1,2,4] *Bizarre infections* such as fungal disease and spinal echinococcosis cannot be easily distinguished from tuberculosis or neoplasms.

The morphologic and pathophysiologic changes encountered in spinal tuberculosis are the most severe among infective spondylitides and are also the most varied. Conventional radiographs are the usual initial imaging investigation. However, early in the disease and in atypical cases such as isolated NAT, plain films may be negative and if the clinical suspicion of tubercular infection is strong MRI which is the modality of choice should be considered. The wider availability of CT, high sensitivity and ability to assist in diagnosis by accurately targeting lesions for guided biopsy make it a useful alternative diagnostic tool for early diagnosis when MR is not available.

A delay in diagnosis may lead to irreversible neurologic sequelae and spinal deformity in a high percentage of cases. Hence, a multidisciplinary approach to tubercular spondylitis is essential to ensure prompt assessment of the location, extent and character of spinal pathology to positively affect the clinical management in a timely fashion.

REFERENCES

1. Yao DC, Sartoris ADJ. Musculoskeletal tuberculosis. Radiol Clin N Am. 1995;35(4):679-89.
2. Moore SL, Rafi M. Imaging of musculoskeletal and spinal tuberculosis. Radiol Clin N Am. 2001;39(2):329-42.
3. Pott P. Remarks on that kind of palsy of the lower limbs which is frequently found to accompany a curvature of the spine. London: J Johnson; 1779.
4. Sharif HAS, Morgan JL, al Shahed MS, al Thagafi MY. Role of CT and MR imaging in the management of tuberculous spondylitis. Radiol Clin N Am. 1995;33(4):787-804.
5. Gupta RK. Tuberculosis and other non-tuberculous bacterial granulomatous infections. In: Gupta RK, Lufkin RB (Eds). MR Imaging and Spectroscopy of Central Nervous System Infection. United States: Kluwer Academic/Plenum Publishers; 2001. pp. 95-146.

6. Resnick D. Osteomyelitis, septic arthritis and soft tissue infection: mechanism and situations. In: Resnick D (Ed). Diagnosis of Bone and Joint Disorder, 4th edition. Philadelphia: WB Saunders; 2002. pp. 2377-480.
7. Bhan S, Nag HL. Skeletal tuberculosis. In: Sharma SK, Mohan A (Eds). Tuberculosis. New Delhi: Jaypee Brothers Medical Publishers; 2001. pp. 237-60.
8. Hsu LC, Leong JC. Tuberculosis of the lower cervical spine C2-C7. J Bone Joint Surg Br. 1984;66(1):1-5.
9. Martin NS. Tuberculosis of the spin: A study of results of treatment during the east twenty-five years. J Bone Joint Surg Br. 1970;53:613.
10. Fang D, Leong JCY, Fang HSV. Tuberculosis of the upper cervical spine. J Bone Joint Surg Br. 1983;65(1):47-50.
11. Lal AP, Rajshekar V, Chandy M. Management strategies in tuberculous atlantoaxial dislocation. Br J Neurosurg. 1992;6:529-35.
12. Tuli SM. Tuberculosis of the craniovertebral region. Clin Orthop Res. 1974;104:209-12.
13. Jain R, Sawhney S, Berry M. Computed tomography of vertebral tuberculosis: patterns of bone destruction clinical radiology. 1993;47:196-9.
14. Chapman M, Murray RO, Stoker DT. Tuberculosis of the bones and joints. Semin Roentgenol. 1979;14:266-82.
15. Weaver P, Lifeso RM. The radiological diagnosis of tuberculosis of the adult spine. Skeleltal Radiol. 1984;12:178-88.
16. Kahn DS, Pritzker KPH. Pathophysiology of Bone infection. Clin Orthop. 1973;96:12-9.
17. Sharif HA, Aideyan OA, Clark DC, Madkour MM, Aabed MY, Mattsson TA, et al. Brucellar and tuberculous spondylitis: Comparative imaging features. Radiology. 1989;155:419-25.
18. Golding FC. Tuberculosis of Bone. In: Shanks CS Kerly P (Eds). A Textbook of X-ray Diagnosis by British Authors, 3rd edition; London: H.K.Lewis & Co. Ltd.; 1959. pp. 274-89.
19. Jalleh RD, Kuppuswamy L, Mahayiddin AA, Acob MF, Yusuf NA, Mokhtar A. Spinal tuberculosis—A five year review of cases at the National Tuberculosis Centre. Med J Malaya. 1991;46:269-73.
20. Fam AG, Rubenstein J. Another Look at spinal tuberculosis. J Rheumatol. 1993;20:1731.
21. Jain AK. Afresh look at an old disease. J Bone Joint Surg [Br]. 2010;92-B:905-13.
22. Negi SS, Khan SF, Gupta S, et al. Comparison of the conventional diagnostic modalities, baltec culure and polymerase chain reaction test for diagnosis of tuberculosis. Indian J Med Microbiol. 2005;23:29-33.
23. Jain AK, Jena SK, Singh M, Dhammi IK, Ramachadran VG, Dev G. Evaluation of clinico-radiological, bacteriological, serological, molecular and histological diagnosis of osteoarticular tuberculosis. Indian J Orthop. 2008;42:173-7.
24. Tuli SM. Tuberculosis of the spine: a historical review. Clin Orthop. 2007;460:29-38.
25. Burrill J, Williams CJ, Bain G, Conder G, Hine AL, Misra RR. Tuberculosis: A radiologic review. Radiographics. 2007;27:1255-73.
26. Pandit HG, Sonsale PD, Shikare SS, Bhojraj SY. Bone scintigraphy in tuberculous spondylodiscitis. Eur Spin J. 1999;8:205-9.
27. Desai S. Early diagnosis of spinal tuberculosis by MRI. J Bone Joint Surg Br. 1994;76:863-9.
28. Nocera RM, Sayle B, Rogers C, Wilkey D. Tc 99m MDP and indium 111 chloride scintigraphy in skeletal tuberculosis. Clin Nucl Med. 1983;8:418-20.
29. Lifeso RM, Weaver P, Harder E. Tuberculous spondylitis in adults. J Bone Joint Surg Am. 1985;67:1405-13.
30. Kaila R, Malhi AM, Mahmood B, Saifuddin A. The incidence of multiple level noncontiguous vertebral tuberculosis detected using whole spine MRI. J Spinal Disord Tech. 2007;20(1):78-81.
31. Stabler A, Reiser MF. Imaging of spinal infection. Radiol Clin N Am. 2001;39(1):115-35.
32. Sharif HA, Clark DC, Aabed MY, Haddad MC, al Deeb SM, Yaqub B, et al. Granulomatous spinal infections MR imaging. Radiology. 1990;177:101-7.
33. Palle L, Reddy MB, Reddy KJ. Role of magnetic resonance diffusion imaging and apparent diffusion coefficient values in the evaluation of spinal tuberculosis in Indian patients. Indian J Radiol Imaging. 2010;20(4):279-83.
34. Pui MH, Mitha A, Rae WI, Corr P. Diffusion-weighted magnetic resonance imaging of spinal infection and malignancy. J Neuroimaging. 2005;15(2):164-7.
35. Gupta RK, Agarwal P, Rastogi H, Kumar S, Phadke RV, Krishnani N. Problems in differentiating spinal tuberculosis from neoplasm on MRI. Neuroradiology. 1996;38:S97-104.
36. Alavi A, Lakhani P, Mavi A, Kung JW, Zhuang H. PET: a revolution in medical imaging. Radiol Clin North Am. 2004;42:983-1001.
37. Andronikou S, Bindapersad M, Govender N, Waner JI, Segwe A, Palliam S, et al. Musculoskeletal tuberculosis-imaging using low-end and advanced modalities for developing and developed countries. Acta Radiol. 2011;52(4):430-41.
38. Buxi TB. Computed tomography in spinal tuberculosis. Ind J Radiol Imag. 1993;3:291-3.
39. Maiuri F, Iaconetta G, Gallicchio B, et al. Spondylodiscitis clinical and magnetic resonance diagnosis. Spine. 1997;22:1741-6.
40. Sharif HA. Role of MR imaging in the management of spinal infections. AJR Am J Roentgenol. 1992;158:1333-45.
41. Harkirat S, Anand SS, Indrajit IK, Dash AK. Pictorial essay: PET/CT in tuberculosis. Indian J Radiol Imaging. 2008;18(2):141.
42. D'Souza MM, Sharma R, Tripathi M, Mondal A. F-18 Fluorodeoxyglucose positron emission tomography/ computed tomography in tuberculosis of the hip: A case report and brief review of literature. Indian J Nucl Med. 2011;26(1):31-3.
43. Hustinx R, Smith RJ, Benard F, Rosenthal DI, Machtay M, Farber LA, et al. Dual time point fluorine-18 fluorodeoxyglucose positron emission tomography: a potential method to differentiate malignancy from inflammation and normal tissue in the head and neck. Eur J Nucl Med. 1999;26(10):1345-8.
44. Zhuang H, Pourdehnad M, Lambright ES, Yamamoto AJ, Lanuti M, Li P, et al. Dual time point 18F-FDG PET imaging for differentiating malignant from inflammatory processes. J Nucl Med. 2001;42:1412-7.

45. Mendonca RA. Spinal infection and inflammatory disorders. In: Atlas SW (Ed). Magnetic Resonance Imaging of the Brain and Spine, 3rd edition. Philadelphia: Lippincot Williams and Wilkins; 2002. pp. 1855-972.
46. Rahman NU, Jamjoom A, Jamjoom ZA, Al-Tahan AM. Neural arch tuberculosis: Radiological features and their correlation with surgical findings. Br J Neurosurg. 1997;11(1):32-8.
47. Loke TK, Ma HT, Chan CS. Magnetic resonance imaging of tuberculous spinal infection. Australas Radiol. 1997;41: 7-12.
48. Kumar K. Clinical study and classification of posterior spinal tuberculosis. Int Orthop. 1985;9:147-52.
49. Raglan R, Abdelwahan F, Braffman B, Moss DS. Posterior spinal tuberculosis—a case report. Am J Neuroradiol. 1990;11:612-3.
50. Abdelwahan IF, Camins MB, Hermann G, Klein MJ. Vertebral arch or posterior spinal tuberculosis. Skeletal Radiol. 1997;26:737-40.
51. Rodriguez-Takeuchi SY, Renjifo ME, Medina FJ. Extrapulmonary tuberculosis: pathophysiology and imaging findings. Radiographics. 2019;39:2023-37.
52. Jacobs P, Renton P. Periosteal reaction; bone and joint infections; sarcoid. In: Sutton D (Ed). Textbook of Radiology and Medical Imaging, 4th edition. London: Churchill Livingstone; 1987. pp. 71-2.
53. Richards AS. Non-tuberculous pyogenic osteomyelitis of the spine. J Canadian Assoc Radiol. 1960;11:45-9.
54. Kang M, Gupta S, Khandelwal N, Shankar S, Gulati M, Suri S. CT-guided fine-needle aspiration biopsy of spinal lesions. Acta Radiol. 1999;40:474-8.
55. Mondal A, Misra DK. CT-guided needle aspiration cytology (FNAC) of 112 vertebrallesions. Indian J Pathol Microbiol. 1994;37:255-61.
56. Francis IM, Das DK, Luthra UK, Sheikh Z, Sheikh M, Bashir M. Value of radiologically guided fine needle aspiration cytology (FNAC) in the diagnosis of spinal tuberculosis: a study of 29 cases. Cytopathology. 1999;10:390-401.
57. Gouliamos AD, Kehasgias DT, Lahanis S, Athanassopoulou AA, Moulopoulou ES, Kalovidouris AA, et al. MR imaging of tuberculous vertebral osteomyelitis: Pictoral review Eur. Radiol. 2001;11:575-9.
58. Hong SH, Choi JY, Lee JW, Kim NR, Choi JA, Kang HS. MR imaging assessment of the spine: infection or an imitation? Radiographics. 2009;29:599-612.
59. Danchaivijitr N, Temram S, Thepmongkhol K, Chiewvit P. Diagnostic accuracy of MR imaging in tuberculous spondylitis. J Med Assoc Thai. 2007;90:1581-9.
60. Dunn R, Zondagh I, Candy S. Spinal tuberculosis: magnetic resonance imaging and neurological impairment. Spine (Phila Pa 1976). 2011;36(6):469-73.
61. Kumar R. Spinal tuberculosis: with reference to the children of northern India. Childs Nerv Syst. 2005;21(1):19-26.
62. Trivedi R, Saksena S, Gupta RK. Magnetic resonance imaging in central nervous system tuberculosis. Indian J Radiol Imaging. 2009;19(4):256-65.
63. Boxer DI, Pratt C, Hine AL, McNicol M. Radiological features during and following treatment of spinal tuberculosis. Br J Radiol. 1992;65:476-9.
64. A controlled trial of six-month and nine-month regimens of chemotherapy in patients undergoing radical surgery for tuberculosis of the spine in Hong Kong. Tenth report of the Medical Research Council Working Party on Tuberculosis of the Spine. Tubercle. 1986;67:243-59.
65. Kim SJ, Kim IJ, Suh KT, Kim YK, Lee JS. Prediction of residual disease of spine infection using F-18 FDG PET/CT. Spine. 2009;22(34):2424-30.
66. Cormican L, Hammal R, Messenger J, Milburn HJ. Current difficulties in the diagnosis and management of spinal tuberculosis. Postgrad Med J. 2006;82(963):46-51.
67. Le Page L, Feydy A, Rillardon L, Dufour V, Le Hénanff A, Tubach F, et al. Spinal tuberculosis: a longitudinal study with clinical, laboratory, and imaging outcomes. Semin Arthritis Rheum. 2006;36(2):124-9.
68. Mittal S, Jain AK, Chakraborti KL, Aggarwal AN, Upreti L, Bhayana H. Evaluation of healed status in tuberculosis of spine by fluorodeoxyglucose-positron emission tomography/computed tomography and contrast magnetic resonance imaging. Indian J Orthop. 2019;53(1):160-8.

CHAPTER

7

Nontubercular Infections of the Spine

Sameer Vyas, Manavjit Singh Sandhu, Ujjwal Gorsi

INTRODUCTION

Spinal infections result from several infectious pathologic agents, and have varied and nonspecific clinical presentations.[1-3] Although the spinal infections are rare, there is growing incidence of these due to many factors which make persons more vulnerable to the spinal infections, including immunodeficiency due to human immunodeficiency virus (HIV) infection, chronically debilitated conditions, old age, the extensive use of broad-spectrum antibiotics or corticosteroids and immunosuppressive drugs, parenteral alimentation, and intravenous (IV) drug abuse.[3] The recent developments of medical technologies help in the early detection and appropriate management of spinal infections. Though, these advancements have also increased the occurrence of spinal infections as there are more patients with iatrogenic immunosuppression, increased life expectancy of patients with chronic medical illnesses, and potential infectious complications from the complex spinal procedures. In this chapter, the pathogenesis of spinal infections including the vascular anatomy of the vertebrae, various routes of spread, and anatomic site involved are discussed briefly for better understanding patterns of the spinal infection.

PATHOGENESIS OF SPINAL INFECTIONS

Vascular Anatomy of Vertebrae

The pathogenesis of spinal infections can be explained on the basis of the vascular anatomy of the vertebrae and intervertebral discs.[4] Vertebrae are supplied by the paired segmental arteries which arise from the vertebral arteries, or the aorta, or the iliac arteries depending on the location of the vertebrae. These segmental arteries course along the vertebral body posteriorly, and give rise to multiple small extraosseous anastomotic branches. Each segmental artery gives rise to paired metaphyseal arteries and a single nutrient artery within a vertebral body. These branches are end arteries at the superior and inferior endplates of each vertebral body. The metaphyseal arteries also supply an intermetaphyseal anastomotic arterial network which extends to multiple vertebral body levels. There is significant change in the vasculature of the vertebral bodies and intervertebral discs with age. In children, this arterial network extends to the intervertebral disc and provides vascular supply whereas in adults, these channels involutes and the end arteries end at the superior and inferior endplates of the vertebral bodies. Due to these differences in vascular anatomy in children and adults, intervertebral discs are usually the first site of infection in children followed by involvement of metaphysis, and in adults, the endplates are involved initially followed by disc involvement. Due to multiple extraosseous and intermetaphyseal vascular channels, the spinal infections can extend to multiple vertebrae. The spinal infection can also spread by venous route as there are valveless veins which exit the vertebrae at the dorsal nutrient foramen and communicate with an extradural venous plexus and then drain into the paravertebral venous plexus of Batson. This venous route is responsible for the retrograde spread of infection from abdominal and pelvic organs.

Routes of Spread of the Spinal Infections

The spinal infections can occur principally by three routes of spread: (1) hematogenous route—the arterial route from distant septic foci is more common, though the infections can also spread by venous hematogenous route; (2) contiguous spread from surrounding infected organs such as the pharynx, thoracic or abdominal wall or pleural space of the lung; and (3) direct inoculation (iatrogenically during surgery or interventional procedures).[1,3] The most validated theory for the spinal infection is that it occurs from arterial hematogenous spread from infected microemboli which gets lodged in one of the metaphyseal arteries, causing infarction and resulting in infection. Spondylitis is most common at the endplates because of the more arteries in this region. Anterior subchondral vertebral region is the usual site of infection within the vertebra corresponding to the area rich in arterial supply.[3] The early infectious lesion occurs in the anterosuperior subchondral region of the vertebral body and subsequently extends through the endplate **(Fig. 1)**. Further dissemination may occur via subligamentous spread of infection with resulting anterior vertebral body

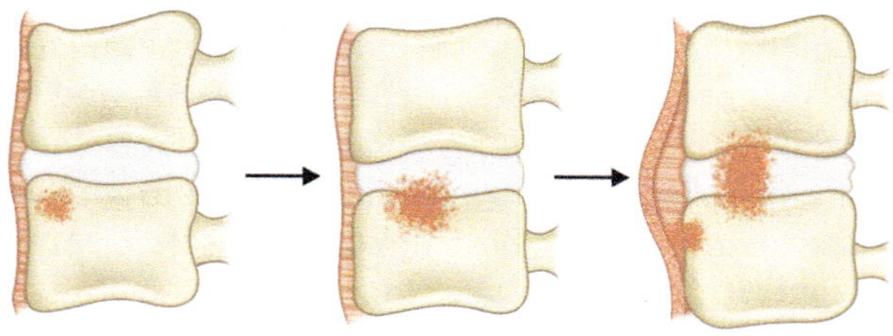

Fig. 1: Pathophysiology of vertebral osteomyelitis: the focus of infection usually begins in the anterosuperior subchondral region and subsequently extends to involve the adjacent disc and vertebral body. Anterior subligamentous spread may also occur.

scalloping or rupture of anterior longitudinal ligament. In children, the intervertebral discs receive nutrition by blood vessels that pass through the cartilaginous endplates of adjacent vertebral bodies. Hence, any infection involving the vertebral endplates easily extends to the adjacent disc space, whereas this is not so in the mature adult spine, where the nutrition of the nucleus pulposus occurs primarily by the process of diffusion. Iatrogenic spinal infections are responsible to 2.5% of all the spinal infections. The infection risk of open surgery is reported to be approximately 3–13%.[3] The spinal infections have also been described with radiological procedures such as myelography, discography, chemonucleolysis, vertebroplasty, and kyphoplasty.

Anatomic Sites of the Spinal Infections

Various anatomic sites involved include discs (discitis), vertebrae (spondylitis), discs and vertebral body (spondylodiscitis), facet joints, and epidural and paraspinal spaces (abscesses). Vertebral bodies and intervertebral discs are commonly involved with extension of the infection to epidural space, posterior elements, and paraspinal (paravertebral or psoas muscle and prevertebral space) soft tissues. Occurrence of the spinal infections in various sites is variable. The spondylodiscitis accounts for majority of all spine infections (95%), with nearly one-third of these cases are complicated by secondary epidural and paraspinal abscesses. Primary septic facet joints infections, isolated discitis, spondylitis, and primary epidural abscesses are less common.

IMAGING MODALITIES OF SPINAL INFECTIONS

The various imaging modalities available for evaluation of patients with suspected spinal infection are plain radiography, computed tomography (CT), and magnetic resonance imaging (MRI).[5-8] In these days, the use of myelography is obsolete and CT myelography is not the preferred imaging modality in patients with suspected spinal infection, though it may be very rarely used where MRI is unavailable or contraindicated. Nuclear medicine imaging studies are also useful in spinal infection.[9,10] A wise selection of the modalities is essential for timely patient management, as untreated spinal infections can lead to crippling and even life-threatening situations. Comparison of various imaging modalities in infections is illustrated in **Table 1**.

Table 1: Comparison of imaging modalities in spinal infections.

Imaging modality	*Advantages*	*Limitations*
Plain radiograph	Readily available and inexpensive	30–50% loss of bone density before becomes abnormal, poor sensitivity
CT	Detects bony changes and surrounding extent	Lacks sensitivity of MRI
MRI	Evaluation of the bone marrow and neural structures	Difficult to distinguish trauma or neoplasm from infection and new from old disease
Nuclear medicine imaging	Scans whole skeleton, sensitive earlier in disease than radiograph and CT	Expensive, long acquisition time, hard to distinguish overlying soft tissue infections

Plain Radiography

Plain radiographs are often done first in patients with suspected spinal pathology. Unfortunately, the changes on plain radiographs appear quite late (2–8 weeks) after the onset of infection. The plain radiographic features of spinal infection **(Figs. 2 to 4)** may include demineralization, loss of definition of endplate margins, narrowing of intervertebral disc space, associated soft tissue swelling (paraspinal or epidural soft tissue masses), and the finally the destruction of the vertebral endplate and the vertebral body (spinal deformity, frank vertebral destruction).[3] Paraspinal extension of the infective process may be appreciated as widened retropharyngeal or retrotracheal space in the cervical region, displacement of paraspinal lines in the dorsal region and evidence of unilateral or bilateral paravertebral psoas abscesses in the lumbar region. It is possible to suggest a positive diagnosis if changes are present on plain radiographs, however, there is a significant overlap of findings on radiographs between various infections. Atypical radiographic features at times make it difficult to differentiate infective spinal conditions from other noninfective causes such as spondylodiscitis degenerative changes and neoplastic diseases.

Healed or healing processes may be seen on plain radiographs as areas of sclerosis, reactive new bone formation, spur formation, bony bridging or vertebral fusion. Limitation of plain radiographs is most evident when it comes to differentiate between chronic vertebral osteomyelitis, discogenic degenerative endplate changes, and the presence of superimposed infection in the setting of chronic degenerative disc disease.

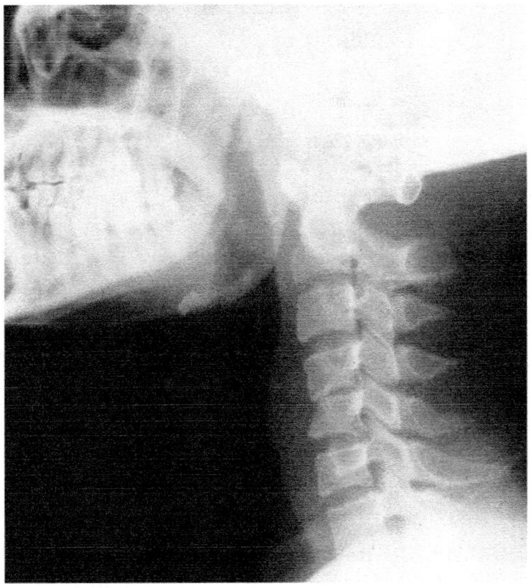

Fig. 2: Bacterial osteomyelitis involving the cervical vertebrae: plain X-ray cervical spine lateral view showing anterior erosion of C5 vertebra, prevertebral soft tissue mass and early loss of disc space height between C4 and 5.

Computed Tomography

Computed tomography entails a much better evaluation of the extent of bone destruction **(Figs. 5A and B)**. Involvement of vertebral body and the posterior elements is easily identified by cross-sectional imaging. In addition, CT also demonstrates destruction of disc space and presence of disc space gas. Identification of pre- or paravertebral soft tissue mass and extent of spread into the epidural space with subsequent thecal sac deformity can be well-appreciated on CT. Chronic stages of infection may reveal extensive osseous destruction, sequestrum, and marked heterotropic bone formation. Contrast-enhanced CT (CECT) allows better evaluation of the paravertebral abscesses with psoas involvement. CECT show peripheral enhancement of an epidural abscess causing compression and displacement of the dural sac. The use of multislice CT scans with reformatted images in the various planes depicts better delineation of the lesion extent. In addition to the diagnostic capabilities, CT and fluoroscopy can be used to guide various diagnostic [fine needle aspiration cytology (FNAC) or biopsy in patients of suspected spinal infections] and therapeutic procedures (percutaneous aspiration or catheter drainage of large paraspinal/psoas abscesses).

Magnetic Resonance Imaging

Magnetic resonance imaging is the imaging modality of choice for evaluating and characterizing the infective lesions of the spine because changes on MRI precede any other radiographic changes, detects marrow inflammation

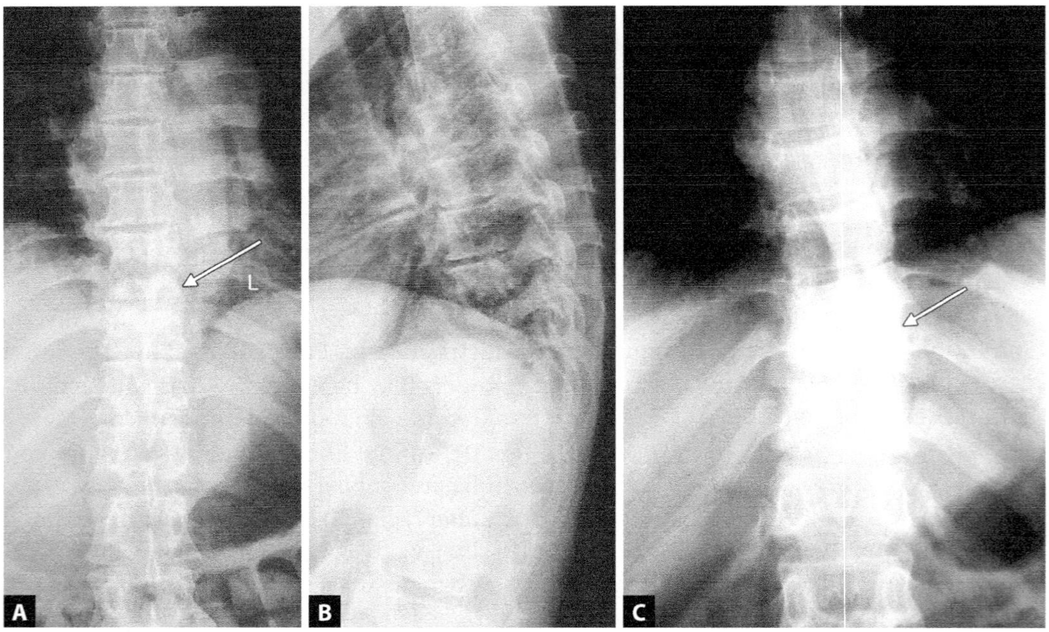

Figs. 3A to C: X-ray dorsal spine anteroposterior (A) and lateral view (B) showing contiguous endplate destruction at D8-9 intervertebral disc space and decrease in height of D9 vertebral body (arrow) features suggestive of pyogenic spondylodiscitis. The follow-up X-ray the dorsal spine anteroposterior view (C) demonstrating healing as evidenced by ankylosis of two adjacent vertebrae (arrow).

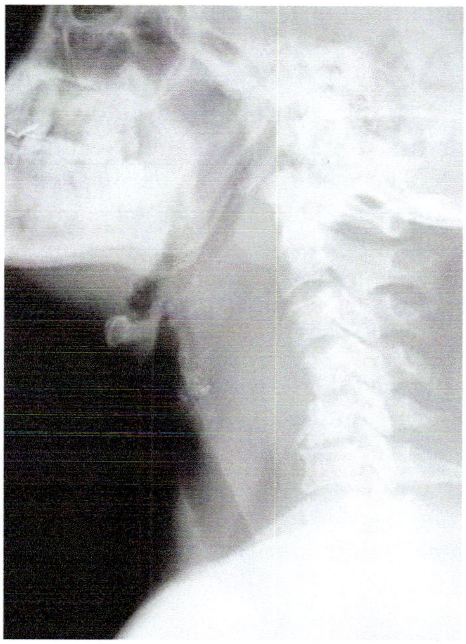

Fig. 4: Case of infective spondylodiscitis in middle-aged female: X-ray cervical spine lateral view showing decreased disc space at C4-C5 level with destruction of anterior vertebral body of C4 vertebra and large prevertebral abscess.

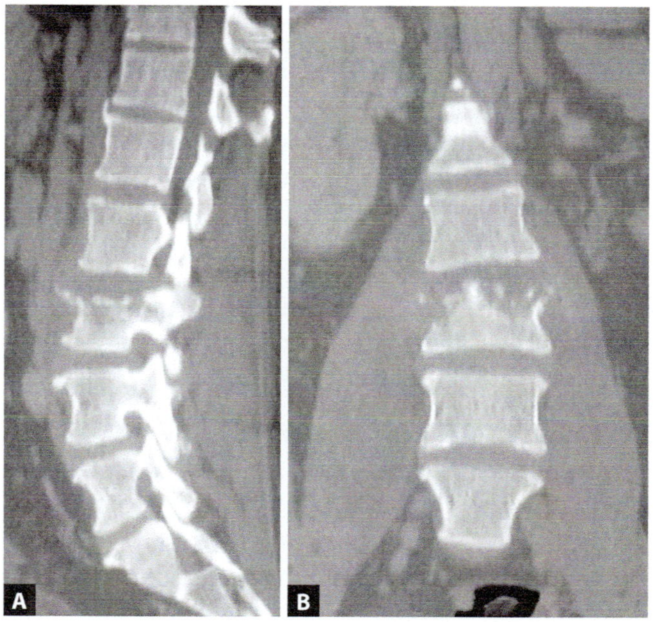

Figs. 5A and B: Noncontrast computed tomography (NCCT) lumbar spine sagittal (A) and coronal (B) reformat images showing better depiction of bony changes. There is superior endplate destruction of the L3 vertebra with involvement of the L2-3 intervertebral disc.

and has superior spatial as well as contrast resolution in imaging the spinal cord and nerve roots.[5-7] MRI has high sensitivity in early stages and with its known multiplanar capabilities and better soft tissue contrast, MRI provides a much better definition of the paravertebral and epidural extension of the disease. Many MRI features have been described for the spinal infection including decreased disc height, altered T1- or T2-signal intensity, enhancement of the disc, effacement of the nuclear cleft, and vertebral endplates erosion on T1-weighted (T1W) MR images.

As in CT, contrast-enhanced MRI allows better definition of the extent of spinal inflammatory lesions. In addition contrast-enhanced images allow better delineation of the paravertebral and intraspinal extension of disease. MRI is also a valuable tool in evaluation of postoperative spinal infections. MRI has a high sensitivity (96%) and a high accuracy (94%) for diagnosing infections.

Though MRI is imaging modality of choice for evaluating the spinal infections, vertebral osteomyelitis may be overlooked in the early course of disease, when there is no exact localization of the disease and when there is sclerosis in or around the lesion.

Nuclear Medicine Imaging Studies

Nuclear medicine imaging studies are important adjunct diagnostic tool to MRI for evaluating the spinal infections. These include radionuclide imaging tests used for detecting inflammatory changes of the spine with technetium-99m (^{99m}Tc) diphosphonate complexes, gallium-67 (^{67}Ga) and indium-111 (^{111}In)-labeled white blood cells (WBC), and ^{18}F-fluorodeoxyglucose (^{18}F-FDG) positron emission tomography (PET) with or without CT.[9,10] The advantages of the radionuclide imaging tests include high sensitivity for early diagnosis of spinal lesions, wide availability, and relatively cheaper. However, main limitation is low specificity as they show increased uptake in cases where there is underlying osseous abnormalities such as trauma, other noninfective inflammatory conditions, and tumors. In addition, the acquisition time for the radionuclide imaging is usually long (hours to days). Gallium-67 scans are mainly used for localization of areas of inflammation, especially for spinal infections. WBC-labeled imaging is not useful for the spinal infections, though it is very useful for diagnosing complicated osteomyelitis.

FDG-PET with or without CT is very useful for imaging of the spinal infections and has evolved as radionuclide modality of choice. Its sensitivity is more than 95% and specificity ranges from 75 to 99% for acute and subacute bone and soft tissue infection. It has a high negative predictive value, and is helpful in differentiating degenerative from infectious vertebral pathologies.

TYPES OF INFECTIONS

Vertebral bodies and intervertebral discs are most frequently involved in the spinal infections. The epidural space, posterior elements, and paraspinal soft tissues are usually involved secondarily due to infection of the vertebrae or discs and, rarely primarily hematogenous route or direct inoculation. In Asia and Africa, majority of the spinal infections are caused by tuberculosis and nontubercular infections are relatively uncommon. These nontubercular infections of the spine can be divided broadly into following subtypes:

- Bacterial [pyogenic and nonpyogenic (e.g., brucellosis, actinomycosis, nocardiosis)].
- Fungal, e.g., coccidioidomycosis, cryptococcosis, blastomycosis, aspergillosis, candidiasis.
- Parasitic, e.g., hydatid disease.

Pyogenic Bacterial Infections

Suppurative infections of the spine comprise only 2–5% of all osteomyelitis.[11,12] A higher incidence is seen in the debilitated, diabetics, and in elderly. *Staphylococcus aureus* is responsible for more than half the cases of infection. Other organisms responsible for infection include *Streptococcus, Pneumococcus*, gram-negative organisms such as *E. coli, Pseudomonas, Salmonella* (in sickle cell disease), and *Klebsiella*.[12] Spine is a common site for infection in IV drug abusers (mainly by *Pseudomonas*) along with sacroiliac and sternoclavicular joints involvement.

Hematogenous spread is common. Infecting organism reach the spine either by arterial antegrade route through the capillary network of the vertebral bodies or by retrograde venous route through the paravertebral Batson venous plexus. There is usually a history of recent primary infection of the skin, urinary tract or the upper respiratory tract, recent surgery or instrumentation. Patients typically present with severe back pain which is constant and aggravated by movement. Other symptoms include fever, malaise, and local tenderness. Development of neurological symptoms usually indicates the spread of infection to the epidural space. Lower lumbar spine involvement may lead to hip pain and contractures. Uncommonly, even radicular pattern of pain may be seen. Examination reveals local tenderness and restriction of movement. Erythrocyte sedimentation rate (ESR) is invariably raised. Diagnosis of spinal infection can be established with blood cultures (positive in less than 25% of cases), image-guided (fluoroscopic or CT guidance) percutaneous FNAC or biopsy sampling of the infected vertebrae or disc (in 68–86% of cases). However, an open surgical biopsy procedure may be performed in cases where percutaneous sampling cannot be performed or fails, or nondiagnostic. Spinal infections are most common in lumbar region (48%), followed by the thoracic spine (35%) and are less common in the cervical spine (6.5%) and sacrum. Infection involves the vertebral body rather than the appendages.

Radiological findings on plain radiographs usually lag behind the symptoms by 2–8 weeks.[11,12] Infection usually starts anteriorly in the subchondral area of the vertebral body, thus, the earliest finding is rarefaction of the endplates. Later frank erosions, scalloping, and destruction of vertebral endplates are noted. Following this, there is a loss of disc space height as the infection spreads to involve the adjacent vertebrae. In most patients, only two vertebrae are involved. Rarely, the infection is confined to one vertebral body. Vertebral destruction occurs and collapse may result with accompanying soft tissue swelling in pre- and paravertebral location. Reparative process can begin as early as 4–6 weeks after the onset of radiologic change and is heralded by increasing sclerosis, reactive new bone going on to spur formation, bony bridging or ankylosis of the adjacent vertebrae. Rarely, ivory vertebrae and soft tissue calcification may be found. Radionuclide scanning may be used to localize the exact site of infection and to search for multifocal lesions.

Computed tomography plays a minor role in cases with bony or soft tissue components. CT findings of vertebral osteomyelitis include: (1) detection of erosion or bone destruction and fragmentation; and (2) presence of adjacent soft tissue swelling with obliteration of fat planes around the vertebral body. CT diagnosis may be problematic if soft tissue lesions are seen in the absence of fragmentation or if fragmentation is seen without associated soft tissue swelling as in the case of previously treated or inactive discitis or hypertrophic degenerative disease. Diagnosis of vertebral osteomyelitis can also be difficult if pathognomonic features of other specific disease entities are present like acute vertebral fractures, metastatic or degenerative disease. Intradiscal or vertebral gas is an extremely uncommon finding in spinal infection and may be detected in clostridial or streptococcal infections. At about 10–12 weeks, an osteoblastic response may occur with sclerotic new bone formation. This is more a feature of pyogenic than tubercular osteomyelitis. Vertebral body ankylosis or fusion may be seen with the process of healing. However, if the therapy is inadequate, collapse with spinal deformity resulting in instability of the vertebral column may occur.

Magnetic resonance imaging is the imaging modality of choice for evaluation of patients with spinal infections. The findings on MR are characteristic and occur early in the disease. A constellation of findings of MR **(Figs. 6 and 7)** indicates pyogenic infection and helps to differentiate it from some of the other disease processes such as TB.[13] These include the following:

- The vertebra usually show homogeneous areas of altered signal intensity (low-signal intensity on T1W images and high-signal intensity on T2W images), but usually at one of the vertebral body metaphyses. These signal alterations mainly represent edema and often precede the destructive changes.
- The intervertebral discs usually show hyperintensity on T2W imaging, with abnormal configuration

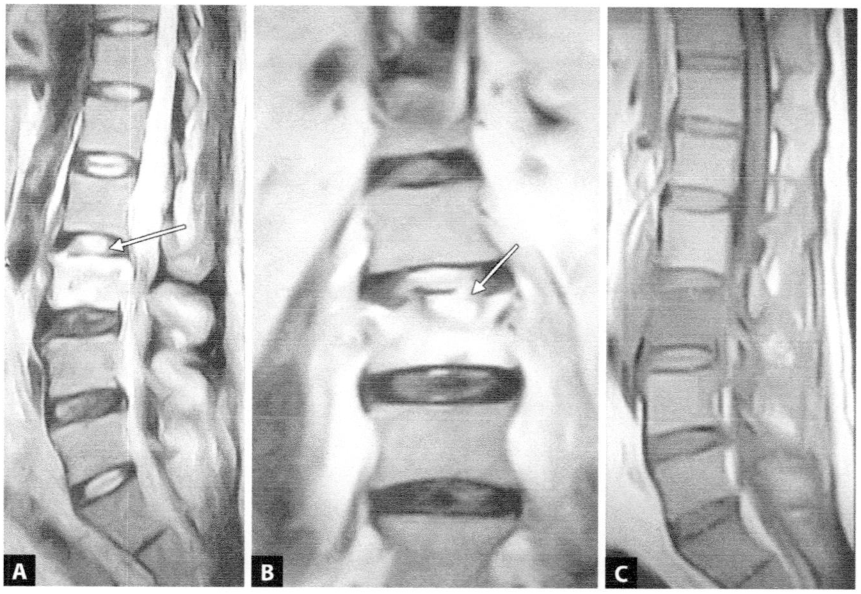

Figs. 6A to C: MRI lumbar spine sagittal (A), coronal (B) T2W and T1W (C) images show abnormal signal intensity (arrow) of L3 vertebra, contiguous L2-L3 intervertebral disc and surrounding soft tissue in a case of pyogenic spondylodiscitis. In addition, there is loss of intranuclear cleft.

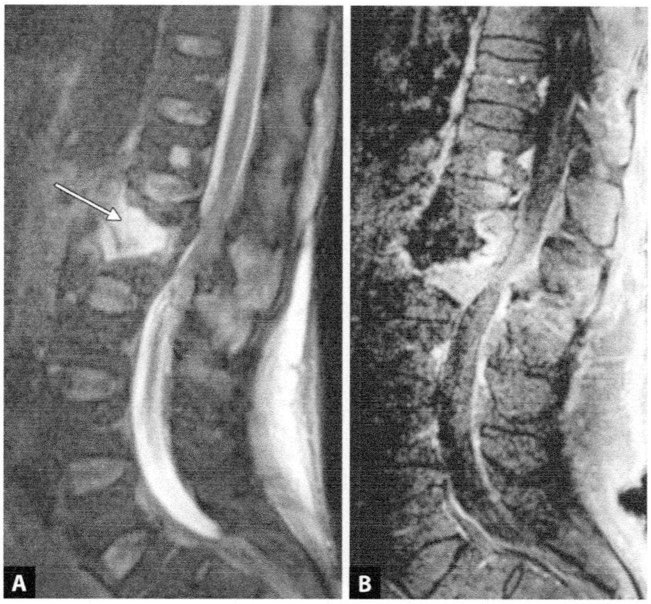

Figs. 7A and B: MRI lumbar spine sagittal T2W (A) and T1 fat saturated postcontrast (B) images show destruction of L1-L2 intervertebral disc (arrow) and contiguous vertebral bodies with T2 hyperintense soft tissue that is showing peripheral contrast enhancement and having intraspinal epidural extension in a case of pyogenic spondylodiscitis.

(absence of the internuclear cleft). The height of the intervertebral disc may be reduced.

- Loss of a margin between disc and vertebral bodies on T2W images.
- Diffuse and homogeneous enhancement is seen in the affected marrow and discs.
- Variable extension of the process into the paraspinal region. The presence of epidural extension and associated meningeal inflammation can be better demonstrated with contrast.
- Osseous and extra-axial abscesses showing restricted diffusion on diffusion-weighted imaging (DWI).

Magnetic resonance imaging may able to differentiate tuberculous spondylitis from pyogenic spondylitis. It is also possible to differentiate between pyogenic infection and other involving the spine, based on clinical and imaging features as described in **Table 2.**[13,14] In tuberculous spondylitis, the paraspinal lesions are more well-defined, abscess wall is thin and smooth, subligamentous spread with multiple vertebral or entire body involvement is seen in contrast to pyogenic spondylitis.

Diffusion-weighted MRI is very useful for the diagnosis of pyogenic spinal infections. It is also helpful for delineating the extent of lesion, treatment planning, and in differentiating the pyogenic spinal infection from nonpyogenic granulomatous infections or malignancy. Pyogenic infection usually shows diffusion restriction due to the pus and the high cellularity. It is important to recognize the MRI artefacts in the spine imaging, like susceptibility artefacts, incomplete fat suppression and volume-averaging artefacts; as these limits the diffusion imaging of the spine.

Pyogenic Disc Space Infections

In adults, since the disc is avascular, hematogenous infection is rare. Most infections occur by contiguous spread from vertebral osteomyelitis or by direct inoculation of bacteria into the disc at the time of surgery

Table 2: Differentiating features of infectious spondylodiscitis.

Features	*Tubercular*	*Pyogenic*	*Brucella*
Associated with pulmonary site	Yes	No	–
Site of predilection	Dorsolumbar	Lower lumbar	Lower lumbar
Onset of symptoms	Insidious	Acute	Acute
Progression	Slow	Rapid	Rapid
Multifocal involvement	Yes	No	Infrequent
Vertebral body height	Destroyed	Destroyed	Preserved
Posterior elements	May be involved	Spared	Spared
Subligamentous spread	Common	May be seen	No
Disc destruction	Late	Early	Early
Intradiscal gas	Infrequent	May be seen	Frequently
Paraspinal and epidural extension	Common	Common	Uncommon
Paraspinal mass	Large	Small	Small
Enhancement of paraspinal mass	Peripheral	Patchy	Patchy
Calcification in paraspinal mass	Yes	No	No
Spinal deformity	Common	Uncommon	No
Bone sclerosis	May be seen	Yes	Yes

or percutaneous procedures such as discography, percutaneous discectomy, and chemonucleosis.[12] *Staphylococcus aureus* is the most common organism implicated and presentation is usually with back pain. ESR is elevated, but this is not a very useful marker especially in postoperative cases where ESR remains elevated even up to 6 months.

Radiographic features include decreased disc space height and reactive sclerosis of adjacent endplates. Isotope scanning may show increased uptake but it may also be due to recent surgery or percutaneous manipulation. MRI has become the modality of choice for evaluating disc space infection. Septic discitis demonstrates disc space narrowing on MRI. The vertebral endplates are indistinct and show low-signal intensity on T1W images and high-signal intensity on T2W images. The vertebral endplates may be of increased signal intensity but the major finding in the disc space is an abnormal high signal. Paraspinal soft tissue thickening and edematous changes in the paraspinal musculature are also seen. In fact the earliest MR finding in pyogenic septic discitis is obliteration of fat planes between the paraspinal musculature and the outer margin of the disc. Diagnosis is usually confirmed by percutaneous disc aspirates which can be cultured for organisms.

Spinal Infections in Children

Spinal infections in children account for approximately 2–4% of all cases of osteomyelitis.[15,16] The clinical features are nonspecific and include fever, malaise, weight loss, and back pain. These features may be intermittent or constant. Sometimes hip contracture may be seen secondary to psoas muscle irritation. In laboratory findings, ESR is raised, however, leukocyte count may be normal and the blood cultures are positive in less number of cases.

The routes of spread of the spinal infections in children are same as in adults.[15] The most common route of spread is by a hematogenous route, usually by an arterial route or rarely by venous system. In the arterial hematogenous route, there is setting of the initial infection in the subchondral region of the vertebral body, where extensive arterial network leads to the involvement of the disc. The spinal infections in children may be seen with urinary tract and other pelvic infections via the venous hematogenous route, as the direction and extent of blood flow through the valveless Batson's paravertebral venous plexus are affected by changes in intra-abdominal pressure. The spinal infection may also occur due to contiguous spread from a neighboring contaminated source or from direct implantation during punctures of the spinal canal or in postoperative period following laminectomy or other instrumentation such as scoliosis repair.

In contrary to the belief that the spine infections in children begin in the discs as the discs are hypervascular; many studies have shown that in children also the spine infection generally starts in the vertebral body adjacent to the endplate with formation of microabscesses.[16] Due to presence of extensive perforating vascular network extending into the endplate and the disc, the infection spread to the disc. Then the infection tends to involve the endplates of the adjoining vertebral bodies. Most common bacteriological agents of the discitis are *Staphylococcus* and

Diplococcus pneumoniae. With the imaging advancements and early diagnosis, discitis is more than spondylitis. Discitis is more commonly seen in the age group of 1–5 years. Most commonly lumbar region is involved, predominantly the L3-4 and L4-5 intervertebral discs. MRI is the modality of choice for early diagnosis and characterizing the discitis or spondylitis, though there is difficulty in localizing the infection to the osseous and articular structures of the vertebrae. Characteristic radiographic finding is disc space narrowing with destruction of the adjoining surfaces (endplates) of vertebral bodies. It is more sensitive than radiography or CT or nuclear medicine imaging studies. MRI helps in better delineation of the soft tissue extension of the spinal infection in the form of epidural abscess or paravertebral abscess **(Figs. 8A to C)**.

Bacterial Spinal Infections in AIDS

The most common bacterial spinal infection in patients with HIV is *S. aureus*, as in immunocompetent patients. The imaging features are also same as in immunocompetent individuals and show involvement of vertebral body, disc, and epidural space in isolation or combination of these. Features which are suggestive of pyogenic spondylodiscitis are the presence of prevertebral soft tissue involvement, absence of posterior elements involvement, diffuse bone destruction, and absence of marginal sclerosis whereas nonpyogenic infection shows presence of focal lytic bone lesions with marginal sclerosis and paraspinal soft tissue lesions.

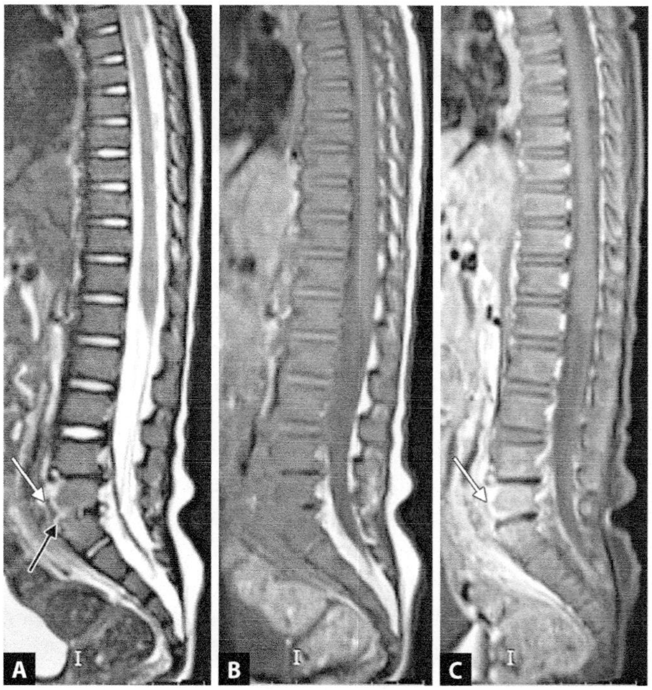

Figs. 8A to C: Sagittal T2 (A), T1 (B) and postcontrast fat sat T1(C) MR images of dorsolumbar spine showing altered signal intensity (T2 hyperintensity and T1 hypointensity) involving L5-S1 intervertebral disc (black arrow) and prevertebral soft tissue (white arrow) overlying the L5 vertebra which is showing mild heterogeneous enhancement (arrow) consistent with spondylodiscitis.

Nonpyogenic Bacterial Infections[17,18]

Brucellosis

Brucellosis (undulant fever or Malta fever) is primarily a zoonotic disease, where affected animals (e.g., camels, sheep, goats) are the primary host and humans are the secondary host.[17] It is a granulomatous nontubercular infection which is caused by small, nonmotile gram-negative facultative intracellular *Coccobacilli* of the genus *Brucella*, most common being *Brucella melitensis*. The organisms are usually transmitted by the consumption of uncooked meat or unpasteurized dairy products. The incidence of spinal infection in brucellosis is 2–65%, with males affected more than the females likely due to occupational risks (males mainly work in the stock industry). The spinal involvement in the brucellosis is more commonly seen in the elderly males. Spine is the most common site for skeletal brucellosis. The clinical features of spinal brucellosis are often nonspecific and the onset of the symptom tends to be subacute. The patients present with focal and diffuse forms in the endemic areas and may involve vertebral bodies, intervertebral discs, facet joints, ligaments, paraspinal soft tissues, and epidural space. In the focal form, common site of the spinal infection is anterior aspect of the vertebral endplate (typically superior endplate of L4 vertebra) at the discovertebral junction. In the diffuse form, the vertebral body is involved initially and then the infection extends to involve the adjoining discs and vertebrae.

The lumbar region is more commonly involved, likely due to rich blood supply and higher incidence of endplate degenerative changes. The diagnosis is often difficult because of the significant overlapping radiologic imaging features of the spinal infections which mimics such as brucellosis like tubercular or pyogenic spinal infections and rarely malignancy. The main problem in the diagnosis is its differentiation from other infective processes particularly tuberculosis which is the most common cause of spinal infection in India. In brucellosis, there occur proliferative changes associated with bony repair, which are not seen in tuberculous infection; and in contrast in tuberculosis there occur deformities of the spine, which are rarely seen with brucellosis.

Laboratory tests may show mildly increased sedimentation rates, altered liver function tests, and decreased WBC and platelet counts. Standard tube agglutination test may be helpful for the diagnosis.

Nuclear medicine imaging studies such as bone scan with ^{99m}Tc or PET scan is helpful and sensitive in demonstrating areas of involvement in patients with *Brucella* infection who have musculoskeletal complaints. Plain radiographs mainly show a focal lesion at the superior endplate with maintained vertebral body architecture. Associated sclerosis is frequently seen. Disc space reduction with presence of gas in disc is a hallmark of brucellosis not seen in tuberculosis. Paravertebral soft tissue abscesses are less commonly associated and spinal deformity is rare when compared with tuberculosis.

Computed tomography confirms the presence of focal or diffuse disease in brucellosis. Findings of bone sclerosis, localized endplate destruction simulating Schmorl's nodes, loss of muscle or fat plane, and disc space gas when seen point to a *Brucella* infection, whereas large paraspinal abscesses with enhancing rim, calcification, or bone fragments suggest tubercular nature of infection. CT-guided percutaneous FNAC or biopsy is helpful for making the definitive diagnosis. On MR, the above findings are further corroborated with evidence of an intact vertebral morphology, normal posterior elements, and a focal lesion which shows decreased signal intensity on T1W images and moderately increased signal intensity or T2W images. Disc destruction is early. There is only a moderate extension into the paraspinal and epidural space by granulation tissue and/or edema and spinal deformity is infrequent.

Actinomycosis

Actinomycosis is a slowly progressive infection caused by gram-positive filamentous bacteria of *Actinomyces* species, most commonly by *Actinomyces israelii*.[19] They are normal commensal of gastrointestinal tract, bronchial, and female genital tracts. Clinical features of the actinomycosis are very nonspecific, and are also referred as the "most misdiagnosed disease". Mandible and spine are most commonly affected. Osseous involvement results from extension of soft tissue infection. Involvement of the spine is rare and usually from the contiguous spread from adjacent sites of infection, especially the lungs and sinuses. Vertebral destruction with deformity is uncommon with *Actinomyces* infection. These infections are usually seen in debilitated persons. Radiological manifestations include lytic lesions with surrounding sclerosis involving several vertebrae and frequently sparing the discs. Posterior elements and ribs are frequently involved, with associated paravertebral abscesses which are not as large as seen in tuberculosis and do not show calcification. Presence of sinus tracts leading to the skin along with above findings suggests the diagnosis.

Nocardiosis

Nocardia are filamentous, branching, gram-positive aerobic bacteria. They are usually associated primarily with pulmonary infection in immunocompromised patients. Spinal involvement is rare with nonspecific radiological findings. There are only about a dozen reported cases of spinal nocardiosis in the literature and occurs both by direct extension of intrathoracic infections and through hematogenous spread.

There are few specific imaging features which have been described for nonpyogenic spondylodiscitis like absence of T2-hyperintensity within the intervertebral discs and the preservation of the intranuclear cleft. However, these finding may also be seen in tubercular spine infections and have been reported in cases of pyogenic spine diseases. In addition, intervertebral discs may also be spared by other nonpyogenic infections caused by *Nocardia*, *Actinomyces*, and *Coccidioides*. The cause of absence of T2-hyperintensity within the intervertebral disc is unclear and may be multifactorial. The imaging findings may be indicative of absence of invasion of the disc, an altered inflammatory reaction within the involved disc, or an intrinsic characteristic of either the disc before infection (e.g., degenerated disc) or of the invading organisms (e.g., paramagnetic elements in fungi).

Epidural Space Infections

Epidural space is usually involved secondarily to contiguous spread of the infections from surrounding infected spinal structures such as adjacent infected vertebrae, disc space or facet joints (spondylodiscitis or facet joint infection). Primary epidural abscesses due to hematogenous spread of bacteria are relatively less common, and account for less than 2% of all the spine infections. Typically, the epidural abscess presents with intense back pain, usually localized over the infected site of spine. The intense pain is more than the concomitant neurologic deficit. Early diagnosis of the epidural abscess is of paramount importance, as neurological sequelae are severe and may lead to cord compression and paralysis.

Contrast-enhanced MRI with DWI provides the best evaluation of patients with the epidural abscess. Main advantages of MRI include its ability to differentiate the cord from the thecal sac, involvement and extension of the infection to paraspinal soft tissues, or vertebral bone marrow. The epidural abscesses can be clearly seen as soft tissue lesion in the epidural space, usually hypointense on T1W and hyperintense on T2W images which displaces the thecal sac away from the vertebrae with delineation from the dural sac as thin T2-hypointense line. Contrast-enhanced MRI demonstrates two types of enhancement pattern, one with a peripheral enhancement a central hypointense area representing true abscess **(Figs. 9A and B)** and other with a homogeneous enhancement pattern representing the inflammatory changes without purulent contents. Fat-suppressed

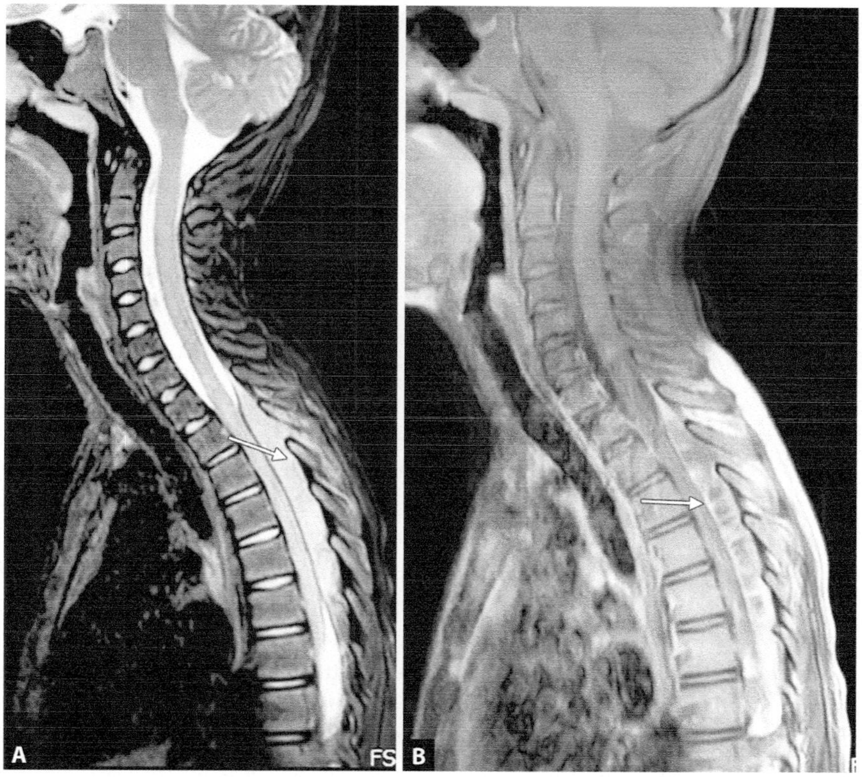

Figs. 9A and B: T2 (A) and contrast enhanced T1 (B) sagittal MR images of the child with large epidural abscess (arrows) in the dorsal region showing peripheral enhancement. Upper dorsal cord is compressed and shows cord edema.

contract-enhanced MRI helps in better delineation of the extent of the lesion and its differentiation from surrounding structures (interspinous and paraspinal region). DWI plays an important role in the diagnosis of epidural abscesses. It helps in delineation of the extension, and differentiating it from epidural hemorrhage and other neoplastic lesion in the epidural space.

Postoperative Spondylodiscitis

Postoperative spondylodiscitis is an uncommon complication of the spine surgeries or interventional procedures.[3] The patients present with recurrent pain after initial postoperative relief, muscular spasm, and fever. Most likely the cause is intraoperative contamination, though rarely hematogenous spread may occur. The imaging findings are nonspecific initially as it is difficult to differentiate from the postoperative changes and may appear several weeks after the symptoms onset. Characteristic MRI findings of the disc space infection include enhancement of the disc space, annulus, and vertebral body. These imaging findings have to be correlated with laboratory findings like an increased ESR as similar findings may be seen in normal postoperative asymptomatic patients. Thus, main role of imaging is to exclude the diagnosis of postoperative spondylodiscitis by showing no abnormal signal changes and abnormal enhancement in the postoperative site rather than looking for characteristic changes because of the significant overlap of the imaging findings.

Facet Joint Infections

The infection of the facet joints are commonly underdiagnosed and frequently overlooked, though they have distinct clinical and imaging features. The facets joints are diarthrodial joints which consist of opposing cartilage surfaces and interlock adjacent vertebral bodies. The joints are enclosed by a firm ligamentous capsule and contain meniscoids. They transfer load and constrain spine movements along with the intervertebral disc. Route of spread of the infection to the facet joints is commonly by hematogenous route, and rarely iatrogenically by facet injections and instrumentations. Clinical features vary and usually present with acute onset of the symptoms such as unilateral back pain with fever. Plain radiographs are nonspecific and imaging features significantly lag behind, so rarely used. Nuclear imaging studies are useful in indicating the infection. CT may show the erosive changes in affected facets, and soft tissue changes in the epidural space, paraspinal region. However, CT is mainly used for image-guided biopsies if required. MRI is very helpful as it shows changes very early on. It demonstrates the infection of the facet joints as intra-articular fluid, joint space destruction, and abnormal surrounding enhancement.

Fungal Infections[20-22]

Infections of the spine by fungus are uncommon. They are more commonly seen in patients with predisposing conditions such as diabetes, prolonged corticosteroid administration, immunosuppression after organ transplantation, prolonged systemic illness associated with malnutrition and multiple antibiotic use, HIV infection, alcohol or IV drug abuse, and parenteral nutrition. Rarely do they occur due to iatrogenic interventions.

Fungal infections of the spine include aspergillosis, coccidioidomycosis, cryptococcosis, *Candida*, and blastomycosis. Following inhalation of spores, these involve the spine by a hematogenous route. Radiologically, each fungal infection does not have any distinctive features of its own. Most of them resemble tubercular infection, but a few characteristic features have been described for some of the infections.

Aspergillosis

Aspergillus, a ubiquitous species of fungus, is usually pathogenic only in immunocompromised patients. The spinal infections from *Aspergillus* usually extend from contiguous site of infection which is mainly pulmonary, but rarely spread hematogenously. Though rare, *Aspergillus* vertebral infections have been reported in immunocompetent hosts as well.[20] Differentiation must be made from tuberculosis, which can closely mimic aspergillosis of the spine, using serologic testing. There are no characteristic radiographic features and resemble other spinal infection. Imaging may show osseous and disc space destruction, and a paraspinal soft tissue lesion.[19] MRI helps in better delineation of the extent of involvement **(Figs. 10A to C)**.

Coccidioidomycosis

Coccidioidomycosis is caused by *Coccidioides immitis*, a filamentous fungus which infects the lung primarily and disseminates throughout the body in about 0.5% of patients. Osseous involvement is seen in 10–50% of which spine is the most common site.[21] Plain radiographs usually reveal multiple erosive defects involving vertebral bodies and appendages. Disc space is usually preserved and spinal deformity is uncommon. Paraspinal masses and adjacent rib involvement is common. Differentiation from tuberculosis can be made by the presence of skull lesions, which although common in coccidioidomycosis, are rare in tuberculosis.[21]

Lumbar spine is commonly affected. MR appearances of the lesion are that of hypo- to hyperintense signal intensity on T1W images and on T2W images, the lesions

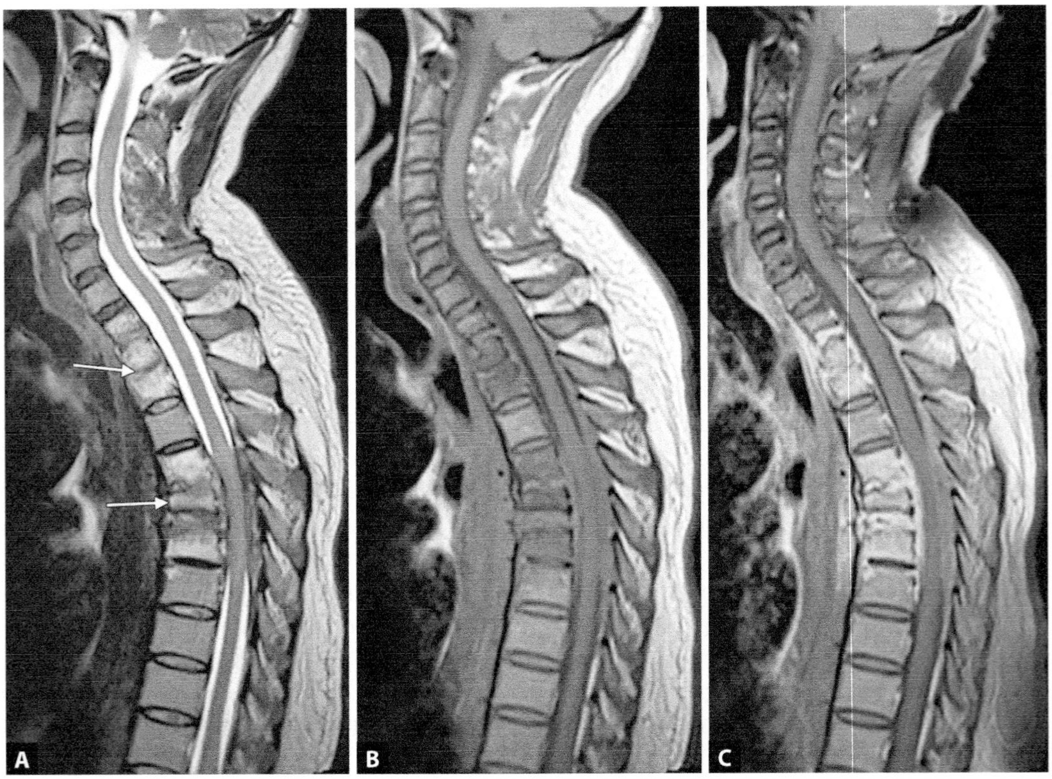

Figs. 10A to C: *Aspergillus* spondylodiscitis in young male. Sagittal T2 (A), T1 (B) and postcontrast T1 (C) weighted MR images of cervicodorsal region showing diffuse altered marrow signal intensity and contrast enhancement of D1-3 and D5-7 vertebral bodies and intervertebral discs (arrows). There are mild epidural and prevertebral soft tissue signal changes.

are almost always hyperintense. Following gadolinium injection, the lesions which are hypo- to isointense on T1W sequence show enhancement.[20] Ring enhancement may be seen in intraosseous abscesses. Presence of paraspinal masses, epidural spread, and subligamentous spread is similar to those seen in tuberculosis.

Cryptococcosis (Torulosis)

Cryptococcosis is caused by *Cryptococcus neoformans*, which has more predilections for the central nervous system. This fungus can be found in soil, pigeon droppings, fruit, and human intestinal tract and skin. The disease is usually acquired by the respiratory route through inhalation of aerosolized spores. This infection tends to occur in immunocompromised patients and is more common in postrenal transplant patients. Disseminated cryptococcal infection may result in osseous involvement in 5–10% of patients and spine is commonly involved. Radiologically, nonspecific well-defined osteolytic areas with sclerotic margins are seen involving the vertebral body and posterior elements **(Figs. 11A to C)**. Again, multifocal involvement and large paraspinal soft tissue abscesses may be present making the picture at times indistinguishable from tuberculosis.

Blastomycosis

This infection caused by *Blastomyces dermatitidis*, which enters the body through skin wound or the respiratory tract. The route of spread to the spine is by hematogenous seeding, or by direct spread from an overlying cutaneous lesion. The vertebra may be involved; however, the radiologic features are not specific. Involvement of the osseous structure is usually secondary, and spine is common site. Common imaging appearance is destructive vertebral lesion with a large paraspinal mass. The lower thoracic and lumbar spine is most often the site of the infection. Features suggestive of blastomycosis of the spine include involvement of the posterior elements of the vertebral body and adjoining ribs, and greater tendency to produce cutaneous fistulae.[20] The definitive diagnosis is typically made by positive cytology or histologic examination of biopsy specimens.

Candidiasis (Moniliasis)

Candidiasis is most commonly caused by *Candida albicans*. Musculoskeletal infections by *Candida* are more common in immunocompromised, especially in IV drug addicts. Osteomyelitis can occur in one or more sites. Spinal involvement is uncommon and seen as involvement of two consecutive vertebral bodies. Usually, the lumbar spine is the region affected and imaging features are nonspecific.[20] The definitive diagnosis as in other spinal fungal infection is typically made by positive cytology or histologic examination.

Parasitic Infections

Echinococcosis or Hydatid

The principal host of echinococcosis is the dog, whereas the intermediate hosts are sheep and humans. The route of transmission is ingestion of ova and then absorption by the bowel. Echinococcosis or hydatid disease of the bones is rare, accounting for approximately 0.5–4% of all patients.[20]

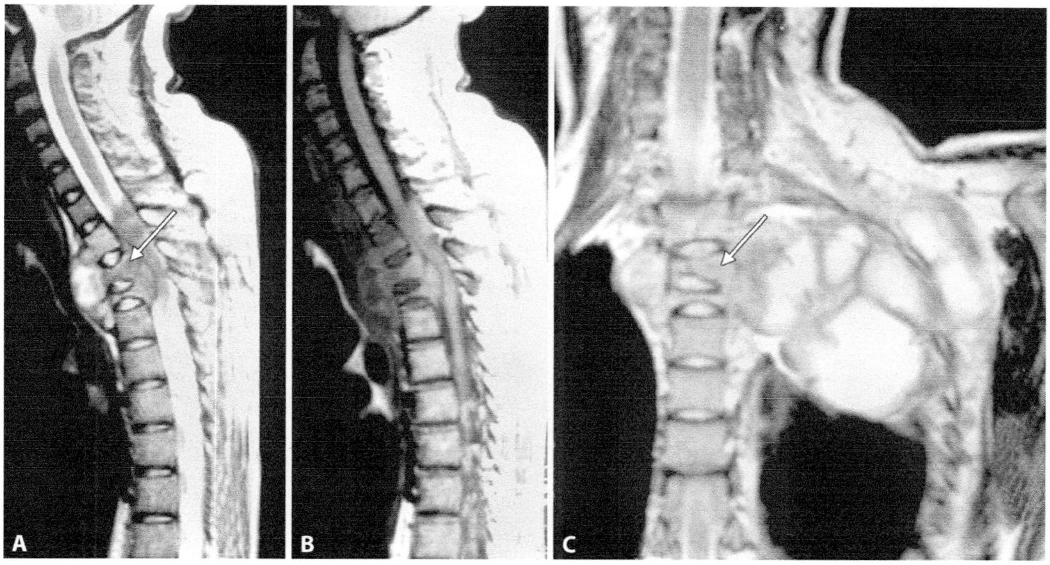

Figs. 11A to C: T2 (A), T1 (B) sagittal, and T2 (C) coronal MR imaging in a case of cryptococcosis of the dorsal spine showing multiple contiguous vertebral involvement of the upper dorsal spine (arrows) with vertebral destruction and prevertebral, epidural and posterior paraspinal abscesses with compression of the adjacent cord and relatively preserved disc spaces.

Spinal involvement by hydatid disease is seen in about half of these patients. In the spine, sacrum and lower dorsal vertebra are commonly involved. The primary infection from the medullary cavity in the vertebral body spreads to involve the pedicles and laminae. Hydatid disease in the bones differs from disease elsewhere in the soft tissues in that the cysts are always multilocular. Growth occurs along the line of least resistance particularly along the intertrabecular spaces with the formation of diverticulated cysts that may form by exogenous vesiculation. Enlargement of the larvae results in dilatation of the bony spaces of spongiosa and resorption of cancellous bone. Expansion is relatively slow with a smooth well-defined sclerotic margin. Erosion through the periosteum into the adjacent soft tissues proceeds without subperiosteal new bone formation. Extension into extradural space or paraspinal tissues may occur. Contiguous involvement of the rib is a feature.

Spinal hydatid has been classified into: (1) primary cyst in the cord; (2) intradural cyst; (3) extradural cyst; (4) hydatid disease of the vertebrae; and (5) paravertebral hydatid disease. Mid-dorsal and lumbosacral levels are most commonly affected. Plain film findings include a uni- or multiloculated lytic expansile bone lesion with marginal sclerosis involving the vertebral body, posterior elements, and even the adjacent ribs with paraspinal soft tissue mass. Disc space is preserved as the disease propagates beneath the periosteum and ligaments. The findings are at times nonspecific and indistinguishable from other benign cystic bone lesions or metastatic disease.

Computed tomography signs are nonspecific and often reveal bone lysis extending into the posterior elements, adjacent vertebrae, disc space and epidural space, creating a picture of spondylitis. However, costal involvement and lack of enhancement following contrast administration suggest hydatid disease. CT is superior to MR in demonstrating calcified lesions.

On MR, cysts demonstrate inhomogeneous low-signal intensity on T1W images and high signal on T2W images **(Figs. 12A to D)**. T2W images are not helpful in differentiating quiescent from active stage of the cysts. MRI may demonstrate intradural extension to better advantage than CT without the need for subarachnoid contrast.

DIFFERENTIAL DIAGNOSIS OF SPINAL INFECTION[23,24]

Imaging features of the various spinal infections are nonspecific and may mimic other spinal diseases. Imaging features such as signal intensity changes and enhancement patterns seen in various conditions may cause significant overlap with the spinal infection, so it is very important to exclude which mimic like the spinal infections. Important masquerader of the spinal infections include degenerative and inflammatory spinal pathologies such as discogenic vertebral body degeneration in the inflammatory phase (Modic type 1 degeneration), acute cartilaginous node, ankylosing spondylitis, neuropathic spine, dialysis-related spondyloarthropathy, and rarely neoplasm. Modic type 1 disc degeneration is characterized by presence of altered signal intensity in the vertebral endplates (in

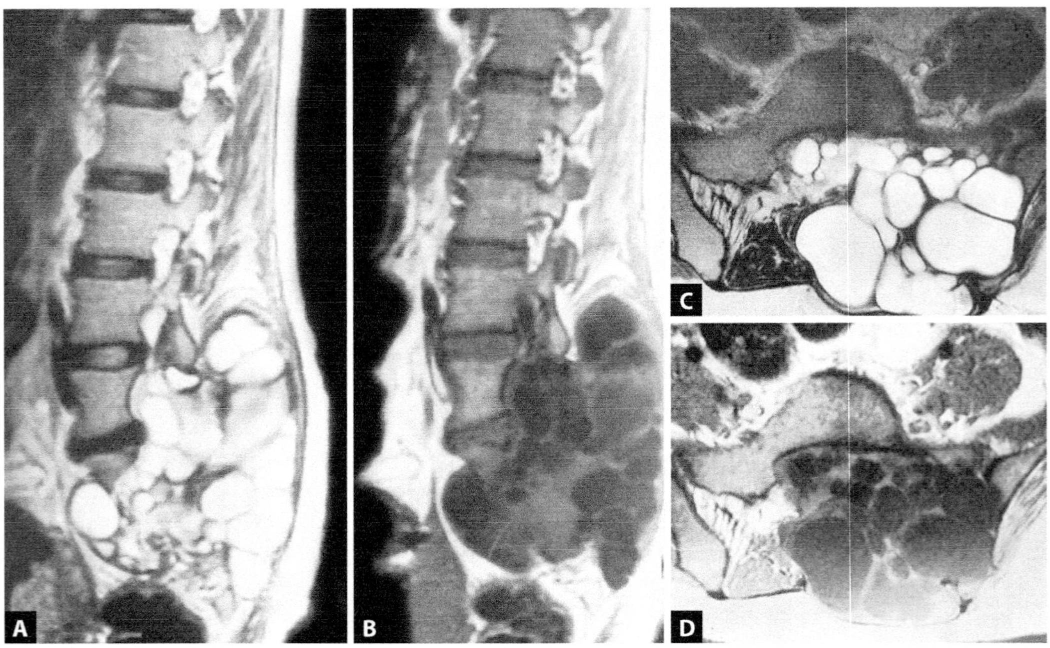

Figs. 12A to D: MRI lumbosacral spine parasagittal T2W (A), T1W (B), axial T2W (C), T1W (D) images show large multiloculated, cystic, expansile lesion involving posterior arch elements of L5 and sacrum demonstrating a having both osseous and extraosseous components. The cysts show peripheral T2 hypointense wall and central fluid signal in a case of spinal hydatid.

form of hypointensity on T1 and hyperintensity on T2) with absence of increased T2-signal intensity of the intervertebral disc and absence of soft tissue involvement whereas infectious spondylitis is characterized by endplate destruction, increased disc T2-signal intensity, or a paravertebral or epidural involvement (abscess). In addition, DWI is very useful in differentiating Modic type 1 degenerative changes from infection. Patients with Modic type 1 signal changes show well-marginated, linear region of high signal within the adjacent vertebral bodies at the interface of normal and abnormal marrow, which is referred as "claw sign".

Acute cartilaginous node may be distinguished by concentric ring of high T2-signal intensity around the node, involvement of only one endplate and no signal intensity changes of the disc. Ankylosing spondylitis can be differentiated by presence of spinal ankylosis and fracture that extends into the posterior column (Andersson lesion). Neuropathic spine is characterized by vacuum phenomenon, facet involvement, lower signal intensity of disc and bone marrow on T2W images whereas in dialysis-related spondyloarthropathy vertebral marrow shows hypointense signal on both T1W and T2W images.

CONCLUSION

Imaging of the spine plays a pivotal role in the early and accurate diagnosis and management of the patient with spinal infection. Imaging helps in delineation of the extent of disease and potential infectious agents; thereby reducing the associated morbidity and mortality. MRI is the imaging modality of choice for the diagnosis and characterization of spinal infection because of the better spatial and contrast resolution. It allows direct evaluation of the bone marrow changes, and simultaneous visualization of the neural structures. However, spinal infections are often indistinguishable on imaging and there is frequent overlap of radiological findings in different types of infections. So it is essential to recognize atypical MRI findings of spinal infection; and imaging features of other noninfectious inflammatory diseases and degenerative disease that may mimic like spinal infections to avoid misdiagnosis and inappropriate treatment.

REFERENCES

1. Babic M, Simpfendorfer CS. Infections of the spine. Infect Dis Clin North Am. 2017;31(2):279-97.
2. Go JL, Rothman S, Prosper A, Silbergleit R, Lerner A. Spine infections. Neuroimaging Clin N Am. 2012;22(4):755-72.
3. DeSanto J, Ross JS. Spine infection/inflammation. Radiol Clin North Am. 2011;49(1):105-27.
4. Esendagli-Yilmaz G, Uluoglu O. Pathologic basis of pyogenic, nonpyogenic, and other spondylitis and discitis. Neuroimaging Clin N Am. 2015;25(2):159-61.
5. Diehn FE. Imaging of spine infection. Radiol Clin North Am. 2012;50(4):777-98.
6. Torres C, Zakhari N. Imaging of spine infection. Semin Roentgenol. 2017;52(1):17-26.
7. Prodi E, Grassi R, Iacobellis F, Cianfoni A. Imaging in spondylodiscitis. Magn Reson Imaging Clin N Am. 2016;24(3):581-600.
8. Moritani T, Kim J, Capizzano AA, Kirby P, Kademian J, Sato Y. Pyogenic and non-pyogenic spinal infections: emphasis on diffusion-weighted imaging for the detection of abscesses and pus collections. Br J Radiol. 2014;87(1041):20140011.
9. Palestro CJ. Radionuclide imaging of musculoskeletal infection: a review. J Nucl Med. 2016;57(9):1406-12.
10. Gemmel F, Dumarey N, Palestro CJ. Radionuclide imaging of spinal infections. Eur J Nucl Med Mol Imaging. 2006;33(10):1226-37.
11. Boody BS, Tarazona DA, Vaccaro AR. Evaluation and management of pyogenic and tubercular spine infections. Curr Rev Musculoskelet Med. 2018;11(4):643-52.
12. Tali ET, Oner AY, Koc AM. Pyogenic spinal infections. Neuroimaging Clin N Am. 2015;25(2):193-208.
13. Harada Y, Tokuda O, Matsunaga N. Magnetic resonance imaging characteristics of tuberculous spondylitis vs pyogenic spondylitis. Clin Imaging. 2008;32(4):303-9.
14. Chang MC, Wu HT, Lee CH, Liu CL, Chen TH. Tuberculous spondylitis and pyogenic spondylitis. Comparative magnetic resonance imaging features. Spine. 2006;31(7):782-8.
15. Tyagi R. Spinal infections in children: a review. J Orthop. 2016;13(4):254-8.
16. Rossi A. Pediatric spinal infection and inflammation. Neuroimaging Clin N Am. 2015;25(2):173-91.
17. Butler JS, Shelly MJ, Timlin M, Powderly WG, O'Byrne JM. Nontuberculous pyogenic spinal infections in adults. A 12 year experience from a tertiary referral center. Spine. 2003;31:2695-700.
18. Tali ET, Koc AM, Oner AY. Spinal brucellosis. Neuroimaging Clin N Am. 2015;25(2):233-45.
19. Young WB. Actinomycosis with involvement of the vertebral column: case report and review of the literature. Clin Radiol. 1960;11:175-82.
20. Chhem RK, Wang SC, Jaovisidha S, Schmit P, Friedman L, Bureau NJ, et al. Imaging of fungal, viral, and parasitic musculoskeletal and spinal diseases. Radiol Clin North Am. 2001;39(2):357-78.
21. Erly WK, Carmody RF, Seeger JF, Lund PJ. Magnetic resonance imaging of coccidioidal spondylitis. Int J of Neuroradiol. 1997;3(5):385-92.
22. Williams RL, Fukui MB, Meltzer CC, Swarnkar A, Johnson DW, Welch W. Fungal spinal osteomyelitis in the immunocompromised patient: MR findings in three cases. Am J Neuroradiol. 1999;20(3):381-5.
23. Hong SH, Choi JY, Lee JW, Kim NR, Choi JA, Kang HS. MR imaging assessment of the spine: infection or an imitation? Radiographics. 2009;29(2):599-612.
24. Ledermann HP, Schweitzer ME, Morrison WB, Carrino JA. MR imaging findings in spinal infections: rules or myths? Radiology. 2003;228(2):506-14.

SECTION

3

Inflammatory, Metabolic and Degenerative Conditions

CHAPTER

8

Imaging in Rheumatological Disorders

Mandeep Kang, Gita Devi, Mahesh Prakash

INTRODUCTION

Rheumatological diseases are the conditions characterized by inflammation affecting connecting or supporting structure of the body, which includes joints, tendons, ligaments, bones, and muscles. Rheumatological disorders are a heterogeneous group which includes inflammatory, autoimmune diseases, degenerative diseases, etc.[1] There is a predilection for the female gender[1] (more common during childbearing age group). Few decades ago, these conditions were grouped under the umbrella term of rheumatism. At present, more than 200 different rheumatic diseases are identified. The common conditions grouped as per etiology are:

- Noninfective inflammatory
  - Rheumatoid arthritis (RA)
  - Juvenile RA
  - Ankylosing spondylitis (AS)
  - Reiter's syndrome (RS)
  - Enteropathic spondyloarthropathy
  - Psoriatic arthropathy (PA)
- Autoimmune
  - Systemic lupus erythematosus (SLE)
  - Systemic sclerosis (scleroderma)
  - Sjögren's syndrome
  - Other connective tissue disorders
- Crystal deposition arthropathy
  - Gout
  - Calcium pyrophosphate dihydrate (CPPD) crystal deposition disease
- Degenerative
  - Degenerative joint disease
  - Diffuse idiopathic skeletal hyperostosis
  - Ossification of the posterior longitudinal ligament
  - Erosive osteoarthritis (OA)
  - Neurotrophic arthropathy
  - Synoviochondrometaplasia
  - Osteoporosis
- Others
  - Idiopathic inflammatory myopathy (IIM)
  - Tendinitis
  - Bursitis
  - Polymyalgia rheumatica (PMR)
  - Behçet's disease
  - Infective arthritis.

Noninfective inflammatory arthritides comprise a group of different, mostly systemic disorders that have one important feature in common; inflammatory granulation tissue eroding and destroying articular cartilage. The noninfective inflammatory arthritides include RA (seropositive) and the seronegative spondyloarthropathies (SSAs), namely—AS, PA, RS and enteropathic arthritis. Although radiologic manifestations of the arthropathies reflect pathologic alterations, joints can react to disease only in limited ways and therefore different pathologic conditions may exhibit similar radiologic features. Many of these are nonspecific, but certain combinations are more likely than others to occur in a particular disease; thus one may consider the "predictive value" of a radiologic feature relative to the clinical condition.[2] A systematic approach with evaluation of various radiological abnormalities helps in arriving at the correct diagnosis. Various features to be evaluated include:

- Distribution of affected joints
- Presence of soft tissue swelling
- Bone density
- Cartilage space narrowing
- Reactive bone formation
- Site and character of erosions
- Subarticular cystic lesions
- Presence of soft tissue calcification
- Joint deformities.[3]

RHEUMATOID ARTHRITIS

Rheumatoid arthritis is the most common inflammatory arthritis, which affects about 0.5–1% of the world's adult population. It is a progressive, chronic, systemic inflammatory disease affecting primarily the synovial joints, which can lead to considerable disability and morbidity. RA may develop at any age, but the peak age of onset is between the 4th and 6th decades. Women are three times more likely to be affected than men.[4] The exact etiology is not known but multiple factors appear to be involved. There is definitely a genetic predisposition with over 70% of the patients expressing HLA-DR4. A role for factors such as smoking and infectious agents has also been suggested in the etiology.[5] Although any synovial joint in the body may be affected, the classical presentation is of a symmetrical polyarthritis affecting the small joints of the hands and feet. However, it may be asymmetrical in 20–25% of cases.[2] Large joints which are commonly involved include the ankle, knee, and shoulder. The axial skeleton is later and less often affected, with the exception of the cervical spine. Characteristically, joints which communicate with one another tend to be affected together, e.g., uniform tricompartmental involvement in the knee joint and simultaneous involvement of the distal radioulnar and radiocarpal joints.[3]

Over the past couple of decades, there has been a fundamental change in the management of RA, which has resulted in significantly improved prognosis. Presently, the management involves two main strategies: first, to initiate treatment as soon as possible which basically translates into early detection and diagnosis of disease and second, to frequently gauge disease activity to monitor response to therapy. New biologic therapies have also emerged such as the antitumor necrosis factor drugs to supplement the conventional disease-modifying antirheumatic agents.[6]

The spectrum of disease manifestations of RA is protean. The diagnostic criteria proposed by the American College of Rheumatology in 1987 were commonly used for the diagnosis of this disease **(Box 1)**.[7] However, these criteria were not fulfilled early in the course of the disease, hence in recent years, the role of imaging like magnetic resonance imaging (MRI) and ultrasound has gained in importance.[8,9]

In 2010, the American College of Rheumatology along with the European League Against Rheumatism (EULAR) revised the diagnostic criteria for RA highlighting features present early in the disease. They included anti-citrullinated protein antibodies (ACPAs) which are a biomarker predicting aggressive disease. Patients with disease of <6 weeks duration are included while patients who already have a bony erosion on radiographs as a sign of structural damage are categorized as RA without applying this scoring system. Four domains are considered, namely (1) the number of joints, (2) serological markers, (3) acute phase reactants and (4) duration of disease **(Table 1)**.[10]

The positive findings in the domains are added according to points appointed and the total is the score assigned. A score of 56 is required to designate RA as the diagnosis.[10] Joint involvement is defined as joint having synovitis on imaging which on clinical examination is swollen and tender.

Box 1: The 1987 diagnostic criteria for the diagnosis of rheumatoid arthritis of the American College of Rheumatology.

- Morning stiffness in and around joints that lasts at least 1 hour before maximal improvement
- Soft tissue swelling of at least three joints that is observed by a physician
- Swelling (arthritis) of the metacarpophalangeal, proximal interphalangeal or wrist joints
- Symmetrical swelling (arthritis)
- Subcutaneous rheumatoid nodules
- A positive test for rheumatoid factor
- Radiographic signs: erosions or periarticular osteopenia in hand or wrist joints

Table 1: The American College of Rheumatology (ACR)/European League Against Rheumatism (EULAR) classification criteria for rheumatoid arthritis: domains, categories and point scores.[10]

Domain	*Category*	*Point score*
A	*Joint involvement (0–5 points)*	
	1 large joint	0
	2–10 large joints	1
	1–3 small joints (large joints not counted)	2
	4–10 small joints (large joints not counted)	3
	>10 joints including at least 1 small joint	5
B	*Serology (at least one test needed for classification) (0–3 points)*	
	Negative rheumatoid factor (RF) and negative anti-citrullinated protein antibodies (ACPAs)	0
	Low-positive RF or low-positive ACPA	2
	High-positive RF or high-positive ACPA	3
C	*Acute-phase reactants (at least one test needed for classification)*	
	Normal C-reactive protein (CRP) and normal erythrocyte sedimentation rate (ESR)	0
	Abnormal CRP or abnormal ESR	1
D	*Duration of symptoms*	
	<6 weeks	0
	>6 weeks	1

Pathophysiology

Rheumatoid factors (RFs) are antigammaglobulin antibodies, which are elaborated by the synovium in response to unknown antigens. These antibodies are believed to be the initiating factors, which trigger RA. Deposition of immune complexes in the synovium activates the complement system with influx of inflammatory cells. This leads to synovial proliferation, pannus formation and ultimate cartilage and subchondral bony destruction. In advanced cases, there may be fibrous ankylosis with subsequent bony ankylosis.[11,12]

Rheumatoid factors are present in the serum and synovial fluid in 70–80% of patients with a clinical diagnosis of RA. They may be found in the synovial fluid even when the serum is negative. However, they may also be present in the synovial fluid of cases with nonrheumatoid disorders; therefore, only high titers of RF in a joint effusion suggest RA. The RFs may initially be negative and later in the course of disease become positive.[4]

Imaging

The radiologic features of RA may be separated into "early" and "late" changes. The detection of early changes is important because new disease-modifying therapies are more effective when used before severe disability has occurred. Since initial changes are nonosseous in character, sonography and MRI imaging can detect disease earlier than conventional X-rays and computed tomography (CT). Secondly, in the present scenario, RA is treated aggressively with disease-modifying drugs, hence osseous changes are delayed.[5]

Radiographic Features

The earliest changes include joint space widening and soft tissue swelling.

Joint space widening is the earliest but a transient radiographic abnormality, sometimes lasting for only a few weeks. This finding is due to edema and swelling of the synovium and joint effusion. Joint space widening is best detected at the metacarpophalangeal (MCP) joints, especially in the 5th digit.[13] *Soft tissue swelling* results from an amalgam of joint effusion, synovial edema and proliferation, and tenosynovitis which invariably precedes cartilaginous and osseous changes. In the hand, periarticular fusiform swelling may be seen over the proximal interphalangeal (PIP) and 2nd and 5th MCP joints. Soft tissue swelling over the 3rd and 4th MCP joints may be appreciated as a local increased density. Swelling of the soft tissues over the styloid process of the ulna may be better detected on radiographs rather than clinical examination and is due to involvement of the extensor carpi ulnaris sheath. Soft tissue swelling over the styloid process of radius can be seen due to involvement of the radiocarpal joint.[14] In the feet, the soft tissue changes are less evident radiographically but may be seen over the 1st and 5th metatarsal heads. There may be blurring and obliteration of the pre-Achilles fat pad and blurring and thickening of the Achilles tendon.[3]

In the knee, there may be lateral bulging of the fat lines over the distal femur on anteroposterior (AP) radiographs. On lateral views, there is distention of the suprapatellar bursa with blurring of its surrounding fat lines. In the elbow, the anterior and posterior fat lines are displaced away from the joint on the lateral view.[14]

Osteopenia in RA is of two types: (1) local juxta-articular osteopenia is due to synovial inflammation and hyperemia and is a feature of early changes and (2) generalized osteopenia is due to limitation of movement due to pain, muscle wasting or steroid therapy and is therefore seen late in the disease.[3] Osteopenia is seen more often as the disease progresses and 80% of patients demonstrate osteopenia by 2 years after onset of symptoms. It is a precursor of erosive disease and may mask early erosions. Assessment of osteopenia may be difficult and comparison between normal and abnormal joints in the same patient is helpful. However, it is subjective and there may be interobserver as well as intraobserver variability in the assessment. Generalized or solitary terminal phalangeal sclerosis may be seen in up to 35% of patients with RA and other arthropathies and may be seen before any other abnormality.[14]

Joint space narrowing results from damage to the articular cartilage and is virtually always uniform **(Fig. 1)**. It may be more apparent than real in the presence of flexion deformities, and an oblique view may be required

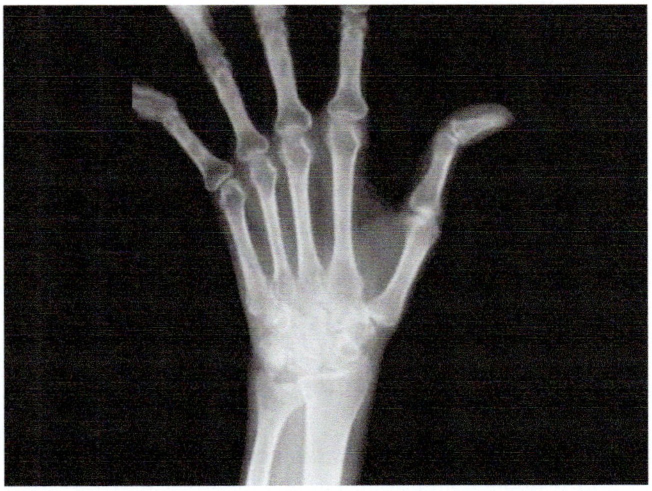

Fig. 1: X-ray of hand reveals the early changes of rheumatoid arthritis with classical juxta-articular osteopenia and uniform narrowing of the distal radioulnar, radiocarpal and intercarpal joints. Subluxations at the 1st metacarpophalangeal (MCP) and interphalangeal (IP) joints cause the classical "Hitchhiker's" deformity.

to assess the space. Uniform narrowing with an intact subchondral cortex is however not specific for RA as it can also be present in the SSAs or connective tissue diseases. Presence of uniform narrowing on the other hand is an important feature of RA that helps to differentiate it from OA in which the joint space narrowing is characteristically nonuniform or segmental.[2]

Subperiosteal bone apposition is uncommon in adult RA and is almost always subtle. When present, it may be seen at the site of capsular or tendon attachments and probably reflects the effect of tenosynovitis. This relative lack of periosteal reaction, despite advanced and often dramatic joint destruction is a distinctive feature of the disease and is so characteristic that the existence of exuberant periosteal reaction should suggest an alternate diagnosis.[3]

Erosions are the most important diagnostic feature of RA but may not be seen when the patient presents initially. Their incidence rises from <40% at 3 months from symptom onset to 90–95% at 10 years of disease.[14] The detection of erosions indicates irreversible joint damage. The earliest sites of cortical surface erosions are at the bare areas of bone between the margin of the articular cartilage and the attachment of the joint capsule and therefore their distribution is related to the anatomy of the joint.[15]

In the hands, erosions usually involve the wrist, MCP and PIP joints. The distal interphalangeal (DIP) joints are usually spared. Erosions involve a wider area on the proximal side of the PIP joints due to the larger bare areas on this side of the joint. At the MCP joints, the metacarpal heads develop the first and most extensive erosions, which are most evident at the radiovolar aspect of the 2nd and 3rd MCP joints. The 5th metacarpal may demonstrate the earliest erosions on its lateral aspect. In the interphalangeal (IP) joint of the thumb, erosions generally develop at the volar aspect on the ulnar side of the base of the distal phalanx. The ulnar styloid is commonly eroded due to inflammation in the prestyloid recess. There may be large erosions of the distal radius at the radioulnar joint. Erosions occur throughout the carpus and may be followed by fusion. However, bony ankylosis is uncommon in other joints in adult RA.[4]

In the feet, erosions appear earlier and are most often seen at the 5th metatarsophalangeal (MTP) joint. The heads of the metatarsals erode before the bases of the proximal phalanges, especially on the medial plantar aspect, although the lateral side of the 5th metatarsal head may be eroded. A characteristic site for erosion in the tarsus is at the posterosuperior aspect of the calcaneum above the insertion of the Achilles tendon. However, tarsal erosions are less often seen in RA as compared to the SSAs.[14] Bone erosions can also appear at extra-articular sites including the upper posterior ribs and ischial margins.[3]

Radiologically, early marginal erosions appear as cortical defects or an indistinctness of the subchondral cortex. This erasure or blurring of the white line of the cortex is first visualized on the radial side of the 4th and 5th metacarpal heads. If seen *en face*, erosions appear entirely within the bone giving a cystic appearance **(Fig. 2)**. Some may be deep or pocketed.

Erosive change is less common in the large joints. There may be a superficial surface irregularity in the presence of diffuse joint narrowing **(Fig. 3)**. In the hip, the medial joint space is characteristically involved with medial migration of the heads of the femora causing protrusio acetabuli. This is distinct from OA, which generally involves the superior compartment of the hip joint.[2]

Rarely, large intraosseous defects or pseudocysts may be seen in patients who have massive proliferation of the synovium. It has been hypothesized that these form due to the high intra-articular pressure, which exceeds the intraosseous pressure resulting in the movement of the synovial fluid into the adjacent subchondral bone. Invariably, there is destruction of the adjacent joint cartilage. Pseudocysts may attain sizes up to 2–3 cm, are usually oval to round, with regular outlines or slightly scalloped margins.[15]

Late Changes

Alignment deformities at joints may result from local synovitis weakening the capsule and tendinitis preventing normal musculotendinous actions causing subluxations and dislocations. Tendons may also rupture in the region of eroded bone. Thus, rotator cuff tears result in upward subluxation of the eroded humeral head. Subluxation at the MCP joints leads to ulnar deviation, which is seen in 50% of patients with chronic disease. There is

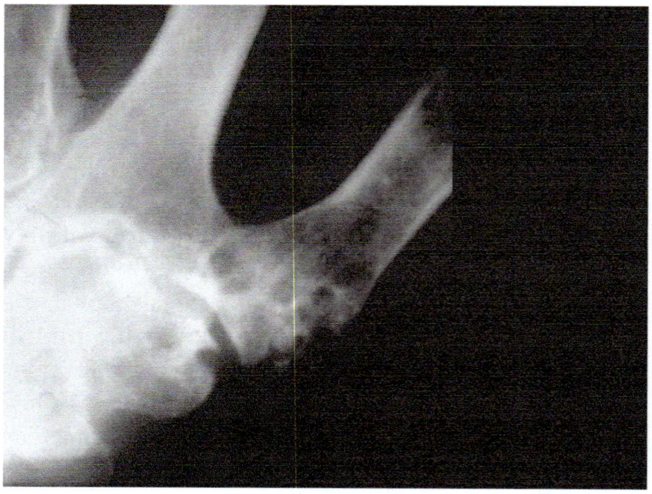

Fig. 2: Rheumatoid arthritis. Magnified view of the carpometacarpal (CMC) joints demonstrates multiple erosions in the bases of the metacarpals and trapezium giving a cystic appearance.

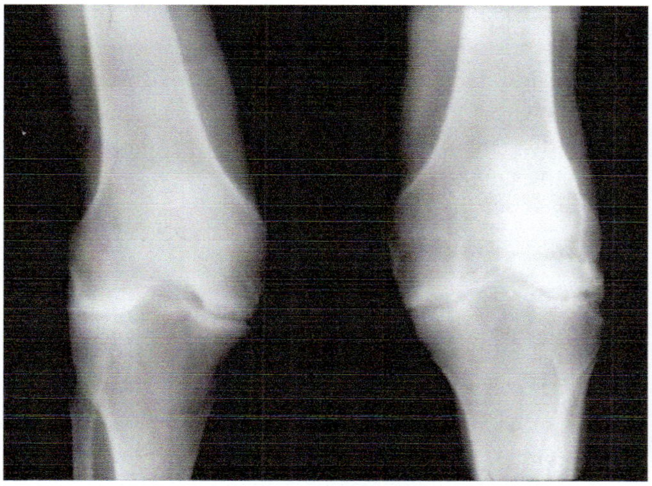

Fig. 3: X-ray of both knee joints in a case of rheumatoid arthritis (RA) reveals diffuse osteopenia with uniform narrowing of the joint spaces. Note the lack of irregularity of the articular margins.

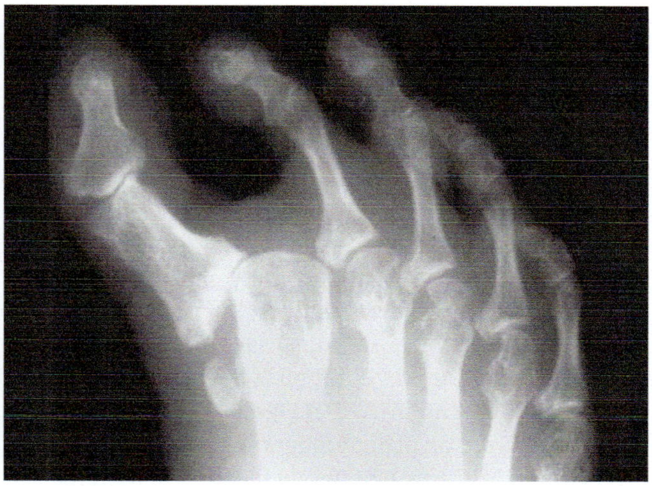

Fig. 4: X-ray of the forefoot shows more advanced changes of rheumatoid arthritis with gross erosions of the metatarsal heads with subluxations at the metatarsophalangeal (MTP) and interphalangeal (IP) joints with hallux valgus.

also increasing palmar flexion due to ulnar deviation of extensor tendons. Other classical deformities in the hands are the "boutonnière" deformity due to flexion at the PIP joint with extension at the DIP joint. The reverse is seen with the "swan-neck" deformity due to PIP joint extension and DIP joint flexion. Flexion at the 1st MCP joint with extension at the IP joint results in the "Hitchhiker's thumb". There may also be dislocation of the carpus causing a bayonet deformity at the wrist.[4]

In the feet, there may be lateral deviation of the toes, especially hallux valgus **(Fig. 4)**. The hallux sesamoids sublux between the 1st and 2nd metatarsal heads and the transverse arch flattens due to ligamentous laxity.[14]

Severe erosive change leads to marked *destruction and narrowing of the joint spaces* with extreme irregularity and destruction of the subchondral bone **(Fig. 5)**. In the hands, the bone ends are often reciprocally eroded and there may be telescoping of the fingers. There is resultant arthritis mutilans, which may also be seen in other conditions such as erosive OA and multicentric reticulohistiocytosis.[3]

Gross *loss of bone* at the femoral head results in a "bird's beak" appearance. There may be pointing of the adjacent bone ends at the acromioclavicular joints with resorption of the distal clavicles.

Stress fractures may occur due to normal stress on bone with decreased elastic resistance. *Giant synovial* cysts may develop, particularly originating from the knee joint and presenting in the calf. They may also occur around the shoulder, elbow and hip where they may protrude into the pelvis. RA can attack any synovial joint and there may be involvement of the laryngeal joints, sternomanubrial or temporomandibular joints.[3]

Pulmonary involvement may lead to pleural effusions, pulmonary nodules (30%) or interstitial fibrosis (predominantly lower lobe). Pulmonary nodules are usually associated with subcutaneous nodules present at the extensor surfaces of the elbows or other joints. Secondary OA may complicate RA in weight-bearing joints. Reactive sclerosis and new bone formation is not marked in these joints.[14]

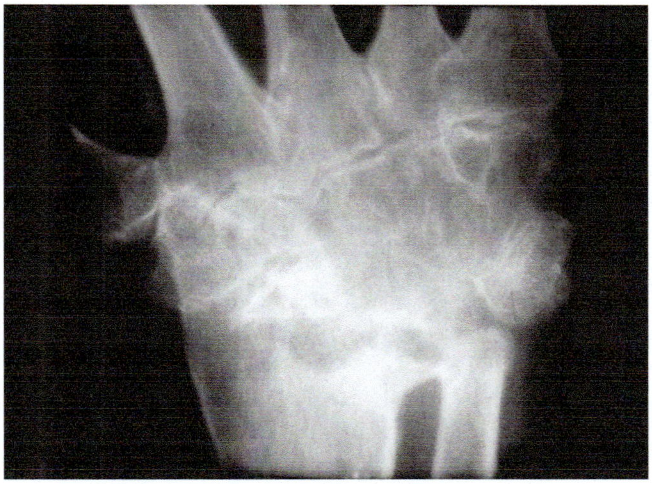

Fig. 5: Magnified view of the wrist joint demonstrating late changes of rheumatoid arthritis with severe osteopenia, gross destruction of the distal ends of the radius and ulna with ankylosis of the carpal bones.

Axial Skeleton Involvement

The spondylitis associated with RA is peculiar in that it usually involves the cervical region. Thoracic or lumbar involvement is distinctly uncommon. Osteoporosis, narrowing of the disc along with endplate irregularity are present in the upper cervical vertebrae with minimal reactive new bone formation. This is in sharp contrast to OA which usually involves the lower cervical spine. Erosions at the facet joints can lead to multilevel subluxations in the upper cervical spine giving a step-ladder appearance.[4]

Atlantoaxial (AA) subluxation may be present in up to 20–25% of patients with chronic RA and is primarily due to looseness of the transverse ligament (which is responsible for maintaining the integrity of the AA joint) with/without erosive changes in the odontoid. A gap of >2.5 mm in adults or 4 mm in children between the anterior border of the odontoid and the posterior surface of the anterior arch of the atlas in flexion in children is deemed diagnostic of atlantoaxial dislocation (AAD) **(Figs. 6A and B)**. Although it can be visualized on plain radiographs, three-dimensional (3D) CT and MRI give a better delineation of both the soft tissue and bony involvement **(Figs. 7A to D)**.[15] The eroded odontoid may at times fracture. Resorption of bone at nonarticular surfaces occurs at the spinous processes which become short, sharp and tapered.[3]

Occasionally, the sacroiliac joints exhibit minimal erosions with joint space narrowing; however, reactive sclerosis as seen in AS is typically absent. Rarely, there may be ankylosis of the sacroiliac joints.

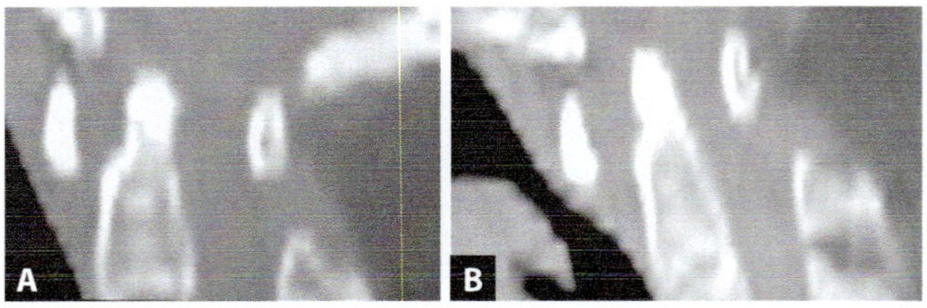

Figs. 6A and B: Sagittal reformatted three-dimensional (3D) CT images of the craniovertebral junction in (A) extension and (B) flexion show increase in the atlantoaxial distance on flexion with erosion of the odontoid peg due to rheumatoid arthritis.

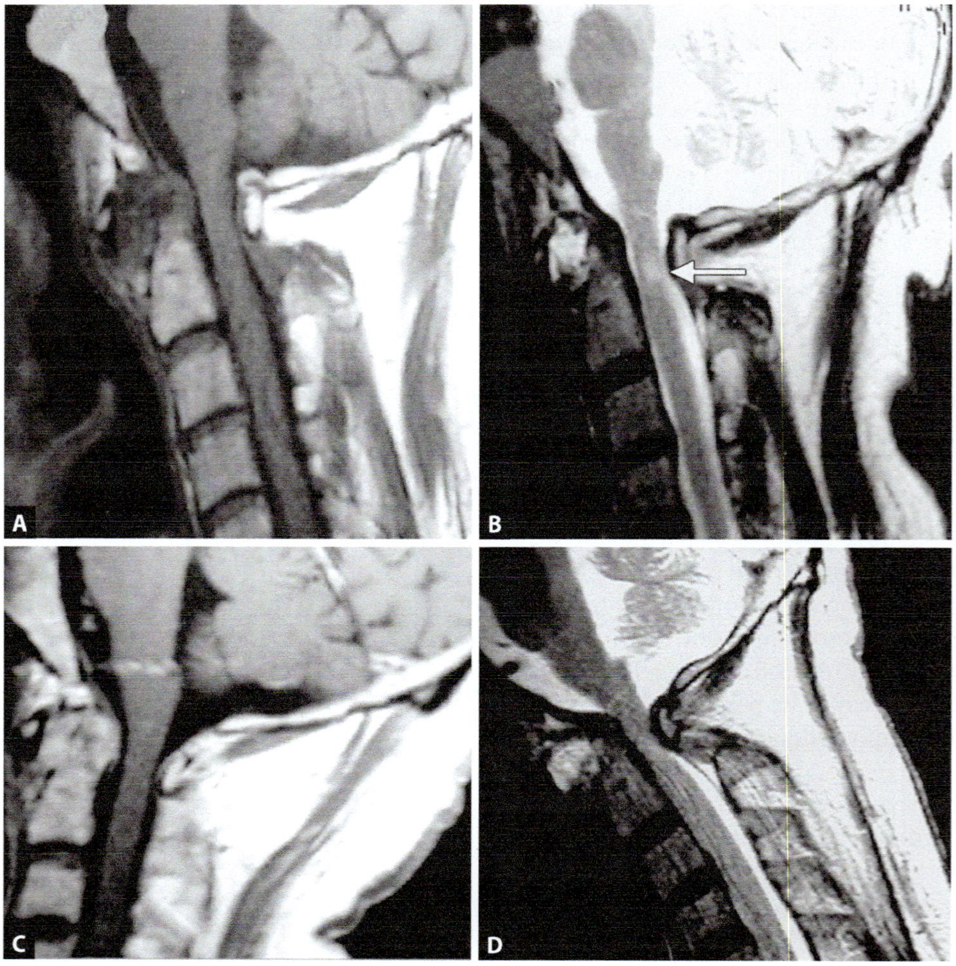

Figs. 7A to D: Magnetic resonance (MR) of the craniovertebral junction in a case of rheumatoid arthritis with atlantoaxial dislocation (AAD). (A) T1- and (B) T2-weighted images in neutral position reveal erosion of the odontoid with pannus which appears hypointense on T1 and hyperintense on T2-weighted sequences. Hyperintense signal is seen within the cord at this level due to ischemia/edema; (C) Postgadolinium, there is significant enhancement of the pannus; (D) T2-weighted image in flexion demonstrates compression of the cord due to posterior displacement of the odontoid peg.

Other Imaging Modalities

Ultrasonography

The introduction of high-resolution linear transducers led to the widespread use of ultrasonography (USG) in musculoskeletal imaging. USG may be used for the detection as well as monitoring of the inflammatory changes and osseous damage. A number of studies have demonstrated the ability of USG to identify early synovial inflammation in the form of synovial thickening and joint effusion. Power Doppler has the capacity to discern and measure alterations in the vascularity of the synovium due to inflammation **(Figs. 8A and B)**. USG contrast agents have the capability to enhance the sensitivity of power Doppler by increasing the signal from the synovial vessels.

The joint margins can be assessed for the presence of erosions. It has been established that USG has higher sensitivity than conventional radiography for detection of erosion in the small joints.[16] The internal structure of the tendons can be assessed and their integrity or rupture demonstrated by dynamic scanning. Leakage of synovial fluid may also be demonstrated, e.g., a ruptured Baker's cyst which needs to be distinguished from other causes of pain in the calf, such as deep vein thrombosis or muscle tear. USG can also be used to evaluate the response to therapy. Following treatment, USG can detect reduction in the synovial inflammation and vascular flow parameters.[17] Several studies have compared power Doppler with MRI for the detection of early arthritis. A prospective study that included 60 patients demonstrated that USG showed a higher sensitivity than MRI for the detection of synovitis.[18] In another study, sonography was found to be a valuable tool; however, contrast-enhanced magnetic resonance (CEMR) was found to be superior for the evaluation of synovial proliferation as well as erosions.[19] Disadvantages of USG include the user-dependent nature of the modality and the long time required to evaluate multiple joints.

Computed Tomography

Computed tomography is not frequently used routinely in RA as it is inferior to MRI and USG for the detection of early disease along with the disadvantage of using ionizing radiation. It can demonstrate the presence of erosions, particularly in the carpal and tarsal bones. It can also show joint space narrowing or ankylosis. A recent study has reported comparable performance of CT with MRI for the evaluation of synovitis and tenosynovitis using contrast-enhanced CT with digital masking of the bone.[20] However, its main use lies in the diagnosis and management of upper cervical spine abnormalities, particularly for the evaluation of AA subluxation.[15]

Radionuclide Scanning

Scanning with ^{99m}Tc-methylene diphosphonate (MDP) is quite sensitive for detection of the inflammatory changes of arthritis but shows poor specificity. In RA, isotopes are at least 70% more sensitive than conventional films and may be used to monitor response to therapy.[11] Findings include increased flow in the synovium in the early or blood pool phase and increased uptake in the delayed 3 hours scans.

Magnetic Resonance Imaging

Over the last two decades, MRI has consolidated its position as the best imaging modality for RA, despite being expensive and time consuming. The Outcome Measures in Rheumatoid Arthritis Clinical Trials (OMERACT) MRI study group was an international, multidisciplinary group which was set up for the purpose of standardizing imaging techniques and definitions of joint pathologies in RA.[6] According to their recommendations, an MRI scan for RA should comprise of the minimum following sequences: (1) imaging in two planes (axial and coronal), (2) T1-weighed sequences before and after gadolinium, and (3) a fat-saturated T2-weighted or a short-tau inversion recovery

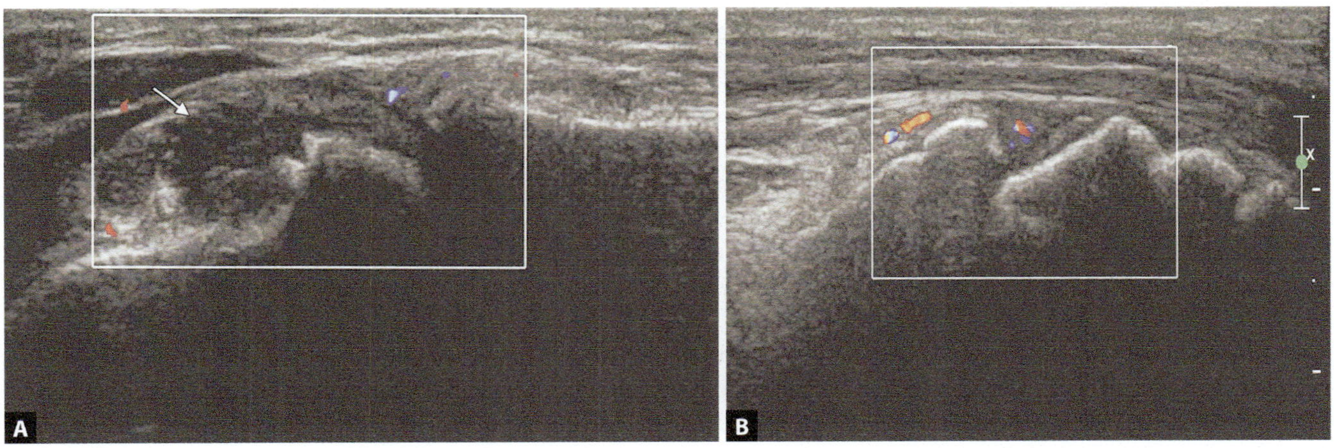

Figs. 8A and B: (A) Ultrasound image of the metacarpophalangeal joints shows diffuse synovial thickening (arrow) with convex margin, loss of articular cartilage, fluid and erosions in a case of rheumatoid arthritis; (B) Power Doppler in the same case showing increased vascularity in the synovial thickening.

(STIR) sequence. MRI is also a useful imaging modality for the follow-up of RA to evaluate progression or remission. The typical progression in RA from the stage of synovitis followed by edema of the bone marrow to bony erosion is well demonstrated on MRI.[6]

Synovial imaging: Magnetic resonance imaging is now believed to be the gold standard for synovial imaging. Inflammatory changes within the soft tissues of the joints which precede the development of erosions and which are not detectable on plain radiographs are well demonstrated on MRI.[21] It has been reported that using the enhancement of MCP and PIP joints as a positive diagnostic criteria, it is possible to diagnose RA with a high sensitivity of 96% and accuracy of 44%.[8] The OMERACT group defines synovitis as an area in the synovial compartment which shows enhancement following contrast administration with thickness which exceeds the width of the normal synovium.[6] MRI depicts irregular thickening of the synovium which is of intermediate signal intensity (SI) compared to darker fluid on T1 and high SI on T2-weighted spin echo sequences. Fat-suppressed T2-weighted sequences more clearly delineate disease extent. Postgadolinium, there can be significant rapid enhancement of the inflamed synovium in contrast to joint effusion which does not show enhancement in the early phase. Images obtained > 10 minutes after gadolinium show diffusion of gadolinium into the synovial joint fluid resulting in increased SI.[6] The activity of the synovitis is best assessed on postcontrast fat-suppressed T1-weighted images and there is indirect evidence suggesting that the amount of postcontrast enhancement correlates with the degree of inflammation.[15] Fibrotic pannus and pannus with hemosiderin deposition show low SI on T1- and T2-weighted images and do not enhance on postgadolinium images.

Quantification of synovial volume has been shown to have a significant role to play in the diagnosis as well as follow-up of RA. The baseline synovial volume has been found to correlate significantly with the number of new bone erosions at 1-year follow-up.[6,21]

Bone marrow edema: Edema of the bone marrow has been described as a characteristic finding in RA, especially in the early phase. It manifests as ill-defined, high SI on fat-suppressed, T2-weighted and STIR images with enhancement following gadolinium **(Fig. 9)**. It has been reported in up to 39–75% of patients with RA with disease duration of below 1 year.[6] It is commonly found in the subchondral bone and can be seen as an isolated finding or surrounding areas of bone erosions. It is presently considered to be a forerunner of erosions. Some studies have shown the high association of bone marrow edema at baseline with development of erosions later in the course of the illness at 1 and 6 years.[22]

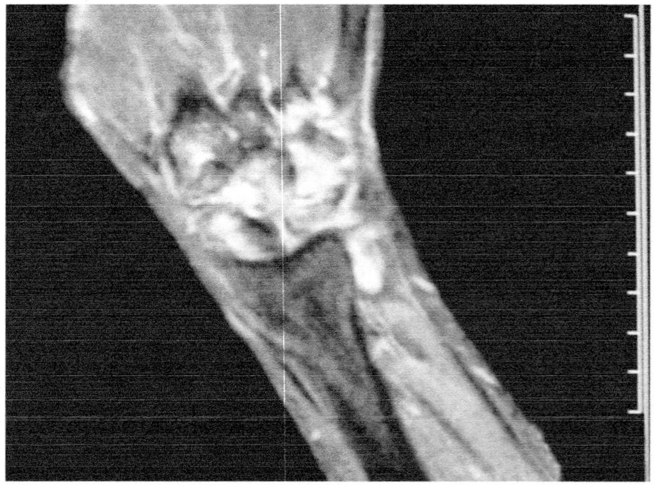

Fig. 9: Coronal short tau inversion recovery (STIR) image shows ill-defined areas of high signal intensity in the carpal bones due to bone marrow edema.

Erosions: On MRI, erosions are seen as focal areas of loss of normal SI from cortical or subchondral bone on T1 with high SI on T2-weighted or STIR images **(Figs. 10A and B)**. Erosions replace marrow fat and contain inflamed synovium which enhances with gadolinium and are thus easily differentiated from other interosseous fluid-filled cystic lesions.[23]

In early RA, MRI can detect bone erosions in 45–72% of patients with early disease (<6 months duration), in contrast to 8–40% on radiography.[6,9] This is important as MRI can expedite the early diagnosis of RA, allowing treatment to be instituted early in the progression of disease. It is also important to identify those patients in whom progressive disease does not occur as these patients do not require aggressive treatment protocols. In one study, 82% of patients who did not show erosions at the baseline MRI did not develop any radiographic erosions at 2-year follow-up.[6]

Tendons and ligaments: Rheumatoid arthritis can involve the ligaments or tendons directly which results in predisposition to rupture. Increased signal on T2-weighted spin echo and STIR sequences indicates tendon involvement and may be due to erosion, invasion by pannus or partial tear. Any alterations in the thickness of the tendon are also abnormal.

Tenosynovitis can be diagnosed by the detection of fluid in the tendon sheath, thickening of the tendon sheath or enhancement. The most commonly involved tendon is the extensor carpi ulnaris.[23] Inflammation of the flexor tendons of the wrist results in a greater carpal tunnel volume, which in turn leads to increased mechanical pressure and compression of the median nerve which can also be inflamed resulting in carpal tunnel syndrome. Axial images are most useful for evaluating the anatomy of the carpal tunnel.

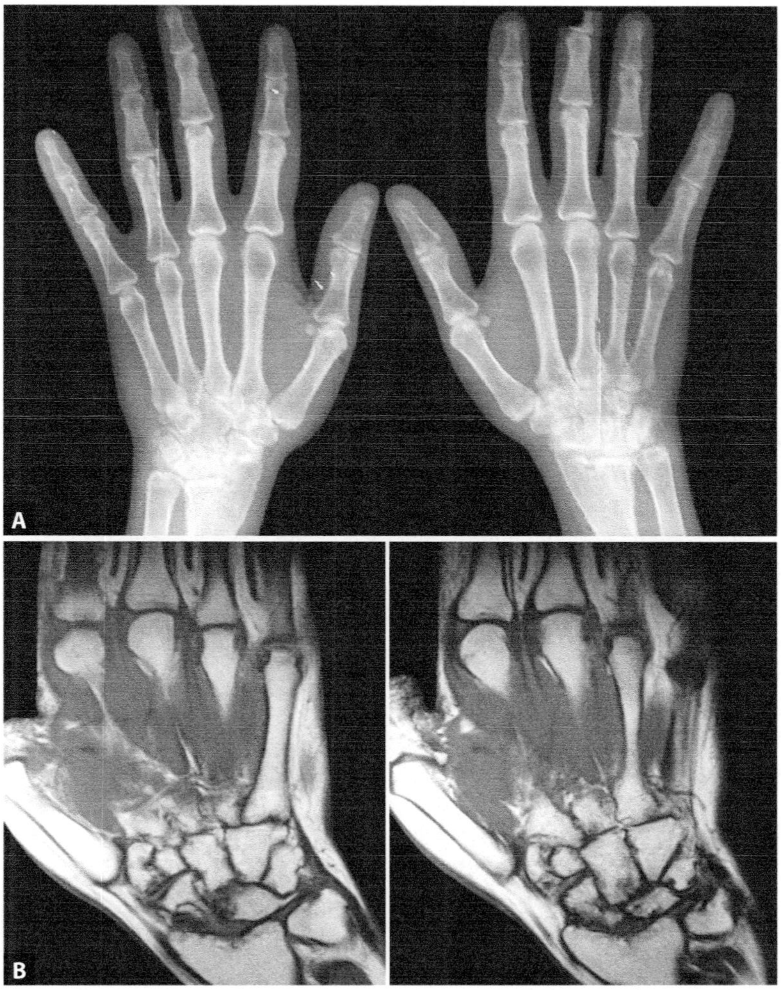

Figs. 10A and B: Patient with rheumatoid arthritis: (A) X-ray of both hands posteroanterior (PA) view shows diffuse loss of the joint spaces at the radiocarpal, intercarpal and CMC joints; (B) T1-weighted coronal image demonstrates multiple erosions in the carpal bones, distal ulna and radius.

Intraosseous cysts show decreased SI on T1 and increased SI on T2- weighted images and may not enhance in the immediate postcontrast phase.[5]

Intra-articular loose bodies are frequently seen due to the destructive inflammatory process and include cartilaginous and osseous fragments. A subset of loose bodies is called "rice bodies" as they resemble polished rice. They are now recognized as a distinctive feature of RA. They may contain various tissues such as collagen, fibrinogen and its products, mononuclear cells, and blood cells along with amorphous material.[5]

Large joints: Though involvement of large joints usually occurs after established disease elsewhere, MRI is more sensitive in picking up early change. In the glenohumeral joint, rotator cuff tears, joint effusion, giant synovial cysts and early erosions are best evaluated on MRI. Similarly, involvement of the hip joint with detection of joint effusion, pannus, erosions and articular cartilage destruction is well depicted on MRI **(Figs. 11A and B)**.[22]

Scoring Systems for Rheumatoid Arthritis

Radiographic images establish the degree of structural damage of the joints at a given point in time. Radiographic abnormalities were initially used to develop an index of the damage that was used to assign patients to four stages. However, by the early 1960s, it was realized that assigning a single score for all radiographic abnormalities lacked sensitivity for detecting disease progression and various scoring systems were developed which rated the severity of bony erosion and degree of joint space narrowing separately. Larsen developed a global scoring system which incorporated the presence of erosions, soft tissue swelling and osteoporosis into a single score. Multiple different modifications and variations of the global or composite methods were extensively used in an attempt to delineate the progression of disease in RA and to effectively assess response to therapy.[24] However, the scoring systems are not exact measurements as they reflect individual readers and so, the error of individual scores can be considerable.

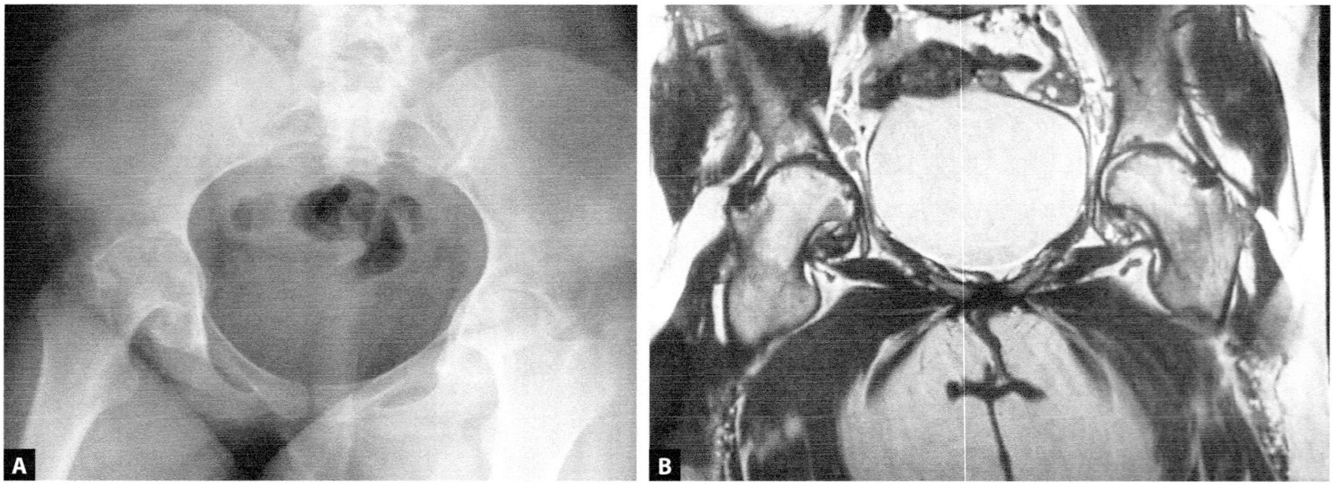

Figs. 11A and B: (A) X-ray pelvis of a patient with rheumatoid arthritis (RA) shows uniform loss of joint space with irregularity of the articular surface in bilateral hip joints. Note the medial migration of the femoral heads; (B) Coronal T2-weighted image better demonstrates the erosions. Note the bone marrow edema manifesting as ill-defined hyperintense signal.

Also, the expected progression of bony or soft tissue damage in untreated disease is not possible to ascertain. Development of an accurate, easily reproducible and easily carried out quantitative measurement of bony erosion and cartilage destruction is required.

On MRI at present, the most commonly frequently used method is the Rheumatoid Arthritis Magnetic Resonance Imaging Score (RAMRIS) proposed by OMERACT. In this, the synovitis is rated in three wrist regions: (1) the distal radioulnar joint, (2) the radiocarpal joint, and (3) the intercarpal, carpometacarpal and MCP joints on a scale of 0–3. An assigned score of 0 is normal, while score of 1 (mild), 2 (moderate) or 3 (severe) reflect the increasing volume of enhancing synovium. Similarly, bone marrow edema is scored from 0 to 3 according to the volume: 0 is no edema, 1 is 1–33%, 2 is 34–66%, and 3 is 67–100% of bone that is edematous. Erosions in the bones of the wrist are scored separately. The scores range from 0 to 10 according to the volume of erosions in the assessed bones in increments of 10%. The maximum score in the wrist is 150.[25] However, using the RAMRIS score is difficult, requiring years of dedicated work, is subject to high interobserver variability and is not practical in clinical practice.

Scoring methods have been shown to be effective in determining the benefit from drug treatment and will continue to evaluate the advantages of new drugs in the coming years. Development of a simple, easy to use, accurate and reproducible method would be a powerful tool for both the physician and the clinical investigator.

At present, the aim of the management of RA is to avert disability and damage evident on radiology with early and persistent remission. Treatment efficacy is measured by ACR/EULAR and Disease Activity Score (DAS) which is the first step in disease management.[26]

JUVENILE IDIOPATHIC ARTHRITIDES

A number of separate disorders can lead to chronic arthritis in children; however, there is as yet no uniformly accepted classification for these diseases. The International League of Associations of Rheumatologists (ILAR) Task Force did attempt to establish classification criteria;[27] however, they are not in universal use.

- *Juvenile-onset adult type (seropositive) rheumatoid arthritis*: Seropositive juvenile rheumatoid arthritis (JRA) accounts for 5–15% of juvenile idiopathic arthritis (JIA). The onset is during adolescence and there is a strong female preponderance. It is a peripheral erosive polyarthritis which is nearly identical with adult RA. Large joints like the knee and hips may be affected.
- Seronegative *chronic arthritis*: In this subgroup, systemic or articular symptoms and signs develop in the absence of positive serology for RF.
  - *Classic systemic disease* represents 20% of children with JIA. It affects children below the age of 5 years. Both sexes are equally affected. These children present with an acute febrile onset with anemia, hepatosplenomegaly, lymphadenopathy, anorexia, weight loss, and chronic recurrent arthralgias. Erosive arthritis is uncommon.
  - *Pauciarticular* type is the most common type of JIA responsible for nearly half the cases. Four or less joints are involved, generally the large joints like the knee, elbow and ankle. It typically affects young girls.
  - *Polyarticular* type represents approximately 20% of JIA. It may occur at any age and is commoner in females. It is symmetric and involves the large and small joints as well as the cervical spine. Growth retardation is common due to premature fusion of the epiphyses and there may be associated mandibular hypoplasia with antegonial notching.

Generally, the prognosis in JIA is good with fewer than 20% children having progressive destructive disease. The pathophysiology is virtually identical to the adult form with inflammation of the synovium and greater production of joint fluid with effusion. Pannus is less extensive than adult RA but still produces significant cartilage and bony destruction.[4,12,28]

Radiologic Features

The knee is the most common joint to manifest radiographic abnormalities followed by the other large joints, wrist, hand, cervical spine, sacroiliac joints, and sternoclavicular joint.[28] Early changes include soft tissue swelling and osteopenia which may be juxta-articular or diffuse. In early stages, it is probably due to hyperemia, but later, disuse atrophy and steroids contribute to it. Band-like metaphyseal lucent zones (growth arrest lines) may be evident. Pathological fractures may occur.[13] Periostitis appears within weeks following the onset of symptoms and is usually seen along the shafts of the metacarpals, metatarsals, and proximal phalanges.[4]

Later, there is uniform loss of joint space and articular erosions **(Figs. 12A to C)**. Progressive destruction can lead to bony ankylosis. Joining together of the carpometacarpal joint of the middle and index fingers is typical as are multiple, fused cervical vertebrae.[4]

The most distinctive radiographic findings are seen as a result of altered growth patterns. There is accelerated bone maturation with early fusion of epiphyses and bone shortening secondary to hyperemia.[12] This results in large expansile (ballooned) epiphyses while the adjacent metaphysis and diaphysis appear gracile and constricted.[4] Muscle atrophy is generally a prominent feature **(Fig. 13)**.

In the carpus and tarsus, the bones show accelerated maturation, crowding with joint space narrowing and an abnormal angular shape (squashed carpi). The cervical spine is often affected with erosions at the apophyseal joints (usually at C2-3) leading to ankylosis. The associated vertebral bodies fail to develop. AAD is said to occur rarely in children with seronegative disease. The intervertebral discs are narrowed and fusion may occur. There may be ankylosis of the sacroiliac joints. Secondary degenerative changes may occur later.[14]

Radiographs are useful for making the initial diagnosis, and also for staging the disease and for follow-up. They are also useful for excluding other causes of pain like congenital disorders, fractures or tumors. However, they mostly illustrate late changes and indirect signs of synovial disease. USG is a rapid and safe modality which does not utilize ionizing radiation which can directly image the synovium for evidence of proliferation or hypervascularity and joint effusion.[29] USG can also be used as a guidance modality for performing joint aspiration, the sample can be cultured to exclude septic arthritis. In a study on 30 patients, USG demonstrated a higher sensitivity than clinical assessment for the detection of synovial effusion and thickening in cases of JIA.[30] In another study, it was found that power Doppler sonography was highly accurate in monitoring the therapeutic response in cases of JIA.[31]

Magnetic resonance imaging remains the imaging modality of choice for evaluating the early changes of JIA because of its ability to allow direct visualization of nonossified portions of epiphyseal cartilage.[12] It clearly depicts joint effusion, cartilage changes, synovial proliferation, bony erosion or synovial cysts. With long-standing JIA of the knee, chronic inflammation involving the meniscal surfaces can lead to meniscal hypoplasia or even atrophy.[28,32] Radiographic evidence of synovitis may be seen in trauma-induced synovitis or infective arthritis. These disorders are monoarticular in contrast to JIA and history of trauma or acute onset may serve to differentiate them from JIA. If tubercular arthritis involves multiple large joints, it may be indistinguishable from JIA. In hemophilic arthropathy, multiple episodes of bleeding into the joint cavity induce synovial inflammation with hypertrophy resulting in a radiologic picture closely resembling JIA.

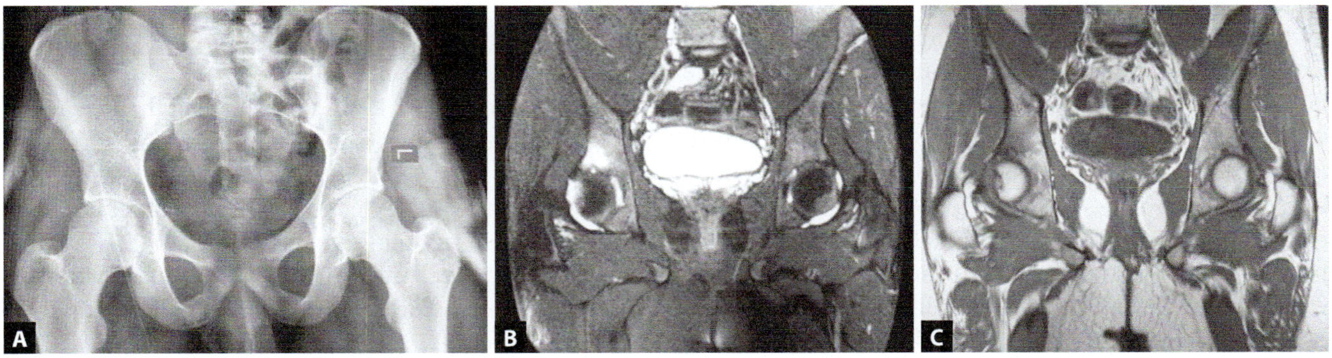

Figs. 12A to C: A 12-year-old boy with juvenile idiopathic arthritis (JIA). (A) X-ray of the pelvis shows mild narrowing of the joint spaces in bilateral hips; (B) Coronal T2-weighted image demonstrates the presence of joint effusion and ill-defined hyperintense signal in the acetabulum signifying bone marrow edema; (C) Coronal T1-weighted image shows bone erosions in bilateral hip joints.

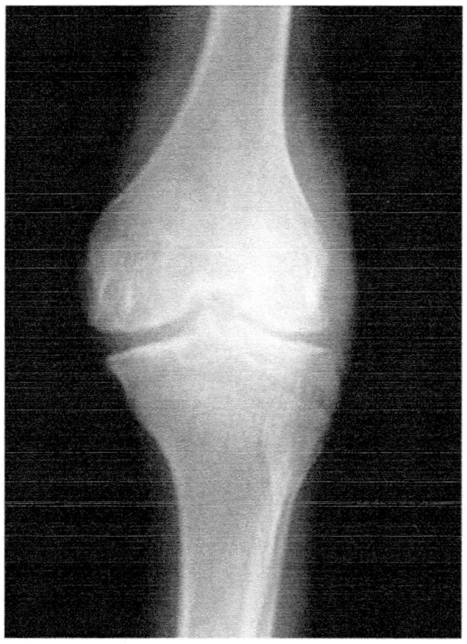

Fig. 13: Juvenile rheumatoid arthritis—X-ray knee joint anteroposterior (AP) view reveals diffuse osteopenia with large squared femoral condyles, widening with irregularity of the intercondylar notch and subchondral lucencies. Note the reduction in the soft tissue bulk.

SERONEGATIVE SPONDYLOARTHROPATHIES

Seronegative spondyloarthropathies are a category of seronegative arthritic diseases affecting multiple organ systems with clinical and radiological overlap and a significant genetic component. They are characterized by the absence of RF, peripheral arthropathy and sacroiliitis with or without spondylitis. A classification criterion for the entire group of SSA has been developed. These criteria are inflammatory spinal pain or synovitis, in conjunction with minimum one of the following criteria: a positive family history, urethritis, inflammatory bowel disease, psoriasis, acute diarrhea, enthesopathy, alternating buttock pain or radiographically evident sacroiliitis.[33]

ANKYLOSING SPONDYLITIS

Ankylosing spondylitis is a chronic, progressive inflammatory arthritis which chiefly involves the synovial joints of the spine along with the adjacent soft tissues as well as the sacroiliac joints, although peripheral, large joints such as the hips, shoulders and knee can also be involved.[4] There is a strong association with HLA-B27 with >90% of patients with AS having this antigen. It has been shown that AS will develop in 0.6–1.3% of persons who are positive for HLA-B27. Approximately 65% of patients of psoriasis with spondylitis or inflammatory bowel disease with spondylitis also have HLA-B27 and it has been postulated that the antigen is essentially related to spinal changes.[14]

The disease is common in males (4:1) though recently it has been realized that women may be more commonly affected than thought earlier. Women more often have only clinical manifestations without radiographic evidence of disease. The onset of disease is generally between 15 and 35 years.[12]

The archetypal clinical description of AS is of an insidious onset with low back pain which carries on for >3 months. Back stiffness is worse after periods of inactivity and there may be pain over the gluteal and sacroiliac regions. Radiographic evidence of sacroiliitis is mandatory for the definitive diagnosis of AS, but may take several years to appear. Various extra-articular features may be present of which the most common is acute anterior uveitis. Others include aortitis, aortic regurgitation, pulmonary fibrosis, cardiac conduction defects, arachnoiditis, and amyloidosis.[34] Pulmonary involvement can result in cavitation with fibrosis in bilateral lung apices mimicking tuberculosis.[10]

Pathophysiology

Histologically, the synovitis of AS is identical to that of RA. There is a predisposition to develop ankylosis due to metaplasia of the cartilage, endochondral ossification, formation of woven bone and fibrosis. The enthesopathy consists of destruction of ligaments, tendons and local bone with inflammatory infiltrate. This heals by the deposition of new bone at the interface between the tendons and ligaments. This causes bone proliferation at nonarticular sites, syndesmophytes and capsular ossification.[14] It has been suggested that there is a genetic predisposition which permits an antigen or other triggering factor to enter the synovium and evoke an inflammatory response. This inflammatory response causes activation of the lymphocytes which liberate tumor necrosis factor-alpha (TNF-α) and other cytokines leading to destruction of tissue.[34]

Radiologic Features

Sacroiliac Joints

The classic sacroiliitis is bilateral and symmetrical. In about 10% of cases, the sacroiliitis may be unilateral or asymmetrical at presentation but eventually becomes bilaterally symmetrical. Changes occur in both the synovial along with ligamentous (superior and posterior) parts of the sacroiliac joints. The earliest radiographic findings occur in the subchondral cortex which appears blurred or lost. Later, small (rat-bite) erosions appear which are worse along the iliac aspect of the joint. These cause widening of the joint space with hazy margins **(Figs. 14A and B)**. This is followed by larger erosions, subjacent sclerosis and joint space narrowing as irregular new bone bridges the joint space with eventual ankylosis and resolution of the sclerosis.[2,12,14]

The modified New York criteria for grading sacroiliitis established in 1994 are:[35]

- Grade 0: Normal findings
- Grade 1: Suspicious changes
- Grade 2: Minimal abnormality (small localized erosions or sclerosis without alteration in joint width)
- Grade 3: Unequivocal abnormality
- Grade 4: Total ankylosis

Joint changes are assessed using prone views with cephalad angulation or oblique views. However, CT is more sensitive than radiographs in depicting small and early erosions and joint space changes.[34] Recently, it has been suggested that dynamic CEMR shows a higher sensitivity than CT for the detection of sacroiliitis.[36] MRI findings include erosions, subchondral sclerosis, bone marrow edema, intra-articular hyperintensity on T2- and T2*-weighted images with postcontrast enhancement within the joint cavity **(Figs. 15A and B)**. Radionuclide scanning shows nonspecific increased uptake in the presence of active sacroiliitis.

Spine

Spinal involvement classically starts at the dorsolumbar or lumbosacral junction with subsequent progressive involvement of the rest of the spine in an ascending

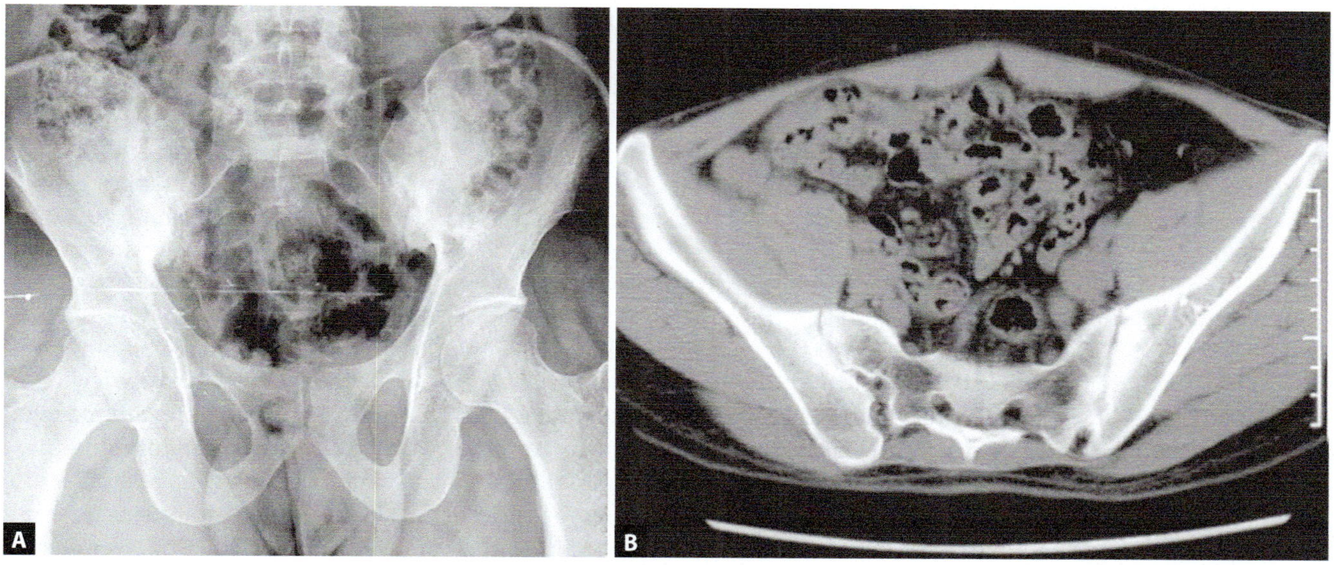

Figs. 14A and B: Sacroiliitis in ankylosing spondylitis. (A) X-ray pelvis anteroposterior (AP) view shows mild irregularity with subarticular sclerosis in both sacroiliac (SI) joints; (B) Axial CT section of the SI joints of the same patient shows irregularity of the articular surfaces with subarticular sclerosis which is more marked in the iliac blades.

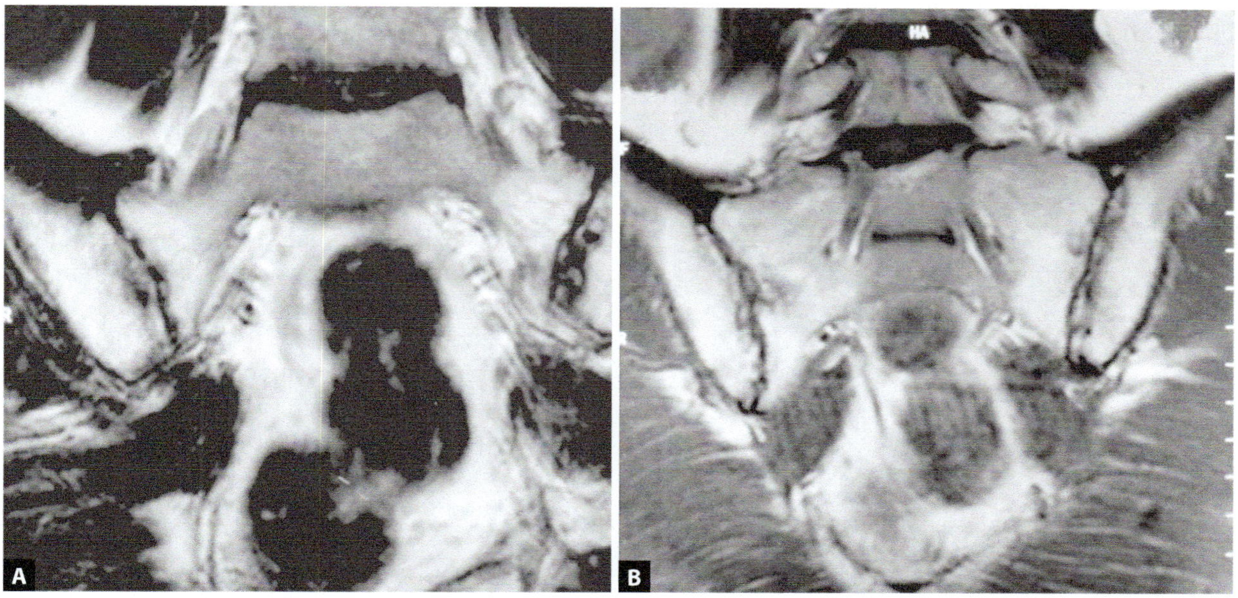

Figs. 15A and B: Ankylosing spondylitis. (A) T1- and (B) T2-weighted coronal images show irregularity of the cortex, discrete subchondral erosions, irregular thinning of the articular cartilage and reactive subarticular bone marrow edema and fatty change.

manner. In females, the cervical region may be initially affected. Erosions initially occur at the vertebral margins at the site of attachment of the outer fibers of the annulus fibrosus (Romanus lesions) with adjacent sclerosis (shiny corner sign). In adolescents, these erosions may be quite large mimicking an infectious process (erosive spondylitis). Healing of these erosions or laying down of bone beneath the anterior longitudinal ligament causes "squaring" of the vertebral bodies, best appreciated on lateral radiographs of the lumbar spine. Exuberant new bone formation may even cause anterior convexity of the vertebral body (barrel-shaped vertebrae).[4,14,34] As the disease progresses, there is syndesmophyte formation along the anterior and anterolateral aspects of the body due to ossification in the annulus. Syndesmophytes are paravertebral in location and vertically oriented in contrast to the osteophytes seen in degenerative disease which are horizontally directed. The syndesmophytes seen in AS are classically marginal, symmetrical, fine and delicate. Ankylosis of multiple vertebrae by syndesmophytes gives the bamboo spine appearance. Similar ossifications may be seen in the interspinous ligaments and facet joints causing the dagger and tram-track signs respectively **(Figs. 16A and B)**. Facet joint ankylosis is the major factor causing loss of spinal mobility.[2-4,12]

Studies have demonstrated than MRI can identify active enthesitis in the spine much before Romanus lesions are seen on radiographs. MRI shows an abnormal area of low SI on T1-weighted image which is hyperintense on T2-weighted image and enhances postcontrast.[34]

Spinal fractures are common in the spine through the porotic bone just beneath the endplates. Two categories have been described: (1) the traumatic fractures and (2) stress fractures. Traumatic fractures occur after spinal fusion even with trivial trauma and are of the unstable category with involvement of all three columns. Stress fractures characteristically occur near the cervicothoracic or thoracolumbar junctions, with development of sclerotic pseudoarthrosis with destruction of the disc and vertebral endplates (Andersson lesion) resembling an infective discitis.[14,34]

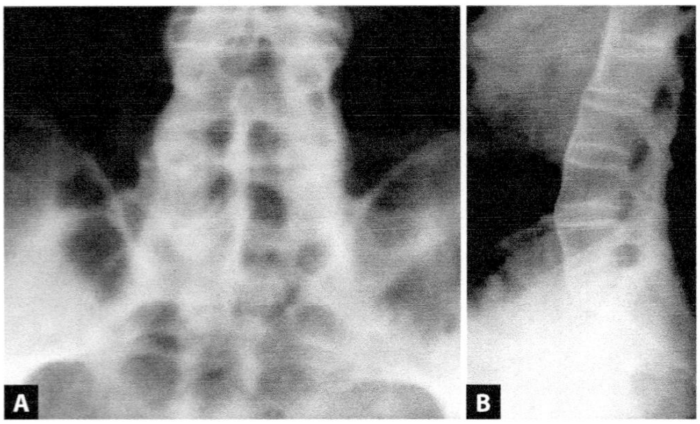

Figs. 16A and B: Ankylosing spondylitis: X-rays lumbosacral spine (A) anteroposterior and (B) lateral views reveal the classical appearance of the bamboo spine on the lateral view and the dagger and tram-track signs on the AP view with bilateral ankylosis of the sacroiliac (SI) joints.

Cauda equina syndrome can result from arachnoiditis with large posterior dural diverticula causing osseous defects in the laminae. Both CT and MRI may delineate peripheral clumping of the nerve roots, laminar erosions, prominent arachnoid diverticula and dural calcifications.[14,34]

Atlantoaxial subluxation can occur but it is much less common than RA. There may be dramatic resorption of bone from the anterior aspects of the lower cervical vertebral bodies.[3]

Peripheral Joints

Ankylosing spondylitis is the only SSA where large joint involvement is not so uncommon. In general, the arthropathy resembles RA with a few differences. Shaggy periostitis and ankylosis are more common, whereas osteoporosis, erosions and joint space narrowing are less prominent.[14]

The hip joints are involved in up to 50% of patients with AS. Radiographic changes include concentric joint space narrowing, axial migration, cuff-like osteophytes on the femoral head and protrusio acetabuli with eventual joint fusion **(Figs. 17A to C)**. The shoulder is the next commonly involved joint and shows narrowing of the acromioclavicular and glenohumeral joint spaces and a hatchet deformity on the humeral head due to enthesitis of the rotator cuff tendon.[34] Small joint involvement is rare and is characterized by an asymmetric distribution, subtle erosions and proliferative bone changes at the involved joints.

Enthesopathies at tendinous and ligamentous insertions can cause erosions with marked sclerosis.[4] These can be frequently seen at the ischial tuberosity (ischial whiskering), iliac crest and the calcaneum.

PSORIATIC ARTHROPATHY

Psoriasis is a chronic inflammatory disease of the skin, which may be associated with a chronic inflammatory arthritis in 5–8% of cases. The incidence is highest between 20 and 39 years in males with females being affected later in the age group of 40–59 years. There is no gender predominance with both sexes being affected. The etiology is unknown. On histopathology, there is a chronic synovitis, which may cause joint destruction with inflammation of the tendon and ligamentous insertion sites.[34]

Skin lesions are usually seen on extensor surfaces, scalp and lumbosacral areas and are well-defined, dry, erythematous plaques with silvery scales. From a clinical

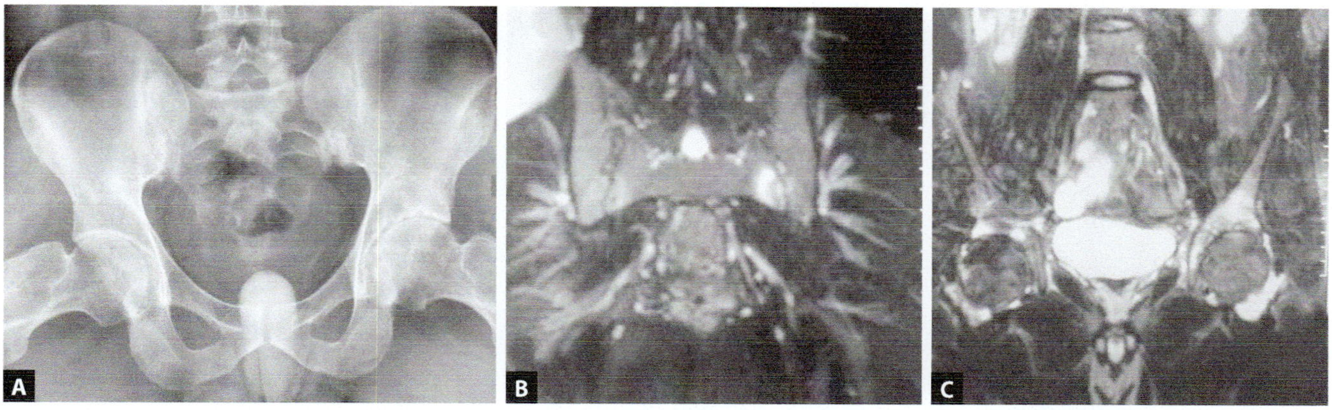

Figs. 17A to C: A 32-year-old male with ankylosing spondylitis. (A) X-ray pelvis shows bilateral sacroiliitis with rat-bite erosions and fuzzy, irregular margins. Note the narrowing of the joint space with erosions in the left hip joint; (B) Coronal short tau inversion recovery (STIR) image shows bilateral sacroiliitis with bone marrow edema; (C) Coronal T2-weighted fat-saturated image demonstrates the narrowing of the left hip joint space, erosions and bone marrow edema.

standpoint, patients with PA can be broadly classified into three groups:[5,14,34]

1. Mono- or oligoarthritis with enteritis
2. Peripheral polyarthritis resembling RA
3. Predominant axial disease resembling AS with or without peripheral joint disease. This is rare, occurring in only 5% of patients.

The skin lesions precede the arthritis in 70% of patients; however, arthritis may precede skin lesions in 15% of cases. In another 15%, the two appear concomitantly.[14] The joints usually involved are the knee, DIP and PIP joints of the hands and feet, MTP and MCP joints and the ankles. Sacroiliitis may be seen in 35–50% and spondylitis in 30–40% of cases.[37]

Radiologic Features

The radiologic features are quite characteristic and the diagnosis can be strongly suggested on the basis of the presence of bone erosions and prominent bone proliferation which is the most characteristic feature in this condition.

The small joints of the hands and feet are most often involved in PA. A fusiform, soft tissue swelling is seen involving the entire digit (sausage digit). The involvement may be unilateral, if bilateral, it is asymmetric. All the joints of a single row may be affected. The bone density is preserved. Bony erosion classically starts at the joint margins. This may then proceed along either the articular surface (surface erosion) or progress along the joint capsule away from the joint along the metaphysis (enthesitic erosion).[34] This leads to a pencil-like tapering of the ends of the small bones. The joint space may be widened due to fibrous tissue deposition and bone resorption due to severe surface erosions resulting in the "pencil-in-cup" appearance. The enthesitic erosions combined with proliferation of bone may provide an irregular outline to the metaphyses or may widen the end of bone (mouse ears' sign) **(Figs. 18A and B)**.[4] Nail changes may be associated with resorption of the terminal tufts or the distal phalanges may become sclerotic. Calcaneal erosions with fluffy periosteal reaction can be seen at both the posterosuperior and posterior plantar aspects. Periosteal reaction commonly occurs along the diaphysis of the short tubular bones. In the advanced stages, there may be "arthritis mutilans" which is a term used to describe severe destruction of the joints of the hands and feet associated with extensive bone resorption.[14]

The sacroiliac joints may be involved in up to 50% of patients with PA and the involvement is usually bilateral. It may be symmetric or asymmetric and ankylosis is relatively uncommon. Involvement of the spine can happen in the absence of sacroiliitis and is commoner in males than females. This is characterized by coarse, asymmetric paravertebral ossification (nonmarginal syndesmophytes) in the dorsolumbar region in contrast to the symmetric, fine marginal syndesmophytes seen in AS.[2,4] These may be unilateral with skip areas. The anterior surface of the vertebral bodies is spared and squaring of the bodies is distinctly uncommon. There may be diffuse, ill-defined, paravertebral ossification. Isolated cervical involvement may be seen with apophyseal fusion and AAD.[34]

On MRI, signal changes are often visualized in the soft tissue as well as bone marrow related to the enthesitis reflecting inflammatory changes.[38]

REITER'S SYNDROME

Reiter's syndrome is a sexually transmitted disease commonly affecting young men which is characterized by arthritis, uveitis, and conjunctivitis. In Europe, a similar syndrome occurs in association with bacillary dysentery.[4,14]

Skeletal involvement may eventually occur in up to 80% of cases. There is a peripheral asymmetric arthritis with a predisposition for the joints of the lower limbs especially the feet where erosions occur at the heels, MTP

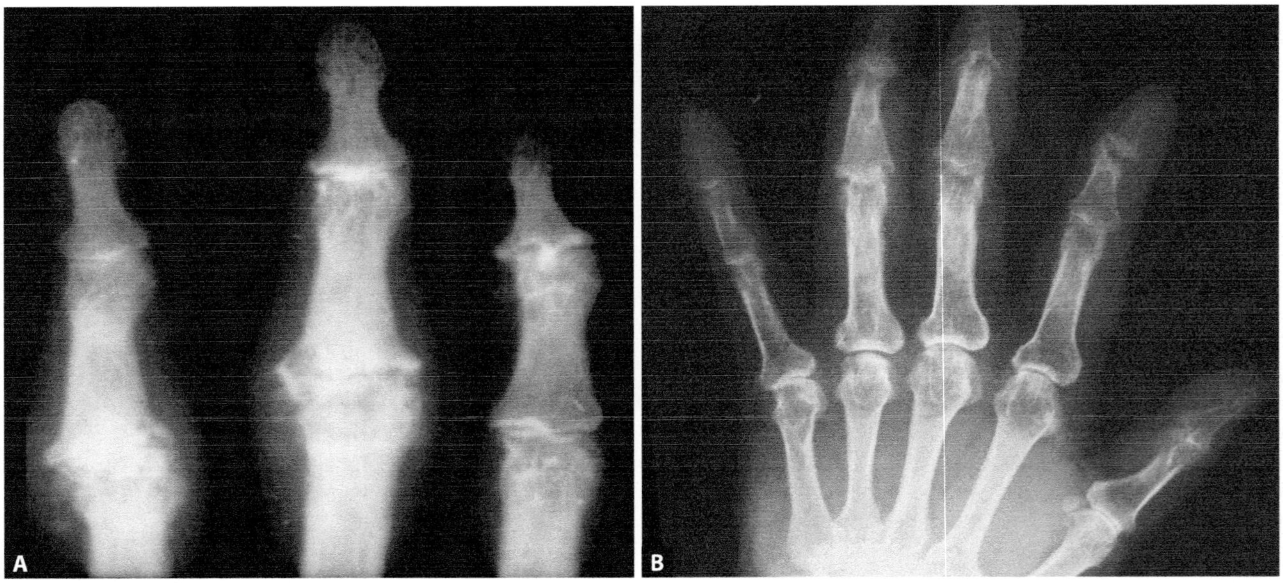

Figs. 18A and B: X-rays of the hands—magnified views reveal (A) fusiform soft tissue swelling with gross erosive changes at the distal interphalangeal (DIP) and proximal interphalangeal (PIP) joints. Note the subperiosteal bone apposition causing widening of the bone ends; (B) Erosive changes at the PIP and DIP joints with a "pencil-in-cup" appearance. These features are characteristic of psoriasis.

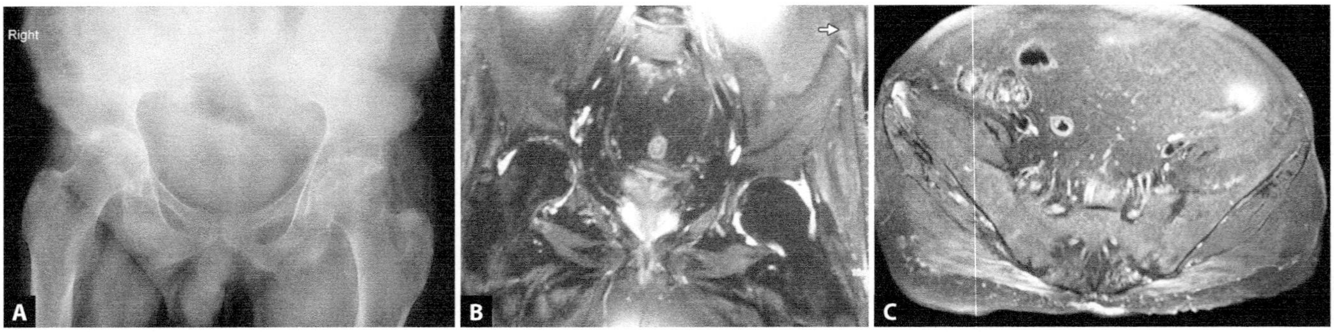

Figs. 19A to C: A 32-year-old male with Reiter's arthropathy. (A) X-ray pelvis shows bilateral sacroiliitis with narrowing and irregularity of the right hip joint; (B) Coronal T2-weighted fat-saturated image shows fluid in bilateral hip joints with erosions and narrowing of the left hip joint; (C) Axial T2-weighted fat-saturated image shows asymmetric ankylosis of the sacroiliac joints.

joints and IP joint of the great toe. The DIP joints are rarely involved (in contrast to PA). Periostitis may be fine and lamellar in acute cases or fluffy and irregular in chronic cases. Reactive calcaneal spurs occur in 20% of patients.[3,14]

Sacroiliitis may develop in about 50% of cases and may be unilateral or asymmetrical in contrast to AS where it is classically bilaterally symmetrical **(Figs. 19A to C)**. Ankylosis is also less common. Coarse, asymmetric syndesmophytes similar to those seen in PA may occur, especially in the thoracolumbar region but occur less frequently.[2,4]

A summary of the joints involved, key features and laboratory parameters of RA and the SSAs are given in **Table 2.**[39]

ENTEROPATHIC SPONDYLOARTHROPATHY

This group comprises arthritides associated with inflammatory intestinal diseases such as regional enteritis (Crohn's disease), ulcerative colitis, and Whipple's disease. HLA-B27 is present in most patients with spinal involvement.[4] There are two distinct types of joint involvement:

1. A spondylitis and sacroiliitis, which cannot be differentiated from AS can be seen in 6% of patients with inflammatory bowel disease and may even precede the development of bowel disease. Syndesmophyte formation, squaring of the vertebral bodies and apophyseal ankylosis are seen similar to AS. The sacroiliitis is bilateral and symmetric. These changes do not correlate with the activity of the gut disease and may continue to worsen even if the gut disease becomes quiescent.
2. A peripheral asymmetrical arthropathy with nonspecific features of soft tissue swelling and local periostitis. The activity of the arthropathy approximates the activity of the bowel disease.[14]

Table 2: Distribution, key signs and laboratory parameters in rheumatoid arthritis and spondyloarthropathy.

Feature	*Rheumatoid arthritis*	*Ankylosing spondylitis*	*Psoriatic arthritis*	*Reiter's syndrome*
Distribution				
Upper extremity	+++	+	+++	–
(hands)	MCP/wrist	–	DIP/PIP	
Lower extremity	+++	+	+++	+++
Sacroiliac	+	+++	++	++
Bilateral	+	+++	++	++ (asymmetric)
Unilateral	+++	+	++	+++
Spine	++ (cervical)	+++	++	+
Key signs				
Osteoporosis	+++	+++	–	+
Joint space	+++ (narrowing)	++ (narrowing)	++ (widening)	+ (narrowing)
Ankylosis	+	+++	++	–
Periostitis	+ (linear)	+++ (fluffy)	+++ (fluffy)	+++ (fluffy)
Tuft resorption	–	–	+++	–
Soft tissue swelling	+++	+	++	++
Laboratory				
ESR	+++	+++	+	++
RA factor	+++	–	–	–
HLA-B27	6–8% (normal)	90%	30–75%	75%

CRYSTAL DEPOSITION ARTHROPATHY

Gout

Gout is a metabolic disorder, which typically presents with recurrent attacks of arthritis. This is because of a disturbance in the metabolism of urates resulting in the deposition of monosodium urate (MSU) crystals within the joints along with soft tissues. Primary gout occurs due to inborn defects, either in the metabolism of purine or the secretion of urates by the renal tubules. Secondary gout can be caused by any acquired disorders that result in the increased turnover of nucleic acids (e.g., myeloproliferative disorders), by acquired defects in renal excretion of urates or due to certain drugs like cyclosporine.[40]

Men in the age group of 40–50 years are traditionally affected; however, gout also occurs in postmenopausal women. Four stages are seen clinically:[41]

1. Asymptomatic gout—presence of hyperuricemia.
2. Acute gouty arthritis—episodes of monoarticular peripheral acute arthritis, involving the 1st MTP joint of the great toe in 75% of cases. Later, the arthritis may be polyarticular and chronic and a phase of chronic gouty arthritis results.
3. Intercritical gout—refers to the symptom-free period between acute attacks.
4. Chronic tophaceous gout—this is characterized by the deposition of MSU crystals (tophi) in tendons, ligaments, cartilage, bone and other soft tissues including synovium or in the subcutaneous tissues in a para-articular location.

Definitive diagnosis involves the demonstration of MSU crystals in the synovial fluid. These are needle-shaped and show strong negative birefringence under polarized light microscopy.[4]

Imaging

Gout has several characteristic radiographic features, but these are seldom seen these days as it takes a few years (4-6) for gout to cause radiographically evident disease. By this time, most patients are correctly diagnosed and treated successfully.[2]

The classic findings are the presence of sharply marginated, round to oval erosions, which are oriented in the long axis of the bone, frequently showing sclerotic borders or overhanging edges **(Fig. 20)**. These are initially periarticular in location, but may later extend into the joint. There is a predilection for the 1st MTP joint; however, other joints such as the ankles, knee, elbow and wrist joint may also be affected. Spinal involvement is unusual but the sacroiliac joints may be involved in 5-13% of cases. The bone density is preserved till the late stages of the disease. Punctate, sclerotic foci may be seen in the bones owing to intraosseous deposition of tophi resembling enchondromas.[15] There is uneven articular space narrowing due to cartilage destruction. Para-articular tophi cause asymmetric "lumpy-bumpy" soft tissue swellings, which frequently show fluffy calcification in the presence of renal disease **(Fig. 21)**. These tophi may saucerize the underlying bone. Chondrocalcinosis may be seen because up to 40% of patients with gout have concomitant CPPD deposition disease. Nephrolithiasis may be present in 20% of cases.[2]

On MRI, an inflamed joint will show joint effusion and para-articular edema with enhancement of the

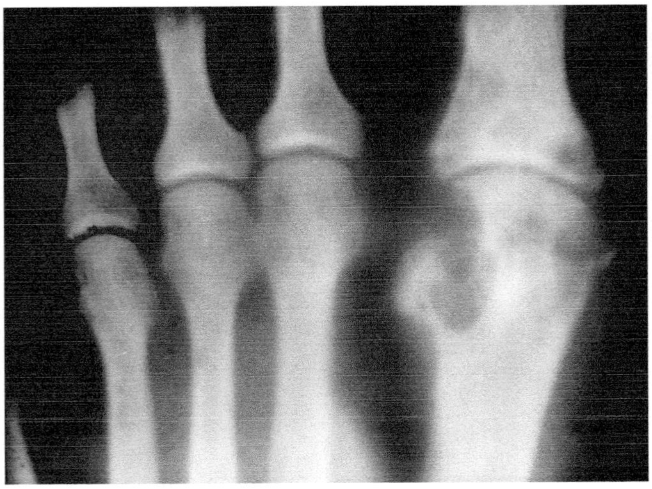

Fig. 20: X-ray of the 1st metatarsophalangeal (MTP) joint shows well-defined periarticular erosions with overhanging edges classical of gout.

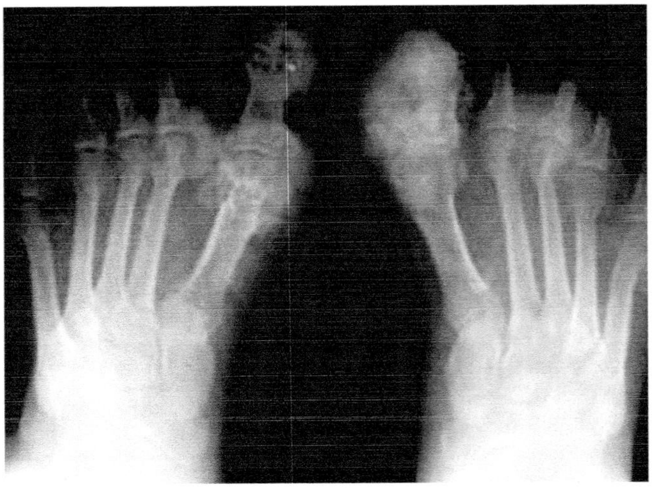

Fig. 21: X-ray of both feet shows advanced changes of gout with multiple soft tissue tophi, some of which are calcified. Gross periarticular erosions are seen in both 1st MTP joints. Note the saucerization of the left 1st proximal phalanx due to overlying soft tissue tophi.

para-articular structures postcontrast. Tophaceous deposits show a low to intermediate SI on T1 with high SI on T2-weighted images. If calcified, the tophi demonstrate low signal on T2-weighted images.[40]

Calcium Pyrophosphate Dihydrate Crystal Deposition Disease

Calcium pyrophosphate dihydrate crystal deposition disease occurs due to the deposition of CPPD crystals in hyaline as well as fibrocartilage along with soft tissues. It is characterized by acute, subacute or chronic joint inflammation. The crystals of CPPD are weakly birefringent on polarized light microscopy. The disease may cause intermittent attacks of acute arthritis when it is called pseudogout.[3]

The classic triad consists of pain, cartilage calcification and joint destruction. Chondrocalcinosis can occur in any joint but usually involves the medial and lateral compartments of the knee, the triangular cartilage and lunotriquetral ligament in the wrist and the symphysis pubis **(Fig. 22)**. When CPPD crystals are found in the soft tissues such as the rotator cuff, they cannot be differentiated from calcium hydroxyapatite crystals, which occur in calcific tendinitis.[2]

The arthropathy of CPPD is a degenerative joint disease caused by the crystals eroding the cartilage. However, CPPD has a tendency to involve the shoulder, elbow, wrist and the patellofemoral compartment of the knee, sites which are not usually involved by degenerative joint disease. Occasionally, CPPD arthropathy may accelerate and severe destruction occurs to such an extent that it mimics a neuropathic joint.[2]

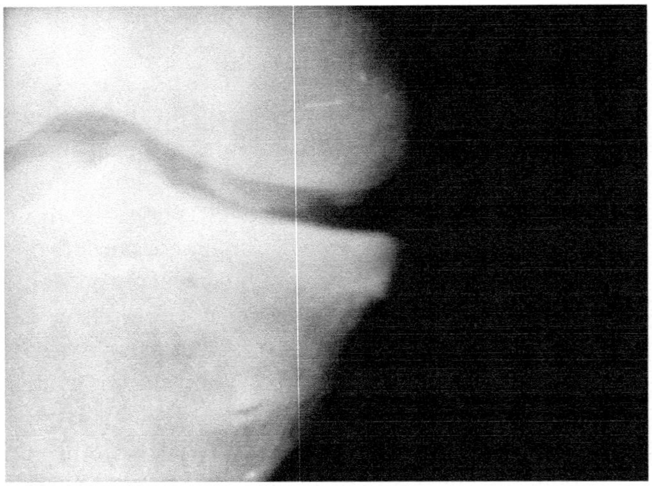

Fig. 22: Magnified view of the knee joint demonstrating chondrocalcinosis.

SYSTEMIC LUPUS ERYTHEMATOSUS

Systemic lupus erythematosus is an autoimmune disease, which can involve multiple organ systems and has a wide age range. Imaging is often done in diagnosed cases to ascertain the extent of the disease and to discover complications. Antiphospholipid antibody syndrome is seen in 27–42% of patients with SLE. Different systems involved in SLE patients would require imaging accordingly like ultrasound or angiography to look for deep venous thrombosis, arterial thrombosis and vasculitis. CT and MRI scans are used to look for strokes, Budd-Chiari syndrome, interstitial lung diseases, arthritis (symmetric and nonerosive), muscle atrophy, insufficiency fractures, etc.[42]

IDIOPATHIC INFLAMMATORY MYOPATHY

Idiopathic inflammatory myopathies are a category of muscle disorders, which are distinguished by proximal muscle weakness as the unique feature. These are rare disorders. Most common of these are dermatomyositis, polymyositis and inclusion body myositis. Biopsy of the muscle should be performed to confirm the diagnosis and exclude other possible causes of proximal myopathy.[43] IIM classification has been improved and according to the recommendation criteria published by EULAR/ACR (2017),[44] the subgroups are: Polymyositis, polymyositis subset includes immune-mediated necrotizing myopathies, inclusion body myositis, amyotrophic dermatomyositis, dermatomyositis, and juvenile dermatomyositis.[44]

Imaging on various modalities shows decrease in the muscle bulk, abnormal attenuation or SI and any destruction of normal muscle morphology, if present. Imaging also helps identifying high-yield biopsy sites to avoid negative biopsies by avoiding fibrotic areas and including inflammation (activity) areas. USG has high sensitivity in detecting myositis, which is comparable with electromyography or serum creatine kinase (CK) activity. Contrast-enhanced USG shows presence of muscle edema and inflammatory hypervascularization, and on follow-up these areas can show normal soft tissue after treatment.[43]

Magnetic resonance imaging shows presence of muscle edema. The most sensitive sequences to differentiate edema from fatty infiltration are the fat-suppressed T2 or STIR sequences. Specific MRI patterns associated with the various subtypes of IIMs have been demonstrated nowadays.[45]

Functional imaging may have a role to play in IIMs but are not yet standardized.[43]

SYSTEMIC SCLEROSIS (SCLERODERMA)

Systemic sclerosis is a chronic autoimmune disease which characteristically causes inflammation of the skin and multiple internal organs.[46] Contractures of the skin are the hallmark of the disease but many patients have joint involvement ranging from mild (arthralgia) to severe (frank arthritis). Joint contractures may occur and tendons can be involved.[47]

Joint involvement may be oligoarticular or polyarticular. Any of the joints can be affected, although there is predominant involvement of the small joints of the hands (in particular the MCP and PIP joints), wrist, and ankle joints.

Fibrinous deposits can occur on the surface of tendon sheaths along with the overlying fascia leading to tendon abnormalities such as a leathery crepitus on palpation of the joints. Bursal involvement may be recurrent. In rare cases, inflammatory proliferative tenosynovitis can result in tendon rupture. RF positivity occurs in up to 30% patients with systemic sclerosis. Presence of anti-citrullinated cyclic peptide (CCP) antibodies helps in the identification of infrequent cases of true systemic sclerosis-RA overlap. On imaging there may be juxta-articular osteoporosis, narrowing of the joint space and even frank erosions involving MCP, PIP and DIP joints (more on the dorsal aspect) and wrist. The 1st carpometacarpal joint may be involved. Pencil-in-cup deformity has also been seen. These articular features occur along with nonarticular features like atrophy of the skin, subcutaneous calcinosis and resorption of the digital tufts on radiography.[48]

FIBROMYALGIA SYNDROME

Fibromyalgia is a syndrome in which patients present with chronic diffuse pain at multiple tendon points along with joint stiffness. Systemic symptoms can occur like mood disorders, cognitive dysfunction, fatigue, and insomnia. Associations with rheumatic pathologies, psychiatric or neurologic disorders, infections and diabetes can be seen.[49]

BURSITIS

Bursae are located where tendons continuously move over bony surfaces or against each other. They are named depending on to their location like subcutaneous, subtendinous, subfascial or submucosal. They are synovial lined sacs that may be communicating or noncommunicating. Bursae near the joints communicate with the joint cavity. Normal bursae cannot be visualized on imaging. They may be seen as cystic, fluid-filled spaces with inflamed walls (thickened and enhancing on imaging) in pathological conditions.[50]

TENDINITIS AND TENOSYNOVITIS

Tendinopathy is a wide term, which is used to describe tendon pain without knowing the specific etiology of the pain. The pain could be due to tears from trauma, inflammatory enthesitis or even chronic degeneration. Tendinitis implies the inflammatory response in arthritis and is associated with decreased function and pain. Tendinosis defines a degenerative state.[51]

Acute tendinitis on imaging presents with increased fluid within the synovial sheath. In chronic tendinitis, there is thickening of the tendon associated with increased fluid in the synovial cavity of the joint. Tenosynovitis is the inflammation of the tendon sheaths caused by various causes like trauma, infections, and RA. Ganglia are the cystic lesions arising from synovial lining of joint or tendon.[52]

BEHÇET'S DISEASE

Behçet's disease is a chronic, systemic disorder distinguished by relapses with recurrent ulcers involving the oral cavity or genitalia, uveitis and involvement of multiple organ systems. Radiologically, its involvement in various body systems shows characteristic features like neuro-Behçet's disease, dural sinus thrombosis, meningitis, vascular occlusions, periaortic pseudoaneurysm, pulmonary thromboembolism, etc.[53]

Arthritis is the most common manifestation of musculoskeletal involvement with the usual pattern being monoarticular involvement. Most commonly, unilateral knee joint involvement is seen. AS without HLA-B5 or HLA-B27 association is seen in around 10% cases.[54]

REFERENCES

1. Østensen M. Drugs in pregnancy: rheumatological disorders. Best Pract Res Clin Obstet Gynaecol. 2001;15: 953-69.
2. Helms CA. Arthritis. In: Helms CA (Ed). Fundamentals of Skeletal Radiology. Philadelphia: WB Saunders; 1989. pp. 135-76.
3. Martel W. Diagnostic radiology in the rheumatic diseases. In: Kelley WN, Harris ED Jr, Ruddy S, Sledge CB (Eds). Textbook of Rheumatology. Philadelphia: WB Saunders; 1982. pp. 580-621.
4. Greenspan A. Inflammatory arthritides. In: Greenspan A (Ed). Orthopedic Radiology: A Practical Approach, 3rd edition. Philadelphia: Lippincott, Williams and Wilkins; 2000. pp. 453-78.
5. Sommer OJ, Kladosek A, Weiler V, Czembirek H, Boeck M, Stiskal M. Rheumatoid arthritis: a practical guide to state-of-the-art imaging, image interpretation, and clinical implications. Radiographics. 2005;25:381-98.
6. Narváez JA, Narváez J, De Lama E, De Albert M. MR imaging of early rheumatoid arthritis. Radiographics. 2010;30:143-65.
7. Arnett FC, Edworthy SM, Bloch DA, McShane DJ, Fries JF, Cooper NS, et al. The American Rheumatism Association 1987 revised criteria for the classification of rheumatoid arthritis. Arthritis Rheum. 1988;31:315-24.
8. Sugimoto H, Takeda A, Hyodo K. Early stage rheumatoid arthritis: prospective study of the effectiveness of MR imaging for diagnosis. Radiology. 2000;216:569-75.
9. Østergaard M, Ejbjerg B, Szkudlarek M. Imaging in early rheumatoid arthritis: roles of magnetic resonance imaging, ultrasonography, conventional radiography and computed tomography. Best Pract Res Clin Rheumatol. 2005;19(1):91-116.
10. Kay J, Upchurch KS. ACR/EULAR 2010 rheumatoid arthritis classification criteria. Rheumatology (Oxford). 2012;51:vi5-9.
11. Imhof H, Nobauer-Huhmann IM, Gahleitner A, Kainberger F, Krestan C, Sulzbacher I, et al. Pathophysiology and imaging in inflammatory and blastomatous synovial diseases. Skeletal Radiol. 2002;31(6):313-33.
12. Resnick D. Rheumatoid arthritis and the seronegative spondyloarthropathies: radiographic and pathologic concepts. In: Resnick B (Ed). Diagnosis of Bone and Joint Disorders, 4th edition. Philadelphia: WB Saunders; 2002. pp. 837-90.
13. Renner WR, Weinstein AS. Early changes of rheumatoid arthritis in the hand and wrist. Radiol Clin North Am. 1988;26:1185-93.
14. Renton P. Diseases of joints. In: Sutton D (Ed). Textbook of Radiology and Imaging, 7th edition. Churchill Livingstone; 2003. pp. 1201-45.
15. Resnick D. Rheumatoid arthritis. In: Resnick D (Ed). Diagnosis of Bone and Joint Disorders, 4th edition. Philadelphia: WB Saunders; 2002. pp. 891-987.
16. Wakefield RJ, Gibbon WW, Conaghan PG, O'Connor P, McGonagle D, Pease C, et al. The value of sonography in the detection of bone erosions in patients with rheumatoid arthritis: a comparison with conventional radiography. Arthritis Rheum. 2000;43:2762-70.
17. Brown AK, Wakefied RJ, Conaghan PG, Karini Z, O' Connor PJ, Emery P. New approaches to imaging early inflammatory arthritis. Clin Exp Rheumatol. 2004;22(5 Suppl 35):S18-25.
18. Backhaus M, Kamradt T, Sandrock D, Loreck D, Fritz J, Wolf KJ, et al. Arthritis of the finger joints: a comprehensive approach comparing conventional radiography, scintigraphy, ultrasound, and contrast-enhanced magnetic resonance imaging. Arthritis Rheum. 1999;42(6):1232-45.
19. El-Miedany YM, Housny IH, Mansour HM, Mourad HG, Mehanna AM, Megeed MA. Ultrasound versus MRI in the evaluation of juvenile idiopathic arthritis of the knee. Joint Bone Spine. 2001;68(3):222-30.
20. Polster J, Winalski CS, Sundaram M, Lieber ML, Schils J, Ilaslan H, et al. Rheumatoid arthritis: evaluation with contrast-enhanced CT with digital bone masking. Radiology. 2009;252(1):225-31.
21. Tehranzadeh J, Ashikyan O, Dascalos J. Advanced imaging of early rheumatoid arthritis. Radiol Clin North Am. 2004;42:89-107.
22. McQueen FM, Benton N, Perry D, Crabbe J, Robinson E, Yeoman S, et al. Bone edema scored on magnetic resonance imaging scans of the dominant carpus at presentation predicts radiographic joint damage of the hands and feet six years later in patients with rheumatoid arthritis. Arthritis Rheum. 2003;48(7):1814-27.
23. McQueen F, Beckley V, Crabbe J, Robinson E, Yeoman S, Stewart N. Magnetic resonance imaging evidence of tendinopathy in early rheumatoid arthritis predicts tendon rupture at six years. Arthritis Rheum. 2005;52(3):744-51.
24. Larsen A. How to apply Larsen score in evaluating radiographs of rheumatoid arthritis in long-term studies. J Rheumatol. 1995;22:1974-75.
25. Østergaard M, Peterfy C, Conaghan P, McQueen F, Bird P, Ejbjerg B, et al. OMERACT rheumatoid arthritis magnetic resonance imaging studies: core set of MRI acquisitions, joint pathology definitions, and the OMERACT RA-MRI scoring system. J Rheumatol. 2003;30(6):1385-6.
26. Ajeganova S, Huizinga T. Sustained remission in rheumatoid arthritis: latest evidence and clinical considerations. Ther Adv Musculoskelet Dis. 2017;9(10):249-62.
27. Petty RE, Southwood TR, Baum J, Bhettay E, Glass DN, Manners P, et al. Revision of the proposed classification criteria for juvenile idiopathic arthritis: Durban,1997. J Rheumatol. 1998;25:1991-4.
28. Buchmann RF, Jaramillo D. Imaging of articular disorders in children. Radiol Clin North Am. 2004;42:151-68.

29. Doria AS, Kiss MH, Lotito AP, Molnar LJ, de Castro CC, Medeiros CC, et al. Juvenile rheumatoid arthritis of the knee: evaluation with contrast-enhanced color Doppler ultrasound. Pediatr Radiol. 2001;31(7):524-31.
30. Kakati P, Sodhi KS, Sandhu MS, Singh S, Katariya S, Khandelwal N. Clinical and ultrasound assessment of the knee in children with juvenile rheumatoid arthritis. Indian J Pediatr. 2007;74(9):831-6.
31. Shanmugavel C, Sodhi KS, Sandhu MS, Sidhu R, Singh S, Katariya S, Khandelwal N. Role of power Doppler sonography in evaluation of therapeutic response of the knee in juvenile rheumatoid arthritis. Rheumatol Int. 2008;28(6):573-8.
32. Lamer S, Sebag GH. MRI and ultrasound in children with juvenile chronic arthritis. Eur J Radiol. 2000;33(2):85-93.
33. Dougados M, van der Linden S, Juhlin R, Huitfeldt B, Amor B, Calin A, et al. The European Spondyloarthropathy Study Group preliminary criteria for the classification of spondyloarthropathy. Arthritis Rheum. 1991;34:1218-27.
34. Bennett DL, Ohashi K, El-Khoury GY. Spondyloarthropathies: ankylosing spondylitis and psoriatic arthritis. Radiol Clin North Am. 2004;42:121-32.
35. van der Linden S, Valkenburg HA, Cats A. Evaluation of diagnostic criteria for ankylosing spondylitis: a proposal for modification of the New York Criteria. Arthritis Rheum. 1984;27(4):361-8.
36. Bollow M, Braun J, Hamm B, Eggens U, Schilling A, König H, et al. Early sacroiliitis in patients with spondyloarthropathies: evaluation with dynamic gadolinium-enhanced MR imaging. Radiology. 1995;194(2):529-36.
37. Boumpas DT, Illei GG, Tassiulas IO. Psoriatic arthritis. In: Klippel JH (Ed). Primer on the Rheumatic Diseases, 12th edition. Atlanta: Arthritis Foundation; 2001. pp. 233-8.
38. Weishaupt D, Schweitzer ME, Alam F, Karasick D, Wapner K. MR imaging of inflammatory joint diseases of the foot and ankle. Skeletal Radiol. 1999;28:663-9.
39. Yochum TR, Rowe LJ. Arthritic disorders. In: Yochum TR, Rowe LJ (Eds). Yochum and Rowe's Essentials of Skeletal Radiology. Philadelphia: Lippincott, Williams and Wilkins; 2005. pp. 951-1136.
40. Monu JU, Pope TL. Gout: a clinical and radiological review. Radiol Clin North Am. 2004;42:169-84.
41. Resnick D. Gouty arthritis. In: Resnick D (Ed). Diagnosis of Bone and Joint Disorders, 4th edition. Philadelphia: WB Saunders; 2002. pp. 1519-59.
42. Lalani TA, Kanne JP, Hatfield GA, Chen P. Imaging findings in systemic lupus erythematosus. Radiographics. 2004;24:1069-86.
43. Gazeley DJ, Cronin ME. Diagnosis and treatment of the idiopathic inflammatory myopathies. Ther Adv Musculoskelet Dis. 2011;3(6):315-24.
44. Leclair V, Lundberg IE. New myositis classification criteria: what we have learned since Bohan and Peter. Curr Rheumatol Rep. 2018;20:18.
45. Kubinova K, Dejthevaporn R, Mann H, Machado PM, Vencovsky J. The role of imaging in evaluating patients with idiopathic inflammatory myopathies. Clin Exp Rheumatol. 2018;36:S74-81.
46. Terenzi R, Karalilova R, Lepri G, Bruni C, Bellando-Randone S, Manetti M, et al. Enthesopathy and involvement of synovio-entheseal complex in systemic sclerosis: an ultrasound pilot study. Rheumatology (Oxford). 2020;59:580-5.
47. Sandler RD, Matucci-Cerinic M, Hughes M. Musculoskeletal hand involvement in systemic sclerosis. Semin Arthritis Rheum. 2019;11:1-6.
48. Avouac J, Clements PJ, Khanna D, Furst DE, Allanore Y. Articular involvement in systemic sclerosis. Rheumatology (Oxford). 2012;51:1347-56.
49 Bellato E, Marini E, Castoldi F, Barbasetti N, Mattei L, Bonasia DE, et al. Fibromyalgia syndrome: etiology, pathogenesis, diagnosis, and treatment. Pain Res Treat. 2012;2012:426130.
50. Hirji Z, Hunjun JS, Choudur HN. Imaging of the bursae. J Clin Imaging Sci. 2011;1:22.
51. Charnoff J, Naqvi U. Tendinosis (Tendinitis). In: StatPearls [Internet]. Treasure Island (FL): StatPearls Publishing; 2019.
52. Kharat AT, Singh A, Ranganath P, Kulkarni VM. Tendinitis and tenosynovitis—a pictorial essay. Ind J Radiol Imaging. 2006;16(2):235-7.
53. Chae EJ, Do KH, Seo JB, Park SH, Kang JW, Jang YM, et al. Radiologic and clinical findings of Behçet disease: comprehensive review of multisystemic involvement. Radiographics. 2008;28(5):e31.
54. Fatemi A, Shahram F, Akhlaghi M, Smiley A, Nadji A, Davatchi F. Prospective study of articular manifestations in Behçet's disease: five-year report. Int J Rheum Dis. 2017;20(1):97-102.

CHAPTER

9

Degenerative Disease of the Spine

Jyoti Kumar, Anju Garg, Anjali Prakash

INTRODUCTION

Degenerative disease of the spine is a ubiquitous collection of conditions that represent some of the most common indications for spine magnetic resonance imaging (MRI). Degenerative changes may arise in the vertebrae, intervertebral discs, facet joints and ligaments. Degeneration at various sites is linked to each other since the main common pathogenetic factor is chronic overload. The intervertebral articulation consists of a three-joint complex consisting of the amphiarthrodial endplate-disc-endplate joint of the anterior column and the two diarthrodial facet joints of the posterior column supported by ligaments and muscle groups. In the cervical spine, uncovertebral joints (joints of Luschka) are the other lateral articulations between the vertebral bodies. The intervertebral disc space consists of the inner nucleus pulposus, outer annulus fibrosus, and hyaline cartilaginous endplates. The ligaments consist of the anterior longitudinal ligament (ALL), posterior longitudinal ligament (PLL), ligamentum flavum (LF), and interspinous ligaments. Since involvement of one site predisposes the other sites to degenerative changes owing to altered biomechanical forces, patients often present with degenerative changes in multiple sites.[1,2]

IMAGING MODALITIES

Back pain requires imaging if it is persistent for >6 weeks or when there is accompanying neurologic deficit, fever, trauma, acute pain in the setting of osteoporosis/cancer/steroid use or history of serious medical condition (e.g., cancer).[3]

Radiographs are often the first imaging modality used to evaluate back pain. However, the role of radiographs is often to exclude other diagnoses than to directly evaluate degenerative disease. The findings that may be seen on radiographs include loss of disc height, irregularity and sclerosis of endplates, osteophytes, Schmorl's nodes (herniation of disc material into the endplate) or intradiscal gas **(Figs. 1A and B)**.

Magnetic resonance imaging is the modality of choice in evaluation of degenerative spine because of its

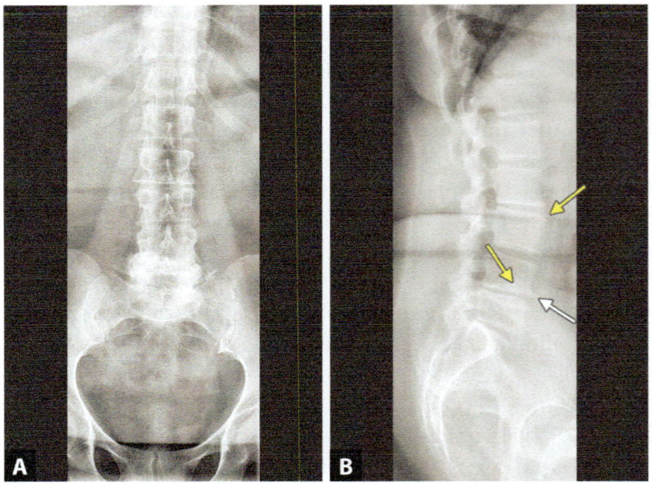

Figs. 1A and B: (A) X-rays lumbar spine anteroposterior and (B) lateral views depict reduced disc spaces most marked at L2/L3, L4/L5 and L5/S1 levels with endplate sclerotic changes (yellow arrows) and osteophyte formation (white arrow).

superior soft tissue contrast. It allows direct visualization of intervertebral discs and neural elements. Contrast MRI is usually not required and is more used in postoperative examinations to differentiate residual and recurrent herniations from scar tissue. It may also be used sometimes in the preoperative setting to detect annular fissures and inflammatory processes that may accompany acute disc desiccation such as facet joint synovitis and radiculitis. MRI can also pick up other alternative causes of back pain such as inflammation, infection, and tumors.

Computed tomography (CT) is unable to detect early disc desiccation. However, it demonstrates superior spatial resolution and improved conspicuity of osseous and calcified structures and intradiscal gas.[4] It can detect advanced changes like disc space narrowing and sclerotic endplate changes. CT is more sensitive than MRI for detecting the presence of transdiscal gas, predominantly nitrogen. This is known as the vacuum phenomenon and is very specific for disc degeneration and is only rarely encountered in infective discitis.[1] CT is also more accurate in detection of discal calcification and posterior osteophytes which may have therapeutic implications.

On MRI, bright T1 signal may be found with mild to moderate intradiscal calcium deposition.[1,2]

Imaging studies with 6–12 months follow-up have demonstrated that nearly 63% of disc herniations may show spontaneous reduction in size. This may be due to dehydration, fragmentation and phagocytosis of the disc material. This is greatest in extrusions and sequestrations.[2] Radiology is also involved in interventional techniques for therapeutic purpose, e.g., automated discectomy, percutaneous laser disc decompression, intradiscal oxygen-ozone injection. Their success rates range from 70 to 80% with minimal potential complications.[2]

Complementary tests in evaluation of degenerative spine include radiography, discography, conventional myelography, CT myelography, and nuclear scintigraphy. Plain films are inexpensive, widely available and give a panoramic view of the entire spine. Bones can be directly visualized and functional information regarding alignment and stability can be obtained with upright dynamic films in flexion-extension and lateral bending. Myelography is reserved only for patients with contraindications to MRI or in whom subtle instability is suspected but not confirmed by other examinations. Discography is reserved for selected patients before intervention or when the diagnosis of discogenic pain must be confirmed.[2]

Upright MRI is advocated by some groups as axial loading in this position owing to gravity, patient's weight, and spine morphology enables MRI evaluation in natural state of loading. This has also been proven to be useful when there is suspicion of dynamic foraminal stenosis and in patients with positional pain difference. However, there is limited availability of upright MRI with additional problems of poor resolution, increased motion artifacts, and higher false-positive rates. Dynamic flexion extension is also possible in these units.[2] Dynamic plain films, weight-bearing CT or MRI have been used for the study of spinal stenosis. Previously occult abnormalities, including disc herniation, ligamentous infolding, subluxations may all be demonstrated using kinematic MRI. Functional information regarding vertebral stability may also be provided on dynamic examination.

PATHOPHYSIOLOGY

Pathogenetic mechanisms are multiple and chronic overload is the most important factor. The other causes are sequelae to acute trauma, metabolic, toxic, genetic, vascular or infectious causes. The distribution of axial load determines the common sites of spine degeneration. In the cervical spine, it is C5-C6 and C6-C7 levels as these are the sites of lordosis inversion. The dorsal spine is rarely involved as it is less mobile and less involved in dynamic load. In the lumbar spine, L4-L5 and L5-S1 are the sites of highest dynamic and static overload and hence most predisposed to degenerative changes.[2]

In patients with degenerative changes of the spine, there are multiple mechanisms that act in combination to produce pain.[6] These are:

- Biochemical mediators of inflammation resulting from disc degeneration and herniation.
- Mechanical compression of nerves by bone, ligament or disc material.
- Instability or abnormal motion with associated disc degeneration and facet arthropathy.
- Disruption of free nerve endings in the outer annular fibers.

ANATOMY OF INTERVERTEBRAL DISC

The intervertebral disc has an inner nucleus pulposus and an outer annulus fibrosus and is bordered by cartilaginous endplates. The nucleus pulposus is made up of >80% water and consists of hydrated proteoglycans supported by network of elastin and collagen type 2 fibers. Over time, the gelatinous proteoglycans are replaced by fibrocartilage. The nucleus is eccentrically located and more closely related to the posterior surface of the intervertebral disc. The annulus is composed of dense collagen type 1 fibers. The collagen in the inner annulus is less plentiful than in the outer ring. The annular fibers become progressively more compact centrifugally. The outermost fibers are the densest, known as Sharpey's fibers.

The nucleus pulposus converts much of the axial force into radial force and functions to spread the load evenly over the adjacent endplate. Cartilaginous endplates are composed of hyaline cartilage. These are usually not well discernible on imaging. Surrounding the cartilaginous endplate is a ring of dense bone, the ring apophysis that fuses to the vertebra in the 2nd decade of life. Fetal and infantile discs are well vascularized but these branches soon atrophy and the adult disc becomes avascular. It obtains its nutrition by diffusion from vertebral endplates.[4] The intervertebral discs in the lumbar region are thicker than those in the cervical and dorsal region.

MAGNETIC RESONANCE APPEARANCE OF INTERVERTEBRAL DISC

The normal intervertebral discs are of slightly lower signal intensity than bone marrow on T1-weighted images (T1WIs) and with higher T2 signal. The annulus is seen as a peripheral region of low signal intensity on T2-weighted images (T2WIs) and nucleus pulposus is hyperintense, owing to high water content of nucleus pulposus. A horizontal internuclear cleft of fibrous tissue containing collagenous, elastic and reticular fibers may normally be seen on T2WI in over 90% of patients over 30 years of age and is considered a paraphysiologic change.[1,2] On T1WI, the distinction between the nucleus and annular fibers is less discernible **(Figs. 2A to C)**, similar to CT. The endplates are well defined and smooth with intact cortical bone.

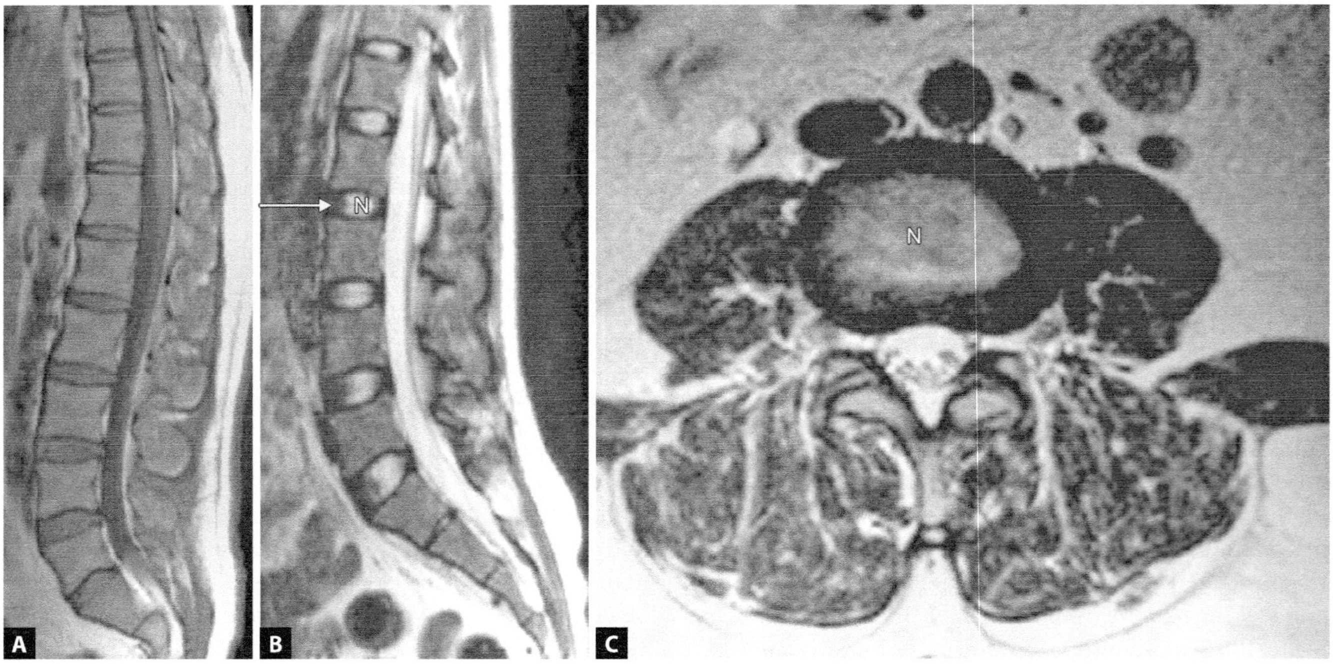

Figs. 2A to C: (A) Sagittal T1W, (B) T2W, and (C) axial T2W MR images of lumbosacral spine show normal intervertebral disc that is slightly lower signal intensity than bone marrow on T1W images and with higher T2 signal. The annulus is seen as a peripheral region of low signal intensity on T2W images (arrow) and nucleus pulposus (N) is hyperintense. A horizontal internuclear cleft is seen on T2W sagittal image.

DEGENERATIVE CHANGES OF THE SPINE

The intervertebral disc undergoes marked changes with aging. With aging, small concentric and transverse tears may develop in the annulus. The composition of the intervertebral disc may change with decrease in glycosaminoglycans and increase in collagen; and hence a decrease in affinity for water. Therefore, aging can reduce the signal intensity of the disc by a few percent. However, it may be confusing to differentiate changes of aging from changes of degeneration. Hence, the term degenerated disc includes the changes of aging as well.[7] Degenerating discs in addition show enhanced inflammatory changes with catabolic metabolism. These undergo desiccation, loss of height, fissures, bulging and herniations. Pfirrmann et al. classified disc degeneration based on the following features—disc structure, distinction between nucleus pulposus and annulus fibrosus, disc signal, and disc height.[8]

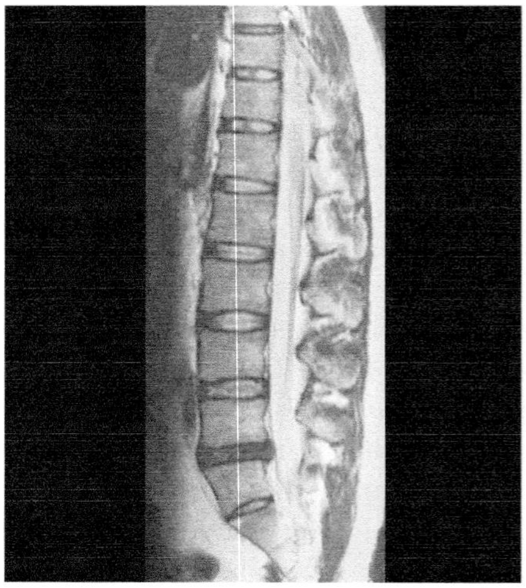

Fig. 3: Sagittal T2W MR image of lumbosacral spine shows decreased T2 signal of L4/L5 disc with loss of differentiation between nucleus and annulus fibrosus suggestive of disc desiccation. Note made of transitional vertebra.

Structural Disc Changes

On MR, the earliest appearance of degeneration of the nucleus is desiccation (progressive loss of water), which manifests as low signal intensity on T2WIs instead of high signal of normally hydrated discs **(Fig. 3)**. Although it is usually asymptomatic, it suggests disc overload and is a precursor to further degenerative abnormalities.[1,2] A feature of interest to remember in the cervical spine is that loss of signal intensity of cervical discs may not be helpful in identification of degenerated disc as cervical discs have lower signal intensity compared to lumbar discs.

There is progressive loss of disc height. Development of annular fissures results in shrinkage of fibrocartilage in the nucleus pulposus and replacement by dense fibrous tissue and cystic spaces. The disc becomes more and more fibrous and disorganized with no clear distinction between nucleus and annulus.[6] Negative pressure produced by abnormal spaces pulls in gas, predominantly nitrogen

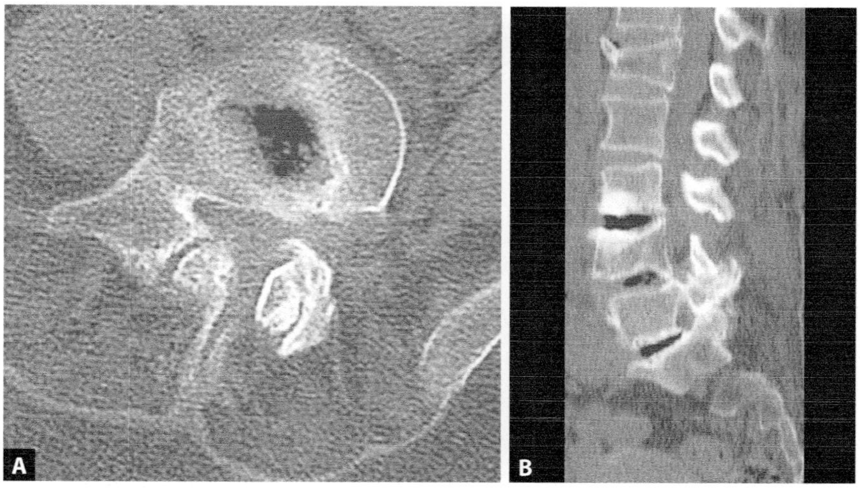

Figs. 4A and B: (A) Axial and (B) sagittal multiplanar reformatted CT images show vacuum phenomenon seen as air within multiple intervertebral discs. Note also made of marked hypertrophy of the left facet joint seen on the axial image and wedge compression fracture of L1 vertebra on the sagittal image.

resulting in vacuum disc phenomenon **(Figs. 4A and B)**. The disc may show linear or patchy low-signal intensity either due to gas or sometimes, calcification. When occasionally fluid may be pulled instead of nitrogen, there may be paradoxical high signal appearance of the disc on T2WI instead of the low signal intensity of desiccated disc. Associated disc narrowing and endplate changes and osteophytes are pointers that this seemingly hydrated disc is a degenerated disc. With progress of degeneration, disc calcification may occur. This can appear as increased or decreased signal on T1WI. Paradoxical high signal on T1WI may be seen depending on the amount and state of calcium.[6,9]

Annular Fissures

Annular disruption is a critical factor in degeneration. Annular fiber degeneration may result in fissures:

- Type 1 circumferential or concentric fissures—run longitudinally along the plane of collagen fibers and precede annular bulging. These are seen as focal hyperintense areas in the external aspect of the annulus.
- Type 2 radial fissures—linear rupture of the annulus fibers extending from the nucleus pulposus traversing the entire inner-to-outer dimension of the annulus and correlate with shrinkage and disorganization of the nucleus.
- Type 3 transverse fissures—rupture of Sharpey's fibers adjacent to the ring apophyses and can be seen in normally hydrated disc.

While concentric fissures can be seen in normal discs, transverse and radial fissures are often associated with degenerated discs. As per the Version 2 of lumbar disc nomenclature,[10] annular tear is not the preferred term to be used as the word "tear" may imply a traumatic origin. Although fissures occur in all degenerated discs, not all of these are seen on MR. Magnetic resonance is less sensitive than cryomicrotomy or discography in detecting radial fissures.[7] Even discography cannot demonstrate all the fissures. On MRI, radial fissures appear as hyperintense transverse band into the annulus on MRI **(Figs. 5A and B)**.[1,2] These either represent fluid and/or granulation tissue within the annulus, the latter showing enhancement on gadolinium administration. However, presence of high-intensity zone (HIZ) or even their enhancement is no more thought to be correlated with the acuity of the fissure.

Disc Herniation

Herniation is the term used most commonly to describe the displacement of disc material. It can involve displacement of the nucleus pulposus, endplate cartilage, fragmented apophyseal bone or annular tissue beyond the normal confines of the disc space. Hence, the term "herniated nucleus pulposus" is inaccurate. Also, "rupture", "protrusion", and "prolapse" are considered nonstandard to describe this general diagnosis.

To bring uniformity to reporting of disc degeneration, the North American Spine Society, the American Society of Spine Radiology, and the American Society of Neuroradiology combined their committees, yielding a consensus paper on nomenclature of disc degeneration in 2001 and this has been updated in 2014.[10,11]

Disc Herniation versus Disc Bulge

Disc herniation is localized displacement of the disc material, involving <25% of the circumference of the disc. Disc space is defined by the vertebral endplates on either side and by the edges of the vertebral ring apophysis (excluding osteophytes) as the circumferential borders.

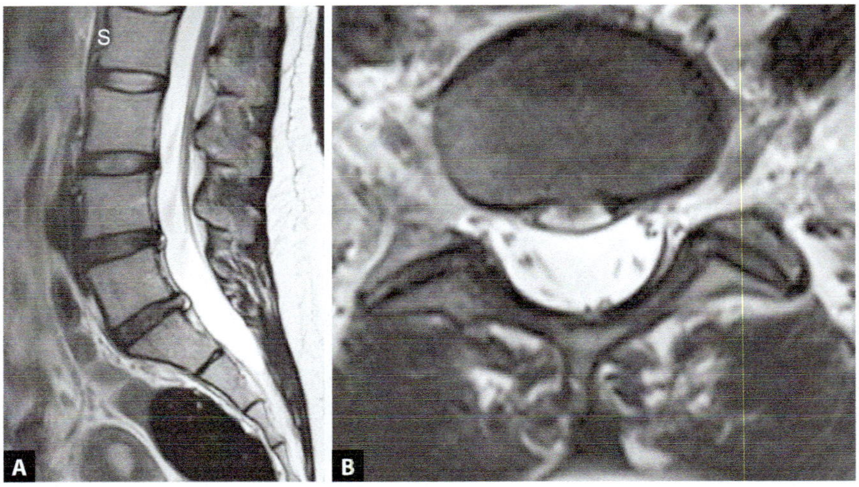

Figs. 5A and B: (A) Sagittal; and (B) Axial T2W MR images of lumbosacral spine depict disc desiccation with annular fissure seen as high-intensity zone at L4/5 and L5/S1 level.

It is also important to remember that for disc to be herniated, there needs to be disruption of the annulus or a defect in the vertebral endplate in case of Schmorl's node. Intra-annular displacement not extending beyond the confines of the disc space is not considered herniation. Also, if the annulus is displaced behind one vertebra as an adaptation to subluxation, it should not be considered herniation.

In contrast, disc bulge by definition is not herniation and is the term used when there is a smooth circumferential extension of the disc margin beyond the boundary of the adjacent vertebral endplates for >25% of the disc circumference **(Figs. 6A to C)**. This is usually <3 mm beyond the edges of the vertebral body. The annulus fibrosus is grossly intact, although weakened due to tears in the oblique collagen bridges between the concentric annular fibers. The concentric fibers are intact. On MR, there is uniform circumferential extension of the outer disc margin. There is usually loss of height of the involved disc space and desiccation/dehydration of the nucleus pulposus **(Figs. 7A and B)**.[1,2,12] Apart from degeneration, disc bulge has several etiologies—normal variation, ligamentous laxity, vertebral body remodeling because of osteoporosis or even partial volume averaging.[9]

The use of the either of the terms "bulge" or "herniation" does not suggest any etiology, symptomatology, prognosis, or treatment.

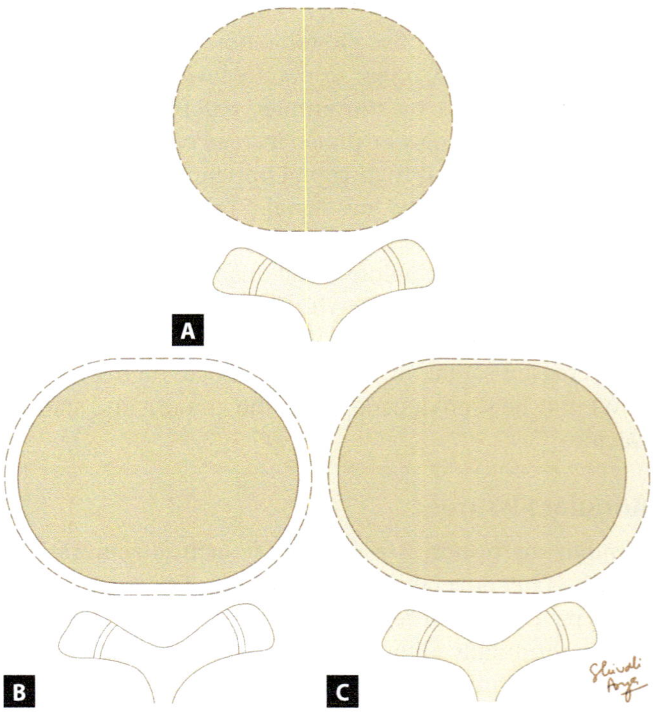

Figs. 6A to C: Schematic representation of (A) normal disc, (B) symmetric bulging disc, (C) asymmetric bulging disc. Disc is represented by the broken line.

Types of Disc Herniation

Disc herniation can be classified into disc protrusion and disc extrusion **(Figs. 8A to C)**.

Disc protrusion: Disc protrusion is the type of disc herniation which has a broad base (when the maximal length of the herniated disc material beyond the disc space in any plane is less than the distance of the edges at the disc base in the same plane) **(Figs. 9A and B)**. The base of the disc is the width of the disc at its outer margin from where the disc herniates. The disc protrudes through a defect in the inner annulus but the outer annular fibers are intact.

Disc extrusion: Disc extrusion is the type of disc herniation with narrow base (when the maximal length of the disc is greater than the base of the disc in the same plane) or when there is no continuity of the herniated disc with the parent disc **(Figs. 10A to C)**.

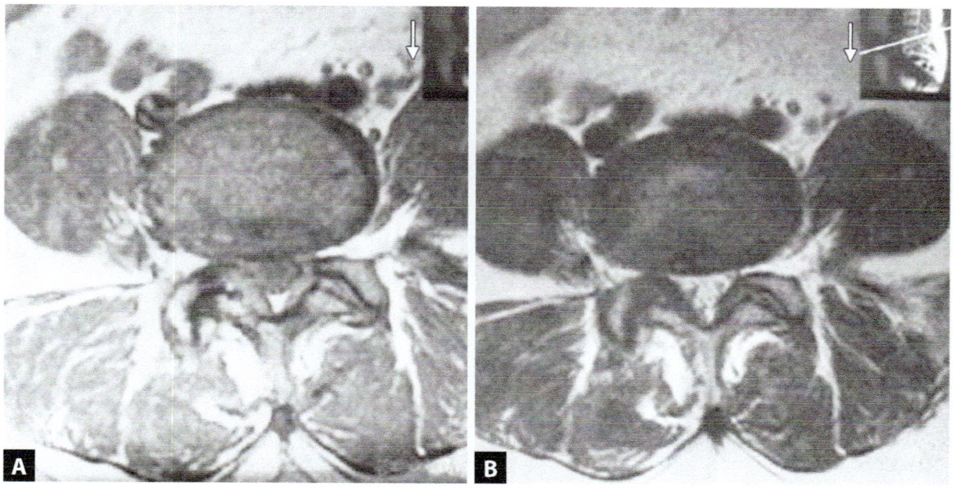

Figs. 7A and B: (A) Axial T1W and (B) T2W images at L4-L5 level show diffuse disc bulge with ligamentum flavum (LF) hypertrophy resulting in canal and lateral recess stenosis. Note that LF is better discernible on T1W rather than T2W image.

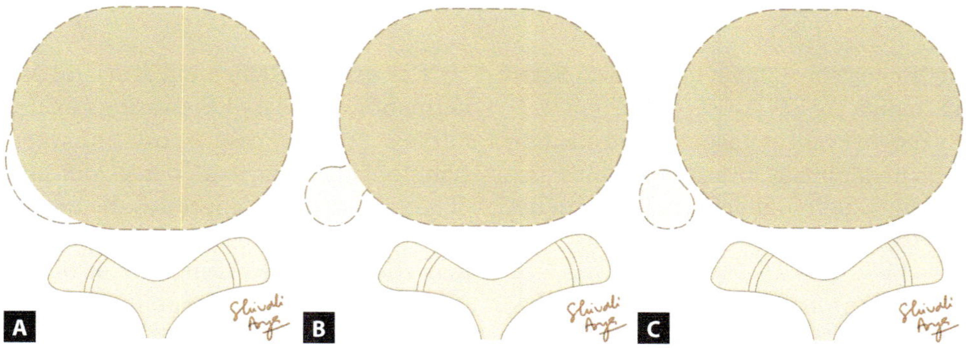

Figs. 8A to C: Schematic representation of (A) disc protrusion, (B) disc extrusion, (C) disc sequestration. Disc is represented by the broken line.

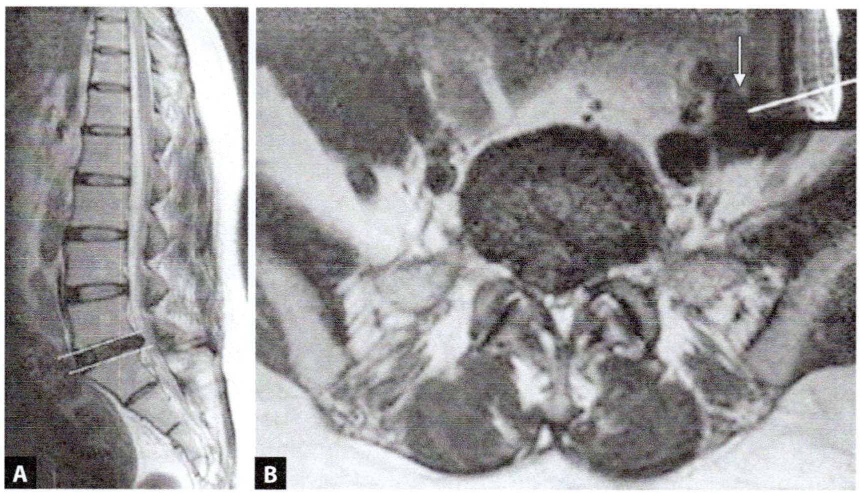

Figs. 9A and B: (A) Sagittal and (B) axial T2W MR images depict central disc protrusion at L5/S1 level. On the sagittal image, the herniated disc is seen to lie within the confines of the disc margins.

Disc extrusions may be further classified into migrated or sequestrated discs:

- *Disc sequestration*: When the fragment of disc separates from the parent disc. It may be seen anteriorly in the spinal canal and less often in the lateral posterior or even intradural compartment of the spinal canal. This is also known as free fragment.[10,13]
- *Disc migration*: This describes the herniated disc which has migrated away from the site of extrusion, regardless of the continuity with the disc. Continuity

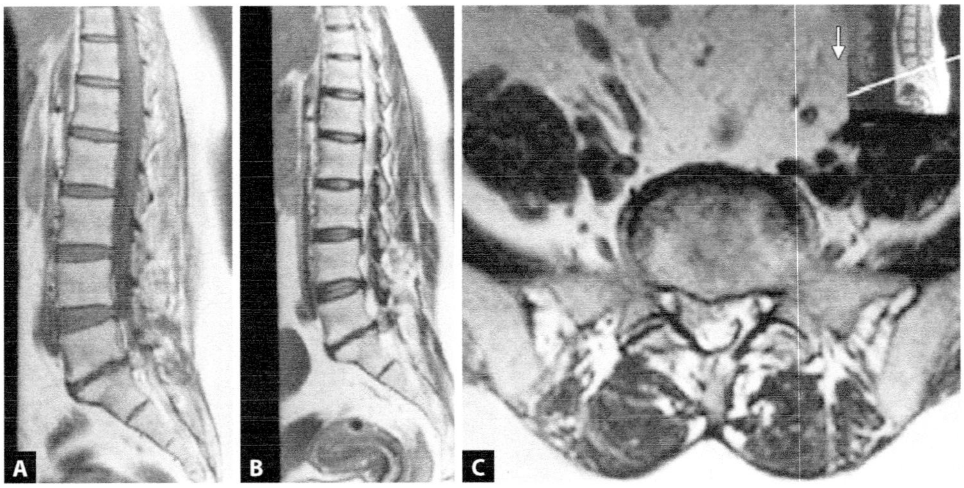

Figs. 10A to C: (A) Sagittal T1W, (B) sagittal T2W and (C) axial T2W MR images reveal markedly decreased disc space between L5/S1 with disc extrusion that is seen to extend beyond the confines of the disc space on the sagittal image. On the axial image, the right central extruded disc is seen to impinge on the traversing S1 nerve root on the right side. Note is made of type 2 endplate marrow changes at L5/S1 level seen as hyperintense signal on both T1W and T2W sagittal images.

with the parent disc may be difficult to establish based on our imaging studies.[10,13]

This is clinically very relevant as a sequestered disc may be a contraindication to minimally invasive therapies such as a microdiscectomies, percutaneous radiofrequency ablations, or the use of intradiscal steroids.[1,2,12]

Contained versus Noncontained Herniation

While protruding discs are contained disc herniations as at least some fibers of the annulus and PLL are intact, extruded discs are uncontained herniations where the annulus and even the overlying PLL is focally disrupted.[10,14]

The differentiation between the two types is often not possible with the current noninvasive imaging techniques (CT and MRI).

The term "subcapsular" is not the preferred term for containment as per the new nomenclature.[10] However, contained herniation may also be referred to as subligamentous and uncontained herniation as transligamentous (when there is extension through the PLL) or transmembranous (when there is extension through the epidural membrane).

Classification of Disc Herniation in the Axial Plane

These disc herniations are classified as central, right/left central, subarticular, foraminal, and extraforaminal in the axial plane. The term "paracentral" disc herniation is not preferred. Instead, the discs should be described as right or left central. However, "extraforaminal disc" can be used exchangeably with the term "far lateral disc". The medial edge of the facet articulations and the borders of the pedicles or the neural foramina are used for anatomic landmarks, although they may be difficult to interpret on axial images as they are curved structures.[12]

The axial classification is useful as it describes the herniation relative to the various exiting and traversing nerves. Lumbar disc herniations generally produce symptoms involving the nerve root inferior to the level of herniation as it compresses the transiting inferior root. However, an extraforaminal or foraminal disc herniation may compress the exiting root at the same level. In the cervical spine, disc herniations tend to involve the nerve root at the same level. This information is important to determine whether the patient's symptoms are attributable to MRI findings, for preoperative planning and to avoid surgery at the incorrect spinal level.[1]

Classification of Disc Herniation in the Sagittal Plane

In the sagittal plane, the disc may be classified as supra-pedicular, pedicular, infrapedicular, and discal as ascertained by the upper and lower borders of the pedicles.

Endplate Changes

These are a reflection of abnormal stresses—loading or motion stresses. According to Michael Modic, endplate changes can be classified into three categories.[6]

Modic type 1 changes (vascular pattern) correspond to active inflammation, showing decreased signal on T1WI and high signal on T2WI. *Modic type 2 changes* (fatty pattern) reflect fatty infiltration and show bright signal on both T1WI and T2WI **(Figs. 10A and B)**. *Modic type 3 changes* (sclerotic pattern) are seen in advanced chronic stage, and correspond to bone sclerosis. This is seen as decreased signal on both T1WI and T2WI. These changes are also apparent on radiographs and CT **(Fig. 4A)**.[1,2] Sometimes, more than one type of Modic change can be seen at the same level.

The relationship with degenerative disc disease is probably caused by multiple factors—common biomechanical factors, raised mechanical stresses on the endplates induced by disc dehydration and disc metabolism changes. Endplate alterations can also induce disc changes as the disc is an avascular structure supplied by metabolite diffusion from endplate cartilage. The relative lack of blood supply and sparse cell population within the nucleus results in limited ability to recover from metabolic or mechanical injury.[2]

The Modic changes do not necessarily progress in an orderly fashion. Type 1 may progress to type 2 changes or may even revert to normal. Type 1 and type 2 changes may occasionally progress to type 3 changes. Modic type 1 and type 3 changes have been more positively correlated with back pain than Modic type 2 changes.[13] According to Chung et al.,[15] asymptomatic type 1 changes when present are generally focal, involve the anterosuperior endplate and involve midlumbar spine. In contrast, in symptomatic individuals, these are confluent changes superior and inferior to a degenerated disc, and usually seen in the lower lumbar spine.

Mimics

Sometimes type 1 changes may be so extensive that the imaging appearance may simulate infective etiology. However, in an infectious process, there is hyperintensity of the disc on T2WI with enhancement, paraspinal or epidural inflammation and erosion or destruction of endplate. Subchondral enhancement may be seen in both cases.[1,2] Sclerotic type 3 changes can be rounded and mimic blastic metastatic disease on radiographs and CT. However, the degenerative endplate changes are seen abutting the endplate and there are associated features of disc degeneration like disc narrowing and vacuum phenomenon.[9]

Schmorl's Nodes

Focal herniations of discs through cartilaginous endplates may produce Schmorl's nodes. In most cases, these are remote occurrences of no clinical consequence. However, some of them may be traumatic in etiology and can be related to episodes of sudden pain when MR may show endplate edema representing endplate fracture.[1]

Most Schmorl's nodes occur after axial loading and result in extrusion of nucleus pulposus through the endplate rather than biomechanically stronger annulus fibrosus. Additional predisposing factors are intrinsic abnormalities of the endplate due to vascular channels or notochordal remnant defects. Patients with straight rather than concave endplates are also more predisposed due to less favorable axial loading.[4]

On CT, Schmorl's nodes are seen as focal indentations in the endplate in continuity with the intervertebral disc.

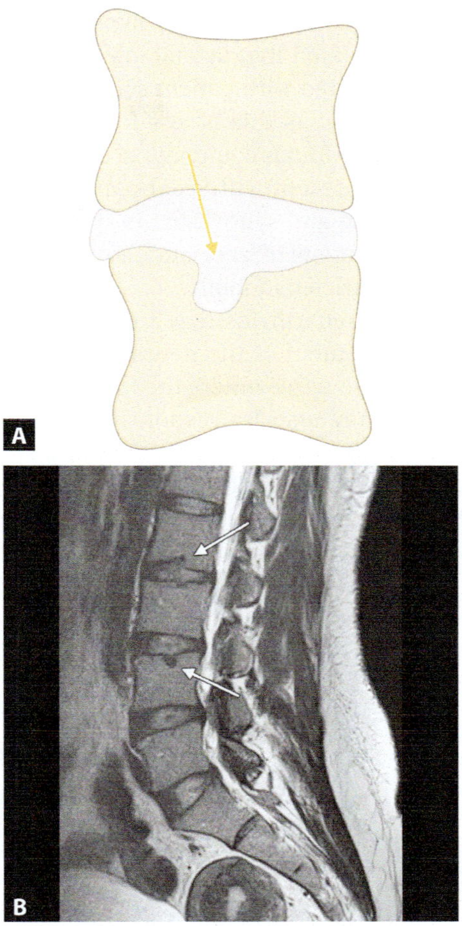

Figs. 11A and B: (A) Schematic representation of Schmorl's node; (B) Sagittal T2W MR image of lumbar spine depicts Schmorl's nodes at superior endplate of L4 and inferior endplate of L2 (arrows), which represent herniation of disc material into the endplates.

There may be surrounding endplate sclerosis. On MR, we can see direct continuity of the disc material into the region of the endplate defect **(Figs. 11A and B)**. In acute/subacute cases, there may be increased T2 signal, typically following the contour of the endplate which may also demonstrate enhancement.[4]

Facet Osteoarthritis

The facet or zygapophyseal joints are synovium-lined joints. They play an important role in flexion/extension and limiting axial rotation. They are oriented nearly in the sagittal plane in the cervical spine and approximately 40° in the sagittal plane in the lumbar spine. Like other synovial joints, these are predisposed to arthropathy with alterations of articular cartilage.

Facetal joint changes may be primary or secondary to disc degeneration. The latter is believed to be the main inciting factor for facet osteoarthritis. Secondary to disc degeneration, increased loading on facets and increased mobility at a segment can contribute to facet arthropathy. Facet tropism (asymmetry) and more sagittal orientation of facets >45° are other hypothesized causes. It has been postulated that facetal joint degeneration is more likely associated with patient symptoms, especially in the lumbar area, as this is less frequently found in asymptomatic individuals compared to disc degeneration. Patients usually present with axial pain as the capsule, subchondral bone and synovium are highly innervated structures. Involvement of facet joints is rare at the thoracic level owing to restricted mobility.

Facet joint osteoarthritis may trigger radicular pain owing to impingement of the neural foramen or at the site just before the nerve enters the foramen. Facet joint osteoarthritis may also be responsible for instability and spondylolisthesis, with an intact neural arch unlike isthmic spondylolisthesis. In the lumbar spine, facetal degeneration is accompanied by LF hypertrophy and calcification contributing to secondary spinal canal stenosis. This is due to fibrosis and loss of elasticity of the ligament. These ligaments are best assessed on T1WIs as these are difficult to differentiate from cortical bone on T2WI **(Figs. 7 and 12)**. In the lumbar spine, posterior paraspinal muscle atrophy also frequently accompanies facet joint degeneration **(Fig. 13B)**.[1,4]

Computed tomography is more sensitive in detecting early changes than MRI. The imaging findings include joint space narrowing, subchondral sclerosis and cyst formation, osteophyte formation, vacuum phenomenon and hypertrophy of the articular processes **(Figs. 13A and B)**. In addition, MRI can demonstrate congestive edema in the adjacent posterior elements and soft tissues, facet effusion and cysts.[1] MR has the advantage of evaluating the entire spine in a single examination and giving information on the neural and ligamentous components of the spine.

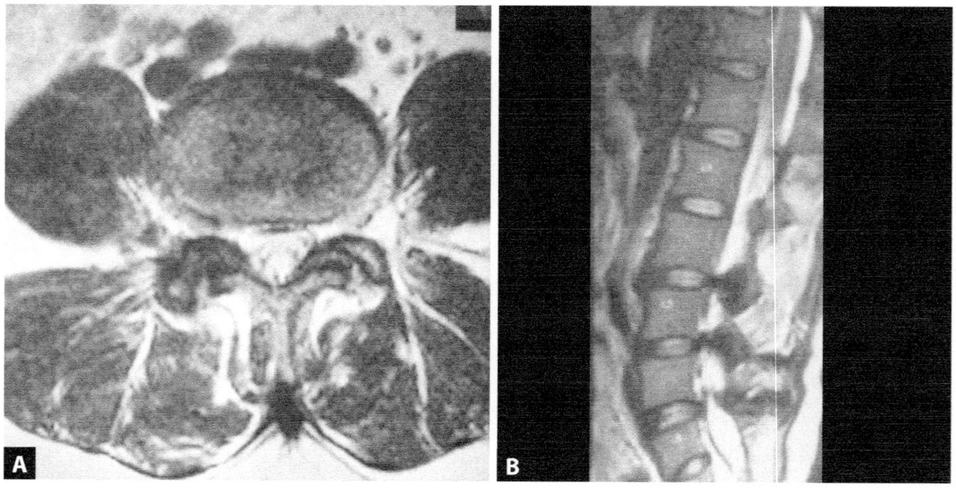

Figs. 12A and B: (A) Axial; and (B) Sagittal T2W MR images show degenerative changes involving the right facet joint in the axial image with evidence of ligamentum flavum hypertrophy resulting in narrowing of the spinal canal at L3-L4 and L4-L5 levels.

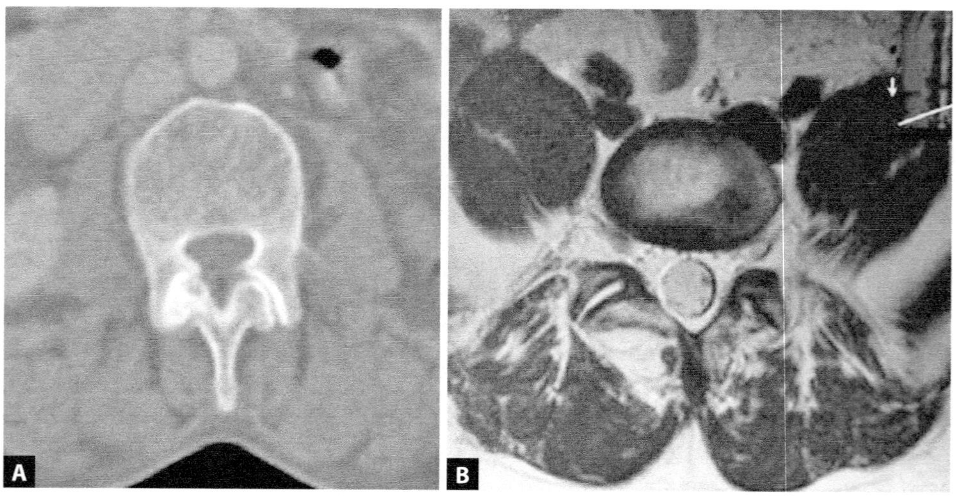

Figs. 13A and B: (A) Axial CT image depicts right facet arthrosis seen as erosions, sclerosis and decreased joint space; (B) Axial T2W image of another patient with facet arthritis shows increased fluid within the right facet joint with accompanying paraspinal muscle atrophy.

Synovial Cysts

Juxta-articular cysts may also be seen accompanying facet degeneration, most commonly at L4/L5, frequently with degenerative spondylolisthesis. These may represent synovial cysts, ganglion cysts or cysts of the LF. They are much rarer at the cervical spinal level. It is often difficult to differentiate between these entities by radiologic, pathologic or surgical means. Although posterior cysts are more common, anterior cysts are more likely to be associated with symptoms than posterior cysts as the former project into the spinal canal or neural foramina.[4]

On MRI, these cysts are generally high signal intensity on T2WI. Some portions may be low SI on T2WI due to calcification or gas. These may be treated surgically or percutaneously, while spontaneous regression is also known.[1,4]

Facet Joint Effusion

This may be seen with and without facet degeneration. It may be observed in healthy individuals without any sign of facet degeneration. It is believed by some that if thickness of fluid is >1.5 mm, it could be predictive of degenerative spondylolisthesis at L4/L5 level, even when there is no anterolisthesis evident on supine MRI.[14]

Uncovertebral Joint Degeneration

In the cervical spine, in addition, uncovertebral joints can undergo degeneration **(Figs. 14A to C)**. These develop between the uncinate processes of the lower vertebrae and the lateral margin of the superior vertebrae and are found from C2-C3 level to C6-C7 level. These are variable joints, not present at all levels and not seen in the infants. These joints are lined with cartilage, which is presumably continuous with the adjacent cartilaginous endplate. Degenerative changes may be seen as hypertrophy, subchondral sclerosis and cyst formation, osteophyte formation and narrowing of joint space. These are clinically important as degeneration of these joints plays an important role in foraminal stenosis and nerve root compromise in the cervical spine.[4]

Interspinous Degeneration

Abnormal contact between spinous processes can lead to degeneration of the spinous processes and interspinous ligaments. This may result in interspinous pseudoarthrosis and cyst formation and has been termed Baastrup's disease or "kissing spine". There is localized tenderness that is exacerbated with extension and relieved with flexion, anesthetic injections or surgical excision. Redundant interspinous ligaments, interspinous bursae, or hypertrophic degeneration may extend anteriorly, contributing to spinal canal stenosis.[4]

The main risk factors in pathophysiology are excessive lumbar lordosis, large spinous processes and degenerative disc disease/fractured vertebra that can lead to decrease in the space within the interspinous joints. The incidence of Baastrup's disease increases as age advances. On CT imaging, there are bone erosions, sclerosis and osteophyte formation with faceted appearance of the spinous processes. On MRI, subchondral edema and bursitis may be seen which are evident as bright signal on T2WIs and enhancement on contrast administration.

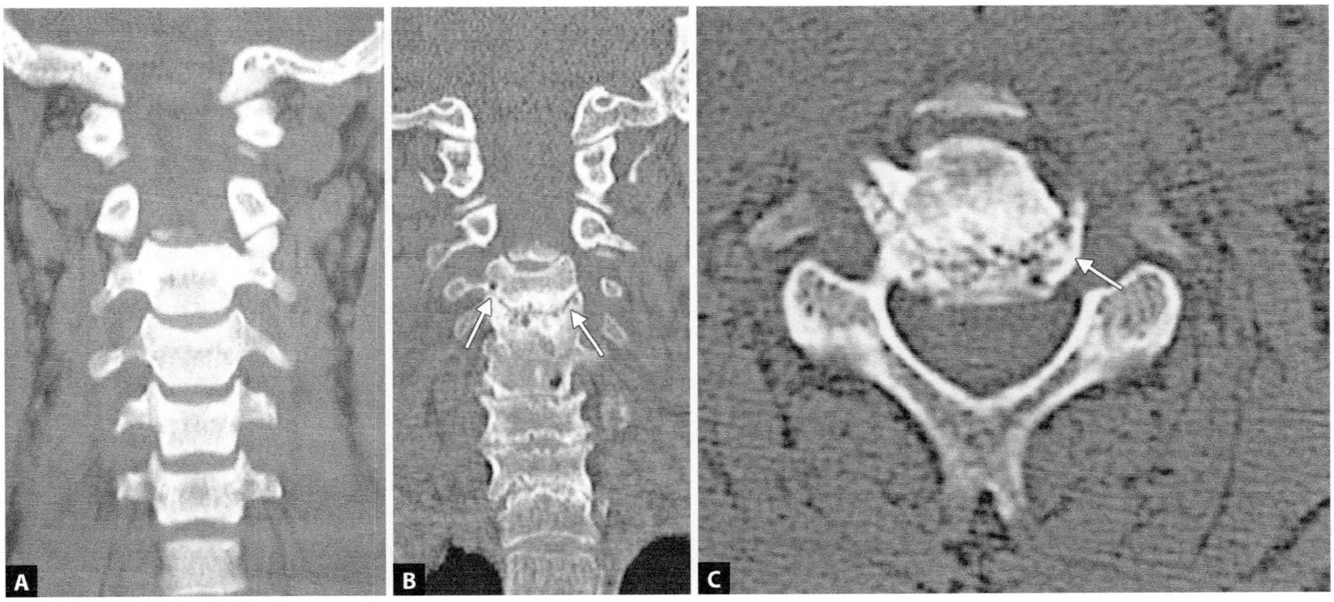

Figs. 14A to C: (A) Coronal reformatted CT image shows normal uncovertebral joints in cervical spine; (B) Coronal reformatted CT image in another patient with extensive spinal degenerative changes depicts marked arthrosis involving uncovertebral joints (arrows) as well as endplate changes; (C) Axial CT image of the same patient depicts uncovertebral arthrosis with neural foraminal narrowing.

Spondylosis Deformans and Intervertebral Osteochondrosis

Degeneration of the disc affects both the nucleus and the annulus simultaneously. The imaging appearance depends on the predominant component.

Spondylosis Deformans

Spondylosis deformans is a degenerative process that essentially affects the annulus fibrosus and adjacent apophyses. The classic sign of spondylosis deformans is osteophytosis where the disc space is essentially preserved or only marginally decreased.[10] Osteophytes are bony spurs that originate from the bone surface and/or ossification of the soft tissue attachment to the bone **(Figs. 15A and B)**. Increased vertebral motility due to weakening and radial degeneration of annular fibers and resultant traction on Sharpey's fibers stimulates osteogenesis. Initially, osteophytes have a triangular horizontal extension (in contrast to syndesmophytes in seronegative arthropathies which are vertically oriented). In more advanced cases, osteophytes become hooked and grow more vertically. These may fuse together on either side of the disc space to form bridging osteophytes. The mucoid matrix of the disc becomes fibrous; however, disc height is normal or only slightly decreased and the disc margins are regular. Posterior osteophytes, although less common, are clinically more relevant because of possible compression of neural structures. They have a triangular shape with marginal location. Large posterior osteophytes may result in spinal stenosis, with compressive myelopathy, especially in the cervical region.[1-4]

Intervertebral Osteochondrosis

In contrast to spondylosis, intervertebral osteochondrosis is a degenerative process that involves primarily the nucleus pulposus and vertebral endplates. There is accompanying fissuring of the annulus fibrosus. Early disc changes seen on sagittal fast spin-echo (FSE) T2WI include loss of normal T2 hypointensity within nucleus. Late changes include further decreasing signal within the nucleus pulposus, loss of distinction between nucleus pulposus and annulus fibrosus, disc space narrowing, disc bulges, vacuum phenomenon and endplate changes. Posterior osteophyte formation may also occur at this stage.[2] CT can detect later changes, including disc calcification, gas within disc space and also aid in differentiating osteophytes from degenerated disc.[4]

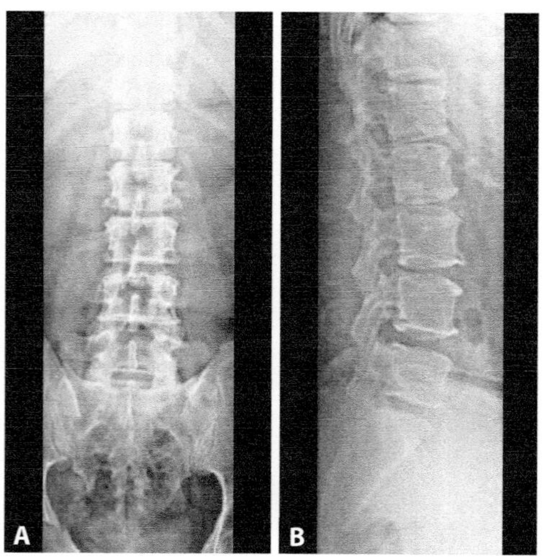

Figs. 15A and B: Lumbar spine anteroposterior and lateral radiographs depict marginal osteophytes at L2, L3 and L4 levels with relatively preserved disc spaces.

Complications of Degenerative Spinal Disease

Spinal and Foraminal Stenosis

Congenital and acquired canal stenosis: Lumbar canal stenosis is the most common acquired disorder in elderly population, caused by degenerative changes and primarily manifesting after the 6th decade of life. Congenital stenosis presents earlier in life with multilevel involvement and fewer degenerative changes.[1]

Congenital stenosis is seen in patients with disorders such as achondroplasia and mucopolysaccharidosis or may be idiopathic. It is usually related to short pedicles, short laminae or sagittal orientation of facet joints. Any superimposed pathological process is much more likely to cause symptomatic compression. Acquired stenosis is most commonly due to degenerative changes and usually involves the cervical and lumbar spine. The central canal may be narrowed anteriorly by degenerated disc, posterior bulging of PLL or posterior osteophytes and posteriorly by facet joints and LF.[1,4] This may get aggravated by spondylolisthesis. Other less common causes of acquired spinal canal stenosis include ossification of the PLL (OPLL) and/or LF and epidural lipomatosis.

Cervical spinal stenosis may present with both upper and lower limb motor/sensory deficits and pyramidal symptoms while the typical presentation of lumbar canal stenosis is neurogenic intermittent claudication. The latter may be provoked by prolonged standing/lumbar extension. Cervical canal stenosis is also aggravated by hyperextension when ligamentum flava may further buckle anteriorly.[14]

Imaging findings: Computed tomography is the gold standard for evaluation of bony abnormalities, and is accurate for identifying posterior osteophytes and calcification of ligaments. It may be more appropriate to evaluate congenital spinal stenosis. MRI depicts the disc pathology and neural structures clearly.[2]

Spinal cord or nerve root compression is a dynamic phenomenon that worsens in erect position or with certain movements. The stenosis can become more evident or sometimes, may only be evident during weight-bearing or dynamic examination.[2,4]

Although absolute measurements may not be clinically relevant in all cases, the diagnosis of spinal canal stenosis should be considered if the anteroposterior diameter of the cervical and lumbar canals is <12 mm and in the thoracic region if it is <10 mm. Stenosis may also be considered if the ratio between canal sagittal diameter and vertebral body sagittal diameter is <0.8. More than objective canal measurements, it is the subjective evaluation of canal morphology and relationship between containing and contained structures that correlates better with patient's symptoms. Epidural fat is reduced or disappears. Multiple anterior and posterior notches can be observed on the dural sac, with disappearance of the subarachnoid space and narrowing of the spinal cord. The stenosis is severe if cerebrospinal fluid (CSF) signal is completely effaced on axial T2WI or CT myelogram images.[1,2]

In severe lumbar canal stenosis, sometimes "redundant nerve root" is seen as enlarged and swollen cauda equina. This may be due to radicular venous congestion, ischemia and edema. The rootlets may not be individually recognizable. In severe stenosis, the epidural fat is not seen posteriorly in addition to unrecognizable roots.[2]

Myelopathy is the most serious complication of canal stenosis. It is thought that continuous pinching of the cord can result in chronic hypoperfusion and result in demyelination and neuronal death. Increased intramedullary signal on T2WI is seen **(Fig. 16)** that indicates the presence of edema, chronic ischemia, myelomalacia or rarely syringomyelic cavitation. Enhancement on T1WI may confirm the abnormality. Low signal on noncontrast T1WI suggests a poor prognosis. However, it must be remembered that absence of abnormal signal does not rule out myelopathy, as clinical and electrophysiological criteria may be more sensitive.

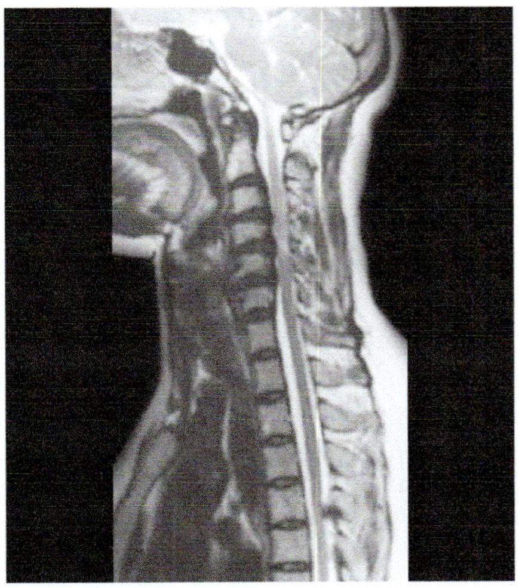

Fig. 16: Sagittal T2W image of the cervical spine shows multiple disc bulges and posterior longitudinal ligament thickening resulting in thecal sac indentation with hyperintense signal within the cord suggesting myelopathy.

Apparent diffusion coefficient (ADC) maps and diffusion tensor imaging may improve the sensitivity in detecting subtle changes, but decrease the specificity.[4]

Facet hypertrophy, PLL thickening or disc herniation can lead to encroachment of lateral recesses. This is best evaluated on axial images and is found most commonly at L4-L5 level **(Figs. 7B and 12B)**. The normal sagittal diameter of the lateral recess is >5 mm; when this space is <4 mm, it is considered stenotic.[2,4]

Foraminal stenosis: Disc and facet degeneration can also project into the neural foramina, causing their narrowing. Remodeling of the endplates secondary to disc degeneration results in wider and shorter vertebral body and this may also cause narrowing of the spinal canal, lateral recesses and neural foramina. Loss of disc height may result in anterosuperior slippage of the facet joint and narrow the craniocaudal diameter of the foramen and hence, contributing to neural foraminal narrowing. In the cervical spine, neural foraminal narrowing is most commonly caused by uncovertebral osteophytes.

Lumbar foraminal herniations are best evaluated on the sagittal plane on T1W images whereas cervical neural foramina are best evaluated on axial MR images.[1,4] On sagittal MRI, foramen is seen as an ovoid structure, filled with CSF and fat. In the lumbar spine, nerve root lies in the superior part of the foramen and the herniated disc may not compress the nerve. When there is clinically significant nerve compression, it is usually due to a multitude of factors that include facetal arthropathy, LF hypertrophy, dorsal spondylophytes in addition to the discal herniation. Mild narrowing is seen as a "keyhole" appearance. Moderate narrowing effaces the inferior portion of the foramen at the level of the disc. Severe narrowing results in effacement of the fat in the foramen. When the fat sleeve around the nerve root is completely lost in this plane, it is consistent with nerve compression.[13] Other signs of nerve compression are contact between the disc and the nerve root with loss of periradicular CSF sleeve, pushed nerve root, increased size of nerve root as well as nerve root enhancement owing to inflammatory changes around the nerve root.[14]

In contrast, the cervical nerve roots lie at the same level or slightly below that of the disc and small herniations can result in nerve compression. At this level, preservation of fat sleeve around the nerve is not considered an accurate sign for ruling out nerve compression. It must be remembered that correlation with symptoms of radiculopathy is essential to diagnose nerve root impingement.[4]

Scoliosis and Kyphosis

Asymmetric degenerative disc changes can result in degenerative scoliosis **(Fig. 17)**. This tends to produce

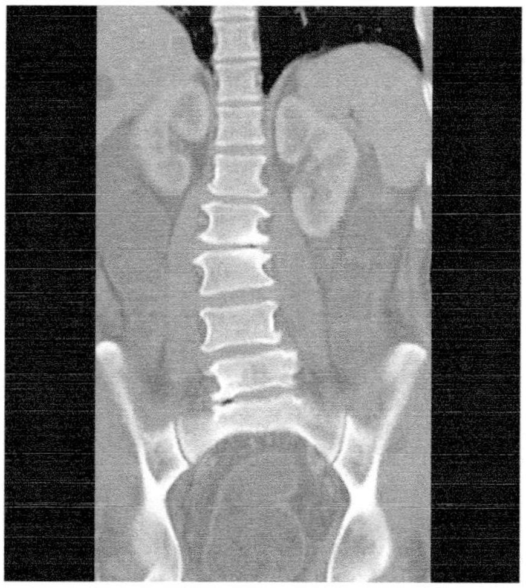

Fig. 17: Coronal reformatted CT image reveals laterally directed osteophytes on the concavity of scoliosis with vacuum phenomenon at multiple levels.

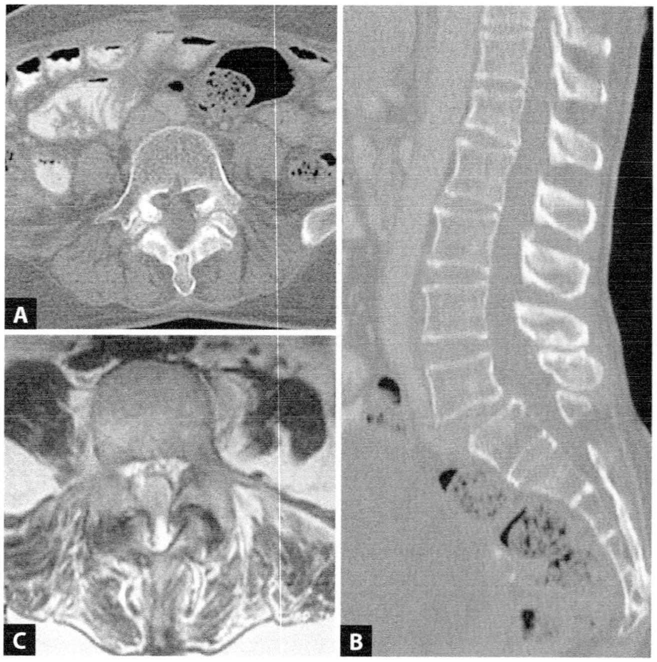

Figs. 18A to C: (A) Axial and (B) sagittal reformatted CT images reveal lysis of pars interarticularis of L4 with spondylolisthesis of L4 over L5 resulting in widening of the anteroposterior diameter of the spinal canal; (C) Axial T2W MR image of another patient shows break involving pars interarticularis of L4 with widening of spinal canal.

a positive feedback loop that tends to accelerate the degenerative changes on one side. Compared to idiopathic scoliosis, degenerative scoliosis is usually short segment and most often occurs in the lumbar spine. Also, loss of lumbar lordosis and spinal and foraminal stenosis are more common with degenerative scoliosis. Thoracic kyphosis in adults is frequently secondary to asymmetric degeneration in the anterior portions of the discs.[4]

Segmental Instability

Disc degeneration can lead to narrow disc space and buckling of LF which can further result in an unstable vertebral segment. Resultant malalignment may result in anterolisthesis, retrolisthesis or lateral spondylolisthesis. Degenerative retrolisthesis occurs classically secondary to disc degeneration and results in canal and foraminal stenosis. It may also occur secondary to asymmetric facet degeneration. Anterolisthesis occurs mostly at L4-L5 level, secondary to facet degeneration. In patients with degenerative scoliosis, lateral and retrolisthesis is often encountered.[4] Posterolisthesis, which is associated with facet and disc degeneration, is frequent at more mobile spine segments such as the cervical and upper lumbar spine.[2] The typical sites of degenerative spondylolisthesis are L3-L4 and L4-L5, because of more sagittal orientation of facet joints.

Spondylolisthesis may also result from pars interarticularis defects (spondylolysis) and the most common is the isthmic type of spondylolysis. This is most commonly seen at L5 and L4 vertebrae and is a defect in pars interarticularis which is considered a fatigue fracture. Other less common causes of spondylolisthesis are acute trauma, congenital dysplasias, tumors and iatrogenic causes. Spondylolisthesis due to pars defect may be distinguished from degenerative spondylolisthesis on imaging. The former depicts canal widening at the involved level **(Figs. 18A to C)** whereas the latter demonstrates canal narrowing at the affected level because of slippage of the posterior arch and facet hypertrophy.[1,2]

Secondary to segmental instability, hypertrophy of the ligaments, facet osteoarthritis, and osteophyte formation may develop which have an additive effect on narrowing of the spinal canal and foramina. These osteophytes may aid in stabilizing the spinal segment, which may be shown on kinematic MRI.[4]

Vertebral body movement may be seen on flexion, extension and lateral bending radiographs where instability may be diagnosed as loss of alignment of one or more vertebral lines. Other radiographic signs are vertebral slippage, variations in pedicle length, narrowing of neural foramina, and loss of disc height. Conventional MRI has a limited role. It may show displacement and pseudobulging of disc at the involved level. Axial loaded CT or MRI or upright MRI can provide functional information regarding vertebral stability.[2]

CLINICAL IMPLICATIONS

Natural history of back pain is poorly understood and causes of low backache remain unknown in majority of cases. Nonspecific imaging findings may often be encountered in asymptomatic subjects and findings seen in symptomatic patients do not necessarily correlate with symptoms.[1] The diagnosis should always be based on combined information from clinical findings and imaging studies for determining appropriate patient management strategy.

REFERENCES

1. Rumboldt Z. Degenerative disorders of the spine. Semin Roentgenol. 2006;41(4):327-62.
2. Gallucci M, Limbucci N, Paonessa A, Splendiani A. Degenerative disease of the spine. Neuroimaging Clin N Am. 2007;17(1):87-103.
3. Shah LM, Ross JS. Imaging of degenerative and infectious conditions of the spine. Neurosurgery. 2016;79(3):315-35.
4. Malfair D, Beall DP. Imaging the degenerative diseases of the lumbar spine. Magn Reson Imaging Clin N Am. 2007;15(2):221-38.
5. Bozzao A, Gallucci M, Masciocchi C, Aprile I, Barile A, Passariello R. Lumbar disc herniation: MR imaging assessment of natural history in patients treated without surgery. Radiology. 1992;185(1):135-41.
6. Modic MT, Ross JS. Lumbar degenerative disc disease. Radiology. 2007;245(1):43-61.
7. Kaplan RT, Czervionke LF, Haughton VM. Degenerative disease of the spine. In: Atlas SW (Ed). Magnetic Resonance Imaging of the Brain and Spine (Vol II), 4th edition. Philadelphia: Lippincott Williams and Wilkins; 2009. pp. 1448-507.
8. Pfirrmann CW, Metzdorf A, Zanetti M, Hodler J, Boos N. Magnetic resonance classification of lumbar intervertebral disc degeneration. Spine (Phila Pa 1976). 2001;26:1873-8.
9. Miller TT. Imaging of disc disease and degenerative spondylosis of the lumbar spine. Semin Ultrasound CT MR. 2004;25(6):506-22.
10. Fardon DF, Williams AL, Dohring EJ, Murtagh FR, Gabriel Rothman SL, et al. Lumbar disc nomenclature: version 2.0: recommendations of the combined task forces of the North American Spine Society, the American Society of Spine Radiology and the American Society of Neuroradiology. Spine J. 2014;14(11):2525-45.
11. Fardon DF, Milette PC. Nomenclature and classification of lumbar disc pathology. Recommendations of the combined task forces of the North American Spine Society, American Society of Spine Radiology, and American Society of Neuroradiology. Spine (Phila Pa 1976). 2001;26(5):E93-113.
12. Costello RF, Beall DP. Nomenclature and standard reporting terminology of intervertebral disc herniation. Magn Reson Imaging Clin N Am. 2007;15(2):167-74.
13. Farshad-Amacker NA, Farshad M, Winklehner A, Andreisek G. MR imaging of degenerative disc disease. Eur J Radiol. 2015;84(9):1768-76.
14. Clarençon F, Law-Ye B, Bienvenot P, Cormier É, Chiras J. The degenerative spine. Magn Reson Imaging Clin N Am. 2016;24(3):495-513.
15. Chung CB, Vande Berg BC, Tavernier T, Cotten A, Laredo JD, Vallee C, et al. End plate marrow changes in the asymptomatic lumbosacral spine: frequency, distribution and correlation with age and degenerative changes. Skeletal Radiol. 2004;33(7):399-404.

CHAPTER

10

Skeletal Disorders of Metabolic and Endocrine Origin

Alpana Manchanda, Jyoti Kumar, Swati Gupta

INTRODUCTION

Metabolic bone disease encompasses a diverse group of disorders associated with altered calcium and phosphorus homeostasis.[1,2] Although many of these disorders are quite common, they may be difficult to distinguish on the basis of history, physical examination, and imaging studies.[1,2]

To the clinician, metabolic bone disease is often silent until the patient presents with fracture, the ultimate complication of many metabolic disorders. Other patients may however present with a clinical history of back pain and a nonspecific radiologic finding of generalized osteopenia.[3] At this stage prior to fracture, accurate diagnosis is crucial. Understanding their diverse manifestations on imaging studies may allow early diagnosis, aid in their management, and in taking appropriate preventive measures.

The manifestations of endocrine derangements in the skeletal system depend on the age of the patient at the time of presentation. In general, skeletal manifestations in childhood and infancy consist of disturbances in growth and maturation, and in adulthood, these manifestations consist of disturbances in maintenance and metabolism.

DISORDERS OF METABOLIC ORIGIN

The most common types of metabolic bone diseases are acquired disorders with nutritional deficiencies being an important cause. Nonetheless, rare forms frequently are genetically based and cause intrinsic alterations in the bone cell population.

The various metabolic bone disorders may be grouped according to their underlying defects:

- Defect in osteoid formation: Scurvy
- Defect in mineralization: Rickets/osteomalacia
- Disorder with increased bone resorption: Hyperparathyroidism
- Disorder with no defect in mineralization and osteoid formation but decreased bone mass: Osteoporosis
- Miscellaneous: Fluorosis, heavy metal poisoning, and hypervitaminosis.

Table 1 lists the metabolic profile with reference values.

Table 1: Metabolic profile–reference values.

Serum calcium	8.7–10.2 mg/dL
Ionized calcium	4.5–5.3 mg/dL
Serum phosphorus	2.4–4.1 mg/dL
Alkaline phosphatase	223–635 U/L
Vitamin D	>25 ng/mL
Serum parathormone	8–51 pg/mL
Serum ascorbic acid	0.6–1.2 mg/100 mL

The imaging manifestations of metabolic bone disease are varied and the same disease process can have a wide range of skeletal findings.

RICKETS AND OSTEOMALACIA

Rickets in children and osteomalacia in adults are a group of bone disorders in which there is incomplete or inadequate mineralization of normal osteoid tissue. Both conditions usually result from an abnormality in vitamin D metabolism. The biochemical and histological abnormalities are identical in the two conditions while skeletal manifestations differ depending upon the age of the patient at the time of onset of disease. Prior to fusion of the growth plate, features of both rickets and osteomalacia can be seen.

Vitamin D is a steroid hormone which is produced by skin exposure to sunlight and also obtained from the diet.[4] To attain its active form, vitamin D must undergo two hydroxylations—first in the liver and second in the kidneys **(Fig. 1)**. The primary function of vitamin D is to maintain calcium and phosphate homeostasis, thereby ensuring normal mineralization of the skeleton. The target areas for vitamin D action include bone, gastrointestinal tract, kidneys, and parathyroid gland.[1,4,5]

Causes

The term rickets has evolved from the old English word wrick, which means "to twist." This twisting or bending of bones has been found to result from more than one cause.

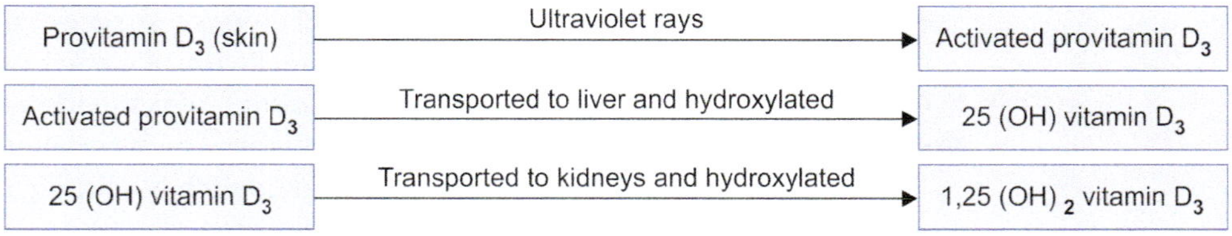

Fig. 1: Pathway for activation of vitamin D_3.

Rickets and osteomalacia occur due to many causes **(Box 1)**, most common being due to dietary deficiency of vitamin D called vitamin D-deficient rickets or nutritional rickets. Many abnormalities in vitamin D metabolism can potentially result in rickets and osteomalacia. These include malabsorption syndromes, hepatobiliary diseases, renal diseases, drugs, and neoplasms.[1,4]

Box 1: Causes of rickets and osteomalacia.

- *Abnormalities of vitamin D metabolism*:
  - Deficiency conditions:
    - Dietary deficiency of vitamin D
    - Lack of exposure to ultraviolet light
  - Absorption defects:
    - Gastrointestinal malabsorption
    - Biliary atresia
    - Small bowel bypass surgery
  - Hepatic diseases:
    - Cirrhosis
    - Hepatitis
  - Anticonvulsant therapy
  - Renal insufficiency:
    - Type I VDDR
    - Type II VDDR
- *Rickets and osteomalacia secondary to phosphate loss*:
  - X-linked hypophosphatemia, genetic (Vitamin D-resistant rickets)
  - Primary hypophosphatemic rickets, acquired
  - Renal tubular acidosis (RTA):
    - Type I (distal) RTA
    - Type II (proximal) RTA
  - Tumor-associated phosphate deficiency
  - Chemotherapeutic drug-induced rickets
- *Syndromes with radiographic appearance or osteomalacia but without abnormalities of vitamin D metabolism or renal tubular dysfunction (phosphate loss)*:
  - Metaphyseal chondrodysplasia (Schmid type)
  - Hypophosphatasia
  - Atypical axial osteomalacia

(VDDR: vitamin D-dependent rickets)

Clinical Features

Clinical findings of rickets and osteomalacia are highly variable and depend on the etiology and severity of the disorder as well as the age of patient at the time of presentation.[1,4,5] In the first 6 months of life, rickets can present with tetany or convulsions. In most children with rickets, skeletal growth is stunted and they present with swollen and tender joints. With advanced disease, they may present with irritability, weakness, and bony deformities. The most notable clinical finding is soft-tissue swelling occurring around the growth plates due to hypertrophied cartilage. Clinically, enlargement of wrists and costal cartilage are most suggestive of the disease with a specificity of 81% and 64%, respectively.[6]

In adults, findings of osteomalacia are more subtle. Initial symptoms include fatigue, malaise, or bone pain. With advanced disease, proximal muscle weakness and abnormal gait may be present.[1,5] Typical manifestations of osteomalacia consist of bone pain, especially in the hips and muscle weakness.

Biochemical Findings

On laboratory evaluation, the serum calcium and phosphorus may be normal or slightly reduced while serum alkaline phosphatase levels are increased.

Pathology

There is remarkable similarity in the biochemical and histologic abnormalities in rickets and osteomalacia. The characteristic changes of rickets are identified in the growth plates prior to closure while abnormalities of osteomalacia are seen in the mature areas of trabecular and cortical bone.

In order to understand the changes of rickets, the general structure and organization of growth plate is discussed briefly. The growth plate is a complex structure which is located at the ends of long bones and situated between the epiphysis and metaphysis.[4] Although, it is adjacent to the epiphysis, functionally it is part of the shaft. Histologically, the cellular arrangement of the normal growth plate is characterized by order with progressive increase in the number and size of cartilaginous cells from the epiphysis to metaphysis. The normal epiphysis has four zones. From the epiphyseal ossification center toward the shaft the various zones are—the resting zone, proliferating zone, hypertrophic zone, and zone of primary and secondary spongiosa. The hypertrophic zone is further subdivided into zones of maturation, degeneration, and provisional calcification **(Fig. 2)**.

In rickets, there is disorganization of the growth plate and adjacent metaphysis. The resting and proliferative zones of the cartilaginous growth plate are not significantly

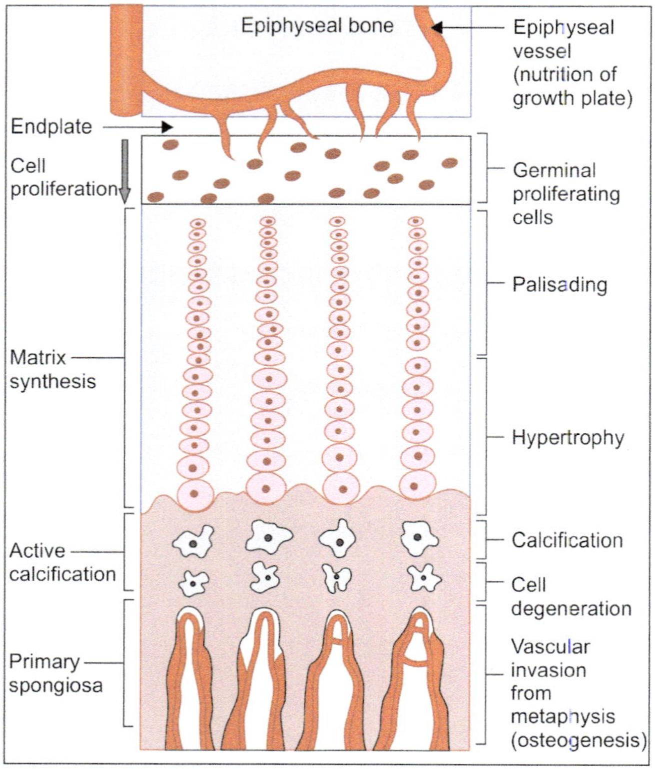

Fig. 2: Structure of the growth plate showing normal cellular organization.

altered from the normal pattern. However, the zone of maturation is grossly abnormal with a disorganized increase in the number of cells and a loss of normal columnar pattern. This cell mass results in an increase in length and width of the growth plate. Overall, there is diminished quantity of calcified osteoid and an increase in uncalcified osteoid, which casts increased radiolucency on the radiographs.

Osteomalacia results from insufficient, delayed, or defective mineralization of cortical and spongy bone. Histologically, it is characterized by abnormal quantities of inadequately mineralized bone matrix called osteoid, coating the surfaces of trabeculae, and lining the haversian canals in the cortex. These layers of osteoid are often referred to as osteoid seams. Osteoid seams are not pathognomonic of osteomalacia and may be found in other active metabolic states associated with high bone turnover. However, there is an increase in both the number and width of the osteoid seams in osteomalacia.

Etiologic Considerations

- *Abnormalities of vitamin D metabolism:*
    - *Deficiency of vitamin D*: It results from a diet which is inadequate in vitamin D or a defect in the synthesis of vitamin D due to poor exposure to sunlight.
    - *Malabsorption of vitamin D*: Defect in absorption of vitamin D may result from small bowel disease, small bowel bypass surgery, rapid intestinal transit, pancreatic insufficiency, or biliary atresia.
    - *Abnormal vitamin D metabolism*: This may occur due to liver diseases such as hepatitis, cirrhosis, or kidney disorders such as chronic renal failure and nephrotic syndrome.
    - *Anticonvulsant therapy*: Epileptic patients require long-term antiepileptic drugs (AED) which are associated with abnormal bone mineral metabolism, osteoporosis, and an increased risk of fracture. A reduction in the active level of vitamin D has been seen which is likely due to induction of liver enzymes by AED leading to its conversion to inactive metabolites in the liver microsomes. Hypocalcemia may also be seen due to low absorption from the gut secondary to hypovitaminosis. This may trigger an increase in circulation of parathyroid hormone and increased bone turnover. AED-induced disturbances of bone integrity are influenced by the type, duration, and dosage of the antiepileptic therapy. The risk of AED-induced bone damage is greater with carbamazepine, phenytoin, and phenobarbital than with other antiepileptic agents.[7]
    - *Renal osteodystrophy*: Renal osteodystrophy is a term which is used to describe the bony changes in patients with chronic renal insufficiency. In children, end-stage renal disease is commonly due to loss of renal parenchyma because of structural abnormalities of the urinary tract. While in adults, chronic glomerulonephritis is the main cause.

Due to chronic renal disease, there is phosphate retention along with impaired ability to form 1, 25 dihydroxy vitamin D_3. Low levels of vitamin D and an excess of phosphate stimulate an excess parathyroid hormone resulting in secondary hyperparathyroidism.

Radiographic changes in renal osteodystrophy, therefore, reflect a combination of different processes including rickets/osteomalacia, secondary hyperparathyroidism, and osteosclerosis. Radiological changes in rickets have already been described. The characteristic radiological changes in secondary hyperparathyroidism consist of bone resorption which may be subperiosteal, intracortical, endosteal, or subligamentous; presence of brown tumors; and soft-tissue and vascular calcification. Increased bone density or osteosclerosis is either focal or diffuse **(Fig. 3A)** and is commonly seen in the spine but also occurs in the pelvis, ribs, skull and tubular bones. The characteristic appearance of the spine is called "rugger jersey spine" because of its resemblance to the striped jersey worn by rugby players and is caused by increased bone deposition in the vertebral endplates **(Fig. 3B)**.

- *Hereditary Vitamin D-dependent Rickets (VDDR):* Vitamin D-dependent rickets should be considered when rickets presents in early infancy and other usual causes such as inadequate vitamin D intake, intestinal malabsorption, liver disease or kidney disorders have been excluded.
  Two forms have been described which involve problems with the formation or function of $1,25(OH)_2 D_3$.
  - *Type I VDDR:* Type I disorder results from a deficiency (genetic defect) of the renal enzyme 1-alpha-hydroxylase, which converts 25 (OH) D_3 to $1,25(OH)_2D_3$. Therefore, the blood levels of $25(OH)D_3$ are normal while those of $1,25(OH)_2D_3$ are decreased.
    Clinical presentation is early, often by 3 months of age, with most patients being symptomatic by 1 year of age. The disease is differentiated from X-linked hypophosphatemic rickets by the presence of convulsions and muscular weakness. Rachitic bone changes may be severe, rapidly progressive, and accompanied by pathologic fractures.[4] Healing occurs with physiologic doses of 1,25 dihydroxy vitamin D_3. This disorder is also known as *pseudovitamin D deficiency rickets* as patients with this condition respond to large doses of vitamin D or physiologic doses of 1,25 $(OH)_2D$ with resolution of the clinical, biochemical, and radiographic abnormalities.
  - *Type II VDDR:* In this type of VDDR serum levels of $1,25(OH)_2D_3$ are elevated, thereby indicating an end-organ resistance to $1,25(OH)_2D_3$. It is also known as *calcitrol-resistant rickets* (CRR) and is a rare autosomal recessive disorder characterized by severe rickets, growth retardation, severe dental changes, and alopecia from early infancy. The diagnosis of type II VDDR should be suspected from the unusual association of severe rickets and alopecia.
- *Rickets and osteomalacia secondary to phosphate loss*: A number of rachitic and osteomalacic syndromes have been identified of both congenital and acquired origin, which share one or several renal tubular abnormalities. Rickets or osteomalacia results from hypophosphatemia secondary to impaired renal tubular resorption of phosphate resulting in phosphate loss. These disorders were described by Albright, Fanconi, and associates who also reported that rickets was resistant to vitamin D therapy in these patients.[4] It includes various conditions with different etiologies, of which increased phosphatonins is a common link. Fibroblast growth factor 23 (FGF23) is the most common studied phosphatonin.
  - *X-linked hypophosphatemia*: It accounts for >80% of familial hypophosphatemic rickets. X-linked hypophosphatemia *(or familial vitamin D-resistant/refractory rickets)* is the most common form of renal tubular rickets and osteomalacia. It is genetically transmitted in an X-linked dominant trait. The syndrome is characterized

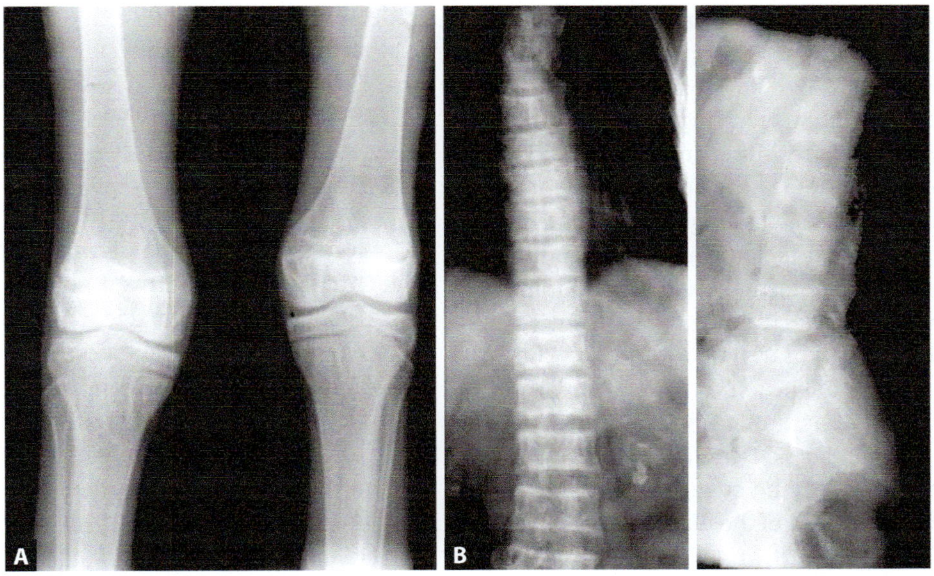

Figs. 3A and B: Renal osteodystrophy: (A) X-ray bilateral (B/L) knees showing knock knee deformity and patchy sclerosis at the distal femoral and proximal tibial metaphysis with slight widening of the growth plate; (B) Characteristic "rugger jersey spine" appearance in a patient of chronic renal failure with nephrolithiasis in the left kidney.

by lifelong hypophosphatemia. The basic defect lies in impaired reabsorption of phosphate from proximal tubules.[4] In addition, the conversion of $25(OH)D_3$ to $1,25(OH)_2D_3$ is also impaired. Serum calcium levels are in the normal range while the serum inorganic phosphate levels are persistently low. Rickets generally develops between 12 and 18 months of age.

- *Clinical features*: Clinical features include bowing of legs, limb deformities, short stature, and premature fusion of cranial sutures leading to skull deformities. Dental abnormalities are also seen.
- *Biochemical findings*: It is characterized by low serum phosphorus, normal serum calcium, normal parathyroid hormone (PTH), and elevated levels of alkaline phosphatase.
- *Radiological features*: Unlike vitamin D deficiency, craniotabes and rachitic rosary are not seen. Frontal bossing is usually the first finding at 6 months. Radiographically, the rachitic changes may be mild to moderate with bowing of long bones seen, particularly in the lower limbs. As the child starts walking, there are progressive limb deformities leading to disproportionate short stature with short lower limbs.[8] Lower limbs are more affected than upper limbs with coxa vera, genu varum, and valgus. Coarsening of trabecular pattern is seen with increasing age. In adults, generalized increase in bone density, especially of the axial skeleton, is characteristic. The spine and pelvis may show changes in the form of calcification and ossification in the paravertebral ligaments, ligamentum flavum, and iliolumbar and sacroiliac ligaments. The spinal changes may resemble to those of ankylosing spondylitis or diffuse idiopathic skeletal hyperostosis (DISH). However, the sacroiliac joints in X-linked hypophosphatemia show no bone erosions in contrast to that seen in ankylosing spondylitis. The appendicular skeleton also shows multiple sites of new bone formation at various muscle and ligament attachments. Osteoarthritis is common, particularly in the ankle, knees, wrists, and sacroiliac joints.

  The above radiographic findings in the axial and appendicular skeleton are distinctive and the diagnosis may be suggested prior to the clinical recognition of the disorder.

- *Primary hypophosphatemic rickets*: It is a form of rickets characterized by low serum phosphate levels and resistance to treatment with UV radiation or vitamin D therapy.
- *Renal tubular acidosis*: Renal tubular acidosis (RTA) comprises a group of tubular transport defects characterized by inability to appropriately acidify the urine with resultant metabolic acidosis. The underlying abnormalities consist of an impairment of bicarbonate resorption or excretion of hydrogen ions or a combination of both. Detailed biochemical tests are essential for reaching at a correct diagnosis in RTA.[9]
  - *Type I (distal) RTA*: It is characterized by persistent severe metabolic acidosis with continuous bicarbonaturia and is an important cause of severe rachitic abnormalities.[9] In untreated cases, nephrocalcinosis/renal calculi are formed.
  - *Type II (proximal) RTA*: This type of RTA may occur in children in an isolated form or as part of global proximal tubular dysfunction called *Fanconi's syndrome*. In this condition, phosphaturia of tubular origin is associated with glycosuria and various aminoacidurias in addition to bicarbonaturia. Unlike type I RTA, children with type II RTA do not progressively accumulate acid.[9] Rachitic deformities and nephrocalcinosis are uncommon in isolated proximal RTA but are common in Fanconi's syndrome.
- *Tumor-associated rickets and osteomalacia*: Tumor-associated rickets and osteomalacia (also termed *oncogenic osteomalacia*) is a syndrome characterized by hyperphosphaturia, with resultant hypophosphatemia, decreased levels of $1,25(OH)_2D_3$ (refractory to vitamin D_3 administration), and various neoplasms.

  The syndrome is more common in adults than children. The tumors are benign, of connective tissue origin, located either in soft tissues or bones. They are typically vascular and often show foci of new bone formation.

  Patients with this syndrome frequently have long-standing generalized muscle weakness and proximal myopathy. Radiographic changes of rickets and osteomalacia may be advanced at the time of initial presentation.

  The cause of rickets in association with these tumors has been attributed to the secretion of a humoral agent termed "phosphatonin" which directly inhibits the absorption of phosphates in the proximal tubule.[10] The tumors are usually small, benign, and of vascular origin (hemangiopericytoma), but there is now known to be a wide spectrum of tumors, some of which may be malignant.[11]

Biochemically, serum calcium is normal with marked decrease in serum phosphate. These patients are resistant or refractory to vitamin D. However, resection of the tumor results in the reversal of metabolic, clinical, and osseous abnormalities.

- *Chemotherapeutic drug-induced rickets:* High doses of a chemotherapeutic agent, *"ifosfamide"* used in the treatment of solid tumors, especially in children have been known to result in Fanconi syndrome with hypophosphatemic rickets. This complication is seen as a result of nephrotoxic metabolites of the drug and may be irreversible.[10] Renal toxicity is predominantly tubular, although glomerular abnormalities may also occur. Any part of the nephron may be damaged by ifosfamide. The major cause of rickets and osteomalacia is hyperphosphaturia with resultant hypophosphatemia.

- *Syndromes with the radiographic appearance of rickets or osteomalacia but without abnormalities of vitamin D metabolism or renal tubular dysfunction (phosphate loss)*:
  - *Metaphyseal chondrodysplasia (Schmid type)*: It is a disorder in which there is generalized symmetric disturbance of endochondral bone formation, primarily at the metaphysis.[4] It is manifested in childhood as short stature and bowing of the long bones, having a benign course. The radiographs show widening of the growth plate. Multiple, small, and bony projections extend from the metaphysis into the growth plate. In contrast to the usual rickets, the metaphysis is well mineralized and may show increased density.[4] There is absence of Looser's zones. The serum calcium, phosphorus, and alkaline phosphatase levels are normal. Spontaneous improvement occurs and patients do not respond to vitamin D therapy.
  - *Hypophosphatasia*: Hypophosphatasia is a rare disorder that is genetically transmitted that may resemble rickets both clinically and radiologically. However, the serum calcium and phosphorus levels are normal. The characteristic diagnostic features are:
    - Defective skeletal mineralization, resembling rickets radiologically
    - Low serum alkaline phosphatase level (in contrast to rickets in which it is increased)
    - Increased amounts of phosphoethanolamine, an amino acid, in the blood and urine.

    A wide spectrum of clinical severity is noted with most patients being diagnosed in infancy and childhood. The most severely affected neonates usually die soon after birth. *Radiologically,* there is reduced mineralization. Fractures with deformity and shortening may suggest a dwarfing syndrome. Radiographic changes at the growth plate may be seen soon after birth, and are similar to those of rickets but show characteristic multiple radiolucent extensions into the metaphysis that represent uncalcified bone matrix.[4] Coarse trabecular pattern, bowing deformities with or without healing fractures may be present. Wormian bones and craniosynostosis may be present.
  - *Atypical axial osteomalacia*: It is a rare condition in which the radiographic abnormalities are confined to the axial skeleton, with sparing of appendicular sites. A dense, coarse trabecular pattern is most marked in the cervical region. The lumbar spine, pelvis, and ribs are also involved. Looser's zones have not been identified in this condition.[10] The biochemical findings are normal with no response to vitamin D therapy.

Radiological Features

Although there is a significant overlap between rickets and osteomalacia, their radiologic findings are quite different and hence, they will be discussed separately.

Rickets

Rickets occurs when the orderly development and mineralization of the growth plate is interrupted. In the earliest stage, rachitic changes are not detectable radiologically. Biochemical and histologic changes develop several weeks prior to the appearance of the conclusive changes in the radiographs.[12]

The most common and nonspecific radiologic finding in patients of rickets is osteopenia.[1,4,5] Characteristic changes occur at the open growth plate.[5] The findings are seen on the metaphyseal side of the growth plate as the unmineralized osteoid is concentrated there. These changes are best seen in those areas showing most active growth. The distal ends of radius and ulna are the optimal sites for the demonstration of the earliest lesion.[11] Significant changes are often seen in the ulna when the radius appears to be normal as the distal ulnar growth plate grows more rapidly than the distal radius. Therefore, the ulna is a more sensitive indicator of rickets at the wrist.

Radiographic abnormalities reflect the disordered proliferation of cartilaginous cells in the zone of hypertrophy along with the deficient mineralization in the zone of provisional calcification.[4,5] The zone of provisional calcification is a band of calcification which marks the end of the radiolucent growth plate and beginning of the radiographically calcified metaphysis.

As the rachitic changes are more advanced at the fastest growing growth plates, radiographs of the most active sites should be undertaken. In order of decreasing activity, the most active growth plates are costochondral junction of the middle ribs, the distal femur, the proximal humerus, both ends of tibia, and the distal ulna and radius.

The characteristic radiologic features of rickets seen at the end of long bones in order of occurrence the radiologic findings are:

- *Widening of the growth plate* is the *earliest specific radiologic change* which occurs as a result of increase in cartilaginous cell mass.[4]
- *Irregular metaphyseal margins* (paint brush metaphyses) occurs due to fraying and disorganization of the spongy bone in the metaphyseal region.
- Further progression of the disease leads to *widening and cupping* of the *metaphysis* **(Figs. 4A and B)**. This can be explained by the protrusion of the bulky mass of cartilaginous cells in the zone of hypertrophy into the poorly mineralized metaphysis. Cupping of the distal end of the ulna in younger infants is not necessarily abnormal as it has been observed in some nonrachitic infants during the first months of life.[12] Cupping is common in both ends of the fibula and the distal ends of the ulna and tibia. Metaphyseal cupping is however never found in the bones of the elbow.[13]
- Similar process occurs on the epiphyseal side of the growth plate. The defective maturation and mineralization result in an *epiphysis* that is *osteopenic* and has irregular, indistinct borders and shows *delayed appearance of ossification centers.*
- The shafts of long bones may appear normal when changes are first detected in the metaphysis. *Rarefaction* of the *shaft* becomes evident a few weeks later due to loss of mineral content. The cortex becomes thin with a coarse texture.
- *Skeletal deformities* are the most common complication detected radiologically, the appearance and location of which depend on age and the part in which disease develops.[4]
  - *Skull*: It is particularly affected in the early months of life as it has to accommodate the rapidly growing brain. There is excess osteoid deposition in frontal and parietal regions and posterior flattening due to supine posture of the infant. This results in squared configuration of the skull known as "craniotabes" **(Fig. 5A)**.
  - *Long bones*: In early childhood, more rapid growth occurs in the long bones and bowing deformities of arms and legs are common which can be related to the sitting position assumed by infants and children. Bowing also is a result of displacement of the growth centers owing to the asymmetrical musculotendinous pulls on the weakened growth plate[14] **(Fig. 5B)**. Bulbous enlargement of the costochondral junctions, particularly those of the middle ribs can be seen (rachitic rosary **Fig. 5C**), which can indent the pleural surface or even the thymic shadow.[6]
  - *Spine*: Scoliosis and vertebral end plate deformities may develop in older children as the effects of weight bearing become more important. Scoliosis coupled with bending deformities of long bones results in an overall decrease in height of the child.
  - *Pelvis*: The protrusion of the hip and spine into the soft pelvis produces a triradiate configuration of the pelvis. Such a pelvic deformity may cause considerable difficulty during parturition.
  - *Fractures*: In long-standing cases of rickets, trivial trauma may result in fracture of the weakened undermineralized bone **(Figs. 6A and B)**.

In severe malnutrition, rickets may be associated with scurvy and protein deficiency.

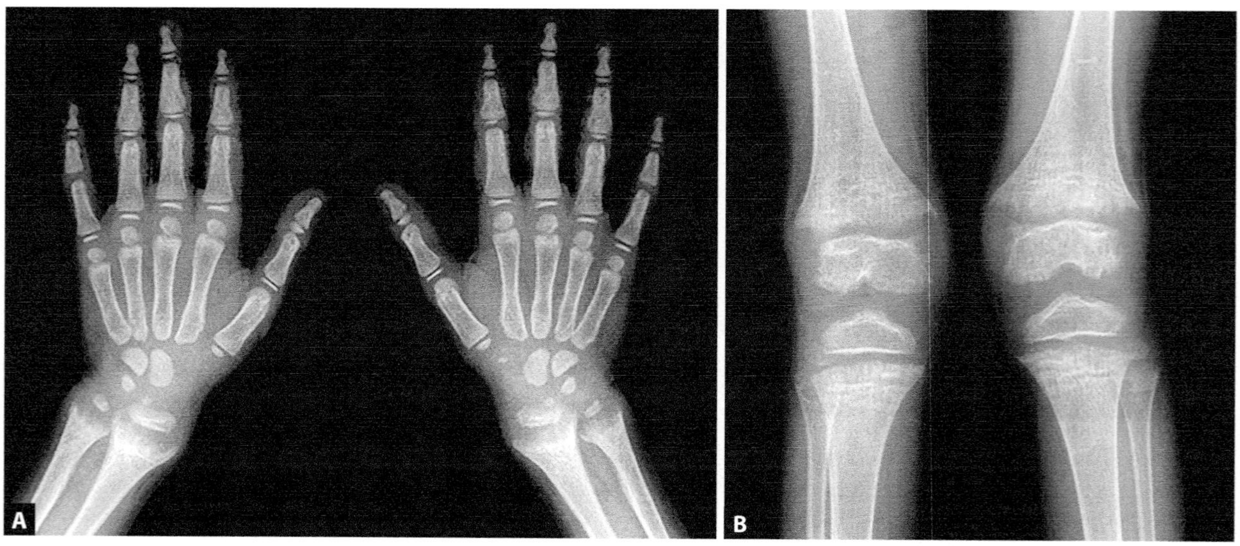

Figs. 4A and B: Rickets: X-ray bilateral wrists (A) and knees (B). Anteroposterior (AP) view: Typical changes of active rickets consisting of fraying, irregularity of distal radius and ulnar metaphysis and distal femoral and proximal tibial metaphysis with widening of the growth plates at the wrists and knees. The adjacent epiphysis and diaphysis are osteopenic.

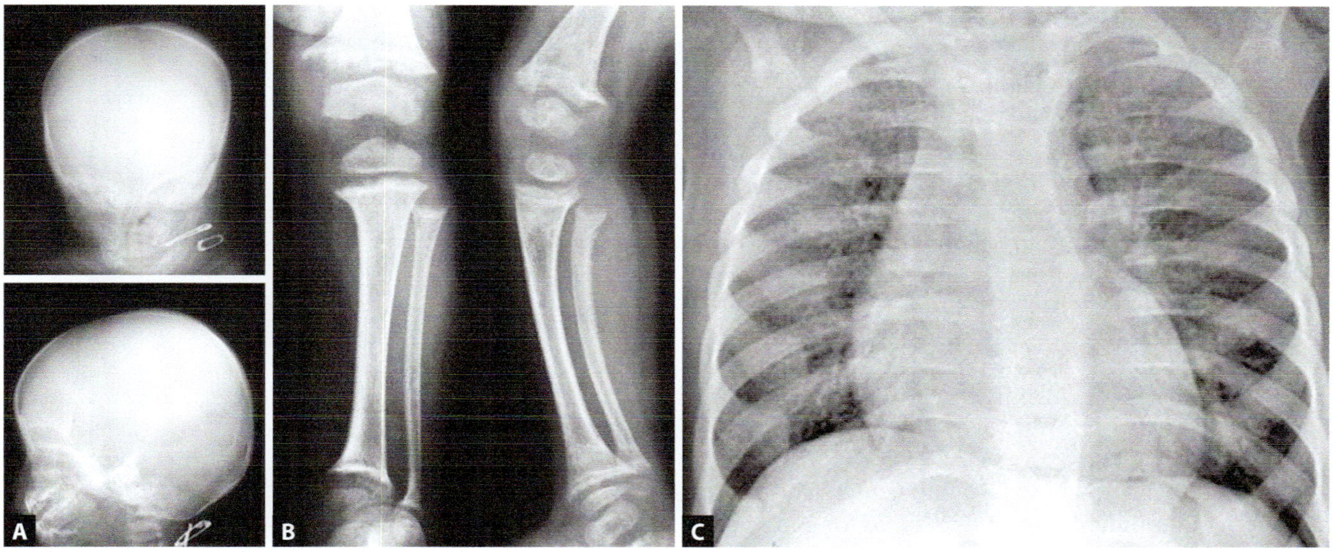

Figs. 5A to C: Skeletal deformities in rickets: (A) Squared configuration of the skull in the neonatal period: "Craniotabes"; (B) Marked anterior bowing of the tibia and fibula with rachitic changes. The visualized bones are osteopenic; (C) "Rachitic rosary": Widened anterior ends of ribs due to hypertrophy of costochondral junction.

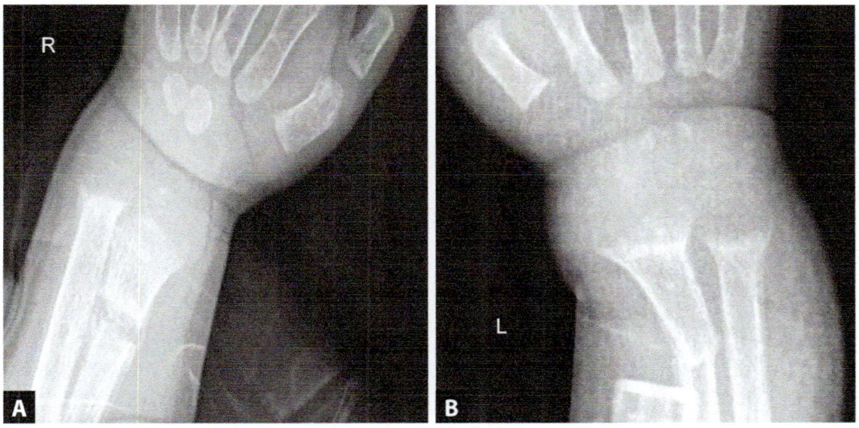

Figs. 6A and B: X-ray wrists of two infants with rickets. The bones are markedly osteopenic with fracture of distal ends of radius in both.

Signs of Healing

Radiological evidence of healing is seen within 2–3 weeks of adequate therapy and total recalcification is usually complete in 2 months.[15] The signs of healing rickets are:

- Reappearance of the dense zone of provisional calcification: This is the first evidence of healing and is seen radiologically as a transverse line of increased density, which appears beyond the visible end of shaft with a metaphysis interposed between the two radiolucent areas **(Fig. 7)**. Further mineralization of the osteoid unites this with the metaphysis.
- Increase in cupping of the healing metaphysis is seen as compared to the cupping seen in the active stage of rickets.
- Recalcification of the subperiosteal osteoid may produce a thick envelope of cortex that surrounds the shaft. This thick, opaque envelope along the shaft may be of uniform density or lamellated.

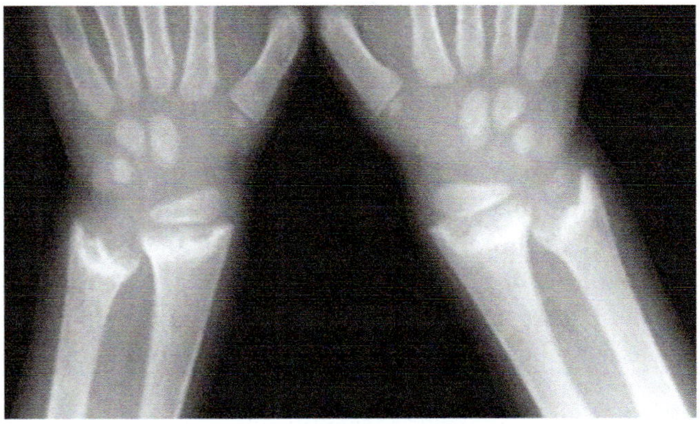

Fig. 7: Healing rickets: X-ray bilateral (B/L) wrists showing reappearance of the dense zone of provisional calcification at the metaphysis.

- Epiphyseal ossification center which were ill-defined and osteopenic in the active stage of rickets become sharply defined in the healing stage. In severe cases, the ossification centers may become invisible during the active stage of rickets and reappear when they are recalcified during healing, erroneously suggesting a rapid advance in skeletal maturation.

When the patient is on intermittent or inadequate treatment, the process of calcification and repair is irregular. Radiologically, patchy sclerosis of the metaphysis is seen, sometimes with alternating sclerotic and lucent bands.

Sequelae

Complete healing and restoration of normal structures is the rule in rickets even when severe changes are present during the active stage.[12]

Central rarefaction of ossification centers and cortical thickening of tubular bones may remain for a long time. Bowing and angulation deformities are not uncommon due to weakened bones.

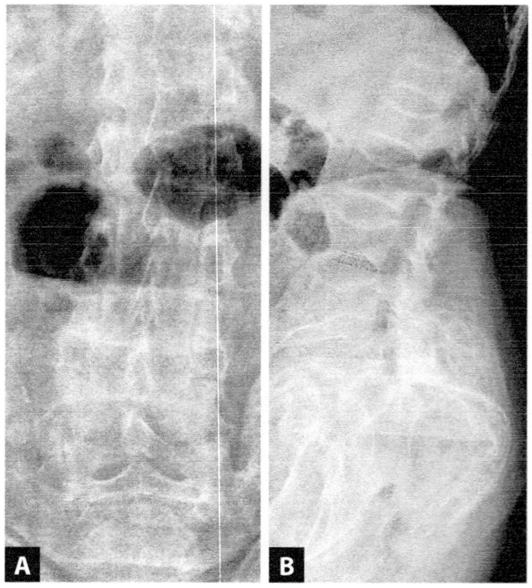

Figs. 8A and B: X-ray lumbosacral spine anteroposterior (AP) and lateral views reveal marked diffuse osteopenia with reduced vertebral height with biconcave appearance giving cod fish appearance. The sacral spine is acutely kyphotic: Osteomalacia.

Osteomalacia

The term osteomalacia literally means *"soft bones."*

Radiological changes: The radiological findings of osteomalacia are often nonspecific.[4] Correlation with appropriate laboratory and clinical data are often required for reaching a correct diagnosis. The major skeletal changes observed are:

- *Osteopenia:* It is the most common radiologic sign due to decreased bone mineral content.[4] It is usually uniform involving all the bones.
- *Coarse indistinct trabecular pattern:* It is in combination with generalized osteopenia and suggests osteomalacia.[4] An overall decrease in number of bony trabeculae within all the bones enhances the contrast of the remaining trabeculae giving a coarse, mottled appearance **(Figs. 8A and B)**.
- *Cortical involvement:* The cortices of long bones become thin, with indistinct definition, especially on the endosteal surface.
- *Pseudofractures or Looser's zones:* These are a more specific but less common manifestation of osteomalacia.[16] Looser's zones are linear radiolucent bands of undermineralized osteoid that occur in a bilateral and symmetric distribution[16,17] **(Figs. 9A and B)**. They are oriented at right angles to the cortex, i.e., perpendicular to the long axis of the bone.[15] The characteristic sites include:
  - Axillary margins of scapula
  - Superior and inferior pubic rami
  - Medial femoral necks
  - Posterior margins of the proximal ulna
  - Ribs.[4,17]

  Looser's zones are considered to be either insufficiency type stress fracture or due to vascular pulsations acting on the softened bone.[6,14] However, in contrast to fatigue type stress fractures, pseudofractures do not necessarily involve weight-bearing bones and may remain unaltered over long periods of time. True fractures may develop later at these sites because they represent areas of weakened bone[14] **(Fig. 10)**. In addition, Looser's zones show mild-to-moderate sclerosis with an absence of callus. Radiolucent areas similar to pseudofractures may be seen in bones affected by Paget's disease and fibrous dysplasia.[14,16]

  The terms *Milkman's fracture, increment fracture and umbauzonen* have also been used to describe osteomalacic pseudofractures.[4,6] Pseudofractures occur at sites of increased stress and therefore, accelerated bone turnover. They are classically seen at the concave (compressive) side of a bony deformity.[31] The osteoid which is laid down in the replacement process is inadequately mineralized, which accounts for its radiolucent appearance **(Fig. 11)**.[4,14]

  Pseudofractures may be identified by radionuclide bone scan or MR imaging before being evident on radiographs.[14]

  Bone scintigraphy has been found to be more sensitive than blood biochemistry and radiographic findings in the detection of osteomalacia. The typical features of osteomalacia seen on whole-body scintigraphy are widening of mandible, rachitic rosary sign, the tie sign of the sternum, pseudofracture sign, and prominent epiphysis of the knees.[18]
- *Bony deformities:* These occur mainly in weight-bearing joints. In the pelvis, there is medial acetabular migration (protrusio acetabulae) and inferior displacement of sacrum thereby producing a triradiate

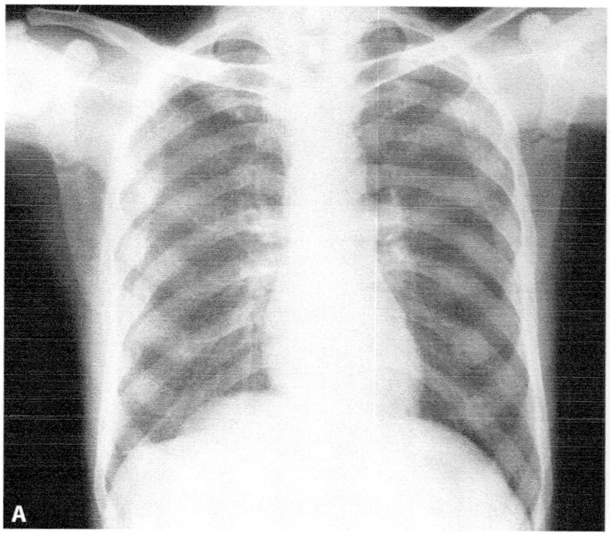

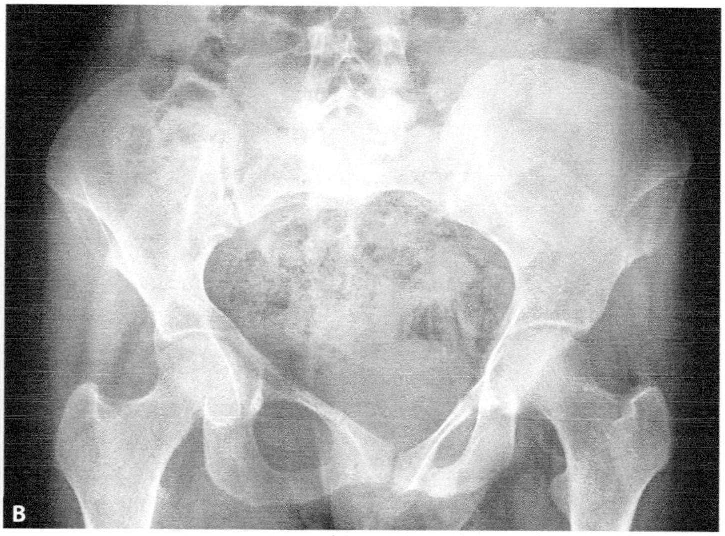

Figs. 9A and B: (A) Chest radiograph showing typical appearance of Looser's zone in bilateral lateral and medial borders of scapulae and ribs; (B) X-ray pelvis [anteroposterior (AP)] showing characteristic appearance of Looser's zones in bilateral superior pubic rami and mild right protrusio acetabuli with resultant asymmetric shape of the pelvic cavity.

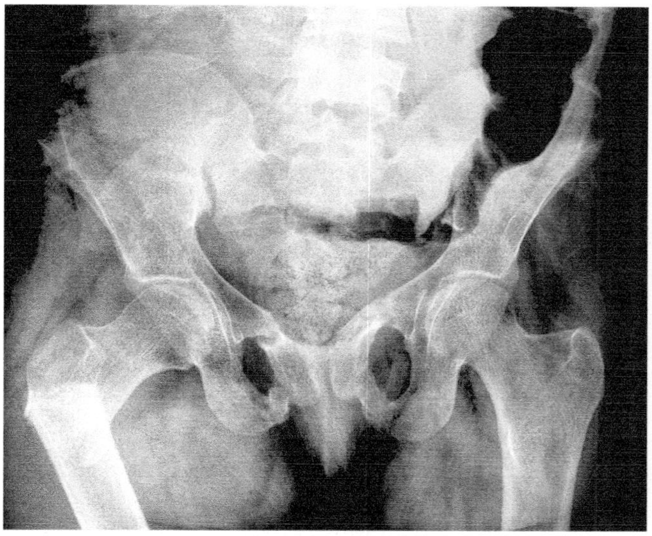

Fig. 10: X-ray pelvis [anteroposterior (AP)] in a 28 years' female with sudden-onset pain over right thigh following trivial trauma reveals fracture of upper end of the right femur. The visualized bones are osteopenic with coarse trabecular pattern. Looser's zones are seen in bilateral superior and inferior rami: Osteomalacia.

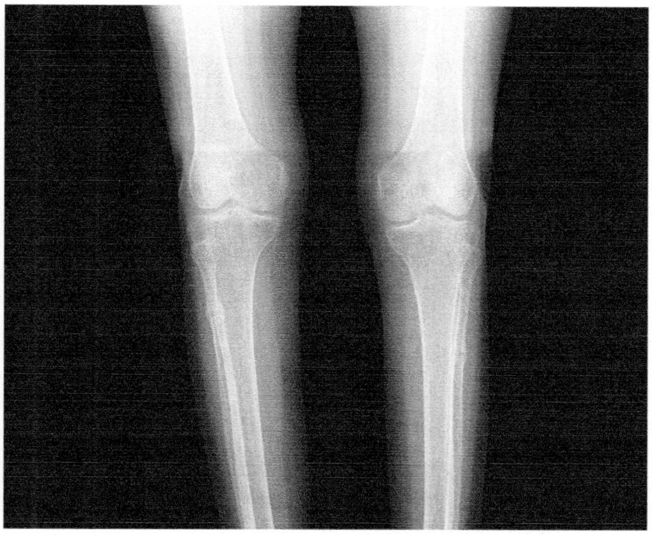

Fig. 11: Radiograph bilateral legs [anteroposterior (AP)] showing Looser's zone in upper one-third bilateral fibula with surrounding sclerosis. There is osteoporosis with cortical thinning of the bones.

shape of the pelvis[9] **(Figs. 12A and B)**. Both the femur and tibia show bowing deformity, vertebral bodies may develop a biconcave shape ("codfish" vertebrae), and kyphoscoliosis is not an uncommon finding. Basilar invagination of the skull may occur.[9]

Radiographs of the spine in osteoporosis (characterized by decrease in bone mass but there is no defect in mineralization) and osteomalacia may appear to be similar but they can be differentiated on the basis of coarse and indistinct trabeculae in osteomalacia while the trabeculae are thin and sharp in osteoporosis. Also, the spinal deformity in osteomalacia is uniform unlike osteoporosis wherein it is nonuniform.[4]

HYPERPARATHYROIDISM

Hyperparathyroidism (HPT) is a pathological state characterized by excessive production of parathyroid hormone (PTH). In the normal state, parathyroid hormone promotes release of calcium into the blood from the bone. It also stimulates extensive bone remodeling. Alterations of parathyroid function cause a breakdown in calcium homeostasis leading to increased renal

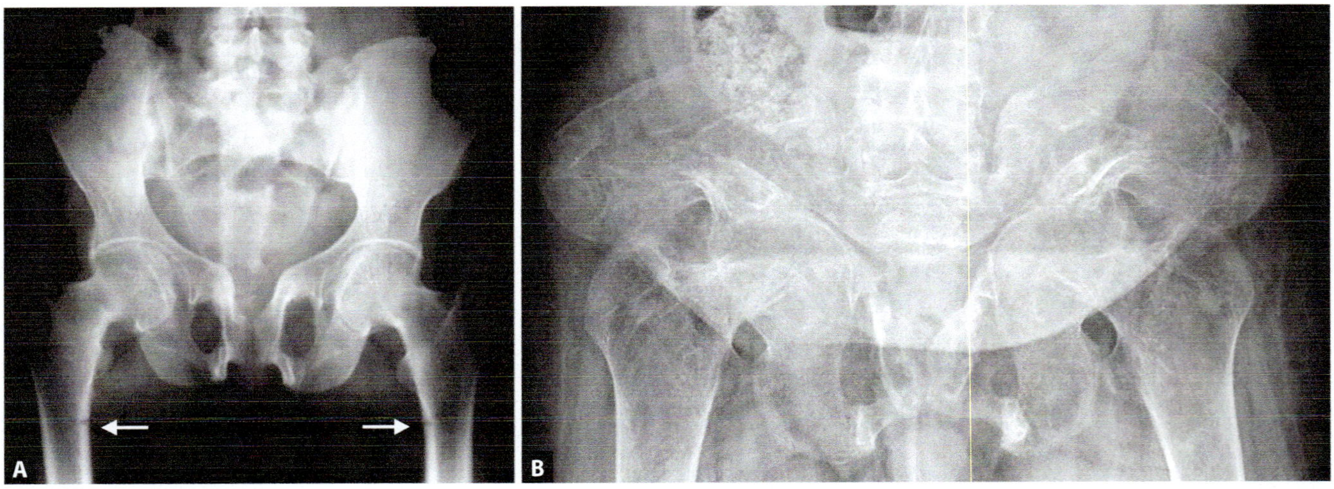

Figs. 12A and B: Pelvis [anteroposterior (AP)] in two different patients of osteomalacia: (A) Looser's zones in bilateral symmetric distribution in inner margins of proximal femora and superior and inferior pubic rami; (B) Severe osteomalacic changes with triradiate pelvis due to bilateral (B/L) protrusio acetabuli and inferior displacement of sacrum. The visualized bones are markedly osteoporotic. Old healed Looser's zones are seen in B/L superior and inferior pubic rami.

absorption of calcium, phosphaturia, increased synthesis of 1,25-dihydroxy vitamin D_3, which increases intestinal calcium resorption, and increased bone turnover, thereby resulting in characteristic pathologic and radiologic abnormalities.[19] Hyperparathyroidism is divided into primary, secondary, and tertiary types.

Primary Hyperparathyroidism

Primary HPT refers to inappropriate or unregulated overproduction of PTH occurring as a result of abnormality in one or more of the parathyroid glands. The cause in most cases is a single parathyroid adenoma (90% of cases); less common causes include double adenomas (4%), hyperplasia of multiple glands (6%), and parathyroid carcinoma (<1%).[20] Hyperplasia of the parathyroid glands can occur as an isolated finding or as part of multiple endocrine neoplasia (MEN) syndromes.

Secondary Hyperparathyroidism

Secondary HPT is more common than primary HPT. It is associated with abnormalities in function of the parathyroid glands induced by a sustained hypocalcemic stimulus. The most common cause is chronic renal failure in which chronically elevated serum phosphate levels depress the serum calcium level leading to compensatory hypertrophy of the chief cells of the parathyroid gland. Occasionally, malabsorption states and dietary abnormalities leading to hypocalcemia may be responsible.[21]

Tertiary Hyperparathyroidism

Tertiary HPT occurs in patients with long-standing secondary HPT who develop autonomous parathyroid function and hypercalcemia.

Pathophysiology

The clinical, pathological, and radiological manifestation of HPT can be understood by understanding the interrelated roles of parathyroid hormone (PTH) and vitamin D in the regulation of calcium metabolism.

Parathyroid hormone influences many tissues in the human body and is essential for the proper transport of calcium and other ions in bone, intestine, and kidney. The synthesis and secretion of PTH is regulated by the ionized serum calcium level. The normal serum calcium levels are maintained within a normal physiologic range by the intestines and kidneys which balance intake and excretion. Ninety-nine percent of the elemental calcium is bound to the skeleton and PTH works to increase the serum calcium by increasing the resorption with liberation of calcium and phosphorus.

In the kidneys, PTH inhibits resorption of phosphate in the proximal and distal tubules. This causes a decrease in the plasma phosphate concentration which in turn helps to maintain the serum calcium level. PTH also increases the renal tubular reabsorption of calcium.

Parathyroid hormone has no documented direct effect upon intestinal calcium absorption. PTH along with a decreased serum calcium and phosphate stimulates synthesis of 1,25 dihydroxy vitamin D the primary mediator of intestinal calcium and phosphorus absorption, and also acts on bone to produce resorption. Thus, functioning renal tissue is critical to the metabolism of both PTH and vitamin D and is a major target organ for the action of these hormones **(Fig. 13)**.

Therefore, there exists a negative feedback loop between serum calcium and PTH. An abrupt fall in calcium will actively stimulate PTH secretion **(Fig. 14)**.

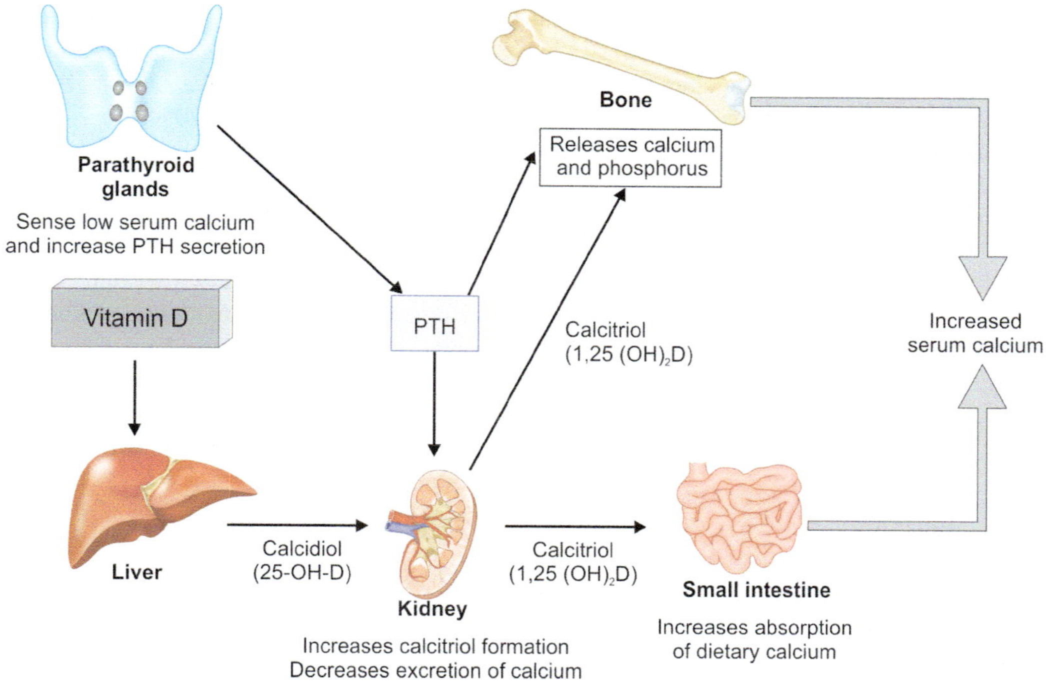

Fig. 13: Overview of vitamin D metabolism. (PTH: parathyroid)

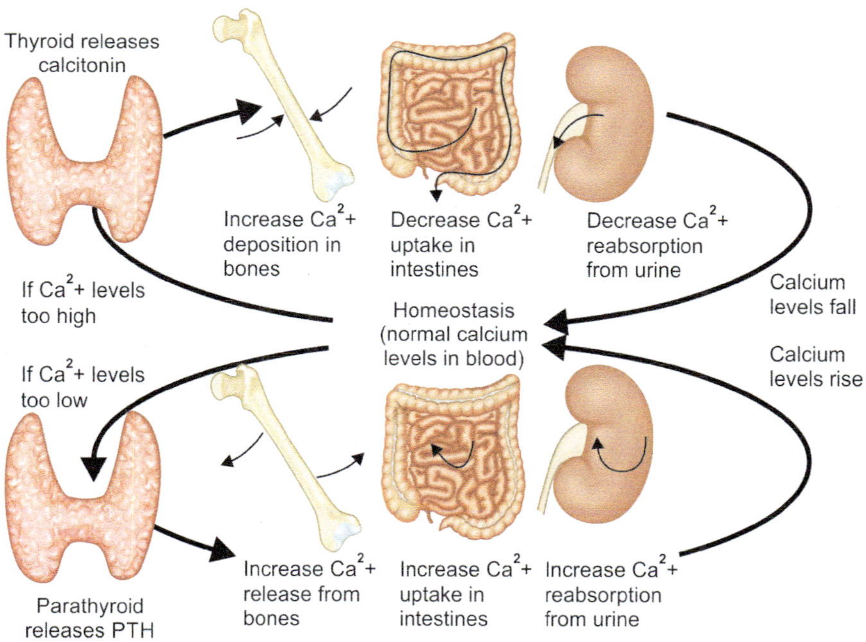

Fig. 14: Role of parathyroid (PTH) and calcitonin in the regulation of calcium metabolism.

Clinical Features

The clinical features of primary HPT relates to hypercalcemia which results from:

- Increased intestinal absorption of calcium
- Increased bone turnover
- Increased tubular resorption of calcium.

Patients may present with tiredness, lethargy, polyuria, anorexia or nausea, or to bone or renal complication.

The true incidence of primary HPT is not known but biochemical screening identifies the condition in unsuspected persons. It is found at all ages from birth to old age, with the highest incidence between 20 and 60 years, with women being affected two to four times more often than men.[15]

There appears to be a relationship between the severity of the disease and the type of symptoms that predominate. Patients with renal calculi are younger, have a chronic course, and are associated with hyperplasia of the parathyroid gland. Those with bone changes have a subacute progressive course characterized by a marked elevation in serum calcium levels, and these patients generally have adenomas.[21]

Nephrolithiasis is the most common clinical manifestation, followed by hypertension, peptic ulcers, pancreatitis, psychiatric disorders, and bone pain.[22]

Biochemical Findings

In most cases, the diagnosis of hyperparathyroidism can be made on the basis of clinical symptomatology and laboratory tests. Sustained elevation of serum calcium and serum parathormone levels are the most accepted means for the establishment of diagnosis of primary HPT.[19] Multiple measurements of serum calcium are often recommended due to the variations in the amount of circulating parathyroid hormone at any given time. Also, hypercalcemia is a feature of other disease states such as malignancy, endocrinological disorders, secondary to drugs, granulomatous disorders, etc. **(Box 2)**.

Box 2: Differential diagnosis of hypercalcemia.

- *Malignancy*:
  - Solid tumors (primarily breast cancer)
  - Hematologic disorders
  - Myeloma
  - Lymphoma
  - Leukemia
- *Enocrinological disorders*:
  - Primary hyperparathyroidism
  - Multiple endocrine neoplasias (types I and II)
  - Ectopic hyperparathyroidism (malignancy predominantly lung cancer)
  - Secondary hyperparathyroidism (renal failure)
  - Hyperthyroidism
  - Hypoadrenalism
- *Drugs*:
  - Vitamin A intoxication
  - Vitamin D intoxication
  - Thiazides
  - Calcium
  - Milk alkali syndrome
  - Dialysis
- *Granulomatous disorders*:
  - Sarcoidosis
  - Tuberculosis
  - Histoplasmosis
  - Berylliosis
  - Rheumatoid arthritis
- *Pediatric disorders*:
  - Infantile hypercalcemia
  - Hypophosphatasia
- *Miscellaneous*:
  - Immobilization
  - Paget's disease

About 10–20% of patients with malignancy have elevated serum calcium levels (normal reference range = 9–11 mg%) with majority of these patients having direct involvement of the skeleton by a malignant lesion.[23]

The term pseudohyperparathyroidism is referred to the syndrome consisting of hypercalcemia of malignancy in the absence of demonstrable skeletal metastasis or primary hyperparathyroidism.

Elevated urinary cyclicAMP and elevated alkaline phosphatase levels signify increase in bone turnover and skeletal involvement.

In secondary HPT, the plasma calcium levels are normal or low and the serum inorganic phosphate levels are high (chronic renal failure) or low (intestinal malabsorption).

Radiological Approach

The value of radiological studies in primary and secondary HPT lies not in the initial diagnosis, but in assessing the severity of the condition, and in noninvasive localization of the parathyroid glands prior to surgery as well as in the follow-up of the patient.[21]

Radiological Findings

The skeletal changes in HPT are characteristic and reflect the histologic changes of increased resorption of cortical and cancellous bone with substitutive fibrosis. Conventional radiography can assess the extent of bone involvement and the presence of bone changes is an accepted indication for parathyroid surgery in primary HPT.[21] The bone changes of primary and secondary HPT are identical, except for the associated changes of renal osteodystrophy in secondary HPT.

In the past, for earlier diagnosis of subtle osseous abnormalities, magnification radiography was done. But now, with advances in digital radiography routine hand radiographs are considered the most effective method.

Bone Resorption

The incidence of bone lesions varies from 30 to 40%.[21] The initial bone changes may not be seen on radiographic or gross pathologic examination, although, microscopic evaluation shows osteoclastic activity.[19] Bone resorption is a hallmark of HPT and is one of the effects of increased PTH production. The bone resorption is due to increased osteoclastic activity and can be detected on the subperiosteal, intracortical, endosteal, subchondral, and trabecular surfaces. Overall cortical bone is affected more severely than cancellous bone. These changes are reflected radiologically by poor definition of cortical surfaces, increased cortical striations ("tunneling"), cortical thinning, and distortion and blurring of trabecular bone.[21]

Subperiosteal resorption: Subperiosteal resorption of cortical bone is considered pathognomonic of HPT.[19,21] Although it may be seen at various skeletal sites, the earliest and best recognized changes are seen in the hands.[24] The earliest site of subperiosteal resorption is the radial aspect of middle phalanges of middle and index fingers **(Figs. 15A and B)**. Some authors have cited the earliest radiographic evidence of subperiosteal resorption to occur in the terminal tufts of the fingers.[21,24] Loss of fine cortical outline around the tufts results in a lace-like irregular appearance of external surface of bone with significant erosion of tufts being more obvious in advanced cases. A distinctive pattern of band-like appearance of acroosteolysis may be seen in the terminal phalanges of the hands (less commonly the feet), consisting of band-like radiolucent areas that may separate the tuft and the base of the phalanx separately.

Other sites of subperiosteal resorption include the medial aspect of the proximal end of tibia, humerus and femur, superior and inferior margins of the ribs, and lamina dura surrounding the teeth[24] **(Fig. 16)**. Loss of lamina dura once considered pathognomonic of HPT is now considered as nonspecific as it may accompany dental sepsis, fibrous dysplasia, Paget's disease, osteomalacia, and other endocrine disorders.[19,24] Subperiosteal resorption may also occur in the marginal areas of joints, particularly in the hands and feet, and may mimic erosive changes of rheumatoid arthritis or other inflammatory arthropathies. A feature to differentiate the erosions in HPT from that of rheumatoid arthritis is that they are located slightly away from the joint margin and are almost always associated with typical subperiosteal resorption of the adjacent phalangeal tufts.

Intracortical bone resorption: Intracortical bone resorption or cortical tunneling is one of the hallmarks of rapid bone turnover wherein groups of osteoclasts tunnel through the Volkman's and haversian canals.[21] This finding is also not specific for HPT and may be seen in hyperthyroidism, acromegaly, and disorders causing rapid osteoporosis. They are radiographically seen as subtle linear striations or scalloping within the cortex parallel to the long axis of the bone, best seen in the tubular bones of the hand and feet, especially in the cortex of the second metacarpal. Intracortical resorption of bone is almost always associated with subperiosteal resorption **(Fig. 17)**.

Richardson et al. quantified the degree of intracortical tunneling in the metacarpal shafts and found it to be a sensitive indicator of the extent of bone disease in HPT.[21,24,25] This method known as the "cortical striation index" requires detailed magnification radiographs.[21,24] A grading system is used to determine the degree of cortical striation present in the first and second metacarpals of each hand.

- Grade 0 Solid cortex with up to one striation
- Grade 1 Mild increase in striations
- Grade 2 Increased striations, but with involvement of <50% of the cortex
- Grade 3 Extensive striations throughout the cortex

The second and third metacarpals of each hand are graded separately. In normal individuals, the "mean cortical index" is 1 or <1. Increased striations are seen in patients with primary HPT, renal osteodystrophy, and osteomalacia. The importance of cortical striation measurement in patients with HPT is in monitoring the response to treatment.[21]

Endosteal bone resorption: It leads to cortical thinning, scalloping, and irregularity of the endosteal surface and may obscure the corticomedullary junction, especially in

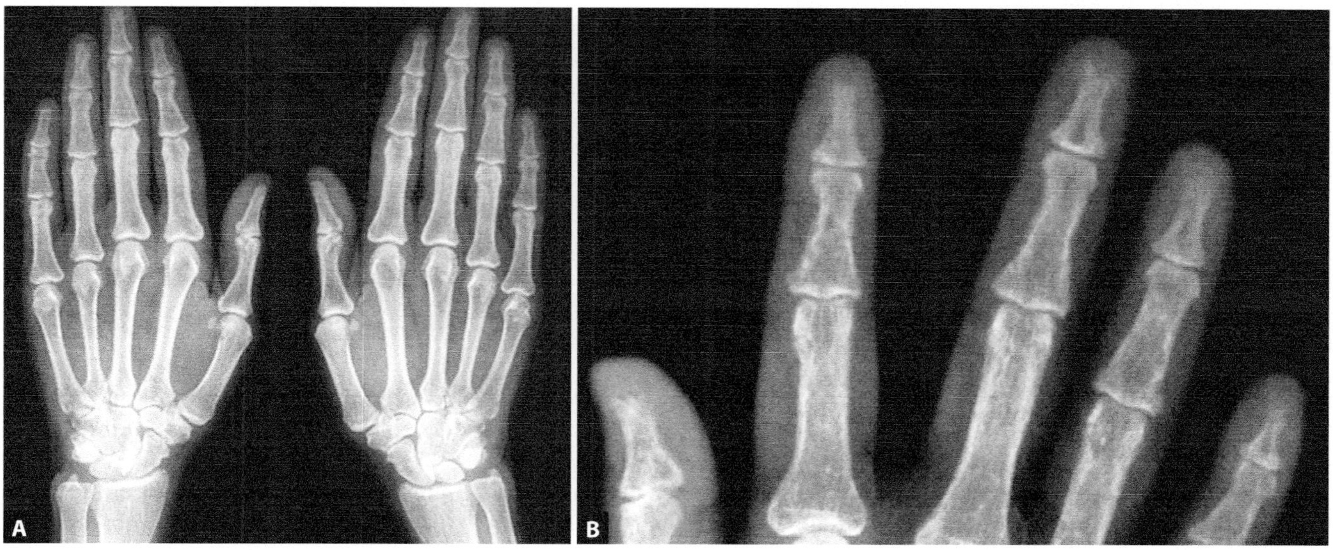

Figs. 15A and B: Hyperparathyroidism: (A) Hands showing resorption of the subperiosteal bone on the radial aspect of the middle phalanges of the index and middle fingers with magnified view; (B) Resorption of the tufts of terminal phalanges as well.

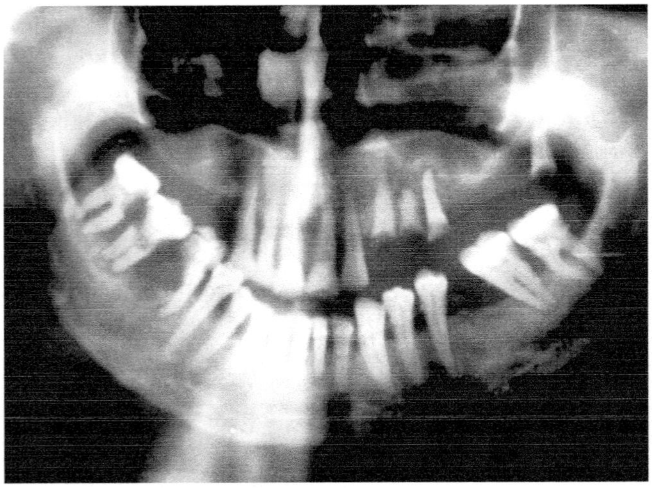

Fig. 16: Pantomogram showing extensive subperiosteal resorption with loss of lamina dura in a patient with parathyroid adenoma.

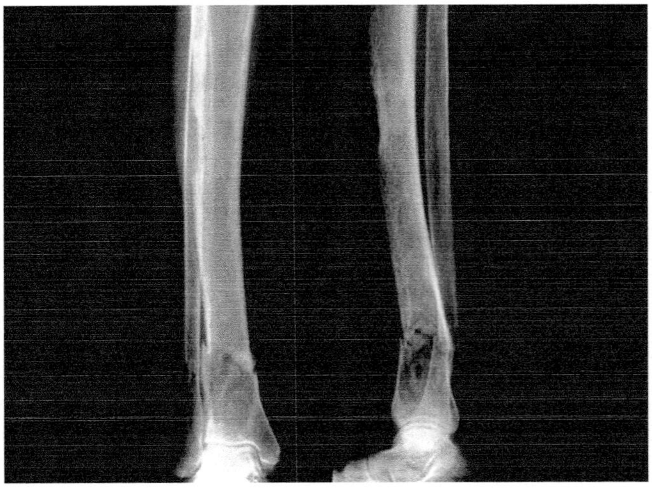

Fig. 17: Anteroposterior and lateral radiograph of leg shows resorption of anterior tibial cortex, intracortical striations, and brown tumor with pathological fractures: Hyperparathyroidism (HPT).

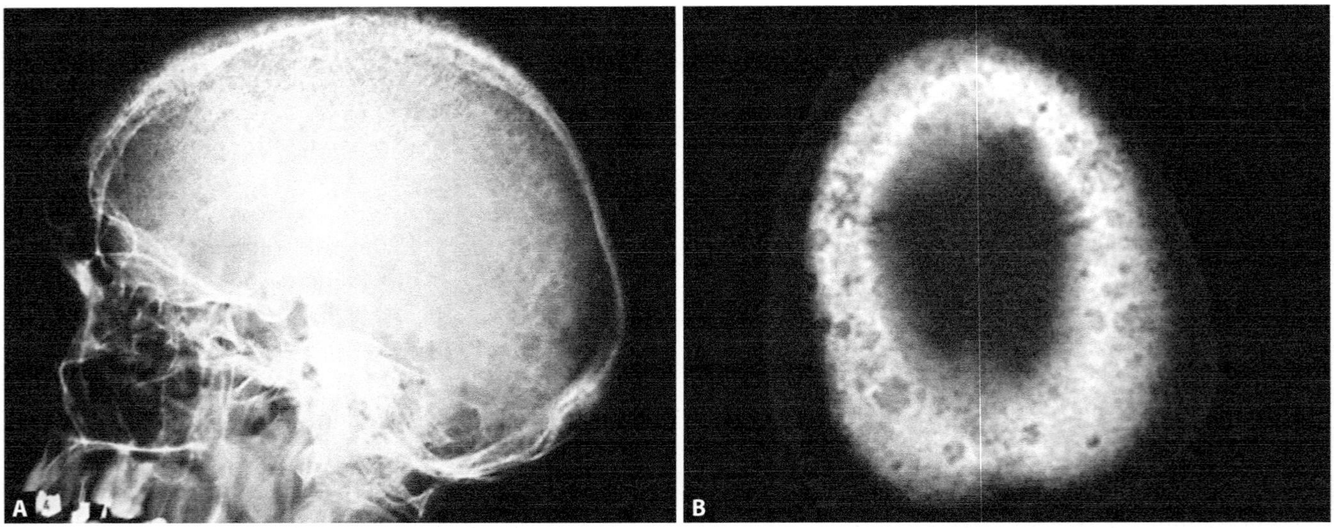

Figs. 18A and B: (A) Osteoporosis with loss of definition of inner and outer tables of the skull causing a classical mottled appearance of the skull vault: "salt and pepper skull"; (B) Computed tomography (CT) bone window reveals multiple variable-sized lytic lesions scattered throughout the calvarium with loss of differentiation of outer and inner tables.

the bones of the hand. Endosteal bone resorption may occur more commonly in conjunction with subperiosteal and intracortical resorption rather than an isolated finding.

Subchondral bone resorption: Subchondral bone resorption is a common manifestation of hyperparathyroidism, particularly in the joints of the axial skeleton, such as the sacroiliac, sternoclavicular, acromioclavicular joints, pubic symphysis, and discovertebral junctions causing surface irregularity and increase in joint space.[21,24] The changes are most severe in the distal clavicles. The peripheral joints may also show subchondral bone resorption, and these changes may mimic infective arthritis.

Subphyseal bone resorption: In children with primary or secondary HPT, irregular radiolucent areas may appear in the metaphysis adjacent to the growth plate. This finding is reminiscent of the abnormalities accompanying rickets.[23]

Subligamentous and subtendinous bone resorption: Resorption of bone occurs at sites of tendon and ligament attachment to bone. The frequently involved sites are greater and lesser trochanter, ischial, and humeral tuberosities, elbow, inferior surface of calcaneus, and inferior aspect of distal end of clavicle.

Trabecular bone resorption: Trabecular resorption occurs throughout the skeleton in HPT, especially in the advanced stages of the disease, though changes in the skull vault are characteristic.[19,21] Osteoclasts on the surface of bone dissect through the center of trabecula, with loss of sharp trabecular pattern giving a stippled, mottled, and granular appearance termed radiologically as *"salt and pepper skull"*[19,21] **(Figs. 18A and B)**. The definition of outer and inner table is lost. Focal areas of osseous thickening in the cranial vault may be observed on radiographs as well-defined or poorly defined radiopaque areas.

Brown Tumors

They are also known as *osteitis fibrosa cystica or osteoclastomas*. Brown tumors are cyst-like well-circumscribed lytic lesions within bone and are an end result of extensive bone resorption.[19] They have initially been described characteristic of primary hyperparathyroidism, but seen with increasing frequency in secondary hyperparathyroidism as well.[24] They represent hemorrhage and deposition of breakdown products of hemoglobin. Brown tumors may cause swelling, pathological fracture, and bone pain in the skeletal system. Histologically, the cavities are filled with fibrous tissue and osteoclasts with necrosis and hemorrhagic liquefaction. *Radiographically,* brown tumors are seen as lytic, expansile, and cystic lesions which are solitary but are often multiple. They appear as well-defined lesions of the axial or appendicular skeleton, and are frequently eccentric or cortical in location, can be central **(Figs. 19A and B)**. The common sites of involvement are the mandible, clavicle, ribs, pelvis, and tubular bones.[19,21,25] Other manifestations of HPT are generally present, although occasionally a brown tumor may be the only finding radiologically. With removal of the parathyroid adenoma, brown tumors may demonstrate healing with sclerosis.[21,25]

The presence of multiple osteolytic lesions in an elderly patient with complaints of bone pain is suggestive of a mitotic/metastatic etiology. However, other etiologies such as multiple myeloma or brown tumor should be considered and serum phosphate, calcium, and PTH levels and serum protein electrophoresis should also be checked.

Brown tumors with hemorrhagic or cystic component in weight-bearing bones are associated with a higher risk of pathological fracture. MR imaging can aid in determining hemorrhage and cystic component and indirectly in estimation of fracture risk.[26]

It has been seen that there is a risk of pathological fracture when the brown tumor involves more than two-thirds of the cortex of the long bone, especially in the weight-bearing area. Preventive internal fixation is indicated if the tumor involves more than two thirds of the cortex of the weight-bearing long bone.[27]

In the past, advanced cases of hyperparathyroidism presenting with severe bone resorption was not an uncommon finding. However, use of more sophisticated diagnostic techniques along with an increased awareness of this condition, have led to an earlier diagnosis, when the degree of bone resorption is somewhat limited.[17] Fine detail and magnification skeletal radiography in primary HPT will not only detect mild disease but will also reveal intracortical, endosteal, and trabecular resorption.[19]

The combined effect of all the patterns of bone resorption is generalized osteopenia in a majority of patients.[19,24] On radiographs, osteopenia is frequently a subjective finding that is difficult to interpret and is identifiable only after 30–50% of mineral content is lost. This difficulty can be overcome by using quantitative bone mineral analysis which will indicate not only the degree and rate of bone loss in the disease but also partial recovery of the loss that is seen after successful parathyroidectomy.[19]

Joint Disorders

Erosive arthropathy of the hands, wrists, and shoulders may occur in patients with HPT, simulating rheumatoid arthritis. These changes are almost always associated with typical subperiosteal resorption of the phalanges and occur on the ulnar aspect of metacarpal heads unlike rheumatoid arthritis.

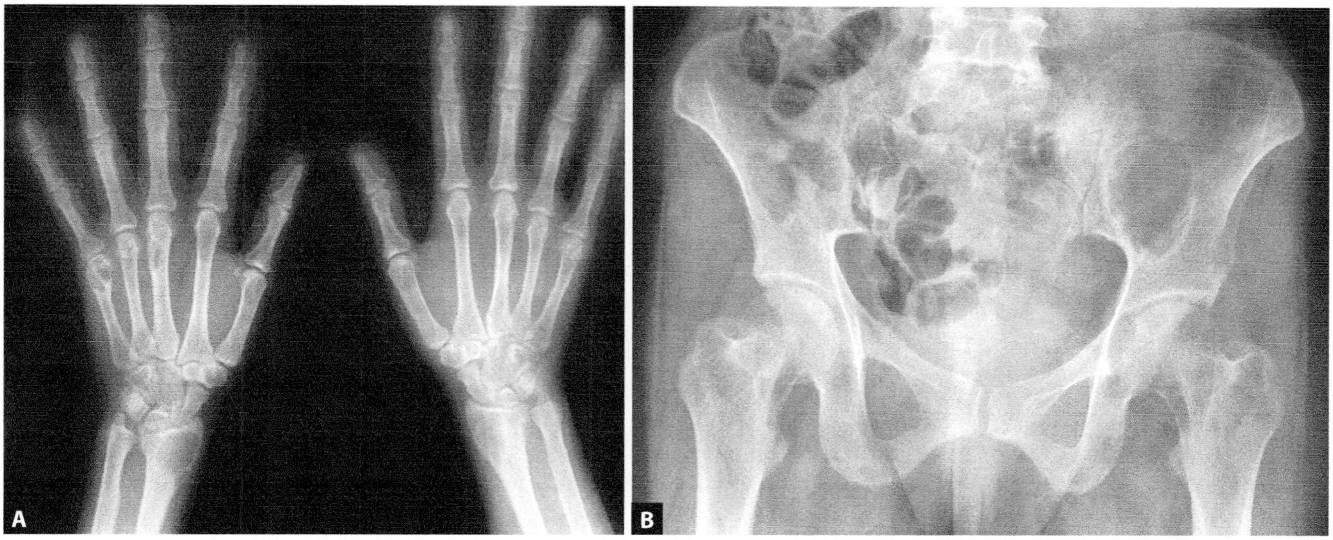

Figs. 19A and B: (A) X-ray bilateral hands in primary hyperparathyroidism (HPT) showing multiple, well-defined, expansile lytic lesions in lower end of radius, head, and distal ends of third and fifth metacarpals of right hand; (B) A large well-defined, oval lytic lesion with sclerotic rim in left iliac bone with multiple smaller ill-defined lesions in bilateral ischium: Brown tumors.

Another feature that is more common in primary hyperparathyroidism is chondrocalcinosis or calcification in hyaline cartilage or fibrocartilage. This occurs due to calcium pyrophosphate dihydrate (CPPD), calcium hydroxy apatite, or calcium oxalate crystal deposition. It may also occur in chronic renal disease, although its frequency is much lower than in primary HPT. Radiologically, chondrocalcinosis is seen in 18–40% patients with primary HPT.[19,24] Chondrocalcinosis may be seen in hyaline cartilage and fibrocartilage of the knee, symphysis pubis, and triangular cartilage of the wrist.[22] The deposition of crystals may lead to episodes of pseudogout. In contrast, soft-tissue and vascular calcification is more common in secondary HPT than in primary HPT.

Osteosclerosis

Increased bone density or osteosclerosis may be seen due to stimulation of osteoblastic activity by PTH in addition to its osteoclastic activity. The bone sclerosis can be either focal or diffuse.[24] Even though the bone shows increased density, it is structurally weak and prone to stress fractures.[30] In patients with secondary HPT, a diffuse increase in bone density is seen while in patients of primary HPT bone sclerosis is localized or patchy. Focal bone sclerosis is apparent in the metaphyseal regions of the long bones, the skull or the vertebral endplates. In the evaluation of hyperparathyroidism, one must keep in mind that osteosclerotic changes may also occur as a manifestation of healing, either spontaneous or as a result of treatment.[28]

Renal Osteodystrophy

Renal osteodystrophy is a term applied to the bone changes present in patients with chronic renal failure. In chronic renal failure, secondary HPT often coexists with rickets, osteomalacia, osteosclerosis, and osteoporosis as part of spectrum of findings called renal osteodystrophy. The skeletal changes of primary and secondary HPT are identical, except for associated changes of renal osteodystrophy seen in secondary HPT. **Table 2** highlights the features differentiating primary from secondary HPT.

Table 2: Primary versus secondary HPT.

Primary HPT	*Secondary HPT*
• Consists of skeletal features of HPT only	• Skeletal features of HPT with features of renal osteodystrophy (rickets/osteomalacia and osteosclerosis)
• Skeletal changes are less florid	• More florid
• Sclerosis rarely seen	• Commonly seen
• Brown tumors are more common	• Less common
• Chondrocalcinosis more common	• Less common
• Soft-tissue and vascular calcification are less common	• More common

The most common cause is chronic glomerulonephritis.[29] It can also result from bilateral chronic pyelonephritis, often associated with vesicoureteric reflux. In both conditions, small contracted kidneys are an evidence of the end-stage renal disease. The findings in renal osteodystrophy in children and adults are distinctive.

The most common finding in secondary HPT of renal osteodystrophy is subperiosteal resorption although other manifestations may be seen. The osseous resorption has shown to increase from 10% in the early stage of disease to 50–70% after 3–9 years of dialysis.[29] Conversely, following parathyroidectomy, bone resorption has shown to regress. Calcification of arteries, articular cartilage, and periarticular tissues also occur in renal osteodystrophy.

Osteosclerosis may occasionally be the only manifestation of renal osteodystrophy. It has a predilection for the axial skeleton **(Figs. 20A and B)**, with deposition of bone in the subchondral areas of the vertebral bodies.[30] This results in the appearance of radiodense bands across the superior and inferior vertebral margins known as "rugger jersey" spine appearance similar to stripes on an English rugby shirt. Other sites of osteosclerosis include the pelvis, ribs, and clavicles **(Fig. 21)**. It also involves the metaphysis of long bones and the skull. Post renal transplantation, the osteosclerosis may regress.[31]

Osteopenia has been reported in up to 85% of patients in renal osteodystrophy and is the end result of effect of osteomalacia, bone resorption, and a decrease in bone quantity (osteoporosis).[29]

In children, metaphyseal changes resembling rickets are seen. This together with cortical erosions can give rise to the "rotting fencepost" appearance, particularly in the femoral neck. Slipped capital epiphysis may also be seen as a complication, most commonly involving the proximal femur.

Renal Lesions

Renal tubular dysfunction results from the direct effect of parathyroid hormone on the kidney and is corrected by parathyroidectomy. Renal calculi have been reported in 50% patients. These calculi are often small and the patient often presents with a renal colic.

Nephrocalcinosis

This is less common than renal calculi. Deposition of calcium is generally in the region of the renal pyramids **(Fig. 22)**, but forms no diagnostic pattern. Uremia is a major cause of death in untreated HPT.

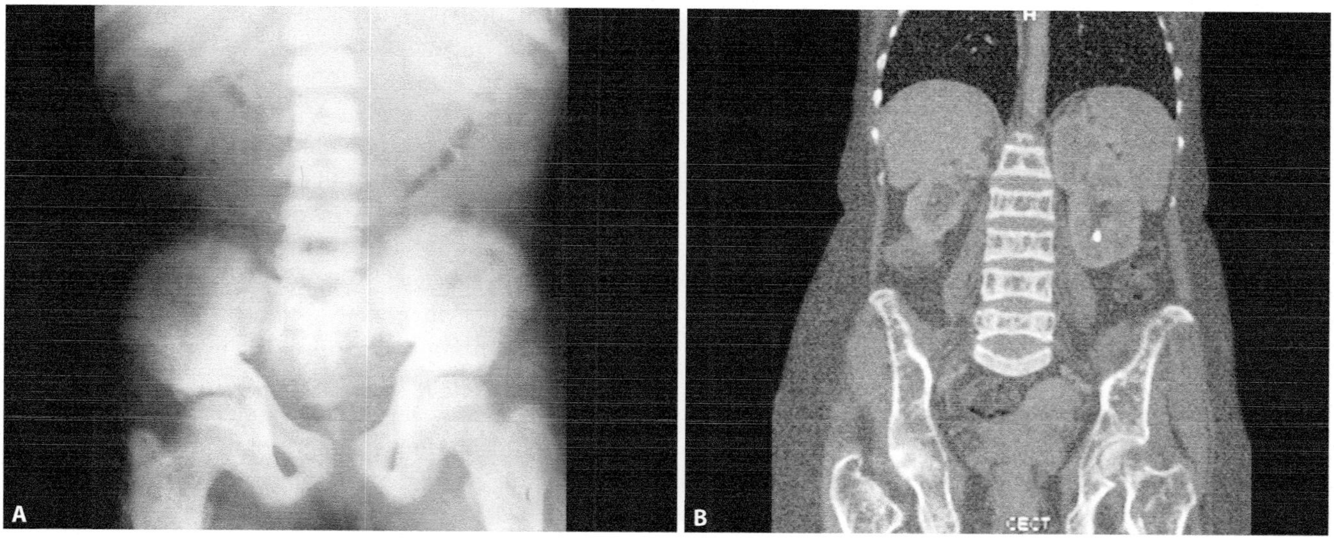

Figs. 20A and B: Renal osteodystrophy: (A) Diffuse increase in bone density of the pelvis and lumbar vertebrae with coarsened trabecular pattern; (B) Computed tomography (CT) abdomen bone window in another patient of secondary hyperparathyroidism (HPT) reveals diffuse osteopenia with coarsened trabecular pattern, loss of height of multiple lumbar vertebrae with mild sclerosis of superior and inferior end plates, patchy areas of sclerosis in the right ilium. Renal calculus noted in lower pole of the left kidney.

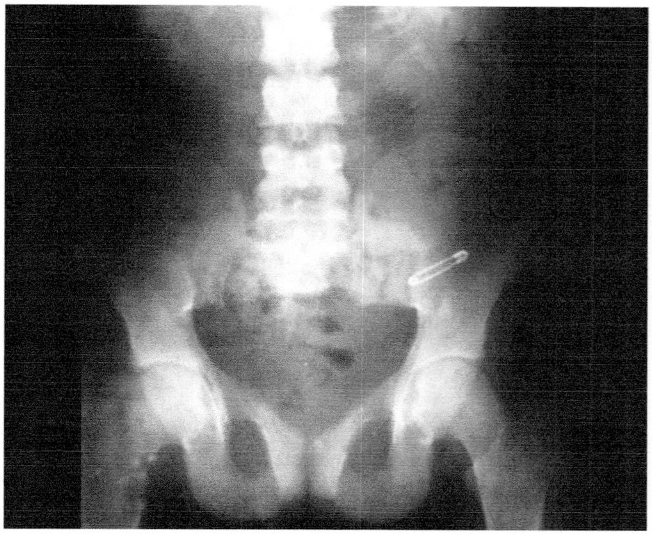

Fig. 21: Typical features of renal osteodystrophy in form of osteosclerosis of the axial skeleton with osteomalacic changes in the pelvis.

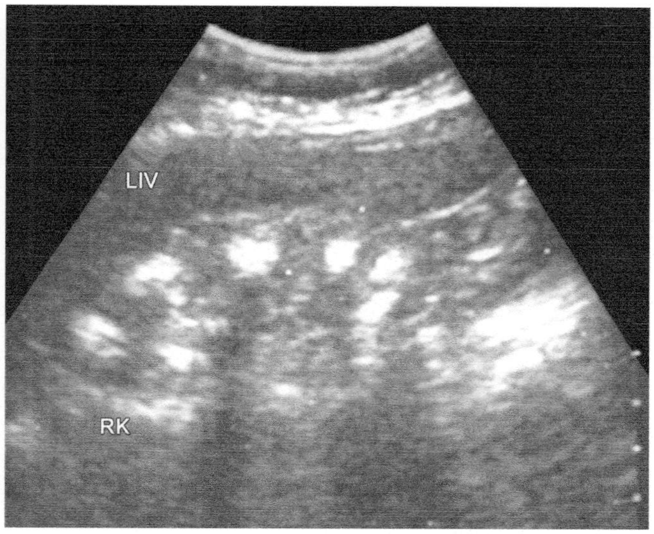

Fig. 22: Ultrasound of the right kidney (RK) shows medullary nephrocalcinosis in a patient of secondary hyperparathyroidism (HPT).

Parathyroid Localization

The standard treatment for primary hyperparathyroidism is surgical removal of the abnormal parathyroid gland or glands.[21,32] This is because untreated HPT leads to bone loss, renal calculi, and nephrocalcinosis. The presence of bone changes is an accepted indication of parathyroid surgery in primary HPT.[21]

Following parathyroidectomy, the subperiosteal resorption resolves, bone turnover decreases, and bone density improves. Patients with nephrolithiasis develop fewer newer stones and renal function improves. Patients with peptic ulcer disease improve and symptoms of depression, weakness, and fatigue often disappear.[21]

Preoperative localization of abnormal parathyroid is not routinely advocated by all surgeons due to a high success rate of 90–95% in localizing the lesion in previously unoperated patients.[32] However, imaging can assist the surgeon in preoperatively identifying a persistent or ectopic parathyroid adenoma or parathyroid hyperplasia, thereby increasing surgical success from 60–90%.[32]

Preoperative Localization Techniques

The noninvasive tests for parathyroid localization are:

- High-resolution ultrasound
- High-resolution computed tomography (HRCT)
- Magnetic resonance imaging (MRI)

- Dual isotope thallium-201 chloride-^{99m}Technetium subtraction scanning
- ^{99m}Technetium sestamibi scintigraphy
- Single-photon emission computed tomography (SPECT)
- Parathyroid digital subtraction angiography
- Selective venous sampling.

The success of all these techniques, except venous sampling depends to a varying degree on the size of the abnormal gland.

Anatomical and Pathological Considerations Important for Localization

Embryology and anatomy: In the majority of population (84%), the parathyroid glands are four in number—two superior and two inferior. The glands are symmetrical, with the superior parathyroid glands usually lying behind the superior third of the two thyroid lobes and the inferior parathyroid glands just below the inferior poles of the thyroid. About 3–5% population has five glands, and 1–3% have three glands. Supernumerary glands are seen approximately 3–5% of time.[33]

The superior parathyroid glands are derived from the fourth branchial pouch along with the lateral lobes of the thyroid. The inferior glands arise from the third branchial pouch along with thymus gland. These embryologic relationships help to explain the normal and variable anatomic location of the superior and inferior parathyroid glands. The superior parathyroid glands being closely related to the thyroid gland undergo minimal descent and their position are relatively constant.[20] More than 90% glands are located deep in relation to the mid portion of the superior pole of the thyroid near the cricothyroid junction.[33]

The incidence of ectopic parathyroid glands is 20%. Ectopic superior parathyroids may be found within the thyroid gland (1–2%), in retrotracheal or retroesophageal location (1% cases), within the carotid sheath (1% of cases) or may descend into the posterosuperior mediastinum (5% of cases). The inferior parathyroid glands along with the thymus descend a greater distance and therefore are more variable in location but most commonly are located inferior, posterior, or lateral to the lower thyroid pole (69%). Ectopic inferior parathyroid glands are more common and can lie anywhere from the angle of the mandible to the pericardium, i.e., along the path of migration of the thymus.[34] They can be found more inferiorly in the neck, in the thyrothymic ligament, in the thymic tongue, or in the cervical portion of the thymus gland (29%). Persistent hypercalcemia after parathyroid surgery can be due to mediastinal parathyroid glands in as many as one third of cases.

Surgical treatment: Definitive treatment of primary hyperparathyroidism involves the surgical excision of hyperfunctioning parathyroid glands. In the past, this was achieved with bilateral neck exploration and removal of the enlarged gland or glands. Improved presurgical imaging localization, intraoperative PTH assays, and hand-held gamma detectors have made the selective excision of hyperfunctioning parathyroid glands possible.[20]

Over the past decade, the development of minimally invasive techniques to parathyroid surgery has made accurate preoperative localization of parathyroid disease absolutely critical for effective surgical treatment.

Currently practiced minimally invasive techniques include unilateral open parathyroidectomy, video-assisted parathyroidectomy, and videoscopic parathyroidectomy. All of these techniques involve a more focused approach wherein the procedure is limited to the abnormal parathyroid gland, thereby reducing the operating time substantially.[33] The extent of minimally invasive parathyroidectomy is often guided by rapid intraoperative PTH testing. A greater than 50% drop in the serum PTH to normal or near-normal levels 10 minutes after parathyroid resection is suggestive of a single parathyroid adenoma as the cause of primary HPT.[20] Thus, the primary benefit of preoperative imaging studies is the accurate determination of uniglandular disease to help select patients most appropriate for unilateral and minimally invasive approaches.

The Guidelines for the Management of Asymptomatic Primary Hyperparathyroidism from the Fourth International Workshop were formulated in 2014. As per the committee, the following are the recommendations for surgery in asymptomatic patients with primary HPT:[35]

- Serum calcium >1 mg/dL
- Peri- or postmenopausal women and men >50 years with T score ≤ –2.5 on bone mineral density (BMD)
- Premenopausal women and men <50 years with Z score ≤ –2.5
- Creatinine clearance <60 mL/min
- If renal stones or nephrocalcinosis is present
- 24-hour urinary calcium >400 mg/dL.

Parathyroid Imaging

High-resolution sonography and ^{99m}Tc sestamibi scintigraphy are the main imaging techniques for preoperative location of parathyroid adenomas with similar sensitivities and specificities for solitary adenoma detection by these techniques.

Localization accuracy improves when both sonography and scintigraphy are obtained preoperatively. Contrast-enhanced CT and MRI can also effectively locate parathyroid adenomas but are less commonly used for preoperative location and are more commonly used in the setting of failed parathyroidectomy for the detection of suspected ectopic (mediastinal) glands.[33]

Sonographic Evaluation

Ultrasonography is the modality of choice for preoperative localization of the pathological gland in all patients of proven HPT. Transducers of 12–15 MHz are used for imaging giving a tissue resolution of 1–2 mm. Solid lesions can be differentiated from blood vessels. High-resolution sonography is an established procedure with a sensitivity of 80% and specificity of 90% in detecting cervical parathyroid adenomas.[21]

Normal parathyroid glands are 2–7 mm in length, 2–4 mm in width, and 0.5–2 mm in thickness and weigh 35–55 mg.[34] They are normally not visible on ultrasound, CT, or MRI.

Most cases of primary hyperparathyroidism are caused by a single parathyroid adenoma (90%). Hyperplasia of all four glands (6%), double adenomas (4%), and rarely parathyroid carcinoma are the other causes. Parathyroid adenomas are benign neoplasms, composed of chief cells, oncocytic cells or transitional oncocytic cells, with frequently a mixture of cell types being seen. Adenomas are considerably larger, having a mean mass of greater than 10 times the normal parathyroid gland and are thus often identified at cross-sectional imaging.[29]

At sonography, *parathyroid adenomas* are typically seen as homogeneously hypoechoic solid masses. This is due to the compact cellularity of the gland that is characteristic of adenomas at sectioning.[33] They may sometimes have a hyperechoic capsule. The echogenicity of vast majority of parathyroid adenomas is substantially less than that of thyroid tissue; normal thyroid parenchyma having a characteristic sonographic appearance of homogeneous medium to high level echoes. Around 90% of adenomas are found at the poles of the thyroid gland and are easily discernable sonographically **(Figs. 23A and B)**. Imaging of the lower poles can be enhanced by asking the patient to swallow, which momentarily raises the thyroid gland in the neck. They are usually oval or bean shaped, but larger adenomas can be multilobulated.

Parathyroid carcinomas are usually larger than adenomas, on an average measuring >2 cm as compared to 1 cm for adenomas. Carcinomas generally have a lobulated contour, heterogeneous echotexture, and cystic components. However, they may be indistinguishable from parathyroid adenomas in all imaging studies except when local invasion of neighboring structures is present.[21]

When parathyroid gland enlargement is not found in the region of the thyroid, the entire neck from mandible to suprasternal notch should be examined sonographically, including the retrotracheal region via a lateral approach.[32] However, ectopic parathyroid glands in the neck may be missed on ultrasonographic evaluation. Ultrasonography cannot be used to identify mediastinal parathyroid adenomas. Rarely, parathyroid adenomas may be intrathyroid in location. These are completely surrounded by thyroid tissue and are oriented with their greatest dimension in the cephalocaudal direction. Sonographically, they are well visualized because they are hypoechoic in contrast to the echogenic thyroid parenchyma. However, percutaneous biopsy may often be required to reliably differentiate an intrathyroid adenoma from a thyroid nodule.

Gray-scale imaging should be supplemented by color and power Doppler imaging to look for feeding vessels and vascularity of suspected adenomas seen at initial gray-scale imaging. As per literature, color and power Doppler

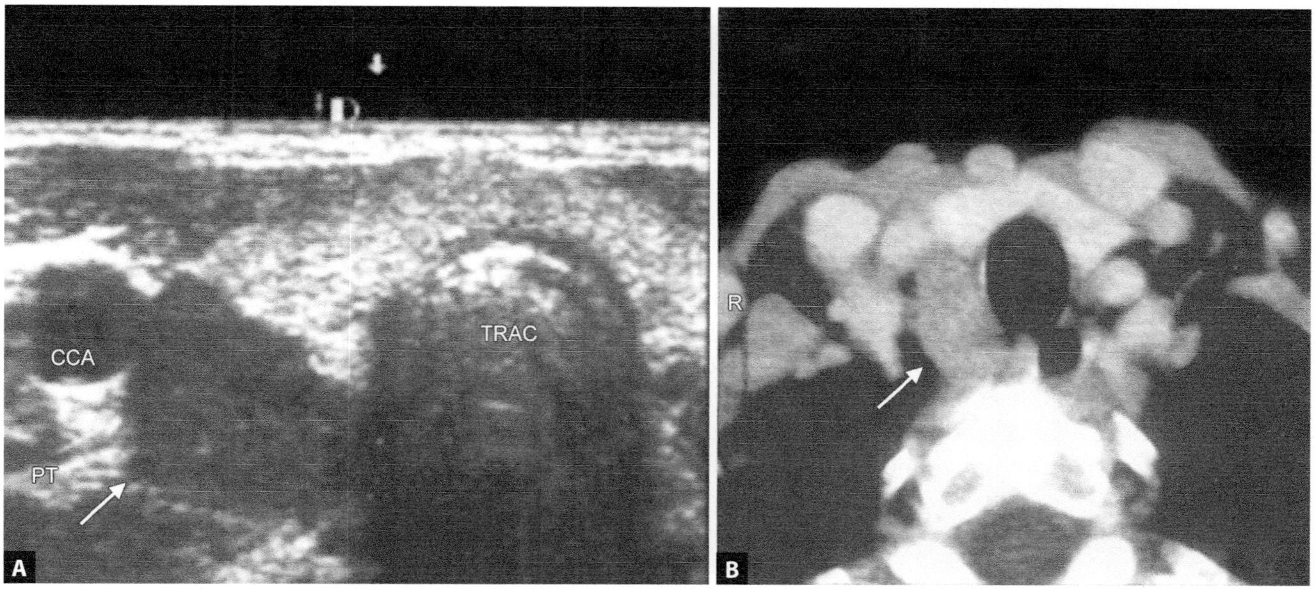

Figs. 23A and B: (A) Transverse ultrasound scan reveals a hypodense mass posteroinferior to the right lobe of thyroid (arrow) in a patient with parathyroid adenoma; (B) Contrast-enhanced computed tomography (CECT) also shows a hypodense solid mass in the same location (arrow).

imaging commonly show a characteristic extrathyroidal feeding vessel (typically a branch of the inferior thyroidal artery), which enters the parathyroid gland at one of the poles. Internal vascularity is also commonly seen in a peripheral distribution. The artery feeding the adenoma tends to branch around the periphery of the gland before penetrating deeper, resulting in a characteristic arc or rim of vascularity. In addition, color Doppler sonography of the overlying thyroid gland may show an area of asymmetric hypervascularity that may help to locate an underlying adenoma. When gray-scale and Doppler imaging fail to show an abnormal parathyroid gland, graded compression of subcutaneous tissues and strap muscles may show a relatively incompressible gland which may help differentiate an adenoma from surrounding soft tissue. This technique is often helpful in detection of ectopic glands in the lower neck.[33]

Hyperplasia is also a more difficult diagnosis to make sonographically because the single gland size is generally much smaller than an adenoma. However, similar to adenomas, compact cellularity may render hyperplastic glands hypoechoic relative to the overlying thyroid.

Pitfalls in Interpretation

Normal cervical structures such as perithyroid veins, esophagus, and Longus colli muscles of the neck can simulate parathyroid adenomas, producing false-positive results during neck sonography. Performing real-time sonography in multiple planes, color Doppler flow imaging, and use of certain maneuvers by the patient help to differentiate the above normal structures from a suspected parathyroid adenoma. Pathologic structures that are potential causes of false-positive results include thyroid nodules and cervical lymph nodes.

Several features may help in distinguishing lymph nodes from adenomas. An echogenic fatty hilum usually indicates a benign lymph node. At color Doppler examination, lymph nodes are supplied by small hilar vessels, whereas a polar, peripheral distribution of color flow is commonly seen with parathyroid adenomas.

Concomitant thyroid disease also contributes to imaging pitfalls. Enlarged multinodular thyroid gland can limit the sonographic evaluation of parathyroid adenomas. Anatomy is distorted and posterior nodules may mimic parathyroid disease. Posterior thyroid nodules can have a similar sonographic appearance to intracapsular parathyroid glands, although the typical vascular pattern of a parathyroid adenoma is uncommonly seen in thyroid nodules.[33]

Thyroid nodules more often show a heterogeneous echotexture with calcification and or cystic changes;[32] while parathyroid adenomas are of a homogeneous, hypoechoic echogenicity. A hyperechoic capsule favors a parathyroid adenoma. However, these sonographic features are inconsistent and it may not be always possible to differentiate abnormal parathyroid glands from lymphadenopathy and thyroid masses.

Percutaneous Aspiration/Biopsy

Fine-needle aspiration cytology (FNAC) of the parathyroid masses has increased the specificity of sonography by reliably differentiating parathyroid pathology from thyroid nodule and cervical lymph nodes. In addition to the cytologic or histologic analysis of the specimen, the aspiration can be diluted with 1 mL of saline and analyzed for parathyroid hormone (PTH) by radioimmunoassay.[21]

Although PTH aspiration is rarely necessary for routine cases, this procedure can be particularly helpful in cases in which prior thyroid or parathyroid surgery has distorted neck anatomy or when preoperative confirmation of unusual-appearing or ectopic glands is needed. A theoretic complication of the procedure is seeding of abnormal parathyroid tissue along the biopsy track resulting in an entity known as parathyromatosis. This has been described in cases of recurrent hyperparathyroidism after parathyroidectomy in which the capsule of the parathyroid gland was disrupted during the procedure.

Although it is primarily used as a therapy to treat tertiary hyperparathyroidism (most often in the setting of renal failure), sonographically guided parathyroid ablation with ethanol is a potential treatment option for patients with primary hyperparathyroidism. The procedure involves placement of the needle in the parathyroid gland and slowly injecting a volume of ethanol equal to approximately 50% of the volume of the gland until the absence of blood flow to the gland is confirmed on color Doppler sonography.[33]

Contrast-enhanced Computed Tomography

Contrast-enhanced computed tomography (CECT) has a sensitivity of up to 87% in detecting parathyroid adenoma. It is superior to sonography in patients with failed parathyroidectomy, in cases of altered anatomy and in delineating ectopic mediastinal parathyroid masses, thereby aiding in operative planning. Computed tomography has the advantage of larger field of view and ability to image all areas of neck and mediastinum. Spiral CT has enabled excellent visualization of neck vasculature and their separation from other neck structures[21] **(Figs. 24A and B)**.

Four-dimensional Computed Tomography

Four-dimensional computed tomography (4D CT) of the parathyroid is a technique for preoperative localization of parathyroid adenomas which was introduced as an alternative to conventional CT by Rodgers et al. in 2006. The technique consists of CT performed in multiple

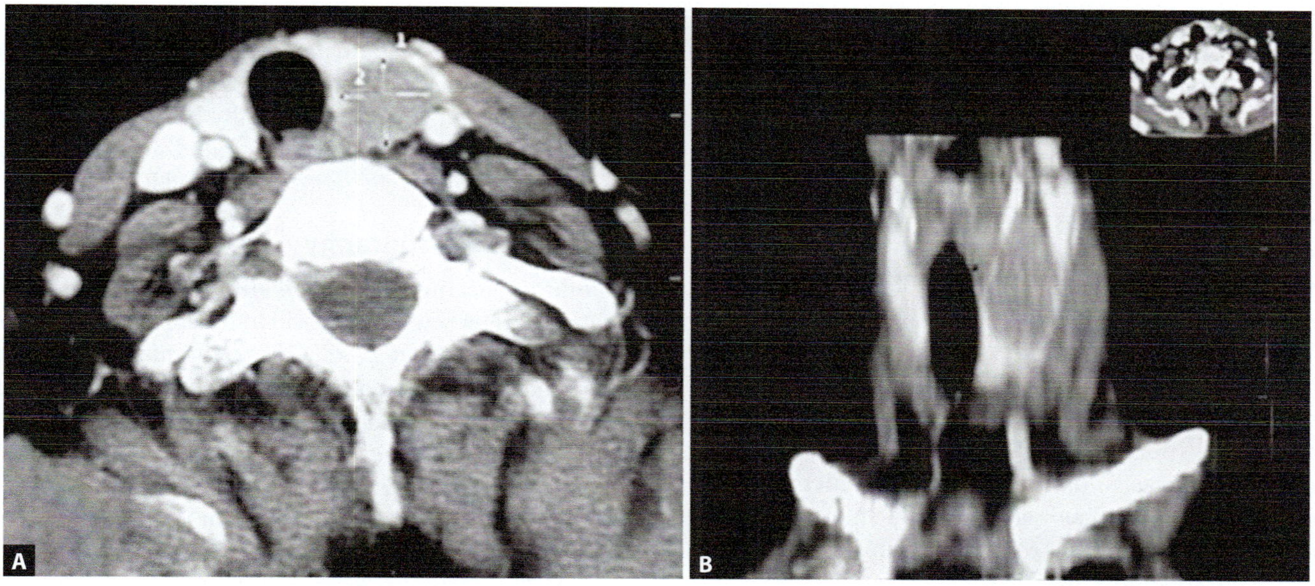

Figs. 24A and B: Axial computed tomography (CT) section (A) and coronal reconstruction (B) showing a solid mass posterior to the left lobe of thyroid extending to the inferior part of neck in a patient of multiple parathyroid adenomas.

Table 3: Phases of 4D CT protocol.

Number of phases	*Phase of CT*	*Region scanned*	*Scan timing after start of contrast injection*
First phase	NCCT	From hyoid bone to clavicular head (to cover thyroid gland)	-
Second phase	Arterial phase	From angle of mandible to carina (so that ectopic parathyroid is not missed)	25 seconds
Third phase	Delayed (venous phase)		80 seconds

(NCCT: noncontrast computed tomography)

phases and reformatted images in three planes, i.e., axial acquisition with coronal and sagittal reformations combined. The "fourth dimension" of 4D CT consists of change in contrast enhancement over time.[36] Thus, it provides both functional and anatomic information enabling localization of eutopic and ectopic parathyroid adenomas and can also depict multiglandular disease which may be missed on other imaging modalities.[37]

The protocol for 4D CT involves a noncontrast multiple detector computed tomography (MDCT) of the neck followed by two or more contrast-enhanced phases. The multiple phases are performed to determine the pattern of enhancement as this is one of the main features which enables identification of a parathyroid adenoma and its differentiation from thyroid nodules and lymph nodes which it can mimic.[38]

The first phase is a nonenhanced scan acquired with a smaller z-axis that only covers the thyroid glands so as to reduce the radiation exposure. Two contrast-enhanced phases are then acquired from the angle of mandible to the carina after intravenous administration of 75 mL of nonionic contrast (300 mg of iodine per mL) followed by a 25 mL-saline chase.

Table 3 depicts the various phases of 4D CT protocol described by Hoang et al.

On the noncontrast phase, a parathyroid adenoma appears as a lesion with lower attenuation than the thyroid gland. On arterial phase, the characteristic enhancement pattern is avid enhancement with peak enhancement greater than that of the thyroid and a washout of contrast in the delayed phase.

The peak enhancement has been described between 25 and 60 seconds after contrast injection, ranging from 138 to 180 HU, while lymph nodes show a peak enhancement at 90 seconds corresponding to the delayed phase.

The morphologic features of a parathyroid adenoma should also be evaluated on CT. It appears as an oval or rounded soft-tissue lesion with smooth or slightly lobulated margins in the typical locations around the thyroid gland. When large, an adenoma can have a low attenuation component due to either cystic degeneration, fibrosis, or hemorrhage.

The vascular imaging features on 4D CT have been described as the "polar vessel sign" depicted on the arterial phase. It consists of a feeding artery which is usually a branch of the inferior thyroid artery and typically enters the parathyroid gland at the upper or lower pole. On a 4D CT scan, the "polar vessel sign" may be seen in around 63% of adenomas.

The 4D CT has shown to be useful in many clinical situations such as:

- In patients with previous neck surgery
- Mild hyperparathyroidism
- Multigland disease
- Patients in whom sestamibi and USG examinations are negative.

Studies have compared 4D CT with sestamibi and ultrasound in recent years and have found 4D CT to be superior to both in accurately lateralizing the parathyroid adenoma, thereby allowing the surgeon to perform minimally invasive parathyroidectomy. Such a directed surgical approach has been adopted since the last two decades because of improved preoperative imaging and use of intraoperative parathyroid hormone assay.[39]

An intraoperative parathyroid hormone (IOPTH) measurement is used to confirm the complete resections of abnormally secreting parathyroid tissue. When IOPTH decreases >50% within 10 minutes of resection, it confirms the removal of hyperfunctioning parathyroid tissue.[40]

There is considerable radiation exposure to the patient due to the multiple phases of 4D CT. Reported effective doses for 4D CT is 10.4 mSv compared to 7.8 mSv for nuclear scintigraphy. However, the radiation organ dose to the thyroid has been found to be >50 times higher with 4D CT. Hence, 4D CT should be used with caution, especially in young patients and the benefit of detecting an adenoma and curing the patient following resection as well as the advantage of minimally invasive surgery over bilateral neck exploration along with radiation risk should be considered.[36]

Magnetic Resonance Imaging

Magnetic resonance imaging is less commonly used for preoperative localization than sonography and scintigraphy though it has similar sensitivity to other techniques in the detection of abnormal parathyroid tissue. MRI is the accepted modality for localizing parathyroid lesion in persistent or recurrent hyperparathyroidism, despite previous parathyroidectomies with a sensitivity of 88%.[34] MRI has an equally high sensitivity when the gland is in the mediastinum.[34]

On MR scans, parathyroid adenomas are soft-tissue masses that are of low-to-medium signal intensity on T1-weighted images, are medium-to-high signal intensity on T2-weighted images, and show moderate enhancement on gadolinium-enhanced images. Approximately 10–35% of enlarged glands do not have high-signal intensity on T2-weighted images. This may be due to fat content, hemorrhage, or fibrosis. The size of the gland is the most important factor affecting detection on MRI.[34]

The typical signal intensities of abnormal parathyroid gland on T1-weighted and T2-weighted images may not be distinguishable from lymph nodes. This differentiation is more often based on topography and shape of the structures. A location medial to the carotid sheath is mostly due to parathyroid while nodes are located laterally.[21]

Parathyroid Scintigraphy

Nuclear medicine computer subtraction images of thallium and technetium can aid in the localization of the abnormal parathyroid gland. This technique relies on the differential uptake of the two isotopes by the thyroid and parathyroid glands. Thallium-201 chloride accumulates in tissues with high blood flow which includes both thyroid and parathyroid glands as well as in thyroid nodules and parathyroid adenomas. ^{99m}Technetium accumulates only in the thyroid. Digital images are produced with each isotope. The technetium scan is then subtracted from the thallium leaving an image of only the parathyroid concentration of thallium.

The primary disadvantage of nuclear medicine techniques is limited spatial resolution. The maximum resolution of thallium-technetium scanning is 7–8 mm and it is very difficult to detect glands weighing <500 mg with this technique.[32]

The *radiopharmaceutical of choice* for imaging parathyroid enlargement is *^{99m}Tc sestamibi*. ^{99m}Tc sestamibi has replaced ^{201}Tl for parathyroid scintigraphy because of superior image quality, more favorable dosimetry, and improved detection sensitivity with its use. Three general techniques of radionuclide scintigraphy are commonly used for the detection and visualization of hyperfunctioning parathyroid glands: Single-phase dual isotope subtraction imaging, dual-phase single-isotope imaging, and a combination of the two. In *dual-isotope subtraction imaging technique*, one radiopharmaceutical (^{99m}Tc sestamibi) is used for visualization of the hyperfunctioning parathyroid gland and the thyroid gland, and a second (^{123}I or ^{99m}Tc pertechnetate) is used for visualization of the thyroid gland only. The second set of images is then digitally subtracted from the first set. Evidence of residual radioactivity on the subtraction image represents a hyperfunctioning parathyroid gland **(Fig. 25)**. Disadvantages of this subtraction method include the necessity of two radionuclide injections and of a cooperative and immobile patient, identically positioned for the two studies. In addition, there is an increased likelihood of artifacts on images obtained with digital subtraction. Dual agent studies with ^{99m}Tc sestamibi and iodine 123 or ^{99m}Tc pertechnetate subtraction have produced a sensitivity of 95 percent for adenomas and 64–80% for hyperplastic glands.[32] The *single-isotope dual-phase imaging technique* was proposed on the basis of the frequently observed difference between the rate

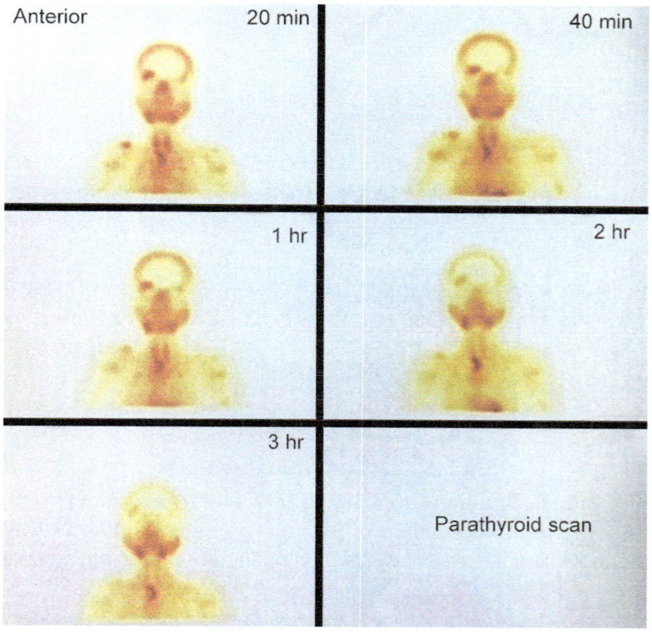

Fig. 25: Sestamibi scan: There is evidence of increased uptake of 99-Tc-Sestamibi in the region of right parathyroid gland which persists on delayed phase image (3 hours). Increased uptake is also seen in the region of right orbit due to a brown tumor.

of ^{99m}Tc sestamibi washout from the thyroid gland and the rate of washout from hyperfunctioning parathyroid glands, which is typically slower. This technique requires a single injection of ^{99m}Tc sestamibi, followed by imaging at approximately 10–15 minutes and 1.5–3 hours after the injection. Increased mitochondrial content in parathyroid adenomas is believed to be responsible for the observed sestamibi concentration. Due to the high sensitivity of sestamibi scintigraphy (82–100%), it is generally considered the standard initial imaging modality to detect a parathyroid adenoma.

Single-photon Emission Computed Tomography

Single-photon emission computed tomography is a technique whereby images of diseased glands which have absorbed a radioactive marker can be obtained. It increases the sensitivity and specificity by 2–3% over routine sestamibi scanning. SPECT can be performed anytime within the first several hours after a patient is injected with sestamibi. SPECT is used with increasing frequency as it provides three-dimensional information (lateral, superoinferior and anteroposterior). The major reason for the superiority of SPECT is the improved contrast resolution (target to background). The fusion of CT images with SPECT images, either by using software or by performing the studies sequentially on hybrid SPECT/CT imaging systems, has the advantage of combining the physiologic three-dimensional information from SPECT and anatomic information from CT. The most important use for SPECT scanning is when ordinary sestamibi scans are inconclusive or when a more detailed anatomic localization is required such as when patients are being reoperated.[21]

HYPOPARATHYROIDISM

The most common cause of hypoparathyroidism is excision or trauma to the parathyroid glands during thyroid surgery.[19] It can also occur as idiopathic hypoparathyroidism in which the parathyroid glands are absent or atrophied.

It usually occurs in childhood with girls being affected more commonly than boys. The disorder may be characterized by the presence of circulating antibodies to the parathyroid, adrenal, and thyroid glands supporting the concept that idiopathic hypoparathyroidism may be part of a generalized autoimmune disease.

Rare forms of hypoparathyroidism are seen after radiation damage to the gland and as a response of an infant to hyperparathyroidism in the mother owing to transplacental transport of calcium with suppression of fetal parathyroid activity.

Clinical Presentation

Patients with hypoparathyroidism usually present with neuromuscular dysfunction precipitated by hypocalcemia.[16] Premature closure of the growth plate may lead to short stature. Dental abnormalities may occur in the form of delay or failure of tooth eruption.

Biochemical Findings

Laboratory findings in hypoparathyroidism consist of decreased serum levels of parathyroid hormone (PTH) and calcium with elevated phosphate levels.

Radiological Findings

- The most common finding in hypoparathyroidism is bony sclerosis, which may be focal or generalized.[16,19] Localized osteosclerosis is more common, reported in 23% of patients while generalized osteosclerosis is seen in 9%.[23] Bones involved more commonly are pelvis, proximal femur, and vertebral bodies.
- Other findings include calvarial thickening and hypoplastic dentition.
- Band-like areas of increased radiodensity in the metaphysis of long bones may also be seen in hypoparathyroidism.
- The abnormalities in the spine resemble those of diffuse idiopathic skeletal hyperostosis (DISH) including calcification and ossification of the anterior longitudinal ligament and spinal osteophytes. The sacroiliac joints are generally spared. This feature

along with lack of erosive arthropathy differentiates it from ankylosing spondylitis.
- Subcutaneous calcification may be seen around the hip and shoulder joints.
- Calcium deposition in the basal ganglia is a characteristic finding and occasionally also seen in the cerebrum and cerebellum. It is also a feature of pseudohypoparathyroidism. It is also seen in infectious disorders such as toxoplasmosis and cytomegalic inclusion disease, in Fahr's syndrome (ferrocalcinosis), after radiation therapy and exposure to toxic substances such as carbon monoxide.[23]

PSEUDOHYPOPARATHYROIDISM

Pseudohypoparathyroidism (PHP) is an inherited disorder that manifests as end-organ resistance to parathyroid hormone rather than from deficient secretion of the hormone. This may be due to a defect in the adenyl-cyclase-cyclic AMP system in the renal tubules and bones. It is transmitted as an autosomal dominant trait and shares many features with hypoparathyroidism.

Clinical Findings

The patients are usually short, obese, mentally retarded, and may have brachydactyly.[16,19]

Pseudohypoparathyroidism is more frequent in women than men and is usually diagnosed in the second decade of life.

Biochemical Findings

Hypocalcemia and hyperphosphatemia are seen similar to that in hypoparathyroidism. However, the levels of serum parathyroid hormone (PTH) are elevated.

Radiological Findings

- The best known sign of PHP is *shortening of the fourth metacarpal*. Although not specific for PHP as it is also seen in pseudopseudohypoparathyroidism (PPHP), this is a characteristic finding **(Fig. 26)**.
  - The metacarpal sign has been used to determine whether this shortening is present. To use the sign, a line is drawn tangential to the heads of the fourth and fifth metacarpals. Normally the line does not intersect the third metacarpal bone or just contacts its distal aspect. The sign is considered positive if the line intersects the third metacarpal, indicating disproportionate shortening of the fourth and fifth metacarpal bone. Other congenital conditions with positive metacarpal sign are basal cell nevus syndrome, multiple epiphyseal dysplasia, Beckwith-Wiedemann syndrome as well as acquired conditions such as juvenile chronic arthritis, sickle cell anemia with infarction, trauma, and neonatal hyperthyroidism. This sign may be unreliable in diagnosing PHP and PPHP as the third metacarpal may also be short in these conditions.[23]
  - Other radiological findings in PHP are similar to those of hypoparathyroidism and consist of bony sclerosis, soft-tissue calcification, dense metaphyseal bands, calvarial thickening, and basal ganglia calcification. Basal ganglia calcification is more common than in idiopathic hypoparathyroidism **(Fig. 27)**.[29]
- *Soft-tissue calcification and ossification.* This occurs in approximately 55% of patients with PHP and is seen commonly in the hands and feet. The calcifications may be present at birth and are superficial in location and usually periarticular in distribution.

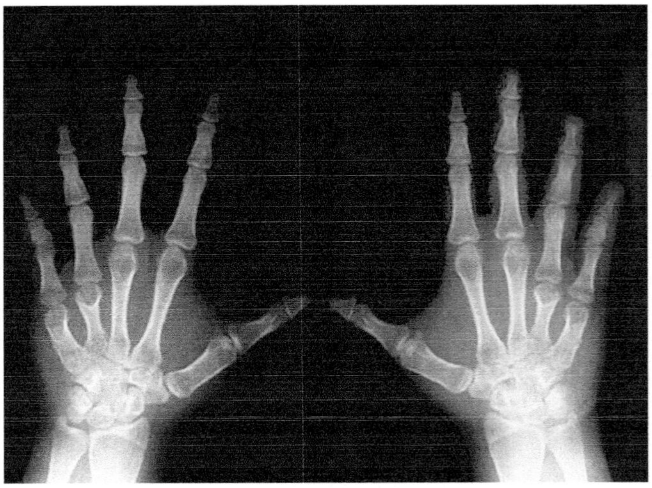

Fig. 26: Shortening of fourth and fifth metacarpal bones seen in both hands in a patient of pseudohypoparathyroidism (PHP) along with shortening of the middle phalanges of the fifth fingers.

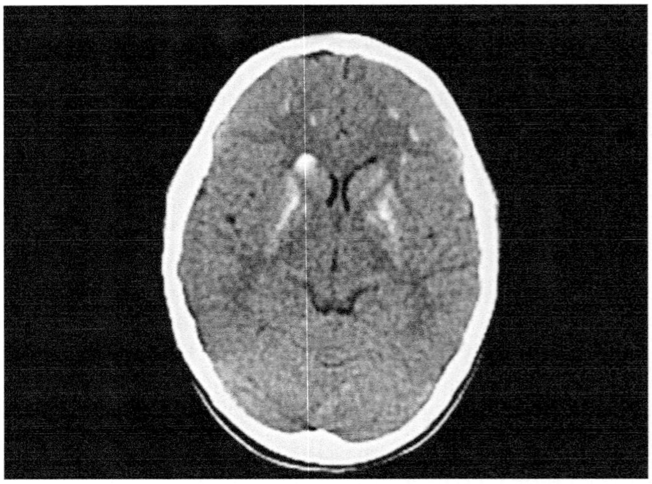

Fig. 27: Pseudohypoparathyroidism (PHP): Axial computed tomography (CT) section of the cranium reveals calcification in bilateral basal ganglia and frontal lobes in a 13-year-old child.

- Radiographic findings of secondary hyperparathyroidism may be seen in some patients with PHP.
- In addition to short metacarpals, metatarsals; phalanges may be short and exostoses and cone shaped epiphysis may be seen. The exostoses are frequently located centrally and project at right angles to the bone and differ from the appearance of multiple hereditary exostoses in which the outgrowths are usually directed away from joints.
- Growth deformities in the form of bowing of long bones may be seen.

PSEUDOPSEUDOHYPOPARATHYROIDISM

This is the result of incomplete genetic manifestation of PHP and like PHP is caused by an end-organ resistance to parathyroid hormone. PHP and PPHP share most of their clinical and radiological features. The main difference between the two is that patients with PPHP are normocalcemic.

Radiographic abnormalities of the hand in PHP and PPHP are almost identical, except for a relatively higher rate of occurrence of short distal phalanges in PHP and relatively shorter metacarpals in PPHP.[19]

The differential diagnosis of short fourth metacarpal includes Turner's syndrome and physeal trauma. Other radiologic features of PHP may resemble fibrodysplasia ossificans progressiva or multiple hereditary exostoses syndrome.

DISORDERS OF ENDOCRINE ORIGIN

Normal skeletal maturation requires the presence of certain hormones in addition to vitamin D and other metabolites. The principal endocrine glands that influence this process are pituitary, thyroid, adrenals and gonads. Deficient production of hormones from any of these glands may disturb normal skeletal maturation and ossification (**Table 4** lists the normal reference values).

The various skeletal disorders of endocrine origin may be grouped as:

- *Disorders due to excessive corticosteroids*:
  - Hypercortisolism
- *Growth hormone disorders*:
  - Acromegaly
  - Gigantism
- *Thyroid disorders*:
  - Hypothyroidism
  - Hyperthyroidism
- *Gonadal disorders*:
  - Hypogonadism
  - Hypergonadism.

Table 4: Endocrine profile–reference value.

• Serum cortisol	Fasting: 8 am–12 noon: 5–25 g/dL; 12 noon–8 pm: 5–15 g/dL; 8 pm–8 am: 0–10 g/dL
• Serum ACTH	6–76 pg/mL
• Serum TSH	0.34–4.25 µIU/mL
• Free T3	2.4–4.2 pg/mL
• Total T4	5.4–11.7 µg/dL
• Serum growth hormone	0.5–17 ng/mL
• Serum LH:	
– Follicular phase	2–15 IU/L
– Ovulatory phase	22–105 IU/L
– Luteal phase	0.6–19 IU/L
• Serum FSH:	
– Follicular phase	3–20 IU/L
– Ovulatory phase	9–26 IU/L
– Luteal phase	1–12 IU/L
• Serum free testosterone:	
– Male	47–244 pg/mL
– Female	0.6–6.8 pg/mL
• Serum calcitonin (male/female)	3–26 pg/mL; 2–17 pg/mL

(ACTH: adrenocorticotropic hormone; FSH: follicle-stimulating hormone; TSH: thyroid-stimulating hormone; T3: triiodothyronine; T4: thyroxine)

HYPERCORTISOLISM

Hypercortisolism or *Cushing's syndrome* is the clinical manifestation of exposure to excessive amounts of cortisol-like corticosteroids (glucocorticoid). It is caused by a tumor of the adrenal glands (adenoma and carcinoma), ectopic ACTH production by a tumor (bronchial carcinoma), or iatrogenically by treatment with glucocorticoids. Cushing's disease caused by a basophil pituitary adenoma is an uncommon cause of hypercortisolism. Hypercortisolism is most frequently the result of excessive administration of exogenous corticosteroids.[41]

The effects of glucocorticoids on the skeleton are numerous and complex and consist of inhibition of bone formation, stimulation of bone resorption by osteoclast, decrease in intestinal absorption and increase in renal excretion of calcium, and decrease in synthesis of collagen. The net result of hypercortisolism on the musculoskeletal system is osteoporosis, osteonecrosis, and muscle wasting.[41]

Radiological Findings

- Generalized loss of bone density (osteoporosis) occurs which is more prominent in the spine, pelvis, ribs, and cranial vault as trabecular bone is affected more severely than cortical bone.

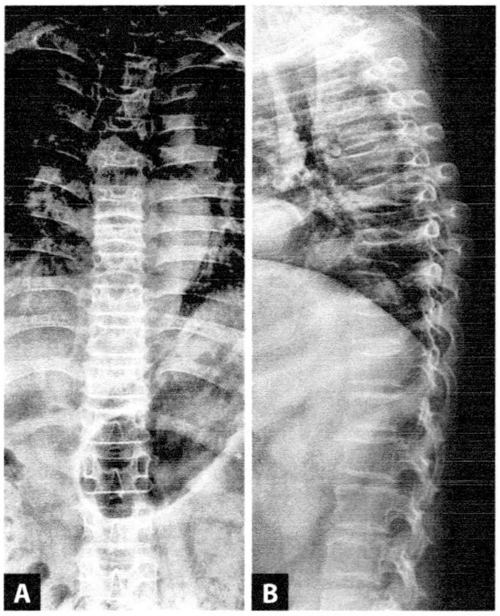

Figs. 28A and B: Cushing's syndrome due to increased adrenocorticotropic (ACTH) production in a 16-year-old. X-ray dorsolumbar spine [anteroposterior (AP)] and (lateral) views reveal reduced height of vertebral bodies with endplate sclerosis and osteoporosis.

- There is accentuation of primary trabeculae, with central endplate depressions in the vertebral bodies giving them a biconcave fish-like appearance.
- Increased radiodensity of the superior and inferior margins of compressed or collapsed vertebral bodies is a characteristic feature due to exuberant callus formation called marginal condensation, resulting, from combination of insufficiency compressive microfractures and subsequent healing **(Figs. 28A and B)**. Exuberant callus may also be seen at fracture sites in long bones and ribs. Although the vertebral end-plate sclerosis with osteoporosis is typical of hypercortisolism, in most cases it may be indistinguishable from generalized osteoporosis resulting from other causes such as hyperthyroidism, hyperparathyroidism, acromegaly, and hypogonadism.
- Local regions of osteonecrosis may be seen especially after treatment with exogenous corticosteroid. The typical sites of avascular necrosis are femoral and humeral heads which may be involved months or years after the corticosteroid treatment has begun or end.
- Hypercortisolism during skeletal immaturity suppresses growth, resulting in a short child with osteoporosis, truncal obesity, and delayed bone age. Osteonecrosis at growing epiphyses may lead to abnormal development at the ends of bone and eventually result in early development of degenerative osteoarthropathy.

HYPOPITUITARISM

This is due to deficiency of anterior pituitary hormones, particularly growth hormone resulting from damage to the pituitary gland by neoplasms, infections, vascular insults or post-therapeutic ablations. If the deficiency in growth hormone occurs in combination with deficiencies in other pituitary hormones, it is called panhypopituitarism.[41]

Radiological Findings

- There is delay in skeletal maturation manifested radiologically by a delay in appearance and closure of epiphysis.
- Skeletal growth is retarded.
- There is overall loss of bone density due to decreased bone formation.

HYPOTHYROIDISM

Deficiency of thyroid hormones (T3 and T4) produces a spectrum of musculoskeletal abnormalities termed "cretinism" in infants, "juvenile myxedema" in children, and "myxedema" or "hypothyroidism" in adults.[22] The deficiency may result from disorders that affect the thyroid gland (primary hypothyroidism) or from a deficiency of thyroid stimulating hormone (secondary hypothyroidism). Primary hypothyroidism occurs as a result of thyroiditis, neoplastic disorders, thyroid ablation, or disturbances in iodine metabolism.

Clinical Findings

Clinical manifestations of hypothyroidism vary according to the age of the patient at the time of presentation.[16] In infants, there is mental retardation and developmental abnormalities as thyroid hormone is essential for postnatal growth. In children, mental retardation, obesity, developmental delay, growth retardation, lethargy, and constipation may be seen. The clinical presentation in adults includes fatigue, lethargy, paresthesias, dry coarse skin and hair, constipation, and bradycardia.

Radiological Findings

The radiologic findings also depend on the patient's age at presentation.

Congenital hypothyroidism is characterized by delayed skeletal maturation with bone age lagging behind the chronological age. This is evident by short stature and the late appearance of epiphyseal ossification centers. Bone age can be assessed by getting a plain radiograph of the knee.[41] Normally, the distal femoral epiphysis is usually ossified at 36 weeks' gestational age and the proximal tibial epiphysis at 38 weeks' gestational age. Decreased size or absence of distal femoral or proximal tibial epiphyses is a marker for intrauterine hypothyroidism. When they appear, the ossification centers are deformed and irregularly shaped (*epiphyseal dysgenesis*). These changes are bilateral and symmetrical. Such changes in the hip must be differentiated from bilateral Perthes disease and multiple epiphyseal dysplasia. There is also delayed closure of the epiphyseal plates in hypothyroidism.

In the *skull,* the sutures may remain open and show the formation of intrasutural (Wormian) bones. The sella is either small and bowl shaped in young children or large, rounded in older children. The paranasal sinus are underdeveloped.

In the *spine,* anteriorly wedged bullet-shaped vertebral bodies are seen, especially at the thoracolumbar junction, where kyphosis may develop.

In the *pelvis,* the incidence of slipped capital femoral epiphysis is increased. The pelvis is often narrow with coxa vara deformities.

In adult or acquired hypothyroidism, skeletal manifestations are usually mild compared to severe skeletal abnormalities in congenital hypothyroidism. Generalized osteoporosis is the most common finding.

HYPERTHYROIDISM

Hyperfunction of the thyroid gland usually occurs as a result of Graves' disease (toxic diffuse goiter) or toxic multinodular goiter.[22] Excessive production of thyroid hormones, both triiodothyronine (T3) and thyroxine (T4) by the overactive gland cause a hypermetabolic state. This results in increase in both formation and resorption, with bone resorption being dominant.[16] Catabolism of protein and loss of connective tissue manifests as muscle wasting.

Hyperthyroidism in children causes accelerated skeletal maturation and advanced bone age. In adults, it causes generalized osteoporosis leading to vertebral fractures and kyphosis.

Clinical Findings

Patients may present with weakness, fatigue, nervousness, weight loss, tachycardia, palpitations, diarrhea, or intolerance to heat.[16] Myopathy is a common clinical feature of hyperthyroidism whose symptoms may mimic that of arthritis. Muscle wasting is also known to occur, especially in the proximal muscle groups.[41]

Biochemical Findings

Biochemical findings show elevated levels of calcium, phosphorus and alkaline phosphatase and elevated urinary calcium.

Radiological Findings

Skeletal finding in hyperthyroidism are more common in men and patients with radiologic abnormalities have had the disease for at least 5 years.

- *Osteoporosis* is the most common radiological finding particularly in the spine, pelvis, skull, hands, and feet. Older patients show rapidly progressive generalized osteoporosis. It has been seen that the progression of thyrotoxic osteoporosis is much more rapid than postmenopausal osteoporosis,[41] even though the two are radiologically indistinguishable. An overall decrease in bone density is seen as a result of bone resorption. Changes in the spine are more common in the dorsal and lumbar vertebrae and consist of biconcave vertebral bodies, wedge deformities, and resultant kyphosis. Fractures may also occur, especially in femoral neck.
- The predominant radiographic pattern of increased osteoblastic and osteoclastic activity consists of *cortical tunneling or striations.* This is more evident in the tubular bones of the hand and feet occurring in up to 50% of patients.[22]
- *Thyroid acropachy* is a rare complication that occurs in 0.5–1%of patients after treatment for hyperthyroidism by surgery or antithyroid medication.[16,41] It may appear years after the initial presentation of hyperthyroidism and the patients are often euthyroid but may be hypo or hyperthyroid. The cause is unknown with no apparent age or gender predilection. Patients may present with exophthalmos, soft-tissue swelling of the fingers and toes, pretibial myxedema, or clubbing.[16,41]

The radiologic findings of thyroid acropachy are virtually diagnostic and consist of dense, solid, and periosteal new bone formation with feathery margins. The periostitis is commonly seen in an asymmetric distribution and is most prominent along the radial margin of metacarpals and phalanges in the diaphyseal region. Uncommonly, long bones may be involved. The bony changes are not progressive.[41]

Thyroid acropachy must be distinguished from hypertrophic osteoarthropathy, a very painful condition wherein the long bones are considerably more likely to be involved than are hands and feet, and the feathery contour is absent. Another differential of thyroid acropachy is pachydermo-periostitis where the periostitis affects the long bones more than the hands with extension of the periosteal new bone to the metaphysis and epiphysis. There is associated soft-tissue prominence of the hands with bilateral symmetrical periosteal bone formation in tibia, fibula, radius, and ulna.[42] The radiological appearance of venous stasis, leukemia, and osteomyelitis may mimic thyroid acropachy but differentiation is usually possible on the basis of characteristic clinical presentation of these disorders.[16] Fluorosis is associated with more extensive abnormality of the axial skeleton and long bones, while leukemic acropachy is particularly prominent in the terminal phalanges.[42]

HYPERGONADISM

Hypergonadism may be caused by overproduction of sex hormones by the testes or ovaries or by the overproduction by the adrenal cortex. In congenital adrenal hyperplasia, a deficiency in the synthesis of cortisol leads to high levels of ACTH. A secondary effect of high ACTH leads to excessive levels of adrenal sex steroids. A central nervous system lesion may also lead to gonadotropin excess and hypergonadism.

The skeletal manifestation of hypergonadism in the child is precocious growth and maturation. The epiphyseal ossification centers appear early. The long bones grow rapidly and the growth plates close early. Although there is initial precocious growth spurt, the early closure of the growth plate results in short stature, with a tall child becoming a short adult.[41] The morphology of the skeleton is otherwise normal.

HYPOGONADISM

Hypogonadism may be secondary to low production of gonadotropins (luteinizing hormone and follicle-stimulating hormone) from the pituitary, or deficient production of hormones by the gonads themselves.[22] The latter is termed "primary gonadal deficiency" and, when present in growing boys is referred to as *eunuchoidism*. *Turner's syndrome* is a female sex-linked disorder in which there is ovarian dysgenesis due to an XO genotype. In older women, primary gonadal deficiency occurs with menopause.

Radiological Findings

The radiographic features of hypogonadism in males consist of:

- Generalized decrease in bone density.
- Delay in skeletal maturation which manifests in the form of delayed closure of epiphysis. This results in long extremities with relatively short trunks.

Turner's Syndrome

- More than 50% of the patients do not have any radiographic abnormalities. In the remaining patients, skeletal maturation is usually normal until 15 years of age, following which delayed epiphyseal closure becomes evident, particularly in the apophysis of the iliac crests[22] and unusually long and slender tubular bones in the extremities.
- There may be depression or slanting of the medial tibial plateau with concomitant overgrowth of the medial condoyle of the femur.
- The fourth and fifth metacarpals are often short producing a positive metacarpal sign. The heads of the third and fourth metacarpals may appear flattened and cubitus valgus may be seen. This is seen in 50% of patients.
- Other findings include narrow ribs, small sella turcica, hypertelorism, and android pelvis.

GROWTH HORMONE DISORDERS

Growth hormone disorders occur as a result of excess or deficient production of growth hormone.

Acromegaly

Acromegaly results from excessive production of growth hormone (somatotropin) in a skeletally mature individual. It is usually caused by a pituitary adenoma that produces growth hormone autonomously. Elevated serum growth hormone reactivates endochondral bone formation, stimulates periosteal bone formation along with connective tissue proliferation leading to characteristic clinical and radiological features.

The overgrowth of bone in association with enlargement of soft tissue is particularly prominent in the acral parts (hands, feet, and lower jaw) of the skeleton leading to the term acromegaly for this condition.[43]

Clinical Findings

Acromegaly is typically seen in the third or fourth decade of life with an equal incidence in men and women.

The clinical features are distinctive and include coarse facial features, thick skin, poor dental occlusion, thick calvarium, deepening of voice, lantern jaw, prominent tongue, broad hand and feet, and organomegaly.[16] Rheumatologic complaints like backache and arthropathy are common.

Definitive Diagnosis

The definitive diagnosis of acromegaly is made by measurement of 24-hour serum growth hormone levels and demonstration that growth hormone secretion is not suppressed by an oral glucose challenge. Measurement of serum levels of insulin-like growth factor 1 (IGF-1 or somatomedin C) is a sensitive screening test.[41]

Radiological Findings

The radiographic findings of bony and soft-tissue overgrowth are quite characteristic in patients of acromegaly.

- Collagen tissue demonstrates a marked response to excessive amounts of growth hormone which manifests in the form of thickening of the skin. *Soft-tissue thickening* is classically seen in the heel pads and digits. The measurement is obtained by calculating the shortest distance between the calcaneus and plantar surface of the skin **(Fig. 29)**. According to Kho and associates, the thickness of the heel pad in acromegaly is related to the severity and chronicity of disease and is correlated with serum levels of growth hormone (GH).[43] Values >23 mm in men and 21.5 mm in women are suggestive of acromegaly and values >25 mm in men and 23 mm in women are diagnostic, if local causes of skin thickening are excluded.[43]

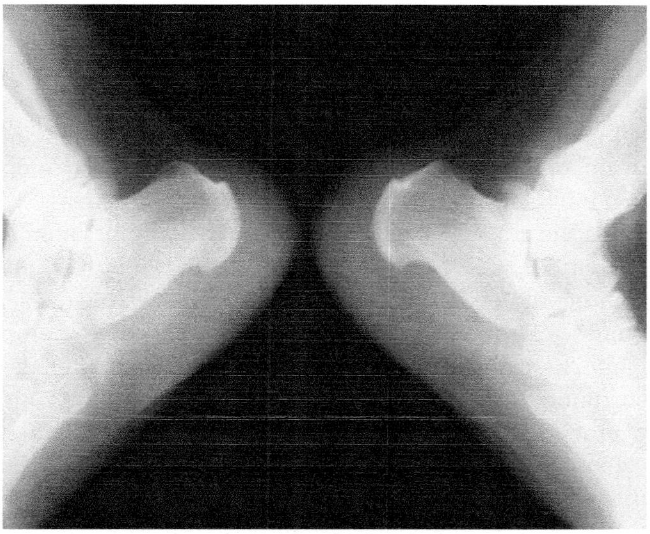

Fig. 29: Acromegaly with increase in soft-tissue thickness of the heel pad.

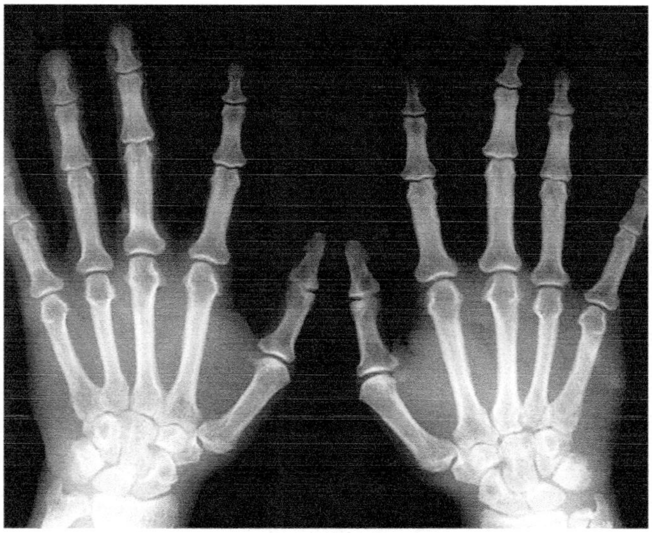

Fig. 30: Acromegaly. There is enlargement of the soft tissues with thickening of fingers and prominent joint spaces due to cartilage hypertrophy. The distal phalanges show the characteristic arrow-head appearance, more marked in the first finger.

- In the *skull, changes* include:
  - Thickening of the cranial vault
  - Prominence of the supraorbital ridges and zygomatic arches
  - Prominence of the external occipital protuberance
  - Enlargement of the sella turcica with distinctive changes
  - Prominence and enlargement of the frontal and maxillary sinuses
  - Excessive pneumatization of the mastoid
  - Enlargement and elongation of the mandible with widening of the mandibular angle.
- *Abnormalities in the hands and wrists* include soft tissue thickening of fingers, thickening, and squaring of the phalanges and metacarpals, tubulation, or overconstriction of the shafts of the phalanges, abnormally wide articular spaces, bony excrescences at sites of tendon and ligament attachment to bone and prominence of the ungual tufts which may assume a spade-like appearance.[43] An increase in soft tissue **(Fig. 30)** and bony measurements at certain specific sites has been described. One such measurement in the *Sesamoid index* which is the greatest product of the medial first metacarpophalangeal sesamoid and its maximum perpendicular diameter. This index >40 mm in men and 32 mm in women is suggestive of acromegaly. No single measurement is specific for acromegaly and the concomitant findings which are suggestive of acromegaly include:
  - Increased phalangeal soft tissue thickness
    ≥27 mm (men)
    (at proximal mid phalanges)
    ≥26 mm (women)
  - Widening of second metacarpophalangeal joint >2.5 mm in men and women
  - Bone excrescences and marginal spurs
  - Increased width of phalanges
  - Large sesamoid index >40 mm (men) >32 mm (women)
  - Increased interstyloid distance.
- The abnormalities in the *vertebral column* in acromegaly consist of:
  - Elongation and widening of vertebral bodies
  - Anterior and lateral osteophytes
  - Increased height of intervertebral disc
  - Scalloping of the posterior margins of vertebral bodies
  - Increased thoracic kyphosis
  - Exaggerated lumbar lordosis.
- *Thoracic cage abnormalities* consist of an enlarged thorax due to elongation of ribs and prominence of costochondral junction.
- In *pelvis*, in addition to articular alteration in sacroiliac joints and hip, enlargement and beaking of symphysis pubis is seen.
- In the *feet*, the radiographic changes resemble those in hands with:
  - Soft-tissue enlargement
  - Prominence of tufts and base of terminal phalanges
  - Bone proliferation at sites of tendon and ligament attachment like under surface of calcaneum.
- *Articular abnormalities* are most frequently seen in the knees, hip, and glenohumeral joints. Proliferation of chondrocytes in the articular cartilage result in widening of articular space seen at metacarpophalangeal, metatarsophalangeal, and interphalangeal joints.

In the later stages of the disease, cartilaginous and osseous degeneration occurs leading to secondary degenerative changes. Superficially, the appearance of acromegalic arthropathy is similar to osteoarthritis, but the joint spaces tend to be widened rather than narrowed. The distribution of involvement usually includes the large joints and the lumbosacral spine which are normally spared by osteoarthritis.

Gigantism

Excess of growth hormone during skeletal development results in gigantism, which is a rare condition. The direct hormonal stimulation of activity at the growth plates and other sites of bone formation by growth hormone leads to progressive enlargement of length and width of the bones. The most striking feature of patients with gigantism is extreme height with normal body proportions.[41] An autonomously functioning pituitary adenoma is the most common cause of gigantism. Unless treated, the growth hormone excess continues after growth plate closure with patients of gigantism developing progressively more striking features of acromegaly.[41]

SCURVY

Scurvy, also known as Barlow's disease, is the result of long-term deficiency of vitamin C. Infantile scurvy is found in infants fed on pasteurized or boiled milk formula since the pasteurization and boiling processes destroy the vitamin C content.[12,22] Children with developmental or psychological disorder, who have a vitamin C-poor diet, are at a risk of developing scurvy. Scurvy is rare before 6 months of age as for scurvy to manifest itself the deficiency must be present for at least 4–6 months.[22] It is seen much less frequently than rickets.[44]

Clinical Findings

Scurvy usually occurs in the age group of 6 months to 2 years. Child presents with progressive irritability, with tender, edematous limbs, and weakness of lower limbs resulting in pseudoparalysis. Musculocutaneous manifestations are seen in 80% of patients with scurvy, such as arthralgia, myalgia, hemarthrosis, and muscular and subperiosteal hemorrhage. Lower extremities are more commonly involved than the upper extremities with knee being more commonly involved. Subcutaneous and mucous membrane hemorrhages occur and a secondary anemia may develop. Scurvy is rare in adults, being seen in patients suffering from chronic severe malnutrition.

Biochemical Findings

Serum ascorbic acid: 0.6–1.2 mg/100 mL (normal range).

Pathophysiology

The pathological changes seen in scurvy are the result of depression of normal cellular activity.[22] There is suppression of osteoblastic activity resulting in cessation of normal bone formation. However, bone resorption continues leading to the development of osteoporosis.

At the growth plate, although cartilage proliferation is decreased, mineralization is unimpaired, resulting in the zone of provisional calcification becoming wide and dense. Similar changes occur around epiphyseal ossification centers, resulting in a thin ring of *increased* density surrounding the *epiphysis*. Vascular invasion of the zone of provisional calcification is arrested and with suppressed osteoblastic activity there is decreased formation of bony matrix. Thus, the trabecular bone mass is decreased in the zone of primary and secondary spongiosa. This is seen radiographically as a *transverse band* of *radiolucency* adjacent to the zone of provisional calcification. This zone, called Trümmerfeld zone represents an area of weakened bone and shows a tendency to fracture. The zone of provisional calcification extends beyond the margins of the metaphysis, resulting in periosteal elevation and marginal spur formation. Large subperiosteal hemorrhages resulting in soft tissue edema occur in late stages of the disease.

The optimal sites for detection of scurvy in the skeleton are bones of the lower extremities. Diagnostic changes may be demonstrable at the knees when minimal changes are present at the wrists.[12]

Radiological Findings

Radiographically, characteristic signs are seen which reflect the pathological changes occurring as a result of lack of vitamin C.

- Osteoporosis.
- *White line of Frankel* is the dense, white line in the zone of provisional calcification at the growing metaphysis.
- Beneath the Frankel's line, there is a radiolucent zone in the metaphysis called *Trümmerfeld zone or Scorbutic zone*, due to lack of mineralization of osteoid **(Fig. 31)**.
- The epiphysis is small, sharply marginated by a sclerotic rim while the central portion is more radiolucent, called *Wimberger's sign.*
- Finally, as the metaphysis is weakened, it is prone to fractures, which manifest themselves at the cortical margin, giving rise to *Pelkan spur*, that project perpendicular to the long axis of the shaft.
- In addition, due to capillary permeability, *subperiosteal hemorrhages* occur which may give rise to periosteal elevation and subsequent new bone formation, particularly following treatment. The hemorrhages appear as soft-tissue density adjacent to the cortical

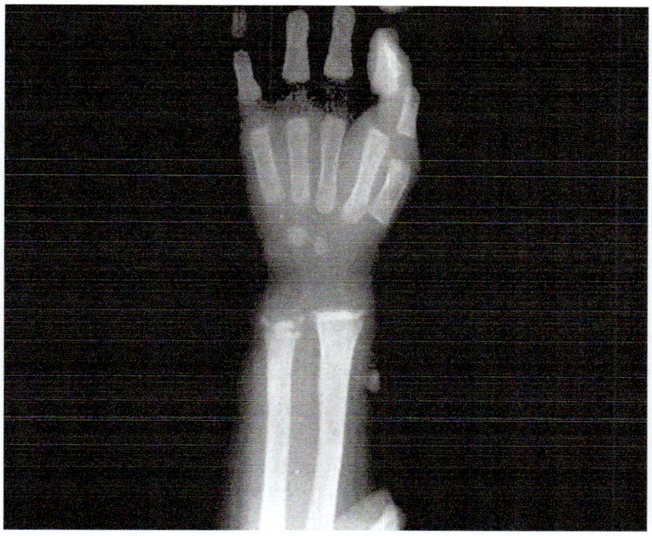

Fig. 31: Scurvy. X-ray wrist anteroposterior (AP) view reveals increased density of the zone of provisional calcification (Frankel's line) with a lucent zone beneath it (Trümmerfeld zone) in the distal radial and ulnar metaphysis.

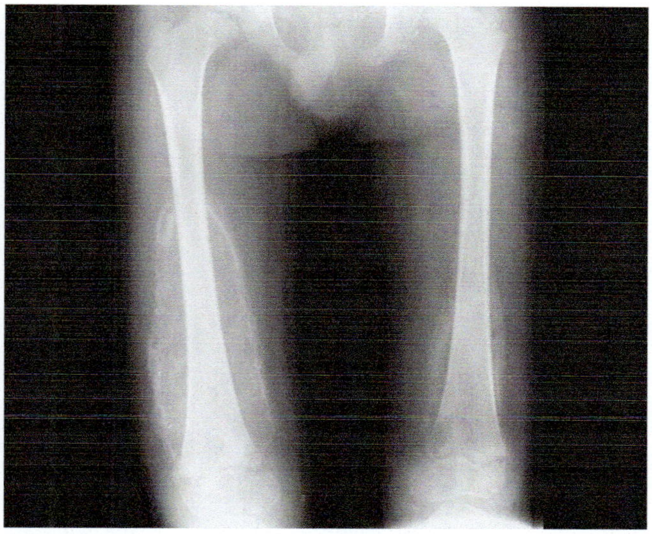

Fig. 32: Calcified subperiosteal hemorrhages seen along bilateral femoral shafts, more extensive on the right side: Healing scurvy.

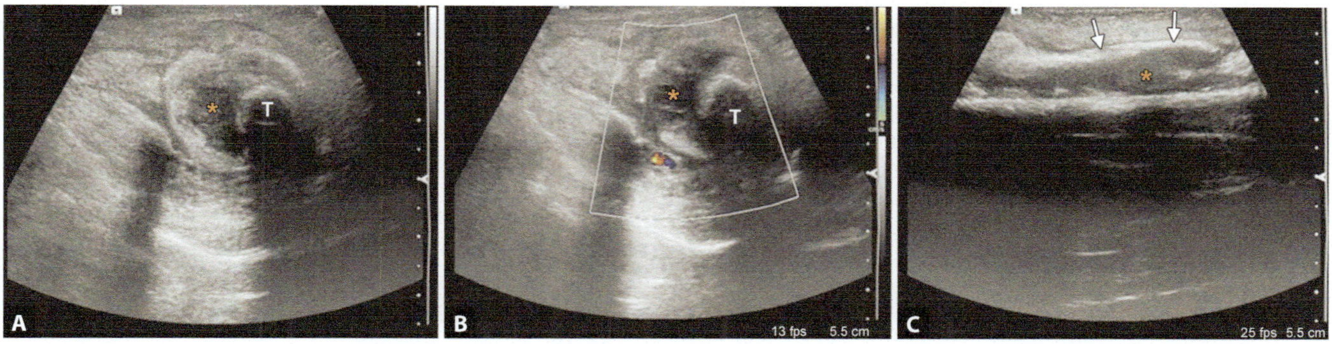

Figs. 33A to C: (A) Ultrasound left leg in a 5-year-old child with mixed cerebral palsy with cellulitis reveals heterogeneous hypoechoic areas (*) beneath the periosteum of left tibial (T) shaft, with no vascularity within on color Doppler (B) suggestive of subperiosteal hemorrhage due to scurvy. Arrows in the longitudinal image (C) depicts the elevated periosteum.

bones such as femur, tibia, and humerus. Upon healing, the subperiosteal hemorrhages calcify, and cast shadows of increased density in the soft tissues surrounding the bone **(Fig. 32)**.

The above findings constitute the classic signs of infantile scurvy. These changes are less apparent as the patient ages. On healing, all changes are reversible on vitamin C therapy though a single growth arrest line may remain in the metaphysis as a residual of Frankel's line, an indicator of prior vitamin C therapy.

Diagnosis

The diagnosis of scurvy is by clinical and radiographic findings and may be supported by additional findings of low level of vitamin C in the serum or Buffy coat of leukocytes.

Ultrasound Evaluation

Though the clinical and radiological changes described in scurvy are the best diagnostic tool, effective use of ultrasonography in pediatric patients has been described, both in diagnosis and follow-up as it does not involve any ionizing radiation. High-resolution ultrasonography of the affected limb very well depicts the recurrent and multiple subperiosteal hemorrhage as heterogeneous hypoechoic lesions beneath the periosteum with absence of vascularity on color Doppler, thereby ruling out the likelihood of a malignant process[45] **(Figs. 33A to C)**.

Magnetic Resonance Imaging

Magnetic resonance imaging findings of scurvy have also been described in the literature. It consists of heterogeneous signal of the marrow on T1- and

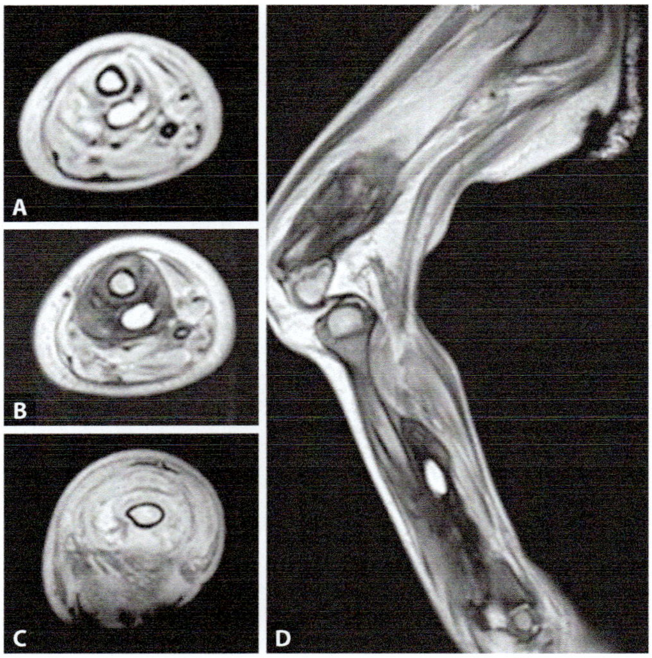

Figs. 34A to D: Magnetic resonance imaging of the lower limb of the same child was done. T2 sagittal, T1 and T2 W axial images and post contrast T 1 W FS images show elevation of distal femoral periosteum with altered signal in the subperiosteal space extending from epiphysis to midshaft appearing isointense on T1 W images (A) and iso- to hypointense on T2 W/STIR images; (B) showing no enhancement on postcontrast images; (C) suggestive of hematoma of varying stage; (D) Similar findings are seen along the tibial diaphysis. Overlying muscles appear atrophic with heterogeneous signal intensity suggestive of fatty infiltration; features suggestive of nutritional deficiency likely scurvy.

T2-weighted sequences, subperiosteal hemorrhage and surrounding edema **(Figs. 34A to D)**. These findings can also be seen in osteomyelitis, subperiosteal abscess, or leukemia which need to be excluded. However, an increase in the subperiosteal hemorrhage on follow-up scans due to recurrent hematoma is a pointer toward the diagnosis of scurvy.[46]

Treatment

Since scurvy is rare with nonspecific symptomatology, the best evidence in diagnosis is the improvement in symptoms that usually start within few days of start of vitamin C therapy.

Oral vitamin C supplementation with a dose of 100–300 mg in children should be given until the serum level improves. Spontaneous hemorrhages stop in 24 hours while muscle and body aches disappear in a few days with complete relief from symptoms observed within 3 weeks.[45]

FLUOROSIS

It is a chronic metabolic bone disease caused by chronic ingestion of excessive amounts of fluoride.

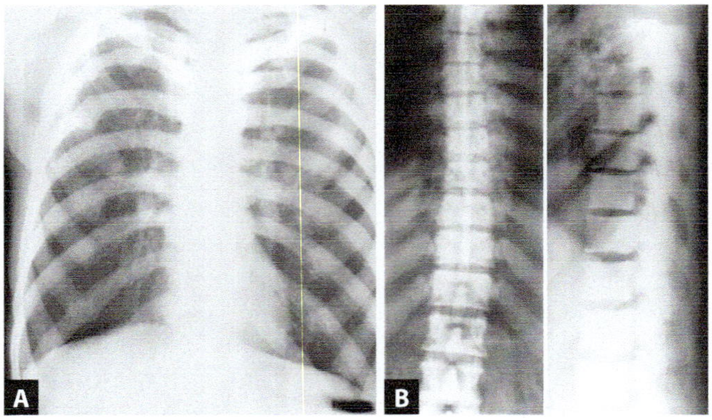

Figs. 35A and B: Fluorosis: (A) Frontal chest X-ray reveals diffuse osteosclerosis; (B) Osteosclerosis and osteophytosis of the dorsal vertebral bodies with posterior longitudinal ligament ossification.

The alterations in bone metabolism in fluorosis are not clearly understood but seem to be multifactorial. A generalized increase in bone density is seen which is due to osteoclastic response to the fluorine rather than fluorine deposition *per se*.[15] The synthesis of normal collagen is also disturbed.

Clinical Findings

Clinically, there is marked variation in presentation. The most pronounced feature is mottled dental enamel. Bone changes produce few symptoms. However, exceptionally high levels of fluorine may be associated with crippling stiffness and pain.[15] Criteria for diagnosing fluorosis clinically consist of:[47]

- Residing in endemic area for >10 years
- Mottled tooth enamel
- Urine fluoride levels >10 mg/L (normal level <1.5 mg/L)
- Typical symptoms and findings on clinical examination
- No evidence of any other metabolic bone disease on clinical evaluation.

Radiographical Findings

Radiological evaluation is considered the best method for diagnosing fluorosis, especially when the patient is asymptomatic.

Radiographically, the changes are diffuse increase in bone density (osteosclerosis), osteophytosis, and calcification/ossification of the attachments of tendons, muscles, and ligaments.

- *Osteosclerosis* is a common finding in fluorosis and involves all bones, but is most marked in the spine, pelvis, and ribs **(Figs. 35A and B)**. Initially, there is a thickening of the bony trabecular pattern which then progresses to a dense, uniform, symmetrical sclerosis that obliterates the bony architectural landmarks. The skull and tubular bones of the appendicular skeleton are relatively spared in the sclerotic process. The only change in the calvarium may be a sclerosis of the base of the skull and posterior clinoids.[44] One needs to remember that osteosclerosis alone is a nonspecific finding seen in many conditions such as metastasis, myelofibrosis, Paget's disease, renal osteodystrophy, etc.

- Thickening of the cortex of the affected bones occurs at the expense of the medullary cavity.
- The inferior margins of the ribs may show characteristic irregularity/fringed appearance called "rose-thorn appearance."
- *Ligamentous calcification* and *ossification*, particularly of sacrospinous and sacrotuberous ligaments, is another characteristic radiographic feature.
- *Ossification* in the *interosseous membranes* of paired bones is *diagnostic* **(Fig. 36)**.
- *Osteophytosis* of the vertebrae can be severe and at times encroach on the spinal canal and intervertebral foramina. Paraspinal and intraspinal ligament ossification is known to occur and may cause compressive myelopathy **(Fig. 37)**.

Magnetic resonance imaging is a useful imaging modality in the early diagnosis of fluorosis and in planning surgical intervention in a symptomatic patient as the extent of soft tissue, spinal cord changes and associated abnormalities are well visualized. Typical MRI findings in fluorosis of spine consist of diffusely sclerotic bones, ossification of posterior longitudinal ligament and ligamentam flavum, and spinal canal and neural foramina narrowing. Osteosclerosis is typically seen as low-signal intensity on both T1- and T2-weighted images. In endemic

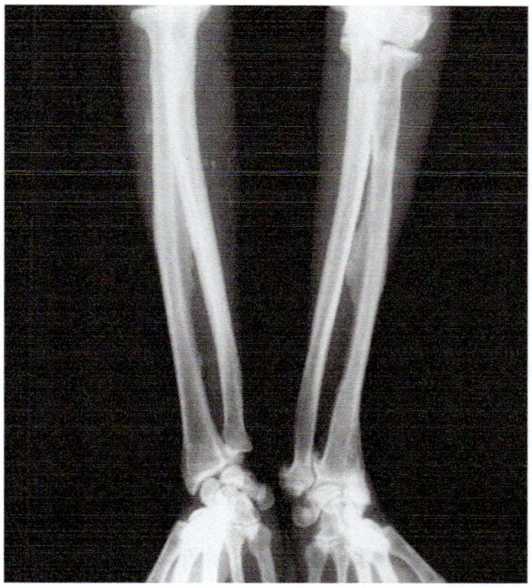

Fig. 36: Interosseous membrane ossification—diagnostic of fluorosis.

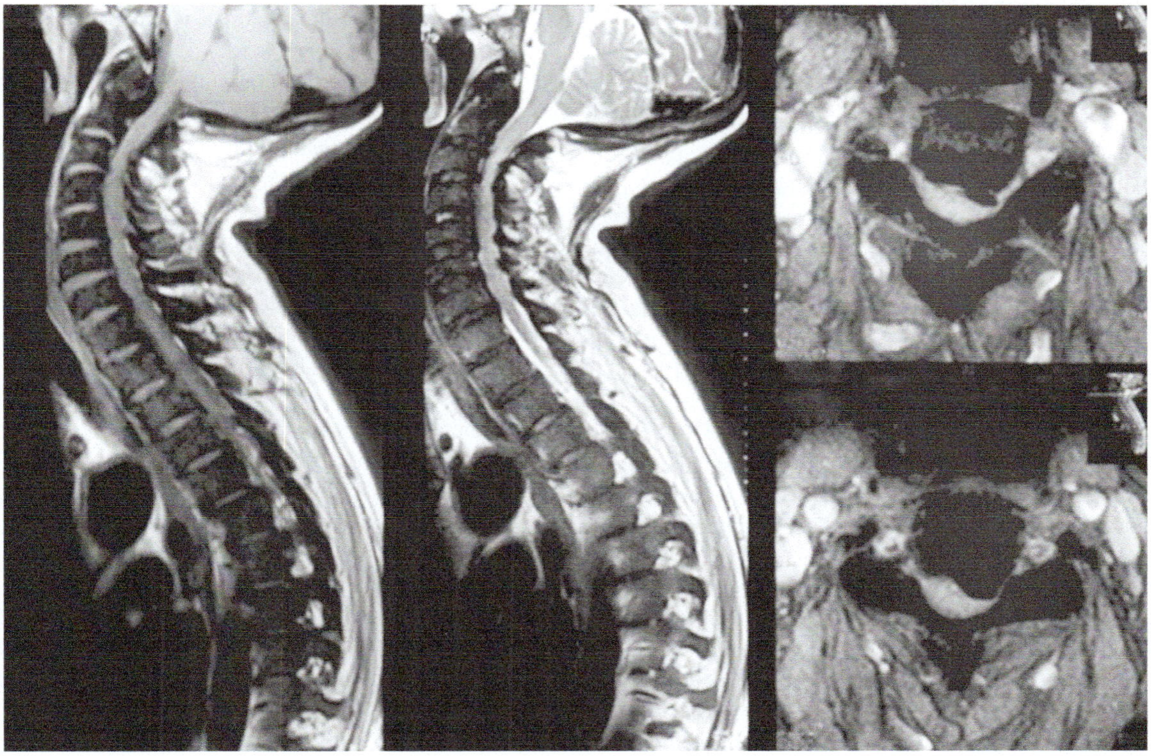

Fig. 37: Fluorosis: T1W and T2W sagittal MR scans of cervicodorsal spine reveals diffuse decrease in marrow signal intensity of vertebral bodies, appearing more hypointense than intervening intervertebral discs consistent with sclerosis. The vertebral bodies show osteophytic changes. Axial images depict ossification of posterior longitudinal ligament with resultant spinal canal stenosis.

regions, MRI may show diffuse low signal on all pulse sequences and help in early detection of fluorosis and save the patients from serious manifestations such as fluorotic myelopathy which may require surgical decompression.

Diagnosis is based on characteristic ligament calcification, history of long-term heavy exposure to fluoride, and high urinary fluoride levels.

CONCLUSION

To conclude, plain radiographs are the primary imaging tools for the evaluation of suspected skeletal disorders of metabolic and endocrine origin. By and large, these disorders involve the skeleton as a whole. The radiographic changes are therefore predominantly diffuse or at least multifocal involving many areas of the skeleton. An understating of the diverse manifestations of these disorders including their findings on imaging helps in reaching an early diagnosis. Imaging also plays a role in evaluation of severity of disease, assessment of disease activity, and in monitoring the effect of treatment.

REFERENCES

1. Mankin HJ. Metabolic bone disease. J Bone Joint Surg Am. 1994;76:760.
2. Reynolds WA, Karo JJ. Radiologic diagnosis of metabolic bone disease. Orthop Clin North Am. 1972;3(3):521-43.
3. Pitt M. Osteopenic bone disease. Orthop Clin North Am. 1983;14(1):65-80.
4. Pitt MJ. Rickets and osteomalacia are still around. Radiol Clin North Am. 1991;29(1):97-118.
5. Mankin HJ. Rickets, osteomalacia and renal osteodystrophy: Part I. J Bone Joint Surg Am. 1974;56:101.
6. Rowe LJ, Yochum TR. Nutritional metabolic and endocrine disorders: In: Yochum, Rowes (Eds). Essentials of Skeletal Radiology, 3rd edition. Philadelphia: Lippincott Williams and Wilkins; 2005. pp. 1497-545.
7. Chaudhari JR, Mridula KR, Rathnakishor C, Balaraju B, Bandaru VS. Association of 25-Hydroxy vitamin D deficiency in pediatric epileptic patients. IJCN. 2017;11(2): 46-56.
8. Jagtal VS. Hypophosphatemic rickets. IJEM. 2012;16(2): 177-82.
9. Gupta AK. Rickets and osteomalacia. In: Berry M, Chowdhury V, Suri S, Mukhopadhyay S (Eds). Diagnostic Radiology-Musculo-skeletal and Breast Imaging, 1st edition. Delhi: Jaypee Brothers Medical publishers (P) Ltd.; 1998. pp. 162-75.
10. Pitt MJ. Rickets and osteomalacia. In: Resnick D (Ed). Diagnosis of Bone and Joint Disorders, 4th edition. USA: WB Saunders Company; 2002. pp. 1901-45.
11. Judith EA. Metabolic and endocrine skeletal disease. In: Adams A, Dixon AK (Eds). Grainger and Allison's Diagnostic Radiology: A Textbook of Medical Imaging, 5th edition. London: Churchill Livingstone Elsevier; 2008. pp. 1083-113.
12. Silverman FN. Dysostoses, miscellaneous syndromes and metabolic abnormalities. In: Silverman FN, Kuhn JP (Eds). Caffey's Pediatric X-ray Diagnosis, 9th edition. USA: Mosby. 1993. pp. 1746-81.
13. Kottamasu SR. Metabolic bone diseases. In: Silverman FN, Kuhn JP (Eds). Caffey's Pediatric X-ray Diagnosis, 10th edition. USA: Mosby; 2003. pp. 2242-68.
14. Pitt MJ. Rickets and osteomalacia. In: Resmick D, Krausdorf MJ (Eds). Bone and Joint Imaging, 3rd edition. USA: Elsevier Saunders; 2005. pp. 563-75.
15. Murray RO, Stoker DJ. Skeletal disorders of metaboloic and endocrines origin. In: Sutton D (Ed). Textbook of Radiology and Imaging, 4th edition. London: Churchill Living Stone. 1987;1:229-63.
16. Lenchik L, Sartoris DJ. Orthopaedic aspects of metabolic bone disease. Orthop Clin North Am. 1998;29(1):103-34.
17. Steinbach HL, Noetzli M. Roentgen appearance of the skeleton in osteomalacia and rickets. AJR. 1964;91:955.
18. Chuang TL, Kuo JL, Chang XY, Chiu JS, Wang YF, et al. Scintigraphic evidence of osteomalacia: Usefulness and typical signs. Ann Nucl Med Sci. 2007;20:115-20.
19. Resnick D. Parathyroid disorders and renal osteodystrophy. In: Resnick D (Ed). Diagnosis of Bone and Joint Disorders, 4th edition. Philadelphia: WB Saunders Company. 2002;2:2043-111.
20. Eslamy HK, Ziessman HA. Parathyroid Scintigraphy in patients with primary Hyperparathyroidism: ^{99m}Tc sestamibi SPECT and SPECT /CT. Radiographics. 2008;28:1461-76.
21. Chowdhury V. Hyperparathyroidism. In: Berry M, Chowdhury V, Suri S, Mukhopadhyay S (Eds). Diagnostic Radiology: Musculoskeletal and Breast Imaging, 1st edition. Delhi: Jaypee Brothers Medical Publishers (P) Ltd; 1998. pp. 186-200.
22. Volger JB, Kim JH. Metabolic and endocrine disease of the skeleton. In: Grainger RG, Allison DJ, Adam A, Dixon AK (Eds). Diagnostic Radiology. A Textbook of Medical Imaging, 4th edition. London: Churchill Livingstone; 2001. pp. 1925-66.
23. Resmick D. Parathyroid disorders and renal osteodystrophy. In: Resmick D, Krausdorf MJ (Eds). Bone and Joint Imaging, 3rd edition. USA: Elsevier Saunders. 2005;2:603-22.
24. Hayes CW, Conway WF. Hyperparathyroidism. Radiol Clin North Am. 1991;29(1):85-96.
25. Richardson ML, Pozz-Mucelli RS, Kanter AS. Bone mineral changes in primary hyperparathyroidism. Skeletal Radiology. 1986;15:85-95.
26. Sahan MH, Guner S, Guner SI. Radiological findings in the primary hyperparathyroid case with multiple brown tumors: a case report. Eastern Journal of Medicine. 2008;13:30-4.
27. Su AW, Chen CF, Huang CK, Chen PC, Chen WM, Chen TH.. Primary hyperparathyroidism with brown tumor mimicking metastatic bone malignancy. J Chin Med Assoc. 2010;73(3):177-80.
28. Greenspan A. Hyperparathyroidism. In: Greenspan A (Ed). Orthopaedic imaging: A practical approach, 4th edition. USA: Lippincott Williams and Wilkins; 2004. pp. 837-42.

29. Young WR. Metabolic and Endocrine disorders affecting bone. In: Sutton D (Ed). Textbook of Radiology and Imaging, 7th edition. London: Churchill Livingstone. 2003;1:1351-69.
30. Chang CY, Rosenthal DI, Mitchell DM, Handa A, Kattapuram SV, Huang AJ. Imaging findings of metabolic bone disease. Radiographics. 2016;36:1871-87.
31. Patel AA, Ramanathan R, Kuban J, Willis MH. Imaging findings and evaluation of metabolic bone disease. Hindawi; 2015.
32. Larson TC, Smith MM, Chong WK, Martin WH. Imaging of the thyroid and parathyroid glands. In: Hagga JR, Lanzieri CF, Gilkeson RC (Eds). CT and MR Imaging of the Whole Body, 4th edition. USA: Mosby. 2003;1:663-90.
33. Johnson NA, Tublin ME, Ogilvie JB. Parathyroid imaging: Technique and role in the preoperative evaluation of primary hyperparathyroidism. AJR. 2007;188(6):1706-15.
34. Mc Dermott VG, Spritzer CE. Parathyroid and thyroid glands. In: Stark DD, Bradley WG Jr (Eds). Magnetic Resonance Imaging, 3rd edition, volume III. USA: Mosby, Inc; 1999. pp. 1807-20.
35. Bilezikian JP, Brandi ML, Eastall R, Silverberg SJ, Udelsman R, Marcocci C, et al. Guidelines for the management of asymptomatic hyperthyroidism: Summary statement from the 4th International workshop. J Clin Endocrinol Metab. 2014;99(10):3561-9.
36. Hoang JK, Sung W, Bahl M, Philips CD. How to perform parathyroid 4D CT: Tips and traps for technique and interpretation. Radiology. 2014;270(1):15-24.
37. Bann DV, Zacharia T, Goldenberg D, Goyal N. Parathyroid localization using 4D-computed tomography. Ear Nose Throat J. 2015;94(4-5):E55-7.
38. Bahl M, Sepahdari AR, Sosa JA, Hoang JK. Parathyroid adenomas and hyperplasia on four-dimensional CT scans: three patterns of enhancement relative to the thyroid gland justify a three-phase protocol. Radiology. 2015;277(2): 454-62.
39. Yeh R, Tay YD, Tabacco G Dercle L, Kuo JH, Bandeira L. Diagnostic performance of 4D CT and Sestamibi SPECT/CT in localizing parathyroid adenomas in primary hyperparathyroidism. Radiology. 2019;291(2):469-76.
40. Lundstroem AK, Trolle W, Soerenses CH, Myschatzky. Preoperative localization of hyperfunctioning parathyroid glands with 4D-CT. Eur Arch Otorhinolaryngol. 2016;273: 1253-9.
41. Chew FS. Radiologic manifestations in the musculoskeletal system of miscellaneous endocrine disorders. Radiol Clin North Am. 1991;29(1):135-47.
42. Resnick D. Pituitary disorders. In: Resnick D (Ed). Diagnosis of Bone and Joint Disorders, 4th edition. USA: WB Saunders Company; 2002. pp. 2003-25.
43. Resnick D. Pituitary disorders. In: Resnick D (Ed). Diagnosis of Bone and Joint Disorders, 5th edition. USA: WB Saunders Company; 2005. pp. 589-96.
44. Greenfield GB. Epiphyseal region. In: Greenfield (Ed). Radiology of Bone Diseases, 5th edition. Philadelphia: JB Lippincott Company; 1990. p. 235.
45. Polat AV, Bekci T, Say F, Bolukbas E, Selcuk MB. Osteoskeletal manifestations of scurvy: MRI and ultrasound findings. Skeletal Radiology. 2015;44(8):1161-4.
46. Choi SW, Park S, Kwon YS, Oh IS, Lim MK, Kim WH, et al. MR imaging in a child with scurvy: a case report. Korean J Radiol. 2007;8(5):443-7.
47. Nair N, Gupta N. Radiology of skeletal fluorosis: A review. Annals of Orthop Rheumatol. 2016;4(2):1069-71.

CHAPTER

11

Osteoporosis

Chirag Kamal Ahuja, Mukesh Kumar Yadav, Vikas Bhatia, Ajay Kumar

INTRODUCTION

Osteoporosis, one of the common metabolic bone disorders, is a manifestation of compromised bone strength. It is defined by the World Health Organization (WHO) as "a skeletal disease, characterized by low bone mass and microarchitectural deterioration of bone tissue, with a consequent increase in bone fragility and susceptibility to fracture."[1] The strength of the bone is a constituent of two features, namely, its quality and density (mass/volume). Bone quality is a composite of bone architecture, turnover, mineralization, and damage incurred. The bone mineral density (BMD) can be subject to measurement and has been used in the quantitative WHO definition of osteoporosis, with bone density <2.5 standard deviations (SD) qualifying for the diagnosis of osteoporosis.[2] Histologically, there occurs a decrease in cortical thickness along with reduction in the size and number of the trabeculae of cancellous bone. There may be fractures of the trabecular as well as compromise of the trabecular connectivity. The structure of organic matrix (osteoid) is preserved with no obvious defect in mineralization. Thus, osteoporosis is histologically distinguishable from osteomalacia, in which mineralization of osteoid matrix is impaired with an increase in the ratio of organic matrix to mineral.

PATHOGENESIS

Bone remodeling (its production and resorption) is a continuous process, which is regulated by systemic and locally produced agents. A number of metabolic, nutritional, and mechanical factors are also involved in the procedure. A fine balance in bone formation and resorption maintains the skeletal mass. Tipping of the balance toward resorption results in reduced bone mass resulting in osteoporosis.[2]

Aging also leads to reduced bone mass. Although skeletal growth ceases by the end of adolescence and there occurs closure of the endochondral growth plate, bone mass continues to increase by radial growth until peak is achieved at about the age of 35 years. Thereafter, a balance is achieved for a few years when there is an equivalence of new bone formation and bone resorption. After a few years of growth, in around fourth to fifth decade, bone resorption starts to increase more than bone formation and skeletal mass decreases. Different areas of the skeleton show different bone loss. There is progressive reduced rate of loss of cortical bone of about 0.3–0.5% per year subsequently in both genders. The rate of bone loss in women may be accelerated around the time of menopause, which is attributable to estrogen deficiency. The cumulative loss of bone mass ranges from 20 to 30% in men and 40 to 50% in women over the last four to five decades of life.[2,3]

ETIOLOGY

Table 1 highlights the various causes, which may contribute to osteoporosis. The various types and causes are briefly discussed in the following text.

Primary Osteoporosis

Type I (Postmenopausal) Osteoporosis

It occurs in women between 51 and 75 years of age in which there is disproportionate accelerated loss of trabecular bone.[4] Fractures of vertebral bodies and distal forearm are common. Biochemically, both circulating parathormone and 1,25$(OH)_2$ vitamin D are reduced.

Type II (Senile) Osteoporosis

It occurs in both sexes over 70 years of age. There is proportionate loss of both cortical and trabecular bone, and the fracture sites are also those which contain both types of bone, i.e., femoral neck, proximal humerus, proximal tibia, and pelvis. Biochemically, circulating parathormone is increased but 1,25$(OH)_2$ vitamin D is reduced.

Juvenile Osteoporosis

Juvenile osteoporosis is a rare disease, which occurs in children between 8 and 15 years of age. Clinical features include bone pain, fractures with minimal trauma (mostly metaphyseal fractures of distal tibia and vertebral crush

Table 1: Various causes of osteoporosis.

Cause unknown	*Causes known*	*Miscellaneous causes*
• Primary osteoporosis (senile, postmenopausal)	*Endocrine disorders:*	• Ankylosing spondylitis
• Juvenile osteoporosis	• Acromegaly	• Chronic obstructive pulmonary disease
	• Adrenal atrophy in Addison's disease	• Congenital porphyria
	• Cushing's syndrome	• Epidermolysis bullosa
	• Eating disorders	• Hemophilia
	• Endometriosis	• Idiopathic hypercalciuria
	• Gonadal insufficiency (primary or secondary)	• Idiopathic scoliosis
	• Hyperparathyroidism	• Multiple sclerosis
	• Hyperprolactinemia	• Rheumatoid arthritis
	• Hyperthyroidism	• Immobilization
	• Hypogonadism	*Genetic disorders:*
	• Type 1 diabetes mellitus	• Hypophosphatasia
	• Nutritional disorders	• Osteogenesis imperfect
	• Tumor secretion of parathyroid hormone-related peptide	• Homocystinuria
	Gastrointestinal disease:	• Ehlers-Danlos syndrome
	• Alcohol-related liver diseases	• Marfan syndrome
	• Celiac disease	*Drugs associated with bone loss:*
	• Chronic active hepatitis	• Aluminum
	• Chronic cholestatic diseases	• Anticoagulants
	• Gastrectomy	• Anticonvulsants
	• Inflammatory bowel disease	• Cigarette smoking
	• Jejunoileal bypass	• Cytotoxic drugs
	• Malabsorption syndromes	• Excessive alcohol
	• Pancreatic insufficiency	• Excessive vitamin A
	• Parenteral nutrition	• Glucocorticoids and adrenocorticotropin
	• Primary biliary cirrhosis	• Gonadotropin-releasing hormone agonists
	• Severe liver disease	• Heparin
	Marrow-related disorders:	• Lithium
	• Amyloidosis	• Tamoxifen (in the premenopausal patient)
	• Hemochromatosis	• Beta carotene
	• Hemophilia	• Bile-acid binding resins
	• Leukemia	
	• Lymphoma	
	• Mastocytosis	
	• Multiple myeloma	
	• Pernicious anemia	
	• Sarcoidosis	
	• Sickle cell anemia	
	• Thalassemia	
	Organ transplantation:	
	• Bone marrow	
	• Heart	
	• Kidney	
	• Liver	
	• Lung	

fractures), reduced bone density at areas of new bone growth, and loss of height. Spontaneous recovery occurs within 4–5 years, but deformities may persist. Biochemical investigations are normal and most forms of treatment are ineffective.

Endocrine Causes

Glucocorticoid Excess

Cushing's syndrome or glucocorticoid excess from exogenous or endogenous sources results in osteoporosis. There are a number of mechanisms responsible for this, and it has been shown by various studies that both dose and duration of steroid treatment correlate with bone loss. Glucocorticoid-induced bone loss predominantly affects the trabecular bone. Once osteoporosis develops in adults with Cushing's syndrome, the abnormality may persist indefinitely even after the cause is removed.

Hypogonadism

Whether due to primary gonadal failure or secondary to gonadotropin deficiency, hypogonadism is associated with osteoporosis, particularly of trabecular bone. It is a well-known fact that estrogen is important in preventing bone loss in normal premenopausal women, and estrogen deficiency due to any cause can lead to osteoporosis.[5] Similarly, testosterone deficiency appears to be the major factor responsible for reduced bone mass in men.

Thyrotoxicosis

Significant bone loss is rare in thyrotoxicosis due to its early diagnosis and treatment. Both bone formation and resorption are increased in this disorder, but the formation is unable to match the resorption which leads to reduced bone mass.

Hyperprolactinemia

In women with hyperprolactinemia, reduced estrogen secretion is the key factor for osteoporosis. Even in men with hyperprolactinemia, there is reduced bone density due to associated hypogonadism.

Diabetes Mellitus

In insulin-dependent (type 1) diabetes mellitus, there is reduction in the bone mass. The mechanism is not clear. Though the calcium levels are high, there is reduced tubular reabsorption of phosphate that may be a contributing factor for osteoporosis. A primary decrease in bone formation due to reduced insulin action has also been postulated.

Hyperparathyroidism

Generalized loss of bone density is a prominent feature in primary or secondary hyperparathyroidism, which is followed by endosteal resorption. Osteoporosis may be seen in patients with primary hyperparathyroidism who may not have subperiosteal resorption or brown tumor or elevated serum alkaline phosphatase. Increased osteoclastic activity is responsible for osteoporosis.[5]

Malignant Diseases

Several malignant tumors may cause diffuse osteopenia. Multiple myeloma is the most common. Other tumors include lymphoma, leukemia, systemic mastocytosis, etc. The neoplastic plasma cells secrete osteoclast-activating factor which may be involved in mediating bone loss. Heparin or possibly other agents released by mast cells or lymphoma cells may be the effector molecule for osteoporosis.

Immobilization

Increased bone resorption resulting from decreased weight bearing is the cause of bone loss.

Drugs

Long-term heparin administration potentiates parathyroid hormone (PTH)-mediated bone resorption and activation of collagenase, which leads to bone loss. Ethanol may also cause or contribute to bone loss. There is a long list of medications associated with bone loss.

Genetic Abnormalities in Bone Collagen Synthesis

Osteogenesis imperfecta (brittle bone syndrome) is described under four types. *Type I* osteogenesis imperfecta is an autosomal dominant form characterized by mild-to-moderate bone fragility, blue sclerae, and premature deafness. *Type II* is a lethal perinatal disorder. *Type III* is characterized by severe bone fragility, progressive bone deformity, and white sclerae. *Type IV* shows features of type I with white sclerae. Defective gene encoding leading to decreased collagen formation of type I leads to osteoporosis. It is postulated that what is now diagnosed as idiopathic or postmenopausal osteoporosis is due to defect in these genes (*COLIA1* and *COLIA2*) in absence of other features of osteogenesis imperfecta.

Osteoporosis also occurs in patients with homocystinuria due to cystathionine synthetase deficiency, an autosomal recessive trait associated with ectopia lentis, various deformities of the extremities, mental retardation, decreased pigmentation of hair and skin, and thromboembolism. The osteoporosis may be due to the effect of homocysteine or other metabolites in interfering with cross linking of collagen.

In Marfan syndrome, an autosomal dominant disease, osteoporosis is due to defective collagen formation. It is characterized by arachnodactyly, posterior scalloping of vertebral bodies, high arched palate, lenticular subluxation, and dissecting aneurysm.

Gastrointestinal Diseases

In diffuse liver diseases, malabsorption or defective metabolism of vitamin D can cause osteopenia. Primary biliary cirrhosis is a well-known example. In addition, many other gastrointestinal diseases are associated with osteoporosis.[5]

Organ Transplantation

Organ transplantation as the effective therapy for end-stage diseases of kidney, lung, liver, and cardiac patients has shown improved outcomes leading to increase in the number of transplant patients. These patients require lifelong medications such as steroids, immunosuppressant drugs, and anticoagulation. Varying mechanisms are responsible for osteoporosis in these patients.[5]

CLINICAL FEATURES

Osteoporosis becomes clinically significant when bone mass is reduced to the extent that the skeleton is insufficient to perform its normal function. Generalized skeletal pain is uncommon, and between fractures most patients are free of symptoms. Pain usually results from collapse of vertebra, especially in the dorsal and lumbar regions, typically acute in nature, and may radiate along the distribution of the respective intercostal nerve and into the abdomen.[6] These may occur even with trivial trauma. The collapse fractures usually cause anterior wedging of the vertebrae and result in loss of height with kyphosis (dowager's or widow's hump). Scoliosis is also common. There may be recurrent episodes of vertebral collapse at different levels resulting in increasing spine deformity with loss of height.

INVESTIGATIONS

Bone Mineral Analysis

With the advent of bone mass measurement, the fracture risk in osteoporosis can be quantified before the fracture occurs. This is the major advancement in the field of osteoporosis.

The advances in radiological sciences have set in motion the development of various noninvasive, accurate, and sensitive techniques for measuring the mineral content of bone.[7] The various modalities which may be utilized are listed in **Box 1**.

Standard Radiography

Qualitative assessment of bone mineral content from standard radiographs of skeleton is usually based on subjective criteria. The assessment is commonly done on metacarpal, calcaneum, talus, femoral neck, vertebral bodies, etc. The findings are:

- Generalized osteopenia, most prominent in the axial skeleton, especially the vertebral column **(Fig. 1A)**
- Reduces thickness and accentuation of cortex
- Accentuation of primary trabeculae with thinning of secondary trabeculae
- Changes in vertebral body shape—wedge shape, biconcave, and compression **(Fig. 1B)**
- Insufficiency fractures as a result of weakened bone resulting from normal stress. Sacrum, supra-acetabular regions, os pubis, etc., are common sites. The fracture may be occult radiographically and detected on computed tomography (CT) or scintigraphy.
- Fractures at other sites (especially wrist and hip)

The major disadvantage is that it is subjective and gets affected by body habitus, radiographic exposure factors, presence of overlying soft tissue, and patient positioning. Approximately, >30% bone loss must be there to be appreciated on plain radiographs.[3,7]

Magnification radiography by either optical or direct geometric means has a small but significant role in the

Box 1: Various modalities for the detection of osteoporosis.

- Standard radiography
- Radiogrammetry
- Photodensitometry
- Compton scattering
- Neutron activation analysis
- Single and dual photon absorptiometry
- Dual energy X-ray absorptiometry
- Quantitative computed tomography
- Quantitative ultrasound
- Magnetic resonance imaging
- Multidetector computed tomography

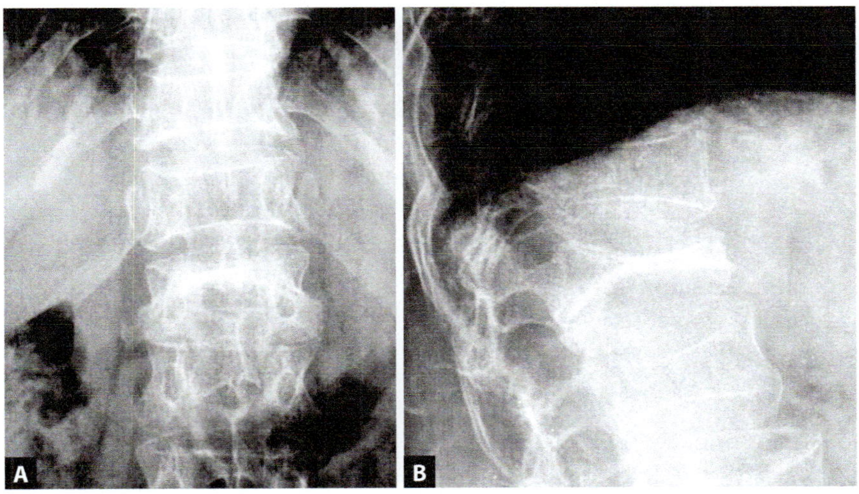

Figs. 1A and B: Radiographs of dorsolumbar spine anteroposterior (A) and lateral (B) views demonstrating decreased bone density with thinning of vertebral endplates, which appear as fine dense lines in contrast to the center of the vertebral body and the presence of multiple biconcave vertebrae.

assessment of osteoporosis. Subperiosteal and intracortical bone absorption, even subtle, may be appreciated on magnification radiography.

Radiogrammetry

Radiogrammetry is one of the simplest methods of quantitative bone mineral assessment. Conventional anteroposterior (AP) radiograph of a tubular bone (like metacarpal) is taken. The cortical thickness on either side of the medullary space is measured with a measuring device, and their sum is expressed as the combined cortical thickness (CCT). This technique is most commonly used at the midshaft of second metacarpal. Cortical bone volume (BV) is calculated from the CCT.[8] This technique is imprecise and insensitive.

Photodensitometry

In this technique, images of bone of interest and of reference aluminum wedge of known density are exposed on the same film. The optical density of the bone is then compared with that of the wedge with a photodensitometer. The information obtained is comparable to that of single-photon absorptiometry but with slightly lower precision, sensitivity, and accuracy.

Neutron Activation Analysis

In this method, neutrons from an accelerator or a reactor bombard a small fraction of the total ^{48}Ca in the body, changing it to ^{49}Ca which is a radioactive isotope. By counting its activity, the total calcium content of the body is estimated. The precision and accuracy are in the order of 2–5%. However, it does not clearly reflect the state of trabecular bone and does not correlate well with spinal mineral measurements. Another disadvantage is a relatively large radiation dose (200–300 mrem).

Compton Scattering

This technique measures the absolute density of a volume of tissue based on its electron density and is the only method other than CT that can measure purely trabecular bone. It is based on the measurement of scattered radiation from a source of 100–700 keV gamma rays and is used for calcaneum, spine, and radius. The precision of this method is about 3–5% and the radiation dose varies from 200 to 2000 mrem. At present, it is largely a research tool.

Single-energy Photon Absorptiometry

Single-energy photon absorptiometry (SPA) technique requires a gamma ray source (^{125}I), a detector, and intervening electronics that measure the beam attenuation through bone and express the result in bone mineral per cm^2 scanned. Usually, the radius is measured at two sites, the mid-diaphysis, which consists of nearly 100% cortical bone, and the distal radial metaphysis, which contains about 75% cortical bone and 25% trabecular bone.

This technique is useful in population studies. The precision of coefficient of variance (CV) of this technique is about 2% and the accuracy about 6% along with low-radiation exposure (<10 mrem). However, because of dosimetric and statistical considerations, the low-energy ^{125}I source cannot be used for body parts thicker than the forearm. A major clinical limitation of this technique, therefore, is that it reflects the status of peripheral long bone and measures primarily the cortex.

Dual-energy Photon Absorptiometry

Dual-energy photon absorptiometry (DPA) technique utilizes a radioisotope that emits photons at two different energy levels. The chief advantage is that the gamma-ray energy of the source is higher (^{153}Gd with photons of 42 and 100 keV) and it has a uniform path length. The lumbar spine from L1 to L4 is usually scanned. This technique yields integral of all minerals within the scan path including the vertebral bodies, endplates, and posterior elements. The major disadvantage is that vertebral compression fractures (VCFs) with callus formation, kyphoscoliosis, articular facet hypertrophy, discogenic sclerosis, marginal osteophytosis, and extraosseous calcification (aorta) are also included in the integral measurement and may result in inaccurate and poorly reproducible vertebral measurements. In healthy subjects, the precision is in the order of 2–3% with accuracy of 4–10% of CV. The usual radiation dose is about 15–20 mrem. It is also used to determine the total body mineral content.

Dual-energy X-ray Absorptiometry

Dual-energy X-ray absorption (DXA) was first described in 1987 and has stood the test of time, representing the most commonly used method of diagnosing osteoporosis in clinical practice. The WHO chose this modality in 1994 for diagnosing osteopenia and osteoporosis. Consequentially, DXA measurements became the standard of reference for the clinical diagnosis of osteoporosis with bone densitometry.[9,10] DXA employs an X-ray beam formed by two different photon energies for generating BMD. Once the high-energy and low-energy photons are transmitted through bones and soft tissue, they are analyzed separately. This is followed by subtraction of the attenuation values of soft tissues with the remainder being the attenuation values of bone. Development in technology has led to significant changes in the DXA equipment. Fan-beam is a wider beam, which has replaced the previously used pencil-thin beam. This, along with a bank of detectors, allows more rapid scanning (approximately 3–5 minutes per site) resulting in better image quality and a high spatial resolution (0.5–0.7 mm).

The variably attenuated X-ray beams received on the detectors are further analyzed and quantified to generate measurements, namely bone mineral content (in grams) at the projected area of the measured site (calculated in square centimeters). BMD is calculated by dividing bone mineral content by the area (expressed in grams/cm^2). BMD is expressed in terms of SD as a T-score and a Z-score.[11] The T-score compares the BMD of the interrogated subject/patient with the mean BMD of a standard young adult individual (between 20 and 30 years of age). The Z-score reflects the difference between the examined BMD of the patient and the mean BMD of age and gender-matched controls. The WHO classifies BMD on the basis of the T-score: with the categories being normal (≥–1.0), osteopenia (<–1.0 but >–2.5), osteoporosis (≤–2.5), and severe osteoporosis (≤–2.5 with a fragility fracture).[12] It should be noted that this definition is applied to DXA measurements made **(Table 2)** in the lumbar spine **(Fig. 2)**, proximal femur **(Fig. 3)**, and forearm. Similar values obtained with other techniques (e.g., quantitative CT) or values similar to DXA measurements made at other anatomic sites (e.g. calcaneus) are not considered in the definition.

Bone mineral density examination serves three principal purposes, namely the diagnosis of osteoporosis, the assessment of patients' risk of fracture, and monitoring response to treatment. BMD is a reasonably strong predictor of fracture risk, reflecting approximately 75–85% of bone strength. It has been found that there is an approximately 1.5 times increase in the fracture risk for each SD decrease of BMD from age-adjusted value.[13,14] Bone density

Table 2: The World Health Organization (WHO) definitions of osteoporosis and osteopenia.

Terminology	*T-score definition*
Normal	$T \geq -1.0$
Osteopenia	$-2.5 < T < -1.0$
Osteoporosis	$T \leq -2.5$
Severe osteoporosis	$T \leq -2.5$ in the presence of one or more fragility fractures

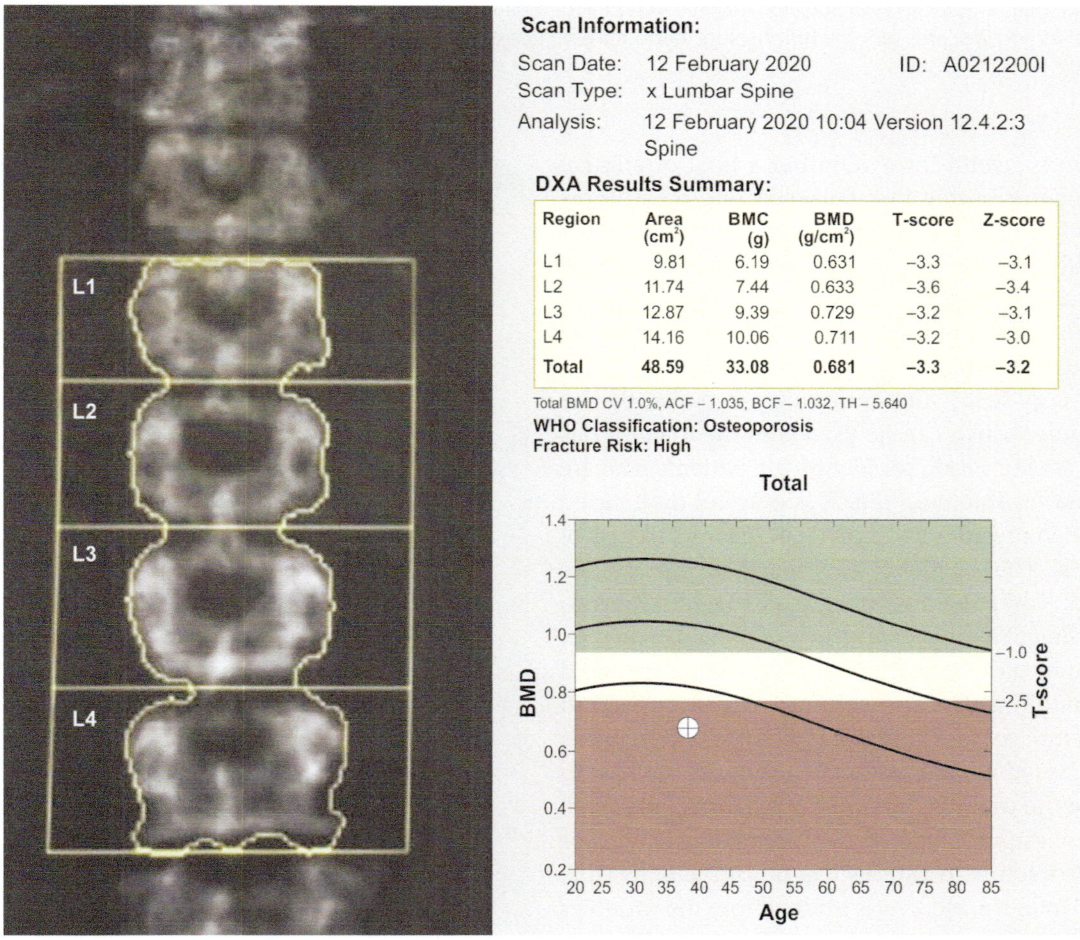

Fig. 2: Axial dual-energy X-ray absorptiometry (DXA) report of a patient demonstrating the L1-L4 vertebrae being interrogated with results generated in the form of T- and Z-scores as well as absolute bone mineral density (BMD) measurements. Graphical display of the BMD serves well for patient understanding. Note that the WHO classification (osteoporosis) and fracture risk (high) have also been interpreted and mentioned based on BMD scores.

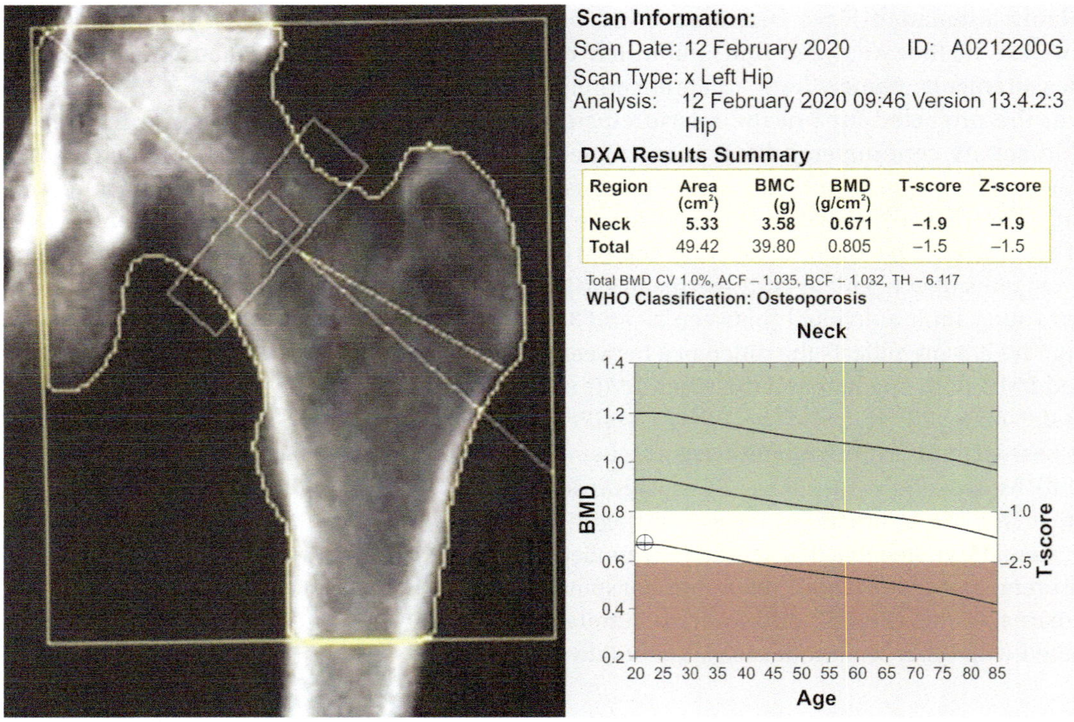

Fig. 3: Femoral dual-energy X-ray absorptiometry (DXA) report of a patient demonstrating the femoral bone being interrogated with generation of T- and Z-scores along with absolute bone mineral density (BMD) measurements. The BMD falls into the category of osteopenia.

examination is useful for evaluating a host of clinical indications contributing to increased bone resorption/faulty bone formation, which has been published by the International Society for Clinical Densitometry (ISCD) and is summarized in **Box 2**.[12]

There are many advantages of central DXA as summarized in **Box 3**.

Dual-energy X-ray absorptiometry is currently the only procedure, which can be used with the fracture risk assessment tool or FRAX, for identifying patients who are at higher risk for fracture.[13] *FRAX* is a useful tool, based on DXA, which provides an estimate of the fracture risk of the individual. The calculation is based on the BMD of the femoral neck;[14] the patient's gender, age, weight, and height; and seven clinical risk factors (history of previous fracture, hip fracture in parent, current smoking, glucocorticoid use, rheumatoid arthritis, secondary osteoporosis, and ingestion of three or more units of alcohol daily). Once this information is fed into the automated software along with the name of the manufacturer of the DXA scanner used, the algorithm estimates the 10-year probability of a major osteoporotic fracture in various regions of the body (hip, spine, distal forearm, etc.). As is evident from the variables used for FRAX generation, FRAX values are different for different ethnicity of population. To cater to our population, Indian data is used to establish age-specified BMD reference range for Indian females and males using

Box 2: Indications for bone mineral density (BMD) testing.[12]

- Women aged 65 years and older
- *For postmenopausal women younger than age 65 years, a bone density test is indicated if they have a risk factor for low bone mass such as:*
  - *Low body weight*
  - *Prior fracture*
  - *High-risk medication use*
  - *Disease or condition associated with bone loss*
- Women during the menopausal transition with clinical risk factors for fracture, such as low body weight, prior fracture, or high-risk medication use
- Men aged 70 years and older.
- *For men <70 years of age, a bone density test is indicated if they have a risk factor for low bone mass such as:*
  - *Low body weight*
  - *Prior fracture*
  - *High-risk medication use*
  - *Disease or condition associated with bone loss*
- Adults with a fragility fracture
- Adults with a disease or condition associated with low bone mass or bone loss
- Adults taking medications associated with low bone mass or bone loss
- Anyone being considered for pharmacologic therapy
- Anyone being treated, to monitor treatment effect
- Anyone not receiving therapy in whom evidence of bone loss would lead to treatment

Women discontinuing estrogen should be considered for bone density testing according to the indications listed above.

DXA.[15] Few studies have shown a lower BMD for Indian population in comparison with age-matched US females, which extends across all age groups.

Apart from axial skeleton (lumbar spine and proximal femur), DXA scan can also be done at peripheral sites such as distal radius and calcaneus. The calcaneus is particularly useful for monitoring changes in BMD secondary to treatment as it contains high percentage (95%) of metabolically active trabecular bone.

Though peripheral DXA (pDXA) is a much easier examination to perform requiring less compact scanners, its fracture predictive ability for vertebral and global fragility fracture risk in postmenopausal women is weaker than central DXA, according to ISCD guidelines. However, pDXA (measurement of radial BMD) in conjunction with clinical risk factors may be useful in screening at the population level for identification of a subset among it with very low fracture probability. This population subset would not require any further diagnostic evaluation. In opposition, central DXA measurements at the spine and femur should be preferentially used for making therapeutic decisions. In conditions where central DXA is not feasible, it is prudent to institute pharmacologic treatment based on radius pDXA if the fracture probability is reasonably high. ISCD has also issued guidelines for use of DXA in children and adolescents.[12] **Table 3** shows comparison of different bone densitometry techniques.

Box 3: Clinical advantages of hip and spine DXA.

- Proven ability to predict fracture risk
- Consensus that BMD results can be interpreted using WHO T-scores
- Proven for effective targeting of antifracture treatments
- Effective for monitoring response to treatment
- Basis of new WHO algorithm for predicting fracture risk
- Short scan times
- Easy patient setup
- Low radiation dose
- Good precision
- Acceptable accuracy
- Availability of reliable reference ranges
- Stable calibration
- Effective instrument quality control procedures

(BMD: bone mineral density; DXA: dual-energy X-ray absorptiometry; WHO: World Health Organization)

Like any other imaging modality, DXA has also got its share of limitations such as limited ability to differentiate cortical and trabecular bone, inability to discriminate between changes due to different bone geometry (e.g., increases in the third dimension), and bone density along with some artifacts. Any hyperdense structure in the immediate vicinity of the bone being interrogated by DXA may induce an artifact and falsely change the generated DXA values, e.g., spinal cord stimulator implant and iodinated contrast in the adjacent colon for a simultaneous CT abdomen examination.[16] Sometimes, a hyperdense foreign structure in immediate contact with the vertebral body may cause it to be mistakenly included in the region of interest (ROI) during estimation of BMD leading to falsely elevated values, e.g., staple and gastric band. A study by Bolotin pointed out inherent fallacies in DXA being contaminated by sizable, unavoidable, inextricable independent soft-tissue contributions leading to erroneous BMD measurements as concerns to the adoption of DXA as a sole medium to describe bone density.[17] Nevertheless, it seems to be the most easily understandable, simple, reproducible imaging modality for BMD estimation currently available.

Quantitative Computed Tomography

Quantitative computed tomography (QCT) is an addition to the field of bone mineral analysis. Quantitative CT differs from DXA in that it has the capability to generate estimates of trabecular and cortical bone BMD as a true volumetric mineral density in mg/cm^3.[18] This method uses a mineral

Table 3: Comparison of different bone densitometry techniques.

	Central DXA	*Peripheral DXA*	*QCT*	*QUS*
Compatible with WHO T-scores	✓	×	×	×
Proven to predict fracture risk	✓	✓	✓	✓
Compatible with new WHO fracture risk algorithm	✓	×	×	×
Proven for effective targeting of treatment	✓	?	?	?
Suitable for patient follow-up	✓	×	✓	×
Stable calibration	✓	✓	✓	×
Good precision	✓	✓	✓	×
Reliable reference ranges available	✓	?	?	?

(DXA: dual energy X-ray absorptiometry; QCT: quantitative computed tomography; QUS: quantitative ultrasound; WHO: World Health Organization)
(✓) Indicates where an alternative technique is known to perform in a comparable manner to central DXA.
(?) Indicates where our knowledge is limited by an absence of suitable studies.
(×) Indicates that alternative types of measurement are definitely unsuitable in these roles.

calibration phantom that is placed in the CT scanner with the patient and provides corrections for machine drifts. A lateral computed radiograph (scout view) is first obtained for localization and then single axial scans are obtained through the midplane of two to four lumbar vertebral bodies **(Figs. 4 and 5)**. Quantitative readings are obtained from a ROI over trabecular bone comprising 3–4 cm^3 of each vertebral body and from four different reference solutions in the phantom. These readings are averaged and used to calculate the mineral density of trabecular bone in mineral equivalents of K_2HPO_4 (mg/cm^3), which subsequently is used for generating T- and Z-scores **(Figs. 6 and 7)**. In addition to estimating the BMD, QCT now can also determine the future risk of osteoporotic fractures.[19]

The precision of this method is 1–3% for single-energy (80 kVp) and 3–5% for dual-energy (80/140 kVp) techniques with an accuracy of 5–10%. The radiation dose is approximately 2 Sv.

The theoretical advantages of QCT[20] over other modalities include: (1) transaxial display of data permitting identification of the anatomy and separate measurement of cortical, cancellous, or integral bone mineral; (2) capability of determining the linear absorption coefficient for a readily defined volume of bone and thereby providing a measure of density, and (3) in the dual-energy mode, the ability to determine mineral content with high accuracy in the presence of variable fat and soft-tissue content.

Quantitative CT serves pretty well for prediction of vertebral fractures in postmenopausal women and for serially measuring bone loss. Its sensitivity is generally considered better than DXA because the trabecular bone located in the center of the vertebral body, which represents the metabolically active bone, is selectively analyzed, unlike in DXA where the entire bone is evaluated. This property of selective assessment of trabecular bone also makes quantitative CT sensitive to detecting BMD changes over short follow-up times. Quantitative CT scores are better than DXA in having the:

- Ability to exclude from the measurement of structures that do not contribute to spine mechanical resistance (which falsely change the DXA values as these cannot be excluded in DXA measurements)
- Capability of selectively measuring various bony segments, namely the trabecular tissue and the most metabolic active tissue which are the main determinants of compressive strength in the vertebrae.[21]

Spine trabecular BMD by QCT can also be used to monitor bone changes related to age, bone disease, and treatment-related changes.[22]

Studies pertaining to fracture prediction using QCT are relatively fewer in number than the ones related to DXA. In postmenopausal females though, QCT of the spine has been found to perform as well as, if not better than, DXA in the prediction of vertebral fractures. However, the prediction of hip fracture by the use of spine QCT is yet not substantiated.[22]

Central DXA measurements in the axial skeleton, namely spine and femur, are the preferred method for making therapeutic decisions and should be used wherever possible.[23] However, high fracture probability as evident on QCT BMD values of the spine in conjunction with clinical risk factors can also be taken into account for instituting pharmacologic treatment. Trabecular BMD of

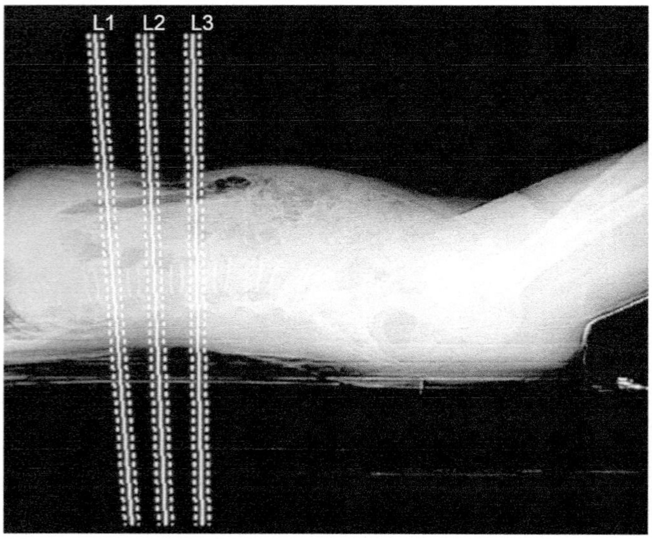

Fig. 4: Lateral topogram (scout view) showing automatic determination of midvertebral slices of L1, L2, and L3.

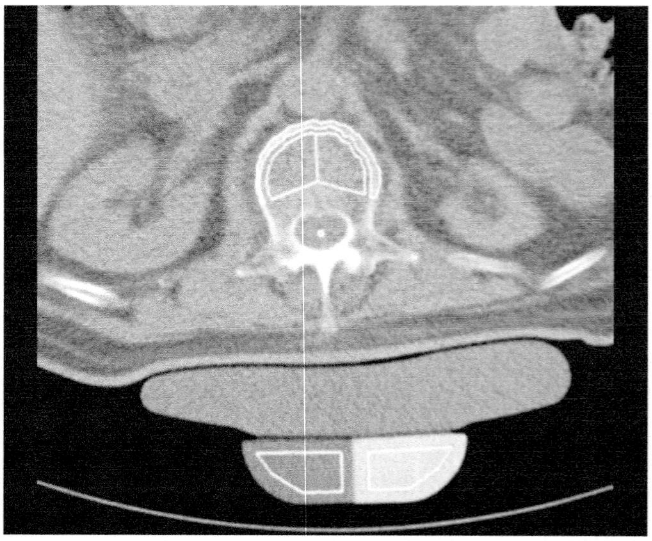

Fig. 5: Midvertebral slice on quantitative computed tomography showing automatic contour determination separating cortical (outer semicircle) and trabecular bone (inner semicircle). Note the phantom and calculation marker.

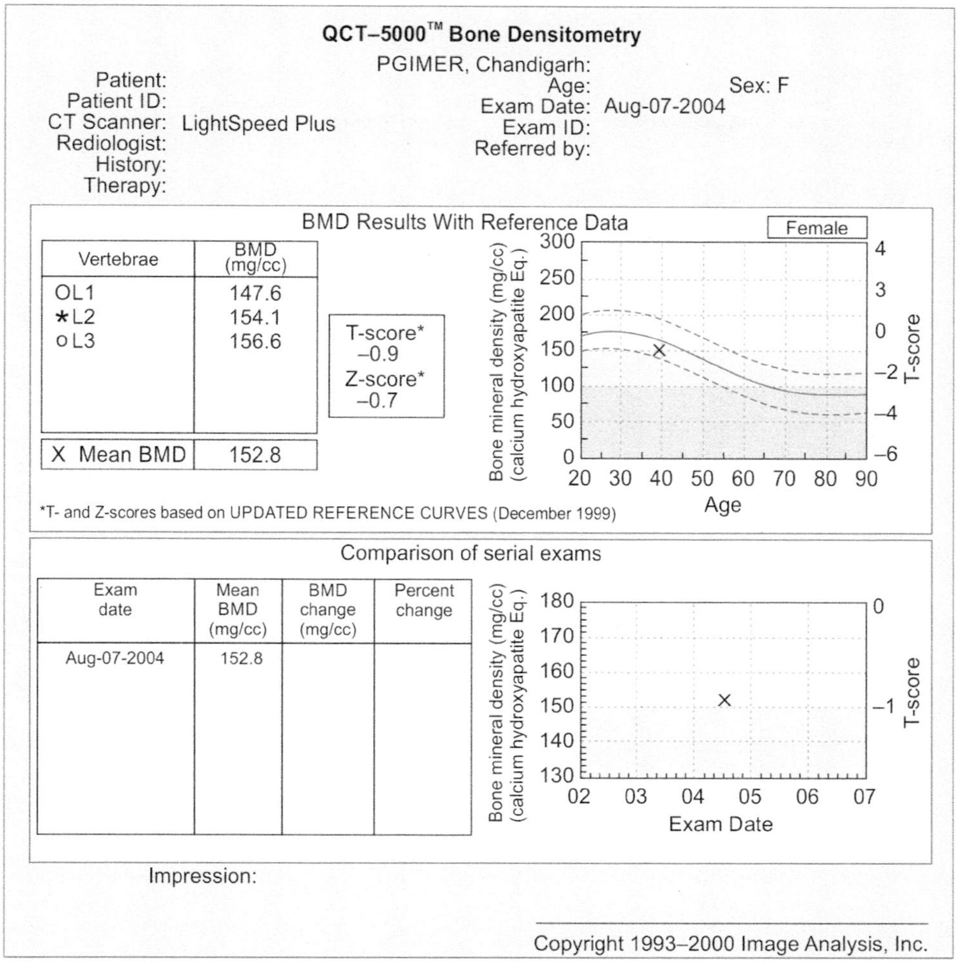

Fig. 6: Quantitative computed tomography (QCT) determination of bone mineral density (BMD) of a normal 36-year-old female with a mean BMD of 152.8 mg/cc with T-score of –0.9 and Z-score of –0.7.

the lumbar spine measured by QCT can be also be used to monitor disease and treatment-related BMD changes and even for assessing the age. The disadvantage of QCT is that the accuracy of BMD decreases to 20–25% in elderly osteoporosis populations.

In a study of 55 patients of prostate cancer who underwent orchidectomy, Agarwal et al. found that a statistical reduction in vertebral trabecular BMD was observed in all patients within 6 months of orchidectomy **(Figs. 8A to C)**.[24] Average BMD decreased by 16.5 ± 8.6 mg/cm^3 (13.8%).

Li et al.[25] evaluated BMD in 140 postmenopausal women for detection of osteoporosis with QCT and DXA in the spine and hip. The detection rate was 17.1% for DXA and 46.4% for QCT ($p < 0.01$). Of the 41 patients with conflicting diagnoses, 7 whose diagnosis by QCT was osteoporosis had vertebral fractures even though their DXA findings did not indicate osteoporosis. QCT thus avoided the overestimation of BMD by DXA. It was thus concluded to have more sensitivity than DXA for detecting osteoporosis in postmenopausal women.

In another study, QCT was compared with DXA in the evaluation of BMD in the lumbar spine. The values generated in both the scanning modalities directly correlated with age. QCT, however, was found to be more efficacious than DXA scan in the diagnosis of osteoporosis, i.e., QCT was better discriminated between normal and osteoporotic subjects than DXA.[26]

Although spinal QCT has many advantages over the DXA technique, it is also fraught with several limitations, the most notable ones being high radiation dose (**Table 4**), poor precision limiting its applicability to longitudinal assessments, higher scanner costs involved, a high degree of operator dependence, and the need for a considerable amount of space. Moreover, it is difficult to assess volumetric BMD of the hip due to its complex shape and inability to generate appropriate phantoms. The WHO definition of osteoporosis of a T-score “at or below” 2.5 applies to DXA of the lumbar spine, femoral neck, total hip, and distal 33% radius. Other sites and modalities are not currently within its ambit due to the fact that DXA provides a composite measurement of integral trabecular and

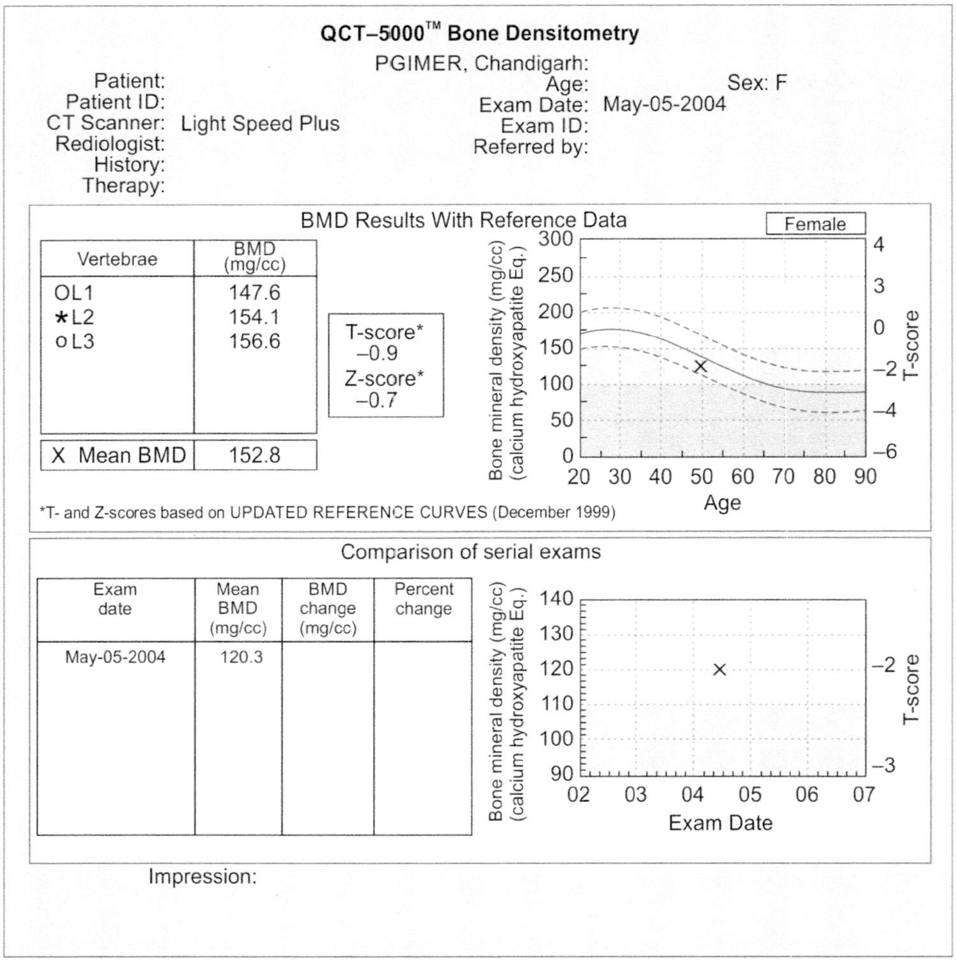

Fig. 7: Quantitative computed tomography (QCT) determination of bone mineral density (BMD) of an osteopenic 50-year-old female with mean BMD of 120.3 mg/cc with T-score of –2.0 and Z-score of –0.7.

cortical bone, while QCT of the lumbar spine measures only the vertebral body trabecular BMD, which is likely to show a more rapid age-dependent decrement than that measured by DXA.[27] Therefore, the WHO criterion of a T-score of "at or below" 2.5 applied to spinal QCT might lead to an earlier diagnosis of osteoporosis and consequently, over-classification of the number of people suffering from the disease.[28] According to one study, individuals with an absolute BMD < 80 mg hydroxyapatite (HA)/cm^3 could be classified as osteoporotic whereas the ones having BMD between 80 and 120 mg/cm^3 may be labeled as having osteopenia.[29]

Over the last decade, technical developments in the CT technique have resulted in development of dedicated peripheral CT scanners, which are smaller, more mobile, and less expensive than whole-body CT scanners to assess peripheral skeletal sites.

A number of bones were assessed previously as part of detection of BMD by peripheral QCT (pQCT). In its current form, it is applied to the nondominant forearm. In view of its lesser radiation-related side effects, pQCT is preferable to central QCT in pediatric patients for assessment of bone development in children.[30,31] Age-related changes can be monitored by pQCT measurement of trabecular and total BMD of the ultradistal radius.

Quantitative Ultrasound

Ultrasound (US) has been successfully used for several years for testing of nonpenetrative materials. Many characteristics, notable ones being scattering capability and US velocity changes, have been used to understand the mechanical competence of various types of material. US variables are speed of sound (SUS) and broadband ultrasound attenuation (BUA). These quantitative ultrasound (QUS) parameters are indirect markers of the material properties of trabecular bone and the degree of fragility of the bones being tested. QUS of bone is performed at substantially lower frequencies, i.e., between 200 and 1.5 MHz, and signals are acquired in the transmission mode. In addition to assessing bone density, these variables reflect parameters such as elasticity and microarchitecture, which are important in assessing fracture risk in osteoporotic subjects. US is currently being

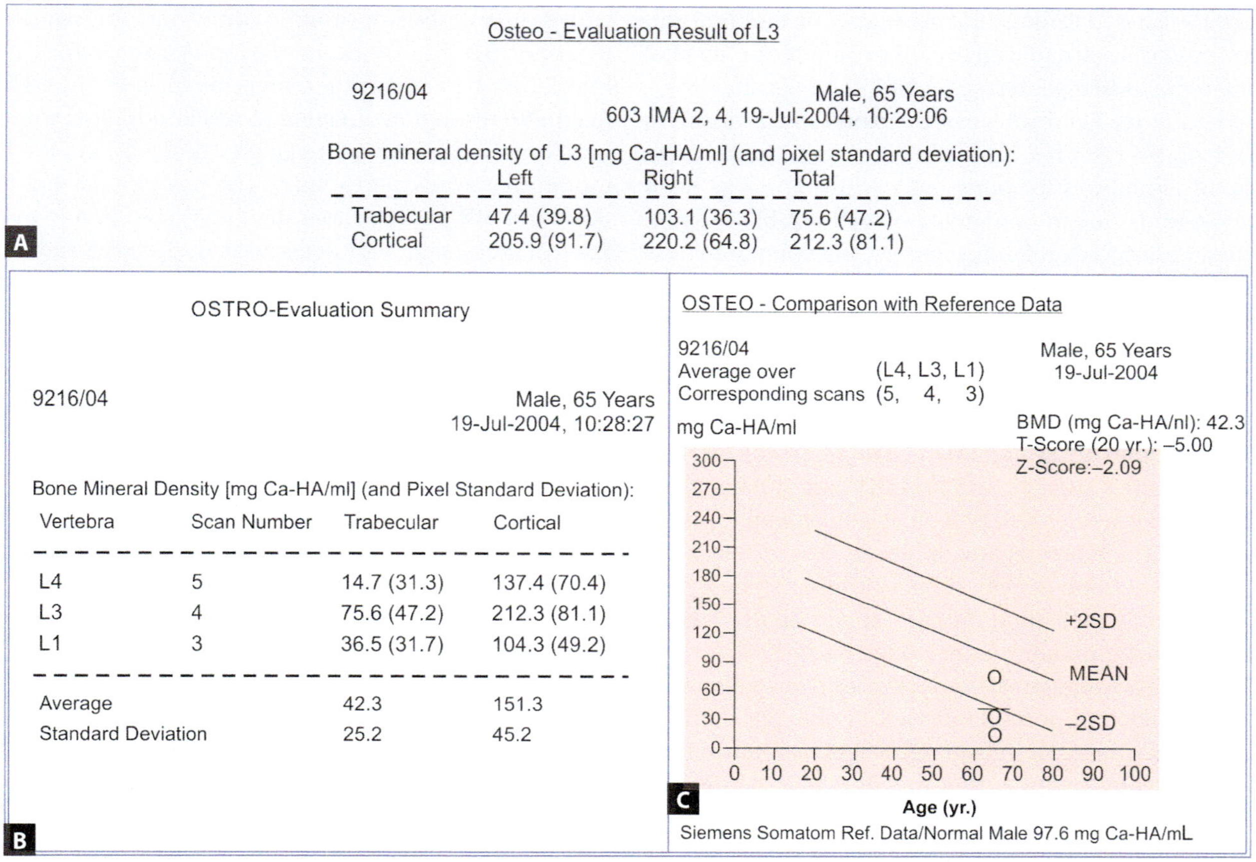

Figs. 8A to C: Quantitative computed tomography determination of bone mineral density of a 65-year-old postorchidectomy male patient at an (A) individual vertebra and (B and C) average of three lumbar vertebrae.

Table 4: Radiation exposure of QCT protocols and other procedures involving ionizing radiation for comparison.

Techniques	*Voltage (kV)*	*Time current product (mAs)*	*Approximate effective dose (mSv)*
Single-slice QCT spine L1–L3 10 mm slice thickness	80	120	<0.2
	120	200	Approximately 1.0
3D QCT spine L1 and L2 (10 cm scan length)	120	100	Approximately 1.5
3D QCT proximal femur (15 cm scan length)	120	200	Approximately 2.5–3
pQCT forearm clinical CT scanner (10 cm scan length)	120	100	<0.01
pQCT forearm/tibia on dedicated single-slice pQCT scanners per slice	<70	<1	<0.003
High-resolution pQCT forearm (XtremeCT) (15 cm scan length)	60	1	<0.005
Annual naturally occurring background radiation (UK)			2.7
Return transatlantic flight			0.08
Chest radiograph			0.02
Lumbar spine radiograph			0.7
CT imaging, e.g., abdomen/pelvis			2.5–4
Radionuclide bone scan			3

(pQCT: peripheral quantitative computed tomography; QCT: quantitative computed tomography)

performed at peripheral sites such as patella, fingers, tibia, and calcaneum. The calcaneum is the most favored site as it is a weight-bearing bone and composed almost entirely of trabecular bone. The US wave is generated by piezoelectric crystals located in the US probe used for scanning, emitted as a sinusoid impulse, and detected once it has passed through the medium. The emitting and receiving probes are placed on either side of the skeletal segment that is being interrogated for bone density.

Quantitative US results can be expressed as absolute values or as T-scores and Z-scores, similar to other forms of modalities for bone evaluation. This has been made possible due to availability of well-established and validated normative reference curves, allowing bone loss to be followed up over time.[32] However, discrepancy has been found in using these parameters for defining bone density according to WHO standards and hence, QUS-related parameters have not found a place in the WHO definition of osteoporosis.

Many studies are available which highlight the fact that the US variables such as SUS and BUA are independent predictors of fractures risk even after adjustment for bone density.[33,34] The false-negative report is up to 10% as the typical sites of bone density such as lumbar spine or hip are not directly measured on QUS. It can be used as an initial screening modality for osteoporosis.[33]

The main advantage of US is lack of ionizing radiation.[35] It is less bulky and portable as well as cheaper than CT or DXA machines. Therefore, QUS has a potential for wider applicability, including preventive screening for osteoporosis. However, the major disadvantage is that there is no standardized method of calibration and expression of measurement results since QUS devices employ diverse technology and different methods of calibration.

Presently, US assessment serves as a screening tool in many centers, with DXA being subsequently done for confirmation of diagnosis in all suspected cases identified. Many studies have demonstrated the utility of quantitative US in predicting osteoporotic fractures of the calcaneus, especially in elderly women aged 65–70 years or older.[36] According to the latest ISCD guidelines for QUS, calcaneus may be used to predict fragility fracture in postmenopausal women (vertebral, hip, and global fracture risk) and men over the age of 65 years (hip and all nonvertebral fractures), independently of central DXA BMD. As highlighted in the recommendations, the combination of heel QUS and clinical risk factors may be used to identify a population at very low fracture probability, which does not warrant any further diagnostic evaluation. In case central DXA is not available as an indicator of BMD, fracture probability information on heel QUS in conjunction with clinical risk factors may be used for instituting pharmacologic treatment. QUS, however, should not be used to monitor the effects of drugs or other forms of therapy on the bony changes in osteoporosis.

High-resolution Bone Imaging

The usefulness of assessing the microarchitectural make-up of bony trabeculae (bone quality) along with mineral density (bone quantity) in the context of osteoporosis cannot be over-emphasized as has been highlighted in a number of publications. Currently, magnetic resonance imaging (MRI) and high-resolution peripheral quantitative imaging (HR-pQCT) are the best modalities available to study the bony make-up. MRI outscores HR-pQCT in that the latter is limited to evaluation of peripheral bony areas, namely the wrist and ankle, while the former can also image other sites, e.g., proximal femur, though with compromised spatial resolution.

Magnetic Resonance Imaging

Magnetic resonance imaging has revolutionized the field of medical imaging with the unique capability of analyzing cortical and trabecular bone in vivo by means of high-resolution images. It is a radiation-free imaging modality and is well-suited for assessing bone structure in a clinical setting. In MRI, bone is usually seen with a negative contrast relative to the high-background signal from bone marrow. Once the images are obtained, segmenting information pertaining to various aspects such as topology, structure, and orientation of the trabecular bone network as well as cortical thickness and area can be done by application of digital postprocessing techniques. The analytical parameters of trabecular and cortical bone are discussed in the following text.

Trabecular bone assessment: Signal-to-noise ratio (SNR) and spatial resolution: Excellent soft-tissue spatial resolution is the hallmark of MRI. Increase in resolution, however, occurs at the expense of SNR, which may compromise the image quality. A balance has to be struck between the two parameters such that the optimal quality of resolution and SNR can be achieved. Li et al. investigated the influence noise and limited spatial resolution on structural parameters.[37] They noted systematic changes in the derived structural parameters with decreasing SNR below a certain threshold. Nevertheless, it became evident that at smaller SNR levels, these errors were correctable by using simple methods such as simple linear transformations. Imaging the peripheral bones has inherent advantages with researchers making considerable efforts to develop trabecular bone imaging of peripheral sites such as the radius, femur, calcaneus, and tibia.[38]

Bone imaging may be performed by using two main types of pulse sequences, namely gradient-echo (GE)-based and spin-echo (SE)-based pulse sequences. Choosing an appropriate sequence depends on the following considerations:

- Higher SNR is provided by a three-dimensional (3D) excitation sequence than a 2D sequence.
- The acquisition of GE should be immediate after the excitation pulse as it would avoid signal loss due to T2 relaxation.
- The acquisition time should be in a clinically feasible range.

The simplest sequence that fulfills the above-mentioned requirements is the basic GE sequence. Further improvements in SNR efficiency are also possible by fully balancing all magnetic gradients during one repetition. The so-called balanced steady-state gradient-echo free precision (bSSFP) pulse sequence optimizes and maximizes SNR efficiency but has a flip side of being susceptible to magnetic field in homogeneities. Krug et al., however, proposed that it may be used to one's advantage.[39] This proved to be a boon for the enhanced visualization of smaller trabeculae, which normally vanish due to partial volume effects. The reason was increased signal cancelation when using bSSFP compared to an SE approach.[40] In the current scheme of things, SSFP has become the sequence of choice among GE-based pulse sequences for trabecular bone imaging due to its high SNR efficiency.[41,42] With the availability of accelerated image acquisition techniques (parallel imaging methods), the imaging time can be remarkably decreased.

Image analysis: The various postprocessing steps involved in image analysis of trabecular bone images in MRI are the correction of the coil sensitivity, outlining of the trabecular bone ROI, and bone/marrow segmentation followed by structural calculations.

Image postprocessing: There are many methods described for extracting structural information from 3D images of the trabecular bone. The final parameter that needs to be determined is bone volume fraction (BVF), which is a ratio of BV to total volume (TV).

Trabecular bone analysis: The various structural parameters required for trabecular bone analysis are topology, scale, and orientation.[43,44] Investigating the plate or rod-like structure of the trabecular network, as is reflective by its name, can assess topology. Scale refers to the volume of bone in a circumscribed ROI with respect to the spacing between the trabeculae or the actual thickness of the trabeculae. The orientation is a marker of the degree of anisotropy of the structure.

The three parameters of scale, topology, and anisotropy can be analyzed by the novel technique of geodesic topological analysis (GTA) described by Carballido-Gamio et al.[45] GTA, which is a measure of bone quality combined with BMD, a bone quantification method, allows for better discrimination than BMD alone [area under the curve (AUC) = 0.95; $p < 0.001$]. It can also be used for treatment monitoring. It should, however, be ensured that the same trabecular sections should be analyzed at baseline and follow-up for detecting microlevel changes in the fine trabecular structure.

Cortical bone assessment using MRI: Cortical bone thickness is an important determinant of the strength of bone as demonstrated by Hyun et al.[46] They have demonstrated significant differences in the cortical thickness of postmenopausal osteopenic versus osteoporotic women, which underscores the importance of geometric measurements of the cortical bone. A study showed that there is an increase in bone water content in the postmenopausal group compared to the premenopausal group.[47] The differential water content may be due to the presence or absence of marrow in the cortical pores. For efficiently imaging the intracortical microstructure, ultra-short echo times (UTE) have to be employed.

Pulse sequences: The 3D fast gradient recalled echo (FGRE) pulse sequence was employed by Hyun et al. for evaluating cortical bone of the distal radius at 1.5 Tesla. They used a slice thickness of 2 mm.[46] Goldenstein et al. used a balanced steady-state free precession (bSSFP) pulse sequence using a dedicated quadrature wrist coil on a 3T MR scanner.[48] The image acquisition resulted in an image resolution of 156 μm × 156 μm × 500 μm. Hyun et al. formulated a semiautomatic segmentation algorithm to measure cortical thickness.[46]

Clinical Applications

Magnetic resonance imaging has found a distinct place in the analysis of almost all regions of the body due to significant technological developments that have taken place in this field in the last couple of decades. Its noninvasive radiation-free nature has added to this effect. Quantitative bone evaluation has proven to be one of its key uses currently and with the ability to provide structural information, it can contribute to fracture discrimination in unison with BMD estimation. Wehrli et al. demonstrated that MRI-based topological bone parameters had better capability to discriminate fracture group from nonfracture group than BMD alone.[49] Many researchers are of the opinion that MRI-based in vivo analysis of trabecular bone can be used as a potential tool for monitoring osteoporosis treatment. However till now, no recommendations are there from ISCD to use it in diagnosis of osteoporosis, prediction of fracture risk, or monitoring of treatment.

High-resolution Peripheral Quantitative Computed Tomography

There has been ongoing work on dedicated peripheral body scanners, being less bulky and possibly more cost-effective in specific scenarios. A dedicated extremity imaging scanner has been designed for trabecular-scale imaging. It is seen to generate higher SNR and spatial resolution compared to multidetector CT (MDCT) and MRI. The radiation is limited to the interrogated body part, namely the extremity not involving critical, radiosensitive organs, and is considerably lower compared to whole-body CT.

However, its major limitation is evaluation of only peripheral skeletal sites. Moreover, presently only a limited number of devices are installed.

Image acquisition scan setup: Due to its limited presence in a clinical setup, a fixed manufacturer-recommended scan protocol needs to be run for generation of optimal results.[50] The protocols have, however, been modified to suit the differences in patient sizes and to avoid radiation exposure to epiphyseal growth plate in evaluating children. Smaller field of view (FOV) (approximately 12–13 cm) is used for optimum imaging. The dataset acquired is reconstructed using a modified Feldkamp algorithm, yielding submillimeter isotropic voxels.[51] The total scan time is around 3 minutes with a significantly attenuated radiation dose (approximately 4.2 μSv), which is remarkably less than a body CT scan and is comparable to DXA.

Image analysis and postprocessing: The dataset obtained is analyzed using a standard manufacturer-provided protocol, which includes segmentation and approximate contour delineation. The cortical bone is segmented using a 3D Gaussian smoothing filter. This component is subtracted digitally from the periosteal contour to generate the trabecular compartment. Using beam-hardening correction and phantom calibration procedures, the linear attenuation values of the tomographic images are converted to HA mineral densities, which are used for designating bone details of that region.

Morphometric analysis: The high isotropic resolution of HR-pQCT (82 μm) permits direct, 3D assessment of important measurements such as intertrabecular distances, trabecular number, average trabecular thickness, and bone volume fraction (BV/TV) which is in contradistinction to CT and MRI, which base the measurements on large-slice thickness relative to the in-plane resolution.

According to ISCD, pQCT of the forearm at the ultradistal radius is a useful predictor of fragility fractures of the hip in postmenopausal females. This value, however, does not hold true for spinal fractures.

Multidetector Computed Tomography

Spiral CT generates densitometric data, which is used to assess mass lesions. Efforts are being made to use this data to assess BMD in the lumbar spine. A recent study calculated BMD from spiral CT data by using equation BMD = 0.77 × mean BMD MDCT, where mean BMD on MDCT is the average of densities of L1 to L3 vertebrae as calculated on spiral CT and 0.77 is the conversion factor. They found significant correlation between BMD data obtained from spiral CT and QCT.[52] Few studies have in fact demonstrated that MDCT depicted trabecular microarchitecture of the dorsal spine outscored BMD obtained by DXA in identifying patients with vertebral fractures from those who did not.[53]

In addition, the advent of MDCT enabled trabecular analysis of the hip (which is a clinically important site of fracture). However, a high radiation dose remains a matter of concern.

MACHINE-BASED ARTIFICIAL INTELLIGENCE IN PREDICTING BONE MINERAL DENSITY

Artificial intelligence has had a significant role to play in the field of medical sciences in the recent past. With the stupendous increase in the performance of machine-learning algorithms, the scope of technology in the diagnosis, prediction, and even management of various disorders in medicine has shown a phenomenal rise. On similar lines, there has been a surge in the models for prediction of BMD using basic imaging modalities such as US and CT by using deep learning methods.[54-56] The bone fragility can be analyzed based upon vertebral bone attenuation on CT done for other indications.[57]

Several newer methods have been described for prediction of fracture risk in osteoporosis along with models to help with the identification and segmentation of bone images from a host of imaging modalities, namely acoustics, MRI, CT, and radiographs.[58]

Radiomics is playing a leading role in developing predictive models to classify osteoporosis, osteopenia, and normal patients in susceptible population. Panoramic dental radiographs,[59] spine radiographs, and CT (lumbar, femoral trochanteric, intertrochanteric, and neck)[60] images have been used as substrates for application of feature selection and classification methods to generate models of osteoporosis classification based on bone mineral densitometry image features.

INTERVENTIONAL MANAGEMENT OF OSTEOPOROTIC COMPRESSION FRACTURES—PERCUTANEOUS VERTEBROPLASTY

Treatment of acute osteoporotic fractures has been largely conservative, with medical therapy emphasizing pain control using various analgesics and anti-inflammatory medications in combination with immobilization.[61] Vertebroplasty aims to alleviate pain and improve mobility, with the secondary goal of stabilizing the vertebral body. Klazen et al. have shown that vertebroplasty outperformed conservative management with significantly greater pain relief.[62] Another large study concluded that percutaneous vertebroplasty was considerably effective in relieving pain associated with osteoporosis-induced VCFs, and the analgesic effect of the procedure was long lasting.[63] The outcome of single-level vertebroplasty is not dependent on the age of the vertebral fracture, with good outcomes noted among acute, subacute, and chronic stages.[64]

Indications

Percutaneous vertebroplasty can be offered for the following indications:

- Painful VCF refractory to medical therapy
- Painful VCF associated with osteonecrosis (Kümmell's disease)
- Unstable VCF that demonstrates mobility at the wedge deformity
- Conditions which warrant reinforcement of the vertebral body or pedicle, before a posterior surgical stabilization procedure or interbody fusion, in patients with osteoporosis
- Although routine prophylactic treatment is not advocated, unaffected vertebra in patients with multiple compressions in whom further collapse may lead to pulmonary compromise as a result of kyphosis may rarely be considered for vertebroplasty

Conservative medical therapy still forms the frontline management of osteoporotic VCFs with intractable pain, in spite of optimum medical management, forming the prime clinical criteria for performing vertebroplasty. Some operators avoid treating patients who have >20–30% spinal canal compromise from retropulsed fracture fragments.[61] Vertebroplasty in such cases may aggravate spinal stenosis and may even lead to compressive myeloradiculopathy.

Procedure

The procedure is done under conscious sedation under fluoroscopy/CT/CT-fluoroscopy guidance. The patient is placed prone on the fluoroscopic/CT table. A vertebroplasty needle (11/13G needle with biopsy set) is introduced under fluoroscopic guidance through the pedicle into the involved vertebral body up to the junction of anterior third and posterior two-thirds and bone cement, an acrylic polymer—PMMA (polymethylmethacrylate), is injected with the aim of almost completely filling the osteoporotic collapsed vertebral body, care being taken not to have any spillage beyond the posterior margin of the vertebral body **(Figs. 9A to F)**.

Postprocedure Care

Nowadays, the procedure is routinely being done on an outpatient basis, with a 2-hour observation period after vertebroplasty. Focal pain at the puncture sites may last 2 for days, which usually responds to analgesics.

Complications

The complication rate of vertebroplasty procedure ranges from 1 to 10% with higher rates being reported in the treatment of neoplastic collapse than the osteoporotic collapse.

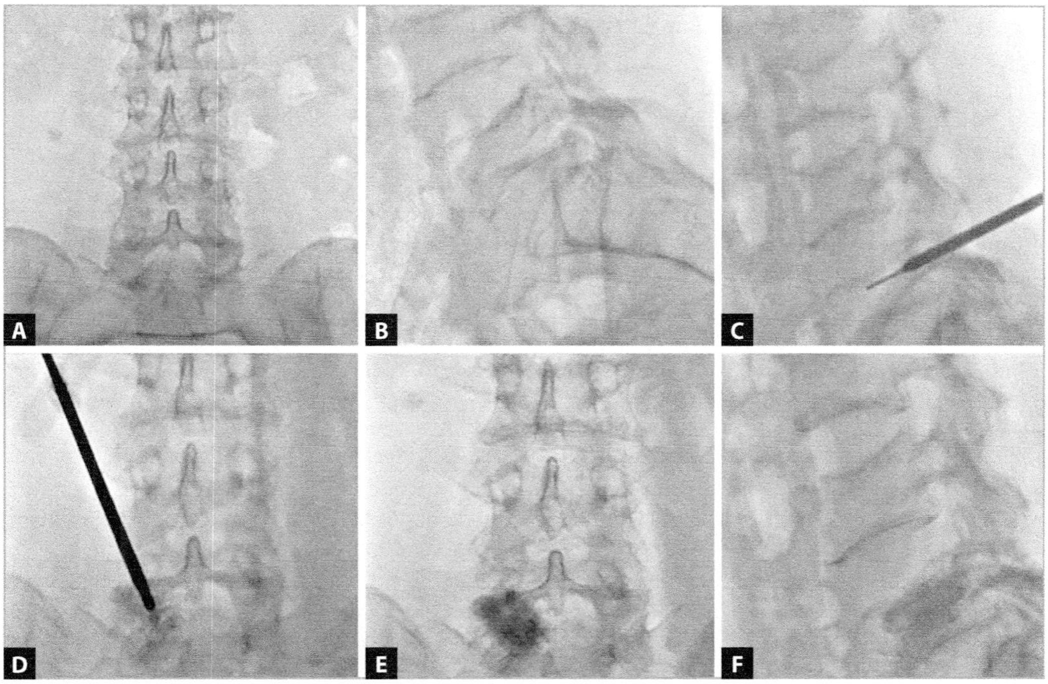

Figs. 9A to F: Vertebroplasty. (A) Anteroposterior; and (B) Lateral lumbar spine radiographs showing L5 vertebral body collapse; (C and D) Percutaneous transpedicular insertion of the cannula with injection of polymethylmethacrylate cement; (E) Anteroposterior; and (F) Lateral radiographs demonstrating the bone cement.

- Extravasation of PMMA into the adjoining structures due to vertebral cortical destruction/fracture, causing nerve root/spinal cord compression
- Injection into vertebral venous plexus leading to pulmonary embolism
- Rib fracture
- Fracture of the pedicle or transverse process
- Paravertebral hemorrhage
- Epidural infection (abscess formation)
- Sedation-related adverse effects, namely seizure/respiratory arrest
- Swallowing difficulties from esophageal compression in a cervical vertebroplasty
- Death from massive PMMA pulmonary embolization

There were initial concerns that there may be a potential for increased risk of fractures at an adjacent level following vertebroplasty. However, many studies have proved otherwise.[65] Many workers postulate that these new fractures are more likely to be the result of natural history of osteoporosis rather than the imbalance created secondary to vertebroplasty.

Bone health is an important component of the overall health of the human body. With the better understanding of the bone morphology and various means to identify reduced bone density, there has been an impetus toward improvement in bone health of the population to prevent the morbidity associated with various fractures.

REFERENCES

1. Assessment of fracture risk and its application to screening for postmenopausal osteoporosis. Report of a WHO Study Group. Geneva, World Health Organization, 1994 (WHO Technical Report Series, No. 843).
2. Kanis JA. Diagnosis of osteoporosis and assessment of fracture risk. Lancet. 2002;359(9321):1929-36.
3. Lane JM, Riley EH, Wirganowicz PZ. Osteoporosis: diagnosis and treatment. JBJS. 1996;78-A:618-31.
4. NIH Consensus Development Panel on Osteoporosis Prevention, Diagnosis, and Therapy. Osteoporosis prevention, diagnosis, and therapy. JAMA. 2001;285(6):785-95.
5. Fitzpatrick LA. Secondary causes of osteoporosis. Mayo Clin Proc. 2002;77:453-68.
6. Jergas M, Gluer CC. Assessment of fracture risk by bone density measurements. Semin Nuclear Med. 1997;27(3):261-75.
7. Sartoris DJ, Resuik D. Current and innovative methods for noninvasive bone densitometry. RCNA. 1990;28(2):257-78.
8. Bach-Mortensen P, Hyldstrup L, Appleyard M, Hindsø K, Gebuhr P, Sonne-Holm S. Digital X-ray radiogrammetry identifies women at risk of osteoporotic fracture: results from a prospective study. Calcif Tissue Int. 2006;79(1):1-6.
9. Kanis JA, on behalf of the World Health Organization Scientific Group. Assessment of osteoporosis at the primary healthcare level: technical report. University of Sheffield, UK: World Health Organization Collaborating Centre for Metabolic Bone Diseases; 2008.
10. Kanis JA. An update on the diagnosis of osteoporosis. Curr Rheumatol Rep. 2000;2(1):62-6.
11. Blake GM, Fogelman I. The clinical role of dual energy X-ray absorptiometry. Eur J Radiol. 2009;71:406-14.
12. International Society of Clinical Densitometry (ISCD) (2013). Official positions of the International Society for Clinical Densitometry. [online] Available from https://www.iscd.org/official-positions/2013-iscd-official-positions-adult/ [Last accessed March, 2020].
13. World Health Organization. FRAX WHO fracture risk assessment tool. [online] Available from https://www.sheffield.ac.uk/FRAX/index.aspx.
14. Kanis JA, McCloskey EV, Johansson H, Oden A, Ström O, Borgström F. Development and use of FRAX in osteoporosis. Osteoporos Int. 2010;21(Suppl 2):S407-S413.
15. Marwaha RK, Tandon N, Kaur P, Sastry A, Bhadra K, Narang A, et al. Establishment of age-specified bone mineral density reference range for Indian females using dual-energy X-ray absorptiometry. J Clin Densitom. 2012;15(2):241-9.
16. Spiro AJ, Hoang TD, Shakir MK. Artifacts affecting dual-energy X-ray absorptiometry measurements. AACE Clin Case Rep. 2019;5(4):e263-6.
17. Bolotin HH. DXA in vivo BMD methodology: An erroneous and misleading research and clinical gauge of bone mineral status, bone fragility, and bone remodelling. Bone. 2007;41(1):138-54.
18. Cann CE. Quantitative CT for determination of bone mineral density—a review. Radiology. 1988;166:509-22.
19. Ryan PJ. Overview of role of BMD measurements in managing osteoporosis. Semin Nuclear Med. 1997;27(3):197-209.
20. Sartoris DJ. Clinical value of bone densitometry. AJR. 1994;163:133-5.
21. Engelke K, Adams JE, Armbrecht G, Augat P, Bogado CE, Bouxsein ML, et al. Clinical use of quantitative computed tomography and peripheral quantitative computed tomography in the management of osteoporosis in adults: the 2007 ISCD Official Positions. J Clin Densitom. 2008;11(1):123-62.
22. Ito M, Hayashi K, Ishida Y, Uetani M, Yamada M, Ohki M, et al. Discrimination of spinal fracture with various bone mineral measurements. Calcif Tissue Int. 1997;60(1):11-5.
23. Grampp S, Jergas M, Wang P, et al. Quantitative CT assessment of the lumbar spine and radius in patients with osteoporosis. AJR. 1996;167:133-40.
24. Agarwal MM, Mandal AK, Khandelwal N, Singh SK. Need for measurement of bone mineral density in patients of prostate cancer before and after orchidectomy: role of quantitative computer tomography. J Assoc Physicians India. 2007;55:486-90.
25. Li N, Li XM, Xu L, Sun WJ, Cheng XG, Tian W. Comparison of QCT and DXA: Osteoporosis Detection Rates in Postmenopausal Women. Int J Endocrinol. 2013;2013:895474.
26. Bansal SC, Khandelwal N, Rai DV, Sen R. Comparison between the QCT and the DEXA scanners in the

evaluation of BMD in the lumbar spine. J Clin Diagn Res. 2011;5(4):694-9.
27. Miller P. Controversies in bone mineral density diagnostic classification. Calcif Tiss Int. 2000;66:317-9.
28. Faulkner R, von Stetten E, Miller P. Discordance in patient classification using T-scores. J Clin Densitom. 1999;2:343-50.
29. Felsenberg D, Gowin W. Bone densitometry by dual energy methods. Radiology. 1999;39(3):186-93.
30. Zemel B, Bass S, Binkley T, Ducher G, MacDonald H, MacKay H, et al. Peripheral quantitative computed tomography in children and adolescents. J Clin Densitom. 2008;11(1):59-74.
31. Brennan BM, Mughal Z, Roberts SA, Ward K, Shalet SM, Eden TO, et al. Bone mineral density in childhood survivors of acute lymphoblastic leukemia treated without cranial irradiation. J Clin Endocrinol Metab. 2005;90:689-94.
32. Ekman A, Michaëlsson K, Petrén-Mallmin M, Ljunghall S, Mallmin H. Dual X-ray absorptiometry of hip, heel ultrasound, and densitometry of fingers can discriminate male patients with hip fracture from control subjects: A comparison of four different methods. J Clin Densitom. 2002;5(1):79-85.
33. Langton CM, Langton DK. Comparison of bone mineral density and quantitative ultrasound of the calcaneus: Site matched correlation and discrimination of axial BMD status. BJR. 2000;73:31-5.
34. Cepollaro C, Gonnelli S, Pondrelli C, Martini S, Montagnani A, Rossi S, et al. The combined use of ultrasound and densitometry on the prediction of vertebral fractures. BJR. 1997;70:691-6.
35. Huda W, Morin RL. Patients doses in bone mineral densitometry. BJR. 1996;69:422-5.
36. Khaw KT, Reeve J, Luben R, Bingham S, Welch A, Wareham N, et al. Prediction of total and hip fracture risk in men and women by quantitative ultrasound of the calcaneus: EPIC-Norfolk prospective population study. Lancet. 2004;363(9404):197-202.
37. Li CQ, Magland JF, Rajapakse CS, Guo XE, Zhang XH, Vasilic B, et al. Implications of resolution and noise for in vivo micro-MRI of trabecular bone. Med Phys. 2008;35:5584-94.
38. Krug R, Banerjee S, Han ET, Newitt DC, Link TM, Majumdar S. Feasibility of in vivo structural analysis of high-resolution magnetic resonance images of the proximal femur. Osteoporos Int. 2005;16:1307-14.
39. Krug R, Han ET, Banerjee S, Majumdar S. Fully balanced steady-state 3D-spin-echo (bSSSE) imaging at 3 Tesla. Magn Reson Med. 2006;56:1033-40.
40. Krug R, Carballido-Gamio J, Burghardt AJ, Kazakia G, Hyun BH, Jobke B, et al. Assessment of trabecular bone structure comparing magnetic resonance imaging at 3 Tesla with high-resolution peripheral quantitative computed tomography ex vivo and in vivo. Osteoporos Int. 2008;19:653-61.
41. Krug R, Stehling C, Kelley DA, Majumdar S, Link TM. Imaging of the musculoskeletal system in vivo using ultra-high field magnetic resonance at 7 T. Invest Radiol. 2009;44:613-8.
42. Kazakia GJ, Hyun B, Burghardt AJ, Krug R, Newitt DC, de Papp AE, et al. In vivo determination of bone structure in postmenopausal women: a comparison of HR-pQCT and high-field MR imaging. J Bone Miner Res. 2008;23:463-74.
43. Wehrli FW, Song HK, Saha PK, Wright AC. Quantitative MRI for the assessment of bone structure and function. NMR Biomed. 2006;19:731-64.
44. Wehrli FW. Structural and functional assessment of trabecular and cortical bone by micro magnetic resonance imaging. J Magn Reson Imaging. 2007;25:390-409.
45. Carballido-Gamio J, Krug R, Huber MB, Hyun B, Eckstein F, Majumdar S, et al. Geodesic topological analysis of trabecular bone microarchitecture from high-spatial resolution magnetic resonance images. Magn Reson Med. 2009;61:448-56.
46. Hyun B, Newitt DC, Majumdar S. Assessment of Cortical Bone Structure Using High-Resolution Magnetic Resonance Imaging. Proceedings 13th Scientific Meeting, International Society for Magnetic Resonance in Medicine; Miami; 2005.
47. Techawiboonwong A, Song HK, Leonard MB, Wehrli FW. Cortical bone water: in vivo quantification with ultrashort echo- time MR imaging. Radiology. 2008;248:824-33.
48. Goldenstein J, Kazakia G, Majumdar S. In vivo evaluation of the presence of bone marrow in cortical porosity in postmenopausal osteopenic women. Ann Biomed Eng. 2010;38(2):235-46.
49. Wehrli FW, Gomberg BR, Saha PK, Song HK, Hwang SN, Snyder PJ. Digital topological analysis of in vivo magnetic resonance microimages of trabecular bone reveals structural implications of osteoporosis. J Bone Miner Res. 2001;16:1520-31.
50. Laib A, Hauselmann HJ, Ruegsegger P. In vivo high resolution 3D-QCT of the human forearm. Technol Health Care. 1998;6:329-37.
51. Feldkamp LA, Davis LC, Kress JW. Practical cone-beam algorithm. J Opt Soc Am A. 1984;1:612-9.
52. Thomas ML, Boris BK, Thomas L, Bauer J, Lu Y, Rummeny EJ. *In vitro* and *in vivo* spiral CT to determine bone mineral density: initial experience in patients at risk for osteoporosis. Radiology. 2004;231:805-11.
53. Ito M, Ikeda K, Nishiguchi M, Shindo H, Uetani M, Hosoi T, Orimo H, et al. Multidetector row CT imaging of vertebral microstructure for evaluation of fracture risk. J Bone Miner Res. 2005;20(10):1828-36.
54. Nakamoto T, Hatsuta S, Yagi S, Verdonschot RG, Taguchi A, Kakimoto N. Computer-aided diagnosis system for osteoporosis based on quantitative evaluation of mandibular lower border porosity using panoramic radiographs. Dentomaxillofac Radiol. 2020;20190481.
55. Pahr DH, Zysset PK. Finite element-based mechanical assessment of bone quality on the basis of in vivo images. Curr Osteoporos Rep. 2016;14(6):374-85.
56. Yasaka K, Akai H, Kunimatsu A, Kiryu S, Abe O. Prediction of bone mineral density from computed tomography: application of deep learning with a convolutional neural network. Eur Radiol. 2020;10.1007/s00330-020-06677-0.
57. Kim YW, Kim JH, Yoon SH, Lee JH, Lee CH, Shin CS, et al. Vertebral bone attenuation on low-dose chest

CT: quantitative volumetric analysis for bone fragility assessment. Osteoporos Int. 2017;28(1):329-38.
58. Ferizi U, Honig S, Chang G. Artificial intelligence, osteoporosis and fragility fractures. Curr Opin Rheumatol. 2019;31(4):368-75.
59. Lee KS, Jung SK, Ryu JJ, Shin SW, Choi J. Evaluation of transfer learning with deep convolutional neural networks for screening osteoporosis in dental panoramic radiographs. J Clin Med. 2020;9(2):E392.
60. Rastegar S, Vaziri M, Qasempour Y, Akhash MR, Abdalvand N, Shiri I, et al. Radiomics for classification of bone mineral loss: a machine learning study [published online ahead of print, 2020 Feb 4]. Diagn Interv Imaging. 2020;pii: S2211-5684(20)30025-5.
61. Jensen ME, Dion JE. Percutaneous vertebroplasty in the treatment of osteoporotic compression fractures. Neuroimag Clin North Am. 2000;10(3):547-68.
62. Klazen CA, Lohle PN, de Vries J, Jansen FH, Tielbeek AV, Blonk MC, et al. Vertebroplasty versus conservative treatment in acute osteoporotic vertebral compression fractures (Vertos II): an open-label randomised trial. Lancet. 2010;376(9746):1085-92.
63. Tanigawa N, Kariya S, Komemushi A, Nakatani M, Yagi R, Kohzai M, et al. Percutaneous vertebroplasty for osteoporotic compression fractures: long-term evaluation of the technical and clinical outcomes. AJR. 2011;196: 1415-8.
64. Rad AE, Kallmes DF. Correlation between preoperative pain duration and percutaneous vertebroplasty outcome. Am J Neuroradiol. 2011;32:1842-5.
65. Yang W, Yang J, Liang M. Percutaneous Vertebroplasty Does Not Increase the Incidence of New Fractures in Adjacent and Nonadjacent Vertebral Bodies. Clin Spine Surg. 2019;32(2):E99-E106.

SECTION

4

Focal Bone Lesions and Bone Marrow Imaging

CHAPTER

12

Diagnostic Approach to Focal Bone Lesions

Shivanand Gamanagatti, Raju Sharma

INTRODUCTION

Plain radiography remains the first-line choice of imaging modality for the initial evaluation of a bone lesion following clinical examination. Radiographs can be obtained quickly, easily, and at low cost. At least two views of the affected bone including anteroposterior and lateral views are usually adequate for the assessment of an osseous abnormality. Computed tomography (CT) and magnetic resonance imaging (MRI) provide complimentary information that is extremely useful in the work-up of focal bone lesion. CT scan is particularly useful in evaluating the cortex and matrix. MRI is useful in determining the intramedullary extent and soft tissue extent of focal bone lesion, and also plays a vital role in detecting skip lesions.[1]

A methodical approach is essential for the evaluation of bone tumors, with particular consideration to the location, multiplicity, margins, zone of transition, type of periosteal reaction, matrix mineralization, cortical integrity, and presence of a soft-tissue component. However, it becomes difficult to define the exact origin of a skeletal lesion in small bones of hand and foot, because whole width of the bone may get involved. It becomes challenging to establish whether the lesion is arising from medullary cavity, cortex, or is juxtacortical.

GENERAL PRINCIPLES OF FOCAL BONE LESION EVALUATION

- Prior to the analysis of the radiographic features of focal bone lesion, certain clinical information is essential to narrow down the differential diagnosis, such as age of the patient, the location of the lesion, and is it single or multiple?
- Within long bones, plane of the lesion must be determined with reference to long axis (epiphysis, metaphysis, and diaphysis) and horizontal axis (medullary, cortical, and juxtacortical). Juxtacortical lesions may be parosteal or periosteal.
- Radiograph is essential for lesion detection and characterization. Radiograph should be systematically assessed for:
  - Type of bone destruction
  - Margins/transition zone
  - Cortical status
  - Type of matrix mineralization
  - Type of periosteal reaction
  - Presence or absence of soft tissue component
  - Lesion number (single or multiple)
- The bone lesion can be classified as nonaggressive or aggressive from its radiographic appearance.
- Nonaggressive versus aggressive pattern on radiograph is not always equivalent to benign versus malignant, e.g., osteomyelitis can have an aggressive pattern on radiograph.
- Do not "overdiagnose" a benign bone tumor and do not "underdiagnose" a malignant bone tumor.
- Do not misdirect the biopsy approach to the lesion so as to convert more conservative operation (compartment resection or limb salvage procedure) into more radical operation (amputation).
- Any skeletal lesion detected on a well-penetrated radiograph rule out infection, eosinophilic granuloma, subchondral degenerative cyst, lesion related to metabolic bone disease such as Brown tumor, post-traumatic changes such as stress fracture or is it normal variant.
- If the lesion is unchanged from old films (at least 2 years old), then consider for a clinical/radiographic follow-up of the patient.
- If there are multiple lesions, rule out metastases, especially in adults or other causes of multiple skeletal lesions such as multiple enchondromas, multiple osteochondromas, fibrous dysplasia, fibrous cortical defects/nonossifying fibromas, and sarcoidosis.
- If there is solitary lesion, characterize the lesion further based on age, location, pattern of destruction, margins, cortical response, matrix, and periosteal reaction.

AGE OF THE PATIENT

Most bone tumors have a predilection for a specific age group; therefore, patient's age is an important clinical information while assessing a bone tumor. Typical peak ages of different lesions are listed in **Table 1**. For example, simple bone cysts (SBCs) and chondroblastomas occur in skeletally immature people, while giant cell tumors (GCTs) occur in skeletally mature people. Ewing's sarcoma typically

Table 1: Bone tumors predilection for specific age groups.

	0–10	10–20	20–30	30–40	40–50	>50
Metastatic neuroblastoma	<2 years					
Simple bone cyst	▨	▨				
Fibrous cortical defect	▨	▨				
Aneurysmal bone cyst	▨	▨				
Ewing's sarcoma		■				
Osteosarcoma		■				
Giant cell tumor			▨	▨		
Chondrosarcoma				■	■	■
Multiple myeloma						■
Metastasis						■

occurs in 10–20-year-old patients, while conventional osteosarcoma has two age peaks, one, arising de novo, in teenagers and the second, arising in background of Paget's disease or previously irradiated bone, in adults older than 50 years. A malignant bone lesion in an adult over 40 years old is much more likely to be metastatic carcinoma, myeloma, or metastatic non-Hodgkin lymphoma rather than a primary bone sarcoma.[2]

LOCATION OF LESION (FIG. 1)

Most bone tumors, regardless of whether they are benign or malignant, often occur in a characteristic location in the skeleton (i.e., axial vs. appendicular skeleton or long vs. flat bone). Thus, some tumors (e.g., osteosarcoma) have a predilection for sites of rapid bone growth, usually the metaphyseal region, while other tumors (e.g., Ewing's sarcoma) tend to follow the distribution of red marrow. Furthermore, lesions such as enchondroma in a long bone are usually located centrally within the medullary cavity, while an aneurysmal bone cyst is located eccentrically in the medullary cavity **(Fig. 1)**. However, in short or thin tubular bones, such as the metacarpals, metatarsals, phalanges, and fibula, the entire diameter of the bone can be involved, sometimes making it difficult to determine in which part of the bone the lesion originated. An apophysis (a growth center that does not contribute to the length of a bone) is the equivalent of an epiphysis (a growth center at the end of a bone that does contribute to length); thus, one should use the "end-of-bone" differential list for a lesion in such sites as the greater trochanter of the femur and the tibial tubercle **(Fig. 1)**. Similarly, other growth centers such as the patella; the small bones of the wrist, hindfoot, and midfoot; and the subarticular portions of flat bones, such as those around the sacroiliac joints and acetabuli in the pelvis, and the glenoid of the scapula are also end-of-bone equivalents.

The differential diagnosis can then be further narrowed by knowing the age of the patient. For example, a lytic lesion in the epiphysis of a long bone of an adolescent is likely to be a chondroblastoma, whereas a lytic lesion at the end of a long bone in a young adult is likely to be a GCT. Ewing's sarcoma and Langerhans cell histiocytosis have a predilection for the diaphysis of long bones in people younger than 20 years and a predilection for flat bones, such as the pelvis and skull, in people older than 20 years, reflecting the normal change in the distribution of red marrow as a person ages.

Some lesions have a predilection for a particular bone and location, such as an adamantinoma and osteofibrous dysplasia for the anterior cortex of the tibia, periosteal desmoids for the posterior distal aspect of the femur, and hemangioma for vertebral bodies.[2]

PATTERNS OF BONE DESTRUCTION

Three patterns of bone destruction have been described as follows **(Figs. 2A to C)**:[3]

1. Type I—geographic bone destruction
2. Type II—moth-eaten bone destruction
3. Type III—permeative bone destruction

Geographic Bone Destruction

This type of bone destruction is the least aggressive form and suggests a slow growing lesion. It is seen as a well-circumscribed lytic lesion with a narrow zone of transition. The slow growth rate results in sharp demarcation between the destructive lesion and adjacent normal bone. The margin of the lesion represents the true histological margin of destruction; however, malignant lesions such as metastasis or myeloma may also demonstrate a similar pattern.

This pattern is further divided into three subtypes:

1. Type IA—geographic lesion with sclerotic margin
2. Type IB—geographic lesion with no marginal sclerosis
3. Type IC—geographic lesion with ill-defined margins

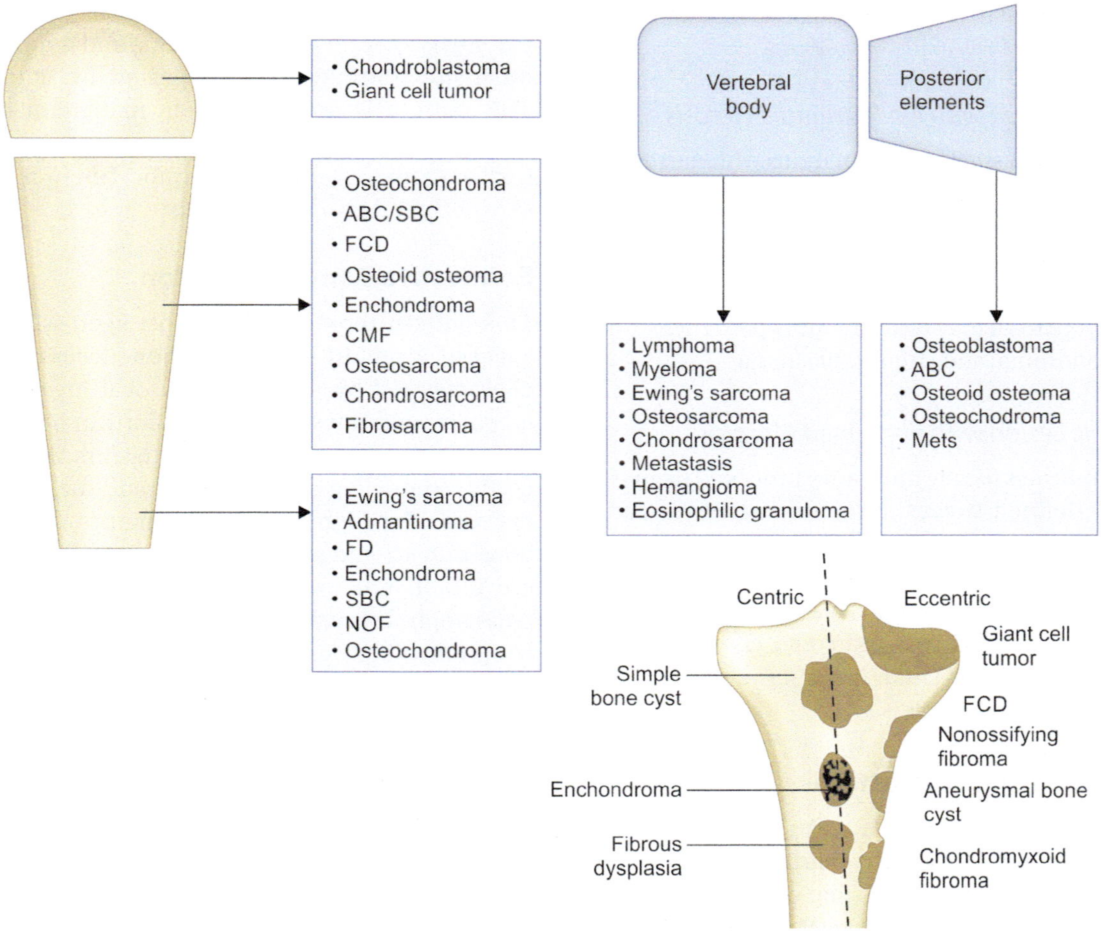

Fig. 1: Diagrammatic representation of the locations of various focal bone lesions. (ABC: aneurysmal bone cyst; CMF: chondromyxoid fibroma; FCD: fibrous cortical dysplasia; FD: fibrous dysplasia; NOF: nonossifying fibroma; SBC: simple bone cyst)

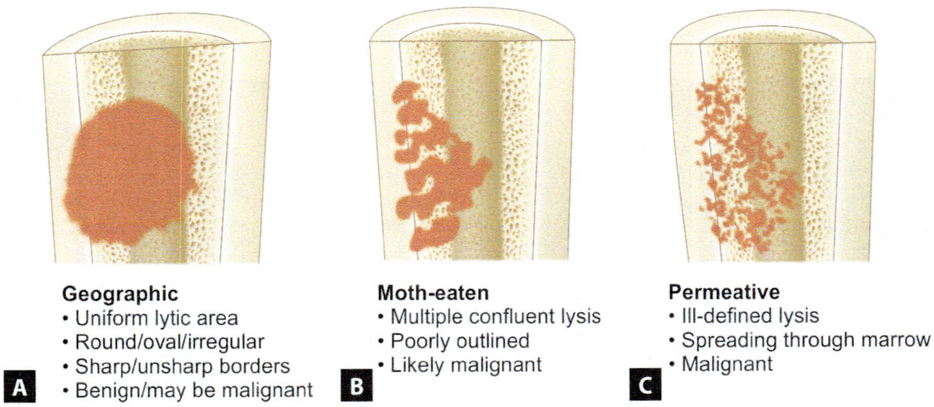

Figs. 2A to C: Patterns of bone destruction.

Geographic Lesion with Sclerotic Margin

The slow growth of the lesion permits the development of a reactive bone around the lesion so as to accommodate the transmission of forces. The sclerotic margin may vary in thickness and is especially thick in lesions occurring in weight-bearing bones such as femur and tibia. This type of lesion is commonly seen in SBC **(Fig. 3A)**, enchondroma, chondromyxoid fibroma, Brodie's abscess, and fibroxanthoma. Fibrous dysplasia often displays a peripheral thick sclerotic rim resembling a "rind" of orange **(Fig. 3B)**. In some lesions such as Brodie's abscess **(Fig. 3C)** and eosinophilic granuloma, the sclerotic rim is rather fuzzy and appears to be fading gradually into adjacent cancellous bone. The sclerotic rim is a mechanical adaptation designed to accommodate forces transmitted around the space-occupying mass.

Geographic Lesion with No Marginal Sclerosis

This type of lesion shows sharp margins with narrow zone of transition, referred to as a punched-out lesion with no sclerosis **(Fig. 3D)**. The margins seen on radiograph reflects the true histological edge of the lesion. GCT typically displays this pattern. Many lesions associated with type IA pattern may also show this pattern, e.g., bone cyst, enchondroma, and chondroblastoma.

Geographic Lesion with Ill-defined Margins

This type indicates locally infiltrative process. The margins are poorly defined suggesting more aggressive pattern than type IB lesions **(Fig. 3E)**. The destructive process extends in the marrow between the trabeculae beyond the radiographic destructive edge. This type of lesion is seen characteristically in GCT, osteosarcoma, chondrosarcoma, fibrosarcoma, aneurysmal bone cyst, eosinophilic granuloma, and osteomyelitis.

Moth-eaten Bone Destruction

This type of lesion is relatively more aggressive, suggesting more rapidly growing lesion. It is characterized by multiple small varying sized lytic lesions that coalesce and involve both cancellous and cortical bone **(Fig. 3F)**. In cancellous bone, normal trabeculae may be seen in between the lytic lesions while in cortical bone, the lytic lesion starts from endosteal surface and extends outward. This may progress to complete cortical destruction with extension into adjacent soft tissues. The lesion has less well-defined margins with wide zone of transition and is more extensive on histopathology than suggested on a radiograph. This pattern is usually seen in malignant neoplasms such as lymphoma, osteosarcoma, chondrosarcoma, fibrosarcoma, round cell tumor (including Ewing's sarcoma), and also osteomyelitis.

Permeative Bone Destruction

This pattern represents the most aggressive form and suggests a rapidly destructive bone lesion. This type is characterized by multiple, tiny oval lucent lesions or lucent streaks, mostly involving cortical bone **(Fig. 3G)**. Progressive cortical destruction occurs with exuberant cortical tunneling by osteoclasts, and the lesions are ill-defined. The highly aggressive nature does not allow bone to react and stop its further progress. These lesions are much more widespread than they appear on a radiograph. This type of lesion is seen in Ewing's sarcoma, lymphoma, high-grade chondrosarcoma, fibrosarcoma, angiosarcoma, leukemia, and metastasis.

Combination and Changing Pattern

This is characterized by combination of type IA, IB, and IC; type II; or type III patterns in a single lytic lesion and suggests more aggressive local growth. This pattern is usually seen in some benign lesions, when they become active, undergo malignant change or fracture. Pressure from tumor growth or active hyperemia are some of the factors that contribute to this pattern. A changing pattern is discernible when a change in the nature of margin is observed radiographically over time.

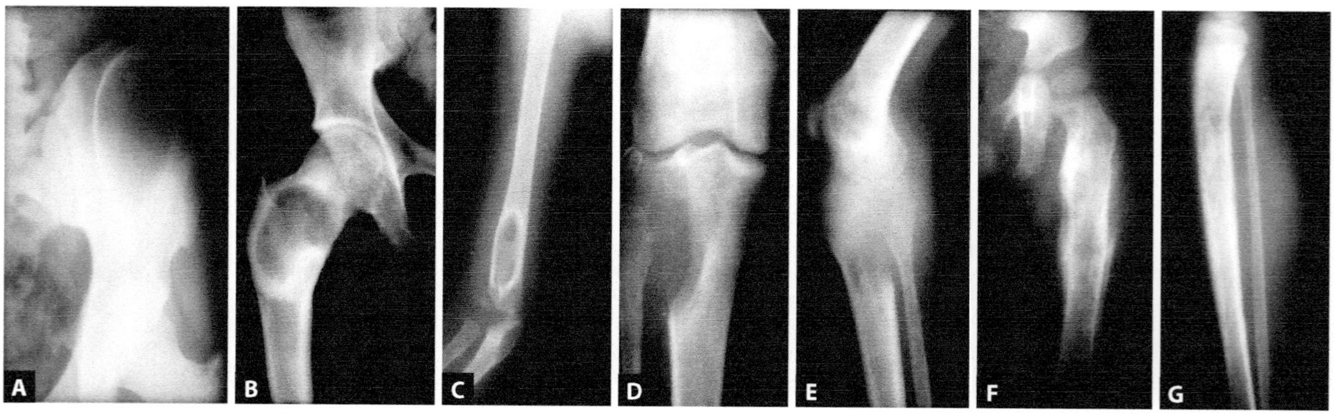

Figs. 3A to G: Patterns of bone destruction: (A) *Type IA*—geographic destruction with sclerotic margins in a simple bone cyst seen in the left iliac bone; (B) *Type IA*—geographic destruction with thick sclerotic margins, "rind sign," seen in fibrous dysplasia involving neck of right femur; (C) *Type IA*—geographic destruction with sclerotic margin which is fuzzy and facing peripherally, in Brodie's abscess involving lower end of humerus; (D) *Type IB*—geographic destruction with punched-out lesion seen in giant cell tumor involving upper tibia—note its typical eccentric subarticular position; (E) *Type IC*—geographic destruction with ill-defined margins seen in another patient of giant cell tumor involving upper tibia; (F) *Type II*—moth-eaten destruction seen in osteomyelitis involving left upper femur in a child—also note associated single lamellar periosteal reaction; and (G) *Type III*—permeative bone destruction involving upper tibia with osteomyelitis, note the tunneling in the anterior cortex.

MARGIN OF THE LESION AND RATE OF GROWTH

The margin of the lesion relates to the radiographic appearance of the interface between the lesion and adjacent normal bone. This is determined by reaction of the host bone to the lesion and rate of growth of the lesion. Well-marginated lesions have a narrow zone of transition **(Fig. 3A)**, while poorly-defined lesions have a wide zone of transition **(Fig. 3G)**. The aggressiveness and rate of growth of the lesion can be assessed from its margin. Sharply-defined margin or a sclerotic margin suggests slow growth rate, while ill-defined margins indicate aggressive lesion and rapid growth rate. Some benign lesions may, however, show a rapid growth rate, and some malignant lesions may be slow growing and have well-defined margins. Therefore, assessment of radiographic margin does not always indicate benign or malignant nature of a lesion.[4,5] Aneurysmal bone cyst, eosinophilic granuloma, majority of GCTs, and chondromyxoid fibroma may display aggressive appearance on radiographs and yet be benign. On the other hand, malignant lesions such as plasmacytoma and juxtacortical osteosarcoma are slow growing and may appear nonaggressive on plain radiograph. Treatment can also alter the appearance of malignant bone tumors; following radiation or chemotherapy, they may exhibit significant sclerosis as well as a narrow zone of transition.[3]

Inflammatory lesions usually produce marked reactive bone formation compared with neoplasms. Typically, these lesions show a sclerotic margin with sharp inner border and hazy outer border. However, osteoid osteoma also shows extensive osteosclerosis around the margin of similar nature. Benign tumors or tumor-like conditions and slow growing malignant tumors usually show sclerotic rim with sharp outer and inner margins **(Fig. 3B)**, while inflammatory lesions show a sclerotic margin with sharp inner border and a hazy outer border **(Fig. 3C)**.

Sometimes, a lesion may demonstrate a scalloped margin. This occurs in lesions of cartilage, fibrous tissue, fat, and vascular tissue, where the cells grow in clumps or lobules at different growth rates. The scalloped margin is seen typically in nonossifying fibroma. The assessment of growth rate on radiographs correlates well with virulence of organisms, host response, degree of spread of infection in inflammatory lesions, and with aggressiveness of the tumors. However, the radiographic rate of growth is not synonymous with actual biological behavior and growth rate of the lesion as seen in acute osteomyelitis and Ewing's sarcoma. Both these lesions may show similar radiographic appearance of aggressive pattern of bone destruction. However, such an appearance develops in a relatively short period of time in acute osteomyelitis in contrast to Ewing's sarcoma, which may take a longer period. Nonetheless, assessment of growth rate may help in narrowing the differential diagnosis.

CORTICAL RESPONSE

Presence of an intact cortex usually suggests nonaggressive nature of the lesion. Cortex responds in different ways (thinning, scalloping, expansion, or complete destruction) to underlying focal lesion. Cortical thinning (trabeculation) implies a slow-growing nature of lesion, usually benign lesion such as SBC and GCT **(Fig. 4A)**. Endosteal scalloping suggests the lobular growth pattern of the underlying tumor seen in chondral **(Fig. 4B)** or fibrous lesion, but does not help to differentiate benign from malignant lesion. Cortical expansion is a misnomer but implies that endosteal bone removal due to tumor growth is occurring at a similar speed to periosteal bone production, again suggesting slow growth. Sometimes, the outer cortical layer may be too thin to be seen on plain radiographs but evident on CT **(Figs. 4C and D)**. Highly aggressive lesions show complete destruction of the cortex with soft tissue component, sometimes saucerization of the cortex may be seen due to pressure erosion by the soft tissue without obvious cortical destruction **(Fig. 4E)**. Destruction of the cortex suggests rapid growth of the lesion. These two features (penetration of an apparently intact cortex and cortical saucerization) are most frequently seen with malignant round cell tumors, particularly Ewing's sarcoma.

MATRIX MINERALIZATION

Matrix refers to the acellular intercellular substance produced by the mesenchymal cells, namely osteoblasts, cartilage cells, and fibroblasts, and this includes osteoid, chondroid, myxoid, and collagen tissue. Matrix becomes visible on the radiograph only when it is mineralized sufficiently with calcium salts.[6]

Evaluation of matrix is valuable for two reasons:

1. Identification of particular configuration of matrix helps in suggesting specific diagnosis.
2. It is an indirect indicator of biological activity, e.g., transition from mineralized to nonmineralized matrix on follow-up radiographs indicates increased biologic activity and suggests this as an optimal site for biopsy.

The plain radiographs remain the best modality for assessing the pattern of matrix mineralization; however, the presence of subtle matrix mineralization can be seen only on CT.

Osseous Matrix

Osseous matrix is produced either by normal or tumor osteoblasts. The presence of bony trabeculae, appearing as thin interlacing radiodense struts within a lesion, is pathognomonic of a bone matrix. This occurs in myositis ossificans produced by normal osteoblasts, and in low-grade parosteal osteosarcoma produced by tumor osteoblasts. The osseous matrix may appear fluffy,

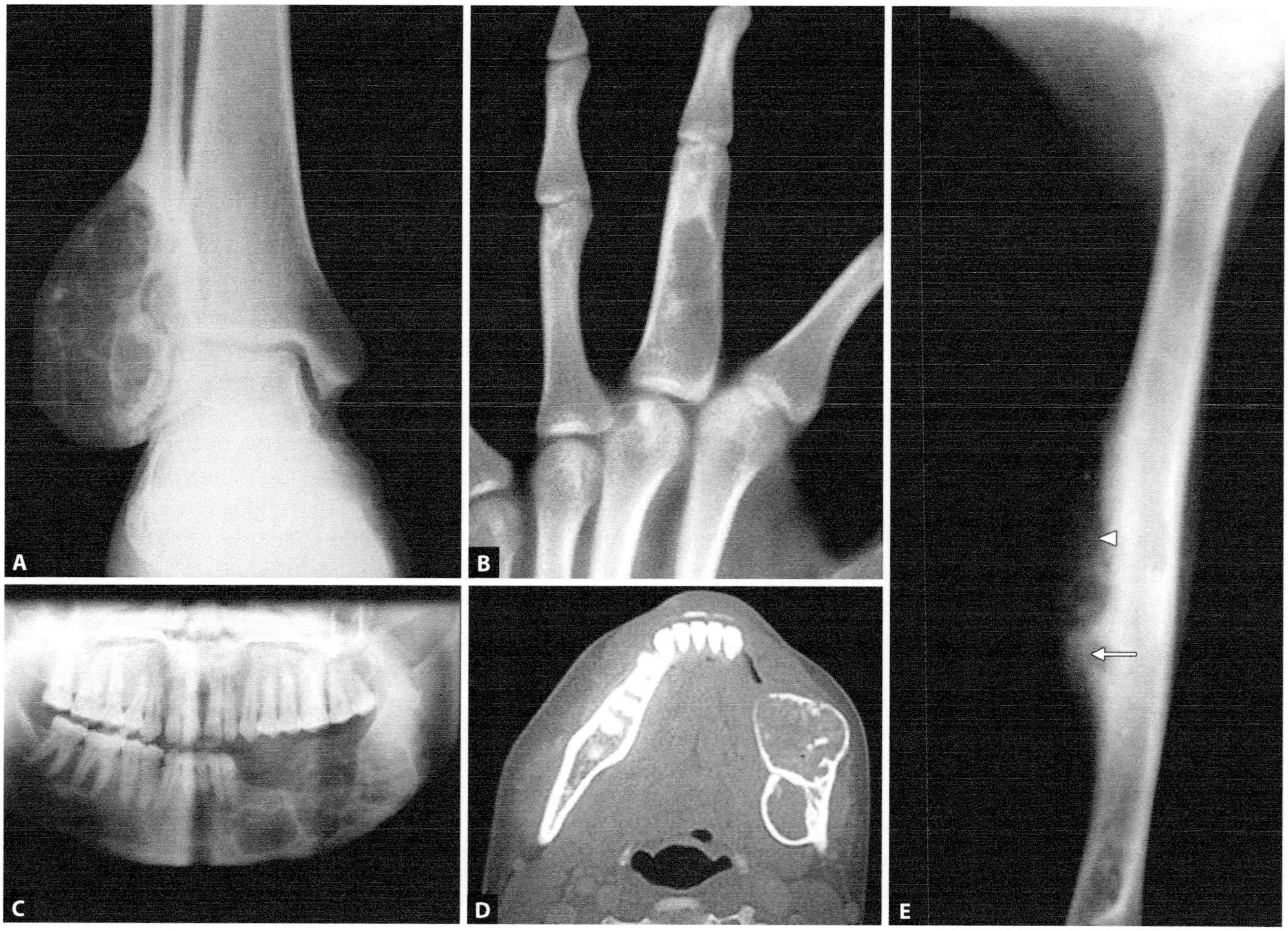

Figs. 4A to E: Cortical response: (A) Giant cell tumor showing expansile lytic lesion with intact cortex in lower end of fibula reaching up to subarticular location suggestive of cortical trabeculation indicating slow growth; (B) Enchondroma showing mildly expansile intramedullary lytic lesion in proximal phalanx causing endosteal scalloping indicating lobular growth; (C and D) Aneurysmal bone cyst showing expansile lytic lesion in body of mandible, cortical integrity is not well seen on plain radiograph, CT section of same patient showing the intact cortex around the expansile lytic lesion; and (E) "Saucerization" (arrowhead) of the medial humeral diaphysis in Ewing's sarcoma caused by the pressure erosion of the soft mass.

amorphous, hazy **(Fig. 5A)**, cloud-like or ivory pattern **(Fig. 5B)** on radiograph, when ossified sufficiently and is seen in high-grade osteosarcoma, parosteal osteosarcoma, and osteoblastoma.

Osseous matrix is also produced by the modulation of fibroblasts into osteoblasts and occurs in fibrous dysplasia and appears diffuse, hazy, or poorly defined but not as radiodense as seen in tumor new bone. Necrosis of fat tissue may result in the development of bone matrix which appears as clumps of radiodensity.

Cartilage Matrix

The cartilage matrix, when sufficiently calcified, is seen as flecks, punctate **(Fig. 5C)**, or flocculated **(Fig. 5E)** in appearance (enchondroma and osteochondroma). When the cartilage matrix is sufficiently ossified, it shows appearance of arcs **(Fig. 5D)** or rings **(Fig. 5D)** hazy, cloud-like or ivory-pattern. The punctate calcification of cartilage occurs in disrupted zone of provisional calcification while ring or arc appearance originates from disrupted enchondral bone formation. Both these patterns may exist alone or in combination. The ossified rings in cartilage tumor suggest low-grade nature of the tumor.

PERIOSTEAL REACTION

Periosteum is like an envelope that separates the bone from surrounding soft tissues. This consists of two layers, the outer fibrous and inner cellular. It is firmly adherent to the underlying bone in adults but less so in children. Normally, periosteum is not visible and even when it is elevated, it cannot be appreciated on radiographs till mineralization occurs. The periosteal reaction can be stimulated by hyperemia, inflammation, or spread of tumor. Its presence is an indicator of biologic activity and reflects the duration and intensity of underlying process.[4]

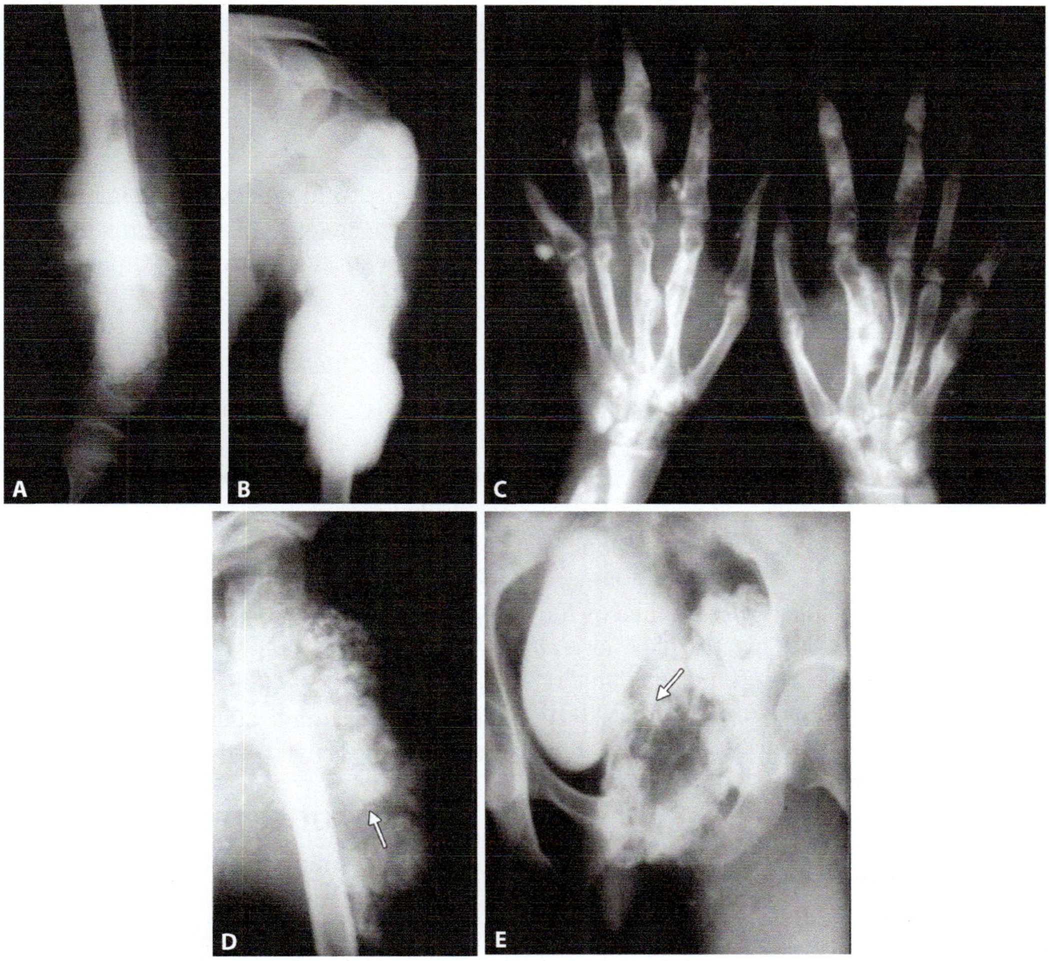

Figs. 5A to E: Patterns of matrix mineralization: (A) Cloud-like pattern of osteoid matrix in mid-diaphysis and ivory-like pattern in metaphyseal region of femur in osteosarcoma—note the single lamellar periosteal reaction along the anterior cortex; (B) Ivory-like pattern of osteoid matrix in a case of parosteal osteosarcoma involving proximal humerus—note that underlying humeral shaft can be seen through the tumor new bone in the lower part; (C) Punctate pattern of chondroid matrix in enchondromas involving multiple bones of hands in Maffucci syndrome—note multiple phleboliths with soft tissue swellings suggestive of cavernous hemangiomas; (D) Flocculent and arc-like (arrow) pattern of chondroid matrix involving upper third of femur with sarcomatous change in diaphyseal aclasis; and (E) Extensive flocculent and ring-like (arrow) chondroid matrix in chondrosarcoma involving left pubic bone, showing mass effect on urinary bladder.

The type of periosteal reaction can be considered under three subgroups **(Fig. 6A)**:

1. Continuous
2. Discontinuous or interrupted
3. Complex

Continuous Periosteal Reaction

Continuous periosteal reaction may occur either with intact or destroyed underlying cortex. It may be solid, single lamellar, multilamellar, or parallel spiculated. An underlying inflammatory or neoplastic process incites hyperemia that activates fibroblasts to osteoblasts that produce osteoid and mineralized layers of new bone. It takes 10–21 days, from the initial insult, for the periosteum to become radiographically visible.

Single lamellar periosteal reaction **(Fig. 6B)** is seen as a thin 1–2 mm faint radiopaque line from the cortical surface and usually occurs in osteomyelitis, histiocytosis, some benign tumors, and healing fractures.

In multilamellated periosteal reaction **(Fig. 6H)**, there are multiple layers of concentric periosteal reaction resembling an onion skin. Repeated insults from underlying disease process with alternating periods of rapid and slow growth first result in ossified layer of periosteum to be elevated, and later subsequent layers of periosteum are formed as the lesion waxes and wanes during its progression. This type of periosteal reaction occurs in osteomyelitis, histiocytosis, aneurysmal bone cyst, Ewing's sarcoma, and osteosarcoma. Interruptions in the lamellated periosteal reaction indicates more aggressive behavior of the lesion.

Solid periosteal reaction **(Fig. 6C)** indicates a slow process and is almost always associated with benign pathology. This occurs as a result of ossified matrix filling the spaces between lamellations and cortex. This is seen as marked thickening of the periosteal surface of the cortex on plain radiographs. It may be smooth or irregular. Lesions that show solid periosteal reaction include osteoid osteoma and eosinophilic granuloma.

Undulating periosteal reaction **(Fig. 6D)** is a variant of solid periosteal reaction, seen in low-grade osteomyelitis, long-standing varicosities, pulmonary osteoarthropathy, and chronic osteitis, but rarely in neoplasms.

Parallel spiculated continuous periosteal reaction represents an underlying malignant pathology. Bony spicules may appear perpendicular to the cortex—"hair-on-end" **(Figs. 6E and F)**, fan out in focal divergent manner—"sunburst pattern" **(Fig. 6G)**, appear to slope in a focal manner ("velvet pattern"), or show an unorganized pattern. The direction of the spicules is determined by the direction in which the tumor grows. This type of periosteal reaction suggests a more rapid process than lamellated or solid reaction. The spicules may show uniform, fine velvet-like pattern to long linear shadows with a gradual reduction in height in each direction along the shaft from the mid-zone of the reaction. *Hair-on-end* periosteal reaction commonly occurs in Ewing's sarcoma, osteosarcoma, metastasis, and thalassemia. These spicules are composed of normal reactive bone. Loose areolar tissue between the spicules may be replaced by tumor tissue in Ewing's sarcoma, osteosarcoma, and metastasis, while these may be replaced by hyperplastic red marrow in thalassemia **(Fig. 6F)** and sickle cell anemia. *Sunburst appearance* is more often seen in osteosarcoma, osteoblastic metastasis, and hemangioma **(Fig. 6G)**. In osteosarcoma, the divergent spicules are composed mainly of tumor bone but may also be composed of reactive bone or a combination of both. In *velvet pattern* of periosteal reaction, the spicules are short and sloped. This is seen rarely in chondrosarcoma. In unorganized form of periosteal reaction, the spicules are seen in various directions and indicate marked aggressive nature of the lesion, seen in Ewing's sarcoma as it extends into soft tissues.

Interrupted Periosteal Reaction

In this type, continuous mineralization of the periosteal reaction does not occur, resulting in the formation of Codman angles, buttresses, or truncated lamellae.

Codman Angles

The periosteal reaction forms an angular configuration with underlying cortex, resembling two sides of an angle **(Fig. 6G)** and indicates an aggressive pathology. This is formed by elevation of the periosteum by tumor, blood, edema, or pus. The angle of the triangle may or may not contain tumor. This is nonspecific, seen in both benign and malignant lesions.

Buttresses

In this type, solid reactive bone is formed at the lateral extraosseous margins of slowly growing bone lesions, the cortex beneath the buttress is frequently intact **(Figs. 6H and 7)**.

Truncated Lamellae

In aggressive neoplasms and virulent infections, the lamellations are sometimes interrupted or truncated **(Fig. 6H)**, because they are resorbed faster than they can be formed.

Complex Periosteal Reaction

Complex periosteal reaction includes combinations of lamellated, divergent spiculated periosteal reaction, buttresses, and Codman angles **(Fig. 6H)**. The more extensive and complex the periosteal reaction, the greater is the biologic activity of the underlying pathology.

SOFT TISSUE EXTENSION

Normally, the soft tissue shadow of muscle bundles when visualized on a radiograph is sharp with no displacement. It appears obscured when there is infiltration of intermuscular fat planes by inflammation, hemorrhage, or tumor. It may show displacement by organized hemorrhage or abscess. Presence of fat density in a soft tissue mass suggests a lipoma **(Fig. 8A)**. The presence of phleboliths indicates low flow vascular malformation or angiomatous lesion **(Fig. 5C)**. In myositis ossificans, focal rounded or streak-like areas of amorphous radiodensity are seen with areas of bone formation in the peripheral part as the lesion matures. Parosteal osteosarcoma also appears as an amorphous mass of increased density, but it matures earliest centrally in contrast to myositis ossificans. Both these lesions may or may not demonstrate a cleavage plane between the mass and underlying bone. Synovial sarcoma shows punctate clumps of calcific density and is usually present around a joint or along a tendon sheath **(Fig. 8B)**.[5]

Soft tissue mass is often associated with primary bone tumor, but less commonly with a secondary deposit. It may displace adjacent intermuscular fat planes **(Fig. 8C)** and may or may not erode the contiguous bony cortex.

MULTIPLICITY

Multiplicity of malignant lesions usually indicates metastatic disease **(Fig. 9A)**, multiple myeloma, or lymphoma. Very rarely, primary malignant bone lesions,

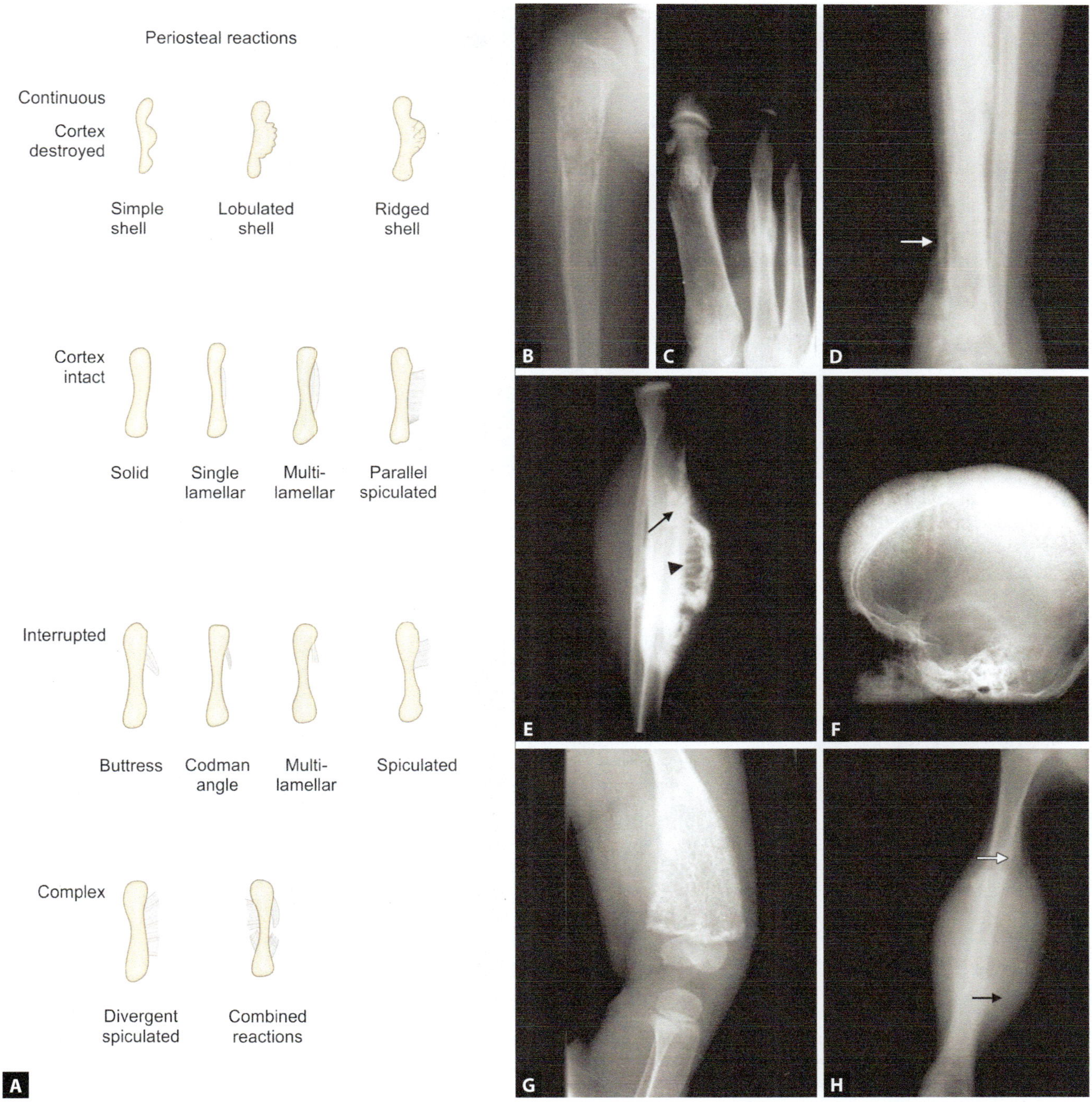

Figs. 6A to H: Various types of periosteal reaction: (A) Schematic diagram showing various types of periosteal reactions; (B) Single lamellar periosteal reaction in osteomyelitis involving upper-half of tibia—note type III—permeative bone destruction; (C) Solid periosteal reaction in stress fracture involving second metatarsal; (D) Undulating periosteal reaction (arrow) in chronic osteomyelitis of tibia; (E) Parallel (hair-on-end) (arrow) and divergent (sunburst) (arrowhead) spiculated periosteal reaction in diaphyseal osteosarcoma of tibia—note ivory pattern of osteoid tumor matrix; (F) Hair-on-end periosteal reaction involving the skull vault in thalassemia with marked thickening of outer table in frontoparietal region; (G) Sunburst periosteal reaction with coarse and striated trabecular pattern seen in hemangioma involving distal femoral metaphysis in a child; and (H) Complex periosteal reaction in Ewing's sarcoma of humeral diaphysis—note interrupted multilamellar (onion skin) reaction, buttress formation (white arrow) in the upper part, and Codman's angles (black arrow) in the lower part of the tumor both on medial and lateral aspects of bone.

such as Ewing's sarcoma or osteosarcoma, present as multifocal disease. Benign lesions, which tend to involve multiple sites, are polyostotic fibrous dysplasia, multiple osteochondromas, enchondromatosis **(Fig. 9B)**, Langerhans cell histiocytosis **(Fig. 9C)**, hemangiomatosis, hemophilia pseudotumors **(Fig. 9D)**, and fibromatosis.[7]

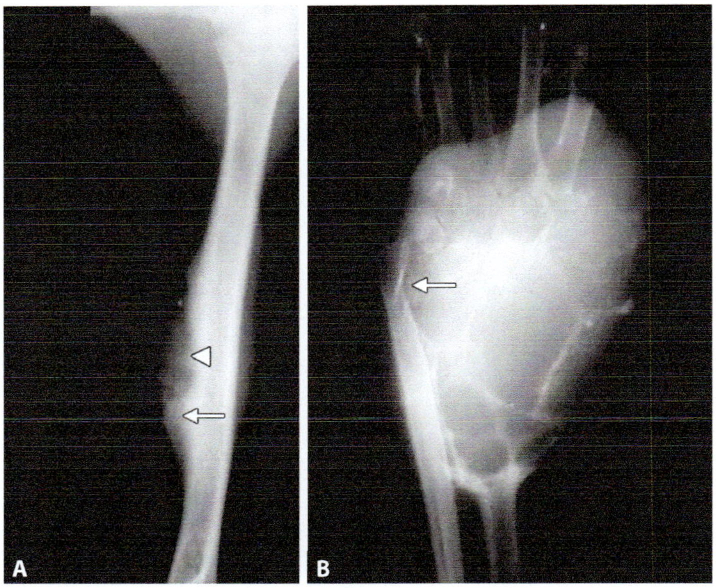

Figs. 7A and B: Saucerization: (A) "Saucerization" (arrowhead) of the medial humeral diaphysis in Ewing's sarcoma—note the buttress type (arrow) of periosteal reaction in the distal part; (B) Expansile, lytic, and multiseptate lesion in a patient with giant cell tumor of lower end of radius—note saucerization (arrow) of lateral ulnar cortex due to soft tissue component of tumor and ridged shell periosteal reaction.

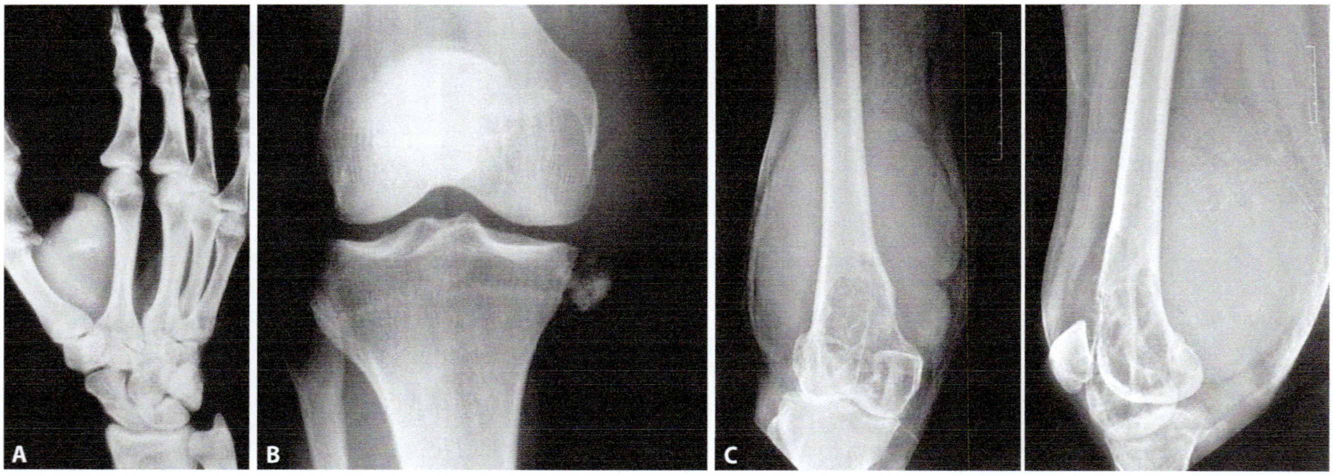

Figs. 8A to C: Soft tissue components: (A) Radiograph of hand showing low-density lesion in first web space (due to presence of fat density) suggests a lipoma; (B) Radiograph of knee joint showing punctate clumps of calcific density around the joint due to synovial sarcoma; (C) Radiograph of thigh including the knee joint showing lytic destructive lesion in the lower end of femur associated with large soft tissue component displacing the adjacent intermuscular fat planes.

MISCELLANEOUS

Septations (Table 2)

Lytic expansile lesions often show septations which represent residual normal bone that has not been resorbed or destroyed. These include aneurysmal bone cyst, GCT, nonossifying fibroma, etc. These septations are left behind by the lobules of growing lesion that advance asymmetrically at a more rapid rate. The septae are thin in GCT **(Fig. 10A)**, while they are thick in nonossifying fibroma and chondromyxoid fibroma **(Fig. 10B)**.[8]

Saucerization

Some tumors invade the cortex of a tubular bone in such a way that the area of bone destruction resembles a saucer when the long bone radiograph is viewed in profile. Ewing's sarcoma and metastasis may show typical saucerization configuration. In Ewing's sarcoma, the tumor breaks through the cortex, extends subperiosteally and erodes from its paracortical location to produce saucerization **(Fig. 7A)**. Metastasis also invades subperiosteal region in the same way as Ewing's sarcoma or may invade cortex

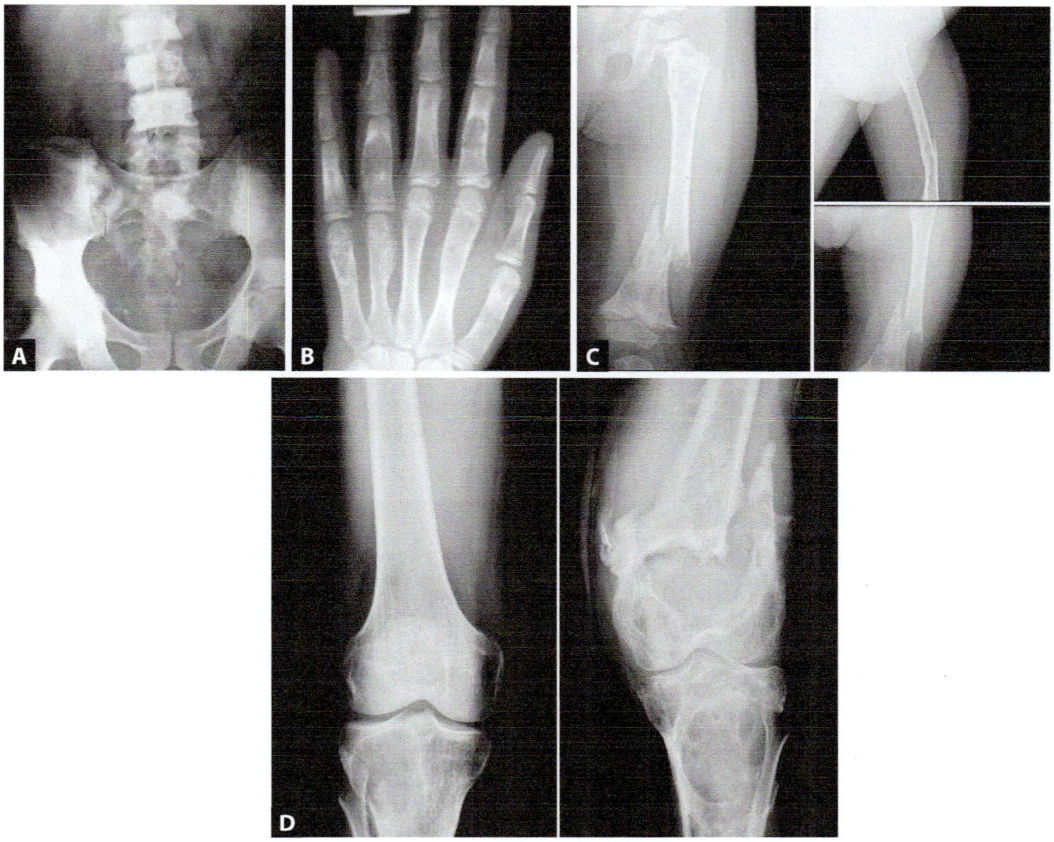

Figs. 9A to D: Multiplicity of lesions: (A) Multiple sclerotic lesions involving pelvis and lumbar spine in elderly patient suggestive of metastases; (B) Multiple intramedullary lytic lesions with chondroid type of calcification in short bones of hand suggestive of multiple enchondromatosis; (C) Multiple lytic lesions involving long bone both metaphysis and diaphysis with pathological fracture in a child suggestive of Langerhans cell histiocytosis; (D) Multiple lytic lesions involving tibia and femur in patient with history of bleeding diathesis suggestive of hemophilic pseudotumors.

Table 2: Examples of septated lesions.

Septations	*Lesions*
Coarse and thick	Chondromyxoid fibroma
Delicate and thin	Giant cell tumor
Delicate and horizontally oriented	Aneurysmal bone cysts
Lobulated	Nonossifying fibroma
Striated and radiating	Hemangioma

directly. Large soft tissue masses may erode bone in a similar manner **(Fig. 7B)**.[8]

Floating Fragment Sign

A fractured fragment may be seen within a radiolucent lesion. This fragment changes its location with change in extremity position, a characteristic feature seen in unicameral bone cyst. This sign is also known as "fallen fragment sign" **(Fig. 11)**. When the fractured fragment remains attached at the fracture site, it is seen in the form of a trapped door due to hydrostatic pressure of the fluid contained within the cyst. This is called "trap door sign". Both these signs are typical of unicameral bone cyst.

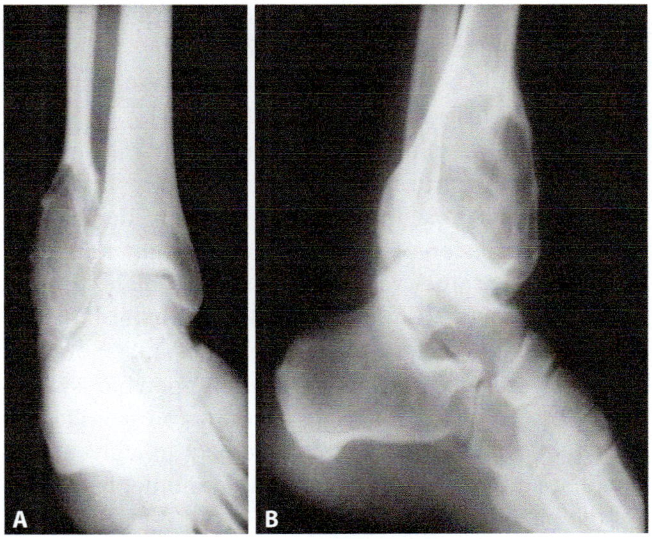

Figs. 10A and B: Septations: (A) Expansile, lytic, and multiseptate lesion in a patient with giant cell tumor of lower end of radius—note saucerization of lateral ulnar cortex due to soft tissue component of tumor and ridged shell periosteal reaction; (B) Eccentric expansile lytic lesion showing thick septa and ridged shell reaction in chondromyxoid fibroma involving the lower end of tibia.

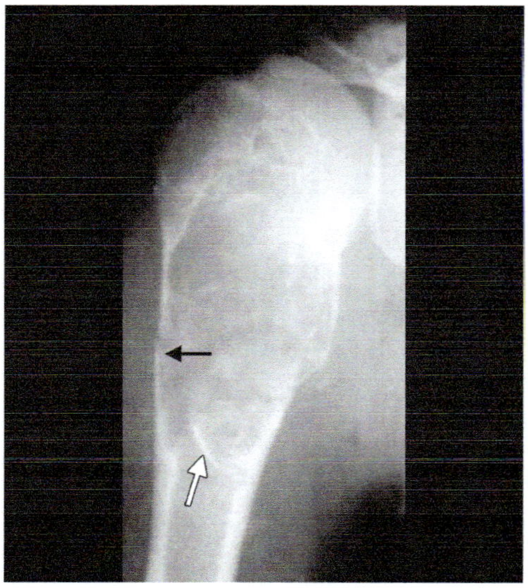

Fig. 11: Simple bone cyst involving humerus showing "fallen fragment" (white arrow) and "trap-door" (black arrow) signs.

BENIGN VERSUS MALIGNANT

Although it is sometimes very difficult to distinguish benign from malignant bone lesions on the basis of plain radiographs alone; however, certain key characteristic features may favor one over the other. Benign tumors usually present with well-defined, sclerotic borders, a geographic type of bone destruction, an uninterrupted solid periosteal reaction, and no soft tissue extension. Malignant lesions, on the other hand, tend to demonstrate poorly-defined borders with a wide zone of transition, a moth-eaten or permeative pattern of bone destruction, an interrupted periosteal reaction of the sunburst or onion-skin type, and an adjacent soft-tissue mass. As noted earlier, it should be kept in mind that some benign tumors can also exhibit aggressive features **(Table 3)**.[9]

When all the clinical and radiographic information concerning a patient with a bone lesion has been analyzed, the most important diagnostic decision is whether the lesion is definitely benign and not to be biopsied, but rather monitored or completely ignored (a "do not touch lesion") **(Table 4)**, or whether it has an ambiguous and an aggressive appearance and should be further investigated via percutaneous or open biopsy. The results of the histopathologic examination would then determine whether further management in a given case would be surgical, chemotherapeutic, radiotherapeutic, or a combination of these.

Table 3: Benign lesions with aggressive features.

Lesion	*Radiographic presentation*
Osteoblastoma	Bone destruction and soft (aggressive) tissue extension similar to osteosarcoma
Desmoplastic fibroma	Expansive destructive lesion, frequently trabeculated
Periosteal desmoid	Irregular cortical outline, mimics osteosarcoma or Ewing's sarcoma
Giant cell tumor	Occasionally aggressive features—osteolytic bone destruction, cortical penetration, and soft tissue extension
Aneurysmal bone cyst	Soft tissue extension, occasionally mimicking malignant tumor
Osteomyelitis	Bone destruction and aggressive periosteal reaction, occasionally, features resembling Ewing's sarcoma
Pseudotumor of hemophilia	Bone destruction and periosteal reaction, occasionally mimics malignant tumor
Myositis ossificans	Features of parosteal or periosteal osteosarcoma
Brown tumor of hyperparathyroidism	Lytic bone lesion and resembling malignant tumor

Table 4: Lesions that should not be biopsied.

Tumors and tumor-like lesions	*Non-neoplastic conditions*
Fibrous cortical defect	Avulsion fracture (healing phase)
Nonossifying fibroma	Bone infarct
Periosteal (cortical) desmoid	Bone island (enostosis)
Small and solitary focus of fibrous dysplasia	Pseudotumor of hemophilia
Myositis ossificans	Degenerative and post-traumatic cysts
Intraosseous ganglion	Brown tumor of hyperparathyroidism
Enchondroma in a short, tubular bone	Discogenic vertebral sclerosis

ULTRASONOGRAPHY

It is of limited utility in the evaluation of primary osseous lesions. In particular, ultrasonography can be used for the initial evaluation of soft-tissue masses in patients with contraindications to MRI. Sonography can confirm the presence of the mass, characterizing it as solid or cystic, and assessing its dynamic features such as compressibility and vascularity. Perhaps one of the most widely used applications of ultrasonography is image-guided intervention. Ultrasonography can be used to guide a minimally invasive technique to guide the placement of the needle during biopsy into an area of solid tissue. Ultrasound also plays an important role in detecting soft issue recurrence in postoperative cases, in patients with metallic implants.

COMPUTED TOMOGRAPHY ANALYSIS OF BONE LESIONS

Computed tomography gives better morphological assessment of the lesion as well as the surrounding area, thereby helping in the evaluation of lesion margin with great advantage. Hence, a lesion with well-defined border and localized within the cortex implies slow growth, while features of cortical destruction suggest aggressive nature of the lesion.

Like radiographic evaluation, CT also has a grading system for evaluating bone lesions:

- *Grade I*: Lesions within the bone or causing thinning of cortex and contained by thick periosteal new bone suggest slow growth process.
- *Grade II*: Lesions with localized destruction of cortex associated with periosteal reaction suggest aggressive nature.
- *Grade III:* Lesions completely penetrate through the cortex but show no localized bone destruction associated with soft tissue, suggest highly aggressive nature.

In the evaluation of focal bone lesion, CT is usually used to get "radiographic" evidence, in areas with complex anatomy, particularly for lesions in vertebrae and flat bones such as ilium, sacrum, and scapula[5] (**Figs. 12A and B**). CT is better than radiography in showing the exact site of the lesion within the bone (medullary, cortical, periosteal, and parosteal). This is very useful for making the diagnosis of certain entities such as nonossifying fibroma and juxtacortical chondroma.

Computed tomography helps not only in defining the margins of the lesion but also helps in detecting subtle cortical alterations and sclerotic reactions. It has the superior ability to show subtle periosteal reactions that may not be visible on radiographs due to superimposition or inadequate contrast resolution. Additionally, CT plays a valuable role in detecting subtle matrix mineralization, making it a very useful modality in confirming the diagnosis of osteoid or chondroid forming lesions.[10]

Computed Tomography Grading System of Bone Lesions

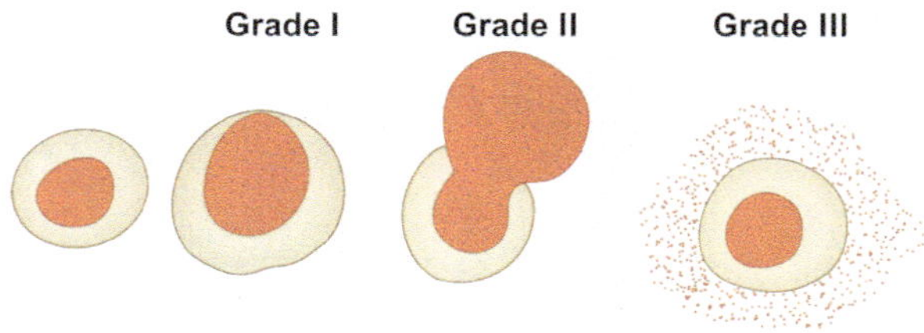

MAGNETIC RESONANCE IMAGING OF BONE LESIONS[11,12]

Magnetic resonance imaging is exquisitely sensitive to lesions that replace marrow and destroy bone. It shows the full extent of lesions and extension into soft tissues. MRI is of minor value in the estimation of the malignant potential of an osseous lesion. Although many bone tumors and tumor-like lesions present similar morphology at MRI, some entities can be diagnosed with good reliability. These include chondrogenic tumors (**Fig. 13A**), solitary (**Fig. 13B**), and aneurysmal bone cysts (**Fig. 13C**); GCTs; lesions containing fatty tissue; and, to a certain extent, osteoid osteomas and osteoblastomas.

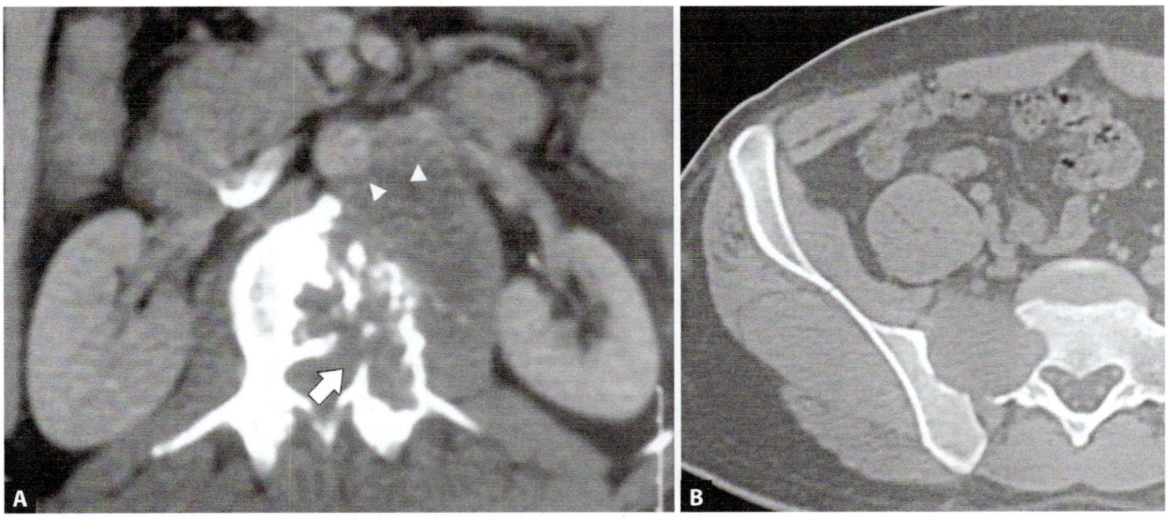

Figs. 12A and B: Role of CT scan in assessment of focal bone lesion: (A) Axial CT of the lumbar vertebra at the level of the renal hilum shows marked tumoral destruction of the left half of the vertebral body and the left pedicle by a proven chondrosarcoma. Matrix mineralization and residual trabeculae are seen inside. The tumor is extending into the left psoas muscle and is lifting the aorta and the left renal vain anteriorly (arrowheads). The fat plane with the aorta is obliterated. Posteromedially, the mass is extending into the spinal canal and causing an impression on the theca (arrow); (B) Axial CT section of sacrum showing expansile lytic lesion in right sacral ala a case of giant cell tumor.

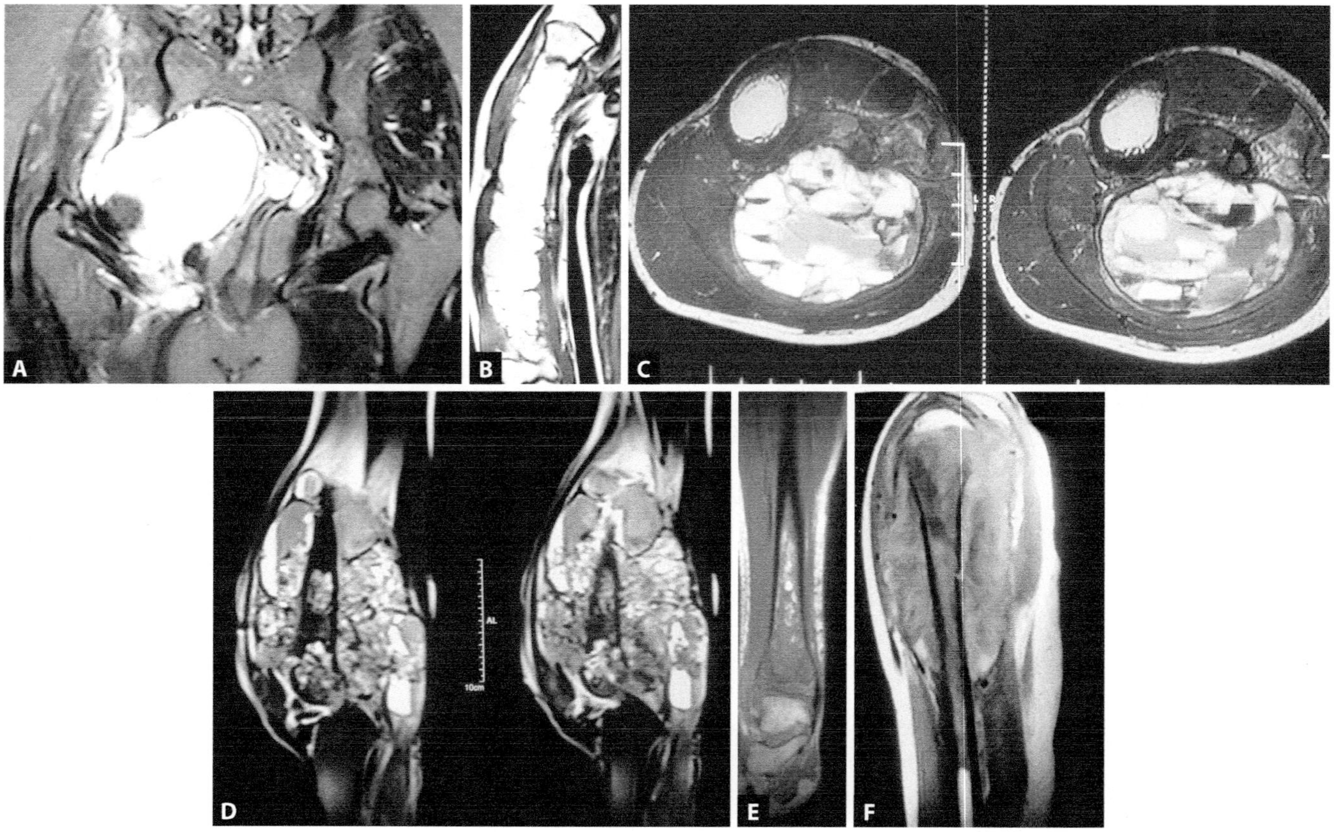

Figs. 13A to F: Role of magnetic resonance imaging (MRI) in assessment of focal bone lesion: (A) Coronal T2-weighted (T2W) MR image showing brightly hyperintense lobulated mass lesion arising from the right acetabulum in elderly patient suggestive of chondrosarcoma; (B) Coronal short tau inversion recovery (STIR) MR image showing elongated hyperintense lesion involving the shaft of humerus in a child suggestive of simple bone cyst; (C) Axial T2W MR image showing expansile lesion with multiple blood fluid levels suggestive of aneurysmal bone cyst; (D) Sagittal T2W MR image of a patient with biopsy-proven case of osteosarcoma showing altered signal intensity involving the metaepiphysis of lower end of femur associated with large soft tissue component which is extending into knee joint; (E) Coronal T1-weighted (T1W) image of a child with osteomyelitis showing heterogenous signal intensity involving the diaphysis, metaphysis, and epiphysis of lower end of tibia suggestive of aggressive lesion; (F) Sagittal T1W MR image of arm in patient with known case of osteosarcoma showing altered signal intensity involving upper end of humerus associated with large surrounding soft tissue component without obvious cortical destruction suggestive of transcortical infiltration.

The differential diagnosis for benign bone lesions surrounded by extensive marrow edema includes osteoid osteoma/osteoblastoma, chondroblastoma, Langerhans cell histiocytosis, and osteomyelitis. As a general (but not absolute) guideline, the greater the extent of surrounding marrow edema, the more likely the bone lesion is benign. Marrow edema may be present around malignant bone tumors, as well, in which case it constitutes the reactive zone of the tumor.

However, its main role is for preoperative staging of tumor extent (precise compartmental localization), involvement of critical structures such as joints and neurovascular bundles and also plays a vital role in detection of skip lesions **(Fig. 13D)**.

Magnetic resonance imaging is particularly useful to evaluate aggressive lesions such as malignant tumors and infective lesions **(Fig. 13E)**. It depicts transcortical infiltration which is a sign of highly aggressive lesions **(Fig. 13F)**. It also depicts intratrabecular infiltration, a sign of infiltrative growth in case of malignant bone tumor. It also shows active tumor growth in periosteal and endosteal extension at tumor margins. Unless it is contraindicated, contrast should be administered when evaluating soft-tissue component of bone tumor. Contrast enhancement delineates areas of necrosis within the lesion.

CONCLUSION

- The guidelines mentioned in this chapter usually permit us to make a correct diagnosis or offer a narrow differential diagnosis **(Flowchart 1)**.
- The pattern of bone destruction, margins, cortical response, location, and site of lesion on radiographs helps in the differential diagnosis of bone tumor and tumor-like lesions.
- Because of high specificity in detecting lesion features, radiography is integrated with clinical findings that allows the differential diagnosis between neoplastic and non-neoplastic lesions including trauma (healing or stress fractures, myositis ossificans), infection (acute osteomyelitis, Brodie's abscess), eosinophilic granuloma, such as Brown tumors of hyperthyroidism.

Flowchart 1: Assessing focal bone lesion.

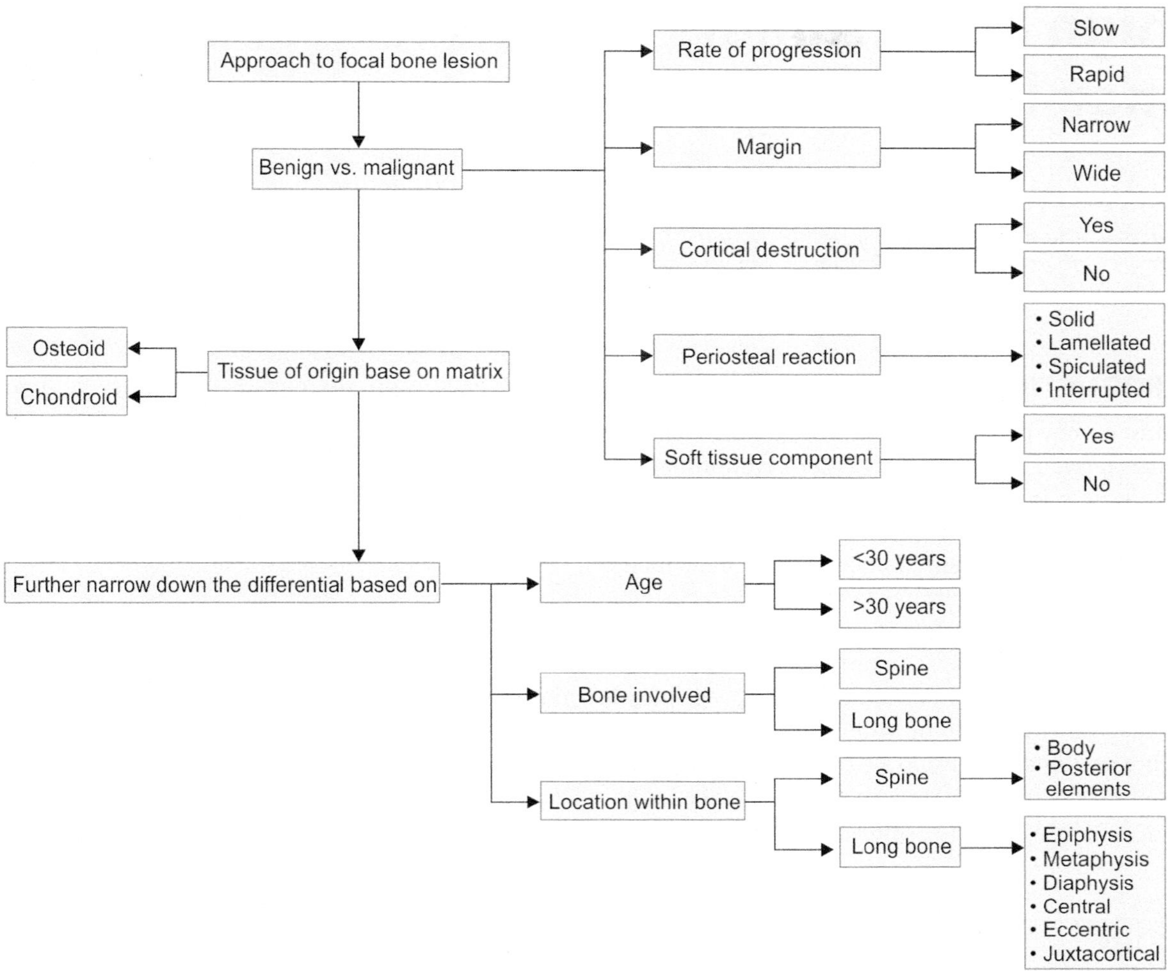

- Radiography is not sufficient to evaluate the lesions in complex anatomical sites such as spine, pelvis, and scapula nor does it define the intra- and extraosseous extent of the tumor. In such cases, cross-sectional imaging such as CT and MRI helps to define the extent of lesions.
- The radiologist should never interpret the CT or MRI of a suspected bone tumor without first reviewing the plain radiographs. The orthopedic surgeon, radiologist, and pathologist must collaborate as a multidisciplinary team to make the diagnosis more accurately and improve patient care.

REFERENCES

1. O'Donnel P. Evaluation of focal bone lesions: basic principles and clinical scenarios. Imaging. 2003;15(4):298-323.
2. Miller TT. Bone tumors and tumorlike conditions: analysis with conventional radiography. Radiology. 2008;246(3):662-74.
3. Madewell JE, Ragsdale BD, Sweet DE. Radiologic and pathologic analysis of solitary bone lesions. I. Internal margins. Radiol Clin North Am. 1981;19(4):715-48.
4. Ragsdale BD, Madewell JE, Sweet DE. Radiologic and pathologic analysis of solitary bone lesions. II. Periosteal reactions. Radiol Clin North Am. 1981;19(4):749-83.
5. Brown KT, Kattapuram SV, Rosenthal DI. Computed tomography analysis of bone tumors: patters of cortical destruction and soft tissue extension. Skeletal Radiol. 1986;15(6):448-51.
6. Sweet DE, Madewell JE, Ragsdale BD. Radiologic and pathologic analysis of solitary bone lesions. III. Matrix patterns. Radiol Clin North Am. 1981;19(4):785-814.
7. Priolo F, Cerase A. The current role of radiography in the assessment of skeletal tumors and tumor-like lesions. Eur J Radiol. 1998; 27(Suppl 1):S77-85.
8. Moser RP, Madewell JE. An approach to primary bone tumors. Radiol Clin North Am. 1987;25(6):1049-93.
9. Ma LD, Frassica FJ, Scott WW, Fishman EK, Zerhouni EA. Differentiation of benign and malignant musculoskeletal tumors: potential pitfalls with MR imaging. Radiographics. 1995;15(2):349-66.
10. Woertler K. Benign bone tumors and tumor-like lesions value of cross-sectional imaging. Eur Radiol. 2003;13(8):1820-35.
11. Pettersson H, Gillespy T 3rd, Hamlin DJ, Enneking WF, Springfield DS, Andrew ER, et al. Primary musculoskeletal tumors: examination with MR imaging compared with conventional modalities. Radiology. 1987;164(1):237-41.
12. Zimmer WD, Berquist TH, McLeod RA, Sim FH, Pritchard DJ, Shives TC, et al. Bone tumors: magnetic resonance imaging versus computed tomography. Radiology. 1985;155(3):709-18.

CHAPTER

13

Benign Bone Tumors and Tumor-like Conditions

Mahesh Prakash, Anindita Sinha, Akshay Saxena

INTRODUCTION

Bone tumors may be defined as a new growth arising in a bone or derived from cells which are components of skeletal tissue.[1] The majority of benign true tumors of bone are detected in children and young adults. Benign bone tumors can be classified according to their matrix production and/or predominant cell type into cartilage forming, bone forming, fibrous, vascular, and other connective tissue lesions.[2,3] The term "tumor-like lesions of bone" denotes various conditions of non-neoplastic nature originating from or affecting the bone and presenting as solitary or multiple bone lesions. A broad classification of benign bone tumor and tumor-like lesions is depicted in **Table 1**. For diagnosis of bone tumors and tumor-like lesion, there is need for close cooperation of radiologist, orthopedician, and pathologists; however, the role of radiologist is most important. The primary aim of imaging should be to make specific diagnosis (if possible) or narrowing of the differential diagnosis which can be a guide for further intervention and management.

Table 1: Benign bone tumors and tumor-like lesions.[4]

Benign bone tumors	*Tumor-like lesions*
Bone-forming tumors • Enostosis • Osteoma • Osteoid osteoma • Osteoblastoma	*Fibro-osseous lesions* • Nonossifying fibroma • Fibrous dysplasia • Osteofibrous dysplasia • Periosteal desmoid
Cartilage forming tumors • Enchondroma • Osteochondroma • Periosteal chondroma • Chondroblastoma • Chondromyxoid fibroma	*Cystic lesions* • Simple bone cyst • Aneurysmal bone cyst • Intraosseous ganglion • Epidermoid cyst • Subchondral cyst
Connective tissue tumors • Desmoplastic fibroma • Benign fibrous histiocytoma • Ossifying fibroma • Myxoma • Lipoma	*Giant cell containing lesions* • Giant cell reparative granuloma • Brown tumor • Pigmented villondoular synovitis
Vascular tumors • Hemangioma • Lymphangioma • Glomous tumor	*Others* • Eosinophilic granuloma • Pseudotumors
Others/Semimalignant • Giant cell tumor • Ameloblastoma	

IMAGING MODALITIES

Before radiological evaluation, consideration of patient's data (age, gender) and clinical information of concerned patient are very useful for diagnosis as many lesions of bone show predilection for particular age group and gender.[2,3]

Radiography

Despite availability of a host of imaging modalities, plain radiographs continue to play a major role in the diagnostic evaluation of bone neoplasms. Plain radiographs demonstrate location of the tumor in the body; segment involved—whether epiphysis, metaphysis, or diaphysis; growth characters of the lesion such as margin—well-defined/ill-defined; presence or absence of periosteal reaction and the appearance of tumor matrix—whether calcified or not, which are all important parameters to arrive at a proper diagnosis.

The pointers to the benign nature of a bone tumor include the following:

- Area of geographic bone destruction which is well-circumscribed and is characterized by a sharp transition between the destroyed area and the normal bone (i.e., narrow zone of transition—less than 1 cm).
- Sclerotic margin indicates slow growth and is generally seen in benign lesions located at the metaphysis. Certain tumors stimulate surrounding sclerosis which may obscure the central lytic area such as osteoid osteoma.
- *Periosteal reaction*: In general, periosteal reaction is not a feature of benign bone tumors unless a fracture has occurred except in a very few lesions such as osteoblastoma, osteoid osteoma, and chondromyxoid fibroma. Periosteal reaction is radiographically

described as solid or interrupted. Solid periosteal reaction is defined as a single layer of new bone >1 mm in thickness which is usually of uniform density. When seen, solid periosteal reaction indicates benign pathology.[1,3] It is seen in osteoid osteoma and osteoblastoma.

- *Tumor matrix*: Presence of calcification in the form of rings, flocculant patches, or stippled flecks point to the cartilaginous origin of the tumor. A ground-glass haze indicates fibrous lesions. Osteoid matrix is seen in bone-forming tumors.

Computed Tomography

Computed tomography (CT) can be used for radiographic information where conventional radiography has limited information such as in the region of complex anatomy and superimposition of bony elements (pelvis, spine, and scapula). CT is superior to radiography in determination of the epicenter of a bone lesion, whether it is in cortex, medulla, or periosteal in location.[3,5,6]

Other advantages of CT over radiography are to detect cortical alteration (breech, scalloping, expansion) and detection of periosteal reaction. CT is most valuable imaging modality in detection of subtle matrix calcifications and therefore it is very useful for diagnosis of a bone- or cartilage-forming benign bone tumor.[3-6]

Magnetic Resonance Imaging

Magnetic resonance imaging (MRI) is the most accurate method for demonstrating extent of tumors especially intramedullary component.[7] MRI has also demonstrated significant potential for tumor characterization. On T1-weighted (T1W) images, most bone tumors show decrease in signal intensity because of marked contrast with hyperintense fat of the marrow. On T2-weighted (T2W) images most of the tumors are of high-intensity making it difficult to separate tumor from fat but easy to differentiate tumor from surrounding muscles. Presence of atypical signal patterns help in predicting a dominant tissue component, e.g., high-signal intensity on T1W images may be due to fat, as seen in lipoma, hemangioma, medullary bone infarct or hemorrhage as seen in aneurysmal bone cyst.[8]

Magnetic resonance is the best technique for demarcating the soft tissue component of bone tumors and its relationship to adjacent joint and neurovascular structures.[7,8]

Generally, only few bone tumors have a classical radiological picture. Similarly, biopsy of the lesion is not always the ultimate answer. On the other hand, some tumors are difficult to diagnose histologically but have a typical radiographic appearance, e.g., osteoid osteoma. Others with unusual radiographic features exhibit a characteristic histological appearance, e.g., aneurysmal bone cysts. Thus, close correlation of clinical history, histology, and radiology are always essential to achieve highest diagnostic accuracy.

BONE-FORMING TUMORS

Enostosis

These lesions are commonly known as "bony islands" are usually asymptomatic. Histologically, bony islands consist of dense intramedullary lamellar bone with normal haversian canals. Enostosis is commonly found in spine, ribs, and pelvis.[9] It is usually seen as oval, densely sclerotic intramedullary lesions. Usually a bone island is aligned in the long axis of trabeculae **(Figs. 1A and B)**. Its only significance lies in the fact that it may be confused

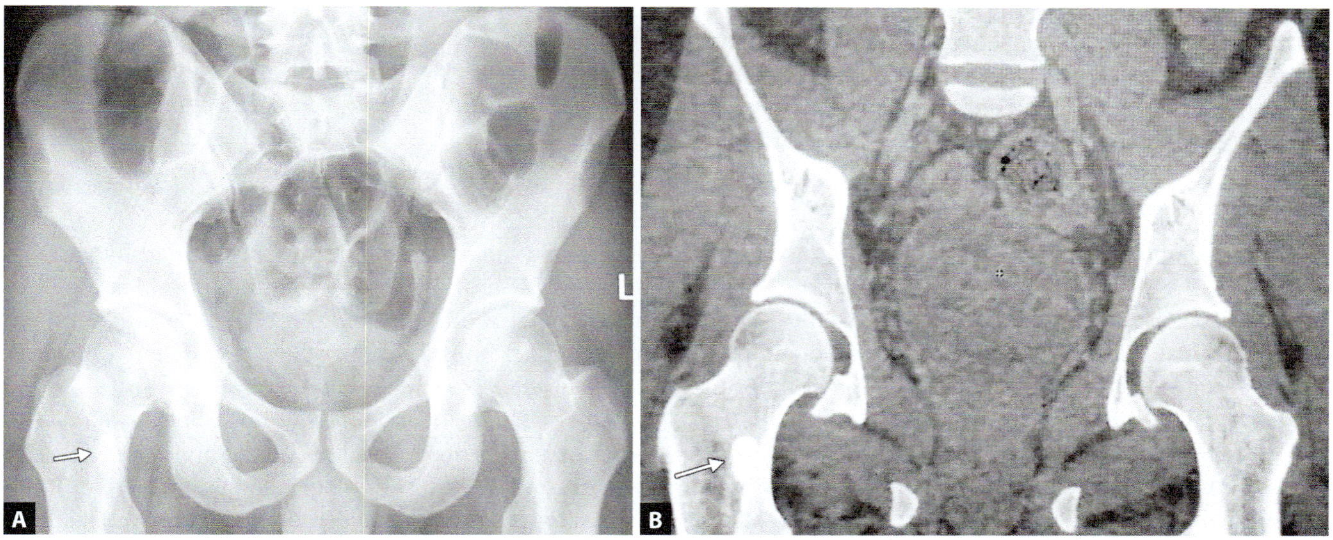

Figs. 1A and B: Enostosis. Radiograph (A) and CT coronal reconstruction (B) of pelvis show well-defined oval sclerotic lesion (arrow) in intertrochanteric region of right femur.

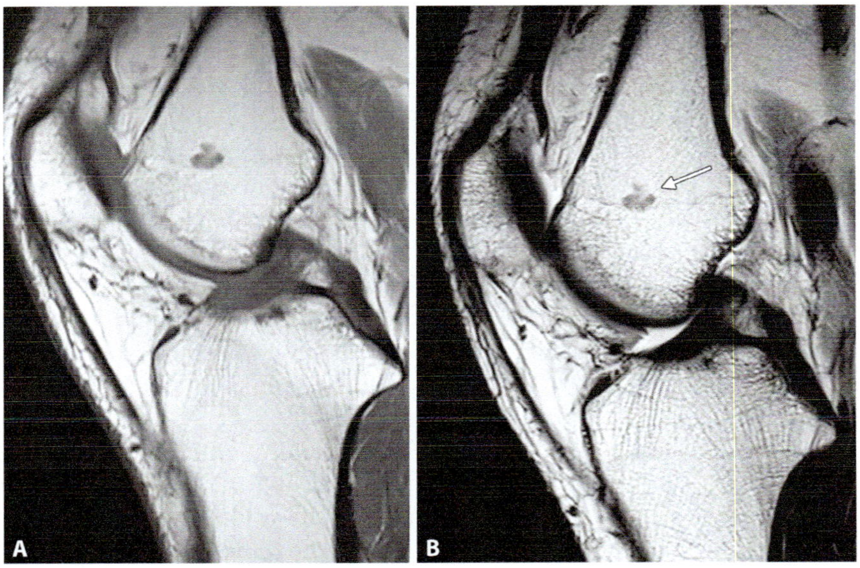

Figs. 2A and B: Enostosis. T1W (A) and T2W (B) sagittal MR images show well-defined lobulated lesion in lower end of femur which shows hypointense signal on both sequences (arrow).

with osteoblastic metastases. Scintigraphy and MRI are helpful in the differentiation, as bony islands usually do not exhibit an increase tracer uptake on bone scans. On MRI, enostosis shows hypointense signal on both T1W and T2W sequences **(Figs. 2A and B)** while sclerotic metastasis shows halo of surrounding marrow edema on fluid sensitive sequences.[10]

Osteoma

Histologically, an osteoma is composed of both dense and woven bone and arises from the cortex. Common sites include outer table of skull, paranasal sinuses (frontal/ethmoid), and mandible. They are generally asymptomatic, but may cause sinus obstruction, proptosis, etc. Radiologically, osteoma is seen as a well-circumscribed lesion arises from the cortex, which protrudes from the surface of the affected bone. It demonstrates same density as cortex on X-ray and CT scan **(Fig. 3)**. On MRI, osteoma shows hypointense signal on both T1W and T2W images.[11] Multiple osteomas occur as a part of Gardner's syndrome.

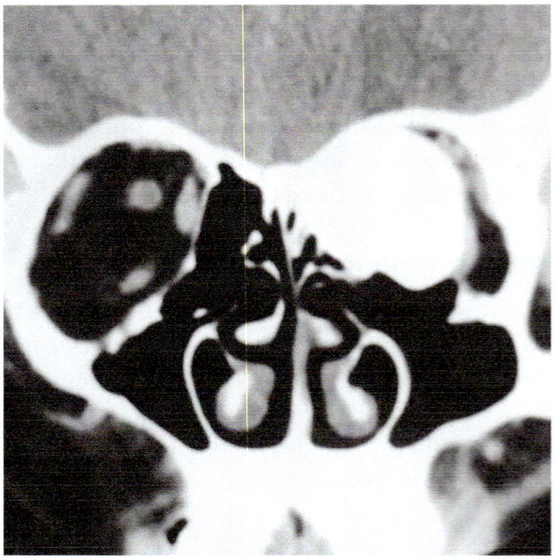

Fig. 3: Large osteoma. CT scan (coronal section) of paranasal sinus shows large well-defined bony lesion arising from ethmoid sinus causing compression of left orbital structures.

Osteoid Osteoma

Osteoid osteoma is a fairly common tumor, accounting for approximately 10–12% of all benign tumors.[12] These tumors usually affects patients between 5 and 25 years of age. Clinically most patients presents with pain that is especially severe at night and relieved by aspirin or other nonsteroidal anti-inflammatory agents.

More than half of tumors are located in proximal femur and tibia. They occur less frequently in the upper extremities than in the lower extremities. Osteoid osteoma also frequently affects the tubular bones of the hands and feet. They are however, less common in the spine, where they affect the posterior arches of the vertebrae. Histologically, the lesion consists of a nidus which is usually less than 1 cm in diameter and surrounded by variable degree of sclerotic bone depending upon location. The nidus contains interlacing trabeculae at various stages of ossification within a stroma of loose, vascular connective tissue. Osteoid osteoma can be cortical (the most common type), cancellous or medullary, and subperiosteal.[11] The latter two types produce less sclerotic bone than those in the cortex do, making radiologic diagnosis difficult.

Radiographically, the lesion appears as well-defined lytic lesion, surrounded by reactive sclerosis **(Figs. 4A and B)**. Nidus may be purely radiolucent or contain a

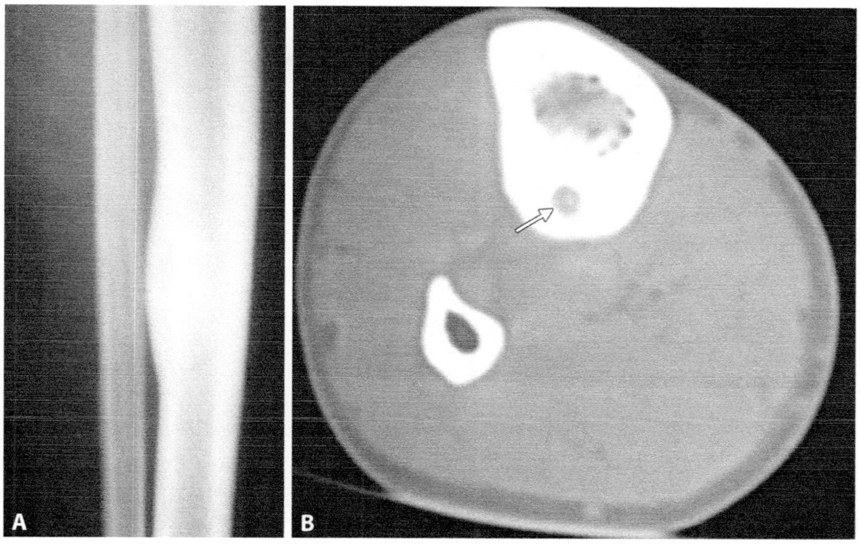

Figs. 4A and B: Osteoid osteoma. (A) Radiograph of leg shows dense sclerosis and solid periosteal reaction in the diaphysis of tibia; (B) CT scan (axial section) reveals well-defined lytic lesion with calcified nidus (arrow) associated with gross adjacent sclerosis.

dense center. Intraarticular osteoid osteomas may be either cancellous or periosteal and have little reactive bone or periosteal new bone formation. [11]

Computed tomography is very useful in showing the nidus, which can vary in its degree of ossification. CT appears to display the nidus better than MRI. Intense bone marrow edema adjacent to nidus is very useful to detect and localized the lesion on MRI **(Fig. 5)**; however, nidus may not readily visible if it is very small.[13] The tumor nidus typically shows hypo- to intermediate signal on T1W images and low to high signal on T2W images. The nidus shows enhancement with gadolinium. Intra-articular osteoid osteomas produce joint effusions and synovial proliferation. Radionuclide bone scans have been used for many years to help diagnosis of osteoid osteomas. Bone scintigraphy, which is a highly sensitive method of detecting osteoid osteoma, typically shows increased flow to the lesion on immediate images and a focus of increased activity on skeletal equilibrium images with double density sign.[14] Many times, osteomyelitis can mimick osteoid osteoma clinically as well radiographically, however, presence of soft tissue extension favors the diagnosis of osteomyelitis.

Osteoblastoma

Osteoblastomas are rare bone-forming tumors and most commonly occurs in patients in the second and third decade of life. This tumor is more common in males than in females. Histologically, the osteoblastoma is closely related to osteoid osteomas except that bony trabeculae are broader and longer with absence of surrounding sclerotic halo. Size is an important consideration in distinguishing between these two types of tumors. If the size of lesion is less than 2 cm in diameter than it is likely of be osteoid osteomas, whereas tumors larger than 2 cm are usually osteoblastoma.[15]

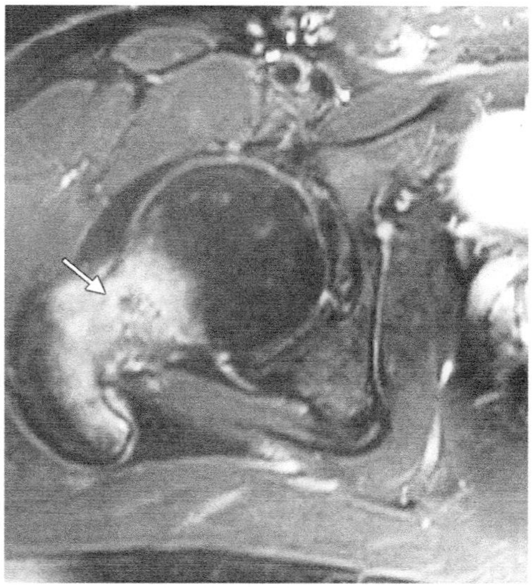

Fig. 5: Osteoid osteoma. T2W fat suppressed MRI (axial section) shows small nidus in neck of femer associated with extensive surrounding edema.

The most common location of osteoblastoma is spine where it classically affects posterior elements **(Figs. 6A to C)**. The other common locations are proximal femur and talus. On plain X-ray, spinal osteoblastoma is osteolytic lesion with destruction of overlying cortex and may extend to in the spinal canal. In the long bones, osteoblastoma appears radiologically as round or oval lucent tumors in the medulla. Periosteal reaction is common. CT demonstrates extent of lesion in complex bony structures such as spine and pelvis better than radiography. MRI features may be

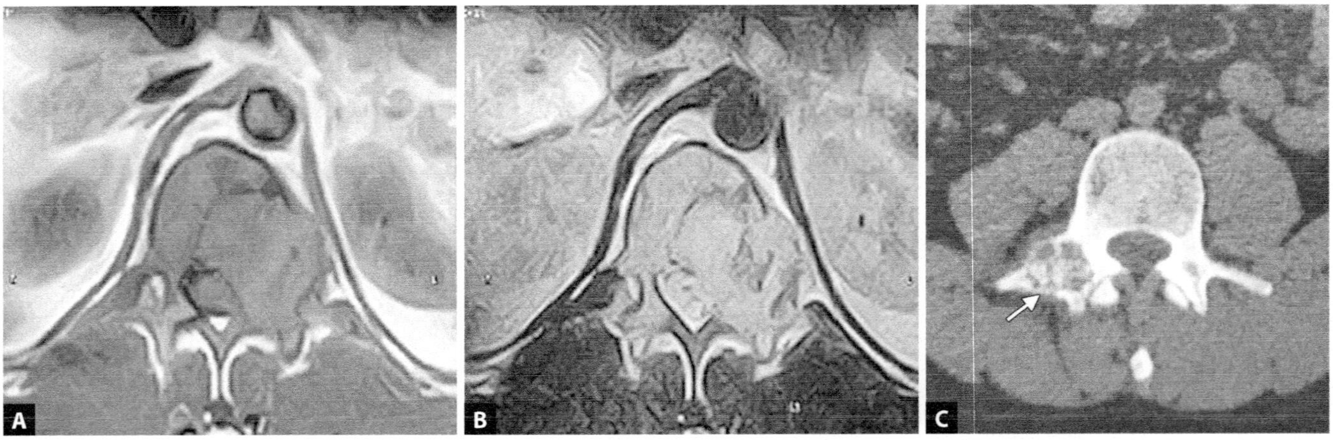

Figs. 6A to C: Osteoblastoma. (A and B) T1W and T2W MR (axial section) images reveal heterogeneous signal mass lesion, predominantly involving posterior elements of vertebra extending into spinal canal; (C) CT scan of spine of another patient shows expansile lytic lesion in right posterior elements with internal matrix mineralization suggestive of osteoblastoma.

nonspecific but helps to determine extension of vertebral lesion into spinal canal and spinal foramina.[16]

CARTILAGE-FORMING TUMORS

Osteochondroma

Osteochondromas are common lesions of the growing skeleton. It is the most common benign neoplasm and constitutes 20–50% of all benign tumors.[17] They arise from bony metaphysis with cartilage cap covering. These tumors are either pedunculated or sessile **(Fig. 7)**. Multiple osteochondroma occur as a manifestation of diaphyseal aclasia, an inherited disorder with autosomal dominance **(Fig. 8)**. The long axis of the osteochondroma pedicle or stalk is almost always directed away from the adjacent joint. The direct communication between the osteochondroma and the cortex and marrow cavity of the bone from which it arises is a distinctive feature, that is particularly well demonstrated on CT and MRI. T2W proton density (PD) MR images are useful to demonstrate a cartilaginous cap **(Figs. 9A and B)**. The cap can be quite thick in early childhood like the normal physis, becomes thinner with age. After epiphyseal closure, growth of the osteochondroma ceases. Because most osteochondromas are asymptomatic, they are usually discovered incidentally. However, mechanical irritation of adjacent soft tissues or nerves, vascular injuries, fracture of the stalk, or malignant transformation can produce symptoms.

Malignant transformation into low-grade chondrosarcoma occurs in 1% of osteochondromas; however, the risk is 10–30% in cases of multiple osteochondromatosis.[17] Malignant transformation should be considered when the osteochondroma grows after epiphyseal closure. Malignancy occurs in the cartilaginous cap, which becomes thickened. After skeletal maturity, the cartilage cap should not be thicker than 2 cm. Pain and cartilage cap growth are the signs of malignant transformation.[18]

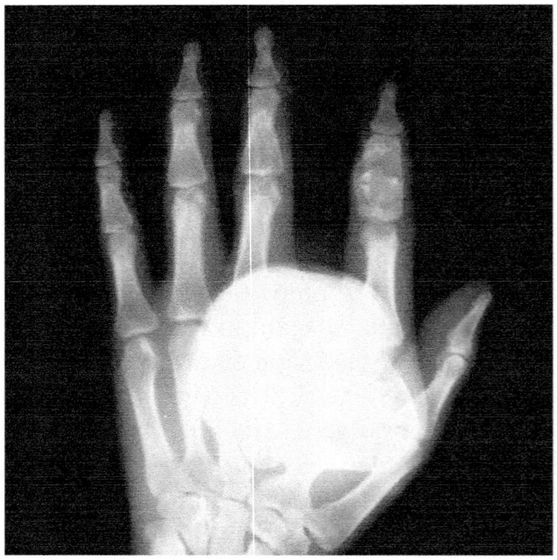

Fig. 7: Sessile osteochondroma. Radiograph of the left hand shows a large well-defined calcified lesion having a broad-based attachment to second metacarpal. An enchondroma showing typical central spotty calcification is also present in the middle phalanx of the index finger.

Enchondroma

Enchondromas accounts for 12% of benign bone tumors.[18] These are most frequently located in the large and small tubular bones of the hands and feet **(Fig. 10)**. Like other cartilaginous tumors, enchondromas exhibit a lobulated growth pattern that results in asymmetric expansion of the medullary cavity and endosteal scalloping. Tumor matrix may be radiolucent or show calcification. Characteristic cartilaginous ring and arc pattern of calcifications is seen on radiographs and CT images. On MRI, the tumor is isointense to muscle on T1W and exhibits a heterogeneous, predominantly high T2W signal.[19] Contrast-enhanced MRI may demonstrate a pattern of thin arcs and rings.

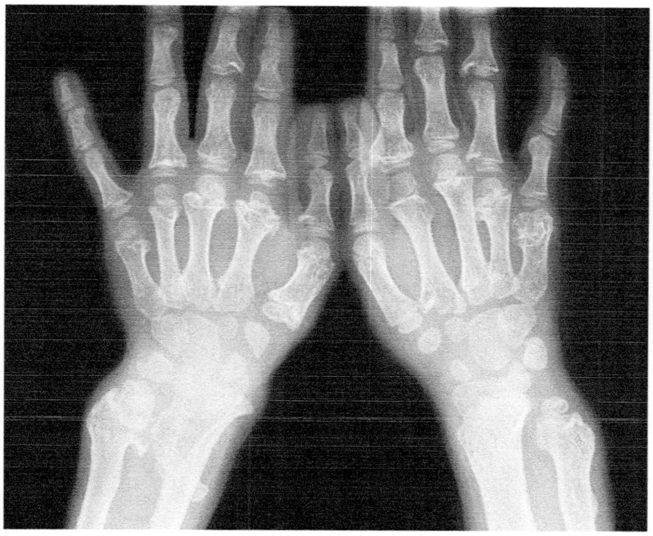

Fig. 8: Diaphyseal aclasia. Radiograph of bilateral hands (PA view) shows multiple osteochondromas and deformities involving multiple bones of hands and forearm.

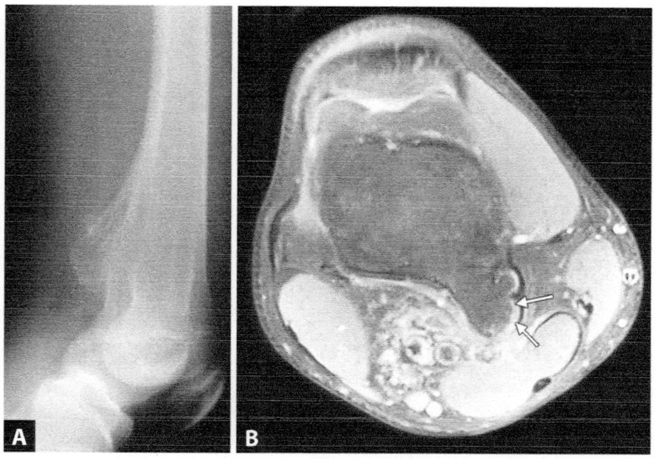

Figs. 9A and B: Pedunculated osteochondroma. (A) Radiograph of lower end of femur (lateral view) shows large well-defined bony outgrowth, with broad-based attachment to femur; (B) MRI (Proton density fat saturation, axial section) of the same patient shows clear demonstration of continuity of marrow and cortex of host bone into osteochondroma with covering cartilage cap (arrows).

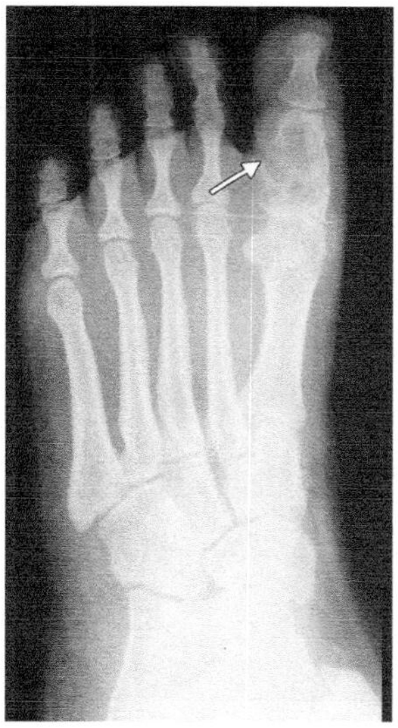

Fig. 10: Enchondroma. Radiograph of foot shows sharply demarcated expansile lesion in proximal phalynx of great toe having endosteal scalloping and cortical breech (arrow).

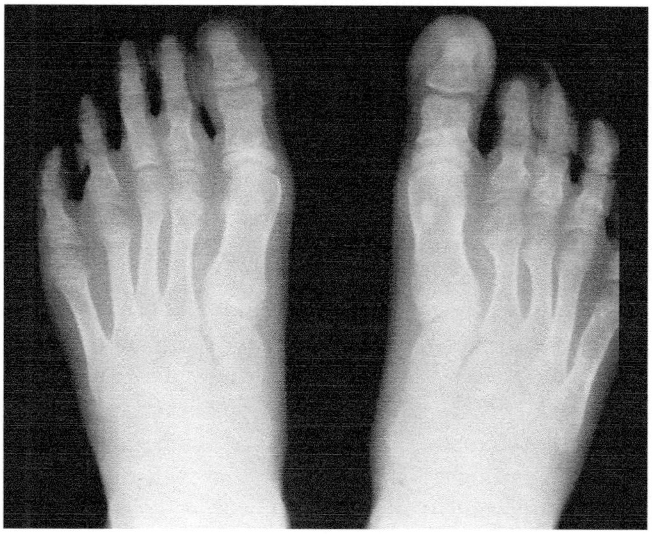

Fig. 11: Ollier's disease. Radiograph of feet shows relatively well-defined expansile lytic lesions involving most of the phalanges, with varying amounts of calcification within them.

Ollier's disease is a nonheritable disorder of cartilage proliferation in which enchondromas involve multiple bones, especially those of the hands and may result in skeletal deformity **(Fig. 11)**. Enchondromatosis accompanied by multiple hemangiomas is known as Maffucci syndrome. Calcified phleboliths may be demonstrated radiographically in the hemangiomatous soft tissue masses. Lesions associated with both Ollier disease and Maffucci syndrome carry a significant risk of malignant degeneration.[20]

Chondroblastoma

It is less common than enchondroma. Chondroblastoma is composed of primitive cartilage cells, usually occurs in the age group of 10–25 years. It is typically located in epiphysis and apophysis of bone, most often the proximal humerus, distal femur, and proximal tibia.[17] On plain X-ray, chondroblastoma is an eccentric, lucent, well-defined lesion with sclerotic borders. Periosteal reaction, far from the lesion is another common feature suggesting an accompanying inflammatory process. Approximately, one-third of chondroblastoma have a calcified matrix which can be better seen on CT scan **(Fig. 12)**.

The tumor shows signal intensity similar to that of muscle on MRI; however, the rim of the tumor has lower signal intensity. On T2W images, the signal intensity of the tumor is low to intermediate. This tumor also shows extensive surrounding inflammation which may

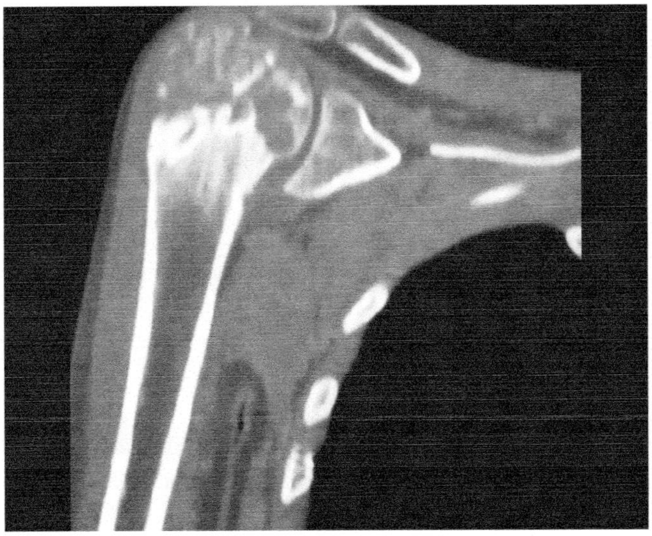

Fig. 12: Chondroblastoma. CT scan (coronal reformation) shows expansile lytic lesion in epiphysis (characteristic location) of upper humerus with matrix calcification.

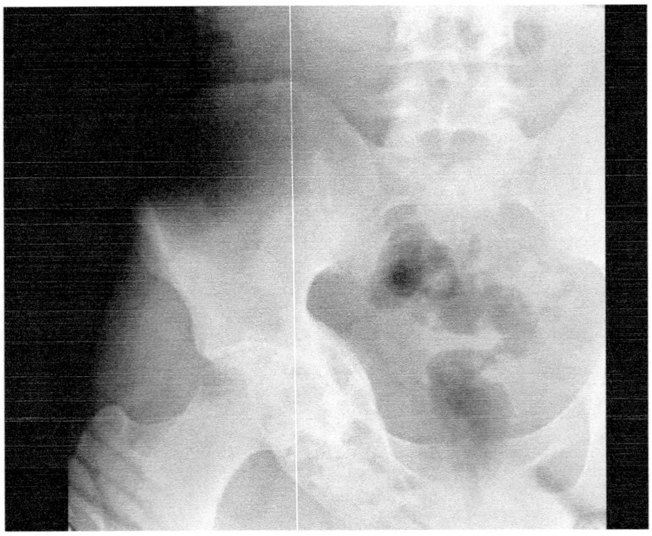

Fig. 13: Chondromyxoid fibroma. Radiograph of right hip shows large expansile lesion with sclerotic border and trabeculations involving right acetabulum.

be confused with more aggressive lesion. Malignant transformation of chondroblastoma is extremely uncommon.[21] The differential diagnosis of epiphyseal lesions includes giant cell tumor (GCT), osteomyelitis, subchondral cyst, and Langerhans cell histiocytosis.

Chondromyxoid Fibroma

Chondromyxoid fibroma is rare and commonly affects males and patients younger than 35 years.[18] Histologically, it is composed of chondroid, myxoid, and fibrous tissue in varying amounts. The common locations of tumor are ilium, tibia, and bones of foot. These tumors are located characteristically in metadiaphyseal location unlike chondroblastoma and do not cross an open growth plate. On plain radiograph, it appears as a well-marginated central or eccentric lucent lesion, with sclerotic margins and cortical thinning **(Fig. 13)**. Half of the lesions may show parallel orientation to the long axis of the involved bone. Matrix calcification and periosteal new bone formation usually do not occur.

FIBROUS TUMORS/LESIONS

Fibrous Cortical Defects and Nonossifying Fibroma

Fibrous cortical defect and nonossifying fibroma are basically similar benign fibrous lesions located slightly differently, nonossifying fibroma being located eccentrically in the medullary cavity **(Fig. 14)**, and fibrous cortical defect seen superficially affecting the cortex **(Fig. 15)**. Pathologically, these lesions are composed of fibrous tissue, xanthoma cells, and giant cells. The common location of lesion is in the bones around the knee joints. These lesions are usually asymptomatic and do not require specific treatment. On plain radiography, the lesion appears as well-marginated eccentric lytic lesion with scalloped margin. Its inner border is often sclerotic and may appear multilocular due to corrugations. Differential diagnosis includes unicameral bone cyst, aneurysmal bone cyst, fibrous dysplasia, and chondromyxoid fibroma. The signal intensity of nonossifying fibroma is equal to or less than muscle on T1W MR images and hypointense on T2W images.[22] Postcontrast images usually show heterogeneous enhancement.

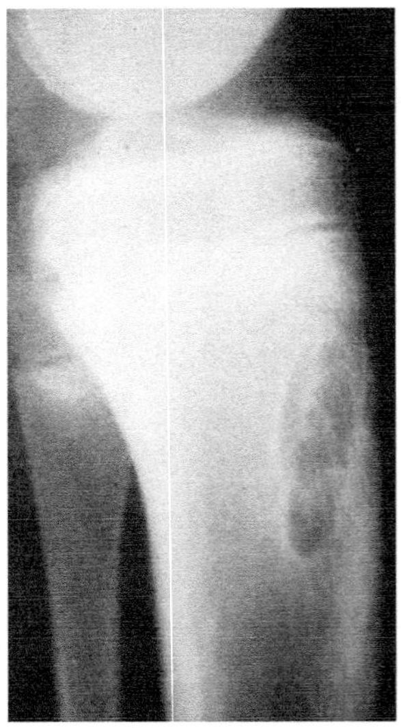

Fig. 14: Nonossifying fibroma. Lateral radiograph of leg shows an eccentric geographic lytic lesion in the medulla of proximal tibial metaphysis.

Fibrous Dysplasia

Fibrous dysplasia is a disorder where bone is replaced by abnormal fibrous tissue. Fibrous dysplasia can be

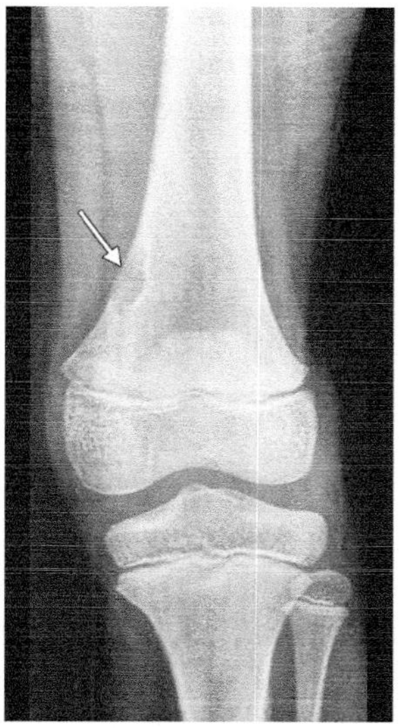

Fig. 15: Fibrous cortical defect. Radigraph of knee (AP view) shows eccentric well-defined lytic lesion in lower end of femur which is limited to cortex (arrow).

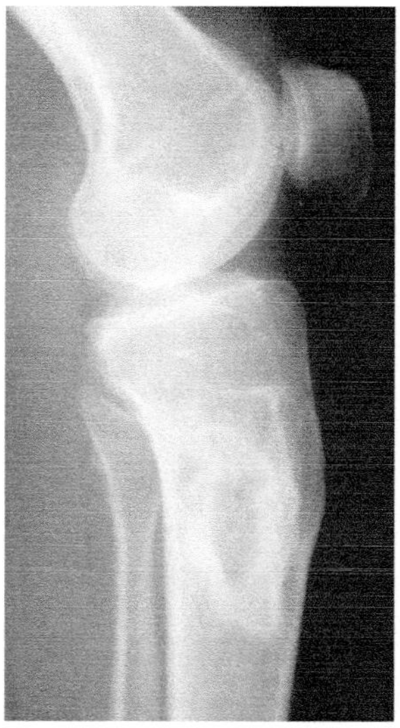

Fig. 16: Fibrous dysplasia. Lateral radiograph of knee joint shows a well-defined lytic lesion in proximal tibial metaphysis with surrounding sclerotic rind which is characteristic of fibrous dysplasia.

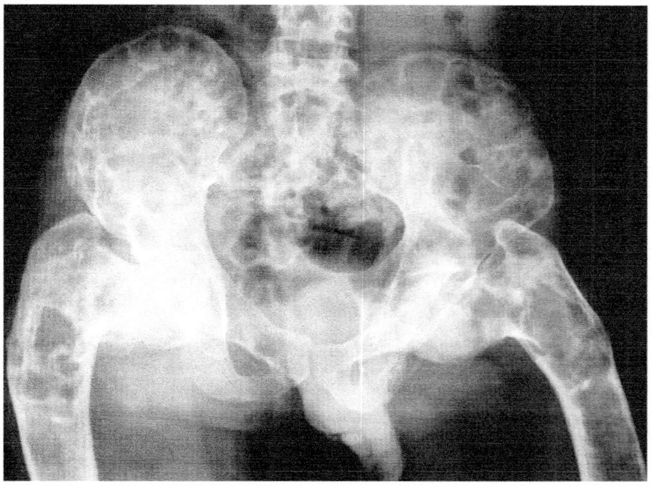

Fig. 17: Polystotic fibrous dysplasia. Radiograph of pelvis shows multiple lytic lesions involving pelvic bones and bilateral femora with characteristic shepherd's crook deformity.

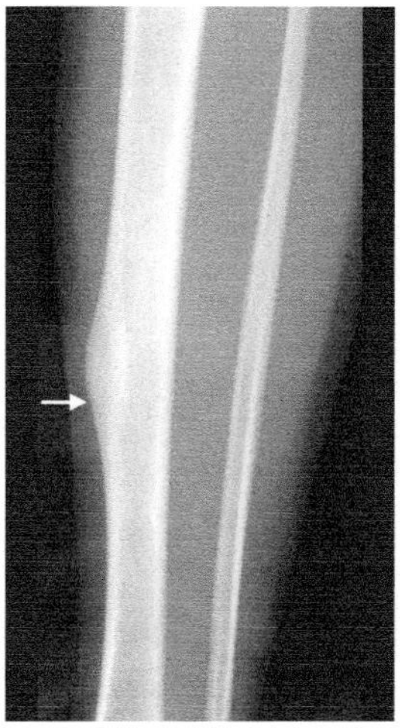

Fig. 18: Radiograph of leg shows well-defined lytic lesion in anterior cortex of tibia characteristic of osteofibrous dysplasia (arrow).

monostotic, polyostotic, monomelic, or polymelic. It is more common in young females. It is occasionally seen in the first decade of life. In a small percentage of cases (2–3%), fibrous dysplasia is associated with endocrine disorders, especially precocious puberty in girls (McCune-Albright syndrome).[23,24] Although it is not a true neoplasm, fibrous dysplasia involving a long bone may mimic a bone tumor or cyst. This type of fibrous dysplasia causes expansion of the medullary cavity of tubular bones, endosteal scalloping, and trabeculation. The margin is sclerotic **(Fig. 16)**. The lesion may appear as ground glass or radiolucent, and this depends upon amount of fibrous tissue within the lesion. Bowing of the affected long bone may occur, when the affected bone is femur, the resulting deformity is called a "shepherd's crook" **(Fig. 17)**. Thinning and destruction of the bony cortex may be seen on CT or MR images. Soft tissue extension of the lesion is unusual. On T1W MR images, the signal intensity of fibrous dysplasia is similar to that of skeletal muscle. Although the signal of pure fibrous tissue is hypointense on T2W images, the signal of fibrous dysplasia is variable.

Osteofibrous Dysplasia

It is a rare lesion that is usually confined to the tibia but can also involve the fibula. Most cases occur during the first decade of life. On plain X-ray, the lesion appears as an eccentric, lucent, solitary, or multiloculated, lesion involving the anterior aspect of tibia **(Fig. 18)**. CT is very helpful in determining its intracortical location, an important feature in distinguishing osteofibrous dysplasia from fibrous dysplasia.[25]

Desmoplastic Fibroma

Desmoplastic fibroma is rare accounting for only 0.1% of benign bone tumors. This lesion is usually seen in the second and third decade of life. Histologically, there is infiltration of abnormal fibrous tissue in the bone and at times it is confused with low-grade fibrosarcoma of bone. They are mostly located in the metadiaphysis of long bones but may invade the epiphysis. Femur, tibia, and humerus are most commonly affected.[26] On radiography, the lesion has aggressive appearance and present as lytic expansile lesion with internal trabeculation and sclerotic margin. CT may demonstrate cortical breech and adjacent soft tissue if any. MRI typically shows intermediate to low signal on fluid sensitive sequences.[27]

VASCULAR AND CONNECTIVE TISSUE TUMORS

Hemangioma

Hemangioma is slowly growing lesions of bone composed of newly formed vascular spaces. About 50% of hemangiomas of bone occur in vertebrae and are most commonly located in lower thoracic and upper lumbar regions.[28] About 20% of hemangiomas occur in skull. Small bones of the hand and feet may also be affected.

Hemangioma of the vertebra has a typical radiographic picture in the form of coarse vertical striations on the plain radiographs and polka dot appearance on CT[29] **(Figs. 19A and B)**. It shows high intensity on both T1W and T2W images. In the skull, hemangioma generally affects the calvarium and is seen as an expansile lytic lesion which has a sunburst appearance with striations radiating from the center. In the short and long bones, the lesion lacks characteristic features and may be difficult to differentiate from other expansile central lesions such as aneurysmal bone cyst, chondromyxoid fibroma, or enchondroma.

Lipoma

Intraosseous lipoma is a rare benign neoplasm that occurs between 5 and 70 years of age. The proximal femur, tibia, and calcaneum are the most common sites of involvement. On plain radiographs lipoma appears as a well-defined osteolytic lesion with a thin sclerotic rim. Bone expansion and trabeculations may be seen within the lesion. Cortical erosion and periosteal reaction are characteristically absent. In the calcaneum, the lesion usually occurs along the plantar margin where a "triangle" is formed by major trabecular groups and there may be a calcified nidus. CT scan shows typical "fat" density (–60 to –120 HU) and lack of contrast enhancement **(Fig. 20)**. On MRI, lipoma typically shows high signal intensity on T1W image and iso to hyperintense signal on T2W image.[30]

OTHER TUMORS

Giant Cell Tumor

Giant cell tumor constitutes about 5% of all bone tumors and slightly less than 20% of all benign tumors.[31] The tumor originates from undifferentiated cells of the supporting tissues of bone marrow. As opposed to other benign tumors, GCT has a female predilection and mostly occurs after the closure of epiphysis, with a peak in the third decade.

Giant cell tumors arise eccentrically in the metaphysis with tendency to approach the adjacent subarticular cortex as they enlarge **(Fig. 21)**. About 40–50% of lesions

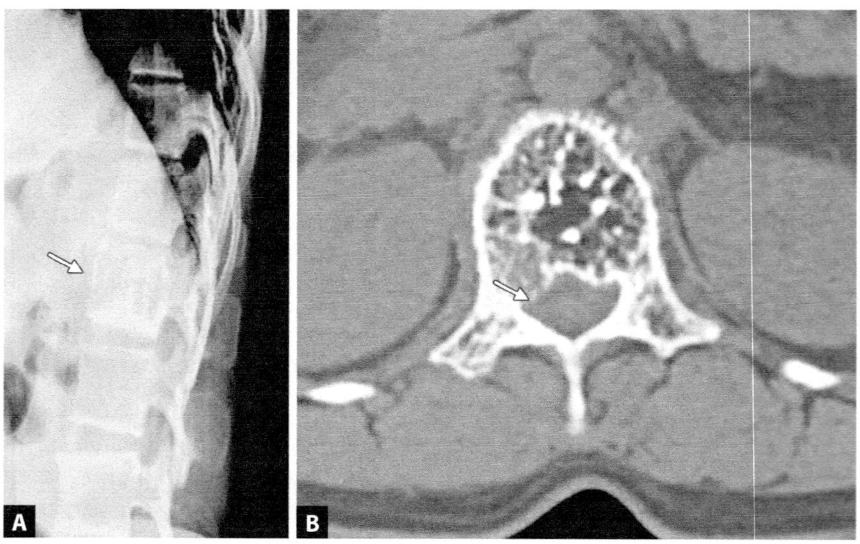

Figs. 19A and B: Hemangioma of vertebra. (A) Lateral radiograph of dorsolumbar spine shows mild expansion of L1 vertebral body with coarse vertical striations (arrow); (B) Axial CT scan of the same patient shows "polka dot" appearance due to vertical trabeculae cut in cross-section. In addition, there is focal disruption of the posterior cortex of vertebral body (arrow).

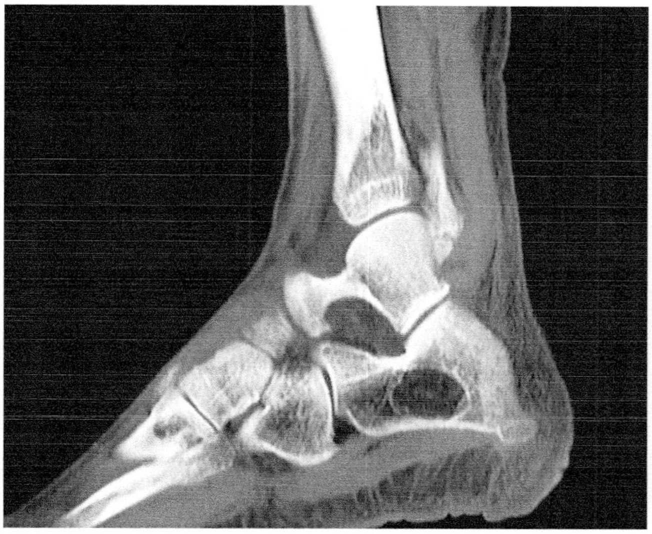

Fig. 20: Sagittal CT (MIP) image of ankle and foot shows well-defined lucent (fatty) lesions in calcaneum suggestive of lipoma.

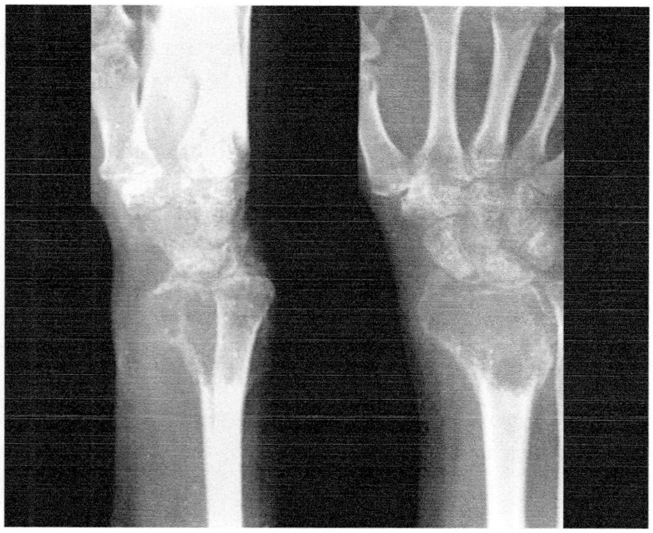

Fig. 21: Giant cell tumor. Radiograph of the left wrist shows an expansile subarticular lytic lesion in the distal end of radius. Cortex appears intact.

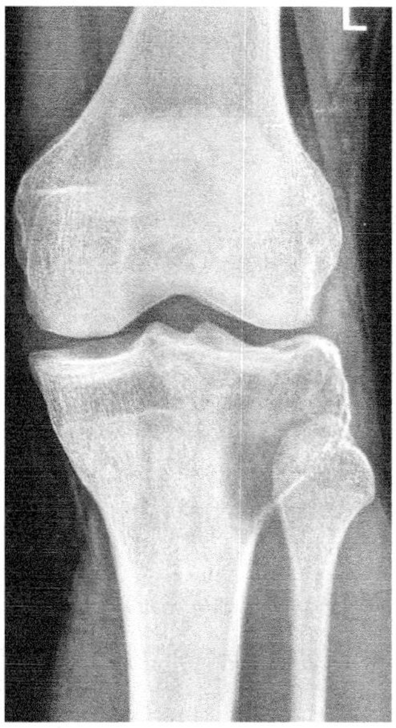

Fig. 22: Giant cell tumor. Radiograph of the knee shows an eccentric expansile subarticular lytic lesion in proximal end of tibia without sclerotic margin.

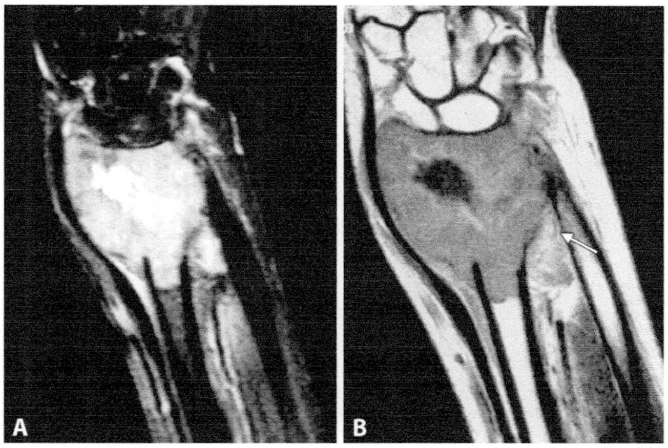

Figs. 23A and B: Giant cell tumor. (A) Coronal MR images of left forearm of the patient (Fig. 19) showing expansile subarticular epiphyseal lesion of radius which is hyperintense on T2W image with central cystic area; (B) Postcontrast image shows homogeneous enhancement of solid component and no enhancement of cystic area. The cortical line on the lateral side is intact but shows disruption with extension of the tumor into the soft tissues on the medial aspect (arrow).

occur around the knee.[31] Involvement of distal radius is seen in 10–12% which otherwise is an uncommon site for bone tumors. Other sites are sacrum, short tubular bones, and vertebral bodies. Classical radiographic picture is that of a well-defined eccentric lytic lesion which expands the bone and is usually not surrounded by a sclerotic rim **(Fig. 22)**. Cortical penetration with or without an associated soft tissue mass is seen in 33–50% of cases. The solid portion of a GCT is usually low to intermediate signal intensity at T1W and T2W images. This has been attributed to its high collagen content, high cellularity, or presence of hemosiderin.[32] GCT is the most common lesion associated with secondary aneurysmal bone cyst. Following contrast administration, there is diffuse enhancement of the solid component and peripheral or septal enhancement of cystic areas **(Figs. 23A and B)**. GCTs are aggressive benign neoplasms with a high rate of recurrence.

TUMOR-LIKE LESIONS

Simple Bone Cyst

A bone cyst is a fluid-filled lesion with fibrous lining. It occurs in metaphysis of long bones and adjacent to physis in children and young adults. Common locations are proximal humerus and femur.[28] Calcaneum and ileum are less common sites. On plain radiograph, the lesion appears as moderately expansile, well marginated with or without sclerosis **(Fig. 24)**. The cortex may be thinned out and may lead to pathological fracture. "Fallen fragment" sign has been described as pathognomonic features of bone cyst when fragment of bone settles at the base of lesion due to simple nature of fluid. "Rising bubbles" sign is also based on similar principles.[33] CT and MRI can confirm the cystic nature of the lesion. The fluid contents are usually of low intensity on T1W images and hypertense on T2W images.[34] However, hemorrhage into the cyst can alter the signal characteristics of the lesion.

Aneurysmal Bone Cyst

Aneurysmal bone cyst is solitary, expansile radiolucent lesion and generally located in metaphysis of long bones. Other sites are dorsolumbar spine, small bones of hand, feet, and pelvis. Pathologically, the lesion contains multiples cystic spaces containing various stages of blood. Radiologically the lesion appears as expansile, lytic sharply circumscribed with thin cortex. The characteristic features are its ballooned out appearance and trabeculated appearance (**Fig. 25**). CT may demonstrate fluid-fluid level and thin rim of bone overlying the lesion. MRI shows the various stages of blood products which appear as layers of different signal intensity on both T1W and T2W images[28] **(Figs. 26A and B)**. The differential diagnosis includes

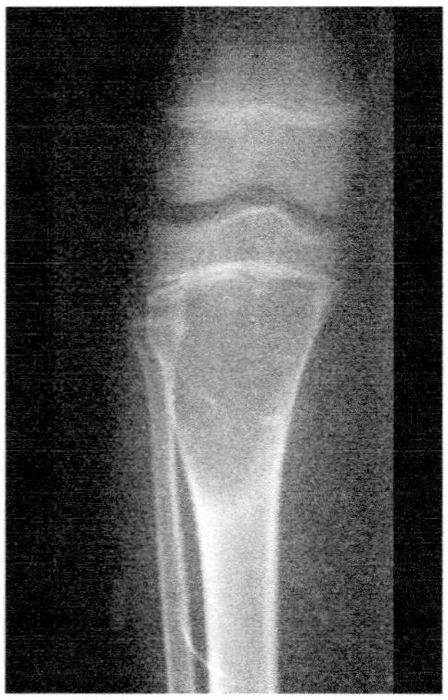

Fig. 24: Bone cyst. Radiograph of knee joint shows mildly expansile lytic lesion in metaphysis of tibia with thinning of cortex and septation.

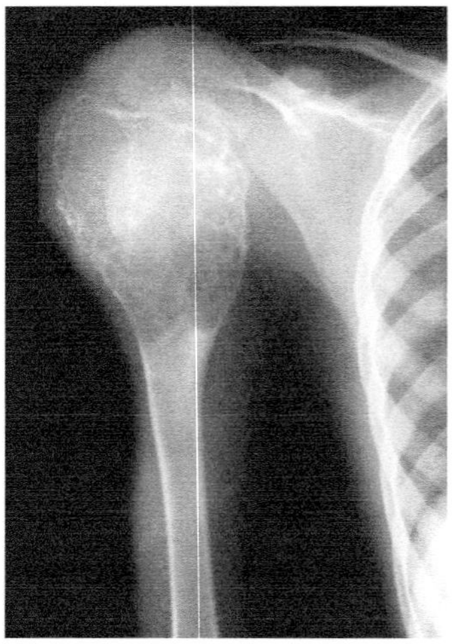

Fig. 25: Aneurysmal bone cyst. Radiograph of shoulder joint shows multiloculated very expansile lytic lesion, involving upper end of humerus.

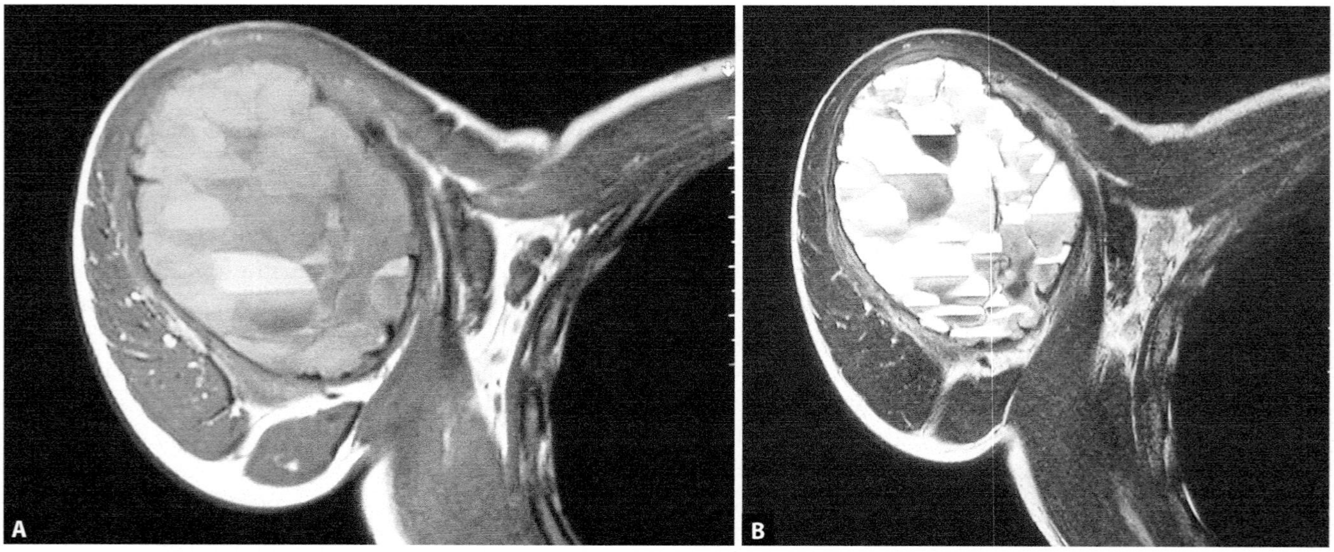

Figs. 26A and B: Aneurysmal bone cyst. MRI of the same patient, axial T1W (A) and T2W (B) images show well-defined multiloculated expansile lesion with extensive fluid–fluid/hemorrhage levels.

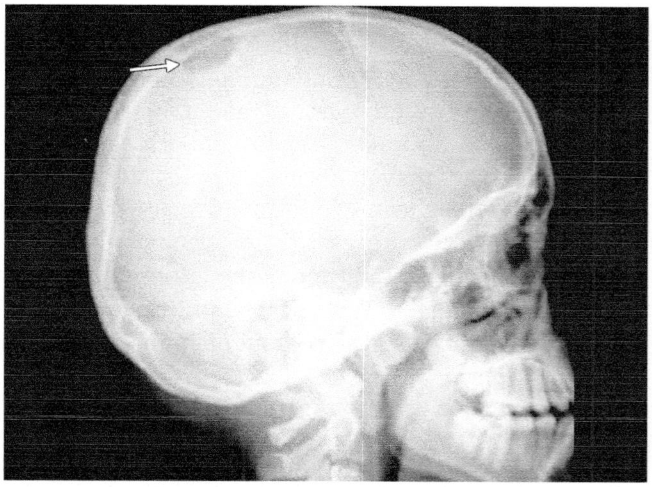

Fig. 27: Eosinophilic granuloma. Lateral radiograph of skull shows a well-defined lytic lesion with bevelled edges in the parietal bone (arrow).

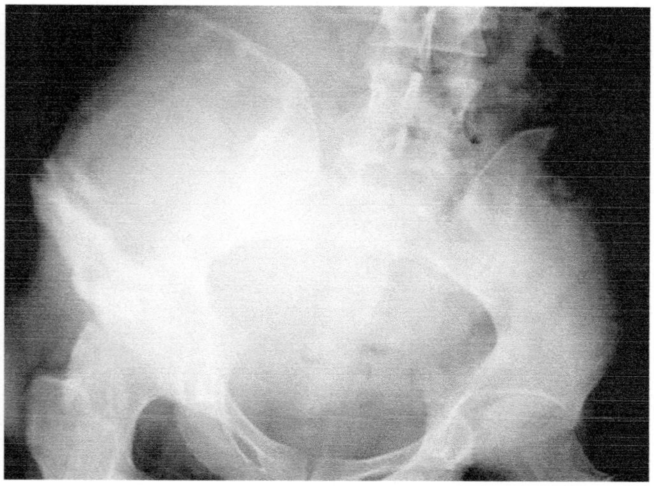

Fig. 28: Hemophilic pseudotumor. Radiograph (anteroposterior veiw) of pelvis reveals a large well-defined lytic lesion in the right iliac bone with an associated soft tissue mass.

GCT, osteoblastoma, chondroblastoma, osteosarcoma, and simple bone cyst.

Eosinophilic Granuloma

Eosinophilic granuloma is the most benign form of histiocytosis X, which is a disease of unknown etiology characterized by proliferation of histiocytes. Eosinophilic granuloma constitutes 60–80% of Langerhans cell histiocytosis. Bone lesion may be solitary (85%) or multiple (20%) with peak incidence between 5 and 10 years.[35] The preferred sites being skull, mandible, spine, and long bones. The skull lesion on radiographs is seen as a punched out lytic lesion having a bevelled appearance due to unequal involvement of outer and inner table, with a variably sclerotic margin **(Fig. 27)**. The center of the lesion has a sclerotic focus which is often termed as a button sequestrum. In the mandible, lytic lesion may cause floating teeth. In the spine, typically the vertebral body is affected, and there may be complete lysis resulting in a solitary collapsed vertebra with a preserved disc space. In the long bones, the lesions are generally diaphyseal or metaphyseal in location and cause endosteal scalloping. Benign type of periosteal reaction is considered typical.

Pseudotumor of Hemophilia

Hemophilia is a bleeding disorder that occurs in males. Repetitive hemorrhage within the bone may result expansile geographic lesion which can simulate neoplasm **(Fig. 28)**. The common locations are femur, pelvis, tibia, and hand. CT scan better demonstrates the bony erosion/destruction with adjacent hematoma **(Fig. 29)**. MRI shows variable heterogeneous signals, in form of various stages of blood products.[36]

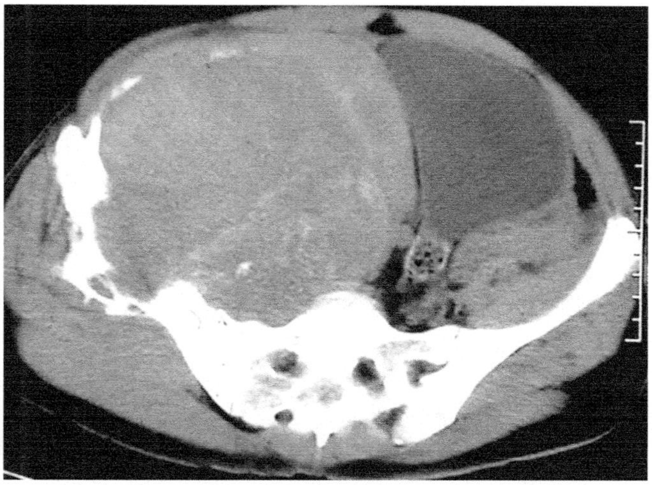

Fig. 29: Axial noncontrast computed tomography (NCCT) scan of the same patient shows erosion of the right ilium with a large soft tissue mass that has a variegated appearance with hyperdense areas within it suggestive of hemorrhage.

Brown Tumor of Hyperparathyroidism

Brown tumors represent focal, bone replacing lesions, encountered both in primary or secondary hyperparathyroidism. They represents hemorrhage and breakdown product of hemoglobin. The lesions most often occur in metaphyses and diaphyses and the common bones involved are mandible, pelvis, ribs, and femur.[37]

On plain radiographs, the lesions are seen as slightly trabeculated, solitary, or multiple expansile lytic lesions with well-defined margins **(Fig. 30)**. Differentiation from a simple bone cyst is difficult when the lesion is solitary. Associated skeletal osteoporosis and biochemical changes, sclerotic appearance of brown tumor after removal of parathyroid adenoma, and the marked activity with scintigraphy are helpful in the diagnosis.[37,38]

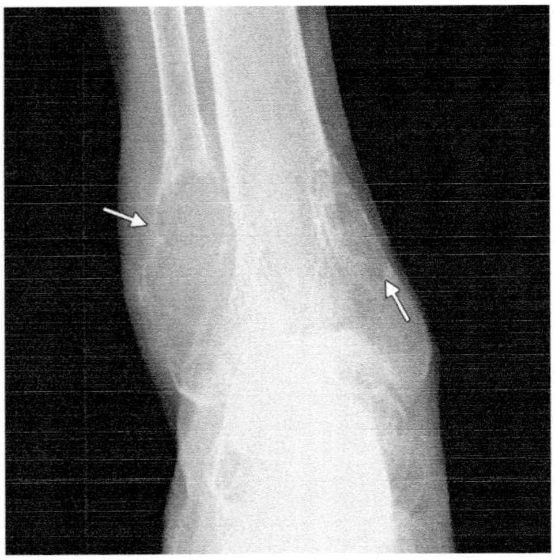

Fig. 30: Brown tumors. Radiograph of left ankle of young man with hyperparathyroidism shows multiple well-defined expansile multiloculated lytic lesions in lower end of tibia and fibula.

ROLE OF ADVANCE MAGNETIC RESONANCE IMAGING

Apart from conventional T1W/T2W MR sequences, there has been advancement in MRI in last two decades with sequences such as diffusion-weighted imaging (DWI), perfusion-weighted imaging, and spectroscopy. Most of them being used in diagnosis and management in malignant bone tumors, however, some authors have tried these sequences in benign bone tumors also.

Diffusion-weighted imaging: DWI is a method of functional imaging.[39] This method measures the Brownian motion of water at a microscopic level. Corresponding ADC (apparent diffusion coefficient) maps provide quantitative assessment of the diffusivity of the lesion. ADC is marker of cellularity and tumor density. High cellularity tumor has low ADC, and low-density tumor shows more ADC. Various authors have tried to differentiate benign and malignant bone tumors by using DWI and reported with good results with some overlap features.[40,41]

Perfusion-weighted MRI: Perfusion sequences provide insight of vascularity of tumor. The most common method of perfusion is dynamic contrast-enhanced MRI (DCMR). This is done by using GRE sequence for particular volume of tumor after injecting intravenous contrast and creating time intensity curve (TIC) and using semiquantitative measurements. Authors have used DCMR to differentiate malignant from benign bone lesions with good sensitivity and specificity.[42] Sometime osteoid osteoma can mimic chronic osteomyelitis on radiographs. Although CT is best to show nidus in osteoid osteoma; however, MRI can help by showing typical TIC curve by using DCMR. Most osteoid osteoma shows arterial enhancement with rapid washout.[43]

MR spectroscopy: Proton MR spectroscopy is noninvasive method form molecular characterization of tumor. Some of the authors have shown choline peaks and different choline ratio for differentiating benign and malignant musculoskeletal tumors.[44,45] The method is technically challenging and may have overlapping features as choline may not be feature of tumor aggressiveness and malignancy.[46]

These advance methods are although promising but should be additional to conventional MRI sequence and should not read in isolation without plain radiographs to avoid misdiagnosis.

CONCLUSION

Some of the bony tumors and tumor-like lesions have characteristic imaging features; however, many others may have overlap imaging findings. Thorough knowledge of radiographic characteristics of these lesions on various imaging modalities (radiography, CT, and MRI) with patient data and clinical information is helpful to make diagnosis or to reach differential diagnosis.

REFERENCES

1. Greenfield BG. The solitary lesion. Radiology of Bone Disease, 5th edition. Philadelphia: JB Lippincott; 1990. pp. 580-732.
2. Forest M, Coindre JM, Diebold J. Pathology of tumors. In: Forest M, Tomeno B, Vanel D (Eds). Orthopedic Surgical Pathology: Diagnosis of Tumors and Pseudotumoral Lesions of Bone and Joints. Epindburgh: Churchill Livingstone; 1997. pp. 71-516.
3. Resnick D. Tumors and tumor-like lesions of bone: Radiographic principles. In: Resnick D (Ed). Diagnosis of Bone and Joint Disorders. Philadelphia: Saunders; 1995. pp. 3613-27.
4. Woertler K. Benign bone tumor and tumor-like lesions: value of cross sectional imaging. Eur Radiol. 2003;13:1820-35.
5. Resnick D, Kyriakos M, Greenway GD. Tumors and tumor-like lesions of bone: imaging and pathology of specific of bone lesions. In: Resnick D (Ed). Diagnosis of Bone and Joint Disorders. Philadelphia: Saunders; 1995. pp. 3628-938.
6. Magid D. Two-dimensional and three-dimensional computed tomographic imaging in musculoskeletal tumors. Radiol Clin North Am. 1993;31:425-47.
7. Berquist TH. Magnetic resonance imaging of primary skeletal neoplasms. Radiol Clin North Am. 1993;31:411-24.
8. Moulton JS, Bvaley SE, Biedel JS. Bone and soft tissue tumors. Clinical Magnetic Resonance Imaging, 2nd edition. Philadelphia: Saunders; 1996. pp. 2042-77.
9. Greenspan A. Bone island (enostotsis): current concept—a review. Skeletal Radiol. 1995;24:111-5.
10. Schweitzer ME, Levine C, Mitchell DG, Gannon FH, Gomella LG. Bull's eyes and halos: useful discriminators of osseous metastases. Radiology. 1993;188:249-52.
11. Cerase A, Priolo F. Skeletal benign bone forming lesions. Eur J Radiol. 1998;27:91-7.

12. Bloem JL, Kroon HM. Osseous lesions. Radiol Clin North Am. 1993;31:261-5.
13. Davies M, Cassar-Pullicino VN, Davies MA, McCall IW, Tyrrell PN. The diagnostic accuracy of MR imaging in osteoid osteoma. Skeletal Radiol. 2002;31:559-69.
14. Brown LM. Bone scintigraphy in benign and malignant tumors. Radiol Clin North Am. 1993;31:731-8.
15. Motamedi K, Seeger LL. Benign bone tumors. Radiol Clin N Am. 2011;49:1115-34.
16. Motamedi K, Ilaslan H, Seeger LL. Imaging of lumbar spine neoplasms. Semin Ultrasound CT MR. 2004;25:474-89.
17. Giudici MA, Moser RP, Kransdorf MJ. Cartilaginous bone tumors. Radiol Clin North Am. 1993;31:237-59.
18. Robbin MR, Murphey MD. Benign chondroid neoplasms of the bone. Semin Musculoskeletal Radiol. 2000;4:45-58.
19. Steven S, Srinivas K, Javicr B. MR imaging of tumors and tumor like lesions of the upper extremity. Magn Reson Imaging Clin N Am. 2004;12:349-59.
20. Holtz P, Sundaram M. Enchondroma. Orthopaedics. 1995;18:509-10.
21. Mermelstein LE, Friedlaender GE, Katz LD. Chondroblastoma. Orthopaedics. 1997;20:67-71.
22. Jee Wh, Choe BY, Kang HS, Suh KJ, Suh JS, Ryu KN, et al. Nonossifying fibroma: Characteristics at MR imaging with pathologic correlation. Radiology. 1998;209:197-202.
23. Hudson TM, Stiles RG, Monson DK. Fibrous lesions of bone. Radiol Clin North Am. 1993;31:279-97.
24. Lucas E, Sundaram M, Boccini T. Polyostotic fibrous dysplasia. Orthopaedics. 1995;18:311-3.
25. Zeanah WR, Hudson TM, Springfield DS. Computed tomography of ossifying fibroma of the tibia. J Comput Assist Tomogr. 1983;7:688-91.
26. Robbin MR, Murphey MD, Temple HD, Kransdorf MJ, Choi JJ. Imaging of musculoskeletal fibromatosis. Radiographics. 2001;21:585-600.
27. Frick MA, Sundaram M, Unni KK, Inwards CY, Fabbri N, Trentani F, et al. Imaging findings in desmoplastic fibroma of bone: Distinctitive T2 characterstics. Am J Roentgenol. 2005;184:1762-7.
28. Conway WF, Hayes CW. Miscellaneous lesions of bone. Radiol Clin North Am. 1993;31(2):339-58.
29. Persaud T. The polka dot sign. Radiology. 2008;246:980-1.
30. Propeck T, Bullard MA, Lin J, Doi K, Martel W. Radiologic pathologic correlation of intraosseous lipomas. Am J Roentgenology. 2000;175:673-8.
31. Manaster BJ, Doyle AJ. Giant cell tumors of bone. Radiol Clin North Am. 1993;31(2):299-323.
32. George N, Murphey M, Kransdof MJ. Primary bone tumors of the lower extremities. Radiol Clin North Am. 2002;40:971-90.
33. Jordanov MI. The "rising bubble" sign: a new aid in the diagnosis of unicarmeral bone cyst. Skeletal Radiol. 2009;38:597-600.
34. Parman LM, Murphey MD. Alphabet soup: cystic lesions of bone. Semin Musculoskelet Radiol. 2000;4:89-101.
35. Marin C, Warrier RP. Langerhans cell histiocytosis. Orthop Clin North Am. 1996;27(3):615-23.
36. Wilson DA, Prince JR. MR imaging of hemophilic pseudotumors. Am J Roentgenol. 1988;150:349.
37. Richardson ML, Pozz-mucelli RS, Kanter AS. Bone mineral changes in primary hyperparathyroidism. Skeletal Radiol. 1986;15:85-95.
38. Hayes CW, Conway WF. Hyperparathyroidism. Radiol Clin North Am. 1991;29:85-96.
39. Einarsdóttir H, Karlsson M, Wejde J, Bauer HC. Diffusion-weighted MRI of soft tissue tumours. Eur Radiol. 2004;14(6):959-63.
40. Pekcevik Y, Kahya MO, Kaya A. Diffusion-weighted magnetic resonance imaging in the diagnosis of bone tumors: Preliminary results. J Clin Imag Sci. 2013;3:63.
41. Rao A, Sharma C, Parampalli R. Role of diffusion-weighted MRI in differentiating benign from malignant bone tumors. BJR Open. 2019;1:20180048.
42. Cao J, Xiao L, He B, Zhang G, Dong J, Wu Y, et al. Diagnostic value of combined diffusion-weighted imaging with dynamic contrast enhancement MRI in differentiating malignant from benign bone lesions. Clin Radiol. 2017;72(9):793.e1-793.e9.
43. Chai JW, Hong SH, Choi JY, Koh YH, Lee JW, Choi JA, et al. Radiologic diagnosis of osteoid osteoma: from simple to challenging findings. Radiographics. 2010;30(3):737-49.
44. Fayad LM, Barker PB, Jacobs MA, Eng J, Weber KL, Kulesza P, et al. Characterization of musculoskeletal lesionson 3-T proton MR spectroscopy. Am J Roentgenol. 2007;188(6):1513-20.
45. Fayad LM, Wang X, Salibis N, Barker PB, Jacobs MA, Machado AJ, et al. A feasibility study of quantitative molecular characterization of musculoskeletal lesions by proton MR spectroscopy at 3 T. Am J Roentgenol. 2010;195(1):W69-75.
46. Ratnaparkhi CR, Tayade KA, Mitra KR. Magnetic resonance spectroscopy of giant cell tumor of bone. J Clin Diagn Res. 2018;12(11):TC07-TC10.

CHAPTER 14

Malignant Bone Tumors

Anju Garg, Radhika Batra, Sapna Singh

Primary malignant bone tumors are rare and they account for only 0.2% of all primary malignancies and 5.0% of all pediatric malignancies.[1,2] Metastatic tumors, benign tumors, and tumor mimics (e.g., bone cysts, nonossifying fibroma, inflammatory lesions, fibrous dysplasia, and Paget's disease) are more commonly seen than primary bone malignancies. There is a peak at the age of 10–20 years, with a second peak seen after the age of 40 years, although primary bone malignancies may occur at any age.[1,3]

The determination of the nature and the extent of the tumor is critical for appropriate decision making regarding the utility of limb salvage procedures, chemotherapy, radiation therapy, or combined therapy in managing skeletal neoplasms. The correct diagnosis and an accurate staging therefore become more than just an academic exercise, as they determine the appropriate therapy and prognosis. Conventional radiography along with cross-sectional imaging modalities, particularly magnetic resonance imaging (MRI), plays a very important role in detecting, establishing the nature, assessing the extent, and in follow-up in all suspected cases of bone tumors.

CLASSIFICATION OF PRIMARY MALIGNANT BONE TUMORS

The bone tumors have been classified according to their cell of origin or histogenesis (e.g., osteogenic, chondrogenic, fibrogenic, fibrohistiocytic, notochondral, and vascular tumors). They have been further broadly divided into benign, intermediate—locally aggressive and rarely metastasizing, and malignant categories. An updated classification of soft-tissue and bone tumors has been published by the World Health Organization (WHO) in 2013. The updates have been established on the identification of new genetic findings in different tumors. This revision has led to reproducible and reliable classification of the tumors enabling more effective treatment stratification. Hemangiopericytoma and malignant fibrous histiocytoma (MFH) have been removed from the 2013 WHO classification with the recognition that these groups include tumors which can be classified as specific sarcoma types.[4,5] **Table 1** gives a modified version of malignant tumors of the WHO classification.

Hematopoietic neoplasms include plasma cell myelomas, solitary plasmacytoma of bone, and primary non-Hodgkin lymphoma of bone which have been discussed elsewhere in the book.

GENERAL PRINCIPLES OF DIAGNOSIS

A reasonable differential diagnosis can be achieved for most bone tumors using the patient's age, location of the lesion and its imaging appearance. However, the final diagnosis is histological, often requiring an imaging-guided biopsy.

The *age* of the patient plays an important role in establishing the diagnosis and may lead to the correct histological diagnosis even when the tumor is radiographically atypical. The preferential time of origin of the various tumors is summarized in **Table 2**. In very young patients, malignant bone tumors are likely to be metastases from neuroblastoma or leukemia. In the first decade, the most likely primary bone tumors are Ewing sarcoma and, later, osteosarcoma. In adolescence and adult life, various primary tumors are probable. In older age groups, most bone tumors are metastatic carcinomas. Multiple myeloma also occurs in this age group.

The *site of origin or location* of a lesion is also of diagnostic significance with respect to which bone is involved and which portion of the bone, i.e., epiphysis, metaphysis, or diaphysis, is the tumor situated in. **Table 3** summarizes the preferential sites of origin of various malignant bone tumors. Many primary osseous neoplasms develop in the areas of rapid bone growth, especially the distal femur, proximal tibia, and proximal humerus. As the tumors of a given cell type typically arise in a location where the homologous normal cells are most active, the predilection of many bone tumors for the metaphysis and physeal regions of an enlarging tubular bone is not unexpected.[6] Furthermore, the vascular anatomy peculiar to this region, consisting of looped vessels and sinusoidal channels, promotes sluggish blood flow and, with it, metastatic seeding of tumor (and infection).

Table 1: WHO classification of malignant bone tumors.

Osteogenic tumors	• Low-grade central osteosarcoma • Conventional osteosarcoma • Chondroblastic osteosarcoma • Fibroblastic osteosarcoma • Osteoblastic osteosarcoma • Telangiectatic osteosarcoma • Small cell osteosarcoma • Secondary osteosarcoma • Parosteal osteosarcoma • Periosteal osteosarcoma • High-grade surface osteosarcoma
Chondrogenic tumors	• *Chondrosarcoma*: Grade II and III • Dedifferentiated chondrosarcoma • Mesenchymal chondrosarcoma • Clear cell chondrosarcoma
Fibrogenic tumors	Spindle cell sarcoma (fibrosarcoma)
Fibrohistiocytic tumors	Malignant fibrous histiocytoma of bone was removed from the current classification and renamed undifferentiated high-grade pleomorphic sarcoma of bone
Ewing sarcoma	
Osteoclastic giant cell rich tumors	Malignancy in giant cell tumor of bone
Hematopoietic tumors	• Plasma cell myeloma • Solitary plasmacytoma • Primary non-Hodgkin lymphoma of bone
Notochordal tumors	Chordoma
Vascular tumors	• Epithelioid hemangioendothelioma • Angiosarcoma
Myogenic, lipogenic, and epithelial tumors	• Leiomyosarcoma • Liposarcoma • Adamantinoma
Undifferentiated high-grade pleomorphic sarcoma	

Table 2: Age and malignant tumors.

Age (years)	*Tumors*
<1	Neuroblastoma
1–10	Ewing sarcoma—tubular bones
10–30	Osteosarcoma and Ewing sarcoma—flat bones
30–40	Spindle cell sarcoma (fibrosarcoma), undifferentiated pleomorphic sarcoma, parosteal sarcoma, malignant giant cell tumor, and lymphomas
>40	Metastatic carcinoma, multiple myeloma, and chondrosarcoma

Table 3: Preferential site of origin of various malignant tumors of bone.

Epiphysis	Giant cell tumor (after fusion of growth plate)
Metaphysis	• Osteosarcoma • Parosteal sarcoma • Chondrosarcoma • Spindle cell sarcoma (fibrosarcoma) • Giant cell tumor (before fusion of growth plate)
Diaphysis	• Ewing tumor • Myeloma • Reticulum cell sarcoma • Adamantinoma • Undifferentiated pleomorphic sarcoma

Certain tumors, because of their derivation, predominate in one or more particular areas of the skeleton, e.g., chordomas, developing from the remnant of the primitive notochord, are typically seen at the cranial and caudal limits of the vertebral column, whereas a variety of neoplasms related to dentition are virtually confined to the mandible or maxilla.

The *morphological features* of the bone tumors generally reflect their tissue of origin. The pattern of bone destruction, the growth rate of the lesion, the presence and the nature of the visible tumor matrix, internal trabeculation, cortical erosion, penetration, expansion, and the periosteal response are some of the features which need to be analyzed.

Predisposing conditions: Certain benign lesions can transform into bone malignancies. Radiation to healthy bone and radiation of preexisting lesions can lead to malignancy. Osteosarcoma can be seen in 10–29% of children <5 years of age who receive 1,500–5,000 cGy of radiation with a latent period of 3–18 years. Osteosarcoma or spindle cell sarcoma can also occur after radiation exposure. The tumors develop in the periphery of the radiation field where cell mutation occurs without cell death.

Malignant transformation can be seen with Paget's disease, more commonly seen in men in the sixth to seventh decades of life. The most common sarcoma to develop is osteosarcoma followed by spindle cell sarcoma and chondrosarcoma. These tumors occur most commonly in the femur, pelvis, and humerus. Lymphoma and leukemia can also arise in the bone in Paget's disease.

Bone infarction is also a predisposing factor for the development of sarcomas. Malignancy can arise sporadically in patients with fibrous dysplasia, most common being osteosarcoma followed by fibrosarcoma. Most cases of malignancy from fibrous dysplasia are secondary to radiation.

Other predisposing factors include chronic osteomyelitis, orthopedic implants, aneurysmal bone cysts (ABCs), giant cell tumors (GCTs), and neurofibromatosis 1.

Determining the *histological type* of the tumor, by fine-needle aspiration cytology or by biopsy, should be the last step in the patient's pretreatment evaluation as the reaction of tissue to the biopsy alters the imaging appearance of tumor obscuring its true anatomic extent and local aggressiveness. Also, if the biopsy is done at the final stage of evaluation, the definitive surgical procedure can be done at the same operation setting with the diagnosis made on the frozen section. Imaging studies can be of value in identifying the specific area of a tumor that should be biopsied and in planning how to get there without undue tissue contamination.

STAGING OF BONE TUMORS

Enneking system for staging malignant musculoskeletal tumors and the American Joint Committee on Cancer (AJCC) system for staging bone sarcomas are the commonly used staging systems for malignant bone tumors.[7] The universal TNM staging system used for most carcinomas is not commonly used for bone sarcomas because of the rarity with which these sarcomas metastasize to lymph nodes.

Enneking and coauthors described a staging system that gained acceptance in which malignant bone tumors are staged by the assessment of the histological grade (G), the local extent (T), and the presence or absence of regional or distant metastases **(Table 4)**.

Grade

The grade of a tumor is a measure of its potential to metastasize. It is based primarily on histological features and therefore requires a preoperative biopsy. A sarcoma is classified as either low-grade or high-grade. Low-grade lesions are well differentiated, have less mitoses, display only moderate cellular atypia, and have low risk of metastases (<25%). They require a relatively conservative surgical procedure. High-grade lesions are poorly differentiated and show high mitotic rate and high cell-to-matrix ratio. Conversely, a high-grade lesion usually necessitates a more radical procedure, because of its more aggressive nature.

Local Extent

The anatomic extent is either intracompartmental (A) or extracompartmental (B). A "compartment" is defined as an anatomic structure or space bounded by natural barriers to tumor extension. Tumors confined to the compartment of origin usually are less aggressive and require less radical surgery than those extending into the adjacent compartment. Small nodules of tumor may be found separate from the main body of the tumor, but usually remain within the same anatomic compartment. Extracompartmental spread may occur via direct tumor invasion of an adjacent compartment or by contamination

Table 4: Enneking surgical staging of musculoskeletal sarcoma.

Stage (M)	*Grade*	*Site (T)*	*Metastasis*
IA	Low (G1)	Intracompartmental (T1)	No (Mo)
IB	Low (G1)	Extracompartmental (T2)	No (Mo)
IIA	High (G2)	Intracompartmental (T1)	No (Mo)
IIB	High (G2)	Extracompartmental (T2)	No (Mo)
III	Any (G)	Any (T)	Yes (M1) Regional/distant

Table 5: American Joint Committee on Cancer system for staging bone sarcomas.

Stage	Grade	Size	Metastasis
IA	Low	<8 cm	None
IB	Low	>8 cm	None
IIA	High	<8 cm	None
IIB	High	>8 cm	None
III	Any	Any	Skip metastasis
IVA	Any	Any	Pulmonary metastases
IVB	Any	Any	Nonpulmonary metastases

resulting from fracture, hemorrhage, or an operative procedure, such as an unplanned resection or poorly planned biopsy.

Metastases

The third component of the staging system is the presence or absence of nodal or distant metastases. Regional lymph node involvement is much less common with musculoskeletal sarcomas than are pulmonary metastases, but both are equally poor prognostic factors.

The AJCC system for bone sarcomas is based on tumor grade, size, presence, and location of metastases **(Table 5)**. Stage I includes low-grade tumors and stage II includes high-grade tumors, which are subdivided based on tumor size; stages IA and IIA are 8 cm or less in their maximum linear dimension and stages IB and IIB are more than 8 cm. Stage III tumors show skip metastases, which are defined as discontinuous lesions within the same bone or within the immediately adjacent bone. Stage IVA has pulmonary metastases and stage IVB has nonpulmonary metastases. There is subdivision in stage IV as patients with nonpulmonary metastases have worse prognosis than patients with only pulmonary metastases.

IMAGING MODALITIES

Conventional radiographic techniques still remain the mainstay in initial diagnosis and work-up of a patient suspected to have any bony pathology. Cross-sectional studies are required following conventional radiography, in cases of suspected malignant bone tumors for (1) staging of tumor, (2) determining the site and route of biopsy, (3) providing measurements needed for an anticipated surgical procedure, and (4) evaluation of residual and/or recurrent disease after therapy.

Conventional Radiography

Plain radiographs can demonstrate the location of the lesion, the pattern of bone destruction, size and shape of the lesion, presence and nature of the visible tumor matrix, trabeculation, periosteal response, and the presence and characteristics of the adjacent soft-tissue mass. This information combined with the site of the lesion and the age of the patient allows formulation of a reasonable diagnosis in most cases. Malignant lesions are generally poorly defined lesions with a wide zone of transition, a moth-eaten or permeative pattern of bone destruction, an interrupted periosteal reaction of the sunburst or onion-skin type, and an adjacent soft-tissue mass. However, some aggressive benign lesions may also show the same pattern on plain radiographs.

Chest radiographs should be obtained in all cases of malignant skeletal tumors to evaluate for pulmonary metastases, particularly in patients with osteosarcoma.

Magnetic Resonance Imaging

Due to its excellent contrast resolution and multiplanar capabilities, MRI has now virtually replaced computed tomography (CT) as the imaging modality for assessing the local extent, local staging, and follow-up of malignant bone tumors. MRI is the best imaging modality (1) in assessing intra- and extracompartmental extent of bone tumors, (2) in assessing neurovascular and juxta-articular involvement, and (3) in detecting skip lesions, leading to a more accurate staging.[8] Evaluation for intra-articular extension needs careful interpretation. When the lesion is far from the joint or obviously within the joint, the diagnosis is easy, but when the tumor abuts the joint, involvement of the joint is often overevaluated. Involvement is suggested when the hyaline cartilage is penetrated or more commonly when the tumor extends through the capsule. Joint effusion does not necessarily mean involvement.[9]

The MRI protocol for bone tumor evaluation should include an initial large field of view T1 or inversion recovery sequence to detect any skip lesions and for planning subsequent sequences. T1 and T2 or inversion recovery sequences of the involved area should then be acquired in axial, coronal, and/or sagittal planes, using the surface coil, to show the complete extent of the tumor in all three dimensions, along with its relation to the adjacent joint and neurovascular bundle.

Magnetic resonance imaging features are usually nonspecific in differentiating benign from malignant tumors. Both benign and malignant tumors are generally seen as low signal on T1-weighted (T1W) and high signal on T2-weighted (T2W) images. Thus, intraosseous extent and skip lesions are well evaluated on T1W images due to the contrast between the high signal marrow and the low signal tumor, whereas the extraosseous extent is better assessed on T2W images due to the contrast provided by the low signal muscles to the high signal tumor. Fat-suppression techniques can suppress the adjacent bright fat to further increase the contrast on T2W images **(Figs. 1A to C)**. Contrast enhancement delineates the exact extent of the tumor, defines viable tumor and necrotic areas, and helps in differentiating edema from tumor tissue and identifying residual/recurrent tumor from scar or fibrotic tissue in treated cases.

Dynamic contrast-enhanced (DCE) perfusion MRI provides physiologic information that cannot be determined from conventional anatomic MRI, including information regarding tissue vascularization and perfusion, capillary permeability, and the volume of the interstitial space. DCE perfusion MRI has been frequently used in the evaluation of musculoskeletal tumors as it helps in tissue characterization, staging of local extent, identification of areas of viable tumor to guide biopsy, monitoring of preoperative chemotherapy, detection of residual or recurrent tumor, and differentiating tumor from fibrosis. Time-intensity curves can be obtained, type IV curve may be seen in malignant tumors (e.g., synovial sarcoma and leiomyosarcoma) and type V curve can be found in tumors after radiation or chemotherapy treatment or in tumors with a large interstitial space such as myxoid tumors.[10]

Dynamic contrast-enhanced MRI can be used to obtain pharmacokinetic parameters, such as the volume transfer constant (Ktrans), the volume rate constant (Kep, which represents the transfer of the contrast agent from the extravascular extracellular space to the blood plasma), and the extravascular extracellular volume fraction (Ve). In a study done by Oh et al., Ktrans and Kep showed significant differences between benign and malignant bone tumors; however, a significant difference could not be found for Ve. This is the first report using a composite parameter derived from DCE-MRI and diffusion-weighted imaging (DWI) to evaluate musculoskeletal tumors. The Ktrans, Kep, and Ktrans/apparent diffusion coefficient (ADC) were significantly higher and the ADC value was significantly lower in the malignant bone lesions than in the benign bone lesions. These findings suggest that the multiparametric approach with a hybrid parameter derived from DCE MRI and DWI could be potentially useful.[11]

Diffusion-weighted MRI: Densely cellular areas with restricted diffusion have lower ADCs as compared to less cellular areas with higher ADCs. ADC values are significantly higher in benign than in malignant tumors.

Diffusion-weighted MRI has also been found useful in assessing tumor response to therapy. Effective therapy in bone tumors leads to breakdown of tumor cell membranes resulting in increased diffusion of water in the tumor on diffusion-weighted images. Even though the tumor bulk

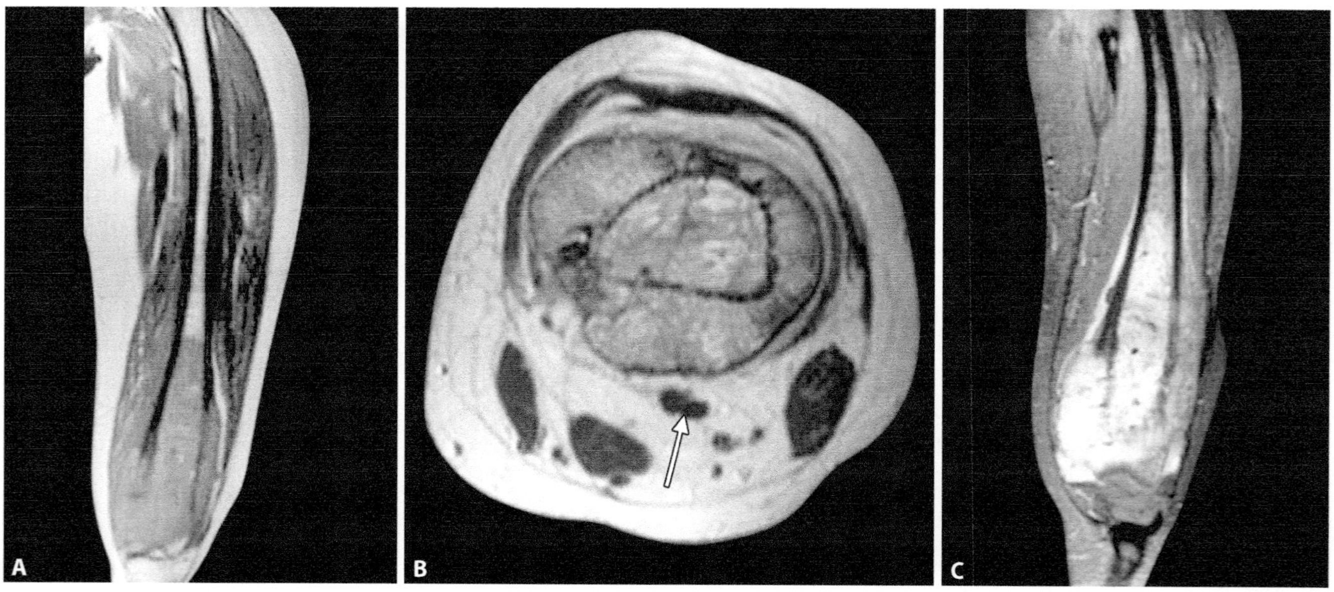

Figs. 1A to C: MRI (magnetic resonance imaging) showing local staging of distal femoral osteosarcoma. Coronal T1-weighted (T1W) sequence (A) demonstrates the intraosseous extent and axial T2-weighted (T2W) sequence (B) demonstrates the extraosseous extent. The periosteum is intact and the neurovascular bundle (arrow) is well separated from the tumor. Coronal short tau inversion recovery (STIR) image (C) shows the soft tissue extension well; however, the intramedullary extension is not well appreciated.

may not reduce significantly, increase in the ADC value indicates a response to treatment.[12]

^{1}H magnetic resonance spectroscopic imaging (MRSI) can be used as a noninvasive approach to the evaluation of musculoskeletal tumors, providing a means of molecular characterization of bone and soft-tissue malignancies. This method can characterize lesions based on their metabolic constituents, such as choline, a phospholipid constituent of cell membranes. Diagnostically, ^{1}H MRSI is used to detect increased levels of choline compounds, which are markers of increased cell membrane turnover, a feature of malignancy.

Multivoxel ^{1}H MRSI has been shown to be feasible for characterizing musculoskeletal tumors. The choline peak is used to differentiate benign and malignant tumors. The presence of a choline peak (identified visually at 3.2 ppm in a spectrum obtained with TE = 135 ms) is supportive of malignancy, although some metabolically active benign tumors and abscesses may also show a choline peak.[10]

Computed Tomography

With the easier availability of MRI, the role of CT in the evaluation of malignant bone tumors has reduced considerably. However, CT still remains superior to MRI in detection and characterization of matrix mineralization (osteoid or chondroid), in picking up subtle calcification, and in the assessment of cortical involvement, bone trabeculation, and periosteal reaction. CT can be used to demonstrate the morphological features of the tumor in areas which are not well evaluated by plain radiography, e.g., pelvis, shoulder, and vertebrae and where MRI is contraindicated. CT is also the investigation of choice for detecting pulmonary metastases.

It helps to evaluate treatment response as bone tumors ossify as they heal. CT-guided procedures allow accurate placement of biopsy needles. It also guides probes for tumoral ablation with ultrasound radiofrequency, microwave, chemical, or cryoablation.[13]

Fluoroscopy

Fluoroscopy is used for localization of bone tumors at the time of surgery and for angiography used in chemoembolization treatments and preoperative embolization of vascular tumors.[13]

Nuclear Medicine

Radionuclide scanning using both traditional technetium-labeled phosphonate compounds and newer positron emitters is an important adjunctive modality.

^{99m}Technetium methylene diphosphonate (^{99m}Tc MDP) bone scan has traditionally been used as the first additional investigation in most instances to detect whether the lesion is monostotic or accompanied by other skeletal lesions. The major limitation of bone scanning is its lack of specificity as a number of bone disorders may have similar scintigraphic appearances. These lesions need to be characterized further by other imaging modalities. The role of ^{99m}Tc MDP bone scan for monitoring response to treatment is limited because it is not always possible to distinguish active disease from healing.

Assessment of tumor response to therapy can be affected by flare phenomenon. An increased uptake of the radioactive substance can be detected up to 6 months after the treatment of metastases and distinguishing this phenomenon from disease progression is difficult and requires additional evaluation with other imaging modalities such as MRI.

Fluorodeoxyglucose positron emission tomography (FDG-PET) is assuming an increasingly important role in the evaluation of skeletal metastatic disease. FDG accumulation in skeletal lesions reflects direct uptake by tumor, in contrast to ^{99m}Tc MDP activity on conventional bone scans, which reflects increased new bone formation in response to destruction of bone by tumor. The role of FDG-PET in the imaging algorithm of primary musculoskeletal tumors is not well defined. Its role in the initial diagnosis is limited. It cannot replace biopsy because it cannot consistently differentiate benign from malignant bone tumors. In the patient with a documented bone tumor, it can (1) guide a biopsy to the most active tissue, (2) predict overall survival, (3) distinguish recurrent tumor from post-therapeutic changes, (4) monitor response to neoadjuvant chemotherapy, and (5) may also identify poorly responding patients earlier in therapy.[14]

Recently, another positron emitter fluorine-18 sodium fluoride (NaF) has been used as a PET bone imaging agent. The bone uptake of this agent is twofold higher and blood clearance is much faster than ^{99m}Tc MDP which makes it much more sensitive and selective than conventional bone scan for diagnosis and detection of bone metastases.[15] It has higher spatial image resolution as compared to ^{99m}Tc MDP bone scan. It is potentially useful in staging and follow-up of bone forming malignancies such as osteosarcoma and osteoblastic osseous metastases.[13]

The use of low-dose CT or MRI in conjunction with PET improves the sensitivity and specificity of the PET imaging techniques.

Angiography

Angiography has limited specificity in differentiating between benign and malignant tumors as there are no characteristic angiographic features of malignancy. However, two signs, i.e., encasement of normal vessels and presence of tumor vessels, occur with greater frequency in malignant tumors.

Currently, conventional angiography has been largely replaced by noninvasive CT and magnetic resonance (MR) angiography techniques. Conventional angiography still remains useful for pretherapy planning in selected cases and in therapeutic interventions. In planning limb salvage procedures, it can be used to map the vascular supply of a potential vascularized bone graft. Preoperative selective arterial embolization can substantially lower the risk of hemorrhage from hypervascular bone tumors, such as GCT and metastatic renal cancer. Conventional angiography also has been used to deliver intra-arterial infusion chemotherapy to some malignant bone tumors.

Ultrasonography

With the advent of CT and MRI, ultrasonography (USG) has been relegated to the role of an adjunct imaging modality in the evaluation of musculoskeletal tumors. USG plays no useful role in diagnosis or staging but has proven to be of value in guiding needle biopsy of those lesions with a large extraosseous component.[14] It can also help detect the solid/cystic nature of the soft-tissue component.[13] Color Doppler flow imaging with duplex analysis has a role in monitoring tumor response to chemotherapy in patients with high-grade sarcomas, provided there is a soft-tissue component. Response is predicted on the basis of changes in intratumoral blood flow and changes in resistive indices in the limb arteries. Postsurgery USG can be of value in detecting sarcoma recurrence, particularly when orthopedic hardware is present.[16]

TREATMENT FOR PRIMARY MALIGNANT BONE TUMORS

- *Surgery*: Surgery remains the primary treatment for most of symptomatic or malignant bone tumors.
  - *Wide excision*: This involves removal of the entire lesion along with reactive tissue surrounded by intact cuff of normal tissue.
  - *Radical excision*: The lesion along with the entire muscle, bone, or other involved tissues in the compartment is removed.

Limb Salvage Considerations

Limb salvage should be considered only if functional result is likely which involves restoration of the musculoskeletal and neurovascular structures. Growing children present a special difficulty in that limb salvage may not be sensibly attempted if the growth plate cannot be maintained. Preoperative imaging should provide specific information including:

- Proximal, distal, and transverse extent of osseous and soft-tissue involvement
- Location of either of the proximal or distal end of the lesion relative to a palpable anatomic landmark
- Specific muscles and compartments involved by tumor must be identified
- Major neurovascular involvement
- Joint involvement
- Tumor extension relative to epiphyseal plate; mostly approximately 2 cm of tumor free bone adjacent to metaphyseal side of growth plate for adequate limb salvage surgery seeking to retain the physis.
- *Chemotherapy*: It is the first-line treatment for Ewing sarcoma and lymphoma and serves as an adjuvant therapy for most other malignant bone tumors. Lesions such as low-grade chondrosarcoma, periosteal osteosarcoma, and parosteal osteosarcoma are not responsive to chemotherapy. Chemotherapy can be used for conventional osteosarcoma and other high grade osteosarcomas, prior to definitive surgical treatment which helps in shrinking the soft-tissue mass and allows easier tumor resection, especially surrounding the neurovascular bundles. Chemotherapy may also help in controlling systemic micrometastases. Evaluation of tumor response to chemotherapy helps in directing further postoperative treatment.
- *Radiotherapy*: Radiotherapy with chemotherapy is considered first-line therapy for Ewing sarcoma and primary bone lymphoma. It helps in decreasing and controlling the tumor mass in high-grade lesions. Postoperatively, it can be used for lesions with marginal resection. Radiotherapy can also be used in the treatment of local recurrence. Low-grade chondrosarcomas and low-grade osteosarcomas are not responsive to radiation.
- Radiofrequency ablation may be used for painful bony metastases which are not responding to other treatment.

Image Fusion for Computer-assisted Bone Tumor Surgery

Adequate tumor resection without excessive removal of normal tissue is required for a successful limb salvage surgery. Imaging modalities such as CT, MRI, and PET scans have been adapted for use with computer navigation to provide more accurate intraoperative assessment and resection. The fusion of images obtained with CT and MRI is a software-dependent processing technique that allows integration and analysis of preoperative images for planning complex musculoskeletal tumor resections. Integration of various imaging modalities into one imaging data set facilitates preoperative image analysis and planning of navigation computer-assisted bone tumor resection and reconstruction. CT and MRI are essential for preoperative assessment for complex bone tumor surgery. Fusion of CT and MRI yields hybrid images that combine the key characteristics of each technique, allowing better interpretation and accurate localization of the lesion.[17]

It yields an excellent picture of anatomic tumor location and extent of infiltration into surrounding tissues. Image fusion might not be restricted to plain CT or MRI data sets, CT angiography, and MRI fusion can provide information regarding regional vascular anatomy. Functional imaging such as F-18 FDG-PET scans can also be incorporated into the navigation software. PET images have low spatial resolution; therefore, they should be combined with anatomic CT or MRI data sets for interpretation. Metabolic information regarding the tumor is particularly useful in patients with previous surgery and radiotherapy as it helps in distinguishing tumor from scar tissue or postradiotherapy changes on anatomic imaging data sets. The fusion images are excellent for surgical planning as they provide better intraosseous and extraosseous extent of the tumors. Merging of postoperative with preoperative images and precise fitting of custom tumor prostheses might allow validation of the accuracy of a resection as planned.[17,18]

OSTEOGENIC ORIGIN

Osteosarcoma

Osteosarcoma is the most common primary osseous malignancy excluding malignant neoplasms arising from the marrow (myeloma, lymphoma, and leukemia); it accounts for approximately 20% of bone cancers. It mostly affects patients younger than 20 years of age.[7] It is characterized by the production of osteoid or bone by the tumor cells. The malignant cells also retain the potential to form fibrous tissue or cartilage. Thus, the constituents of the tumor matrix are highly variable and can include osteoid tissue, calcification, fibrous tissue, cartilaginous tissue, or a combination of these tissues. Demonstration of osteoid formation by malignant cells on histopathology is essential for diagnosing osteosarcoma. Defects in RB and p53 genes play an important role in the development of osteosarcoma. Abnormalities in INK4a, which encodes p16 (a cell cycle regulator) and p14 (which aids and abets p53 function), are also seen.[7] They can be classified according to their main tissue component and their site of origin **(Box 1)**.

Osteosarcomas can be associated with various syndromes such as McCune-Albright syndrome, Mazabraud syndrome, familial Paget's disease, retinoblastoma, Li-Fraumeni syndrome, and Bloom syndrome.[19]

Conventional Osteosarcoma

Conventional intramedullary osteosarcoma is the most common subtype of osteosarcoma and accounts for approximately 75–85% of all cases.

Box 1: Classification of osteosarcoma.

- *Primary osteosarcomas*:
  - Conventional intramedullary/central high grade (osteoblastic, chondroblastic, and fibroblastic)
  - Telangiectatic
  - Small cell
  - Low-grade central
- *Surface osteosarcoma*:
  - Juxtacortical/parosteal
  - Periosteal
  - High-grade surface
- Secondary osteosarcomas can occur in Paget's disease and after radiation exposure
- Unusual forms of osteosarcoma given below are viewed as subtypes of conventional osteosarcoma as their biological behavior is similar
- Osteoblastic osteosarcoma—sclerosing type
- Osteosarcoma resembling osteoblastoma
- Chondromyxoid fibroma such as osteosarcoma
- Chondroblastoma such as osteosarcoma
- Clear cell osteosarcoma
- Malignant fibrous histiocytoma such as osteosarcoma
- Giant cell rich osteosarcoma
- Epithelioid osteosarcoma

Clinical Presentation

Age: It is commonly seen in the second and third decades of life with peak incidence seen between 10 and 15 years. Conventional osteosarcoma is rare in patients <6 years or >60 years.[19] The median age of patients with osteosarcoma arising in tubular bones is 17 years. Flat bones are affected at median age of 25 years.

Sex: The male:female ratio is 2:1.

Clinical picture: Most patients present with pain and a palpable mass. Symptoms are usually present for several months, the swelling having been attributed to trauma or infection in the first place. Systemic symptoms and pathological fractures are common. Serum alkaline phosphatase may be elevated with larger tumors.

Site: The typical lesion affects the metaphyseal region of the growing end of a long bone. About 50–75% are found in the distal femur or the proximal tibia. Other common sites include proximal humerus and femur. Rarer sites include the ilium, ribs, vertebrae, and jaw bones. Extension of the tumor into the diaphysis and/or epiphysis is common. About 10% of the tumors arise in the diaphysis. Skip metastases may be seen in approximately 5% of patients.[19] Distant spread is mainly via the bloodstream with early metastases to the lungs.

Imaging Features

On plain radiographs, the tumor may be predominantly osteosclerotic (25%) or osteolytic (25%), but more frequently, it is of the mixed osteosclerotic/osteolytic type (50%). The classical appearance is that of a focal lesion in the metaphyseal end of a long bone showing a moth-eaten or permeative pattern of destruction with a wide zone of transition. The tumor breaks through the cortex early in the course of the disease leading to a soft-tissue mass. This mass is first unmineralized but later shows ill-defined tumor bone within it. Mineralization of the tumor osteoid leads to a cloud-like density in the region known as the *cumulus cloud* appearance. The medullary lesion is predominantly lytic but mineralization leads to a characteristic-associated medullary sclerosis. A Codman triangle may form at the margin of the lesion due to subperiosteal extension of the tumor lifting the periosteum **(Figs. 2A and B)**. Bone spicules can be seen perpendicularly or radially in a "sunburst" or "sunray" pattern following the line of extended Sharpey's fibers **(Figs. 3A and B)**. A lamellated (onion skin) pattern of periosteal reaction resembling that of Ewing sarcoma may sometimes be seen. In contrast to cortical bone, the articular cartilage is more resistant to tumor invasion and is not violated until late in the course of the disease.[20,21]

Magnetic resonance imaging is the investigation of choice following conventional radiographs. The entire bone should be scanned to look for skip metastases. An obvious heterogeneous tumor can be seen within the bone, often associated with a soft-tissue mass, with low-signal intensity on T1W images and high-signal intensity on short tau inversion recovery (STIR) or T2W images **(Figs. 4A to D)**. Areas with increased sclerosis

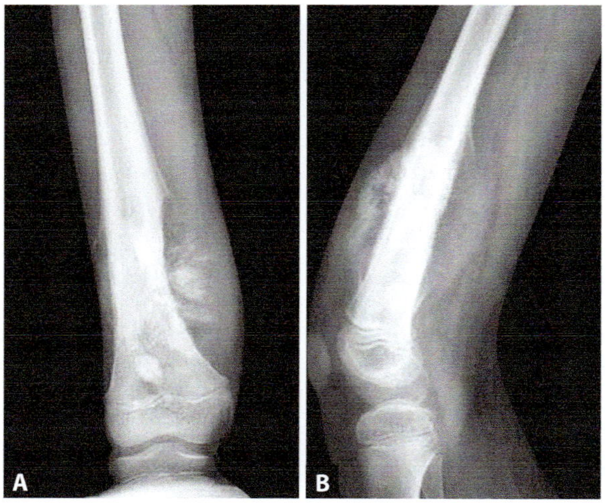

Figs. 2A and B: Conventional central osteosarcoma. Anteroposterior (AP) (A) and lateral (B) radiographs of the distal femur in a 14-year-old boy showing a classical osteosarcoma with mixed lytic and sclerotic areas, extraosseous mass with tumor bone formation, and Codman triangles at the upper and lower margins of the lesion.

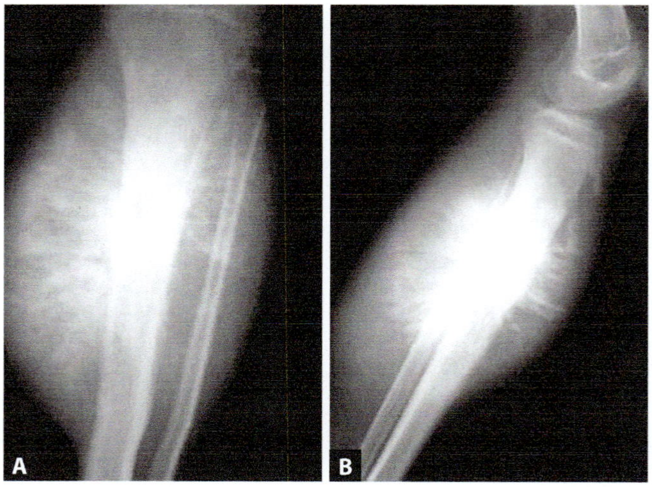

Figs. 3A and B: Osteosarcoma of the tibia. Anteroposterior (AP) (A) and lateral (B) radiographs of the leg show a mixed lesion in metadiaphyseal region of tibia with a large soft tissue component and the characteristic "sunburst" or spiculated periosteal reaction.

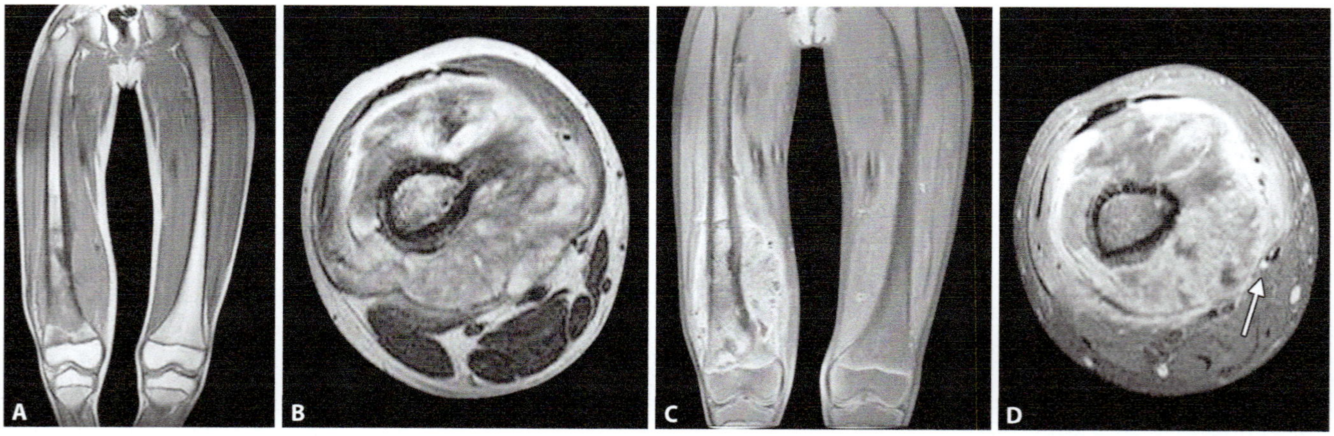

Figs. 4A to D: MRI of the osteosarcoma (same case as in Figure 2). Coronal T1-weighted (T1W) magnetic resonance (MR) image (A) shows the large tumor as a predominantly hypointense mass with evidence of cortical destruction and axial T2-weighted (T2W) image (B) shows the cortical disruption with soft tissue extension of the tumor mass with loss of fat planes with the neurovascular bundle. Contrast-enhanced coronal (C) and axial (D) MR images show heterogeneous enhancement of the tumor mass.

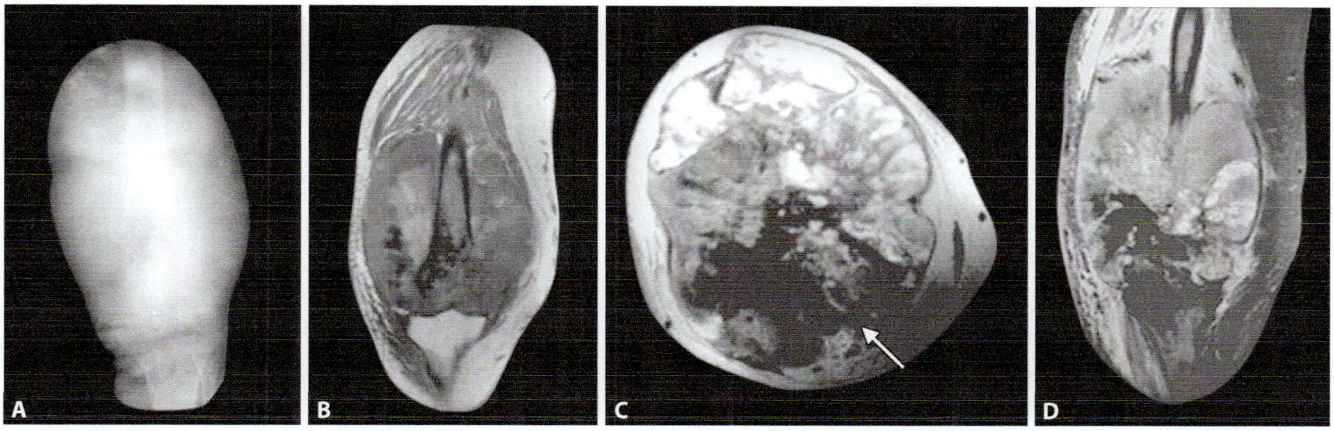

Figs. 5A to D: Osteosarcoma of distal femur. Anteroposterior (AP) radiograph (A) showing a destructive lesion in the distal femur with extensive cloud-like mineralization in the intra- and extraosseous component. Coronal T1-wieghted (T1W) magnetic resonance (MR) image (B) shows the large tumor as a predominantly hypointense mass with evidence of cortical destruction. An axial T2-wieghted (T2W) image (C) shows a heterogeneous mass which is completely encasing the neurovascular bundle (arrow). T2W (fat-suppressed) coronal image (D) shows the intra-articular extension of the tumor into the knee joint.

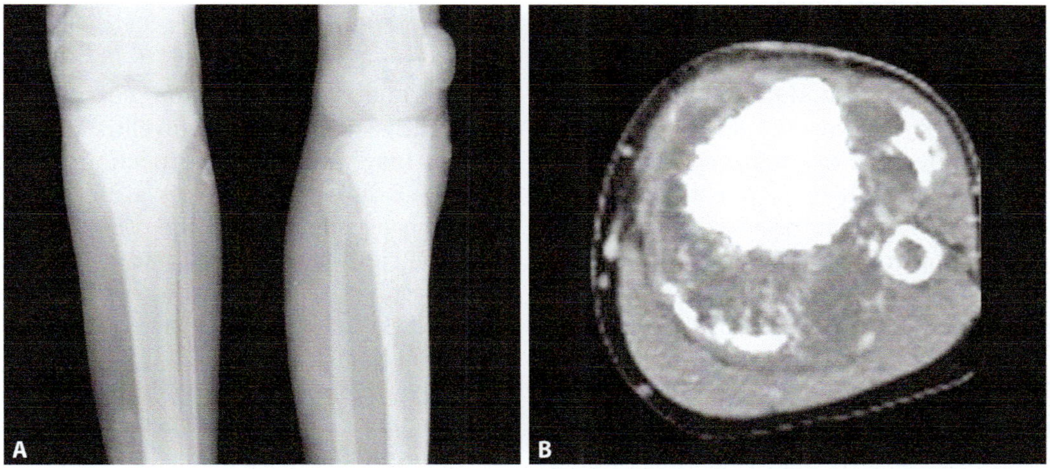

Figs. 6A and B: Osteosarcoma—osteoblastic variety. Anteroposterior (AP) and lateral (A) radiographs show a purely osteosclerotic lesion of the proximal metaphysis of the tibia. Computed tomography (CT) (B) shows mineralization of tumor matrix within the soft tissue component and a spiculated periosteal reaction.

may show lower signal intensity on both T1W and T2W images. Peritumoral edema in the marrow tends to be of an intermediate signal intensity on STIR and T1W images and does not disrupt the normal architecture.[22] Both intramedullary and extraosseous extensions are accurately demonstrated as is the involvement of the neurovascular bundle and extension into the adjacent joint **(Figs. 5A to D)**. Intramedullary "skip" lesions may also be identified.

The classical osteosarcoma has been described above, but a variety of appearances may be observed. The tumor bone may be entirely sclerotic **(Figs. 6A and B)** or the tumor may be entirely lytic when it is difficult to differentiate from Ewing sarcoma. A chondroblastic variety of osteosarcoma may occur when a large part of the tumor is composed of cartilage.

Telangiectatic Osteosarcoma

The rare *telangiectatic osteosarcoma*[23] is characterized by the formation of large septated blood-filled cavities with a rim containing high-grade osteosarcomatous cells. It accounts for 2.5–12% of osteosarcomas and presents usually as a lytic lesion resembling an aggressive ABC.[19] The femur, tibia, and humerus are most commonly involved. It arises frequently in the diaphysis and extends into the metaphysis. It lacks visible bone production. A predominant expansile, lytic lesion with remodelling, cortical destruction, and periosteal reaction is seen on plain radiographs **(Fig. 7A)**. Subtle matrix mineralization may be demonstrated by CT. Extensive hemorrhage and blood-fluid levels can be seen on both CT and MRI **(Fig. 7B)**, mimicking ABC. However, the presence of

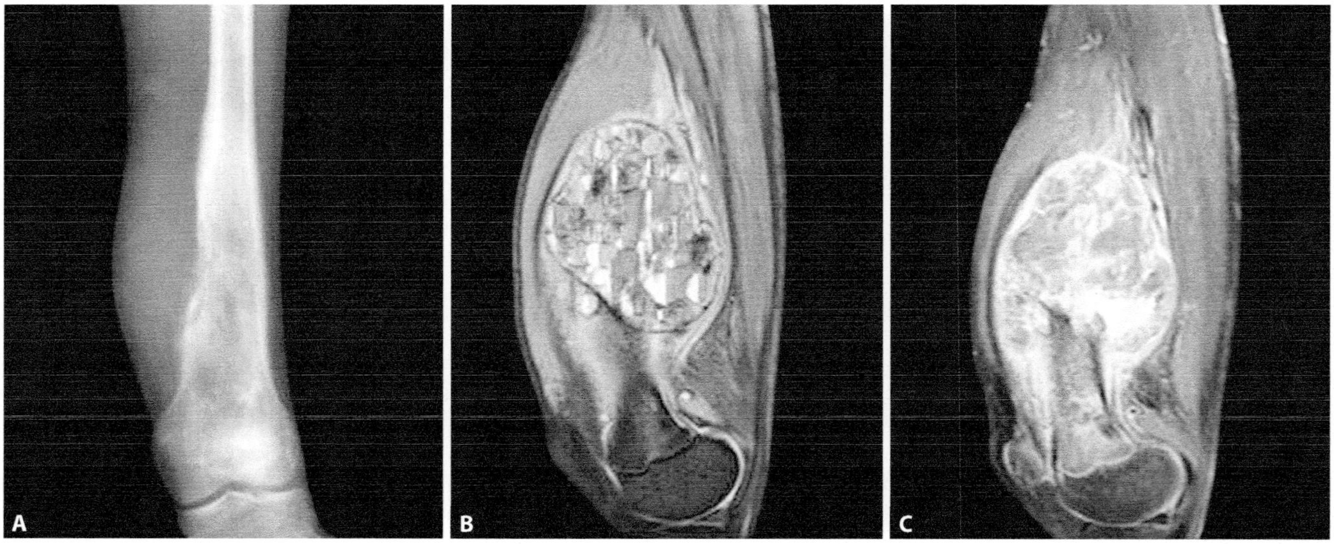

Figs. 7A to C: Telangiectatic osteosarcoma. Anteroposterior (AP) radiograph (A) of the distal femur shows a predominantly lytic lesion in the distal femur with irregular cortical destruction and a large soft tissue component and sagittal T2W fat-suppressed magnetic resonance (MR) image (B) shows the characteristic blood–fluid levels within the tumor. On contrast-enhanced image (C), marked peripheral and septal enhancement is seen.

thick peripheral, septal, and nodular enhancement of solid viable tissue on postcontrast studies **(Fig. 7C)** helps to distinguish telangiectatic osteosarcoma from ABC. Although the prognosis for this type of osteosarcoma is poor as compared to conventional osteosarcoma, effective chemotherapy has improved survival.

Small cell osteosarcoma[24] (approximately 1–4%) is a rare subtype and is similar to conventional osteosarcomas in its clinical presentation and radiographic appearance. Equal number of men and women are affected; lesions are seen in the metaphysis most commonly and may extend into the diaphysis occasionally. Isolated diaphyseal lesions can be seen in 15%.[19] They are seen as intramedullary, permeative lesions with ill-defined margins associated with cortical destruction, periosteal reaction, and soft-tissue mass. Histologically, it contains solid areas of small round cells or spindle-shaped cells resembling those seen in Ewing sarcoma. The significance of this entity is its extremely poor prognosis.

Low-grade osteosarcoma,[25] also referred to as intraosseous well-differentiated osteosarcoma, is a rare type of osteosarcoma (around 1–2%), which presents in an older age group (median age 30 years) with a long-standing history. The radiographic features vary from predominantly osteolytic or ground glass to predominantly sclerotic. The tumor may show geographic destruction and is frequently expansile with regular cortical destruction and solid periosteal reaction. It has a good prognosis. Due to its relatively benign appearance, the tumor may be mistaken for fibrous dysplasia, osteoblastoma, or a low-grade chondroid tumor. However, CT and MRI will show extraosseous extension, which should aid in the diagnosis.

The main *differential diagnoses* of osteosarcoma in its early stages are osteomyelitis and trauma. A long history may indicate that infection is unlikely. Once the plain radiograph reveals a medullary lesion, the diagnosis usually lies between osteosarcomas and other malignancies, including metastasis. Of the benign lesions, osteoblastoma, GCT, osteoid osteoma, and osteomyelitis, particularly the sclerosing variety of Garré, have to be considered.

Osteosarcoma spreads via the bloodstream leading to pulmonary metastases. These contain osteoid, take-up bone-seeking isotopes, and ultimately ossify. The metastases are often subpleural in location and commonly associated with a pneumothorax. It is essential to exclude the presence of lung metastases with CT for purposes of staging before starting therapy **(Figs. 8A to C)**.

The prognosis of osteosarcoma has improved greatly with the use of chemotherapy and limb-preserving surgery. Presently, the treatment requires multiple cycles of chemotherapy before surgical resection. DCE MRI has been used with considerable success in some centers to predict the degree of chemotherapy response and to identify active tumor remnants in recurrences.[26] Biochemical markers such as alkaline phosphatase and lactate dehydrogenase can be used to assess prognosis and treatment response.

Surface Osteosarcomas

Surface osteosarcomas arise from the surface of the bone and account for 4–10% of osteosarcomas. They include the periosteal, parosteal, high-grade surface, and intracortical osteosarcomas.

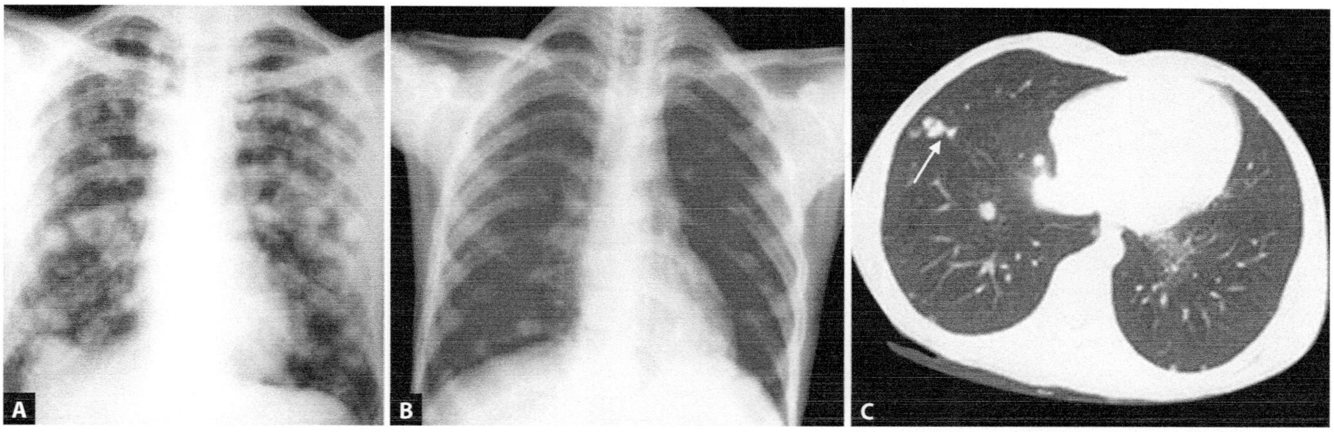

Figs. 8A to C: Pulmonary metastases from osteosarcoma. (A) Multiple dense rounded opacities are seen scattered through both the lung fields suggestive of osteoblastic metastases; (B) In another case, plain radiograph of the chest shows a few ill-defined opacities suspicious of metastases; and (C) Axial computed tomography (CT) scan shows multiple nodular metastatic lesions scattered in both lung fields. Ossification can be seen in some (arrow).

Periosteal Osteosarcoma

Periosteal osteosarcoma is an intermediate-grade chondroblastic osteosarcoma that originates from deep periosteal layer. It accounts for 25% of surface osteosarcomas. It is seen in the second and third decades with a slight male preponderance. This entity is characteristically diaphyseal in location with the involvement of 50% of osseous circumference and the center of the tumor is located on the surface of the bone with a saucer-like shallow area of adjacent cortical bone destruction.[19] The crater contains striated, radiating mineralization. It is found in the tibia and femur followed by ulna and humerus. Tumor mineralization is best shown by CT. Absence of marrow involvement is easily seen on CT/MRI. MRI classically shows hyperintensity on T2W images due to the chondroblastic nature of the lesion. Reactive marrow changes may be seen in >50% cases, appearing hypointense on TIW images and hyperintense on T2W images adjacent to but not contiguous with the lesion.

Juxtacortical/Parosteal Osteosarcoma

Parosteal osteosarcomas account for around 65% of all surface osteosarcomas. They arise from the outer layer of the periosteum and are attached to the surface of the affected bone and have a tendency to encircle it. They occur in the third and fourth decades and are more common in women. This tumor is almost exclusively found in long bones, with 70% occurring around the knee, especially the posterior aspect of the femur.[19]

The characteristic feature is a dense ossific mass abutting or enveloping the distal femoral metaphysis **(Fig. 9A)**. A broad-based soft-tissue mass with perpendicular periosteal reaction is seen on the surface of the bone with cortical thickening and cortical scalloping. Codman triangle can be seen at upper or lower margins. In its early growth, a well-defined radiolucent line separates the tumor from the normal cortex. Cortical thickening without aggressive periosteal reaction may be seen. Medullary involvement needs to be evaluated on CT or MRI **(Figs. 9B to D)**. MRI shows a low signal equivalent to normal cortex in the poorly cellular ossified element with a variable increase in the signal intensity from the peripheral more active element of the tumor.[27] Eventually, both cortex and medulla become involved by the tumor. Most parosteal osteosarcomas are low grade; however, high-grade foci can be seen in 22–64% of cases and appear as nonmineralized soft-tissue components >1 cm^3 on CT and MRI. The differential diagnosis includes a heavily mineralized osteochondroma and juxtacortical

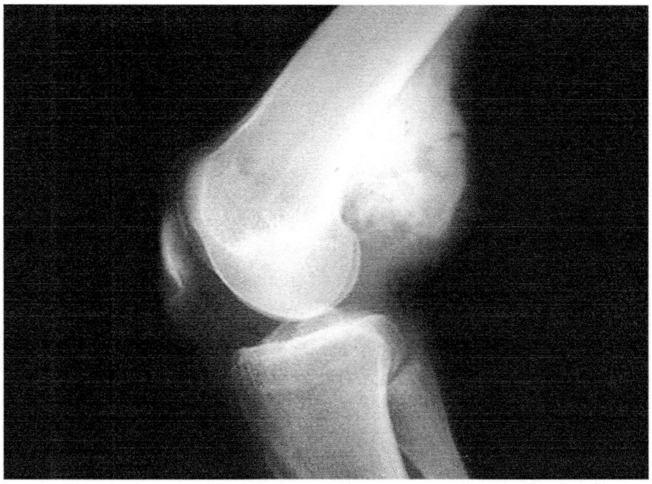

Fig. 9A: Parosteal osteosarcoma. Lateral radiograph of the knee shows a dense, lobulated mass arising from the posterior distal femur. This is the classical location for parosteal osteosarcoma.

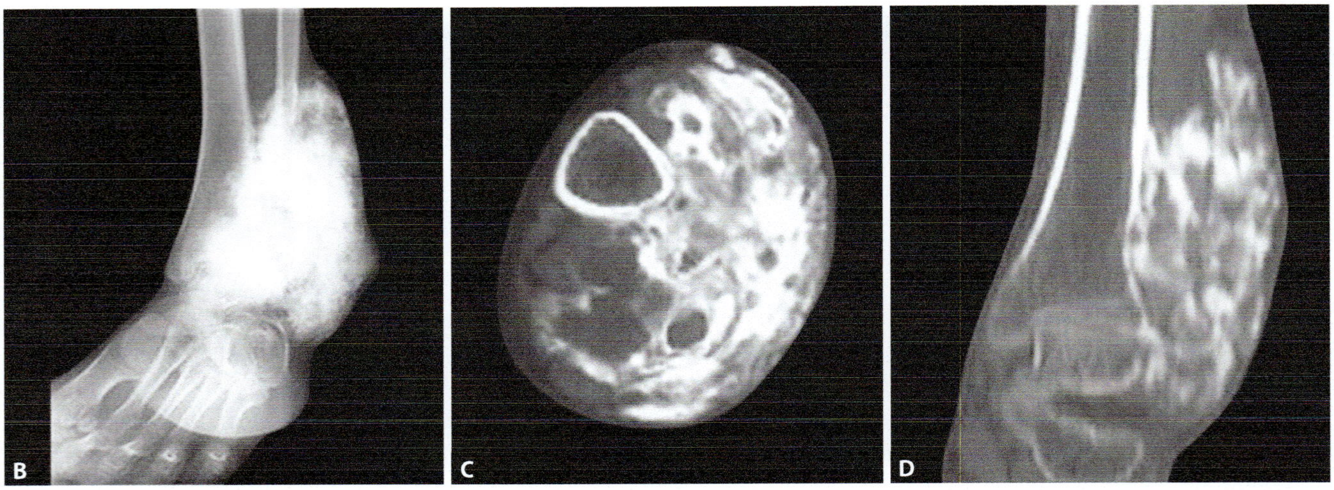

Figs. 9B to D: Parosteal osteosarcoma. In another case, anteroposterior (AP) radiograph of the ankle shows a dense homogeneous mass of bone overlying the distal fibula and tibia (B); Axial and coronal reformatted computed tomography (CT) sections show the cleavage plane separating the lesion from the underlying bone (C and D).

myositis ossificans, which is differentiated by its peripheral mineralization pattern and lack of attachment to the cortex. Parosteal osteosarcoma is associated with an excellent prognosis with a 10-year survival rate of 80%.[19]

High-grade Surface Osteosarcoma

This is a very rare lesion arising from the surface of the bone but having the same histological features as conventional central osteosarcomas. It, therefore, has a very much poorer prognosis than other osteosarcomas. High-grade surface osteosarcoma is more common in second and third decades with male preponderance. It involves diaphysis of long bones (femur, humerus, and fibula). The radiological features are similar to those of periosteal osteosarcoma but more aggressive in that the tumor is usually larger and there is a greater degree of cortical erosion.[28] It involves entire circumference of bone with invasion of medullary cavity.

Intracortical Osteosarcomas

Intracortical osteosarcomas are the rarest form of osteosarcoma, accounting for <1% of cases. They are usually seen in the second decade and in men.[19] All reported cases had arisen in the cortex of femur or tibia. The tumor appears as a small lytic lesion surrounded by thickened cortex, resembling an osteoid osteoma or osteoblastoma. These tumors have a better prognosis than the conventional intramedullary osteosarcoma. Medullary invasion is rare.

Extraosseous Osteosarcoma

Occasionally, osteosarcomas may arise in an extraosseous site. The most common site is the soft tissue of the thigh, but they can also be found in the pleura, dura of brain, heart valves, retroperitoneum, axilla, breast, etc. These rare tumors present the same histological pattern as other osteosarcomas. They usually present as large soft-tissue masses, which may not be close to bone. The radiological appearance is nonspecific. Mineralization of the matrix can suggest the diagnosis, but differentiation from other soft-tissue sarcomas which calcify (e.g., chondrosarcoma, fibrosarcoma, and synovial sarcoma) is difficult.[29]

Multifocal Osteosarcoma

This condition is characterized by multiple intraosseous osteosarcomas that was earlier thought to represent multicentric osteosarcomas, but it is now believed to represent rapidly progressive multicentric metastatic disease. It accounts for approximately 3–4% of all osteosarcomas. It is bilaterally symmetrical in skeletally immature patients but asymmetrical in skeletally mature older patients. The dominant lesion is large and has osteoid, or it may be purely lytic with metastatic foci which are smaller, sclerotic, well-defined with absent periosteal reaction, and cortical destruction **(Fig. 10)**. It is associated with poor prognosis with mean survival being only around 12 months.[19]

Secondary Osteosarcoma

Secondary osteosarcomas occur following malignant degeneration of benign disorders, most commonly seen after radiotherapy and in Paget's disease. Rarely, osteosarcoma develops in the association with osteonecrosis, fibrous dysplasia, osteogenesis imperfecta, metal prosthesis, and chronic osteomyelitis.[29]

Radiation therapy may lead to the development of osteosarcoma. The criteria for diagnosing a *postradiation*

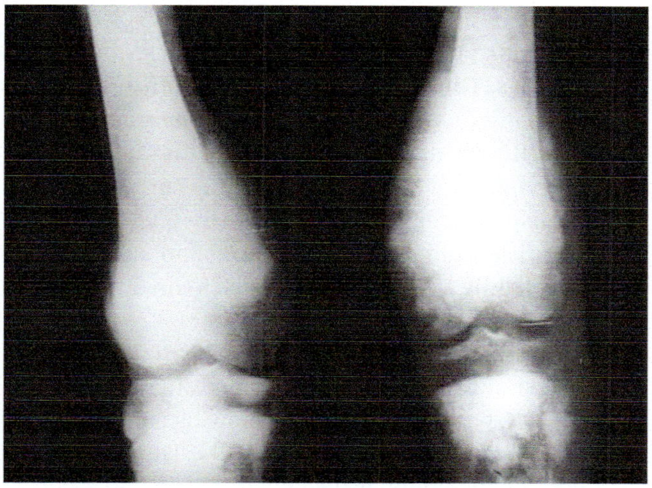

Fig. 10: Multifocal osteosarcoma. Anteroposterior (AP) radiograph of bilateral knees of a 16-year-old boy shows dense osteoblastic lesions involving the metaphyses of both femora and tibia.

sarcoma (PRS) include: (1) a history of radiation therapy, (2) development of a neoplasm in the radiation field, (3) a latent period of several years, and (4) histological proof of a sarcoma, which differs significantly from that initially treated.

Precise threshold dosage is unknown, but it is considered that a minimal dose of 30 Gy is required to induce a PRS and it is also suggested that concurrent chemotherapy increases the risk of sarcoma development. The treated tumors, which most commonly result in the development of PRS, are breast carcinoma, lymphoma, head and neck cancers, and gynecological malignancies. The most common sites are pelvic and shoulder girdle and the most common PRS is an osteosarcoma followed by undifferentiated pleomorphic sarcoma (UPS). Radiologically, there is an evidence of bone destruction, soft-tissue mass, matrix mineralization, and periosteal reaction. There may also be associated features of radiation changes in the underlying bone in the form of radiation osteitis and marrow infarction. The prognosis is usually poor.[30]

Malignant change has also been reported to occur in about 5% patients with Paget's disease. Most common malignancy is osteosarcoma (73–84%), fibrosarcoma (9–16%), chondrosarcoma (14%), or UPS (5%).[19] Radiologically, the most common sites for Paget's disease, the pelvis, and the femur are common locations for malignant change. CT and MRI show an area of bone destruction with a wide zone of transition and a large soft-tissue mass.[29]

CHONDROGENIC ORIGIN

Chondrosarcoma

Chondrosarcoma is a malignant tumor of chondrogenic origin that remains essentially cartilaginous throughout its evolution. It arises from chondroblasts and collagenoblasts, thus producing only cartilage and collagen. It is the third most common primary malignant tumor of bone after multiple myeloma and osteosarcoma, accounting for about 25% of all primary bone tumors.[19] It usually develops later in life than osteosarcoma and carries a much better prognosis because metastases often occur late. A high-grade chondrosarcoma, however, behaves in a fashion very similar to an osteosarcoma.

Chondrosarcoma can be divided into two broad categories: primary and secondary. A primary chondrosarcoma is believed to be malignant from the outset while a secondary chondrosarcoma arises in a preexisting bony lesion, usually an enchondroma or an osteochondroma and rarely in chondromyxoid fibroma or chondroblastoma. A chondrosarcoma may also be classified according to its histological grade as low grade (grade 1: 45–50% of cases), myxoid (grade 2: 30–40% of cases), high grade (grade 3: 8–25% of cases) or dedifferentiated, which refers to the development of an adjacent high-grade nonchondroid neoplasm, typically osteosarcoma or UPS. Chondrosarcoma grade I (now officially termed atypical cartilaginous tumor) is reclassified as an intermediate (locally aggressive) tumor better reflecting its clinical behavior.[5] Other varieties include mesenchymal, clear cell, and dedifferentiated chondrosarcoma on the basis of histology. According to its epicenter, chondrosarcoma can be classified into two types: central, when it is intramedullary, and peripheral, when it arises from the surface of the bone. Rarely, chondrosarcomas may arise in an extraosseous site.

Chondrosarcomas may be associated with osteochondromatosis and Maffucci syndrome.

Central Chondrosarcoma

It is the most common type of chondrosarcoma (approximately 90%).

Clinical Presentation

Age: It is most commonly seen in the sixth decade.[19] It is rare in children and should be differentiated from the chondroblastic variety of osteosarcoma.

Sex: Male:female incidence is 1.5–2:1.

Site: The common sites are the pelvis, the ribs, and the proximal ends of the femur and the humerus. It is relatively rare distal to the knee and elbow joints. In the long bones, chondrosarcoma is located in the metaphysis or metadiaphysis.

Imaging Features

Radiologically, the *central tumors* are seen as large, osteolytic, expansile, round, or oval lesions which are well marginated with endosteal thickening or thinning **(Figs. 11A and B)**. There is evidence of cartilaginous matrix mineralization which may be stippled, nodular, or conglomerate (popcorn), sometimes showing rings or arcs. CT may show calcification of the matrix when it is not visible on plain radiographs **(Figs. 12A and B)**. As chondrosarcomas are slow-growing tumors, reactive changes occur in the normal bone, so that as endosteal resorption takes place, periosteal new bone is laid down and bone expansion occurs. Deep endosteal cortical scalloping (greater than two-thirds) is suggestive of chondrosarcoma as opposed to chondroma. Periosteal reaction is common and is seen in almost 50% of cases.[31,32]

As the tumor grows, tumor margination may be lost and the tumor tissue may invade the overlying cortex to extend into the adjacent soft tissues. A soft-tissue mass out of proportion to the size of the intraosseous lesion may be present **(Figs. 13A to F)**. In the pelvic tumors, this mass is not easily demonstrated on conventional radiography. CT and MRI can demonstrate the soft-tissue extension with much greater accuracy. On MRI, cartilage shows characteristic increased signal intensity on T2W images and a multilobulated and septated appearance. The lesion is slightly hypointense to muscle on T1W images **(Figs. 14A to C)**.

Most chondrosarcomas are poorly vascularized and therefore show minimal enhancement after intravenous contrast on CT and MRI, typically showing a peripheral or septal enhancement pattern **(Fig. 14D)**. The presence of clear cut enhancement, especially if it is only in a part of

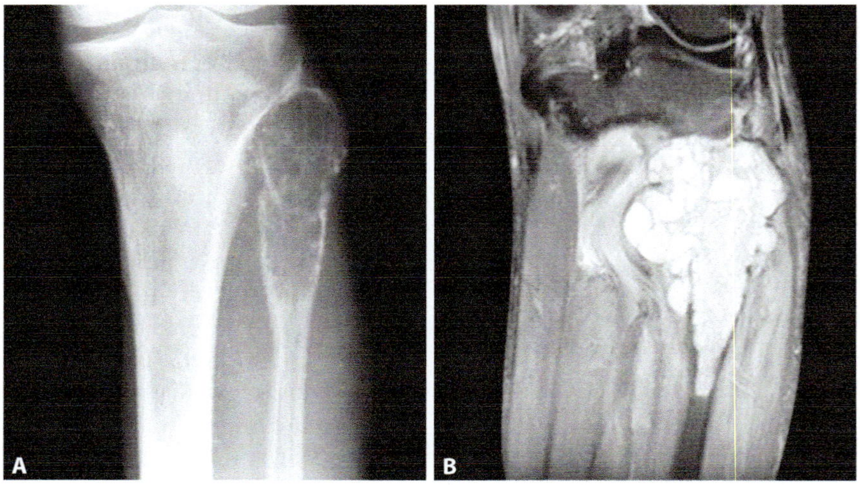

Figs. 11A and B: Conventional chondrosarcoma. Plain radiograph (A) shows an osteolytic, expansile lesion in the upper end of the fibula with faint calcification seen within. Coronal T2-weighted (T2W) fat-suppressed magnetic resonance (MR) image (B) shows the characteristic hyperintense, lobulated lesion with internal septations.

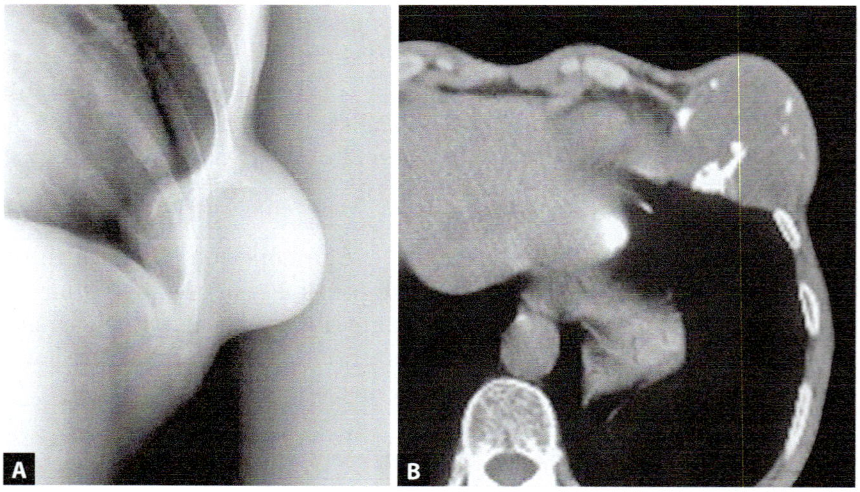

Figs. 12A and B: Chondrosarcoma. (A) A large expansile lesion is noted in the anterior end of the left 7th rib; (B) Computed tomography (CT) shows specks of calcification within the lesion.

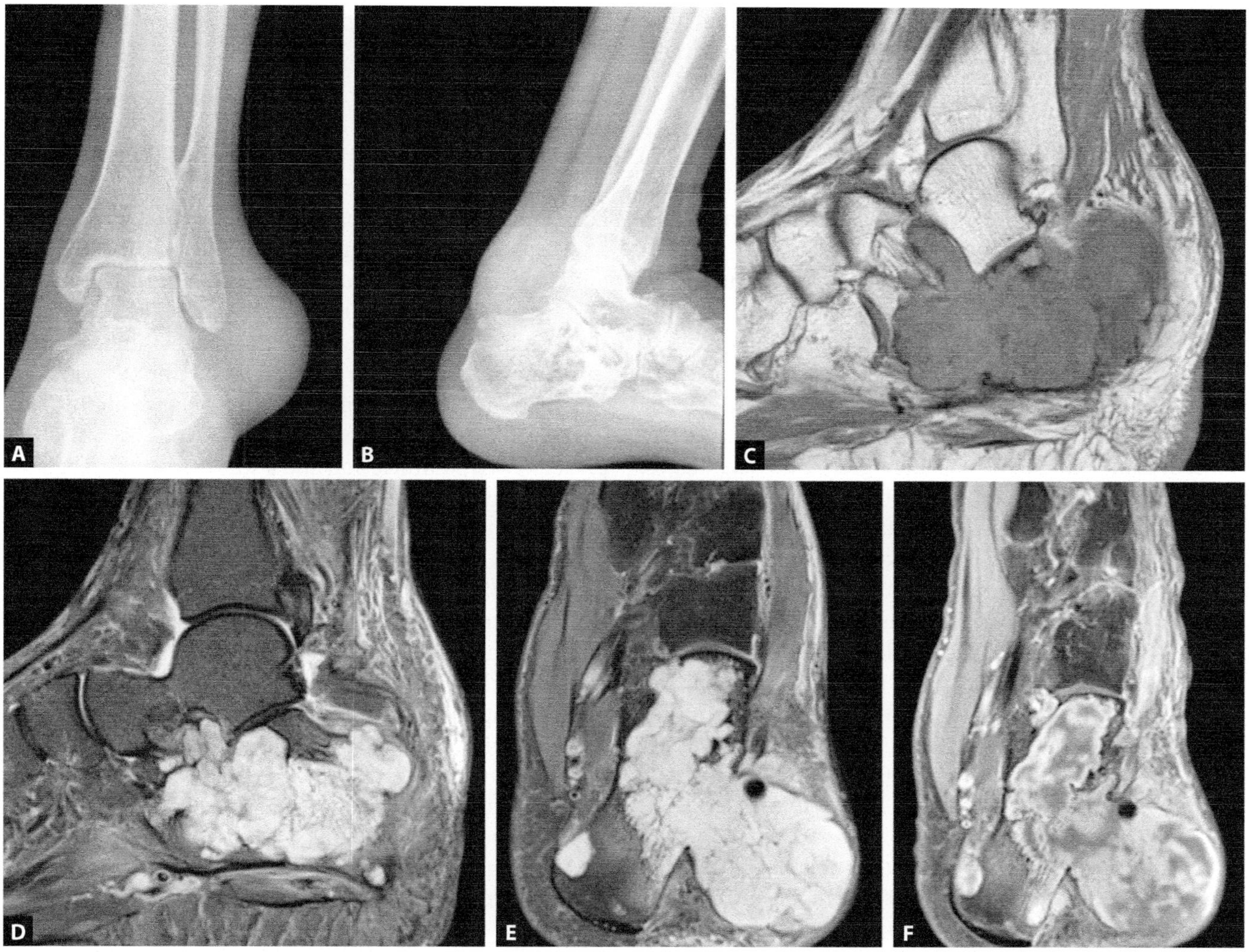

Figs. 13A to F: Chondrosarcoma calcaneum. Anteroposterior (AP) (A) and lateral (B) radiographs of the ankle show an ill-defined lytic sclerotic lesion involving the calcaneum with a large soft tissue swelling along the posterolateral aspect of the ankle joint. T1-weighted (T1W) sagittal (C), short tau inversion recovery (STIR) sagittal (D), and proton density (PD) fat-saturated (FS) axial (E) magnetic resonance (MR) images show a lobulated lesion in the calcaneum with a large extraosseous soft tissue component extending laterally, the lesion appears hypointense on T1W image and hyperintense on STIR and PD FS images with heterogeneous enhancement on postgadolinium image (F). Another smaller similar lesion is seen in the medial aspect of the calcaneum.

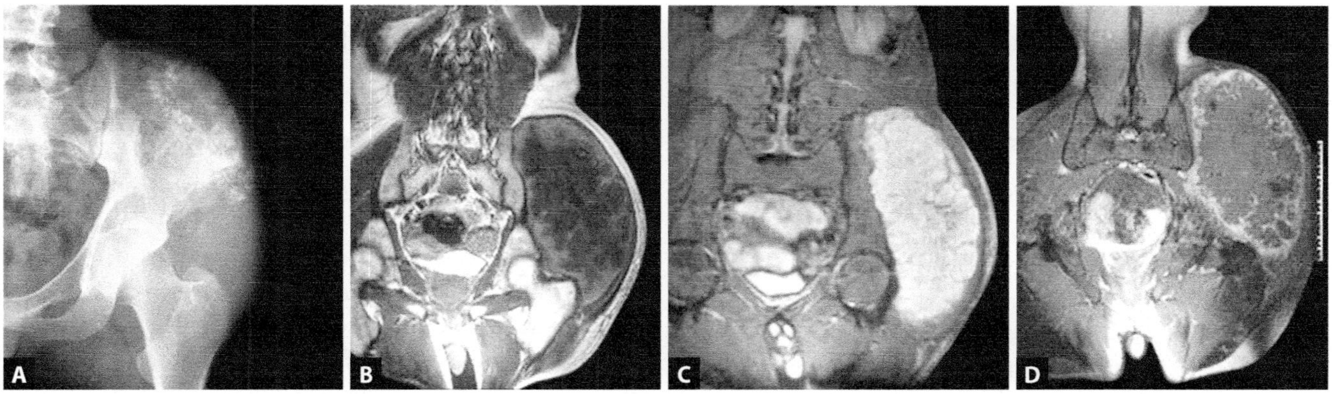

Figs. 14A to D: Conventional chondrosarcoma. Radiograph of the hemipelvis (A) shows a mass extending from the left iliac blade with the characteristic "popcorn" calcification of a cartilaginous matrix. T1-weighted (T1W) magnetic resonance (MR) image (B) shows the large soft tissue component of the chondrosarcoma as a low signal intensity lobulated mass. On coronal T2-weighted (T2W) MR image (C), the tumor is seen as lobulated mass of high signal intensity with septations of low signal intensity. After intravenous administration of gadolinium, a coronal T1W MR image (D) shows irregular peripheral and septal enhancement.

the tumor, is a feature which favors dedifferentiation into a more malignant tumor, usually a UPS, with a more adverse prognosis.

Peripheral Chondrosarcoma

Most of the *peripheral chondrosarcomas* probably arise from benign osteochondromas. Risk of conversion is more in the presence of multiple lesions such as osteochondromatosis (5–25%), enchondromatosis (10–25%), or Maffucci syndrome. It is more common in men and has a younger age distribution as compared to conventional chondrosacrcoma.[19] The distinction between active osteochondroma and low-grade chondrosarcoma can be extremely difficult. Clinical features such as recent onset of pain or presence of an enlarging mass may suggest a malignant transformation. Radiologically, there may be destruction of part of a well-formed calcified cap or ossified stem of such a structure. The thickness of the cartilage cap cannot be assessed radiographically unless it abuts some other structure, e.g., a vessel or viscus filled with contrast medium. It can be readily identified by USG, CT, or MRI, and the thicker the cap, the more likely it is that malignant degeneration has supervened. Most osteochondromas have cartilage caps <5 mm thick, and a cap in excess of 20 mm is likely to be malignant. Unfortunately, the wide separation between these figures makes this observation of limited value.[33]

The prognosis of chondrosarcoma is good when complete resection is achieved before metastatic spread. When metastatic spread occurs, it is generally owing to invasion by the tumor of regional venous channels. Parenchymal metastases to the lungs are therefore not uncommon. Metastases elsewhere, particularly to the skeleton, are rare; similarly, regional lymph nodes are also only rarely involved. The prognosis is better for peripheral tumors in the limbs than with central tumors, e.g., in the pelvis. Failure to remove the complete tumor leads to local recurrence and often breakdown of the overlying skin. The tumor shows a poor response to radiotherapy and cytotoxic drugs.

Other Varieties of Chondrosarcoma

Mesenchymal Chondrosarcoma

Mesenchymal chondrosarcoma is an uncommon entity. It occurs typically in the spine, ilium, or the nonpelvic flat bones (craniofacial bones and ribs) and at a younger age as compared to the conventional chondrosarcomas. Histologically, it has a much more cellular malignant matrix than the conventional chondrosarcoma. Radiologically, it is indistinguishable from a conventional chondrosarcoma. About 75% show chondrogenic calcification. Local recurrence and disseminated metastases occur earlier and more frequently.[19,34]

Clear Cell Chondrosarcoma

Clear cell chondrosarcomas are low-grade, slow-growing variant of chondrosarcomas with a long history. They are seen in third and fourth decades being more common in men and almost always involve the ends of long bones (femur or humerus) after closure of the epiphyseal plate. Less commonly, they may be seen in ribs, skull, spine, hands, and feet. Radiographically, they are usually lytic and may show a loculated or a "soap-bubble" appearance. Lesions may show well-defined margins with thin sclerotic rim or may appear expansive with cortical thinning. One-third may show chondrogenic calcification; periosteal reaction is rare. They may be indistinguishable from chondroblastoma or even chondromyxoid fibroma. The presence of a painful lesion and a soft-tissue mass suggests the provisional diagnosis of chondrosarcoma and makes a biopsy obligatory.[19,35]

Dedifferentiated Chondrosarcoma

Dedifferentiated chondrosarcoma (around 10% of chondrosarcomas) shows a bimorphic pattern of well-differentiated chondrosarcoma and high-grade noncartilaginous lesion. It is seen in fifth to ninth decades with a male preponderance. Dedifferentiated chondrosarcoma is seen in pelvis, femur, and humerus. On imaging, an intramedullary lesion is seen with a bimorphic appearance with a cartilaginous component showing calcification and an aggressive osteolytic component with ill-defined margins and soft-tissue mass.[19]

Juxtacortical Chondrosarcoma

Juxtacortical chondrosarcoma is rare and originates on the surface of long bones. Age of patients varies from 17 to 65 years and it is more common in women. It most commonly occurs in the distal posterior femoral metaphysis. Juxtacortical osteosarcoma is seen as a surface mass causing scalloping of the cortex; it may show matrix calcification. MRI may show reactive marrow involvement and a thick radial periosteal reaction.[19]

FIBROGENIC TUMORS

Spindle Cell Sarcoma (Fibrosarcoma)

Spindle cell sarcomas, originally called fibrosarcomas of bone, are rare malignant tumors that contain spindle-shaped cells that produce no osteoid in either the primary lesion or in any metastatic deposits. They may be primary or can occur secondarily in Paget's disease, chondrosarcoma, bone infarction, following irradiation, and even in the sinus tracts of osteomyelitis.

Clinical Presentation

Age: Most of the tumors occur between 20 and 50 years.

Sex: Equal in both sexes.

Clinical picture: Pain, swelling, and pathological fractures are the common presenting features.

Site: The tubular bones are more frequently involved in younger patients, the flat bones in older patients. Almost 50% of these tumors arise in the lower limbs, particularly around the knee. The femur, tibia, and humerus account for approximately two-thirds of the tumors and the classical locations within these bones are the condyles of the femur and the epicondyles of the humerus. Other frequent sites include the innominate bones, skull, and facial bones. Lesions are mostly seen in the metaphysis but may extend into the epiphysis. The majority develop primarily in bone and may be either medullary or periosteal in location, while a few arise primarily in soft tissue and cause secondary bone changes. Metastases occur to the lungs, central skeleton, and viscera in a large percentage of cases.

Imaging Features

The tumor is essentially osteolytic with moth-eaten pattern of bone destruction and wide zone of transition; it provokes little new bone formation and usually lacks calcification or ossification **(Figs. 15A and B)**. The medullary variety is characterized by an irregular area of radiolucency. With very low-grade tumors, a minimal degree of sclerosis may surround the radiolucency. Slowly growing tumors may thin and expand the cortex, but with a diffuse infiltrative pattern, it is more usual for cortical destruction to occur. The subsequent soft-tissue extensions are without calcification or ossification, and periosteal new bone formation is unremarkable. This feature may differentiate it from osteosarcoma or chondrosarcoma.[36]

Periosteal tumors, however, frequently exhibit shaggy ill-defined periosteal new bone formation. Destruction of the outer side of the cortex frequently takes place, but the erosion is usually clearly defined, almost as though a piece of bone has been removed surgically. In this respect, considerable variance is shown from the poor definition of the edge of most malignant tumors. Secondary involvement of bone may result also from a spindle cell sarcoma arising in the soft tissue.

The major differential diagnoses are lytic osteosarcoma, dedifferentiated chondrosarcoma, and metastases. The more aggressive ill-defined varieties may be indistinguishable from malignant round cell tumors.

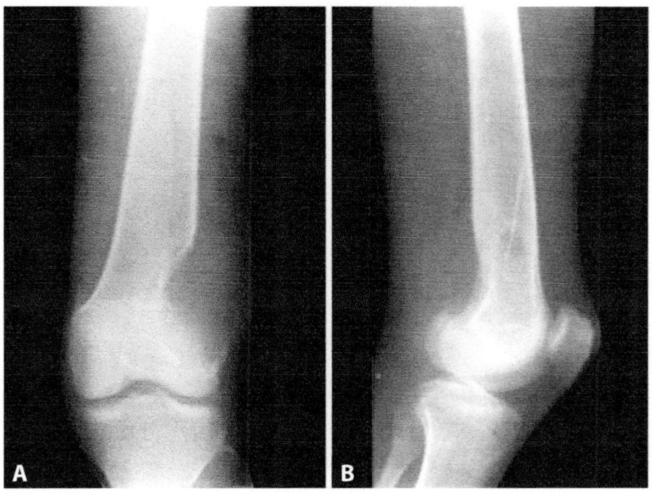

Figs. 15A and B: Spindle cell sarcoma. Anteroposterior (AP) (A) and lateral (B) radiographs of the knee show an osteolytic lesion with a short zone of transition in the distal femur. Note the absence of a periosteal reaction and tumor matrix mineralization.

SMALL ROUND BLUE CELL TUMORS

Small round blue cell tumors (SRBCTs) are comprised of a group of undifferentiated embryonal tumors that show aggressive behavior and include neuroblastoma, rhabdomyosarcoma, non-Hodgkin lymphoma, and the family of Ewing sarcomas. These tumors display similar histologic features and immunohistochemistry, and other molecular techniques are required for their diagnosis.[10]

EWING SARCOMA FAMILY OF TUMORS

The Ewing sarcoma family of tumors includes osseous Ewing sarcoma, extraskeletal Ewing sarcoma, primitive neuroectodermal tumor of bone (PNET), and Askin tumor which share a karyotype abnormality with translocation involving chromosomes 11 and 22. These lesions show sheets of small round blue cells on histopathology.[37]

Ewing Sarcoma

Ewing first identified this tumor in the early 1920s. Ewing sarcoma is the second most common primary malignant bone tumor in children and adolescents after osteosarcoma. It is also the fourth most common malignant bone tumor after multiple myeloma, osteosarcoma, and chondrosarcoma.

Clinical Presentation

Age: It is most frequently seen in the first three decades of life with 95% of cases occurring between 4 and 25 years of age.[37]

Sex: Slight male preponderance is seen (male-to-female ratio of 1.5:1).

Clinical picture: The patient presents with pain and mass or swelling and symptoms are mostly present for >6 months before diagnosis. The presence of fever and raised erythrocyte sedimentation rate (ESR) can simulate an infectious cause. Pathological fractures at presentation are uncommon.

Site: Most commonly affected sites include femur, ilium, tibia, humerus, fibula, ribs, and sacrum. Less frequently involved sites include mobile portion of spine, scapula, hand, foot, radius, ulna, mandible, maxilla, clavicle, calvaria, facial bones, and sternum. Long tubular bone involvement is more common proximally than distally, the lesion is seen in the diaphysis but the involvement can often be metadiaphyseal.

Usually, a single bone is involved, but multiple lesions occur at presentation in 10% of cases and more commonly later in the disease as Ewing sarcoma spreads by direct infiltration and hematogenous route to other bones and the lungs **(Figs. 16A to C)**. About 60% have bone metastases at autopsy.[38]

Imaging Features

On radiography, Ewing sarcoma appears as an aggressive lesion with bone destruction showing a moth-eaten or permeative pattern. The lesion shows a wide zone of transition. Cortical destruction associated with a soft-tissue mass is also commonly seen **(Figs. 17A and B)**. Periosteal reaction is also frequently seen and can be lamellated (onion skin), spiculated (sunburst or hair on end) **(Figs. 18A and B)**, or marginal (Codman triangle).

Sclerotic components can be seen that are often noted in the intraosseous component of lesions, in flat bones and spine; it appears dense, cloud-like, and represents reactive bone formation. Less common imaging features include cortical thickening, pathological fracture, expansile bone remodeling, soft-tissue calcification, saucerization, vertebra plana, or a well-marginated lesion. A soft-tissue mass may be the predominant abnormality with the osseous destruction being subtle at radiography. Saucerization of the outer bone cortex is often seen in cases extending from medullary canal.

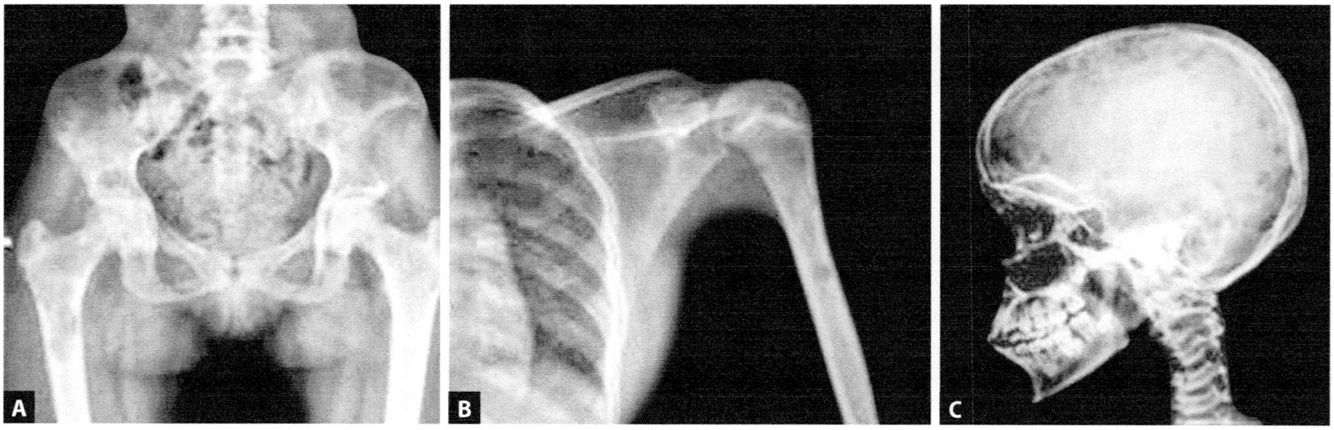

Figs. 16A to C: Ewing sarcoma with skeletal metastases. Pelvic radiograph (A) shows the primary tumor as a large predominantly lytic lesion in the left iliac bone with multiple lytic bony metastases in the right iliac blade and both the femora, humeral shaft (B), and skull (C).

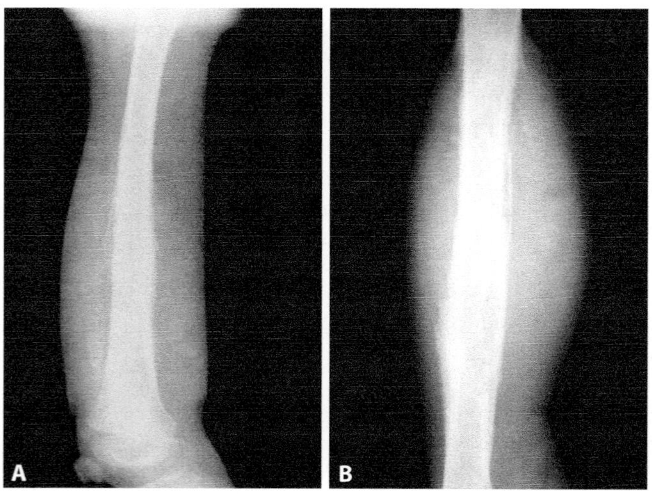

Figs. 17A and B: (A) Ewing sarcoma of the femur shows an ill-marginated, lytic-sclerotic lesion with cortical irregularity, laminar periosteal reaction, with a large soft tissue mass in the metadiaphyseal region; (B) In another case involving the femoral diaphysis, "saucerization" is well seen, with peripheral Codman triangles and a large soft tissue mass.

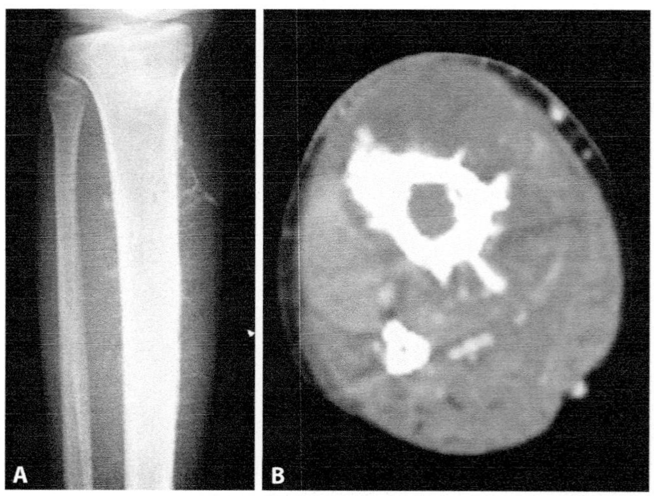

Figs. 18A and B: Ewing sarcoma. (A) Conventional radiograph shows a permeative lesion in the tibial diaphysis with a soft tissue component with spiculated periosteal reaction better appreciated on the axial computed tomography (CT) scan (B).

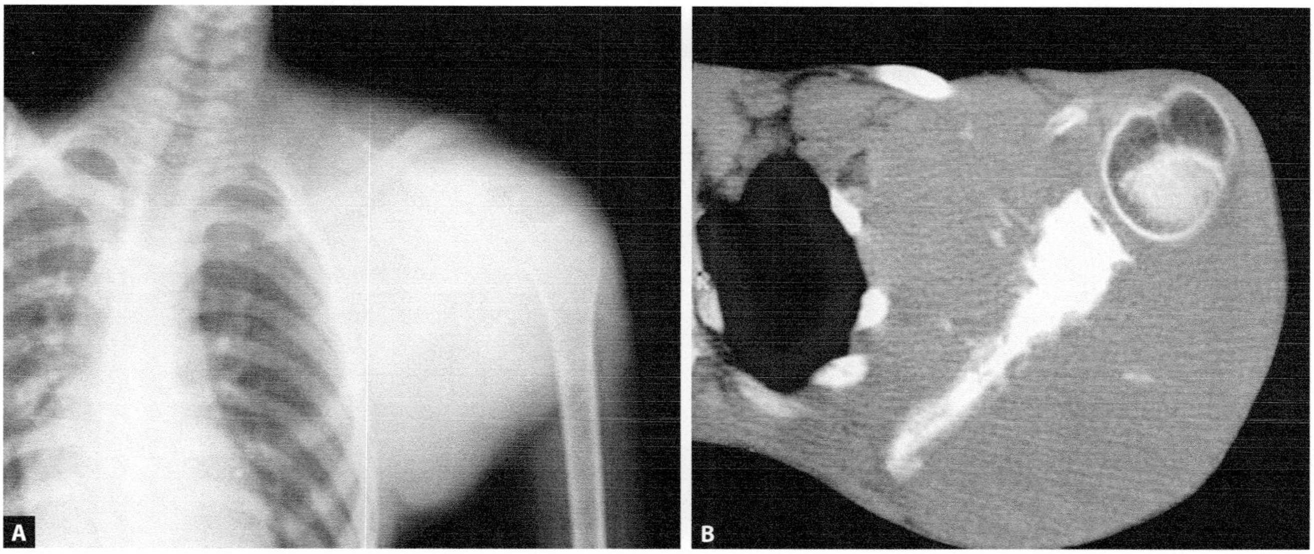

Figs. 19A and B: Ewing sarcoma. (A) Plain radiograph; (B) Axial computed tomography (CT) section of left shoulder shows a dense sclerotic involvement of the scapula with a large soft tissue mass.

Computed tomography demonstrates aggressive bony destruction with soft-tissue mass **(Figs. 19A and B)**, areas of focal cortical destruction with continuity between intraosseous and soft-tissue component can be seen. Hypodense linear channels extending through the high attenuation cortex representing tumor extension along neurovascular channels and haversian canals are also common and indicate subtle cortical involvement.[37]

Magnetic resonance imaging shows marrow replacement, cortical destruction, and soft-tissue mass which is circumferential but asymmetric around the osseous involvement **(Figs. 20A to D)**. It shows homogeneous and intermediate signal on T1W images with homogeneous, low-to-intermediate signal on T2W images. Heterogeneity and high T2W signal intensity can also be seen which are more common in larger lesions due to hemorrhage or necrosis **(Figs. 21A to I)**. Large areas of cortical destruction with continuity between medullary cavity and soft-tissue component are common at MRI **(Figs. 22A to D)**. Subtle cortical involvement as seen on CT is also evident on MRI with intermediate signal intensity channels extending through low signal intensity cortex; this imaging feature strongly suggests an SRBCT such as Ewing sarcoma, lymphoma, or leukemia. Contrast enhancement can be peripheral and nodular or diffuse.[37]

Ewing sarcoma is one of the more aggressive tumors with a tendency toward recurrence and metastases. It is the most common primary malignant tumor to metastasize to bone. Skip lesions are common. Secondary spread to the lungs also occurs frequently involving the lung parenchyma and pleura. FDG-PET is more sensitive than bone scan in the detection of bone metastases, with accuracy similar to whole body MRI.

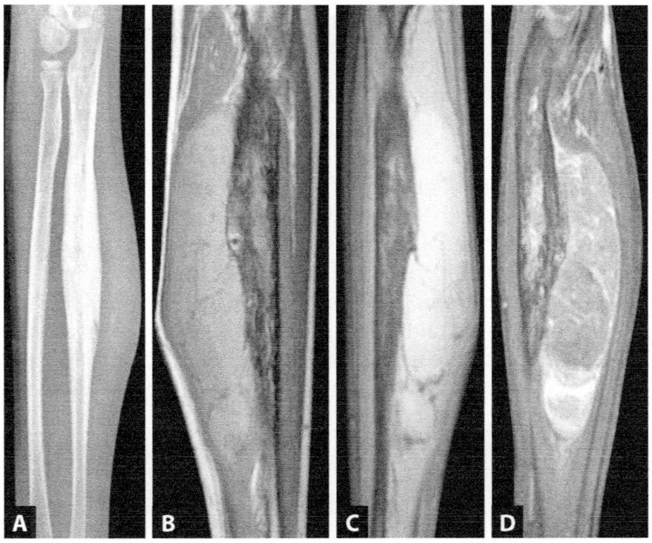

Figs. 20A to D: Ewing sarcoma of ulna. Anteroposterior (AP) radiograph of forearm (A) in a young girl presenting with pain and swelling reveals an aggressive lesion with a wide zone of transition involving the diaphysis of the ulna with cortical thickening and periosteal reaction. T1-weighted (T1W) (B), T2-weighted (T2W) (C), and T1-weighted (T1W) fat-saturated postcontrast (D) images show marrow replacement in the diaphysis of the ulna with a large associated soft tissue component appearing hypointense on T1W and hyperintense on T2W images showing heterogeneous postcontrast enhancement.

Differential diagnosis in the early stages is with osteomyelitis or occasionally trauma. Each of these may produce a periosteal reaction with little bone destruction. In Ewing sarcoma, a well-defined soft-tissue mass is seen, while in infection, the soft-tissue component is ill-defined. In later stages, Ewing sarcoma may be indistinguishable

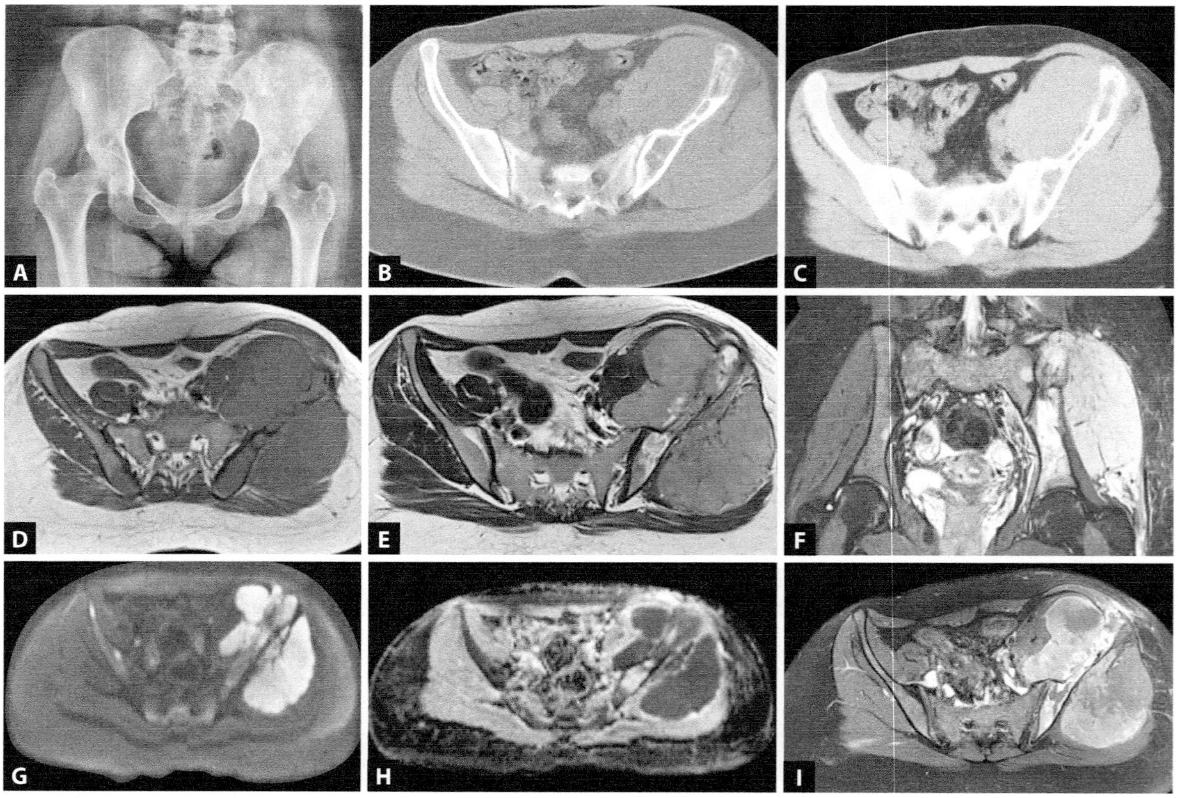

Figs. 21A to I: Ewing sarcoma of left iliac blade. Anteroposterior (AP) radiograph of the pelvis (A) in a young female with complaints of pain and swelling in gluteal region shows a large lytic lesion with permeative pattern of bony destruction involving the left iliac blade. Axial computed tomography (CT) images in the bone (B) and soft tissue (C) windows show the large, ill-defined lytic lesion in the left iliac blade associated with a large soft tissue component. Axial T1-weighted (T1W) (D), axial T2-weighted (T2W) (E), and short tau inversion recovery (STIR) coronal (F) images of the same patient show diffusely altered marrow signal intensity within the left iliac blade with a large soft tissue component seen along both sides of the bone, appearing hypointense to isointense to the surrounding muscle on T1W image and heterogeneously hyperintense on T2W and STIR images. Two small hyperintense focal lesions are seen in the left sacral ala and right iliac bone on STIR images suggestive of metastases. The lesion shows restricted diffusion on diffusion-weighted image (G) and appears hypointense on the corresponding apparent diffusion coefficient (ADC) map (H); heterogeneous enhancement with few nonenhancing necrotic areas are seen within the soft tissue component on postgadolinium scan (I).

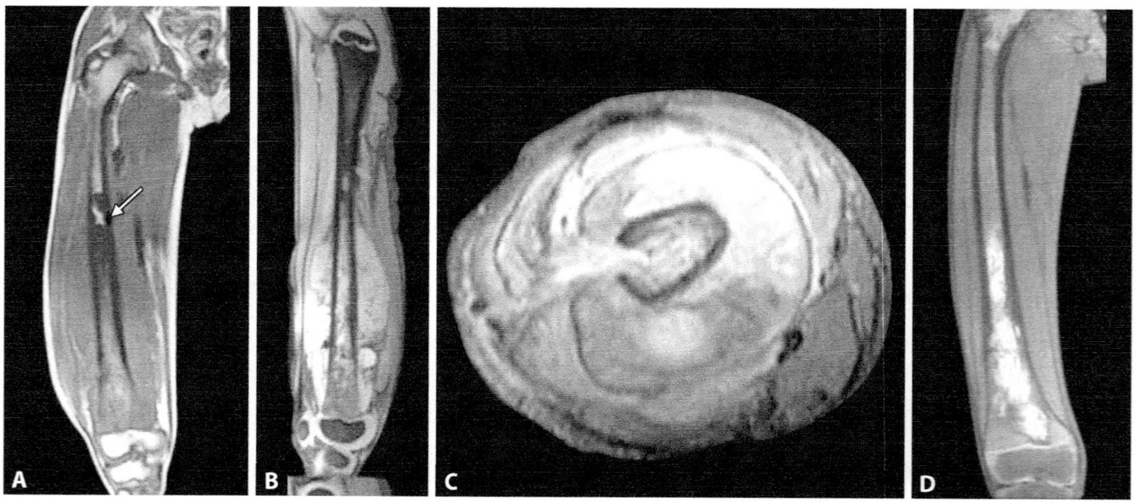

Figs. 22A to D: Ewing sarcoma. A T1-weighted (T1W) coronal scan (A) shows the intramedullary extent of the tumor as low signal intensity of the marrow with a small "skip" lesion proximally (arrow). The extraosseous component is better appreciated on the short tau inversion recovery (STIR) coronal image (B). The axial T2-weighted (T2W) image (C) shows the tumor within the femur as high signal intensity with cortical discontinuity. Soft tissue component can be seen surrounding the femoral diaphysis, displacing the neurovascular bundle posteromedially (D). After radiotherapy, there is marked reduction in the soft tissue mass with well-defined high signal intensity mass within the bone suggesting necrotic change.

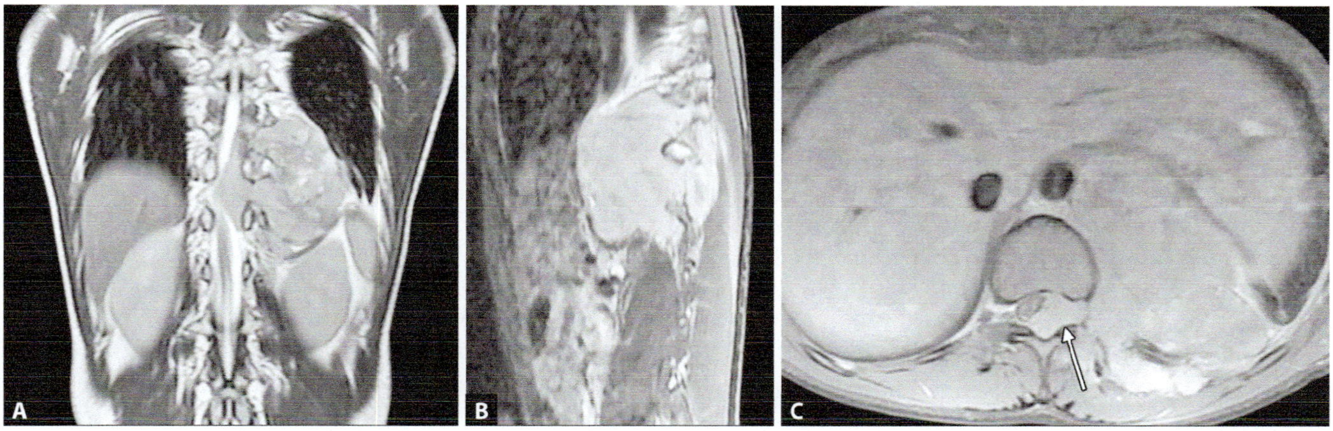

Figs. 23A to C: Askin tumor of chest wall in a young male presenting with lower back pain and difficulty in walking, T2-weighted (T2W) coronal (A) and short tau inversion recovery (STIR) sagittal images (B) show a relatively well-marginated paraspinal mass of high signal intensity in the left dorsolumbar region. Postcontrast axial (C) image shows the enhancing lesion with associated rib destruction, intradural extension, and mass effect on spinal cord (arrow in C).

from a lytic osteosarcoma. Primary lymphoma is differential in patients over the age of 30 years. Langerhans cell histiocytosis may occasionally mimic Ewing sarcoma, especially when presenting at an early destructive stage and involving the pelvis.[29]

Ewing sarcoma is usually treated with multiple cycles of multidrug chemotherapy for local and metastatic disease and radiation therapy or limb salvage for local control of tumor. Resectable lesions in the extremities have a better prognosis than those found in the pelvis or other bones of the axial skeleton.[39] Pretreatment DCE MRI has a potential role for determining the outcome and may be used in the decision to intensify treatment.[40] With treatment, the soft-tissue mass decreases in size and the intraosseous portion becomes necrotic with a higher signal on T2W imaging. MRI is also more accurate than standard radiography, CT, or scintigraphy in the diagnosis of recurrent Ewing sarcoma.

Rarely, extraskeletal Ewing sarcoma (EES) may develop in the soft tissues at any location. The most common sites of occurrence of EES are the trunk, extremities, and retroperitoneum. Although it is a soft-tissue primary tumor, it can cause changes in the cortex of the adjacent bone. EES is more common in adults and is associated with a high incidence of local recurrence and distant metastases.[41]

Primitive Neuroectodermal Tumor of Bone

These rare tumors of bone resemble Ewing tumors clinically except that they are more common in the female sex. They arise in the metaphyses and diaphyses of the lower limbs, humerus, pelvis, and scapula. Radiologically, they resemble Ewing sarcoma in being destructive ill-defined neoplasms which readily spread into the soft tissues. *Askin tumor* is a rare PNET of the thoracopulmonary region occurring in children and young adults. Radiologically, in 70% of patients, it presents as a pleural disorder **(Figs. 23A to C)**. A soft-tissue mass involving the chest wall is seen in about half of the patients and a subpleural pulmonary mass with pleural involvement in about one quarter.[29]

NOTOCHORDAL ORIGIN

Chordoma

Chordoma is a rare, low-to-intermediate grade malignant tumor which arises from ectopic cellular remnants of the notochord which have persisted within the nucleus pulposus of the intervertebral disc or from aberrant cell rests of notochord tissue within the vertebral bodies. This tumor has a predilection for the sacrococcygeal and spheno-occipital regions.[19,42]

Clinical Presentation

Age: It is most common in the fifth and sixth decades.

Sex: Incidence is more common in males with male:female ratio varying from 2:1 to 3:1.

Clinical picture: Patients present with pain. Other symptoms relate to pressure on local structures—rectal/vesical dysfunction in the sacral region and cranial nerve palsies in the spheno-occipital region.

Site: It usually occurs as a solitary lesion and is exclusively seen in the axial skeleton, in midline of sacrococcygeal region, more commonly below S3 level (50%), spheno-occipital region (40%), or vertebrae (5%). Spheno-occipital tumors are seen in younger patients and are smaller in size as compared to sacrococcygeal lesions. Vertebral chordomas can occur equally in both men and women, it can affect children and is more common in cervical region. Distant metastases are rare, mainly involving lymph nodes, liver, and lungs.

Imaging Features

Clinical presentation is delayed due to the slow-growing nature of these tumors and radiologically, these lesions appear advanced. Radiographs reveal a destructive lytic lesion associated with a soft-tissue mass that may show nonspecific, amorphous calcification **(Fig. 24A)**. A sclerotic margin and narrow zone of transition may be present as a result of slow growth, especially in spinal lesions. In the spheno-occipital region, the dorsal aspect of the sella and clivus may be destroyed, with a soft-tissue mass indenting the nasopharyngeal airway.

Computed tomography scans show a destructive expansive lesion and a large lobulated soft-tissue mass containing calcification **(Fig. 24B)**. Due to the gelatinous matrix, the soft-tissue mass shows low attenuation on CT and intermediate-to-low signal intensity on T1W images and high signal intensity on T2W images on MRI **(Figs. 25A to C)**. Hemorrhage, when present, appears as a high T1 signal. Variable contrast enhancement is seen, appearing minimal in myxoid-containing lobules and moderate in vascular septa, which produces a crisscross pattern. Sacral nerve root involvement is best seen on coronal MR images. Assessment should include extension to sacroiliac joints, spinal nerves, and plexus. The differential diagnosis for this condition includes chondrosarcoma, plasmacytoma, metastasis, and lymphoma.

Vertebral chordoma lesions begin in the center of the body and extend to involve the posterior elements, with soft-tissue masses seen anterior, posterior, and lateral to the bodies. With involvement of the epidural space, the soft-tissue mass may extend to involve multiple craniocaudal contiguous levels. Discal involvement is seen very late in the disease and as chordoma and discs show the same signal on MRI, disc involvement is not diagnosed based on MRI signal, but on the loss of end-plate integrity. The differential diagnosis for vertebral chordoma includes tuberculosis, chondrosarcoma, and metastasis from renal adenocarcinoma.

Treatment for chordoma includes wide resection and surgical debulking; rectal involvement necessitates a colostomy. Radiotherapy may be done in operable cases,

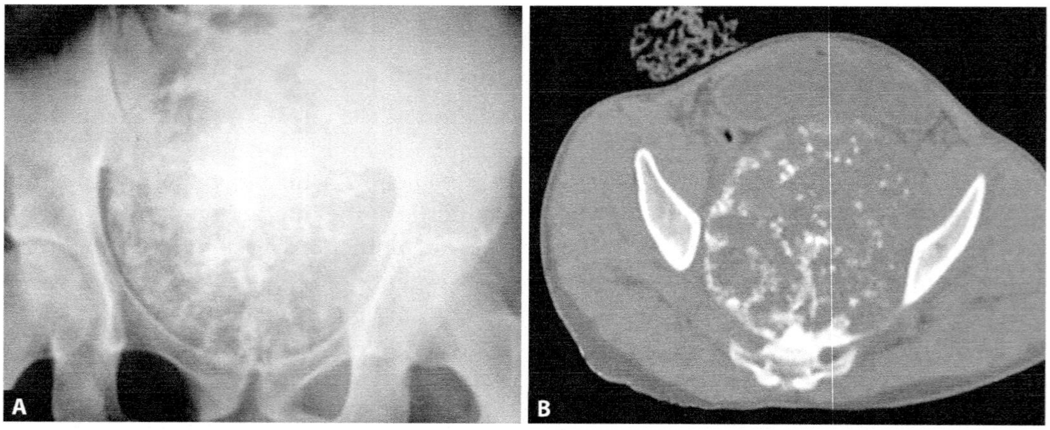

Figs. 24A and B: Chordoma of the sacrum. Plain radiograph (A) and computed tomography (CT) (B) showing a large pelvic mass with calcification.

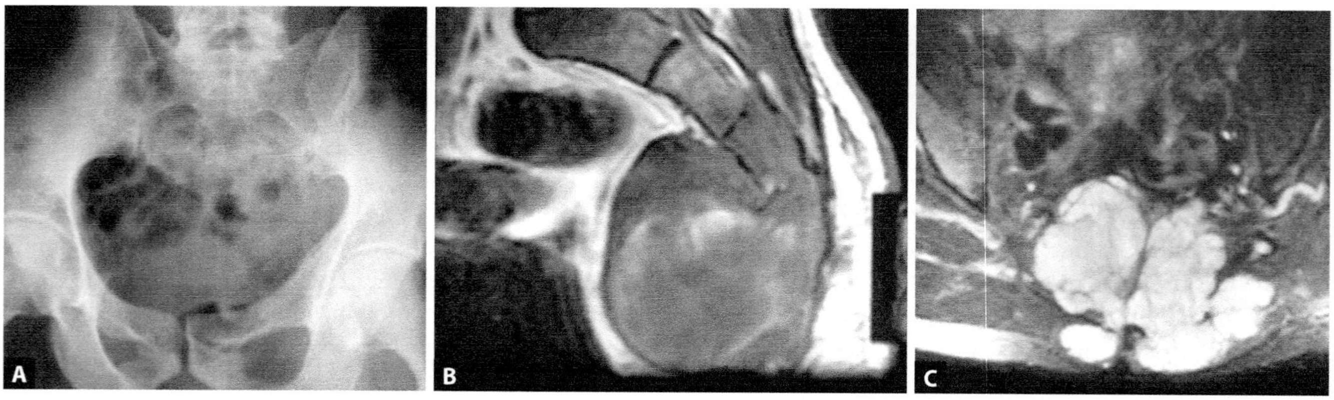

Figs. 25A to C: Chordoma of the sacrum. (A) Plain radiograph shows a lytic lesion destroying the distal half of the sacrum (B) and (C) T1-weighted (T1W) sagittal and T2-weighted (T2W) axial magnetic resonance (MR) images show the large tumor with inhomogeneous signal intensity arising from the distal sacrum.

where wide resection is not possible. Younger patients and those with lesions that are small or sacrococcygeal have a better prognosis. Metastasis occurs late in the disease in 10% of the patients with sacrococcygeal lesions and in 30–40% of patients with spinal lesions. Although metastasis is relatively uncommon, it is locally aggressive, often resulting in severe neurologic symptoms. High rate of local recurrence (around 40%) is noted, especially in the surgical bed, which is treated with radiation.

The chondroid variant of chordoma (approximately 15% of chordomas) contains cartilaginous areas with most present in the skull base. Imaging features for this variant are similar to those of chondrosarcoma. CT and MRI reveal a lobulated tumor, with low attenuation areas and calcification and with low T1 and high T2 signal. Contrast enhancement is not lobular, but there is only mild septal enhancement compared with the lobular, nodular, or diffuse enhancement of chondrosarcomas. Occasionally, a rings-and-arcs pattern of enhancement may be seen.

Chordomas (chondroid and nonchondroid) stain for cytokeratins, epithelial membrane antigen (EMA), and carcinoembryonic antigen (CEA), but these antigens are not expressed by chondrosarcomas.

Dedifferentiated chordomas (around 6–9% of chordomas) can occur in either primary or recurrent chordoma. It is more common in the sacrococcygeal region, particularly after radiation. Extra-axial chordomas have also been reported; patients with these lesions tend to have a better prognosis because the tumors are not near vital structures in the midline. CT and MRI show destructive lesions with internal hemorrhage and cyst formation.[1]

VASCULAR TUMORS OF THE BONE

Malignant vascular lesions of the bone are rare and usually present with nonspecific clinical and radiological features. Tumors in this group include hemangioendothelioma, epithelioid hemangioendothelioma, and angiosarcoma. Vascular tumors of the bone should be considered in the presence of multifocal bony lesions, especially distal to elbow or knee joints in young or middle-aged patients.

Angiosarcoma

Angiosarcoma is a rare, high-grade malignant vascular tumor of bone, affecting all ages, although peak incidence is seen in third and fourth decades. Male:female ratio is 2:1. Any bone can be affected, but the vertebrae and the femur are most commonly involved. Multiple lesions occur in one-third of the cases.[19,43]

Radiologically, a multilocular or "soap bubble" appearance may be seen. The lesion often involves a considerable length of bone. It may be seen as a lytic lesion with ill-defined margins, mixed lytic and sclerotic lesions have also been described. Purely sclerotic lesions are rare. Endosteal erosion, cortical destruction, and extraosseous extension can be seen; however, periosteal reaction and pathological fractures are rare. CT and MRI appearances are nonspecific. This is a highly malignant tumor usually treated by surgery including amputation, limb salvage, radical local resection, and radiotherapy with a 5-year survival rate of under 10%. Differential diagnosis includes primary sarcomas and metastases.

Hemangioendothelioma

Hemangioendothelioma is a rare low-grade endothelial neoplasm that can occur between the ages of 10 and 60 years and is more commonly seen in males. Sites of involvement include lower limb (femur and tibia) followed by vertebrae, upper limb, and flat bones. It is common in diaphysis but may also be seen in metaphysis or metaepiphysis. Twenty-five percent of patients may have multicentric disease.[19] Multiple lesions in one bone or extremity or multifocal lesions in various bones may suggest this diagnosis. Usually, the lesion is lytic, although mixed lytic sclerotic and purely sclerotic lesions may be seen. Osseous expansion, cortical thinning, and endosteal erosions can be present; periosteal reaction, cortical destruction, and soft-tissue masses are uncommon.

In children, differential diagnosis for a multifocal lesion includes Langerhans cell histiocytosis, fibrous dysplasia, brown tumor, and metastasis; and in adults, the differential diagnosis includes metastasis, multiple myeloma, lymphoma, brown tumors, and fibrous dysplasia. A solitary lesion may be confused with fibrous dysplasia, fibrous cortical defect, solitary bone cyst, osteosarcoma, spindle cell sarcoma (fibrosarcoma), or Ewing sarcoma. These patients have variable prognosis which depends on the histologic grade, level of differentiation, and unifocal or multifocal nature of the tumor. Treatment includes surgery and adjuvant therapy for unifocal lesions and radiation for multifocal lesions.

Epithelioid Hemangioendothelioma

Epithelioid hemangioendothelioma is a rare malignant vascular neoplasm that involves multiple skeletal sites; it has nonspecific imaging features. This condition can occur across a wide age range, most commonly in the second and third decades. It is more commonly seen in men. Typical sites of involvement include calvarium, spine, femur, tibia, and feet. In the long bones, it is seen in the metaphysis or epiphysis. Radiographs reveal lytic lesions, 40% of which are multifocal and usually involve a single anatomic site or extremity. Cortical destruction and expansion are commonly seen, whereas periosteal reaction and matrix mineralization are rare. A soft-tissue mass is seen in 40% of cases.[19]

MYOGENIC, LIPOGENIC, AND EPITHELIAL TUMORS

Liposarcoma

Primary intraosseous liposarcoma is extremely rare despite the extensive fatty content of the bone marrow. It is four times as common in males as in females, and is seen between 24 and 45 years of age.[19]

Most tumors affect the long bones of the lower limbs, the femur and the tibia. The lesion can be seen in the epiphysis, metaphysis, or diaphysis. Radiologically, appearance varies from local geographic bone destruction to a permeative pattern. Fluid-fluid levels may be seen. CT and MRI provide characteristic diagnostic information due to the nonhomogeneous fatty content of the tumor. Although fat-containing lesions are usually considered benign, biopsy is essential in the presence of cortical destruction and soft-tissue mass which can indicate malignancy.

Adamantinoma of Long Bones

This is a rare low-grade epithelioid malignant lesion which is characterized by squamous, alveolar, and vascular tissues of unknown origin. It most commonly involves the midshaft of the tibia. Although it has some histological resemblance to maxillofacial adamantinoma, the two conditions are not related.

Clinical Presentation

Age: It is commonly seen in the second and third decades.

Sex: It is more common in men.

Clinical picture: Local pain and tenderness of several months to several years' duration is the most common presenting complaint.

Site: Most commonly seen in tibia (83%) followed by fibula, humerus, and femur. It is classically located in the anterior tibial diaphysis in its mid or proximal portions. Tumors with multiple foci in the same long bone may sometimes occur.

Imaging Features

Adamantinomas can be situated in the cortex or the medullary space. Radiographs reveal an eccentric, intracortical, expansile mixed lytic lesion that can extend longitudinally in the cortex or it can destroy the cortex and extend into the medulla. Soap bubble appearance can be seen with multilocularity and thin walls. A multiloculated appearance and satellite lesions are useful diagnostic features. Periosteal reaction is uncommon. MRI is invaluable in the local staging of adamantinoma for features such as extension into the marrow cavity, extraosseous extension, and multifocal lesions. A lobulated growth pattern is typical, but there are no specific signal characteristics. Intense, uniform enhancement is seen following contrast-enhanced studies.[44]

Differential diagnosis includes metastatic carcinoma, plasmacytoma, ABC, fibrous dysplasia, and osteofibrous dysplasia. However, fibrous dysplasia is seen at a younger age and shows ground-glass opacity with anterior tibial bowing without periosteal reaction or moth-eaten destruction. Unlike adamantinoma, osteofibrous dysplasia occurs in patients younger than 10 years and is typically intracortical with no medullary extension. Age is a helpful differentiating factor when imaging findings overlap.

Adamantinomas grow at a slow rate but are characterized by local recurrences and eventual metastases to the lung. Metastases to the bones and lymph nodes can also occur. Extensive local resection is the usual form of treatment.

Differentiated adamantinoma (osteofibrous dysplasia-like adamantinoma) is a variant of adamantinoma, a diagnosis that is based on histology. It has a prolonged course similar to osteofibrous dysplasia and is treated less aggressively.

UNDIFFERENTIATED PLEOMORPHIC SARCOMA (MALIGNANT FIBROUS HISTIOCYTOMA)

Malignant fibrous histiocytomas were replaced by the term undifferentiated pleomorphic sarcoma (UPS) which denotes the anonymity of the entity but confirms its mesenchymal origin and malignant nature.[45]

Most of these lesions arise de novo; about 22–43% of the lesions arise secondary to preexisting osseous lesions that are caused by previous irradiation, bone infarcts, Paget's disease, chronic osteomyelitis, fibrous dysplasia, ABC, GCT, neurofibromatosis 1, or orthopedic implants.[19]

Clinical Presentation

Age

Most commonly seen in fifth to seventh decades with peak incidence in the fifth decade.

Sex

Males are more commonly affected, with male-to-female ratio of 3:2.

Clinical Picture

The patient presents with localized pain and swelling of insidious onset. Pathological fracture is common.

Site

Lesions involve the ends of long bones commonly, especially the distal diametaphysis of the femur and proximal metaphysis of the tibia. Other bones involved are the humerus, the ribs, the craniofacial bones, and the spine.

Imaging Features

An aggressive lytic lesion with permeative type of bony destruction is seen on radiographs with involvement of soft tissue being a common feature. Periosteal reaction is rare. Occasionally punctate, soft-tissue calcification is present. Most cases present with multiple skeletal lesions and the initial impression is of skeletal metastases rather than of a primary or multifocal bone tumor. The main differential diagnosis is a malignant round cell tumor.

The lesions show variable appearance on MRI, ranging from isointense to slightly hyperintense relative to muscle on T1W images and intermediate to slightly hyperintense relative to muscle on STIR and T2W images, with nodular and inhomogeneous enhancement pattern. This appearance makes it one of the few lytic malignant lesions without a very high T2 signal, similar to lymphoma and leiomyosarcoma, because of the histologic fibrous tissue matrix and variable cellularity in these lesions. Predominantly, hypointense T1 and hyperintense T2 signals in the lesion have also been reported. In secondary cases, the underlying bone lesion is seen along with UPS. Extraosseous disease is seen in almost all patients with UPS. UPS is associated with a high rate of local recurrence and metastasis, particularly to lungs, bones, brain, kidneys, and heart.

MALIGNANT GIANT CELL TUMOR

Malignant GCTs are a heterogeneous group of tumors, which contain giant cells that have aggressive local behavior and systemic metastasis. The malignant GCT classification can be divided into categories of malignancy in GCT, giant cell-containing sarcoma, secondary malignant GCT, and benign metastasizing GCT. Malignancy in GCT and secondary malignant GCT account for about 6% of all GCTs. Malignancy in GCT have sarcomatous areas juxtaposed with typical benign GCT in patients with no history of radiation, resection, or curettage.

When a sarcoma develops in patients with a history of radiation, resection, or curettage of conventional GCT, the lesion is labeled secondary malignant GCT (87%). A history of radiation is present in 76% of these secondary GCT cases, with a latent period of 10 years or longer. Secondary malignant GCT in the absence of radiation is extremely rare. Malignancy in GCT is said to occur in an older population than conventional GCTs. Giant cell-containing sarcoma is an anaplastic variant of the typical benign GCT, but without the evidence of tumor osteoid, bone, or cartilage. It is often associated with Paget's disease and should be differentiated pathologically from giant cell-rich sarcoma variants, such as osteosarcoma and fibrosarcoma.

Benign metastasizing GCT is a term used for skeletal GCT with pulmonary metastasis that is histologically identical to GCT. It is seen in 1.8–5% of GCTs. Local recurrence is seen in 48% of these patients. The prognosis for these patients is good. Metastasectomy is recommended when feasible.[19]

METASTATIC BONE DISEASE

Skeletal metastases are defined as tumors involving bone, which originate from another distal site. Metastases are the most common malignant tumors of the skeletal system. Approximately 70% of all malignant tumors are metastatic in origin, with only 30% being primary in nature.[46] Postmortem studies show that their incidence is much higher than may be detected in vivo. Bony metastases are present in approximately 25% of all deaths from malignant diseases.[47] Most of the osseous metastases are from a primary extraskeletal focus; the majority are epithelial in origin. The most common primary sites are in the breast, lung, prostate, kidney, thyroid, and bowel. With the exception of tumors of the central nervous system and basal cell carcinoma of the skin, almost every malignant tumor can metastasize to bone.

Bone involvement in metastases occurs by means of three main mechanisms: (1) direct extension, (2) retrograde venous flow, and (3) seeding with tumor emboli via the blood circulation which is the most common route of spread. Venous tumor emboli get arrested at a distant capillary bed. As the tumor emboli have to pass through the pulmonary bed, metastatic cancer to bone is a relatively late occurrence and generally occurs after pulmonary metastases have appeared.[48] Retrograde venous embolism is probably the major mechanism when spread from intra-abdominal cancer involves the vertebrae. Increased intra-abdominal pressure causes blood to be diverted from the systemic caval system to the valveless vertebral venous plexus of Batson; this diversion allows the caudal and cranial flow of blood.

Clinical Presentation

Age

Most patients are older than 40 years. In children <5 years, skeletal metastases usually occur from neuroblastoma. Metastases between the age group of 10 and 25 years commonly occur from Ewing sarcoma and osteosarcoma, and between 20 and 35 years, they occur from Hodgkin lymphoma.

Sex

In females, the carcinoma of the breast is responsible for majority of all bone metastases followed by the carcinomas of thyroid, kidney, and uterus. In males, carcinoma prostate is the most common primary focus, followed by the carcinoma of the lung.

Site

They are most often found in the axial skeleton and other sites of residual red marrow. Thus, the common sites for metastases are vertebrae, pelvis, proximal femora and humeri, skull, sternum, and ribs. Metastases to bones of hand and feet are rare and almost 50% of these are due to the carcinoma of the lung.

Clinical Picture

The lesions may be entirely asymptomatic or present with vague bone pains. Occasionally, a pathological fracture through the metastatic lesion may bring it to notice. Weight loss, cachexia, anemia, and even fever may be seen in the later stages.

Imaging Features

Plain Radiographs

Bone metastases may be lytic, sclerotic, or mixed lytic and sclerotic. As a metastatic lesion grows in the medullary cavity, the surrounding bone is remodeled by means of either osteoclastic or osteoblastic processes. The relative degree of resultant bone resorption or deposition is highly variable and depends on the type and the location of the tumor. The relationship between the osteoclastic and osteoblastic remodeling processes determines whether a predominant lytic, sclerotic, or mixed pattern is seen on radiographs. The majority (75%) of metastases is osteolytic. Lesions usually appear in the medullary cavity, spread to destroy the medullary bone, and then involve the cortex, usually without the development of much periosteal reaction. Soft-tissue extension is relatively uncommon. At least 30–50% bone destruction is necessary before the lytic lesions can be detected on plain radiographs.

Some metastases (15%) are predominantly osteoblastic, e.g., from prostate, stomach, and carcinoid. The increased density of the blastic metastases is due to the laying down of new bone, which is non-neoplastic in nature, but is a reactive response of the local osteoid tissue to the presence of the tumor. Mixed osteolytic and osteosclerotic metastasis (10%) occur from carcinoma of the breast and occasionally, lung.

Breast in females and prostate in males are the most common primary tumors metastasizing to bone. Breast metastases are commonly lytic **(Figs. 26A and B)**, but 10% may be osteoblastic and in another 10% can be mixed. Diffuse infiltration of the whole marrow may occur and may only become evident radiologically when sclerosis occurs after therapy. Skeletal metastases from prostate are predominantly blastic or mixed **(Figs. 27A and B)**. Purely lytic lesions are rare. Individual lesions may sometimes show a florid "sunburst' appearance, simulating osteosarcoma **(Fig. 28)**. Metastases from the lung occur most commonly to the axial skeleton **(Figs. 29A to D)**; however, metastases to hand and foot are most commonly from bronchogenic carcinoma **(Fig. 30)**. The squamous cell and oat cell carcinomas of lung produce lytic metastases, while adenocarcinomas and bronchial carcinoid which metastasize to bone in about 10% of cases, produce focal, or diffuse densely blastic lesions.

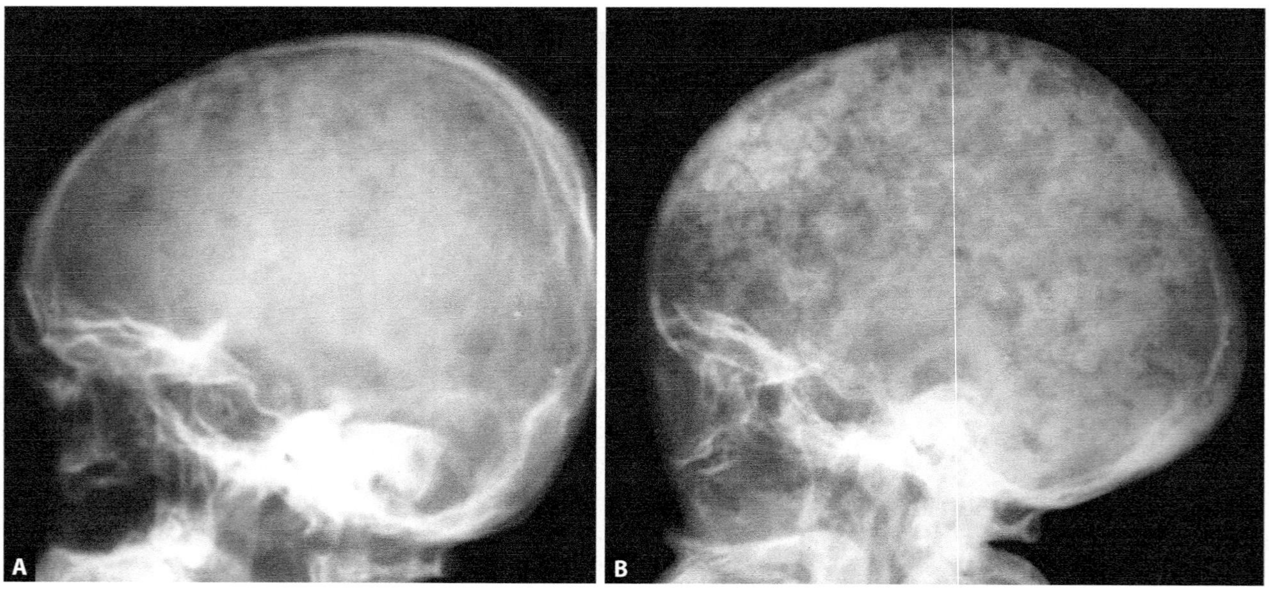

Figs. 26A and B: Skeletal metastases. Lateral radiographs (A and B) of the skull of two different patients show multiple ill-defined lytic lesions of varying sizes in the calvarium.

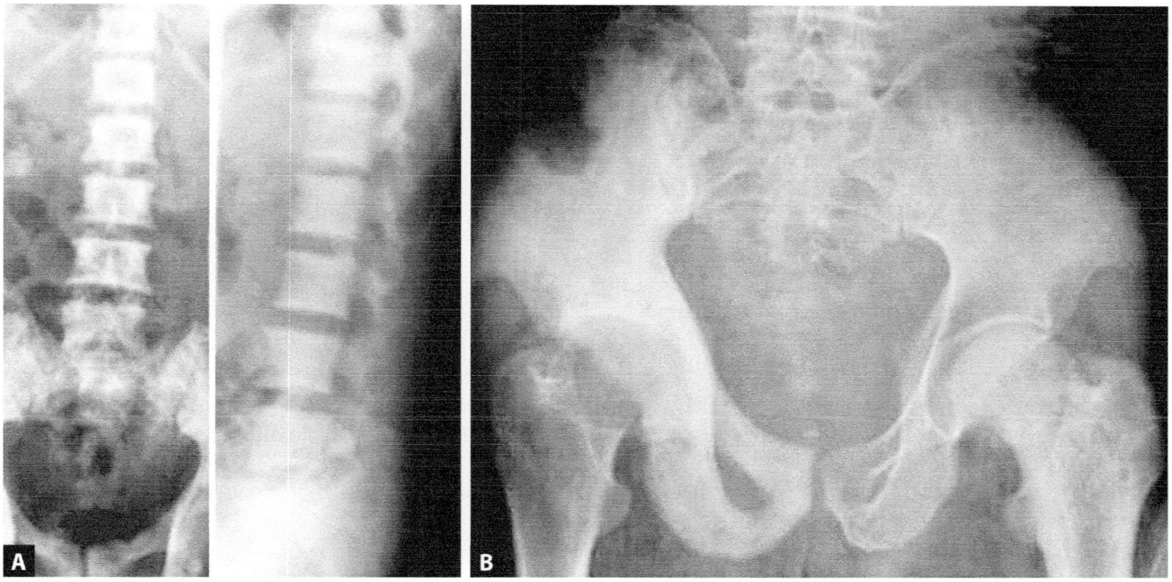

Figs. 27A and B: Metastases from carcinoma prostate. (A) Anteroposterior (AP) and lateral radiographs of the lumbar spine show characteristic osteoblastic metastases; (B) Radiograph of pelvis shows diffuse sclerosis in the right iliac bone and left femoral head.

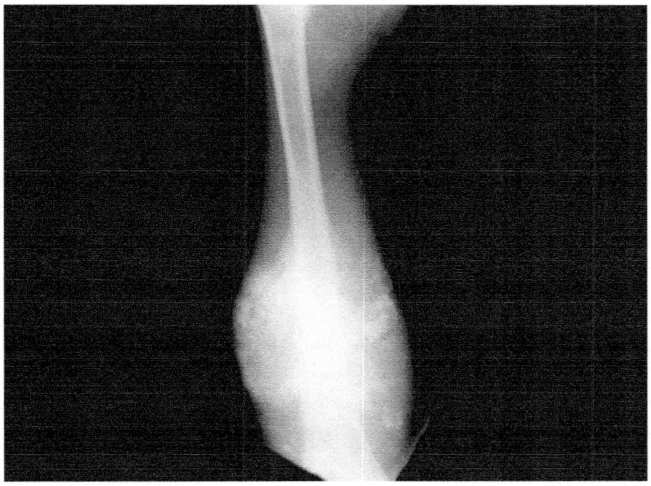

Fig. 28: Metastasis from carcinoma prostate. Anteroposterior (AP) radiograph of the femur shows osteoblastic metastasis with extensive "sunburst" periosteal reaction resembling osteosarcoma.

Hypernephroma and thyroid carcinoma generally show lytic, expansile metastases, also called "blow-out metastases" **(Fig. 31)**. The incidence of skeletal metastases from the gastrointestinal tract is under 7%, but as these malignancies are more common than kidney and thyroid, they are encountered commonly. They are usually lytic, but sclerotic metastases may occur. Calcification is also a feature. Cervical carcinoma usually involves bone by contiguous spread to the bony pelvis. Blood-borne metastases are uncommon and usually lytic, but may rarely be osteoblastic or mixed. Carcinoma of the uterine body is an adenocarcinoma and, like that of the ovary, may produce osteoblastic metastases, particularly of the vertebrae.

Nuclear Medicine

The value of establishing the presence of multiple skeletal lesions cannot be overemphasized, as individual metastatic lesions may mimic primary malignant tumors of bone. For this purpose, bone scintigraphy remains the most cost-effective method.[49] Several patterns of scintigraphic abnormality may be seen. The most common is one of multiple sites of increased skeletal activity typically in the axial skeleton **(Fig. 32)**. The abnormal uptake on scintigraphy depends upon intact local blood flow and increased osteoblastic activity. Lesions which outgrow their blood supply or stimulate no osteoblastic response may appear as photopenic or "cold spots." Occasionally, a combination of both "hot" and "cold" lesions may be seen. A super scan appearance, i.e., generalized increase in skeletal activity with reduced or absent renal activity is typically seen in diffuse osteoblastic metastatic disease from breast or prostate **(Fig. 33)**.

The specificity of bone scintigraphy is generally lower, due to a known increased blood flow and bone remodeling in response to a variety of disease processes, including trauma, infection, inflammation, and osteoarthritis. Therefore, further assessment with other imaging modalities, mainly CT and MRI, and in some cases, histologic confirmation may be required for precise diagnosis.

Single photon emission computed tomography (SPECT) imaging of the skeleton uses ^{99m}Tc-MDP, the same radionuclide used in conventional skeletal scintigraphy; however, images are acquired in a cross-sectional rather than a planar fashion. Whereas planar imaging is limited by superimposition of structures, SPECT can show axial slices through the body, providing better localization of

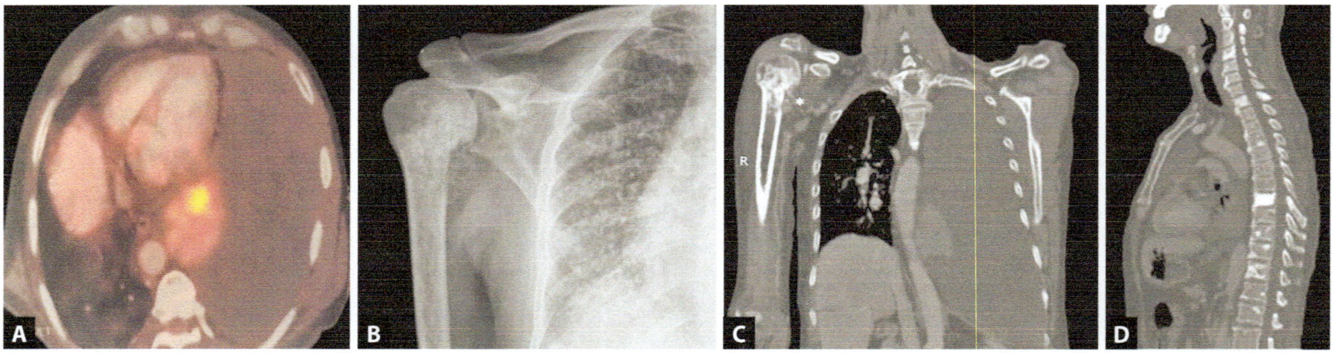

Figs. 29A to D: Carcinoma of the left lung with metastases to right humerus and vertebrae in an adult male patient. Positron emission tomography computed tomography (PET-CT) (A) reveals a malignant lesion showing increased uptake in the collapsed left lung with massive left pleural effusion. Anteroposterior (AP) radiograph of right shoulder (B) shows a sclerotic lesion in the humeral head and proximal shaft with associated irregularity along the medial aspect of the humeral head and neck. Coronal (C) and sagittal (D) CT images in bone window shows the sclerotic lesion in head and shaft of right humerus with associated soft tissue in axilla and multiple sclerotic lesions involving vertebrae at various levels.

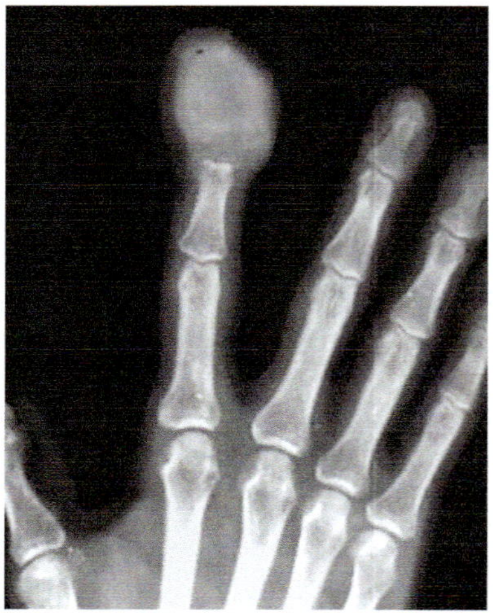

Fig. 30: Metastasis from carcinoma lung. A lytic lesion involves the terminal phalanx of the index finger.

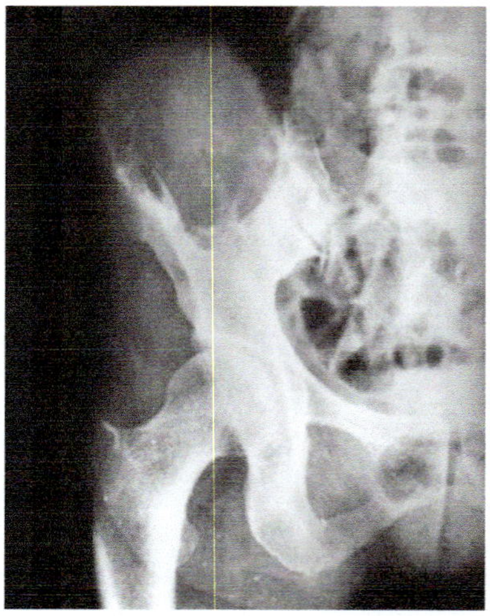

Fig. 31: Metastasis from a hypernephroma. A large lytic lesion is seen in the left iliac blade.

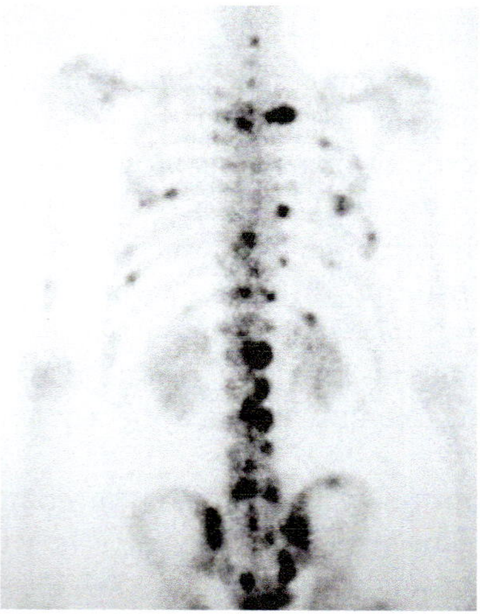

Fig. 32: Skeletal scintigraphy in metastatic disease of the skeleton shows multiple randomly distributed focal lesions scattered throughout the skeleton, particularly the spine, ribs, and pelvis.

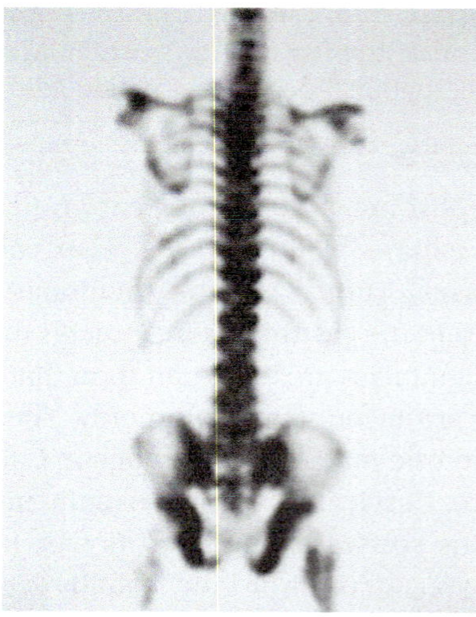

Fig. 33: Technetium-99m bone scintiscan in a case of prostatic carcinoma. This image shows diffuse and intense uptake in most of the bones. Patchy rib lesions are also seen, but renal uptake is absent.

abnormal radionuclide uptake. Addition of SPECT has been reported to detect 20–50% more lesions in the spine compared with planar scintigraphy. It increases both the sensitivity and the specificity of bone scans.

FDG-PET is more sensitive and specific than bone scan for detecting bone metastases. It detects all types of bone metastases; however, it is more sensitive for detecting lytic metastases than sclerotic metastases **(Figs. 34A to E)**. The increased avidity of lytic lesions for FDG is because of the high glycolytic rate and relative hypoxemia that are characteristic of these lesions in contrast to sclerotic lesions, which are relatively acellular, less aggressive, and not prone to hypoxia.[14] FDG-PET has the additional advantage of detecting extraskeletal metastatic disease as well. FDG-PET has also proved to be an effective modality for the assessment of therapeutic response by showing rapid reduction in FDG uptake by the tumors in responders following chemotherapy. The changes in standard uptake value (SUV) with therapy showed good correlation with the overall clinical assessment of response as well as with the change in tumor marker value.

Sodium fluoride PET is very sensitive for detecting both osteolytic and osteoblastic lesions and is superior to bone scintigraphy for diagnosing skeletal metastases. Evan-Sapir et al. compared bone scintigraphy, NaF-PET, and NaF-PET/CT in patients with high-risk prostate cancer and found that NaF-PET/CT was the most accurate modality for detecting bone metastases.[50] Increased FDG activity at the sites of skeletal lesions represents active tumor itself, whereas increased ^{99m}Tc-MDP or 18F-fluoride activity represents a blastic activity/reparative process in response to tumor and destroyed bone.

Gallium-68 prostate-specific membrane antigen (Ga-68 PSMA) PET-CT is a new addition and is useful for prostate cancer staging, particularly for bone metastasis. It shows high sensitivity and specificity for bone metastasis from prostatic carcinoma.

MRI depicts early hematogenous dissemination of the tumor to the bone marrow before reactions in the adjacent bone are detectable on ^{99m}Tc scintiscans. Metastatic seeding in the bone marrow is characterized by long T1 relaxation times, whereas T2 relaxation times are variable, depending on tumor morphology. Lesions are seen as focal or diffuse areas of hypointensity on T1W images and as areas of intermediate or high signal intensity on T2W images. Tumor deposits typically appear hyperintense against a dark background of suppressed signal intensity within fat on STIR images. Osteoblastic metastases may appear hypointense on all pulse sequences. The identification of a "halo" of high signal intensity around

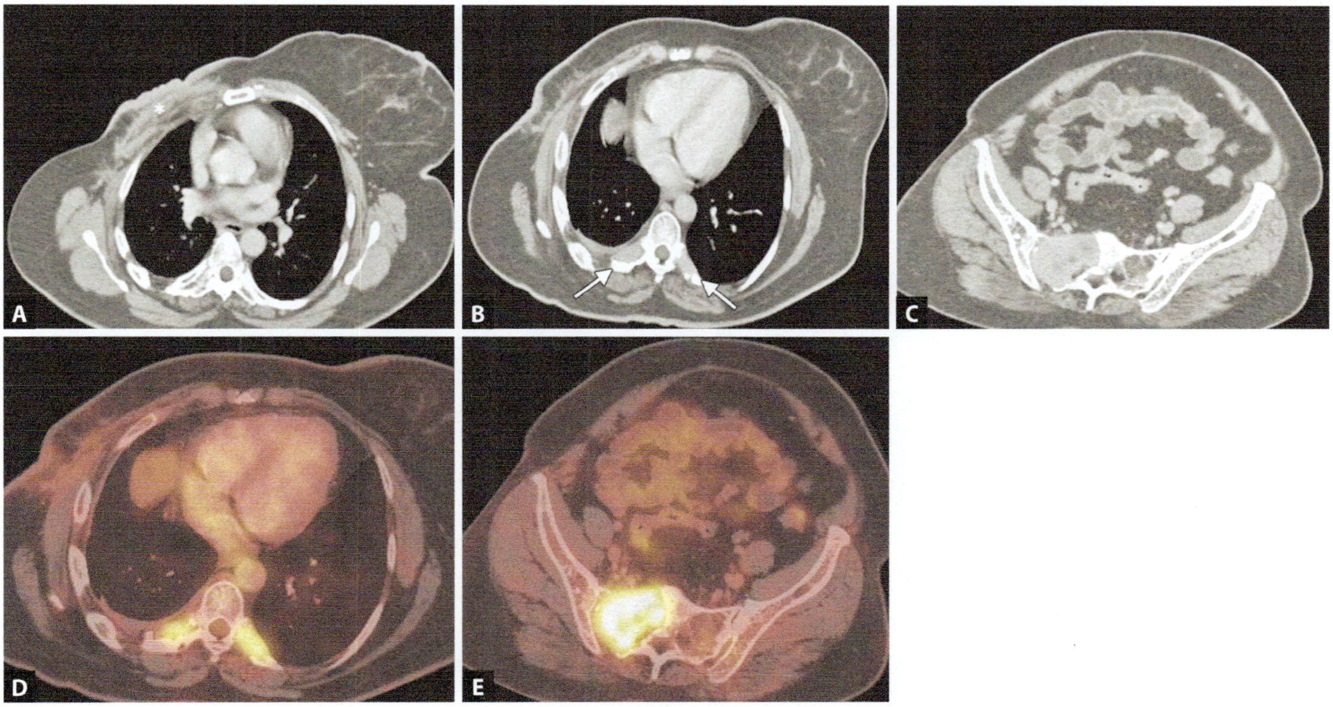

Figs. 34A to E: Bone metastases in a postoperative postradiotherapy case of invasive ductal carcinoma right breast with neuroendocrine differentiation. Axial contrast-enhanced computed tomography (CECT) images of the chest (A and B) show right mastectomy with postradiotherapy changes involving chest wall on the right side, lytic lesions with associated soft tissue noted at the vertebral ends of bilateral ribs (arrows). Axial CECT image at the level of sacrum (C) shows an expansile soft tissue density lesion in the right sacral ala. Axial positron emission tomography computed tomography (PET-CT) images (D and E) show avid fluorodeoxyglucose (FDG) uptake in the lesions involving the ribs and sacrum.

a lesion is a highly specific feature of metastasis on T2W sequences.[51] In vertebrae, additional criteria for malignancy include bulging of the posterior margin of the vertebral body, signal intensity changes that extend into the pedicle, and paraosseous tumor spread **(Figs. 35A to D)**.

Diffusion-weighted MRI is highly sensitive to cellularity and the mobility of free water molecules, which are responsible for the differences between benign and malignant fractures. Using a single-shot echo-planar DWI pulse sequence with a high B factor, Chan et al. showed that ADC values are useful in differentiating benign osteoporotic fractures from malignant vertebral body compression fractures.[52]

Whole-body MRI, using fast pulse sequences over multiple anatomic stations to acquire a survey of the entire body, has resulted in the ability to use unenhanced T1W spin echo and STIR sequences to screen the whole body for marrow abnormalities with a sensitivity and specificity superior to skeletal scintigraphy.[53] One limitation of MRI is that cortical bone, due to its very short T2 relaxation time, is not well seen, and therefore, bones with a low marrow volume such as the ribs are better evaluated with CT. Whole body MRI with diffusion weighting allows qualitative and quantitative evaluation of the focal lesions through signal intensity evaluation on DWI images and the reconstruction of the ADC map.

Differential Diagnosis

A solitary metastasis may resemble a primary malignant bone tumor, a primary benign tumor of aggressive nature, e.g., a GCT, infection, and miscellaneous disorders such

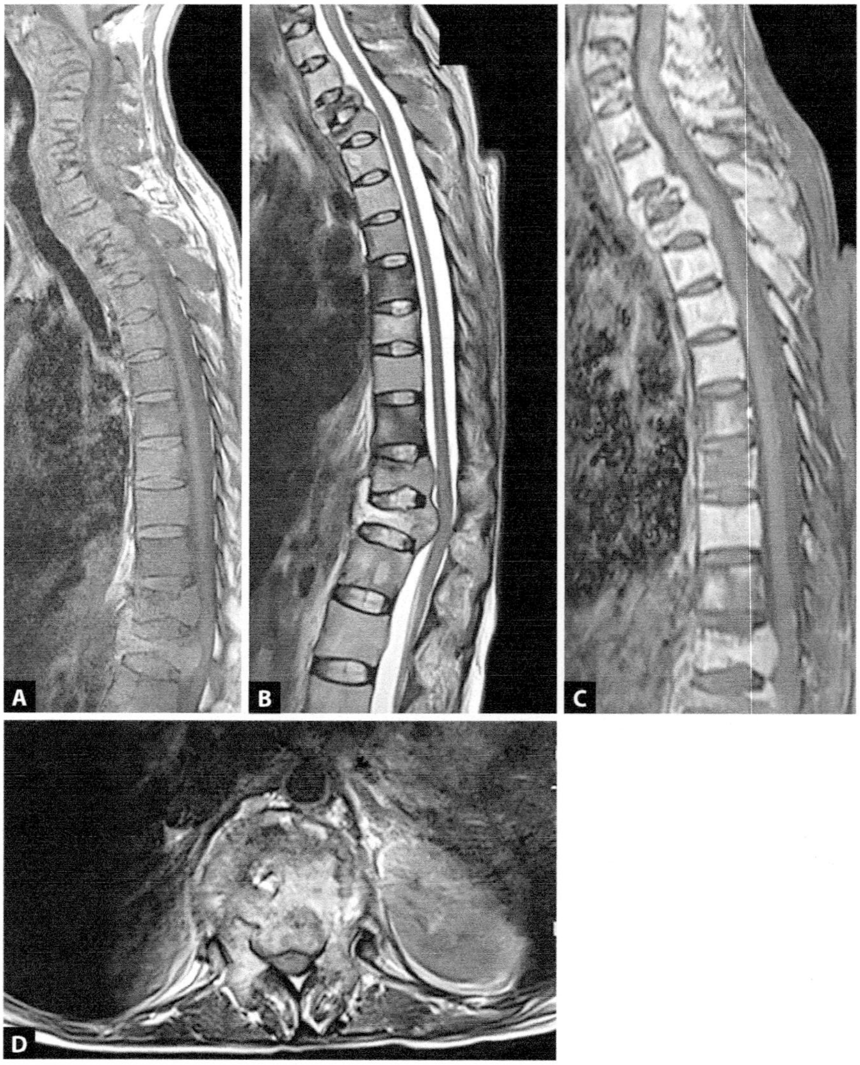

Figs. 35A to D: Skeletal metastases from carcinoma breast. T1-weighted (T1W) sagittal (A), T2-weighted (T2W) sagittal (B), and postcontrast sagittal (C) magnetic resonance (MR) images of the dorsolumbar spine show multiple lesions with collapse of the vertebrae appearing hypointense on T1W and hyperintense on T2W sequences with heterogeneous postcontrast enhancement. The disc spaces are spared and the collapsed vertebral bodies show posterior convexity. Axial T2W MR image (D) shows the presence of paraspinal soft tissue.

as Paget's disease. The most important factor in the differential diagnosis is the patient's age. The second important factor is the presence of multiple bone deposits. Other features are the diaphyseal location, involvement of vertebral bodies and then pedicles, the lack of bone expansion, absence of florid periosteal reaction, and tumor bone or soft-tissue mass. No one investigation, apart from biopsy, can provide a specific diagnosis of a metastasis or its site of origin.

CONCLUSION

Conventional radiographic techniques remain of fundamental importance in the diagnosis and analysis of bone tumors and tumor-like lesions. Radiographic information combined with data concerning the clinical presentation, the site of the lesion, and the age of the patient allows the formulation of a reasonable diagnosis in most cases. CT and MRI are useful in determining the intraosseous and extraosseous spread of the lesions. MRI has virtually replaced CT in its ability to detect the presence of a lesion and demonstrate its extent with respect to compartmental anatomy, i.e., in the staging of the tumor. MRI also plays an important role in prognosticating and follow-up after therapy to look for recurrence or residual disease.

REFERENCES

1. Dorfman HD, Czerniak B. Bone cancers. Cancer. 1995;75(Suppl 1):203-10.
2. Unni KK, Inwards CY, Bridge JA, Kindblom LG, Wold LE. Tumors of the bones and joints. In: AFIP Atlas of Tumor Pathology, Series 4. Washington, DC: American Registry of Pathology; 2005.
3. Kindblom LG. Bone tumors: epidemiology, classification, pathology. In: Davies AM, Sundaram M, James SJ (Eds). Imaging of Bone Tumors and Tumor-like Lesions. Berlin: Springer; 2009. pp. 1-15.
4. Fletcher C DM, Bridge JA, Hogendoorn P, Mertens F. WHO Classification of Tumours of Soft Tissue and Bone, Fourth edition. WHO 2013; IARC WHO Classification of Tumours, No. 5.
5. Doyle LA. Sarcoma classification: An update based on the 2013 World Health Organization Classification of Tumors of Soft Tissue and Bone. Cancer. 2014;120(12):1763-74.
6. Johnson LC. A general theory of bone tumors. Bull N Y Acad Med. 1953;29(2):164-71.
7. Kundu ZS. Classification, imaging, biopsy and staging of osteosarcoma. Indian J Orthop. 2014;48(3):238-46.
8. Nomikos GC, Murphey MD, Kransdorf MD, Bancroft LW, Peterson JJ. Primary bone tumors of lower extremities. Radiol Clin North Am. 2002;40(5):971-90.
9. Stoller DW. Bone and Soft Tissue Tumors in Magnetic Resonance Imaging in Orthopaedics and Sports Medicine, 3rd edition. Philadelphia: Lippincott Williams and Wilkins; 2007.
10. Costa FM, Canella C, Gasparetto E. Advanced Magnetic Resonance Imaging Techniques in the Evaluation of Musculoskeletal Tumors. Radiol Clin N Am. 2011;49(6):1325-58.
11. Oh E, Yoon YC, Kim JH, Kim K. Multiparametric approach with diffusion-weighted imaging and dynamic contrast-enhanced MRI: a comparison study for differentiating between benign and malignant bone lesions in adults. Clinical Radiology. 2017;72(7):552-9.
12. Hayashida Y, Yakushiji T, Awai K, Katahira K, Nakayama Y, Shimomura O, et al. Monitoring therapeutic response of primary bone tumors by diffusion-weighted image: initial results. Eur Radiol. 2006;16(12):2637-43.
13. Mintz DN, Hwang S. Bone tumor imaging, then and now: review article. HSS J. 2014;10(3):230-9.
14. Hwang S, Panicek DN. The evolution of musculoskeletal tumor imaging. Radiol Clin North Am. 2009;47(3):435-53.
15. Evan-Sapir E. PET/CT in malignant bone disease. Sem Musculoskeletal Radiol. 2007;11(4):312-21.
16. Van der Woude HJ, Vandershueren G. Ultrasound in musculoskeletal tumours with emphasis on its role in tumour follow up. Radiol Clin North Am. 1999;37(4):753-66.
17. Wong KC, Kumta SM, Antonio GE, Tse LF. Image fusion for computer-assisted bone tumor surgery. Clin Orthop Relat Res. 2008;466(10):2533-41.
18. Wong KC, Kumta SM. Use of computer navigation in orthopedic oncology. Curr Surg Rep. 2014;2(4):47.
19. Rajiah P, Ilaslan H, Sundaram M. Imaging of primary malignant bone tumors (Nonhematological). Radiol Clin North Am. 2011;49(6):1135-61.
20. Ellis JH, Siegel CL, Martel W, Weatherbee L, Dorfman H . Radiologic features of well-differentiated osteosarcoma. AJR Am J Roentgenol. 1988;151(4):739-42.
21. Kumar R, David R, Madewell JE, Lindell MM Jr. Radiographic spectrum of osteogenic sarcoma. Am J Roentgenol. 1987;148:767-72.
22. Miller SL, Hoffer FA. Malignant and Benign bone tumours. Radiol Clin North Am. 2001;39(4):673-99.
23. Murphey MD, wan Jaovisidha S, Temple HT, Gannon FH, Jelinek JS, Malawer MM. Telangiectatic osteosarcoma: radiologic-pathologic comparison. Radiology. 2003;229(2):545-53.
24. Edeiken J, Raymond AK, Ayala AG, Benjamin RS, Murray JA, Carrasco HC. Small-cell osteosarcoma. Skeletal Radiol. 1987;16(8):621-8.
25. Choong PF, Pritchard DJ, Rock MG, Sim FH, McLeod RA, Unni KK. Low grade central osteogenic sarcoma. A long-term follow-up of 20 patients. Clin Orthop Relat Res. 1996;322:198-206.
26. Van der Woude HJ, Bloom JL, Hogendoorn PC. Preoperative evaluation and monitoring chemotherapy in patients with high grade osteogenic and Ewing sarcomas: A review of current imaging modalities. Skeletal Radiol. 1998;27(2):57-71.
27. Jelinek JS, Murphey MD, Kransdorf MJ, Shmookler BM, Malawer MM, Hur RC. Parosteal sarcoma: Value of MR imaging and CT in the prediction of histologic grade. Radiology. 1996;201(3):837-42.

28. Okada K, Kubota H, Ebina T, Kobayashi T, Abe E, Sato K. High grade surface osteosarcoma of the humerus. Skeletal Radiol. 1995;24(7):531-4.
29. Stoker DJ, Saifuddin A. Bone tumours (2): Malignant lesions. Grainger and Allison's Diagnostic Radiology. London: Churchill Livingstone; 2007. pp. 1059-81.
30. Sheppard DG, Libshitz H. Post-radiation sarcomas: a review of the clinical and imaging features in 63 cases. Clin Radiol. 2001;56(1):22-9.
31. Murphey MD, Walker EA, Wilson AJ, Kransdorf MJ, Temple HT, Gannon FH. From the Archives of the AFIP: Imaging of primary chondrosarcoma: radiologic-pathologic correlation. Radiographics. 2003;23(5):1245-78.
32. Brien EW, Mirra JM, Luck JV Jr. Benign and malignant cartilage tumors of bone and joint: Their anatomic and theoretical basis with an emphasis on radiology, pathology and clinical biology. II. Juxta cortical cartilage tumors. Skeletal Radiol. 1999;28(1):1-20.
33. Lee YK, Yao L Wirth CR. MR imaging of solitary osteochondromas: Report of eight cases. AJR Am J Roentgenol. 1987;149(3):557-60.
34. Nakashuma Y, Unni KK, Shives TC, Swee RG, Dahlin DC. Mesenchymal chondrosarcoma of bone and soft tissue. A review of 111 cases. Cancer. 1986;57(12):2444-53.
35. Collins NS, Koyama T, Swee RG, Inwards CY. Clear cell chondrosarcoma: radiographic, computed tomographic and magnetic resonance findings in 34 patients with pathologic correlation. Skeletal Radiol. 2003;32(12):687-94.
36. Taconis WK, Mulder JD. Fibrosarcoma and malignant fibrous histiocytoma of long bone: Radiographic features and grading. Skeletal Radiol. 1984;11(4):237-45.
37. Murphey MD, Senchak LT, Mambalam PK, Logie CI, Klassen-Fischer MK, Kransdorf MJ. From the radiologic pathology archives: Ewing sarcoma family of tumors: radiologic-pathologic correlation. Radiographics. 2013;33(3):803-31.
38. Eggli KD, Quiogue T, Moser RP Jr. Ewing's sarcoma. Radiol Clin North Am. 1993;31(2):325-37.
39. Sailer SL, Harmon DC, Nakin HJ, et al. Ewing sarcoma: Surgical resection as a prognostic factor. Int J Radiat Oncol Biol Phys. 1988;15(1):43-52.
40. Miller SL, Hoffer FA, Reddick WE, Wu S, Glass JO, Gronemeyer SA, et al. Tumor volume or dynamic contrast enhanced MRI for prediction of clinical outcome of Ewing sarcoma family of tumors. Pediatric Radiol. 2001;31(7): 518-23.
41. Weshi AS, Allam A, Ajarim D, Al Dayel F, Pant R, Bazarbashi S, et al. Extraskeletal Ewing sarcoma family of tumors in adults: Analysis of 57 patients from a single institution. Clin Oncol. 2010;22(5):374-81.
42. Papagelopoulos PJ, Mavrogenis AF, Galanis EC, Savvidou OD, Boscainos PJ, Katonis PG, et al. Chordoma of the spine: clinicopathological features, diagnosis and treatment. Orthopaedics. 2004;27(12):1256-63.
43. Lomasney LM, Martinez S, Demos TC, Harrelson JM. Multifocal vascular lesions of bone: Imaging characteristics. Skeletal Radiol. 1996;25(3):255-61.
44. Van der Woude HJ, Hazelbag HM, Bloem JL, Taminiau AH, Hogendoorn PC. MRI of adamantinoma of long bones in correlation with histopathology. AJR. 2004;183(6):1737-44.
45. Sarode SC, Sarode GS, Ingale Y, Ingale M, Raj AT, Patil S. Malignant fibrous histiocytoma of the mandible—A case report and review of published case reports. J Oral Biol Craniofac Res. 2019;9(2):221-5.
46. Yochum TR, Rowe LJ. Tumors and tumor-like processes. In: Yochum TR, Rowe LJ (Eds). Essentials of Skeletal Radiology, 3rd edition. Philadelphia: Lippincott Williams and Wilkins; 2005. pp. 1137-372.
47. Abrams HL, Sprio R, Goldstein N. Metastasis in carcinoma; analysis of 1000 autopsied cases. Cancer. 1950;3(1):74-85.
48. Galasko CSB. The anatomy and pathways of skeletal metastases. In: Weiss L, Gilbert HA (Eds). Bone Metastasis. Boston: GK Hall Publishers; 1981. pp. 49-63.
49. Rosenthal DI. Radiological diagnosis of bone metastases. Cancer. 1997;80(S8):1595-607.
50. Evan-Sapir E, Mester U, Mishani G, Lievshitz G, Lerman H, Leibovitch I. The detection of bone metastases inpatients with high risk prostate cancer: ^{99m}Tc-MDP planar bone scintigraphy, single and multi-field-of-view SPECT, ^{18}Fluoride PET, and ^{18}Fluoride PET/CT. J Nucl Med. 2006;47(2):287-97.
51. Schweitzer ME, Levine C, Mitchell DG, Gannon FH, Gomella LG. Bull's eyes and halos: Useful MR discriminators of osseous metastases. Radiology. 1993;188(1):249-52.
52. Chan JH, Peh WC, Tsui EY, Chau LF, Cheung KK, Chan KB, et al. Acute vertebral body compression fractures: discrimination between benign and malignant causes using apparent diffusion coefficients. Br J Radiol. 2002;75(891):207-14.
53. Choi J, Raghavan M. Diagnostic imaging and image-guided therapy of skeletal metastases. Cancer Control. 2012;19(2):102-12.

CHAPTER

15

Imaging in Marrow Disorders: Benign and Malignant

Swati Gupta, Sapna Singh, Alpana Manchanda

INTRODUCTION

The bone marrow lies within the skeleton and it provides red blood cells, platelets and white blood cells to meet the requirements for oxygenation, coagulation and immunity. It is composed of a combination of red marrow and yellow marrow, and its composition changes throughout life in response to normal maturation (red marrow to yellow marrow conversion) and stress (yellow marrow to red marrow reconversion).

Normal bone marrow has following three primary components:

1. The osseous component consisting of primary and secondary trabeculae of cancellous bone, which provide the structural framework for myeloid and fat cells.
2. The red marrow is hematopoietically active and supplies red blood cells, white blood cells, and platelets.
3. The yellow marrow contains fat, which is hematopoietically inactive.

The chemical composition and vascular supply of these various components of bone marrow are different from each other.[1-4] Although red marrow and yellow marrow are described as discrete elements for convenience, they are actually intermixed within the medullary space. Their proportions determine the overall distribution of fat and water.[5] **Table 1** describes the composition of marrow.

A variety of imaging techniques can be used in bone marrow assessment which is mentioned here.

Conventional radiographic techniques are insensitive to marrow infiltration and are not helpful in accurate bone marrow characterization. Indirect evidence of pathology may be seen in the form of trabecular destruction or sclerosis.

Radionuclide imaging uses various different tracers to evaluate specific components of bone such as reticuloendothelial system, erythroid precursors, myeloid components or active bone production. This may allow different bone marrow disorders to be distinguished. In addition, positron emission tomography (PET) tracers are useful to assess the metabolic and proliferative activity in the bone marrow.

Hybrid techniques such as PET-CT (positron emission tomography-computed tomography) and PET-MR (positron emission tomography-magnetic resonance), which fuse the functional and morphological data, are playing an increasing role in the evaluation of marrow disorders. PET and magnetic resonance imaging (MRI) are combined either by retrospective spatial registration of data from PET and MRI obtained on separate PET and MR machines or sequential data acquisition on combined PET-MR scanners. PET-MRI is superior to PET-CT because of the improved intrinsic soft-tissue contrast and direct bone marrow depiction using MRI. The SUV_{max} of normal bone marrow is approximately 1.[7] An SUV_{max} ≥4 has been shown to allow distinction between benign and malignant bone marrow lesions.[8]

Computed tomography has a low sensitivity and specificity for detection of marrow disorders. Trabecular destruction can be visualized on CT, and obvious asymmetry in marrow attenuation on visual or quantitative inspection may warrant further evaluation.

Table 1: Cellular and chemical components of bone marrow in adults.[6]

Component of bone marrow	*Cellular composition*	*Chemical composition*
Yellow marrow	95% fat cells 5% nonfat cells	80% fat 15% water 5% protein
Red marrow	40% fat cells 60% hematopoietic cells	40% fat 40% water 20% protein

Characterization of marrow changes is however not feasible on CT.

Magnetic resonance imaging is a useful technique for noninvasive evaluation of pathologic bone marrow conditions.[1,2] MRI with its excellent spatial and contrast resolution, allows direct visualization of the bone marrow. The signal intensity, morphology, and location of pathological findings on MRI can be used to provide more accurate diagnosis, to guide treatment and to follow therapy-related changes. Various MRI techniques are utilized to accentuate chemical and cellular composition of normal marrow and marrow diseases. MRI is more sensitive than specific in marrow disorders but an integration of clinical and radiologic data helps in suggesting an accurate diagnosis.

MAGNETIC RESONANCE APPEARANCE OF NORMAL MARROW

The differences in signal intensities of yellow and red marrow result primarily from differences in their proportional amounts of water and fat. The normal MR appearance of red and yellow marrow includes the following features **(Figs. 1 and 2)**:

- Red marrow demonstrates low-signal intensity on T1-weighted (T1W) images, reflecting its increased water content, and intermediate-signal intensity with progressive T2 weighting. Normal red marrow demonstrates T1 signal that is equal to or higher than adjacent muscle or intervertebral discs.
- With suppression of the signal from fat on short tau inversion recovery (STIR) images, areas of red marrow demonstrate higher signal intensity than areas of yellow marrow.
- On T1W and conventional T2-weighted (T2W) images, yellow marrow demonstrates the bright signal intensity of fat.
- Yellow marrow demonstrates low signal intensity on STIR images, in which signal from fat is nulled. The signal intensity is also reduced on fat-suppressed

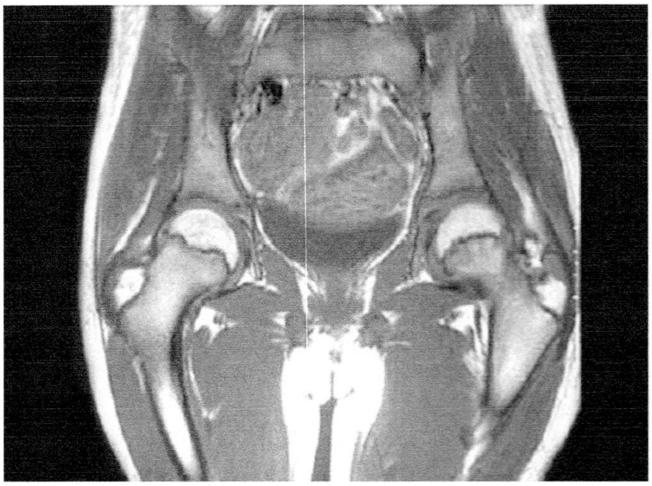

Fig. 1: Normal marrow pattern in childhood (1–10 years). T1-weighted (T1W) coronal magnetic resonance (MR) image of the pelvis showing high-signal yellow marrow (signal identical to subcutaneous fat) in the femoral epiphysis, apophysis, and the femoral diaphysis. Red marrow has intermediate signal intensity (higher than adjacent muscle), is seen present in the proximal femoral metaphysis and in the pelvic bones. Marked symmetry of distribution seen bilaterally.

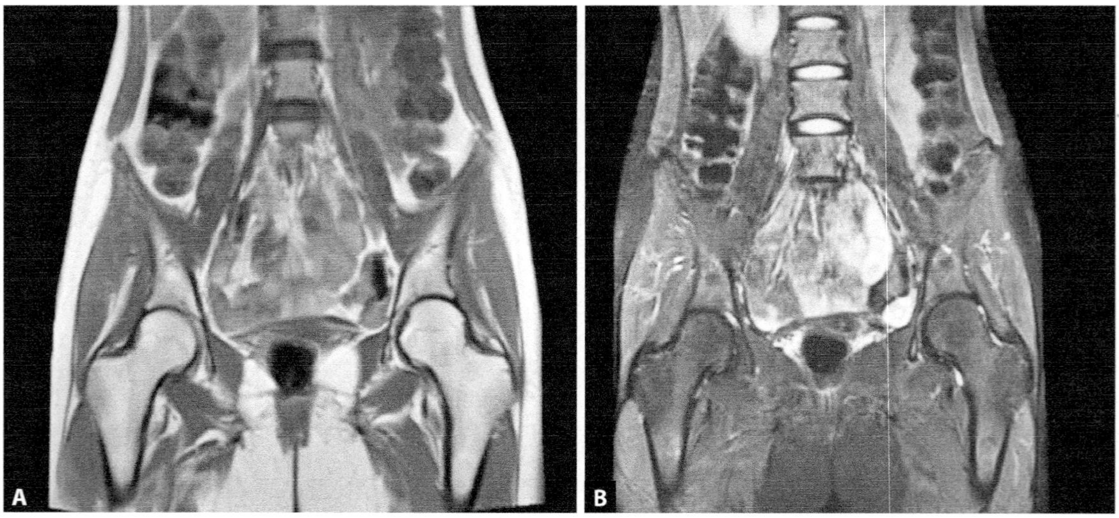

Figs. 2A and B: Normal red and yellow marrow. T1-weighted (T1W) coronal image (A) of the pelvis and the femora. Yellow marrow has signal identical to that of the high signal subcutaneous fat. It is present in the apophyses, the epiphyses, the femoral diaphyses, and the focal regions in the pelvis. Red marrow is intermediate signal and located in the pelvis and the proximal femoral metaphyses. Note the striking symmetry of the distribution of red and yellow marrow bilaterally. Short tau inversion recovery (STIR) coronal image (B) of the pelvis and the femora. Fatty marrow becomes black from fat suppression in this sequence. Red marrow is intermediate signal, similar in appearance to the muscle; this is best seen in the pelvis.

T2W spin-echo (SE) and fat-suppressed T2W fast SE sequences, and it appears darker when using fat-suppression techniques with sequences having longer repetition times (TR) and echo times (TE).[9]
- Red and yellow marrow contrast differences become less distinct on heavily T2W protocols with TR >2,500 ms.

NORMAL DISTRIBUTION OF MARROW

Hematopoiesis begins in utero, at approximately 19 gestational days, within the yolk sac. By week 16 of gestation, the main sites of fetal hematopoiesis are the liver and the spleen. After week 24 of gestation, marrow becomes the main organ of hematopoiesis. At birth, active hematopoiesis (i.e. red marrow) is present throughout the entire skeleton, including the epiphyses. Early in the normal ossification process, yellow marrow replaces the hyaline cartilage template in the epiphysis and the apophysis. Conversion of red to yellow marrow commences in the terminal phalanges of hand and feet. Bone marrow conversion occurs from appendicular to axial skeleton.

Within the long bone, marrow conversion first starts in the diaphysis and progresses bidirectionally toward the metaphyses, faster distally than proximally as described in **Table 2**.

In the femoral diaphysis, on T1W images, high-signal intensity yellow marrow is observed as early as when the subject is 3 months old, with marrow heterogeneity at 12 months, and homogeneous high-signal intensity after the age of 5 years.

In <10 years of age, yellow marrow is seen in most of the diaphysis of long bones of arms and legs.

From the age of 10–20 years, yellow marrow is seen predominantly in the limbs with residual red marrow in the femoral and humeral metaphysis.

Conversion happens continuously from peripheral to central with respect to the skeleton and is complete by the age of 25 years, when the adult pattern is established, characterized by the distribution of red marrow limited to the axial skeleton (skull, vertebrae, ribs, sternum, and pelvis) and proximal aspects of the appendicular skeleton (femora and humeri) **(Figs. 3A to C)**.

At 60 years of age, the percentage of fat in red marrow can be as high as 70% **(Figs. 4A and B)**. These changes are also described in **Table 3 (Fig. 5)**.

This conversion is not entirely symmetric. These changes vary and are dependent on factors such as diseases, athletic activities, and therapies.[11-13] Regional differences between the two sexes have been demonstrated. Small differences in the amount and distribution of red marrow from side to side are normal, but marked asymmetry is indicative of a marrow-infiltrating disease process.

The appearance of vertebral marrow has been explained by Sebag et al.[14] He explains that vertebral marrow remains hypointense before the age of 1 year and hyperintense after the age of 5 years due to progressive red to yellow marrow conversion on T1W images **(Figs. 6A and B)**. Marrow around the basivertebral venous plexus

Table 2: Progression of conversion from red to yellow marrow.[10]

Skeletal segment (extremities to axial skeleton)	*Individual long bones (peripheral to central)*
Hands/feet	Epiphyses/apophyses
↓	↓
Forearms/lower legs	Diaphysis
↓	↓
Humeri/femora	Distal metaphysis
↓	↓
Pelvis/spine	Proximal metaphysis

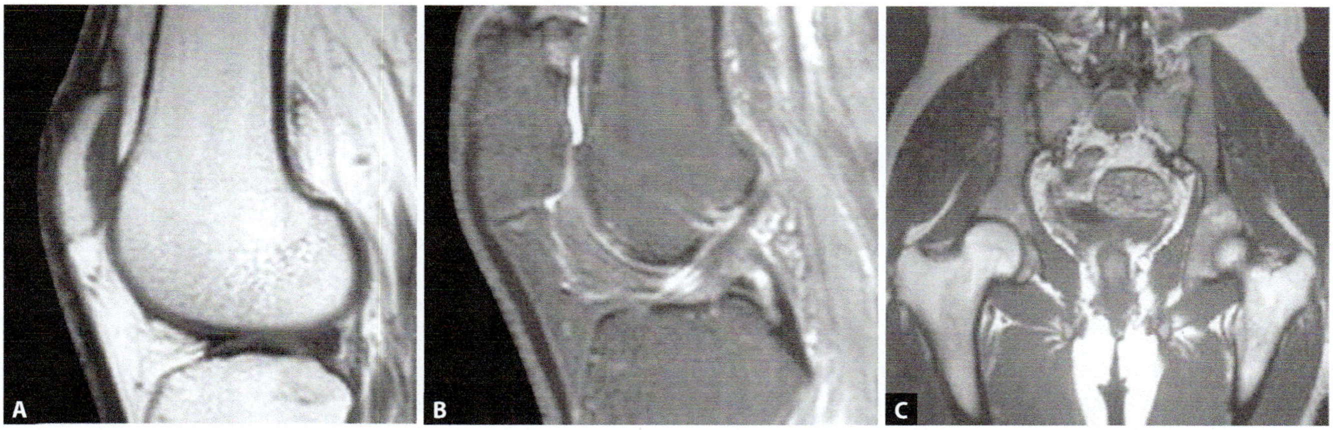

Figs. 3A to C: Normal marrow pattern in an adult >25 years of age. T1-weighted (T1W) sagittal (A), short tau inversion recovery (STIR) sagittal (B) magnetic resonance (MR) images of the knee showing normal yellow marrow in the diaphysis and the distal metaphysis of the femur. T1W coronal image of the pelvis (C) showing intermediate signal intensity red marrow in the proximal femoral metaphysis and the pelvic bones.

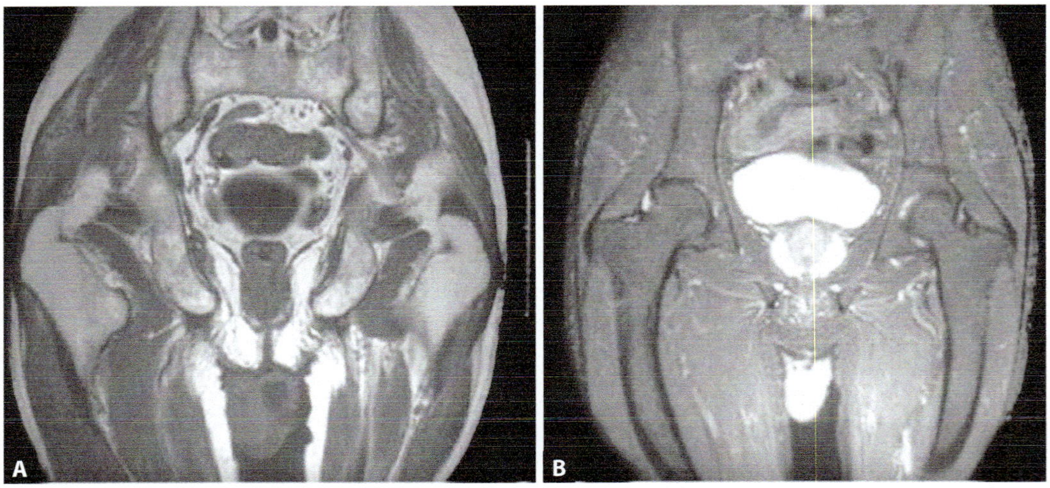

Figs. 4A and B: T1-weighted (T1W) coronal image of the pelvis (A) in a 70-year-old showing high-signal yellow marrow in the proximal femoral metaphyses and foci of yellow marrow in the pelvic bones. Short tau inversion recovery (STIR) coronal image of the pelvis (B) shows complete suppression of the signal indicating fatty marrow. Normal marrow pattern for >60 years of age.

Table 3: Age-related conversion from red to yellow marrow.[10]

Age group	*Marrow findings*
Infants (<1 year)	Diffuse red marrow except for ossified epiphyses and apophysis
Children (1–10 years)	Yellow marrow below knees and elbows, and in diaphysis of femora and humeri
Adolescents (10–20 years)	Progressive yellow marrow in distal and proximal metaphyses of proximal long bones
Adults (>25 years)	Yellow marrow except in axial skeleton and proximal metaphyses of proximal long bones

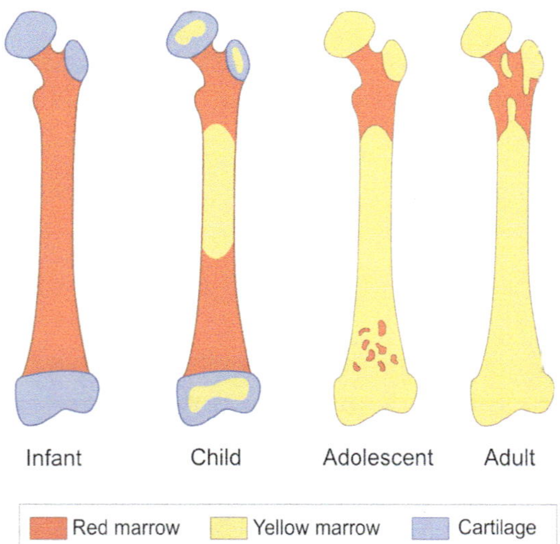

Fig. 5: Diagram of marrow maturation in the long bones from left to right and pattern of reconversion from right to left.

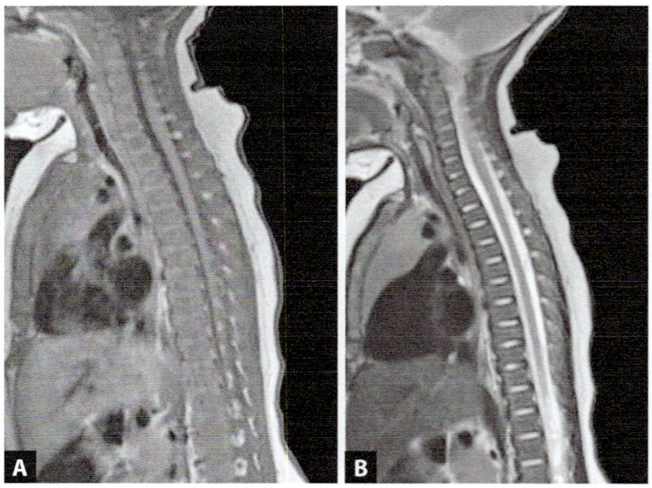

Figs. 6A and B: Marrow signal in a 1-month-old child. T1-weighted (T1W) sagittal (A) and T2-weighted (T2W) sagittal magnetic resonance (MR) images (B) of cervical and dorsal spine showing vertebral marrow that is hypointense to intervertebral disc on both T1- and T2-weighted images.

is first to get converted, followed by subchondral marrow adjacent to end plates **(Figs. 7A and B)**. Focal islands of yellow marrow are common in the spine around the central venous channels in the vertebral bodies.

Heterogeneous pattern of marrow distribution is a normal variant. Chronic stresses and biomechanical stimuli cause a decrease in the vascularity to specific sites in marrow and stimulate conversion of red to yellow marrow, which probably accounts for many focal areas of conversion to fat. A classic example of this phenomenon occurs in the marrow adjacent to vertebral end plates that border on a degenerated disc. A band-like focal alteration

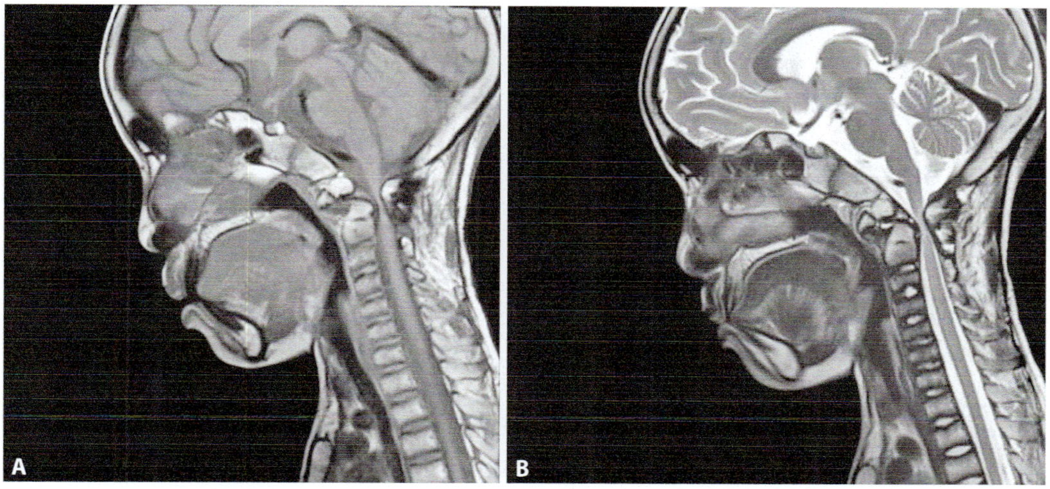

Figs. 7A and B: Marrow signal in a 10-year-old child. T1-weighted (T1W) sagittal (A) and T2-weighted (T2W) sagittal magnetic resonance (MR) images (B) of cervical spine in a patient with craniovertebral junction anomaly showing vertebral marrow that is hyperintense to intervertebral disc on T1W image. The conversion begins around basivertebral venous plexus.

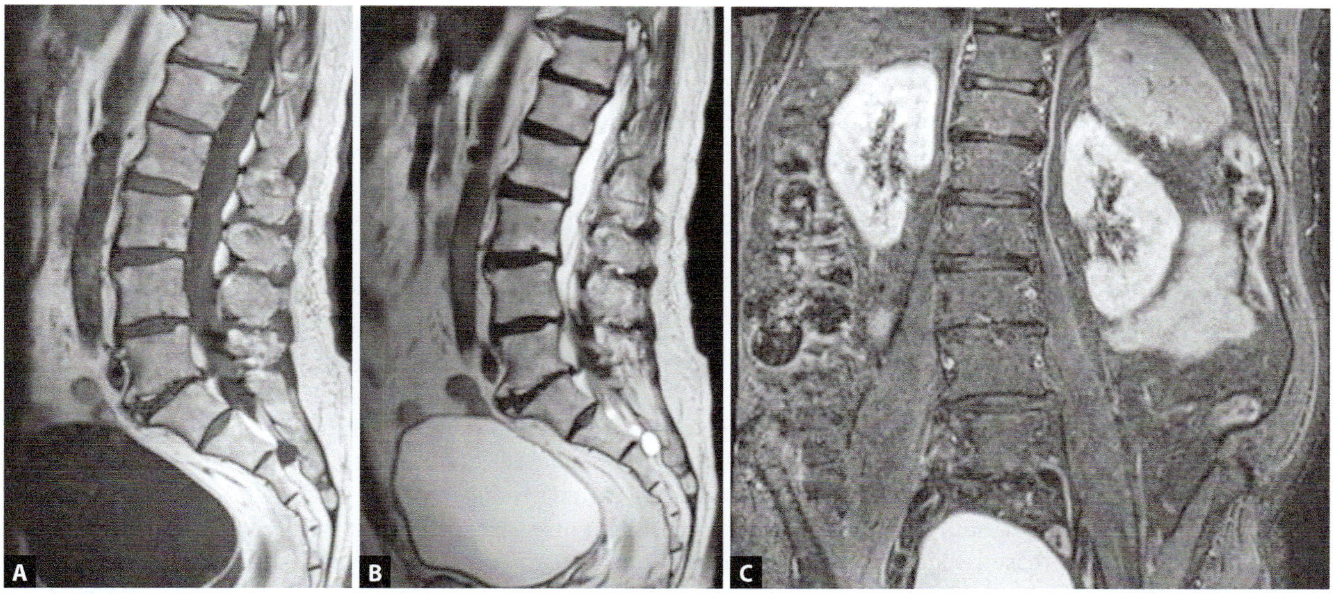

Figs. 8A to C: Degenerative disc disease. T1-weighted (T1W) sagittal (A), T2-weighted (T2W) sagittal (B) and short tau inversion recovery (STIR) coronal (C) magnetic resonance (MR) images showing a band-like focal alteration in marrow signal adjacent to end plates, more prominent at L3 and L4 level which shows suppression on STIR image suggestive of fatty replacement, associated with the disc disease.

in marrow signal occurs as a result of the ischemia associated with the disc disease **(Figs. 8A to C)**. Islands of red marrow may also occur in predominantly yellow marrow **(Figs. 9A and B)**. Presence of yellow marrow within the islands of red marrow, known as the "Bull's eye appearance," indicates benign appearance. Other helpful features in distinguishing heterogeneous red marrow from a pathologic process include higher signal intensity relative to skeletal muscle on T1W images, feathery margins representing red marrow elements interdigitating with the adjacent yellow marrow, relative bilaterality, and the absence of mass effect in red marrow.

Red marrow may extend in the epiphyses and is considered a normal variant as described by Mirowitz.[15]

MAGNETIC RESONANCE IMAGING TECHNIQUES

The MRI protocol includes T1W SE sequences, fat-suppression sequence (STIR-sequences), chemical shift imaging (in-phase image/opposed-phase image), diffusion-weighted imaging (DWI), and T1 SE with fat presaturation (FS) before and after contrast (Gadolinium-Gd) injection with subtraction manipulation, if possible.

T1-weighted Sequence

T1-weighted sequence is the most fundamental sequence in marrow imaging. There is high tissue contrast between

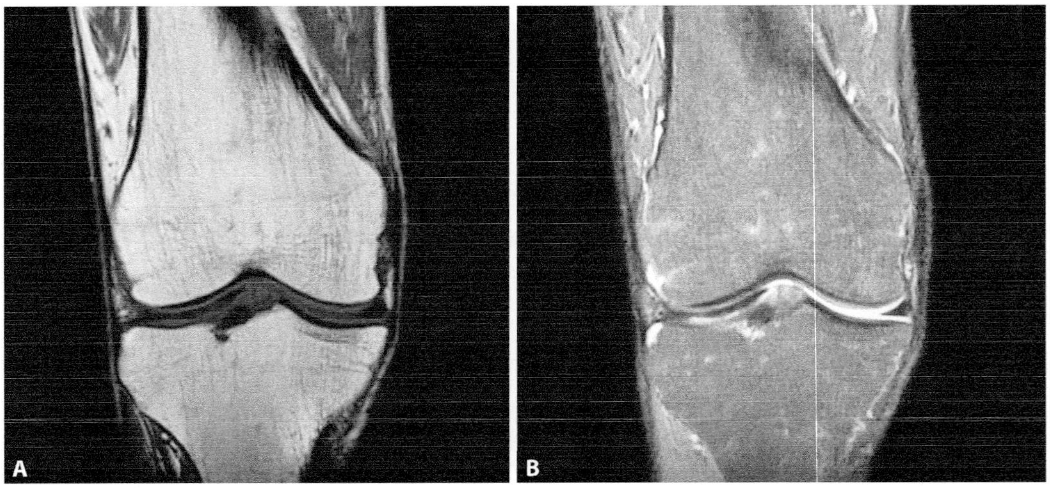

Figs. 9A and B: Heterogeneous marrow in an adult (normal variant). T1-weighted (T1W) coronal (A) and short tau inversion recovery (STIR) coronal (B) magnetic resonance (MR) images of knee show foci of red marrow that are hypointense on T1 and of intermediate intensity on STIR image in distal femur metaphysis on a background of yellow marrow.

yellow and red marrow as well as between yellow marrow and disease on this sequence. Fat has a bright signal on T1W images and pathologic lesions have a low signal; hence, the lesions are easily detected on T1W images as the contrast is maximized on T1W images. There is little contrast between red marrow and pathologic lesions as both have a low-signal intensity. The differentiating feature is that the signal intensity of pathological lesions is usually less than that of the intervertebral discs in the spine and less than that of the muscle in the extremities.

T2-weighted Sequence

On fluid-sensitive images, the signal intensity difference between red and yellow marrow is less apparent. Also, the difference between the pathologic marrow and yellow marrow is minimal as both show a high signal on the sequence. Fat-suppressed sequences are useful to increase the contrast. The two widely used fat suppression techniques are the STIR sequence and the fat-saturated SE sequence.[3,16]

STIR Sequence

The STIR sequence is of great value for pathological lesions associated with prolonged T1 and T2 values. The STIR sequence has a high sensitivity but a low specificity. Pathological lesions have a high-signal intensity due to increased cells, fluid, and edema. Normal yellow marrow is seen as signal void, red marrow as low-signal intensity, and pathological lesions are seen as high-signal intensity. Fibrous tissue, calcification, and hemosiderin deposits are low in signal intensity, whereas fluid, edema, and recent hemorrhage are bright. Muscle remains intermediate in signal intensity.

The main drawback of the STIR sequence is that it cancels every signal identical to fat, e.g., blood in hematoma or contrast-enhanced tissue. Further, a very homogeneous magnetic field is required for this sequence; therefore, it is not efficient on every MR unit. The other disadvantages include a relatively long imaging time and a low signal-to-noise ratio. The combination of T1W SE sequence with an STIR or fat-suppressed fast SE T2W sequence forms the basis of most bone marrow imaging protocols.[16]

Chemical Shift Imaging

Chemical shift imaging uses the difference in resonance frequency between fat and water photons to cancel their signal on out-of-phase images. Since fat is present in both red and yellow marrow but not in neoplastic lesions, neoplastic lesions do not demonstrate the normal loss of signal on out-of-phase images. It has been suggested that a decrease in signal intensity >20% on out-of-phase images compared with in-phase images should be used as a cut-off threshold for normalcy **(Figs. 10A and B)**. Any lesion, which is not composed of fat on T1W images, and which decreases <20% of its signal intensity on out-of-phase images compared to in-phase images, should be considered suspicious for malignancy.[17] A further refinement of this technique is the development of quantitative chemical shift imaging where the quantitative assessment of fat fraction can be done.[3,18,19] Two main families of techniques have been emerging for proton-dependent fat fraction quantification: single-voxel proton magnetic resonance spectroscopy (MRS) and chemical shift encoding-based water–fat imaging.[20]

Diffusion-weighted Imaging

Red marrow has higher apparent diffusion coefficient (ADC) values and signal intensity on high-*b*-value images due to higher cellularity and water content; yellow marrow, on the other hand, has lower cellularity mainly

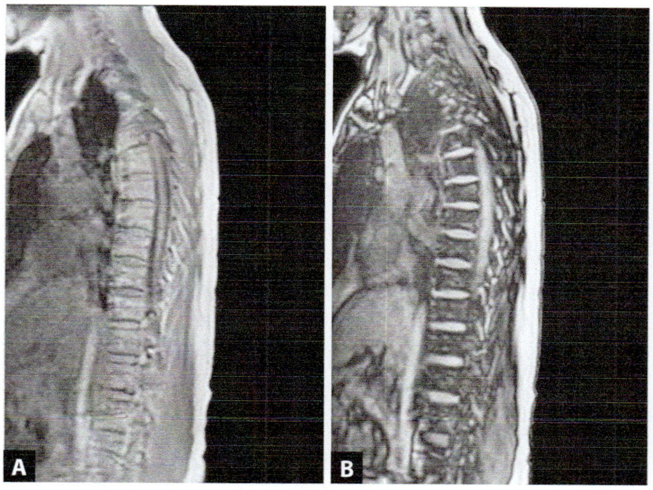

Figs. 10A and B: Normal appearance of marrow on chemical shift imaging. Magnetic resonance (MR) images of the dorsolumbar spine in-phase (A) and opposed phase (B) showing drop of signal on the opposed phase images as compared to the in-phase images due to the presence of fat.

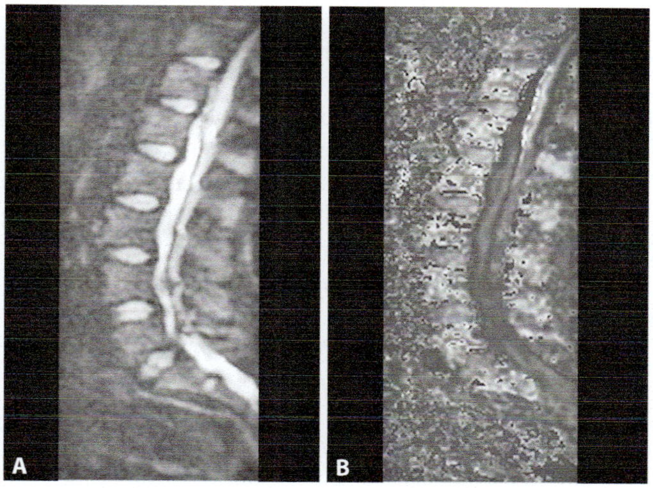

Figs. 11A and B: Normal appearance of marrow on diffusion-weighted imaging. Diffusion-weighted magnetic resonance (MR) images of the spine showing the normal vertebral bodies as hypointense with the normal apparent diffusion coefficient (ADC) map.

represented by large adipose cells, poorer water content, and lower perfusion.

Diffusion-weighted imaging (DWI) has proven to be a useful method in identification of marrow pathology. As red marrow restricts diffusion, DWI must be used with caution in infants and children.[21] ADC values lower than 1.1-1.2 × 10^{-3} mm^2/s are usually seen in cases of high cellularity or malignancy.

Diffusion-weighted MRI is useful in differentiating benign fracture edema and tumor infiltration of the vertebral body **(Figs. 11A and B)**.[3,18,19] DWI is also useful in distinguishing progressive changes in bone marrow among treatment sequelae, fracture, or tumor, which can be difficult on conventional MRI. In addition to the tumor evaluation, DWI may be useful in differentiation of degenerative and infectious endplate abnormalities. DWI showed hyperintensity in patients with infection, and no hyperintensity in degenerative end plates; ADC values of infectious end plates were significantly lower than normal and degenerative end plates. In a study on spine metastasis, decreased DWI signal of the spine was seen after 2 months of therapy in patients with clinical improvement, whereas persistent abnormal hyperintense signal was found when there was no clinical improvement.[22]

Proton Magnetic Resonance Spectroscopy

There is paucity of literature on the use of MRS in the evaluation of marrow due to signal dropout from cortical bone and spectral peak contamination from adipose tissue. In this technique, the global MR signal from bone is divided into the two major segments of water and lipid separated by 3.1 ppm. The spectra of proton MRS have a water peak, originating mostly from red marrow, and a lipid peak, arising from yellow marrow. Signal peaks can vary among subjects, and are influenced not only by the water-lipid proton quantity and the tissue environment but also by the surface coil and the distance between the voxel and surface coil. Because of these variables, instead of measuring the absolute signal peak for signal quantification, a lipid-water ratio is often measured. The fat fraction value determined from MRS has been adopted as a predictor of bone marrow fat content in most studies. It has been shown that a decrease in cancellous bone is accompanied by a corresponding increase in fat cells and decrease in arterial capillaries and sinuses in bone marrow. Data also suggests that an elevated choline signal may be used to discriminate malignant from benign lesions.[23,24]

Contrast Enhancement

The enhancement of the normal marrow in adults is usually <35% from baseline on intravenous gadolinium administration.[25] The uptake is best seen on T1W fat presaturated sequences.[3,4,26] Contrast enhancement is less useful as both normal red marrow and various diseases (infection, inflammation, and tumor) can enhance. It has been stated that in case of normal STIR images no relevant additional information is found with contrast-enhanced T1W images, while in the case of abnormal STIR images, additional information is obtained on administration of gadopentetate dimeglumine.[27]

Dynamic Contrast-enhanced Magnetic Resonance Studies

Dynamic gadolinium-enhanced MR scans show increased enhancement of the neoplastic infiltration compared to normal marrow. They can be used to generate estimates of the volume of normal or pathological marrow before and after treatment. The enhancement is significantly higher in marked marrow infiltration and in lesions with higher vessel density as compared to those with mild or no infiltration. Bone marrow perfusion assessed by dynamic contrast-enhanced MR has also been studied in patients with osteoporosis. Studies have shown that decreasing marrow perfusion and increasing marrow fat content accompany a reduction in bone density.[28]

MAGNETIC RESONANCE PROTOCOL FOR SURVEY OF MARROW

Magnetic resonance imaging of suspected bone marrow abnormalities should be directed to the site of clinical symptoms or where abnormalities or confusing findings are present on other imaging studies. When diffuse marrow disease is suspected, a marrow survey of the entire body or, more commonly, of the entire spine, pelvis, and proximal femora is performed. These areas are surveyed because the bulk of red marrow (and marrow pathology) exists there.

The protocol for an MR survey examination includes:

- T1W coronal images of the pelvis and proximal femori, which are adult sites of red marrow concentration. These images are acquired with large (40 cm) fields of view to include assessment of lumbosacral spine marrow.
- Coronal STIR images are obtained to null fat signal and identify abnormal T1 or T2 prolongation.
- Sagittal T1W and STIR images are routinely acquired to evaluate suspected spinal malignancies.

In addition, components of survey include:

- Axial T1W, STIR images may be obtained at specific sites of suspected pathologic processes and are important in determining cross-sectional marrow involvement. T1W images are particularly valuable in evaluating blastic processes, which are low in signal on STIR images.
- Gadolinium-enhanced axial images, especially in cases with soft-tissue or cord involvement.
- Additional techniques on case-to-case basis.

WHOLE BODY MAGNETIC RESONANCE IMAGING

Whole body magnetic resonance imaging (WBMRI) has demonstrated huge potential for evaluation of malignant marrow disorders because of advantages such as absence of ionizing radiation, superior diagnostic performance, one-step staging, and ability to assess therapeutic response.[29] WBMRI is also useful in targeting marrow biopsy due to the favorable contrast between tumors and normal tissue on the STIR sequences.

Magnetic resonance imaging pulse sequences can be divided into anatomic (or morphologic), i.e., the classic T1W, T2W, and STIR pulse sequences that provide tissue delineation and basic physicochemical information about tissue content; and functional (or metabolic), i.e., DWI and perfusion sequences that provide information on tissue cellularity and/or vascularity.

Whole body T1, STIR is performed in coronal or axial planes. The coronal plane is preferred because of increased coverage. DWI sequences using high-diffusion sensitizing gradients (*b* values) are usually performed in the axial plane at consecutive anatomic stations. Sagittal study of the spine is recommended for detecting small lesions, lesions at risk or responsible for neurologic complications, and vertebral compression fractures. Gadolinium-based contrast scan is performed if liver and brain scanning is planned.

For scanning, it is preferable to use multiple surface coils. Depending upon the indication, WBMR can be limited from "eyes to thighs" or can cover the entire body.

Whole-body magnetic resonance imaging has been shown to be comparable to PET/CT, and better than bone scintigraphy, in detection of neoplastic marrow with sensitivities of 98, 90, and 30%, respectively.[30] WBMRI is useful in lymphomas with poor fluorodeoxyglucose (FDG) avidity and it also detects extramedullary lesions such as lymph nodes in non-Hodgkin lymphoma (NHL).[31,32] In multiple myeloma, consensus statement by the International Myeloma Working Group presents WBMRI as the imaging reference standard for the detection of bone marrow involvement and recommends systematic WBMRI in patients with smoldering myeloma and asymptomatic patients. Interpretation of WBMR is however challenging because of huge amount of information. It is also associated with a high false-positive rate and low sensitivity in early stage of a disease.

BONE MARROW PATHOLOGY

Abnormalities of bone marrow sometimes have a diagnostic appearance, but they are often nonspecific in their features. Five broad categories of marrow diseases can be used to facilitate an approach to evaluate the images and form an appropriate differential diagnosis. These categories are elaborated in **Table 4**. The categories are as follows:

- Marrow proliferative disorders
- Marrow replacement disorders
- Marrow depletion
- Vascular abnormalities
- Miscellaneous marrow diseases.

Table 4: Categories of bone marrow pathology.[10]

Category	*Comment*	*Distribution*	*Causes*
Marrow proliferative disorder	Arises from existing marrow elements	Mostly diffuse except plasmacytoma	• Reconversion • Myelofibrosis • Polycythemia vera • Mastocytosis • Myelodysplastic syndrome • Leukemia • Multiple myeloma • Amyloidosis • Waldenström macroglobulinemia • Langerhans cell histiocytosis
Marrow replacement disorder	Implantation of cells in marrow that do not normally exist there	Mostly focal	• Primary bone tumors • Osteomyelitis • Metastases • Lymphoma
Marrow depletion	Ablation of red marrow elements	Diffuse or regional distribution	• Aplastic anemia • Chemotherapy • Radiation therapy
Vascular abnormalities: Hyperemia	Hyperemia causes bone marrow edema	Focal lesions, often involving epiphyses	• Trauma • Transient osteoporosis of hip • Regional migratory osteoporosis • Complex regional pain syndrome • Infection • Tumors • Joint abnormalities • Early osteonecrosis
Vascular abnormalities: Ischemia	Ischemia causes osteonecrosis in poorly vascularized fatty marrow	Focal lesions in epiphyses or diaphyses	• Trauma • Steroids • Sickle cell anemia • Dysbaric causes • Systemic lupus erythematosus • Gaucher's disease • Alcoholism • Pancreatitis • Idiopathic
Miscellaneous marrow diseases	These abnormalities do not fit neatly into the other categories of marrow disease		• Gaucher's disease • Paget's disease • Osteopetrosis • Hemosiderosis • Serous atrophy (gelatinous transformation) of marrow

MARROW PROLIFERATIVE DISORDERS

Marrow proliferative disorders are diseases that arise from proliferation of cells that normally exist in the marrow. MRI of marrow proliferative disorders can have several appearances. Normal appearance of marrow on MRI does not eliminate the possibility of a significant marrow disease. Proliferation of abnormal cells may be indistinguishable from normal red marrow early in the disease, when the tumor burden is low. This is the situation in about 10–20% of patients with multiple myeloma and leukemia, and it is important to understand this weakness of the imaging technique.

The major abnormalities we look for on an MRI to indicate a marrow proliferative disease are as follows:

- Abnormal signal intensity
- Abnormal distribution of what appears to be normal signal intensity red marrow
- Both abnormal marrow distribution and signal intensity.

Reconversion of Yellow Marrow to Red Marrow

Reconversion of yellow marrow to red marrow takes place when demand of the body exceeds the capacity of the existing red marrow store. It occurs in people with obesity, chronic infection, chronic cardiac decompensation, hyperparathyroidism, endurance athletes, and heavy smokers.[2,33] It also occurs in hematologic disorders such as severe chronic anemia, thalassemia **(Figs. 12A to F)**, sickle cell disease, and hereditary spherocytosis. This happens because of the erythrocytes produced in the bone marrow being either less efficient at transporting oxygen or having a shorter life than normal or due to a combination of both these factors.[1,2,34]

The pattern of reconversion is opposite of that of physiological marrow conversion. Reconversion begins in the axial skeleton in the vertebrae and flat bones of the pelvis and progresses peripherally to the long bones of the extremities, the proximal bones before the distal long bones. Epiphyses are usually spared and reconversion occurs only in the severely affected patients.[1,2,35]

Imaging

On radiography, changes related to expansion of medulla, thinning of cortical bone, and reduction in bone density may be seen in patients with extensive reconversion such as thalassemia. In the skull, widening of diploic space occurs with hair-on-end appearance. Hypopneumatization of sinuses, premature fusion of epiphyses, and coarsened trabeculae may also be seen. Extramedullary hematopoietic soft-tissue masses are common.

Hyperplastic hematopoietic cells lead to a reduction in signal intensity on T1W images although the signal intensity is still equal to or greater than that of muscle. On T2W images, the signal intensity may be equal or hypointense to that of yellow marrow. The reconversion tends to be symmetrical **(Figs. 13A and B)**. It is however difficult to differentiate foci of reconverted bone marrow in an atypical location, e.g., diaphysis of long bones from a malignant process and metastases.

Differentiating criteria between reconversion and malignancy are tabulated in **Table 5**.[1,2,34,36]

Red marrow, being more vascular and active, is more commonly involved by malignancy. Normal red marrow is

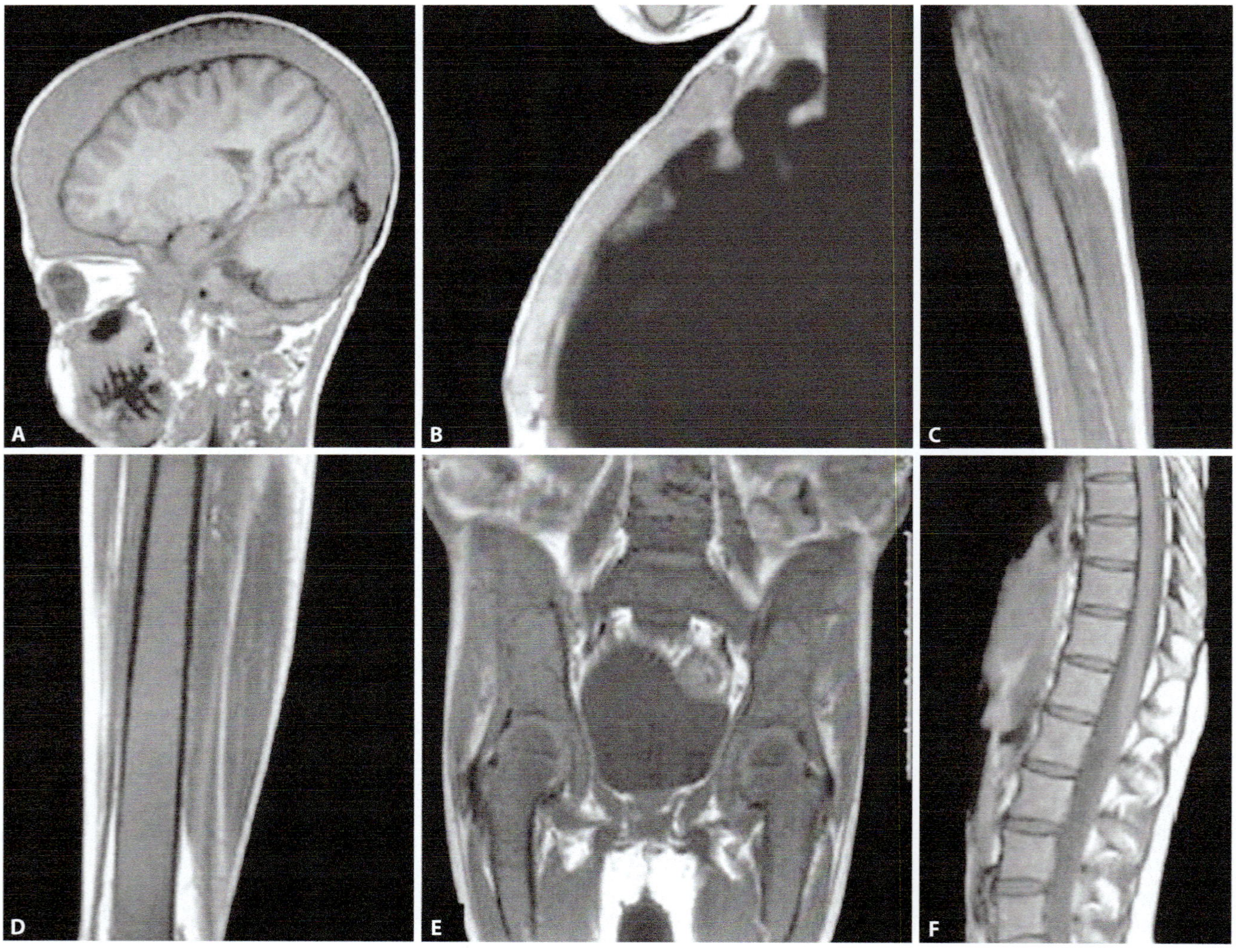

Figs. 12A to F: Thalassemia. T1-weighted (T1W) magnetic resonance (MR) images of skull (A), sternum (B), humerus (C), femur (D), pelvis (E), and dorsolumbar spine (F) showing medullary expansion and red marrow reconversion. The hematopoietic marrow is seen as decreased signal intensity on these T1W images throughout the axial and appendicular skeleton.

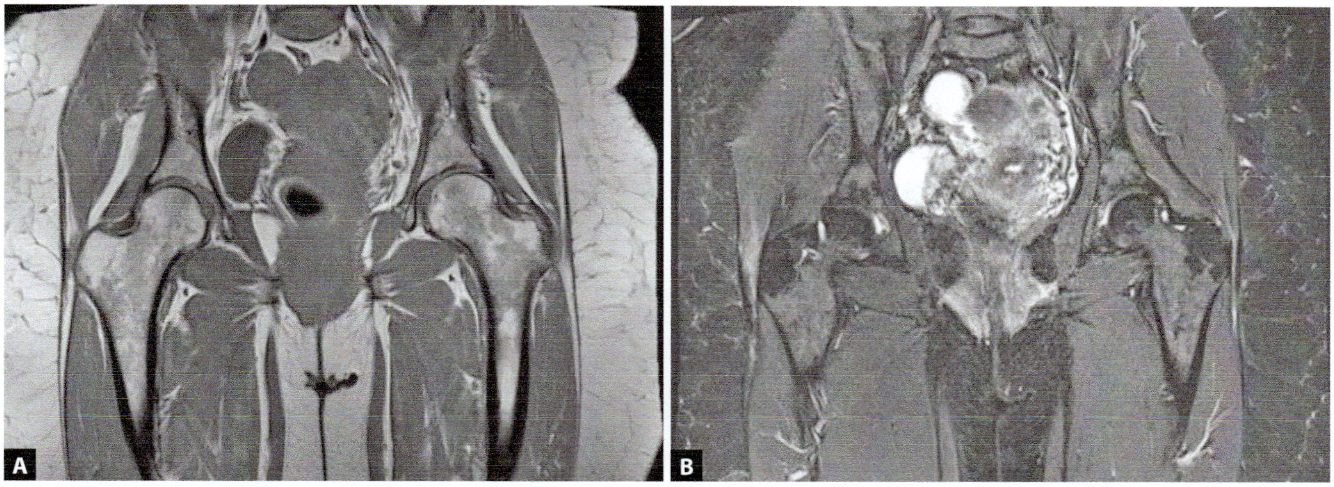

Figs. 13A and B: Reconverted marrow in a 70-year-old female. T1-weighted (T1W) coronal (A) and short tau inversion recovery (STIR) coronal (B) magnetic resonance (MR) images of the pelvis with red marrow in proximal metaphyses, diaphyses of bilateral femori, and pelvis due to chronic anemia. Yellow marrow is hyperintense on T1W image with suppression of signal on STIR image. Red marrow is hypointense on T1W image and intermediate signal intensity on STIR image.

Table 5: Differences between reconverted and malignant infiltration of marrow.

Reconversion marrow	*Malignancy*
Follows the normal pattern of marrow distribution and is bilaterally symmetrical	Asymmetric and geographic in distribution
Signal intensity equal to muscle on STIR and fat-saturated T2W images	Signal intensity more than muscle on STIR and fat-saturated T2W images
No cortical break or soft tissue mass	Cortical break with mass may be seen
Significant contrast enhancement not present; changes do not extend beyond the growth plate line, sparing the articular ends	Contrast enhancement present; changes can extend beyond growth plate line and involve articular ends
On chemical shift imaging, signal drop on out-of-phase image is >20% when compared to in-phase image	Malignancy does not show signal drop on out-of-phase image

mildly hyperintense to muscle and intervertebral disc on T1W images. Hypointensity to muscle has 81% accuracy and hypointensity to vertebral disc has 78% accuracy for identification of an infiltrative process.[36]

Myelofibrosis

Myelofibrosis refers to a spectrum of bone marrow disorders that result in replacement of red marrow with fibrotic tissue. It occurs due to neoplastic process leading to abnormal proliferation of fibroblasts and collagen deposition.

Primary myelofibrosis (PMF) is believed to arise from a somatic mutation of a pluripotent hematopoietic progenitor cell and has an incidence of approximately 0.4–1.4 per 100,000 individuals. Janus kinase 2 *(JAK2)* mutation is believed to play a role in PMF.

Secondary myelofibrosis can be a complication of variety of benign and malignant disorders like acute leukemia, polycythemia vera, essential thrombocythemia, myelodysplasia, and renal osteodystrophy.

The most common signs and symptoms include easy bruising, weight loss, anemia, extramedullary hematopoiesis, and hepatosplenomegaly. Replacement of bone marrow can lead to deficiency of all blood cell lineages and related clinical manifestations. Hemorrhage and infection can be severe and are often the presenting clinical complaint. Primary acute myelofibrosis is a rapidly progressing disease with a high mortality rate. Leukemic conversion can be seen in up to 20% of affected individuals.

Imaging

The predominant radiographic feature of myelofibrosis is osteosclerosis, typically seen in axial skeleton, ribs, proximal femur, and humerus; a finding that occurs in approximately 30–70% of patients. Other features may include hepatosplenomegaly and extramedullary hematopoietic soft-tissue masses.

Bone scan may give superscan appearance.

Magnetic resonance imaging findings include low T1 and T2 signal of bone marrow without associated

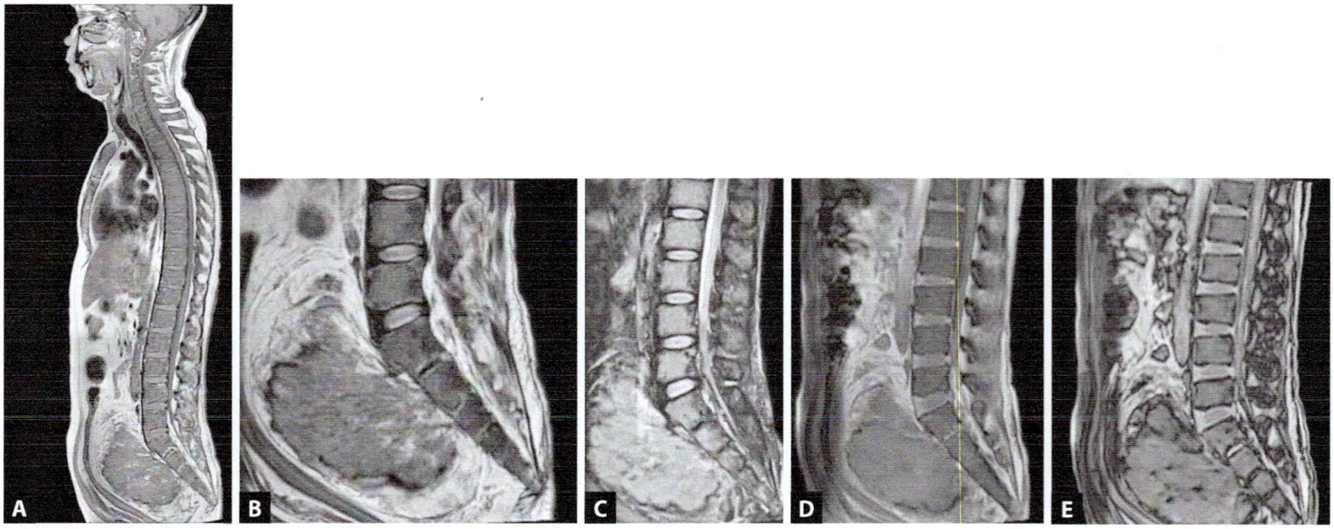

Figs. 14A to E: Myelofibrosis. T1-weighted (T1W) sagittal (A), T2-weighted (T2W) sagittal (B) magnetic resonance (MR) images showing a diffuse low signal in all the vertebral bodies. Presacral lobulated soft tissue with similar signal intensity suggestive of extramedullary hematopoietic mass. Short tau inversion recovery (STIR) sagittal (C) image showing diffuse increase in signal intensity and no drop of signal on opposed phase image (E) as compared to in-phase image (D).

enlargement of the affected bones. On STIR images, the signal intensity is greater than muscle. Opposed-phase imaging does not show a drop in signal as typically noted in normal red marrow; however, drop may be seen in areas of reconverted marrow. Extramedullary hematopoiesis is a common associated finding in the paraspinal soft tissue (**Figs. 14A to E**).

Other causes of low marrow signal are listed in **Table 6**.

In Gaucher's disease (GD), associated bone infarcts may be present; while in hemosiderosis, excessive iron deposition can cause almost a complete signal loss resulting in a "black marrow."[37]

Bone marrow and stem cell transplantation appear to improve prognosis of the disease, with some patients demonstrating long-term remission. Mild cases can be monitored and blood counts managed with medication or transfusions. JAK2 inhibitors appear to be a promising developing treatment option.[38]

Leukemia

Leukemia is a malignant condition arising due to excess production of immature or abnormal leukocytes, which eventually suppresses the production of normal blood cells in marrow. Malignant transformation usually occurs at the pluripotent stem cell level, although it sometimes involves a committed stem cell with limited capacity for self-renewal. Abnormal proliferation, clonal expansion, aberrant differentiation, and diminished apoptosis (programmed cell death) lead to replacement of normal blood elements with malignant cells.

Table 6: Differential diagnosis for low T1 and T2 signal marrow.[10]

	Distribution	
	Focal	*Diffuse*
Conditions	• Bone islands **(Figs. 15A to C)** • Sclerotic metastases • Intraosseous vacuum phenomenon	• Myelofibrosis • Mastocytosis • Hemosiderosis • Osteopetrosis • Gaucher's disease

Classification of Leukemia

The current approach to classifying leukemia is based on the 2016 World Health Organization (WHO) system. The WHO classification is based on a combination of clinical, morphologic, immunophenotypic, and genetic features. Leukemias are commonly also categorized as:

- *Acute or chronic*: Based on the percentage of blasts or leukemia cells in bone marrow or blood.
- *Myeloid or lymphoid*: Based on the predominant lineage of the malignant cells.

  The four most common leukemias are:
  1. Acute myeloid leukemia (AML)
  2. Acute lymphoblastic leukemia (ALL)
  3. Chronic myeloid leukemia (CML)
  4. Chronic lymphocytic leukemia (CLL).

Leukemia comprises one-third of all malignancies in childhood and ALL is the most common. In adults, CLL and AML are the common subtypes.

Risk factors for leukemia include exposure to radiation, chromosomal abnormalities such as Down syndrome, oncoviruses such as human T-cell leukemia virus type 1

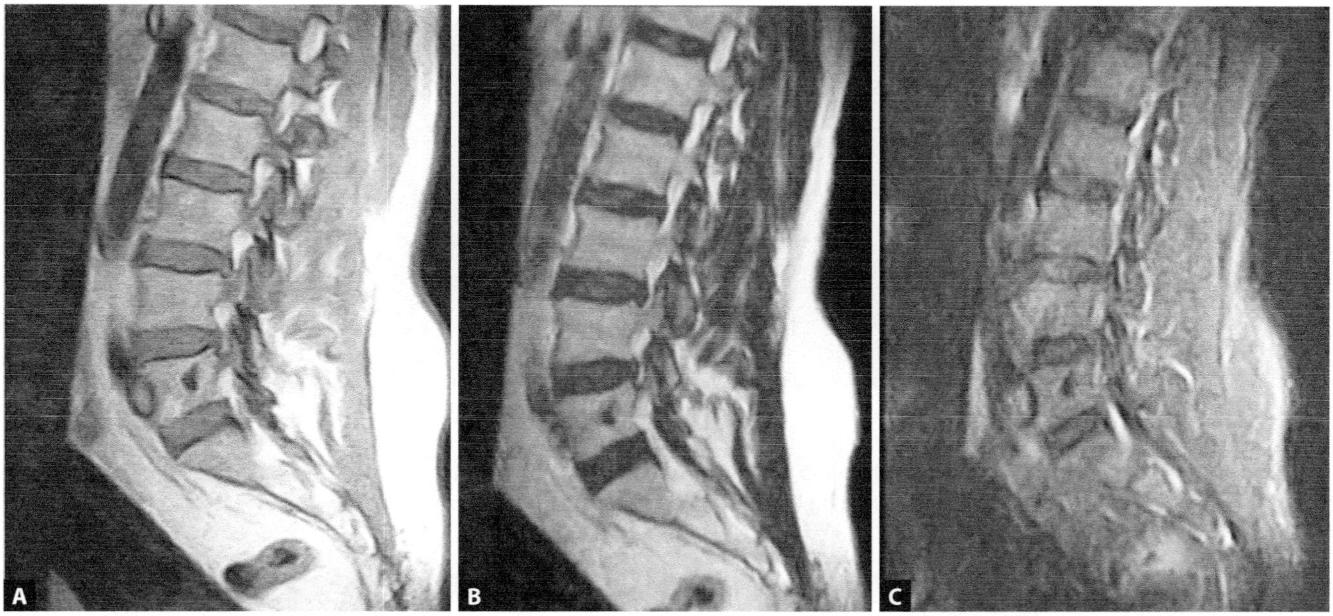

Figs. 15A to C: Bone island. T1-weighted (T1W) sagittal (A), T2-weighted (T2W) sagittal (B) and short tau inversion recovery (STIR) sagittal (C) magnetic resonance (MR) images showing hypointense focus in L5 vertebral body suggestive of bone island.

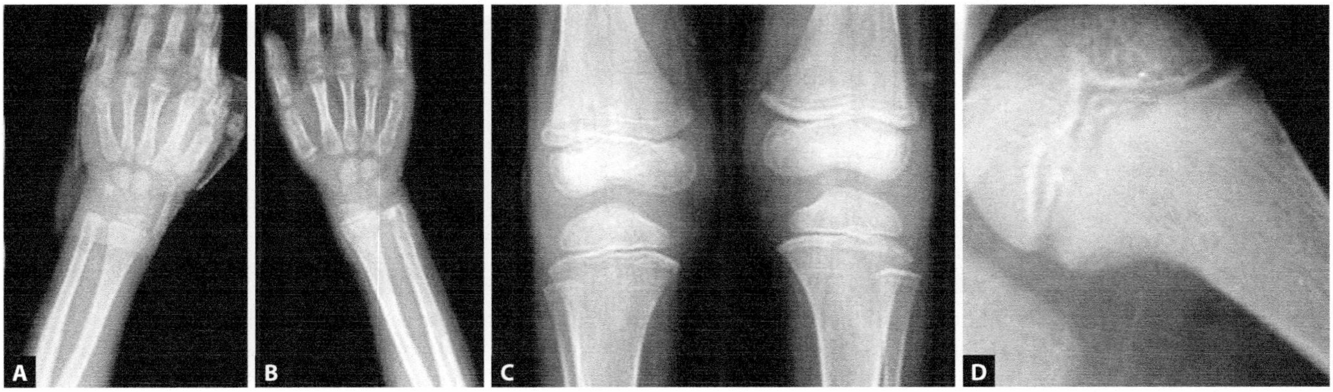

Figs. 16A to D: Leukemia: Radiographs bilateral wrist anteroposterior (AP) view (A and B), bilateral knees AP view (C), and left shoulder AP view (D) reveal diffuse osteopenia with radiolucent metaphyseal bands. Area of osteolysis is seen in the radial aspect of bilateral distal ulnar metaphyses.

(HTLV-1), cigarette smoking (AML), obesity, family history (CLL), and chemical exposures (AML).

Common signs and symptoms of chronic or acute leukemia include pain in the bones or joints, lymphadenopathy, fever, fatigue, bleeding and bruising, frequent infections, hepatosplenomegaly, weight loss, etc.

The red marrow is preferentially infiltrated by leukemic cells ultimately leading to anemia, neutropenia, and thrombocytopenia. The calvaria, spine, flat bones, proximal end of the long bones and subsequently the appendicular skeleton are involved. Extramedullary sites of involvement include lymph nodes, thymus, central nervous system (chronic meningitis), infiltration of salivary glands, skin, lungs, liver, spleen, pleura, pericardium, and testis.

Imaging

The diagnosis of leukemia may be missed on radiographs as the findings are subtle and do not appear till advanced stage of disease. Osteopenia with coarse trabeculation may be seen.[39-42] Other findings include periosteal reaction, radiolucent metaphyseal bands (classically in pediatric cases) **(Figs. 16A to D)**.[42] Leukemic bone marrow infiltration may also cause collapse of vertebral body (vertebra plana).[43]

The pattern of involvement of marrow may be diffuse or multifocal. On MRI, infiltration by leukemic cells is seen as decreased signal intensity on T1W images and increased signal intensity on STIR images[44] **(Figs. 17 to 19)** with increased enhancement of involved areas. The signal

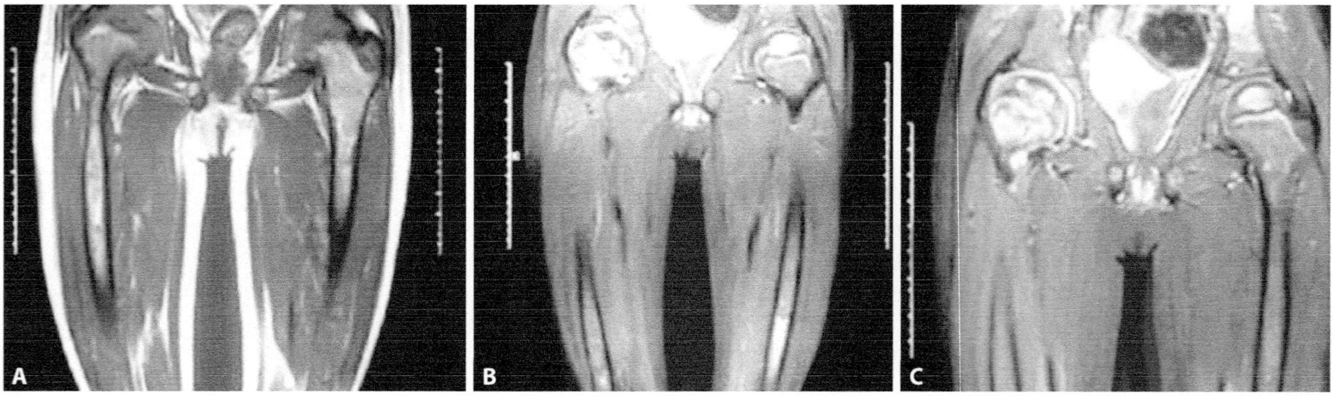

Figs. 17A to C: Leukemic infiltration of marrow. T1-weighted (T1W) coronal magnetic resonance (MR) image of the pelvis (A) in a 5-year-old child showing abnormal low-signal in the femoral head instead of the high-signal fat normally seen at this age. Few foci of abnormal signal are also seen in the femoral diaphysis. Short tau inversion recovery (STIR) coronal images of the pelvis (B and C) show these foci in the femoral head, diaphysis, and iliac blades to be high-signal (higher than muscle) which is abnormal.

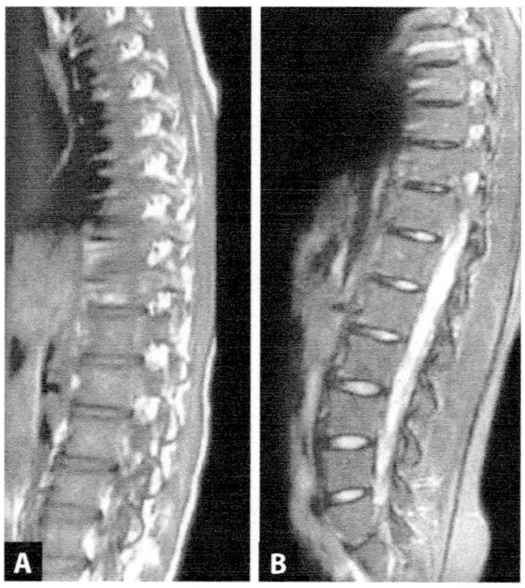

Figs. 18A and B: Leukemic infiltration of marrow. T1-weighted (T1W) sagittal magnetic resonance (MR) image of the dorsolumbar spine (A) showing diffuse abnormal signal in the vertebrae, the signal being lower than the adjacent intervertebral discs. T2-weighted (T2W) sagittal image (B) showing no increase in signal.

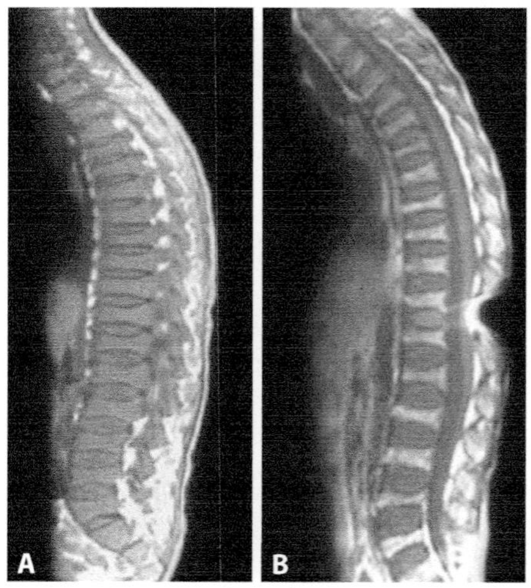

Figs. 19A and B: Acute lymphocytic leukemia (ALL). T1-weighted (T1W) magnetic resonance (MR) images of the spine in a case of ALL showing a diffuse low signal of the vertebral bodies in the active stage. The vertebrae also show reduced height (A). In the stage of remission (B), the vertebral bodies show a replacement of the marrow with fat.

intensity is increased or unchanged on T2W images because of the high water content of leukemic cells. Leukemic marrow shows restriction of diffusion and DWI has been shown to be predictive of leukemia even before bone marrow biopsy.[45-47] Although marrow aspiration or biopsy is required for definitive diagnosis, MRI has been shown to demonstrate leukemic infiltration of the bones even with a negative bone marrow biopsy in pediatric cases.[41]

Bone marrow necrosis (BMN) is an unusual entity that has been reported to occur in close association with malignancy, particularly acute lymphocytic leukemia. BMN is characterized by a loss of myeloid tissue and marrow fat without trabecular destruction which is unlike avascular necrosis (AVN). About 91% of patients with BMN have malignancy, with acute lymphocytic leukemia representing 18% of cases.[48] MR findings of BMN are similar to those of AVN but are more diffuse and involve the axial skeleton without vertebral collapse.

Chloroma (also known as granulocytic sarcoma) is a rare manifestation of AML, but it may also occur with other myeloproliferative and myelodysplastic disorders. It is a solid tumor composed of mass-like *extramedullary* proliferation of primitive cells of myeloid lineage. Most common sites of chloroma are the bone and periosteum, which is explained by the direct spread from the adjoining infiltrated marrow. Other frequently involved sites are skin (leukemia cutis), lymph nodes, and orbit, although any site may be potentially affected. On MRI, it is iso-/hypointense on T1 and mildly hyperintense on T2W images **(Figs. 20A to G)**.

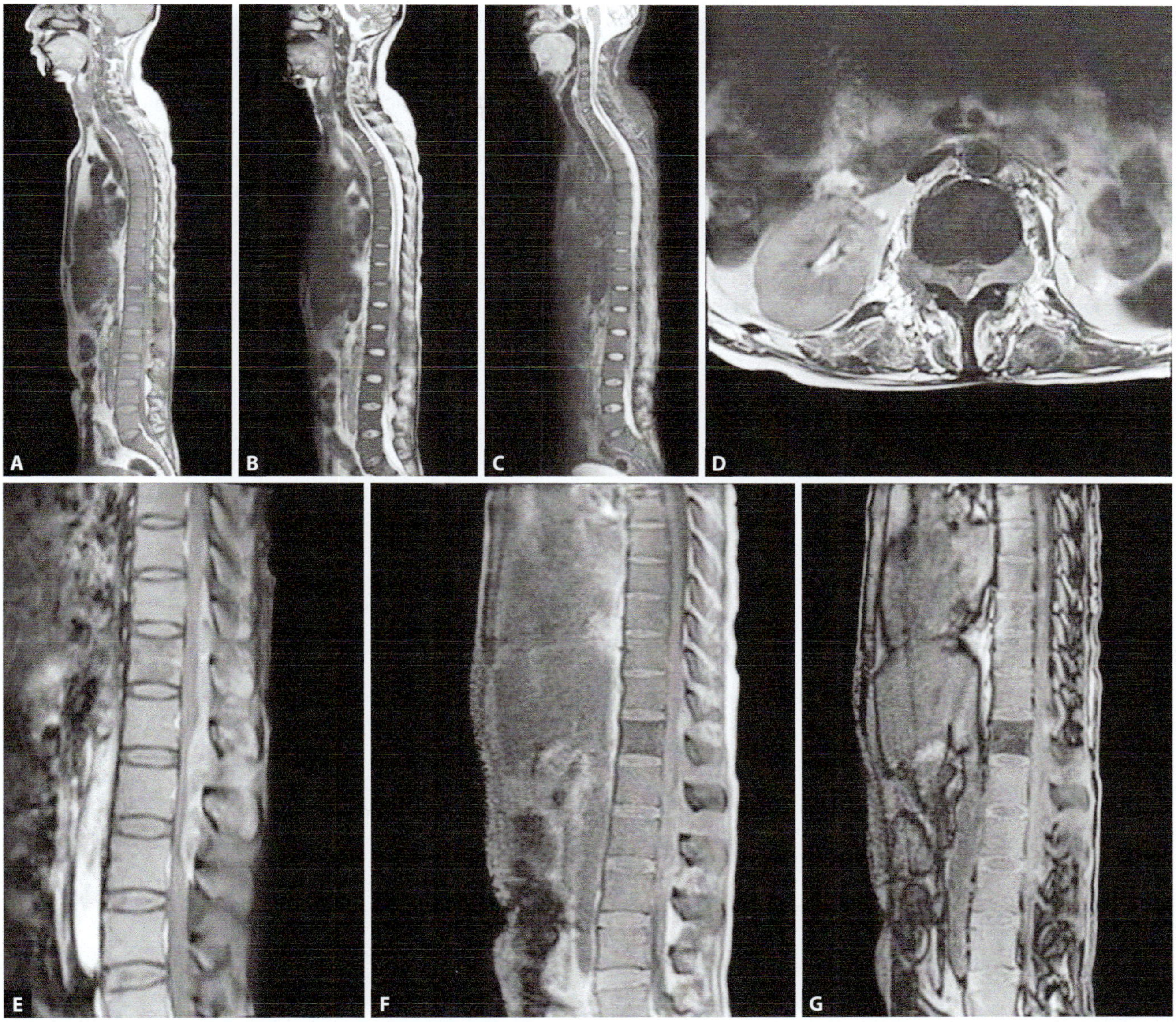

Figs. 20A to G: Chronic myeloid leukemia with granulocytic sarcoma. T1-weighted (T1W) (A), T2-weighted (T2W) (B), short tau inversion recovery (STIR) (C) sagittal magnetic resonance (MR) images show diffuse infiltration of marrow that is hypointense on T1W with hypointense signal on T2W and STIR images. T2W axial (D) and contrast-enhanced sagittal (E) image reveals heterogeneously enhancing soft tissue within the posterior and lateral epidural space causing narrowing of the spinal canal and compressive myelopathy suggestive of granulocytic sarcoma. In-phase (F) and opposed phase (G) images show no drop in the signal of the vertebral marrow except one vertebral body which shows some preserved fatty marrow.

On FDG-PET/CT and FDG-PET/MRI, increase in uptake is seen in involved marrow. Further research needs to be performed before it can be accepted as a staging tool.[49,50]

Treatment options for leukemia include chemotherapy regimens, bone marrow or peripheral blood stem cell transplant, and antibody-mediated medications such as ibrutinib or idelalisib for CLL and imatinib for CML.[51] Although acute leukemia is more aggressive than chronic leukemia, the former responds better to treatment than the latter.

Multiple Myeloma

Multiple myeloma refers to a spectrum of disorders arising due to malignant clonal proliferation of plasma cells of B-cell origin. There is production of an abnormal paraprotein leading to a wide M-band on plasma electrophoresis. Multiple myeloma is the third most common blood cancer in adults.[51] This is a disease of the elderly. About 75% of those affected are over the age of 50 years with a peak over 80 years. A male predominance of up to 2:1 is seen. Risk factors for multiple myeloma include male sex, increasing age, African-American ethnicity, monoclonal gammopathy of undetermined significance (MGUS), and radiation exposure. MGUS often precedes frank multiple myeloma.

Production of light-chain immunoglobulins results in Bence Jones proteinuria in over half the patients. Multiple systemic effects, including hypercalcemia, renal failure and/or hematologic dyscrasias may also occur. Diseases in the multiple myeloma spectrum have been described in **Table 7**.

Persistent bone pain is the most common symptom which is worse during the day, is relieved by rest, and aggravated by weight bearing. Pathological fracture is a common complication. Associated weight loss, anemia and, cachexia occur. Bacterial infections occur in 10% of cases, most of which are respiratory in nature.

Table 7: Definitions of multiple myeloma and related conditions.[52]

	Definition
Multiple myeloma	Monoclonal proliferation of plasma cells with myeloma-defining CRAB* findings
MGUS	Monoclonal proliferation of plasma cells without myeloma-defining CRAB* findings
Solitary plasmacytoma	Monoclonal plasma cells manifesting as a single tumor
Smoldering myeloma	Monoclonal proliferation of plasma cells in bone marrow and/or serum/ urine with abnormal levels of monoclonal protein

*CRAB = calcium level elevation, renal failure, anemia, or bone lesions. (MGUS: monoclonal gammopathy of undetermined significance)

Laboratory findings reveal a normochromic, normocytic anemia, thrombocytopenia, hypercalcemia, hyperglobulinemia with a reversed A:G ratio, hyperuricemia, and Bence Jones proteinuria. Erythrocyte sedimentation rate (ESR) is often raised to over 100 mm/h. Bone marrow biopsy confirms the plasma cell dyscrasia. The spine, pelvis, skull, ribs, and scapula are the most frequently involved bones.

Imaging

On radiography, multiple myeloma may be seen as diffuse or focal osteolysis. The involved bones show well-defined, small, punched-out lytic lesions, most characteristic in the skull **(Figs. 21A to C)**. These lesions can also be seen in the pelvic bones, clavicles, ribs, and long bones. Osteolytic lesions involving long bones tend to show signs of cortical erosion from the medullary side, i.e., endosteal cortical scalloping. These lesions may be differentiated from lytic metastatic lesions by the more uniform size of the lesions in multiple myeloma. Generalized osteopenia is another important form of presentation. A pathological fracture affects about half of the patients at some time or the other. Examples of purely sclerotic myeloma have been occasionally reported. They may take the form of diffuse osteosclerosis, patchy sclerotic areas throughout the

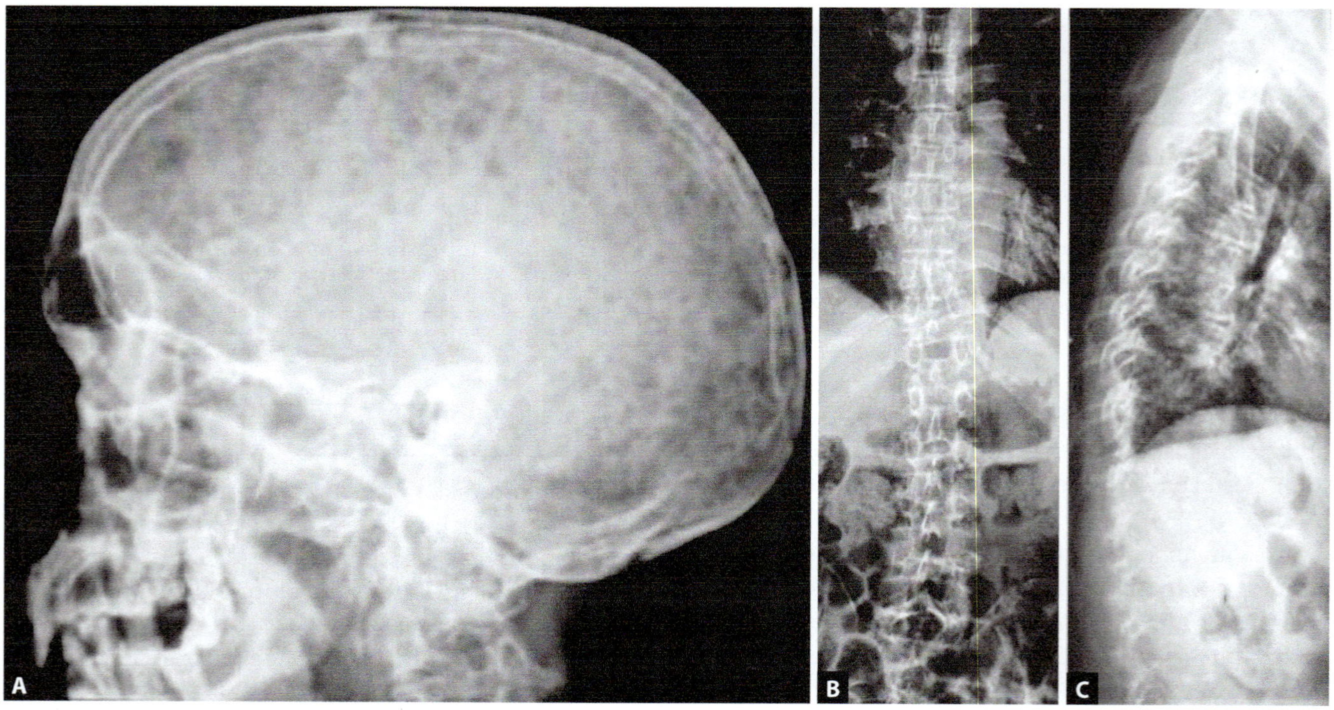

Figs. 21A to C: Multiple myeloma. X-ray of skull lateral view (A), dorsolumbar spine anteroposterior (AP) (B) and lateral view (C) reveal diffuse osteopenia with multiple well-defined punched out lesions in the skull.

skeleton and, very rarely, small numbers of focal sclerotic lesions.

Involvement of the spine is usually in the lower thoracic and upper lumbar regions, and is seen as diffuse osteopenia. Pedicular involvement, although rare, can occur in multiple myeloma patients; and so the usefulness of this feature to differentiate multiple myeloma from metastatic disease appears doubtful.

On CT, well-circumscribed, lytic "soap bubble" osseous lesions, with a narrow zone of transition, are seen. The attenuation of lesions is 40–80 HU of attenuation, similar to soft tissue **(Figs. 22A and B)**.

Multiple myeloma generally has no osteoblastic activity and is thus typically negative on ^{99m}Tc bone scans. FDG-PET/CT has high specificity and sensitivity for multiple myeloma lesions and is especially good at demonstrating extramedullary disease.[53] FDG-PET/CT can be used to monitor treatment response because the ^{18}F-FDG uptake of osseous lesions will decrease with successful treatment.

On MRI, bone marrow in multiple myeloma shows elevated signal intensity on T2W images and decreased signal intensity on T1W images **(Figs. 23 and 24)**. MRI correlates with the clinical severity. Stabler et al. have found five infiltration patterns of multiple myeloma on MRI. These are as follows:

1. Normal appearing marrow with low-grade interstitial infiltration
2. Focal pattern
3. Diffuse
4. Mixed focal and diffuse
5. Salt and pepper appearance.

The infiltration patterns correlated with the clinical staging in their study. They concluded that MR is of prognostic value and can be a supporting pillar in the staging and planning treatment of patients with multiple myeloma.[54]

Vertebral body compression fractures occur frequently in patients with multiple myeloma. The differentiation between osteoporotic vertebral collapse and that due to myeloma may be difficult even on MRI. DWI and opposed-phase (in-phase–out-of-phase) imaging have been advocated to help differentiate insufficiency fractures from pathologic compression fractures.

The most important differential diagnosis in this age group is metastases. Features, which help in distinguishing the two, are summarized in **Table 8**.

Early- or low-grade infiltration of myeloma in the bone marrow may demonstrate normal bone marrow signal intensity at MRI, underlining the importance of correlation with the laboratory tests and bone marrow biopsy. Greater than 40% increase in signal intensity compared with the baseline after contrast administration correlates with diffuse tumor infiltration of marrow.[55]

Despite the widespread use of the radiographic skeletal survey, MRI has been shown to be useful in the assessment of multiple myeloma patients; and considering the increased sensitivity of FDG-PET/CT and MRI in identifying bone marrow infiltration, the staging

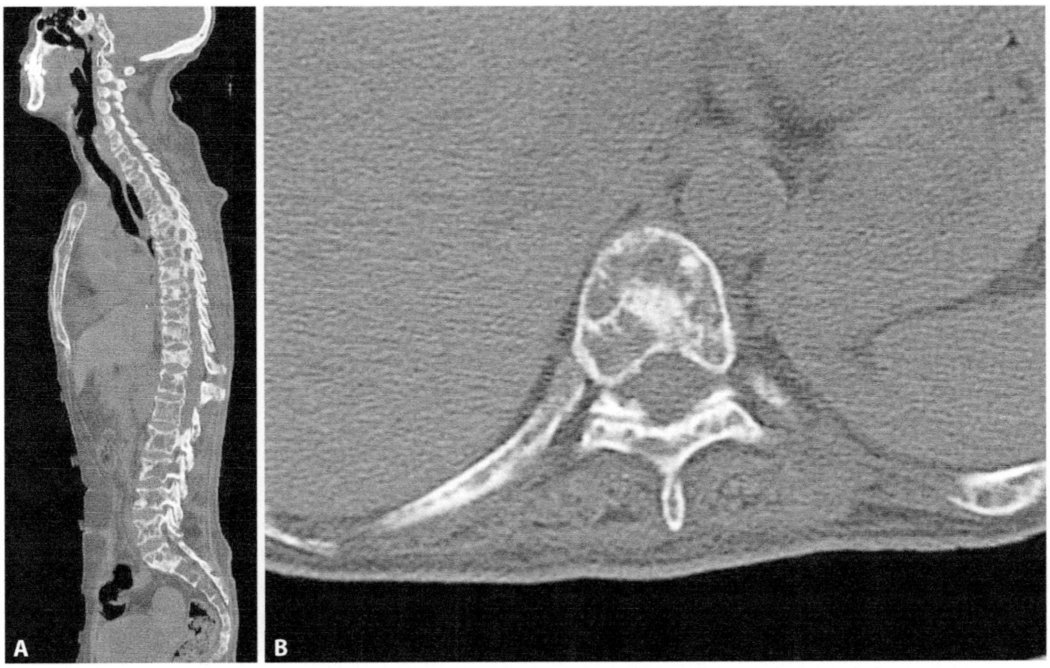

Figs. 22A and B: Multiple myeloma. Computed tomography (CT) bone window sagittal (A) and axial (B) images show multiple well-defined lytic lesions in visualized bones.

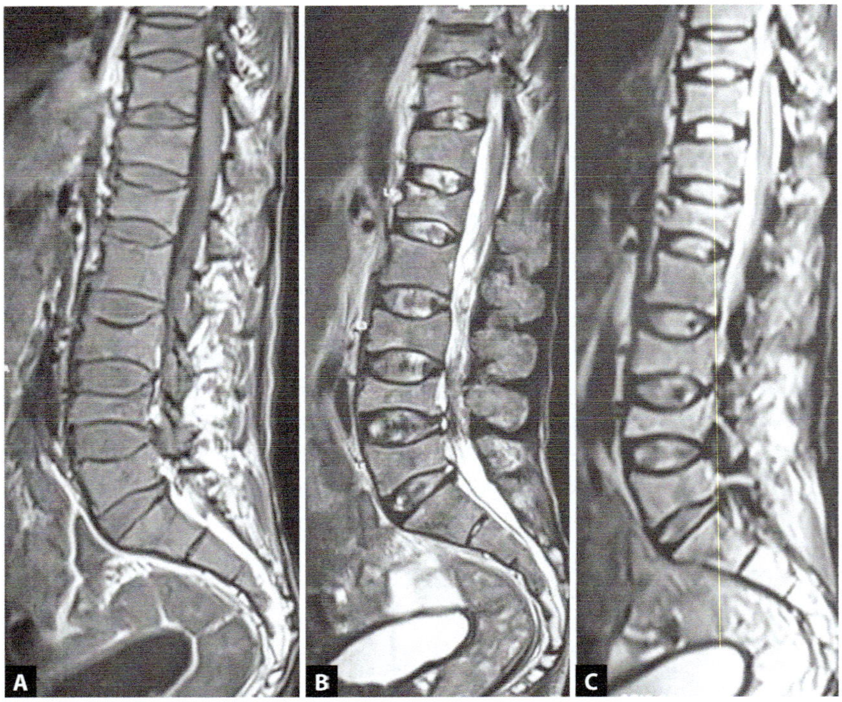

Figs. 23A to C: Multiple myeloma. T1-weighted (T1W) sagittal (A), T2-weighted (T2W) sagittal (B), and short tau inversion recovery (STIR) sagittal (C) magnetic resonance (MR) images of the lumbar spine showing diffuse alteration of marrow signal appearing hypointense on T1W and mildly hyperintense on T2W and STIR images.

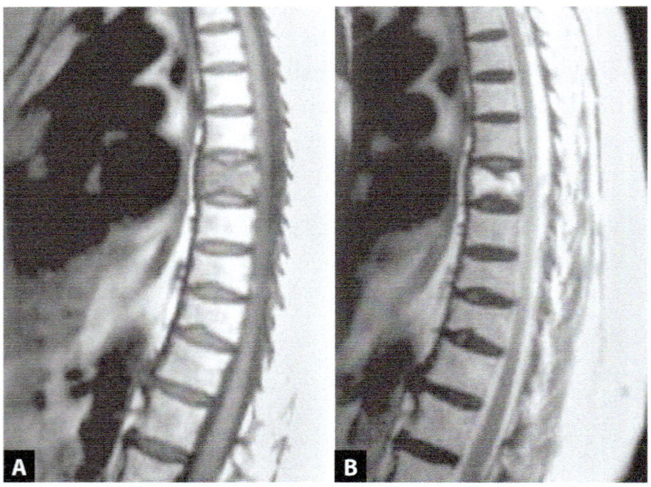

Figs. 24A and B: Multiple myeloma. T1-weighted (T1W) (A) and T2-weighted (T2W) (B) sagittal magnetic resonance (MR) images of the dorsal spine show complete alteration of the marrow signal in the seventh thoracic vertebra, hypointense on T1W and hyperintense on T2W images, with evidence of collapse. A posterior convexity of the involved vertebra suggests a malignant etiology.

system has been revised. The Durie-Salmon PLUS system replaces the radiographic skeletal survey with MRI and FDG-PET/CT.[53] The Durie-Salmon PLUS system divides patients with multiple myeloma into three groups (each of which has two subgroups) on the basis of the number of focal lesions or the severity of diffuse bone infiltration noted on imaging.

Table 8: Distinguishing features between multiple myeloma and metastases.

Multiple myeloma	*Metastases*
Vertebral pedicles and posterior elements less commonly involved; destruction of intervertebral disc may occur	Destruction of vertebral pedicles
Soft-tissue mass associated with a bony lesion	Soft tissue extension is relatively uncommon
Mandible involved commonly	Mandible involved rarely
Radionuclide studies may give false negative results	Radionuclide studies are very sensitive
Serum alkaline phosphatase may be normal	Serum alkaline phosphatase is always raised in disseminated disease

Durie-Salmon PLUS staging system—MRI findings, FDG-PET/CT findings, or both.

MGUS: All negative.

Stage IA, smoldering or indolent: Can have single plasmacytoma or limited disease at imaging.

Stage IB: <5 focal lesions, mild diffuse disease.

Stage IIA or IIB: 5–20 focal lesions, moderate diffuse disease.

Stage IIIA or IIIB: >20 focal lesions, severe diffuse disease.

The criteria for subgroup A classification is a serum creatinine level <2.0 mg/dL and no extramedullary disease, whereas the criteria for subgroup B classification is serum creatinine level >2.0 mg/dL or the presence of extramedullary disease.

Magnetic resonance may also help guide the biopsy and also to confirm the response to therapy. Complete response to chemotherapy includes the following postcontrast enhancement patterns:

- Complete resolution of abnormality
- Persistent abnormality with no enhancement
- Peripheral rim enhancement only.[56]

A partial response to chemotherapy can show conversion of diffuse pattern to a focal or variegated pattern with persistent contrast enhancement. Reconstituted fatty tissue is seen as multifocal, diffuse increase in signal intensity on T1W images with less contrast enhancement[3] **(Figs. 25A to C)**

Treatment options for multiple myeloma include chemotherapy, steroid therapy, stem cell transplant, radiation therapy, biologic therapy, and watchful waiting.

Plasmacytoma

A plasmacytoma represents a localized form of plasma cell proliferation, which is apparently solitary at presentation and may remain localized for many years, but is potentially capable of transition to generalized myelomatosis.

Although few cases present below the age of 40 years, the overall age of presentation tends to be earlier, and the age range wider, than in generalized myelomatosis.

Presentation may be with local pain as a result of fracture, but uncomplicated plasmacytoma may cause no symptoms. The lesion predominantly affects sites containing persistent red marrow. The mandible, ilium, vertebrae, ribs, and proximal femur are the commonly involved bones. Peripheral lesions are rare.

Imaging

A plasmacytoma arises in the medulla and the bone changes usually resemble a benign lesion. The characteristic appearance is that of a geographic, radiolucent lesion which is highly expansile with apparent trabeculation or a "soap bubble" appearance.

Involvement of the vertebral body is common, sometimes leading to early collapse. Sometimes a whole vertebral body is lost, with geographical destruction of the margins of the adjoining vertebral bodies, usually posteriorly. Coarse trabecular strands of increased density may give a network appearance in the area of destruction. Exceptionally, the lesion may be entirely sclerotic. Scintigraphy and CT/MRI do not give any specific information; however, the finding of apparently solitary plasmacytoma in the spine should be investigated

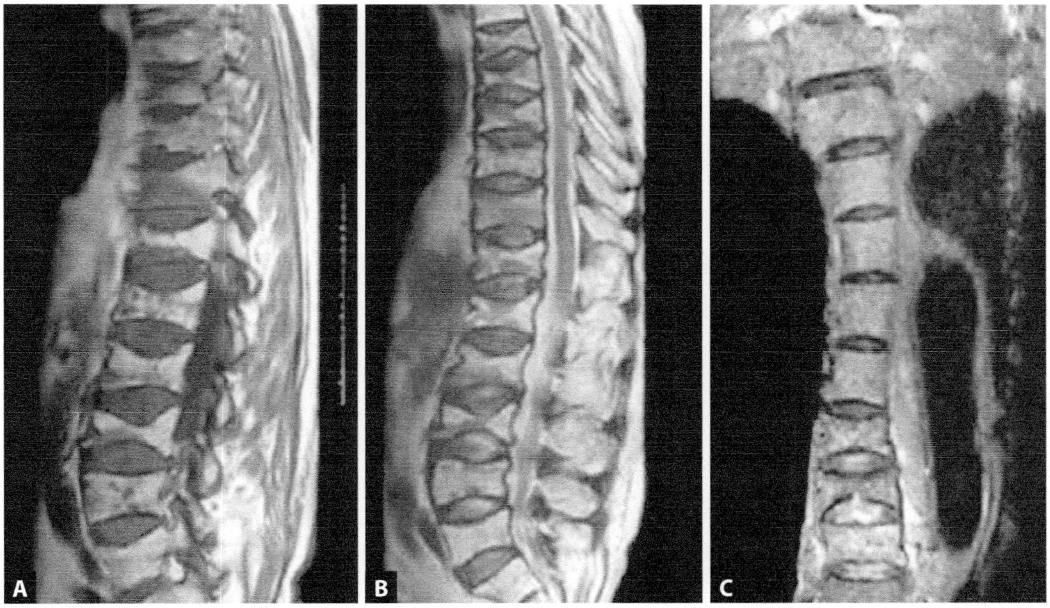

Figs. 25A to C: Multiple myeloma on treatment. T1-weighted (T1W) sagittal (A), T2-weighted (T2W) sagittal (B) and short tau inversion recovery (STIR) coronal (C) magnetic resonance (MR) images showing collapse of multiple vertebrae with heterogeneous marrow signal of vertebral bodies predominantly hyperintense on both T1W and T2W images s/o fatty marrow replacement. Areas of active marrow infiltration/edema are noted involving D11 and few other lower dorsal and lumbar vertebrae seen as hypointense on T1, hyperintense on T2, and STIR images with associated (L) paravertebral mass. Proven case of multiple myeloma on treatment showing fatty marrow replacement with residual active marrow infiltration in few vertebrae.

with whole spine MRI to identify further radiographically occult lesions **(Figs. 26A to D)**.

The most important differential diagnosis is an osteolytic metastasis. In the vertebrae, such metastases are likely to involve the pedicles. Chordoma, brown tumors of hyperparathyroidism, hemophilic pseudotumor, hydatid cyst, fibrous dysplasia, and giant cell tumor can also be considered in the differential diagnosis.

A study of patients initially diagnosed with solitary plasmacytoma found that there was evidence of additional sites of intramedullary involvement in one-third of cases at MRI screening of the thoracic and lumbosacral spine.[57] This is significant, as these cases were initially thought to have only a single focus of disease.

The International Myeloma Working Group has recommended that low-dose whole-body CT, FDG-PET/CT or whole-body, and/or spine MRI be performed in all patients with a clinical presentation of smoldering multiple myeloma and solitary plasmacytoma; equivocal or small lesions should be reassessed with prompt (3–6-month) follow-up MRI.[53]

POEMS Syndrome, also known as Takatsuki Disease or Crow-Fukase Syndrome

An uncommon condition with the acronym POEMS is characterized by a chronic, progressive polyneuropathy, organomegaly (hepatosplenomegaly), endocrinopathy (commonly diabetes mellitus), M-proteins (plasma cell dyscrasia), and skin changes (hirsutism, pigmentation, and edema). In POEMS syndrome, there is also a monoclonal proliferation of plasma cells, but at a lower level than in multiple myeloma.[53] It is usually seen in young men. Imaging findings of POEMS syndrome include organomegaly and sclerotic osseous lesions that can have the same ^{18}F-FDG avidity as a normal bone. Findings include multiple sclerotic lesions, most commonly in the spine and pelvis. The lesions may be uniformly sclerotic or appear target-like, with a peripheral margin of bone sclerosis. Ivory vertebrae and areas resembling bone islands may be seen. Bone proliferation is seen at sites of tendon and ligament attachments. Irregular bony excrescences involving the posterior elements of the spine are characteristically seen. Digital clubbing and periostitis

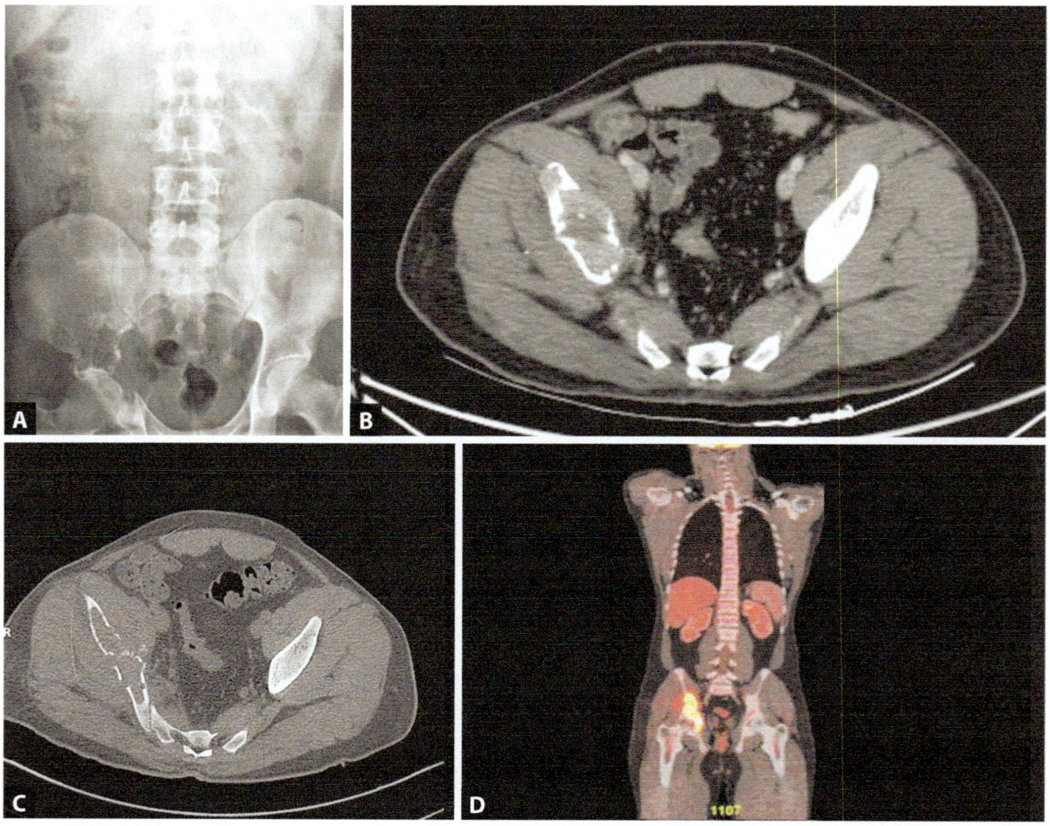

Figs. 26A to D: Plasmacytoma. A 30-year-old male patient presented with pain in right gluteal region. Plain anteroposterior (AP) radiograph (A) of the pelvis shows a lytic expansile lesion in the supra-acetabular region of right iliac bone causing erosion and thinning of overlying cortex. The computed tomography (CT) axial soft tissue (B) and bone window (C) of the pelvis of the same patient show a soft tissue lesion in the right iliac bone causing bony erosion. Coronal positron emission tomography (PET)-CT image (D) shows increased fluorodeoxyglucose (FDG) uptake in the lesion.

in tubular bones simulate the findings of hypertrophic osteoarthropathy.[58]

Langerhans Cell Histiocytosis

Langerhans cell histiocytosis (LCH) is a rare multisystem disease with a wide and heterogeneous clinical spectrum and variable extent of involvement. There is abnormal proliferation of cells derived from myeloid dendritic cells that exhibit the same antigens (CD1a, S100, and CD207) and the same unique intracytoplasmic organelles as in Langerhans cells. The intracytoplasmic organelles appear racquet-shaped on electron microscopy, and are known as Birbeck granules.

Langerhans cell histiocytosis is divided into three groups, on the basis of the number of lesions and systems involved.

1. *The unifocal (localized) form*: Patients usually present between 5 and 15 years of age and involvement is limited to a single bone or a few bones. This form is seen in approximately 70% of LCH cases. Patients may be asymptomatic or may present with focal pain and swelling and are at risk for pathologic fractures. It may involve the lungs. Patients with mandibular involvement may present with gingival bleeding and facial swelling.
2. *The multifocal unisystem (chronic recurring) form*: Patients with this form of disease present between 1 and 5 years of age. The disease involves multiple bones as well as the reticuloendothelial system (i.e., the spleen, liver, lymph nodes, and skin). It comprises approximately 20% of LCH cases and is accompanied by diabetes insipidus when the pituitary gland is involved.
3. *The multifocal multisystem (fulminant) form*: It is typically diagnosed in the first 2 years of life and is characterized by disseminated involvement of the reticuloendothelial system, thrombocytopenia, and anemia.[59] It constitutes approximately 10% of LCH cases and is often fatal.

Eosinophilic granuloma, Hand-Schüller-Christian disease, and Letterer-Siwe disease respectively are older names for the three groups.

Imaging

The most common radiographic manifestation of LCH are bone lesions and occurs in approximately 80% of patients. Any bone can be affected by LCH, but the involvement of flat bones is more common.[60] The skull is the most common flat bone involved. The lesions in skull are well-defined lytic "punched-out" and show beveled margins. This appearance is caused by asymmetric destruction of the inner and outer cortices **(Figs. 27A and B)**.[60] When the skull lesions grow in size, they may coalesce, creating a map-like appearance referred to as a *geographic skull*. The differential diagnosis for calvarial lesions includes lymphoma, multiple myeloma, leukemia, and metastases for multiple lesions and dermoid and epidermoid cysts for single lesions. Osteomyelitis must also be considered in the list of differential diagnoses.

Severe mandibular lesions may destroy the alveolar ridge, resulting in a radiographic appearance of "floating teeth".

The vertebral body is the most commonly affected part of the spine in LCH. Early lesions appear lytic at radiography and computed tomography (CT). As the disease progresses, the early lytic lesions can result in symmetric uniform collapse of the vertebral body with preservation of the intervertebral disc spaces.[60] The flattened vertebral body has been termed *vertebra plana* and may result in substantial neurologic defects and pain. Although vertebra plana can have additional causes in children, such as leukemia, aneurysmal bone cyst, metastatic neuroblastoma, or Ewing sarcoma, the most common cause in children is LCH.

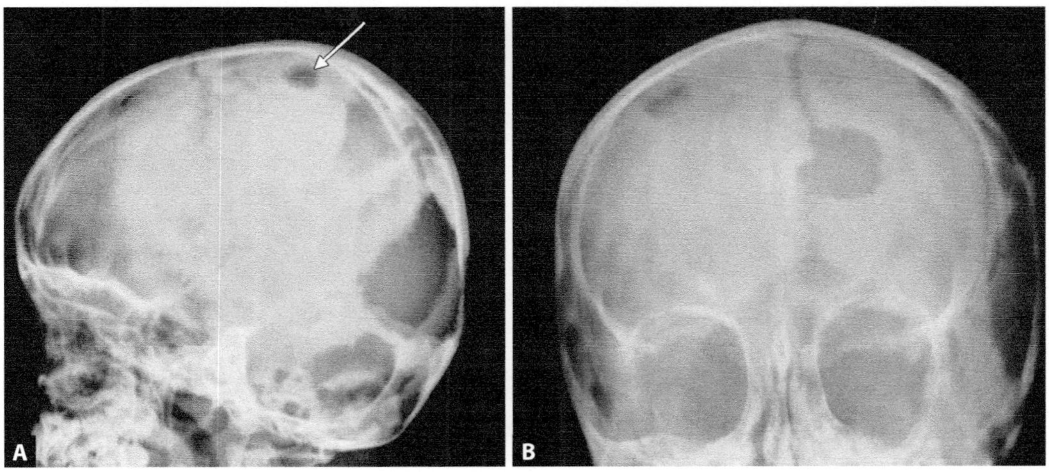

Figs. 27A and B: Langerhans cell histiocytosis. X-ray of skull—lateral (A) and anteroposterior (AP) (B) view showing multiple well-defined lytic areas in skull bones. On lateral view, one of the lesions in parietal bone shows characteristic beveled margin (arrow).

Long bone involvement is more common in children than in adults. Lesions typically occur in the metaphysis or diaphysis, with femur, humerus, and tibia being the most commonly involved long bones. Early lesions often appear expansile, lytic, and aggressive. Less aggressive lesions have been associated with imaging findings of smooth periosteal reaction and cortical thickening. As lesions become chronic, they may resolve or appear sclerotic from periosteal new bone formation.

Bone scintigraphy typically shows increased radiotracer uptake. However, bone scan should be evaluated in conjunction with radiographic findings, as false-negative bone scan findings are common, particularly in patients with older lesions.[60]

Magnetic resonance imaging shows intramedullary lesions with extramedullary soft-tissue components. The soft-tissue component is isointense on T1W images and hyperintense on T2W images, with enhancement after gadolinium-based contrast agent administration **(Figs. 28A to C)**.[60]

Diagnosis of LCH is made by corroborating clinical features, immunohistochemistry, histopathology, and radiologic findings. Treatment of single lesion includes radiation therapy, curettage, or curettage with intralesional steroid injection. Oral systemic steroids and chemotherapy may be used to treat multiple lesions or to prevent central nervous system (CNS) extension in cases of a skull lesion. Radiation therapy is the treatment of choice for vertebral lesions that are at risk for collapse.

MARROW REPLACEMENT DISORDERS

In contrast to marrow proliferative diseases, which are usually diffuse and arise from cells that originate in the bone marrow, the most common marrow replacement diseases are usually focal abnormalities that arise from cells other than those inherent in the bone marrow.

Benign Marrow Replacement Disorder

Osteomyelitis

Osteomyelitis is an infection of medullary bone caused by bacteria and the most common infecting organisms are *Staphylococcus aureus*, *Streptococcus*, and *Pneumococcus*. Less common organisms are *Haemophilus influenzae*, *Escherichia coli*, and *Pseudomonas*. Occasionally fungi, viruses, and parasites are the causative agents.[2,3]

There are three major routes of pathogenesis which are as follows:

1. Hematogenous, beginning in the metaphysis of long bones, juxtachondral portion of flat bones, or spiral end plates. This is commonly seen in infancy and childhood. In neonates, the intact vascular communication between metaphysis and epiphysis leads to epiphyseal involvement in up to 70% cases. Between 1 year and skeletal maturity, the cartilage provides a barrier to joint involvement, except in the hip where the femoral head is intra-articular.
2. Direct inoculation due to trauma/surgery.
3. Via contiguous spread from an adjacent infection.[1-3]

Imaging: Radiographs are insensitive in the first 2 weeks. Routine radiographs are fairly specific in the late stages **(Figs. 29A and B)**. Early changes include soft-tissue swelling and loss of fat planes. Other changes include osteopenia with periosteal thickening and lytic areas.

Osteomyelitis causes marrow replacement with inflammatory cells resulting in increased extracellular water or fluid, which causes a decreased signal intensity on T1W images and increased signal intensity on T2W

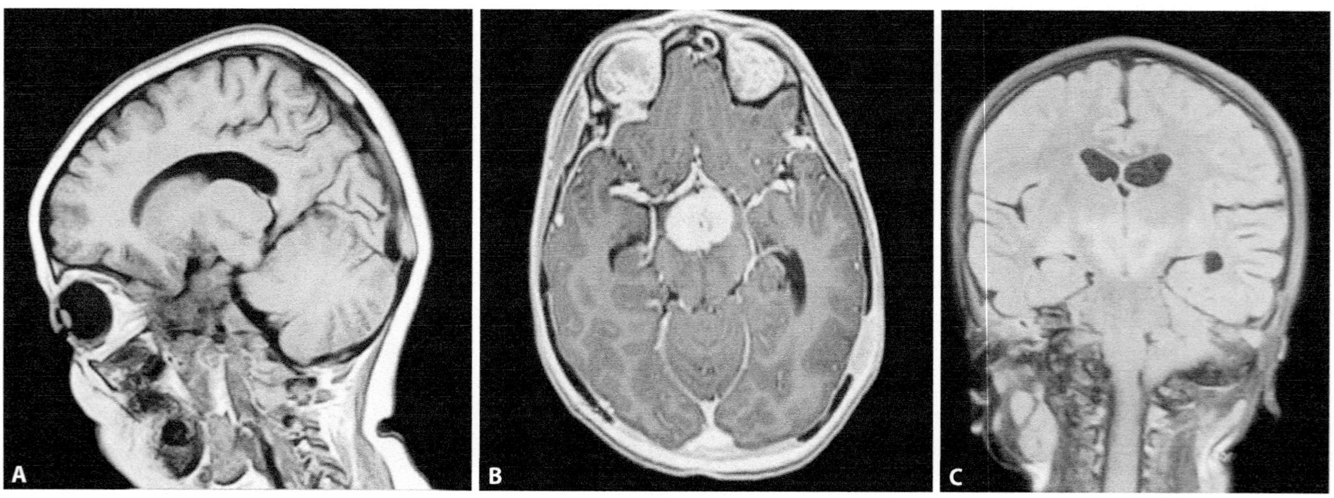

Figs. 28A to C: Magnetic resonance (MR) of same patient as Figure 27 with T1 sagittal image (A) and postcontrast axial MR images (B) showing enhancing T1 hypointense lesion in hypothalamus with multiple enhancing lesions in parietal bones. Coronal fluid-attenuated inversion-recovery (FLAIR) (C) image shows the presence of cervical lymphadenopathy.

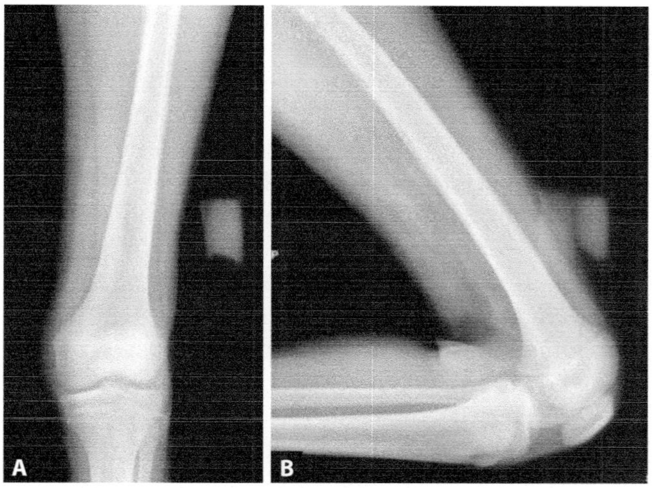

Figs. 29A and B: Acute osteomyelitis. X-ray of the left femur anteroposterior (AP) (A) and lateral view (B) in a 13-year-old girl showing subtle changes of acute osteomyelitis as evidenced by periosteal reaction, areas of osteolysis in the diaphysis, and blurred fat planes.

fat-saturated, STIR images as well as contrast-enhanced images. Fat-suppressed images increase the specificity and conspicuity of bony changes. Edema on STIR images and enhancement on contrast administration are the two most common findings in osteomyelitis **(Figs. 30A to D)**.

Acute osteomyelitis causes marrow replacement due to infiltration by inflammatory cells, hemorrhage, fibrin, debris, and edema. The margins are typically ill-defined against the surrounding marrow. Secondary signs of infection such as cellulitis, cortical disruption, sinus tracts, soft tissue abscesses, and periosteal reaction help establish the diagnosis of osteomyelitis.[2,3,61]

Healed osteomyelitis appears as localized fat replacement within red marrow.

Chronic osteomyelitis is defined as persistent infection after 1 month of treatment. On radiograph, it is seen as thickening and irregularity of cortex with mixed sclerotic and lucent areas. Involucrum and cloacae are also seen. It exhibits the same signal pattern as acute osteomyelitis, but

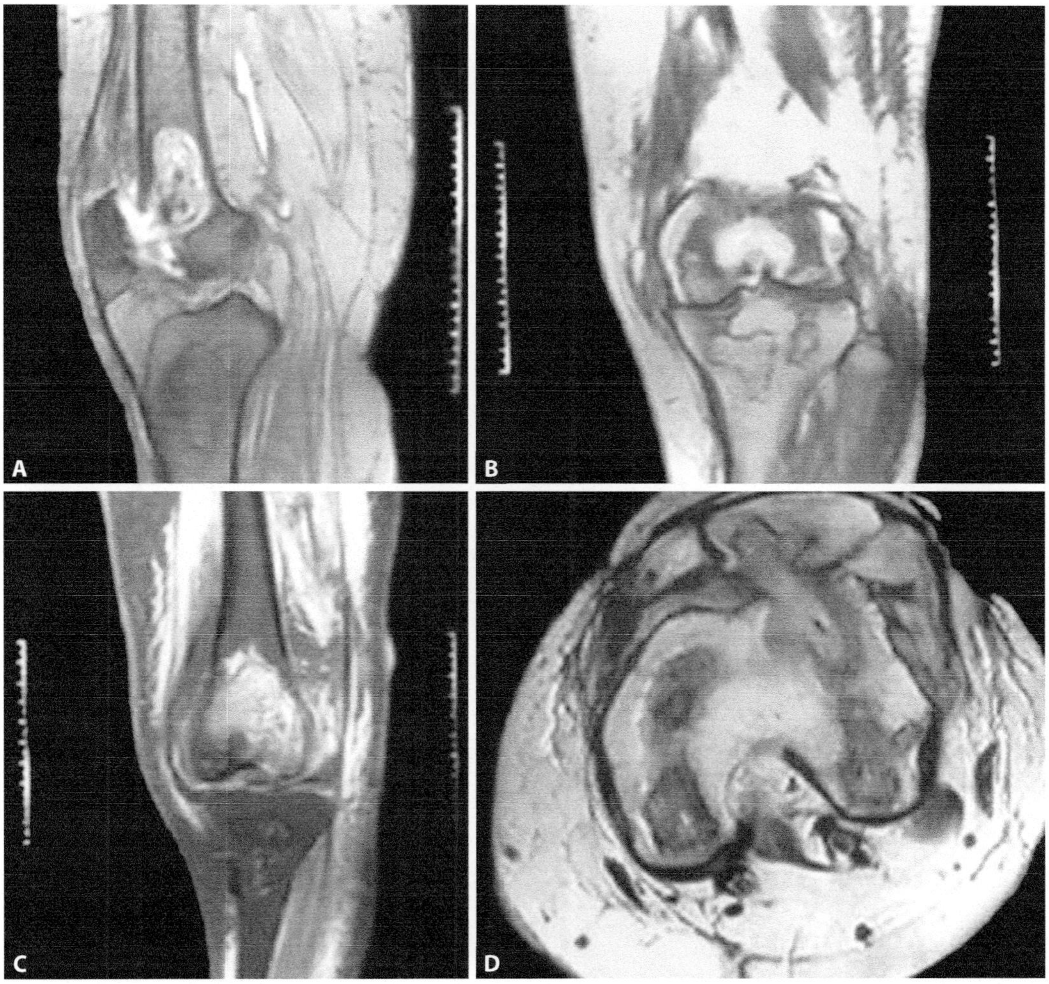

Figs. 30A to D: Chronic osteomyelitis of the femur with intramedullary abscess and associated infective arthritis. Fat-suppressed sagittal (A), T1 coronal (B), short tau inversion recovery (STIR) coronal (C) and T2 axial (D) magnetic resonance (MR) images of the knee showing an area of marrow signal alteration in the metadiaphyseal region of lower femur. Signal alteration is also seen in the patella and the upper end tibia. Cortical destruction with cloacae formation seen in anterior aspect of the femur, posterior aspect of the patella, and joint effusion with edema seen in the muscles.

the foci are surrounded by a sclerotic rim seen as a signal void, which clearly delineates the extent of the lesion. Sequestrated bone appears as a signal void, while infarct is seen as "double line" with associated muscle infarction.[61,62]

Malignant Marrow Replacement Disorder

Metastasis

Metastatic infiltration of the marrow occurs by hematogenous spread. The red marrow is predominantly affected because of its rich vascular supply. The most common metastasis in children are from neuroblastoma, rhabdomyosarcoma, and Ewing's sarcoma; while in adults, they are from the prostate, breast, lung, and kidney **(Figs. 31A to D)**. They are discussed in detail elsewhere in this book.

Lymphoma

Lymphomas are a heterogeneous group of tumors of the lymphoid tissue which can arise anywhere in the body. They arise more commonly from B lymphocytes than T lymphocytes.

Infiltration of bone marrow is found in 20–40% of patients with NHL and 5–15% of patients with Hodgkin lymphoma (HL).[63]

Risk factors for lymphoma include Epstein-Barr virus, immunosuppressant medications, severe autoimmune conditions, obesity, family history [human leukocyte antigen (HLA) subtype] and chronic *Helicobacter pylori* infection in the case of gastric mucosa-associated lymphoid tissue (MALT) lymphoma.[51] HL tends to affect young adults and adolescents, while the median age of diagnosis for NHL is 66 years.

Lymphoma is characterized as *primary osseous lymphoma* when bone is the only known site of disease for 6 months.[64] It accounts for <5% of all bone malignancies.[65] Synonyms for primary osseous lymphoma include reticulum cell malignant lymphoma of bone, sarcoma, and osteolymphoma.[66] Primary osseous lymphoma typically affects the metadiaphysis or diaphysis of long bones in

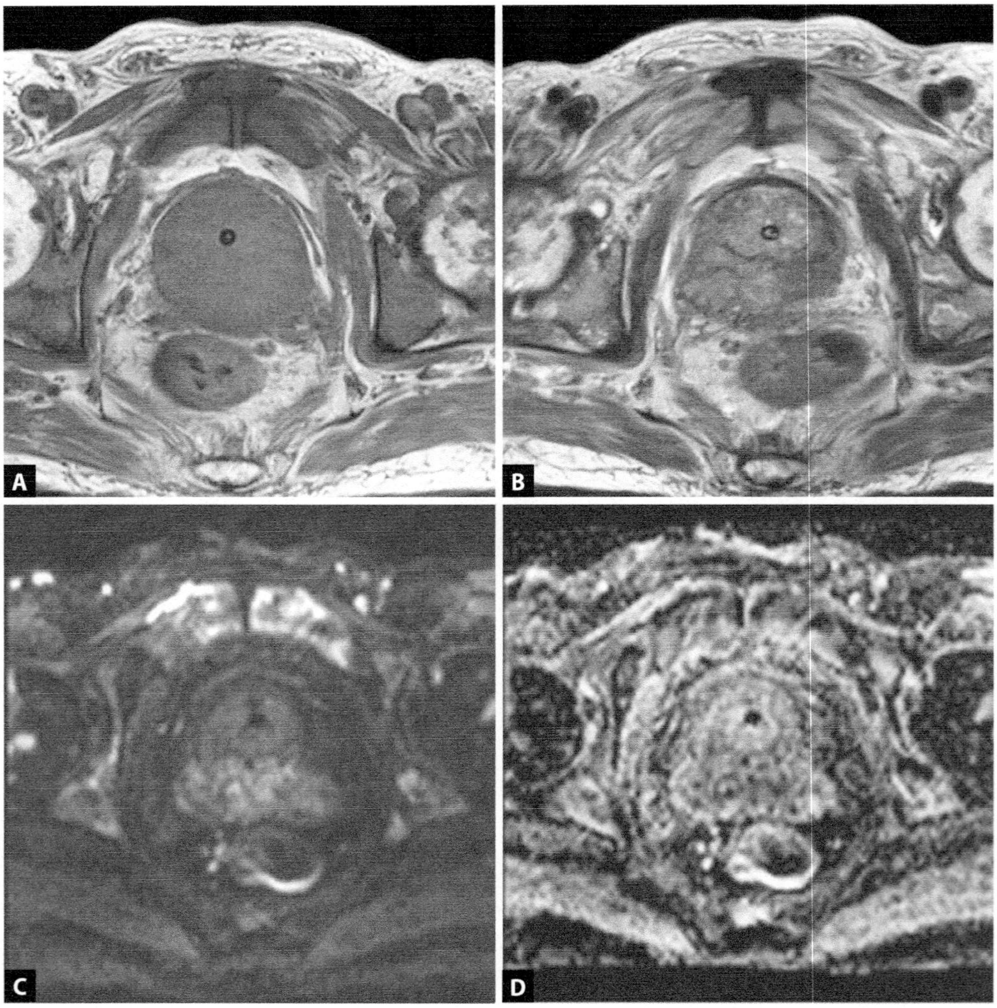

Figs. 31A to D: Metastases. T1 axial (A) and T2 axial magnetic resonance (MR) images (B) show hypointense marrow in the pelvic bones with the presence of restriction of diffusion (C and D) in a patient with skeletal metastases from carcinoma prostate.

the appendicular skeleton or the flat bones of the axial skeleton.

Secondary osseus lymphoma occurs due to metastatic spread from another primary site. Secondary or metastatic osseous lymphoma tends to favor the axial skeleton.[65]

Imaging: The findings on radiography can be subtle, nonspecific, or even inapparent. Osseus lymphoma is seen as the area of permeative osteolysis or mixed lytic sclerotic pattern with broad zone of transition. Periosteal reaction, when present, is usually aggressive and lamellar.[66] In the more common lytic destructive pattern, channels of bone loss can be seen parallel to long axis of bone with focal devascularization and sequestrum formation.[53] However, a bony sequestrum can also be seen in other conditions, such as radiation necrosis, osteomyelitis, osseous tuberculosis, and in tumors such as fibrosarcoma or eosinophilic granuloma. The mixed lytic-sclerotic pattern may be seen after therapeutic intervention and is more common in secondary osseous lymphoma.[66] Lymphoma should also be considered in the differential diagnosis for an ivory vertebrae or sclerotic vertebral lesion. A soft-tissue mass may be seen around an apparent intact or minimally involved cortical bone. This occurs due to spread through the Volkmann and haversian canals of bone cortex and may also be found in small cell malignancies.

At FDG-PET/CT, patterns of multifocal or focal uptake of ^{18}F-FDG on a background of diffuse uptake in bone marrow should be considered positive for bone marrow involvement. HL most commonly shows a multifocal pattern. Higher SUV has been correlated with more aggressive disease.[53] FDG-PET/CT is sensitive in detecting bone marrow involvement; with a pooled meta-analysis sensitivity of 88.7%.[67,68] The concordance rate for bone marrow biopsy and FDG-PET/CT is higher for more aggressive subtypes of lymphoma as compared to more indolent varieties.[69]

On the MR, patterns of bone marrow involvement in lymphoma can be diffuse or focal. These appear as areas of decreased signal intensity of T1W images and increased signal intensity on STIR images **(Figs. 32A to J)**. Contrast-enhanced studies show gadolinium enhancement of the lesions.[66,70] The nodular nature of lymphomatous marrow deposits allows MR mapping to select the site of biopsy because blind bone marrow biopsy may give false negative results.[7,8] In HL, marrow involvement is detected more often with MR than with marrow biopsy. In low-grade NHL, the involvement is diffuse, and biopsy is superior. In high-grade lymphomas, the involvement is more focal, and MRI is more efficient.[65]

The diagnosis of bone marrow involvement by lymphoma can be made by ^{18}F-FDG or with percutaneous biopsy, usually of the posterior iliac bone.[53] Currently, FDG-PET/CT is more widely used due to greater availability, although more research may prove ^{18}F-FDG-PET/MR and WBMRI to be useful, especially in patients who need protection from excess radiation, such as children and young women.[71]

There are many treatment regimens for NHL, including radiation therapy, chemotherapy, targeted drug therapy (e.g., rituximab), and peripheral blood stem cell or bone marrow transplant. Yttrium 90 (^{90}Y)-tagged ibritumomab tiuxetan is a beta-emitting radiopharmaceutical agent that is effective as an adjunct to chemotherapy and autologous stem cell transplant in treating certain cases of refractory NHL. ^{90}Y-tagged ibritumomab tiuxetan binds to the CD20 surface antigen, present in mature B lymphocytes, but not in precursor cells, and causes selective beta radiation-induced cell death.[72] Treatment of HL usually involves a combination of radiation therapy and chemotherapy, directed by the histologic grade and stage of the disease.[69]

MARROW DEPLETION

Myeloid depletion refers to the loss of hematopoietic tissue. Diffuse or regional absence of normal red marrow may occur as a consequence of aplastic anemia, chemotherapy, and/or radiation therapy.

Aplastic Anemia

Aplastic anemia is a pan myelopathy thought to result from suppression of the multipotent myeloid cells. The myeloid depletion manifests as cytopenia of the erythrocytes, leukocytes, and thrombocytes. There is a resultant decrease in the cellularity due to decrease in the hematopoietic marrow, which is replaced by fatty marrow.

Causes of aplastic anemia have not been identified yet but its provoking factors are viral infections, drugs, toxic substances, hepatitis, and unknown causes.[3,73]

Imaging

Two MRI patterns have been seen with aplastic anemia. One pattern is that of diffuse yellow marrow throughout the skeleton in areas where red marrow is expected to exist (**Figs. 33A and B**). This pattern may be difficult to recognize as abnormal in older individuals, in whom large proportions of fatty marrow are normal. The second pattern is seen in patients who have been treated for aplastic anemia and develop focal islands of red marrow regeneration scattered throughout the yellow marrow. These islands of red marrow can be very focal in appearance and may simulate other diseases. The hematopoietically active cell nests return mainly in the marrow space of the vertebral body.[3,73]

Treatment-related Changes

Chemotherapy, radiation, granulocyte colony-stimulating factor, and bone marrow transplant are routinely used in the treatment of neoplasms and can result in temporary or

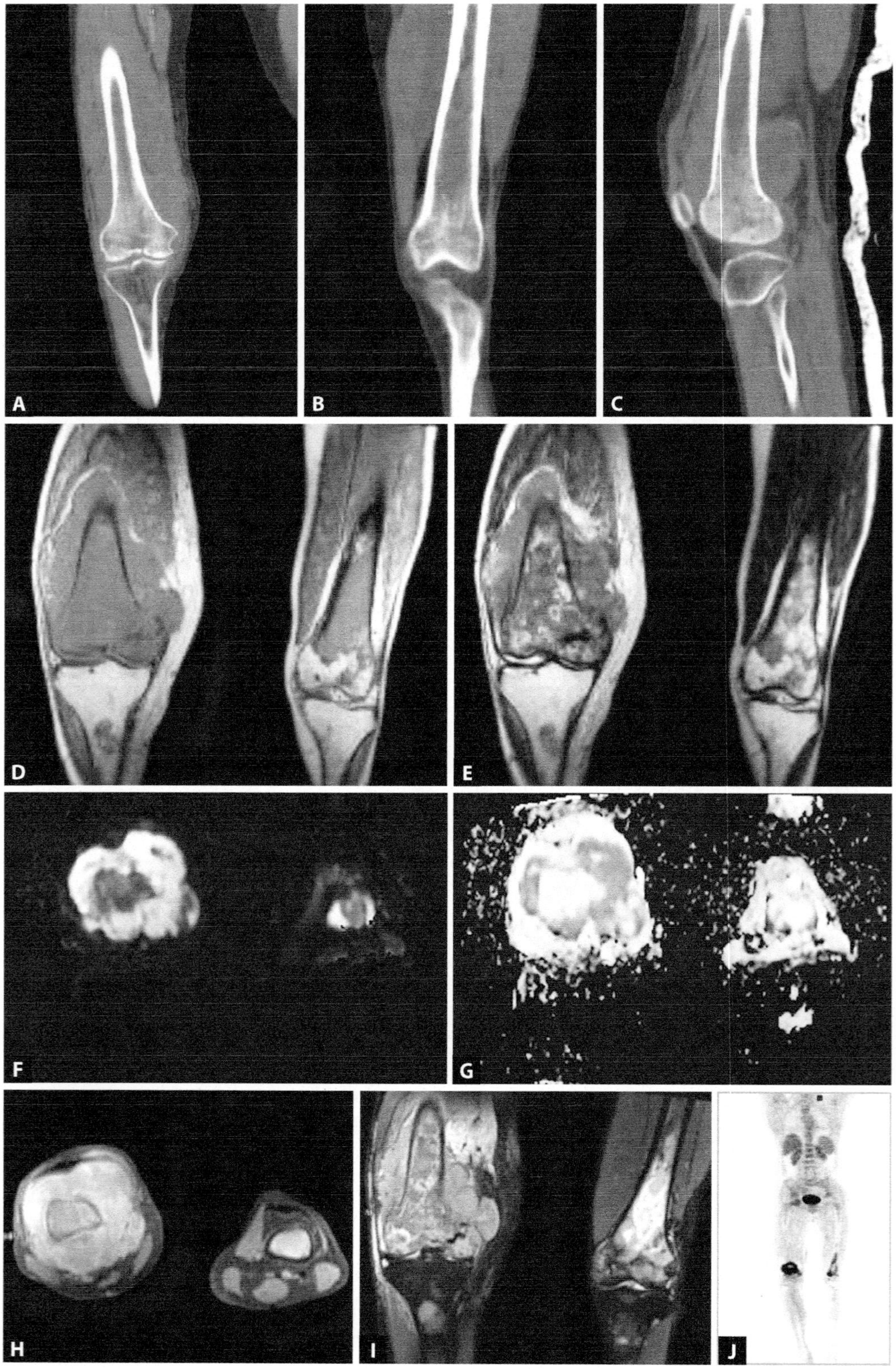

Figs. 32A to J: Lymphoma. Coronal (A and B) and sagittal (C) computed tomography (CT) images of right knee (bone window) show e/o an ill-defined permeative type of bony lesion involving femoral condyles and supracondylar region causing marrow expansion and erosion of the articular margin with heterogeneous soft tissue around the femoral shaft. Coronal T1-weighted (T1W) (D) and T2-weighted (T2W) (E) magnetic resonance (MR) images, respectively, showing the above described lesion appearing isointense on T1W image and hypointense on T2W image. Similar lesion is also noted in the distal left femur. There is associated soft tissue mass involving the muscles of various compartments with edema. The lesion is showing restricted diffusion (F and G). T1 fat saturation postgadolinium axial (H) and coronal (I) MR images show heterogeneous avid postcontrast enhancement in the lesion. Left femoral shaft also shows similar lesion. Coronal positron emission tomography (PET)-CT (J) image shows fluorodeoxyglucose (FDG) avid lesion in the bilateral femori.

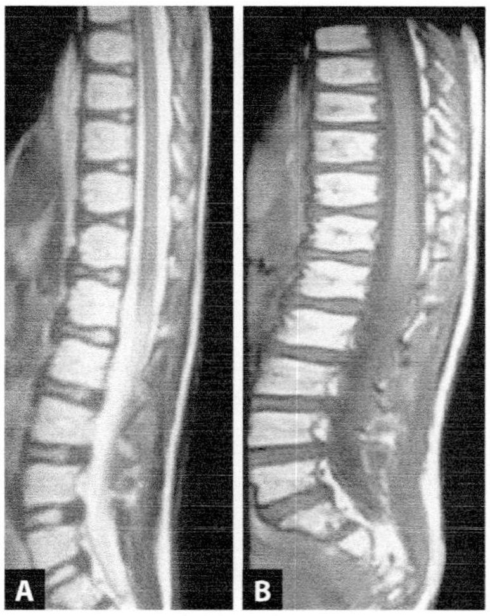

Figs. 33A and B: Aplastic anemia. Sagittal T2-weighted (T2W) (A) and sagittal T1-weighted (T1W) (B) magnetic resonance (MR) images of the dorsolumbar spine showing high-signal of the vertebral marrow on both T1W and T2W images s/o fatty marrow.

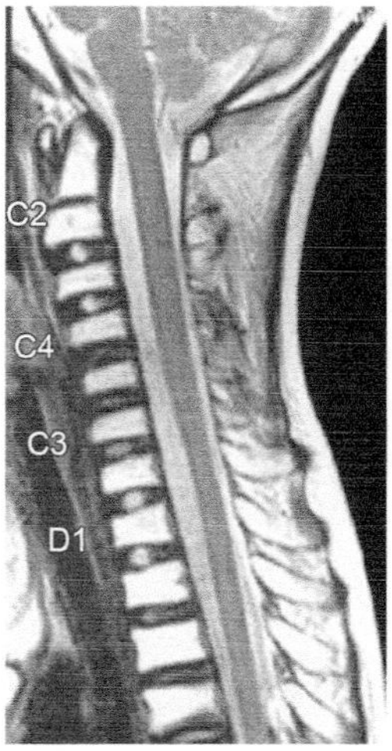

Fig. 34: T2-weighted (T2W) sagittal magnetic resonance (MR) image of the cervical spine in a case of carcinoma breast (postradiation) revealing increased signal in the vertebral marrow s/o fatty replacement.

permanent changes in marrow composition. It is crucial to understand the expected post-treatment changes for identifying recurrent or residual neoplastic marrow involvement.

Chemotherapy changes are diffuse and influenced by time duration since the last cycle. In the first week, increased dilatation and permeability of the sinusoids in marrow leads to edema. In the following weeks, the cytotoxic effect leads to fatty marrow transformation and reduction of myeloid precursors. Within 3–4 weeks, numerous small foci of red marrow may be seen due to regeneration.[74] There may be no changes in the MRI study of some patients receiving chemotherapy.

Granulocyte colony-stimulating factor is administered in conjunction with chemotherapy to stimulate myeloid cell production. Stimulation of red marrow proliferation typically occurs in a diffuse or patchy pattern and can mimic disease. The effect occurs rapidly, maximizes at 2 weeks, and normalizes 6 weeks after discontinuation of the growth factor.

Radiation therapy causes changes restricted to the region covered by the radiation port. Altered marrow signal intensity can occur in adjacent structures due to a combination of indirect effects and/or scattered radiation.[75,76] In the first 2 weeks, hemorrhage and edema is seen leading to a variable imaging appearance. After 3–6 weeks, there is preferential disappearance of the red marrow. After 6 weeks, the fatty marrow transformation becomes more homogeneous **(Fig. 34)**. Recovery of normal marrow signal intensity is largely dependent on the patient's age and the radiation dose. Younger patients and patients receiving <30–40 Gy are more likely to recover with full marrow regeneration. At doses >40–50 Gy, little or no regeneration occurs due to sinusoidal destruction.[77] Complications after radiation therapy include growth disturbance in the skeletally immature, osteonecrosis, insufficiency fractures, and secondary radiation-induced benign and malignant neoplasms, most commonly osteochondroma and osteosarcoma.

Bone marrow transplant involves ablation of the patient's native marrow and infusion of either autologous or allogenic stem cells to reconstitute a new marrow free of neoplastic cells. 2–4 weeks after stem cell infusion, a peripheral band-like pattern of mildly increased T1W signal intensity relative to muscle appears, which reflects regenerating hematopoietic cells repopulating along the subendosteal sinusoids. In other areas, a multifocal pattern with numerous small foci of red marrow can be present. Post-transplant changes typically stabilize by 3 months. In patients with successfully reconstituted marrow, T1W signal intensity often remains increased compared with that of age-matched controls.[74]

Angiogenesis-inhibiting drugs, such as thalidomide, depend on neovascularization to be useful for treating hematologic malignancy; these agents were added to some treatment regimens for patients with advanced myeloma. The antiangiogenesis is intended to stop cancer progression by suppressing tumor recruitment of new blood supply. One sign of a response to this treatment is a rather delayed, less steep, and smaller bone marrow enhancement after intravenous administration of small molecular Gd-chelates, compared to pretreatment studies.

Treatment effects of various chemotherapeutic regimen on the bone marrow in patients with leukemia and lymphoma can be detected with ^{31}PMR spectroscopy. The treatment-induced change in tumor pH with an alkaline shift is related temporally to increases in the phosphodiester/beta-adenosine triphosphate ratio and occurs before alterations in tumor size are documented. The changes in the ^{31}PMR spectral profile can also be detected by investigations of serum of the patients.[74]

VASCULAR ABNORMALITIES (HYPEREMIA AND ISCHEMIA)

The underlying cause of extracellular bone marrow edema is usually hyperemia. Different clinical abnormalities may lead to localized bone marrow edema, including trauma, transient osteoporosis of the hip, regional migratory osteoporosis, complex regional pain syndrome, osteonecrosis (early), infection, tumors, and joint abnormalities.

The MRI appearance of marrow edema is that of intermediate-signal intensity on T1W images, and very high-signal intensity on T2W images. The signal characteristics are the result of yellow marrow cells intermixed with the edema fluid. It has a heterogeneous appearance without a discrete pattern. Tumor and infection generally have edema at the periphery of the underlying lesion.

Trauma

Bone Contusion

Direct or indirect trauma can involve the bone marrow, and mild marrow changes have been termed as bone bruises. These can be caused by edema, hemorrhage, and hyperemia. Conventional radiographs are generally normal. On MR, these are seen as geographic areas of decreased signal intensity on T1W and increased signal intensity on T2W images **(Figs. 35A and B)**. Bone bruises are most often seen in the juxta-articular and subchondral areas of the distal femur and proximal tibia in association with ligamentous and meniscal injuries. Bone bruises resolve within 6–9 weeks.

Occult Fractures

These are trabecular bone microfractures which may be diagnosed on MR in the absence of conventional radiographic signs. The use of STIR or a fat-suppressed T2W sequence is helpful for screening for an occult fracture. These subchondral occult fractures are well seen as a linear signal void on all sequences surrounded by an ill-defined band of decreased signal intensity on T1W, and increased signal intensity on T2W images[78] **(Figs. 36A and B)**.

Stress Fractures

Stress fractures are caused by an imbalance between the strength of the bone and the stress applied. These may be seen after marching, jogging, chronic cough, etc.[79]

Conventional radiographs show a juxtacortical transverse or oblique sclerotic band with a thin radiolucent line within this band. MRI can visualize the pathophysiologic changes accompanying a stress fracture. This consists of a band-like signal void surrounded by marrow edema. The signal void band represents trabecular microfractures and intratrabecular callus formation.

Differentiation of stress fractures from occult intraosseous fractures is difficult. Stress fractures are almost always metaphyseal or diaphyseal, while occult fractures are typically subchondral or epiphyseal and have a precipitating cause.

Transient Osteoporosis

Mainly young and middle-aged men are affected by transient osteoporosis of the hip/painful bone marrow

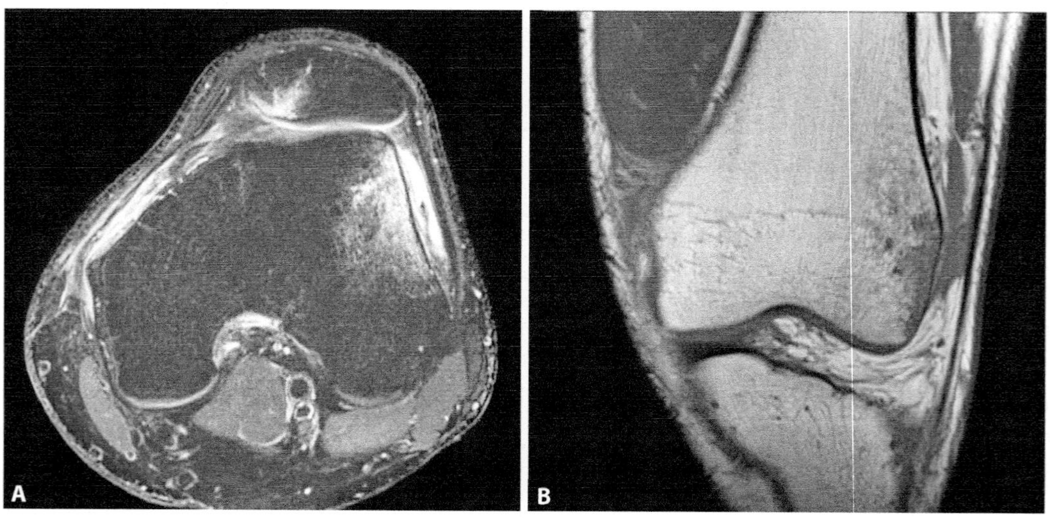

Figs. 35A and B: Contusion. Short tau inversion recovery (STIR) axial (A) magnetic resonance (MR) image showing focal areas of increased signal intensity in lateral femoral condyle and medial aspect of patella due to kissing contusion caused by transient patellar subluxation. T1 coronal image (B) showing area of hypointensity in that area in lateral femoral condyle.

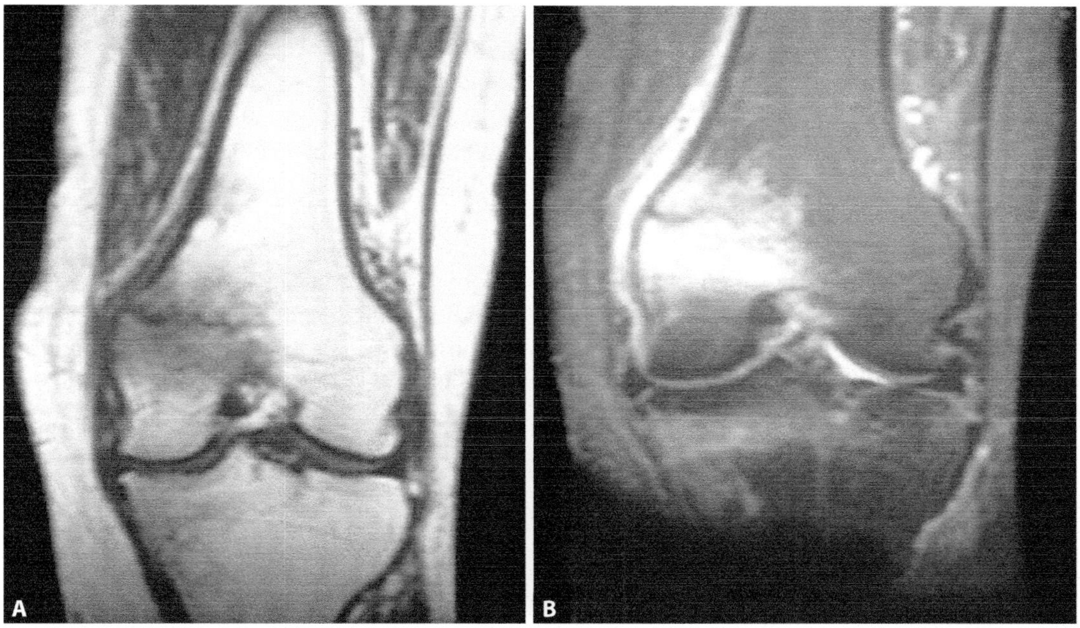

Figs. 36A and B: Occult fracture knee. T1-weighted (T1W) coronal (A) and short tau inversion recovery (STIR) coronal (B) magnetic resonance (MR) images of the knee showing a linear fracture line in the medial femoral condyle with surrounding bone marrow edema in a case where X-ray of knee appeared normal.

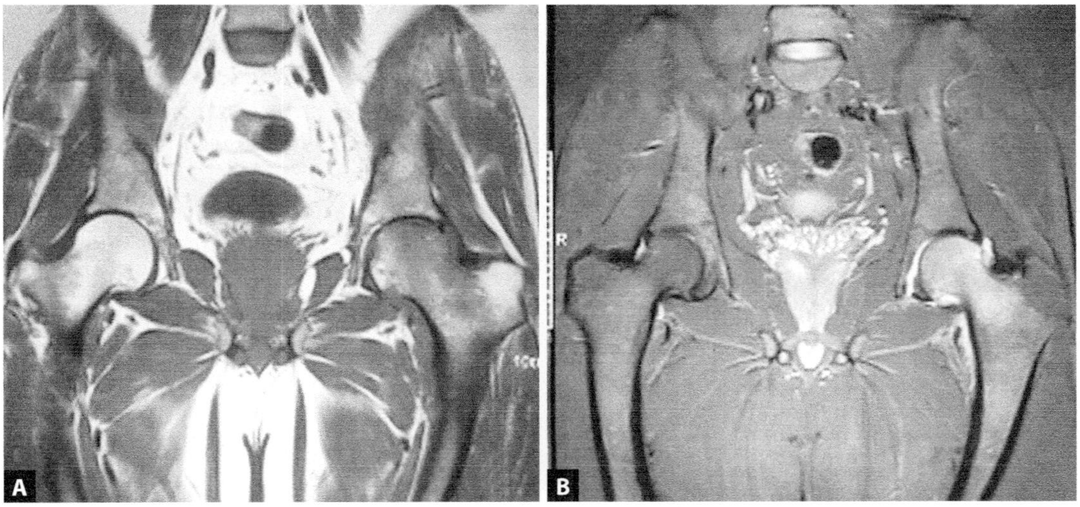

Figs. 37A and B: Transient osteoporosis. T1 coronal (A) and short tau inversion recovery (STIR) coronal (B) magnetic resonance (MR) images showing the area of reduced intensity on T1 and increased intensity on STIR image in proximal metaphysis and epiphyses of left femur.

edema syndrome. Women with transient osteoporosis of the hip are often affected in the last trimester of pregnancy, with a predilection for the left hip. Osteoporosis may also be severe enough to cause fracture.

Imaging: The joint space remains normal, but joint effusions are common. Bone marrow edema usually affects the femoral head and neck, down to the intertrochanteric region. Follow-up studies show resolution of edema and osteoporosis as the clinical symptoms subside in 3–12 months **(Figs. 37A and B)**.[80-82]

Regional Migratory Osteoporosis

Regional migratory osteoporosis has the same MRI and clinical features as transient osteoporosis of the hip. The major difference is that abnormalities are not confined to the hip and are migratory in nature. The subchondral regions of the knee, ankle, and hip, each may be affected in turn, and both extremities may be involved over several years. Spontaneous recovery also occurs in this entity.

The pathogenesis of transient osteoporosis of the hip and regional migratory osteoporosis is unknown, but clinical similarities to reflex sympathetic dystrophy syndrome are striking. The MRI findings for all of these entities are compatible with ischemic changes of the small vessels that supply proximal nerve roots, with a majorly distal loss of control of the normal vascular supply, leading to localized hyperemia.

The relationship between transient osteoporosis of the hip and regional migratory osteoporosis to osteonecrosis is unclear. Biopsy of these lesions shows areas of bone necrosis. There have been reports of typical changes of transient osteoporosis of the hip that, rather than undergoing spontaneous resolution, went on to develop typical MRI and biopsy changes of osteonecrosis in the femoral heads. It is unclear why this should occur and in which patients.

Imaging: MR findings include patchy areas of intermediate-signal intensity (isointense or higher than muscle or disc) on T1W images that become bright on T2W images.

Complex Regional Pain Syndrome

Complex regional pain syndrome affects children aged 5–17 years, and is more common amongst adolescent girls.[44] Inciting events include fracture (in up to 40% of cases), blunt trauma, and surgery. It occurs due to sensitization of nociceptive receptors and subsequent hyperalgesia consequent to an increased inflammatory or immune response. Abnormal sudomotor and vasomotor function in the form of skin discoloration, temperature changes, hyperhidrosis, and edema occurs due to sympathetic dysfunction. Muscle contractures and loss of function may occur in the late stages.

Imaging: Within 2–8 weeks, patchy subchondral and subperiosteal osteopenia can be seen, which progresses to diffuse severe periarticular osteopenia. In adults, upper extremity involvement is more common, whereas in children, the lower extremity is five times more likely to be affected.

Magnetic resonance imaging demonstrates extensive subcortical and patchy marrow edema with occasional articular erosions in the acute stage. Extraosseous manifestations include skin thickening, muscle atrophy, joint effusion, and periarticular soft-tissue edema. In some cases, the abnormal findings may be limited only to the soft tissues.

In the chronic stages, there is periarticular soft-tissue atrophy. The imaging appearance is nonspecific and often overlaps with those of altered and disuse biomechanics. A complex treatment may result in favorable outcome in 1–43% of patients.[38]

Ischemia

The causes of ischemia of bone marrow are numerous and include traumatic disruption of the blood supply, steroids, sickle cell anemia, hyperglobulinemia, GD, alcoholism, pancreatitis, dysbaric causes, systemic lupus erythematosus, and others. Many clinicians refer to ischemic changes in the epiphyses as AVN and to changes in the shafts of bone as bone infarction. The MRI findings are similar, regardless of location of the lesions. Osteonecrosis most commonly affects areas where yellow marrow (with its poor vascular supply) predominates the epiphyses and diaphyses of long bones. Hematopoietic cells die within the first 6 hours of anoxia, while osteocytes, osteoblasts, and osteoclasts survive for up to 48 hours. Fat cells become vulnerable in 2–5 days following the insult. An adequate circulation allows repair to begin with a fibrous demarcation of necrotic area.

Imaging: On radiography, there is initial minor osteopenia. Gradually, microfractures of the subchondral bone accumulate in the dead bone, which is unable to repair leading to collapse of the articular surface. Eventually, the cortex collapses and fragments, with superimposed secondary degenerative change.

The MRI appearance of osteonecrosis varies based on the age and stage of the lesion. The earliest manifestation seen with MRI is a nonspecific focal area of what looks like marrow edema-intermediate-signal intensity on T1W images and high-signal intensity on T2W images, in the typical anatomic locations for infarction, i.e., in the epiphyses and diametaphyses. This pattern rapidly progresses to a distinctive, well-defined pattern that allows a specific diagnosis to be made.

A characteristic, low-signal intensity serpentine rim develops in >90% of cases on T1W and T2W images. This serpentine line represents the interface at the junction between the living and the dead bone. This is the site of active bone repair, where a new bone and an advancing front of granulation tissue is seen histologically. In approximately 80% of cases of osteonecrosis, a high-signal intensity line is present on T2W images, just inside the low-signal intensity serpentine line, producing the *double-line sign* **(Figs. 38A and B)**. This line probably occurs as a result of chemical shift misregistration or perhaps reflects the pathologic changes at the reactive bone interface. A "double line" sign consisting of two parallel stripes of low- and high-signal indicates irreversibility.[2,83]

The area of bone within the infarcted segment usually has signal intensity identical to fat. Occasionally, the infarcted bone has signal that is low intensity on T1W images and high signal on T2W images (edema), or low-signal intensity on T1W and T2W images (fibrosis, sclerosis, and trabecular collapse). Due to partial blood supply to the peripheral marrow cavity, the infarct exhibits a peripheral line, with a subcortical double contour giving the "bone-in-bone" appearance. Symptoms tend to be least severe in lesions that are isointense with fat and most

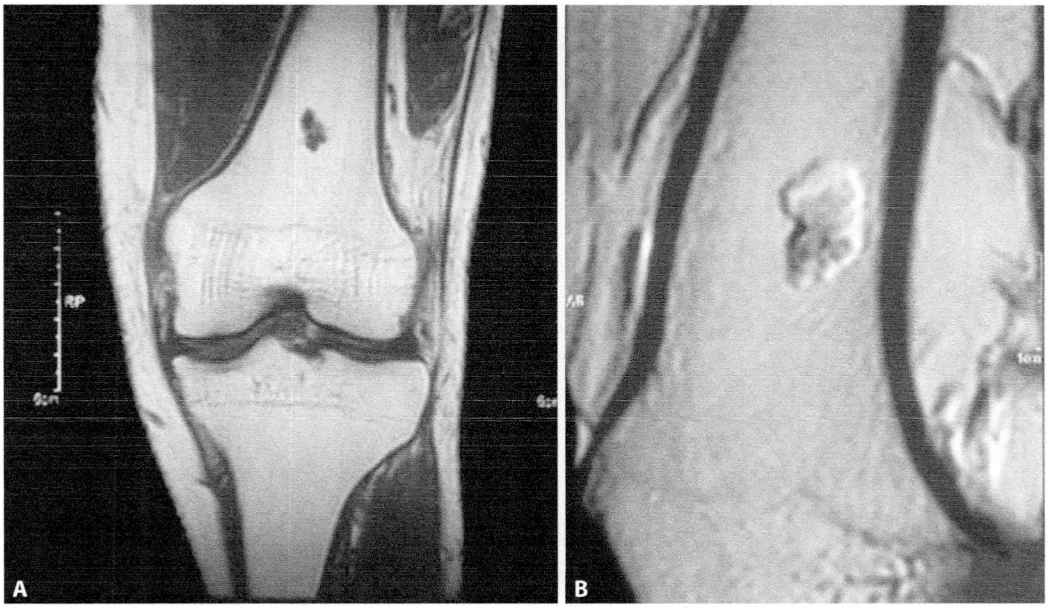

Figs. 38A and B: Osteonecrosis. T1-weighted (T1W) coronal magnetic resonance (MR) image (A) showing a geographic hypointense lesion in distal femoral metaphysis. T2-weighted (T2W) coronal MR (B) image showing hyperintense line inside the low-signal intensity line suggestive of "double line" sign.

severe in lesions with low-signal intensity on all pulse sequences. Joint effusions are usually present in cases of painful osteonecrosis that involve the epiphysis of a bone that makes up the joint.

Magnetic resonance imaging can be used to determine the volume and location of bone involved with osteonecrosis. MRI also can show if there is a collapse of the bone or if degenerative changes are present. Infarcts may become infected leading to osteomyelitis.[83]

MISCELLANEOUS MARROW DISEASES

There is an important group of abnormalities that affect bone marrow, but these abnormalities do not fit neatly into the other categories of marrow disease. This group includes Gaucher's disease (GD), Paget's disease, osteopetrosis, hemosiderosis, and serous atrophy (gelatinous transformation) of marrow.

Gaucher's Disease

Gaucher's disease is the most common lysosomal storage disorder which is caused by a genetic deficiency of glucocerebrosidase, leading to an increase in the deposition of glucosylceramide in macrophages in the brain, spleen, liver, and bone marrow. Consequently, these macrophages get enlarged with a build-up of glycolipids, and are called Gaucher cells. About 80% of patients with GD have skeletal abnormalities.

Imaging

On radiography, an array of bone findings is seen in GD, including growth retardation in children, osteopenia, lytic lesions, pathologic fractures, osteonecrosis, cortical and medullary infarcts. Marrow replacement with Gaucher cells can lead to the expansion of the medullary cavity with thinning of the cortex, endosteal scalloping, and Erlenmeyer flask deformity in distal femori. Nonskeletal manifestations include hepatomegaly and splenomegaly. Focal splenic masses are common and may represent clusters of Gaucher cells or extramedullary hematopoiesis. They may be detected with sonography, CT or MRI.

Magnetic resonance imaging can be used in the early diagnosis of GD and for demonstrating improvement after enzyme therapy. Accumulation of Gaucher cells leads to osteoporosis, localized destruction, and ischemic necrosis. Infiltration of the marrow increases the T1 relaxation time and shortens the T2 relaxation time causing a low-signal intensity of the affected marrow on both T1W and T2W images. These appearances are similar to those in other infiltrative processes but the low-signal intensity on T2W images allows differentiation from tumor processes. This low-signal intensity is due to fibrosis.[1,2,84] Bone marrow infiltration starts proximally and increasingly affects more peripheral areas of the appendicular skeleton. Bone marrow infarction is also a typical finding related to GD and is characterized by a serpiginous pattern with a bright signal in fat-saturated T2W or STIR sequences. Erlenmeyer flask deformities of the distal femora are obvious on MRI.

Other causes of bone marrow changes with osteonecrosis include sickle cell anemia, Waldenström macroglobulinemia, and marrow disorders treated with steroid.

Treatment of GD may consist of administration of an enzyme to break down the glucocerebroside. MRI is often used for monitoring the changes in the liver, spleen, and marrow in these patients. Decreased amounts of marrow infiltration are evident on serial images in patients who respond to the therapy.

Iron Overload (Hemosiderosis)

This disorder occurs due to hemosiderin (iron) deposition in macrophages located in the bone marrow and other organs. Causes include chronic breakdown of red blood cells (sickle cell anemia and thalassemia), chronic blood transfusions, metabolic abnormalities in chronic inflammatory disorders, and acquired immunodeficiency syndrome (AIDS).

Imaging

The iron deposition can be patchy or uniform in distribution involving the pelvis, spine, and metaphysis or diaphysis of long bones. On MRI, the marrow appears hypointense on T2W and gradient recalled echo (GRE) images. In severe hemosiderosis, the signal also decreases on T1W images. Excessive iron deposition can cause nearly a complete signal loss resulting in a "black marrow" **(Figs. 39A to C)**.[26,36] Sickle cell disease can be further complicated by bone infarction. The liver and spleen have the same low-signal intensity as bone marrow, which helps to distinguish this process from similar appearing diseases on MRI.

Paget's Disease

Paget's disease of bone (PDB), also known as osteitis deformans, was originally described by Sir James Paget in 1877. It is a chronic disorder characterized by excessive and abnormal remodeling of bone, often leading to osseous deformities. PDB has osteolytic and osteoblastic phases, with the lytic phase predominating early on in the course of the disease process. It primarily affects the pelvis, spine, skull, and femur. PDB is polyostotic in 66% cases. The etiology is unclear but likely multifactorial. There is epidemiologic data to support an autosomal dominant trait and a possible causative role of paramyxoviral infection.

Paget's disease affects the aging population, with affected individuals usually older than 55 years at diagnosis. Patients younger than 40 years are rarely affected. The prevalence of PDB varies greatly between different countries.

Imaging

On radiography, the classically described radiological appearance is an expanded bone with a coarsened trabecular pattern. Plain radiographic features will depend upon the phase of the disease. The early phase features osteolytic (lucent) regions which are later followed by coarsened trabeculae and bony enlargement. Sclerotic changes occur much later in the disease process.

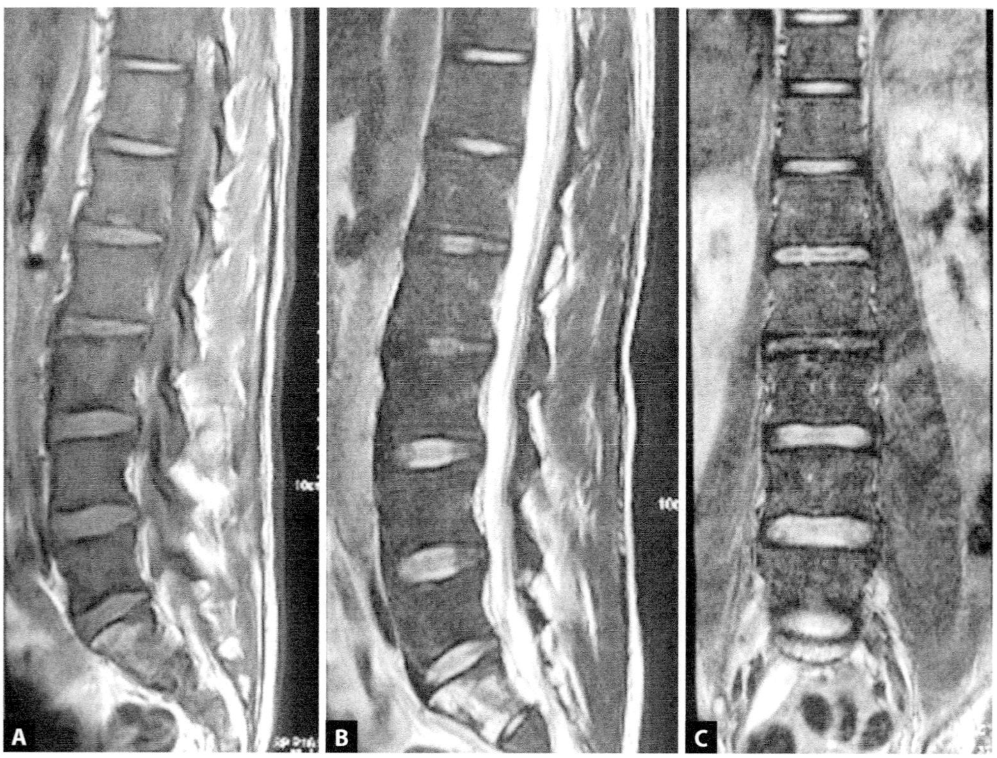

Figs. 39A to C: Hemosiderosis. T1-weighted (T1W) sagittal (A), T2-weighted (T2W) sagittal (B) and short tau inversion recovery (STIR) coronal (C) magnetic resonance (MR) images showing diffuse reduction in signal intensity of marrow.

Additional destructive features may become apparent if malignant transformation occurs.

Characteristic vertebral body findings have been described as "picture frame" appearance secondary to central osteopenia and a peripheral coarse and thickened trabecular pattern. Findings may also include increased size and diffuse sclerosis of the vertebral body, referred to as "ivory" vertebra. Vertebral enlargement could lead to neural foraminal and/or central canal stenosis with associated neurologic symptoms.

Bone scan is highly sensitive but not specific and may aid with polyostotic disease. There is marked increased uptake in all phases of the disease, although in the burnt-out sclerotic quiescent phase uptake may be normal.

Common MRI findings in pagetic bone include areas of normal high-signal intensity from fat and areas of intermediate- or low-signal intensity on T1W images due to fibrovascular connective tissue, dilated vascular channels, or uncalcified osteoid. Thick bone trabeculae and cortical bone can be seen but not as easily as on conventional radiographs or CT. Areas of active lysis demonstrate increased T2 signal intensity. Contrast-enhanced CT or MRI may demonstrate significant marrow enhancement in the active or lytic phase. There is preservation of the normal marrow in unaffected areas.

Secondary complications of Paget's disease include basilar invagination, kyphoscoliosis, fractures due to bone softening, extramedullary hematopoiesis, and congestive heart failure. If there is interval change in imaging characteristics, soft tissue component, or increasing pain, further cross-sectional contrast-enhanced imaging should be performed to evaluate for rare sarcoma formation. Osteosarcoma is the most common type of sarcoma associated with Paget's disease, representing approximately 50% of cases.[85] Sarcomatous transformation is highly fatal, with a 3-year mortality rate >90%.[86]

Differential diagnosis for Paget's disease involving the spine includes metastatic disease and vertebral hemangioma. Although PDB has a distribution similar to metastatic disease, greater involvement of the ribs has been described with the former. There is also typically no enlargement of the affected osseous structures with metastatic disease. However, sometimes the distinction is difficult and biopsy is necessary. Vertebral hemangiomas have a delicate trabecular pattern, in contrast to the coarse and enlarged trabecular pattern seen in pagetoid bone. Additionally, typical vertebral hemangiomas demonstrate high T1- and T2-signal intensity on MRI.

Alkaline phosphatase, which reflects the level of new bone formation, is used as an adjunct in the diagnosis and also plays a role in evaluating treatment response. However, it is nonspecific and values are normal in up to 15% of symptomatic patients with monostotic disease. Disease activity and response to therapy can be followed with measurements of alkaline phosphatase and other serum markers.

Treatment of PDB is mostly targeted at symptomatic relief with analgesic medication. Medications that inhibit osteoclastic activity (e.g., bisphosphonate) also play a role. Surgical intervention is sometimes needed.

MAGNETIC RESONANCE APPROACH TO MARROW DISEASE

An attempt at systematic approach toward categorization of the bone marrow lesions has been made in the past. One of the articles by Del Grande et al.[87] divides the bone marrow lesions into three categories based on the imaging appearances as described in **Table 9**. Category I includes

Table 9: MRI characteristics of various categories of bone marrow lesions.

MR technique	*MR sequences*	*Category 1*	*Category 2*	*Category 3*
Conventional	T1W SE	Signal intensity > muscle	Signal intensity < muscle/disc	Heterogeneous signal intensity
	PD-W/T2W TSE	Signal intensity approaching or similar to fat	Signal intensity approaching or similar to fat	Heterogeneous
	STIR/T2 fat sat	Increased signal intensity—generally no focal lesions	Increased signal intensity, focal lesions	Heterogeneous with or without focal lesions
	Postcontrast T1W	Minimal enhancement	Intense enhancement	Minimal or no enhancement
Problem-solving techniques	CSI	>20% signal loss on out-of-phase imaging	Neoplasm <20% signal loss on out of phase imaging. Infection: signal loss on out-of-phase imaging	>20% signal loss on out-of-phase imaging
	DWI	Usually no diffusion restriction	Neoplasm/pus-diffusion restriction	Usually no diffusion restriction
	MRS	No choline peak	Neoplasm–choline peak	No choline peak

(CSI: chemical shift imaging; DWI: diffusion-weighted imaging; MR: magnetic resonance; MRS: magnetic resonance spectroscopy; PD: proton density; SE: spin echo; STIR: short tau inversion recovery; T1W: T1-weighted; T2W: T2-weighted)

bone marrow lesions related to trauma, insufficiency injury, aseptic necrosis, biomechanical, disuse, CRPS, transient osteoporosis of hip, or degenerative/inflammatory etiologies. Category II includes aggressive processes, such as infections or neoplastic conditions. Category III includes pathologies with complex/mixed phenomena, such as metabolic, hematopoietic, treated infiltrative malignancies, human immunodeficiency virus (HIV) treatment-associated lipodystrophy, serous marrow lesions, and Paget's disease.

CONCLUSION

Imaging characteristics of normal bone marrow change throughout life and familiarity with these changes is important to correctly approach bone marrow pathology. Neoplastic disease of the bone marrow is a frequent pathology and has different morphologic patterns. For standard imaging of bone marrow, T1W and STIR sequences are the fundamental sequences. The addition of newer imaging techniques and advances in MRI has enabled a better characterization of the various pathologies and helped in narrowing the differential diagnosis.

REFERENCES

1. Moore SG, Bisset GS III, Siegal MJ, Donaldson JS. Pediatric musculoskeletal MR imaging. Radiology. 1991;179(2):345-60.
2. Siegel MJ, Luker GD. Bone marrow imaging in children. Magn Reson Imaging Clin N Am. 1996;4(4):771-96.
3. Vogler JB III, Murphy WA. Bone marrow imaging. Radiology. 1988;168(3):679-93.
4. Waitches SG, Zanvin JK, Poznanski AK. Sequences and rate of bone marrow conversion in the femora of children as seen on MR imaging: Are accepted standards accurate? Am J Roentgenol. 1994;162(6):1399-406.
5. Cohen MD, Klatte EC, Baehner R, Smith JA, Martin-Simmerman P, Carr BE, et al. Magnetic resonance imaging of bone marrow disease in children. Radiology. 1984;151(3):715-8.
6. Małkiewicz A, Dziedzic M. Bone marrow reconversion - imaging of physiological changes in bone marrow. Pol J Radiol. 2012;77(4):45-50.
7. Mettler FA, Guiberteau MJ. Essentials of Nuclear Medicine Imaging, 5th edition. Philadelphia: Saunders/Elsevier; 2006.
8. Tian R, Su M, Tian Y, Li F, Li L, Kuang A, et al. Dual-time point PET/CT with F-18 FDG for the differentiation of malignant and benign bone lesions. Skeletal Radiol. 2009;38(5):451-8.
9. Mirowitz SA, Apicella P, Reinus WR, Hammerman AM. MR imaging of bone marrow lesions: Relative conspicuousness on T1-weighted, fat-suppressed T2-weighted, and STIR images. Am J Roentgenol 1994;162(1):215-21.
10. Helms CA, Major NM, Andersson MW, Kaplan PA, Dussault R. Musculoskeletal MRI, 2nd edition. Philadelphia: Saunders Elsevier; 2009. pp. 20-49.
11. Moore DG, Dawson KL. Red and yellow marrow in the femur: Age-related changes in the appearance at MR imaging. Radiology.1990;175(1):219-23.
12. Dooms GC, Fischer MR, Hricak H, Richardson M, Crooks LE, Genant HK. Bone marrow imaging: Magnetic resonance studies related to age and sex. Radiology.1985;155(2):429-32.
13. Taccone A, Oddone M, Dell Acqua AD, Occhi M, Ciccone MA. MRI "road map' of normal age-related bone marrow: Thorax, pelvis and extremities. Pediatric Radiology.1995;25(8):596-606.
14. Sebag GH, Dubois J, Tabet M, Bonato A, Lallemand D. Pediatric spinal bone marrow: Assessment of normal age-related changes in the MRI appearance. Pediatr Radiol 1993;23(7):515-8.
15. Mirowitz SA. Hematopoietic bone marrow within the proximal humeral epiphysis in normal adults: Investigation with MR imaging. Radiology 1993;188(3):689-93.
16. Jones KM, Unger EC, Granstrom P, et al. Bone marrow imaging using STIR at 0.5 and 1-5T. Magn Reson Imaging.1992;10(2):169-76.
17. Zajick DC, Morrison WB, Schweitzer ME, Parellada JA, Carrino JA. Benign and malignant processes: Normal values and differentiation with chemical shift MR imaging in vertebral marrow. Radiology. 2005;237(2):590-6.
18. Glover GH. Multipoint Dixon technique for water and fat proton and susceptibility imaging. J Magn Reson Imaging. 1991;1(5):521-30.
19. Subhawong TK, Jacobs MA, Fayad LM. Diffusion-weighted MR imaging for characterizing musculoskeletal lesions. RadioGraphics. 2014;34(5):1163-77.
20. Karampinos DC, Melkus G, Baum T, Bauer JS, Rummeny EJ, Krug R. Bone marrow fat quantification in the presence of trabecular bone:initial comparison between water-fat imaging and single-voxel MRS, Magn Reson Med. 2014;71(3):1158-65.
21. Herrmann J, Krstin N, Schoennagel BP, Sornsakrin M, Derlin T, Busch JD, et al. Age-related distribution of vertebral bone-marrow diffusivity. Eur J Radiol 2012;81(12):4046-9.
22. Byun WM, Shin SO, Chany Y, Lee SJ, Finsterbusch J, Frahm J. Diffusion weighted MR imaging of metastatic disease of the spine: assessment of response to therapy. AJNR. 2002;23:906-12.
23. Zhang J, Cheng K, Ding Y, Liang W, Ding Y, Vanel D, et al. Study of single voxel 1H MR spectroscopy of bone tumors: Differentiation of benign from malignant tumors. Eur J Radiol. 2013;82(12):2124-8.
24. Fayad LM, Bluemke DA, McCarthy EF, Weber KL, Barker PB, Jacobs MA. Musculoskeletal tumors: Use of proton MR spectroscopic imaging for characterization. J Magn Reson Imaging. 2006;23(1):23-8.
25. Vande Berg BC, Lecouvet FE, Galant C, Simoni P, Malghem J. Normal variants of the bone marrow at MR imaging of the spine. Semin Musculoskelet Radiol. 2009;13(2):87-96.
26. Enlemann R, Vassollo B, Bongartz G, Müller-Miny H, Rummeny E, Stöber U, et al. Musculoskeletal neoplasms with fast low angle shot MR imaging with and without Gd-DTPA. Radiology. 1990;176(2):489-95.
27. Mahnken AH, Wildberger JE, Adam G, Stanzel S, Schmitz-Rode T, Günther RW, et al. Is there a need for

contrast enhanced T1 weighted MRI of the spine after inconspicuous short T inversion recovery imaging? Eur Radiol. 2005;15(7):1387-92.
28. Griffith JF, Yeung DKW, Antonio GE, Lee FKH, Hong AWL, Wong SYS, et al. Vertebral bone mineral density, marrow perfusion and fat content in healthy men and men with osteoporosis: Dynamic contrast enhanced MR imaging and MR spectroscopy. Radiology. 2005;236(3):945-51.
29. Ghanem N, Altehoefer C, Kelly T, Lohrmann C, Winterer J, Schäfer O, et al. Whole body MRI in comparison to skeletal scintigraphy in detection of skeletal metastases in patients with solid tumours. In Vivo. 2006;20(1):173-82.
30. Kumar J, Seith A, Kumar A, Sharma R, Bakhshi S, Kumar R, et al. Whole-body MR imaging with the use of parallel imaging for detection of skeletal metastases in pediatric patients with small-cell neoplasms: Comparison with skeletal scintigraphy and FDG PET/CT. Pediatr Radiol 2008;38(9):953-62.
31. Goo HW. Regional and whole-body imaging in pediatric oncology. Pediatr Radiol. 2011;41(Suppl 1):S186-94.
32. Padhani AR, Koh DM, Collins DJ. Whole-body diffusion-weighted MR imaging in cancer: Current status and research directions. Radiology. 2011;261(3):700-18.
33. Shellock FG, Morris E, Deutsch AL, Mink JH, Kerr R, Boden SD. Hematopoietic bone marrow hyperplasia, high prevalence on MR images of the knee in asymptomatic marathon runners. Am J Roentgenol. 1992;158(2):335-8.
34. Levin TL, Sheth SS, Ruzal-Shapiro C, Abramson S, Piomelli S, Berdon WE. MRI marrow observations in thalassemia: The effects of primary disease, transfusional therapy and chelation. Pediatr Radiol. 1995;25(8):605-13.
35. Emery JL, Follet GF. Regression of bone marrow haematopoiesis from the terminal digits in the foetus and infants. Br J Haematol. 1964;10:485-99.
36. Chan BY, Gill KG, Rebsamen SL, Nguyen JC. MR imaging of pediatric bone marrow. RadioGraphics. 2016;36(6):1911-30.
37. Kaplan KR, Mitchell DG, Steiner RM, Murphy S, Vinitski S, Rao VM, et al. Polycythemia vera and myelofibrosis: Correlation of MR imaging, clinical and lab findings. Radiology. 1992;183(2):329-34.
38. Mesa RA, Tefferi A. Emerging drugs for the therapy of primary and post essential thrombocythemia, post polycythemia vera myelofibrosis. Expert Opin Emerg Drugs 2009;14(3):471-9.
39. Bancroft LW. Hematopoietic tumors. In: Davies AM, Sundaram M, James SLJ (Eds). Imaging of Bone Tumors and Tumor-like Lesions: Techniques and Applications. Berlin: Springer-Verlag; 2009. pp. 351-63.
40. Kim SH, Smith SE, Mulligan ME. Hematopoietic tumors and metastases involving bone. Radiol Clin North Am. 2011;49(6):1163-83.
41. Kato M, Koh K, Kikuchi A, Toyama D, Mochizuki S, Uchisaka N, et al. Case series of pediatric acute leukemia without a peripheral blood abnormality, detected by magnetic resonance imaging. Int J Hematol. 2011;93(6):787-90.
42. Tafaghodi F, Aghighi Y, Rokni Yazdi H, Shakiba M, Adibi A. Predictive plain X-ray findings in distinguishing early stage acute lymphoblastic leukemia from juvenile idiopathic arthritis. Clin Rheumatol. 2009;28(11):1253-8.
43. Desmond R, McDerra J, Kelly K, Smith O. Multiple vertebral collapse as a presentation of childhood acute lymphoblastic leukaemia. Br J Haematol. 2009;144(5):627.
44. Silva JR Jr, Hayashi D, Yonenaga T, Fukuda K, Genant HK, Lin C, et al. MRI of bone marrow abnormalities in hematological malignancies. Diagn Interv Radiol. 2013;19(5):393-9.
45. Nishii T, Kono AK, Akasaka Y, Mori T, Hayakawa A, Iijima K, et al. Bone marrow magnetic resonance imaging of the clivus in pediatric leukemia patients and normal controls. Jpn J Radiol. 2015;33(3):146-52.
46. Wang J, Zhang X, Niu J. Clinical significance of magnetic resonance imaging of bone marrow in patients with leukemia. J Tongji Med Univ. 2001;21(3):242-5.
47. Nöbauer I, Uffmann M. Differential diagnosis of focal and diffuse neoplastic diseases of bone marrow in MRI. Eur J Radiol. 2005;55(1):2-32.
48. Janssens AM, Offner FC, Van Hove WZ. Bone marrow necrosis. Lancet. 2000;88(8):1769-80.
49. Hutchings M, Specht L. PET/CT in the management of haematological malignancies. Eur J Haematol 2008;80(5):369-80.
50. Mauro FR, Chauvie S, Paoloni F, Biggi A, Cimino G, Rago A, et al. Diagnostic and prognostic role of PET/CT in patients with chronic lymphocytic leukemia and progressive disease. Leukemia. 2015;29(6):1360-5.
51. American Cancer Society. Cancer facts and figures 2015. Atlanta: American Cancer Society; 2015.
52. Rajkumar SV, Dimopoulos MA, Palumbo A, Blade J, Merlini G, Mateos MV, et al. International Myeloma Working Group updated criteria for the diagnosis of multiple myeloma. Lancet Oncol. 2014;15(12):e538-48.
53. Navarro SM, Matcuk GR, Patel DB, Skalski M, White EA, Tomasian A, et al. Musculoskeletal imaging findings of hematologic malignancies. RadioGraphics. 2017;37(3):881-900.
54. Stäbler A, Baur A, Bartl R, Munker R, Lamerz R, Reiser MF. Contrast enhancement and quantitative signal analysis in MR imaging of multiple myeloma: Assessment of focal and diffuse growth patterns in marrow correlated with biopsies and survival rates. Am J Roentgenol. 1996;167(4): 1029-36.
55. Hwang S, Panicek DM. Magnetic resonance imaging of bone marrow in oncology part 2. Skeletal Radiol. 2007;36(11):1017-27.
56. Moulopoulos LA, Dimopoulos MA, Alexanian R, Leeds NE, Libshitz HI. Multiple myeloma: MR patterns of response to treatment. Radiology. 1994;193(2):441-6.
57. Moulopoulos LA, Dimopoulos MA, Weber D, Fuller L, Libshitz HI, Alexanian R. Magnetic resonance imaging in the staging of solitary plasmacytoma of bone. J Clin Oncol. 1993;11(7):1311-5.
58. Moulopoulos LA, Dimopoulos MA, Varma DG, Manning JT, Johnston DA, Leeds NE, et al. Waldenström macroglobulinemia. MR imaging of the spine and CT of the abdomen and pelvis. Radiology. 1993;188(3):669-73.
59. Zaveri J, La Q, Yarmish G, Neuman J. More than just Langerhans cell histiocytosis: A radiologic review of histiocytic disorders. RadioGraphics. 2014;34(7):2008-24.

60. Stull MA, Kransdorf MJ, Devaney KO. Langerhans cell histiocytosis of bone. RadioGraphics. 1992;12(4):801-23.
61. Cohen MD, Cary DA, Kleiman M, Smith JA, Broderick NJ. Magnetic resonance differentiation of acute and chronic osteomyelitis in children. Clinical Radiology. 1990;41(1):53-6.
62. Erdman WA, Tamburno F, Jayson HT, Weatherall PT, Ferry KB, Peshock RM. Osteomyelitis: Characteristics and pitfalls of diagnosis with MR imaging. Radiology. 1991;180(2):533-9.
63. Cortés-Romera M, Sabaté-Llobera A, Mercadal-Vilchez S, Climent-Esteller F, Serrano-Maestro A, Gámez-Cenzano C, et al. Bone marrow evaluation in initial staging of lymphoma: 18F-FDG PET/CT versus bone marrow biopsy. Clin Nucl Med. 2014;39(1):e46-52.
64. Coley BL, Higinbotham NL, Groesbeck HP. Primary reticulum-cell sarcoma of bone: Summary of 37 cases. Radiology. 1950;55(5):641-58.
65. Ruzek KA, Wenger DE. The multiple faces of lymphoma of the musculoskeletal system. Skeletal Radiol. 2004; 33(1):1-8.
66. Krishnan A, Shirkhoda A, Tehranzadeh J, Armin AR, Irwin R, Les K. Primary bone lymphoma: Radiographic–MR imaging correlation. RadioGraphics. 2003;23(6):1371-83.
67. Chen-Liang TH, Martin-Santos T, Jerez A, Senent L, Orero MT, Remigia MJ, et al. The role of bone marrow biopsy and FDG-PET/CT in identifying bone marrow infiltration in the initial diagnosis of high grade non-Hodgkin B-cell lymphoma and Hodgkin lymphoma: Accuracy in a multicenter series of 372 patients. Am J Hematol 2015;90(8):686-90.
68. Adams HJ, Kwee TC, de Keizer B, Fijnheer R, de Klerk JM, Nievelstein RA. FDG PET/CT for the detection of bone marrow involvement in diffuse large B-cell lymphoma: Systematic review and meta-analysis. Eur J Nucl Med Mol Imaging. 2014;41(3):565-74.
69. Adams HJ, Kwee TC, Fijnheer R, Dubois SV, Nievelstein RA, de Klerk JM. Bone marrow 18F-fluoro-2-deoxy-D-glucose positron emission tomography/computed tomography cannot replace bone marrow biopsy in diffuse large B-cell lymphoma. Am J Hematol. 2014;89(7):726-31.
70. Vande Berg BC, Lecouvet FE, Michaux L, Ferrant A, Maldague B, Malghem J. Magnetic resonance imaging of the bone marrow in hematological malignancies. Eur Radiol. 1998;8(8):1335-44.
71. Heacock L, Weissbrot J, Raad R, Campbell N, Friedman KP, Ponzo F, et al. PET/MRI for the evaluation of patients with lymphoma: Initial observations. Am J Roentgenol 2015;204(4):842-8.
72. Auger-Quittet S, Duny Y, Daures JP, Quittet P. Outcomes after (90) yttrium-ibritumomab tiuxetan-BEAM in diffuse large B-cell lymphoma: A meta-analysis. Cancer Med. 2014;3(4):927-38.
73. Kaplan PA, Asleson RJ, Klanen LW, Duggan MJ. Bone marrow patterns in aplastic anaemia: Observations with 1.5T MR imaging. Radiology. 1987;164(2):441-4.
74. Daldrup-Link HE, Henning T, Link TM. MR imaging of therapy-induced changes of bone marrow. Eur Radiol. 2007;17(3):743-61.
75. Otake S, Mayr NA, Ueda T, Magnotta VA, Yuh WT. Radiation-induced changes in MR signal intensity and contrast enhancement of lumbosacral vertebrae: Do changes occur only inside the radiation therapy field? Radiology. 2002;222(1):179-83.
76. Blomlie V, Rofstad EK, Skjønsberg A, Tverå K, Lien HH. Female pelvic bone marrow: Serial MR imaging before, during, and after radiation therapy. Radiology. 1995;194(2):537-43.
77. Sacks EL, Goris ML, Glatstein E, Gilbert E, Kaplan HS. Bone marrow regeneration following large field radiation: Influence of volume, age, dose, and time. Cancer. 1978;42(3):1057-65.
78. Lee JK, Yao L. Stress fractures: MR imaging. Radiology. 1988;169(1):217-20.
79. Staffard SA, Rosenthal DI, Gebhardt MC, Brady TJ, Sott JA. MRI in stress fractures. Am J Roentgenol. 1986; 147:553-6.
80. Wilson AJ, Murphy WA, Hardy DC, Totty WG. Transient osteoporosis—transient bone marrow oedema. Radiology. 1988;167(3):757-60.
81. Pory NT, Singer WS, Bartel E. Hip pain in three children accompanied by transient abnormal findings on MR images. Radiology.1989;171(1):147-9.
82. Bloem JL. Transient osteoporosis of the hip: MR imaging. Radiology.1988;167(3):753-5.
83. Imhof H, Breitenseher M, Trattnig S, Kramer J, Hofmann S, Plenk H, et al. Imaging of avascular necrosis of bone. Eur Radiol. 1997;7(2):180-6.
84. Rosenthal DI, Scott JA, Barianger J, Mankin HJ, Saini S, Brady TJ, et al. Evaluation of Gaucher's disease using magnetic resonance imaging. J Bone Joint Surg Am. 1986;68(6):802-8.
85. Hadjipavlou A, Lander P, Srolovitz H, Enker IP. Malignant transformation in Paget disease of bone. Cancer. 1992;70(12):2802-8.
86. Smith SE, Murphey MD, Motamedi K, Mulligan ME, Resnik CS, Gannon FH. From the archives of the AFIP. Radiologic spectrum of Paget disease of bone and its complications with pathologic correlation. RadioGraphics. 2002;22(5):1191-216.
87. Del Grande F, Farahani SJ, Carrino JA, Chhabra A. Bone marrow lesions: A systematic diagnostic approach. Indian J Radiol Imaging. 2014;24(3):279-87.

SECTION

5

MRI of Joints

CHAPTER 16

Magnetic Resonance Imaging of Shoulder and Temporomandibular Joints

Mahesh Prakash, Paramjeet Singh

SHOULDER JOINT

INTRODUCTION

Various imaging modalities have been used to assess the shoulder joint, like radiography, computed tomography (CT), ultrasonography (USG), and magnetic resonance imaging (MRI). Although each modality has its own advantages and disadvantages, MRI provides the comprehensive and accurate assessment of shoulder.[1] Clinical examination is important and usually help in providing the proper choice of subsequent investigative modality. Radiographs and CT are useful to demonstrate osseous structures of shoulder girdle; however, they provide poor or limited evaluation of soft tissue anatomy. USG has also been used to visualize pathology of rotator cuff and bursae of the joint with variable success.[2-4] This technique however is operator dependent and needs high end equipment.[5] The MRI, because of its excellent soft tissue contrast and imaging capability in any desired plane and nonionizing noninvasive nature, is an ideal modality for evaluation of shoulder joint.[6]

MAGNETIC RESONANCE IMAGING PROTOCOLS

Improved coil designs have helped to improve the signal-to-noise ratio and provide adequate spatial resolution in MRI of shoulder. Proper immobilization and comfort of the patient, off axis small FOV imaging capability, high matrix size, and elimination of phase wrap are desirable requisites for imaging the shoulder.

During MRI of shoulder, patient is placed in supine position with their arm on the side of body in partial external rotation. After localizer images, joint should be imaged in axial, coronal-oblique, and sagittal-oblique planes.[7] Coronal-oblique plane is selected parallel to the course of supraspinatus tendon (SST). The sagittal-oblique images are done parallel to glenoid surface. The imaging sequences may vary in different institution and depends on available hardware and other factors and have seen changing over the years. Previously we had used proton/T2 turbospin-echo (TSE) and gradient-echo sequences in axial planes, T1 SE and proton/T2 TSE sections oblique coronal planes, and oblique sagittal sections using T1 SE and T2 TSE sequences. An STIR, turbo inversion recovery or fat suppressed T2 TSE sequence, was additionally used in one of the planes. The basic sequences presently done in our institution on 3 Tesla MR machine are listed in **Table 1**.

MAGNETIC RESONANCE ARTHROGRAPHY

Magnetic resonance arthrography with intra-articular contrast is performed by injecting 12–15 cc mixture of gadolinium dimeglumine (2 mmol/L), normal saline, lidocaine, and iodinated contrast media into joint cavity with a 20G spinal needle through either anterior or posterior approach under fluoroscopic guidance.[8,9] The gadolinium concentration of 2 mmol/L is achieved by mixing 0.5 mL of contrast in 50 mL of saline. T1 fat suppressed sections are taken in axial, oblique coronal, and sagittal planes. Additional imaging in an abducted externally rotated (ABER) arm may also be done to assess capsule-labral pathology. Some people are comfortable using USG guidance for injecting contrast in the joint cavity.

Table 1: Standard pulse sequences for MRI examination of the shoulder at 3 Tesla.

Pulse sequence	*FOV (cm)*	*Slice thickness (mm)*	*Matrix*	*TR/TE*
Axial PD with fat saturation	14	3	256 × 256	3,000/43
Sagittal oblique PD with fat saturation	14	3	256 × 256	3,000/43
Coronal oblique T1	14	3	256 × 256	650/24
Coronal oblique T2 with fat saturation	14	3	256 × 256	3,000/89
Sagittal oblique T1	14	3	256 × 256	650/24

NORMAL ANATOMY

Shoulder joint is a ball and socket joint formed by articulation between head of humerus and glenoid of scapula. Structurally, it is a weak joint because of disparity of articulating surface area between small and shallow glenoid cavity in comparison to the humeral head. However, this arrangement provides the glenohumeral joint with the greatest range of motion of any articulation in human body. Stability to this unstable joint is provided by following structures.

- Coracoacromial arch (CCA) consisting of acromian, coracoacromial ligament (CAL), coracoid process, and the acromioclavicular joint (AC joint).
- Musculotendinous cuff of shoulder.
- Glenoid labrum along with capsule and glenohumeral ligaments (GHL).
- The muscles attaching the humerus to pectoral girdle, i.e., long head of biceps and triceps, coracobrachialis, teres major, etc.

Osseous Structures

The osseous structures of shoulder joint include proximal humerus, scapula, and clavicle. The proximal humerus consists of head, neck, and greater and lesser tuberosities. The humeral head is typically round with slight flattening of posteroinferior surface. This flattening should not be confused with Hill-Sachs lesion which is seen at or above the level of coracoid process.[10] The anatomic neck forms the oblique circumference and separates head from tuberosities. The acromian and glenoid of scapula makes articulation with humeral head and clavicle to become components of shoulder joint. The acromian is posterior landmark and articulates with clavicle. The coracoid process is anterior landmark of shoulder with variable morphology.[11] The glenoid is important structure, which articulates with humeral head to form shoulder joint. The glenoid is pear or oval shaped in coronal plane.[12] The lateral end of clavicle articulates with acromian to form AC joint.

Ligaments

The joint capsule is loose and permits free movements. It is least supported inferiorly where dislocations are common. Medially the capsule is attached to the scapula beyond the supraglenoid tubercle and margins of the labrum and laterally to the anatomical neck of humerus. The capsule is reinforced anteriorly and inferiorly by several thickenings, namely the anterior and posterior bands of inferior glenohumeral ligament (IGHL) with an inferior axillary recess, the more variable middle GHL (MGHL) and the smallest superior GHL (SGHL). They all extend to the anatomical neck of humerus and stabilize the joint variably. The coracohumeral ligament (CHL) extends from lateral aspect of coracoid process to the neck of humerus and is a key structure in impingement and instability syndromes. Transverse humeral ligament bridges the bicipital groove and holds tendon of long head of biceps brachii. The glenoid labrum is a fibrocartilaginous ovoid rim attached to the margins of the glenoid cavity. It is often deficient anterosuperiorly. It functions to deepen the glenoid cup and is a site of capsuloligamentous attachment. It is more mobile superiorly and functions with biceps tendon as a mobile "biceps labral complex" that slides over the superior glenoid.

MUSCULOTENDINOUS ANATOMY

From anterior to posterior, subscapularis muscle (SCM), biceps, supraspinatus muscle (SSM), infraspinatus muscle (ISM), and teres minor (TM) muscles together with their tendons form the rotator cuff. All originate from the scapula and insert on the humerus. Of these tendons, the SST, infraspinatus tendon (IST), and teres minor insert on their respective notches on the greater tuberosity while subscapularis tendon (SCT) attaches to the lesser tuberosity. The SST and IST fibers may partially fuse posteriorly to form a conjoint tendon (an area sometimes referred to as posterior rotator interval). The gap between SCT and SST, named anterior rotator cuff interval (RCI), is filled with fibrofatty tissue. The CHL, SGHL, and biceps tendon (BT) lie beneath it in that order. The long head of BT originates from the supraglenoid tubercle, crosses the joint obliquely through RCI, attaches to superior labrum, and exits the joint into bicipital groove. The bicipital groove is hooded by transverse humeral ligament.

Bursae

Numerous bursae are related to shoulder joint, which can be communicating or noncommunicating with the joint. The subscapularis, subcoracoid, infraspinatus, and peribicipital bursae are communicating bursae. Bursa superior to AC joint and those related to coracobrachialis, teres major, long head of triceps, and lattisimus dorsi do not communicate with the joint. The subacromial-subdeltoid bursa (SASDB), the largest bursa in the body, is lined with areolar tissue and synovium, which allow free sliding motion of adjacent structures. They are fused and considered as one and do not communicate with the joint.

NORMAL MAGNETIC RESONANCE APPEARANCE

(*Refer to Abbreviations in Table 2*)

Axial Sections (Figs. 1 and 4)

The cuff muscles appear as intermediate signal intensity structures on T1W. Highest sections show SSM, followed posteriorly by ISM and TM and their tendons. The tendons

Table 2: Abbreviations used for figures 1 to 4.

1. AC	Acromian process	13. IST	Infraspinatus tendon
2. BT	Biceps tendon	14. MGHL	Middle glenohumeral ligament
3. CAL	Coracoacromial ligament	15. QS	Quadrilateral space
4. CCL	Coracoclavicular ligament	16. RCI	Rotator cuff interval
5. CHL	Coracohumeral ligament	17. SASD	Subacrominal subdeltoid bursa
6. CL	Clavicle	18. SCT (m)	Subscapularis tendon/muscle
7. CP	Coracoid process	19. SGHL	Superior glenohumeral ligament
8. D	Deltoid muscle	20. SST(m)	Supraspinatus tendon/muscle
9. GL	Glenoid	21. TM	Teres minor
10. HH	Humeral head	22. TMj	Teres major
11. IGHL	Inferior glenohumeral ligament	23. TR	Trapezius
AB—	anterior band, PB—posterior band	24. PL	Post labrum
12. ISM	Infraspinatus muscle		

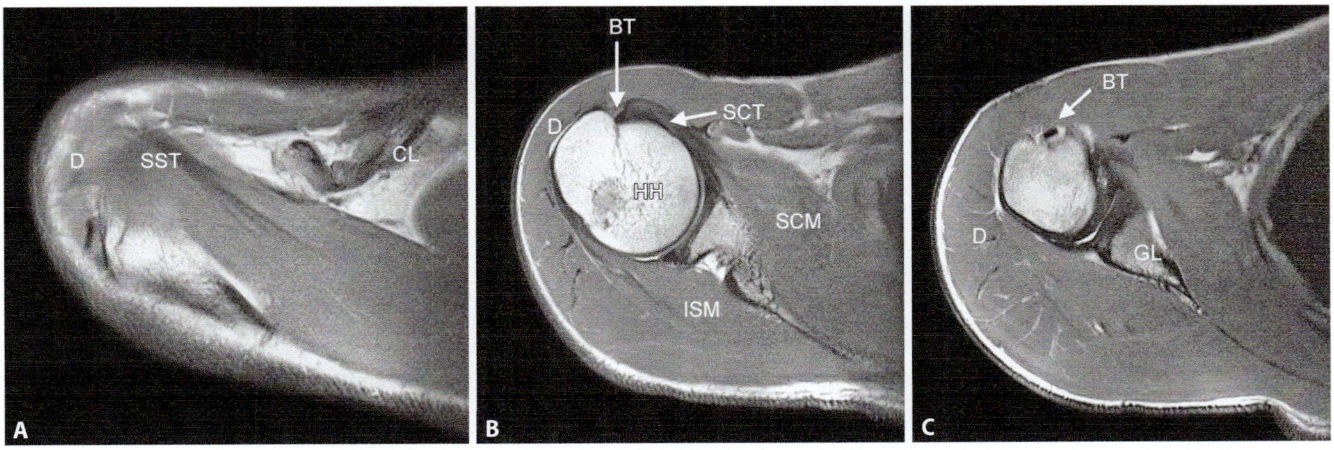

Figs. 1A to C: Axial T1-weighted sections of shoulder (normal anatomy).

appear darker than muscles and can be traced to greater tuberosity. Biceps tendon is seen anterosuperiorly and SCT anterior to the scapula at midsuperior head level. Bicipital groove is best seen on these sections lateral to lesser tuberosity. Anterior and posterior labra are particularly well seen on axial sections. The GHLs are low-intensity structures and better seen in presence of fluid in the joint or on MR arthrogram. The SGHL lies superiorly and follows the concavity of coracoid on its lateral aspect. The MGHL closely follows posterior margin of SCT and IGHL lies at lower head level. The articular cartilage appears bright on T2 and gradient images and best evaluated in axial sections.

Coronal Sections (Figs. 2 and 4)

The rotator cuff tendon structures are best evaluated on oblique coronal sections. The mid to anterior sections show the SST (along with AC joint). The sections posterior to this show conjoint tendons of SST and IST and TM. The tendons can be traced to greater tuberosity. The SASDB appears as a thin bright line beneath the deltoid muscle on T2W. The anterior sections also show SST and biceps tendon passing beneath it as well as coracohumeral, coracoacromial, and coracoclavicular ligaments. The superior labrum is best evaluated in the coronal plane. Axillary pouch is seen medial and inferior to humeral head.

Sagittal Sections (Figs. 3 and 4)

These sections provide a cross-sectional view of all the muscles of shoulder. Mid and lateral sagittal images show the SST/IST conjoint tendon as a low signal structure between humeral head and acromion. The morphological abnormalities of acromion (i.e., anterior sloping) are best shown on these images. The long head of biceps can be seen passing anteroinferiorly between SST and

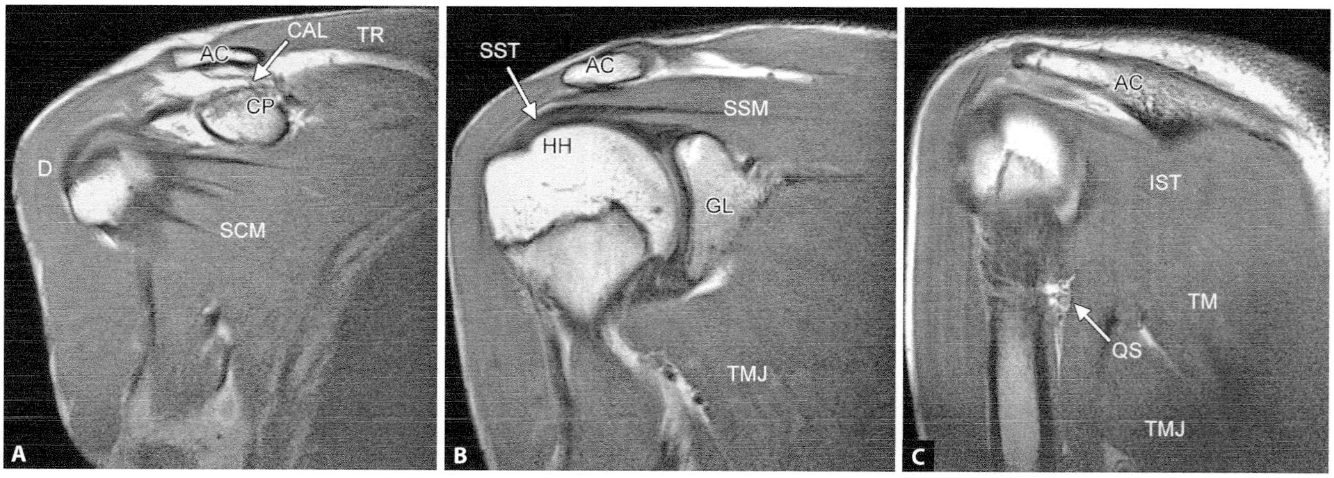

Figs. 2A to C: (A to C—anterior to posterior) Oblique coronal T1-weighted sections (normal anatomy).

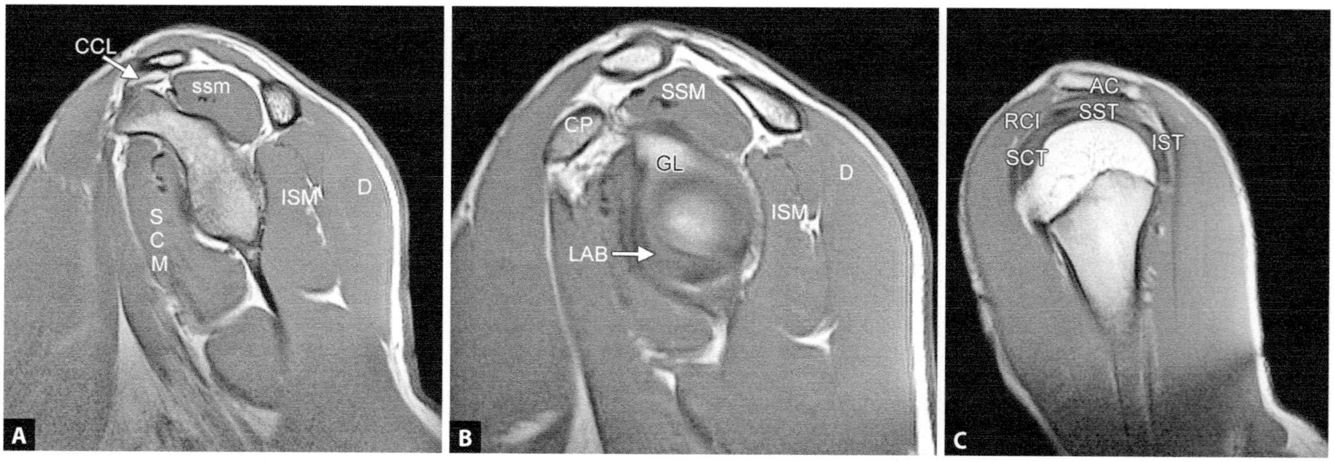

Figs. 3A to C: Oblique sagittal T1-weighted sections (normal anatomy).

SCT through the rotator cuff interval. More medially coracoacromial ligament can be seen arching over the rotator cuff interval along with AC joint in profile. The SGHL can be seen lying beneath the long head of biceps, the MGHL anterior to medial humeral head, and IGHL along with a thick inferior labrum along the inferior aspect of the glenoid cavity.

SHOULDER IMPINGEMENT SYNDROME

Impingement syndrome is a clinical diagnosis in which pain is felt in shoulder due to encroachment of the rotator cuff and associated soft tissues between the humeral head and overlying CCA. The CCL is a triangular strong structure limiting the space available to rotator cuff during abduction. Abnormalities involving one or more of the components of CCA results in narrowing of the acromiohumeral distance.

Rotator cuff impingement can be classified as:

- Primary extrinsic impingement
- Secondary extrinsic impingement
- Intrinsic impingement.

Primary Extrinsic Impingement

This is due to the abnormalities of the CCA and can be subacromial or subcoracoid types.

Possible etiologies of subacromial impingement are:

- Subacromial spur
- Hypertrophic changes in AC joint
- Unstable os acromial (failure to fuse by 25 years)
- Subacromial subdeltoid bursitis
- Thickening of the coracoacromial ligament
- Laterally downsloping acromian process (type 3).

As seen on oblique sagittal plane (outlet view on plain radiographs) the anterior acromion is straight in type I, curved in type II, and anteriorly hooked in type III morphology **(Figs. 5A to C)**.[13] Type II configuration is most common and type III is most commonly associated with rotator cuff pathology. Anterior part of SST is most commonly affected in subacromial type impingement alone or along with other tendons in 95% cases. The cuff along with subacromial bursa is entrapped along the undersurface of CCA.

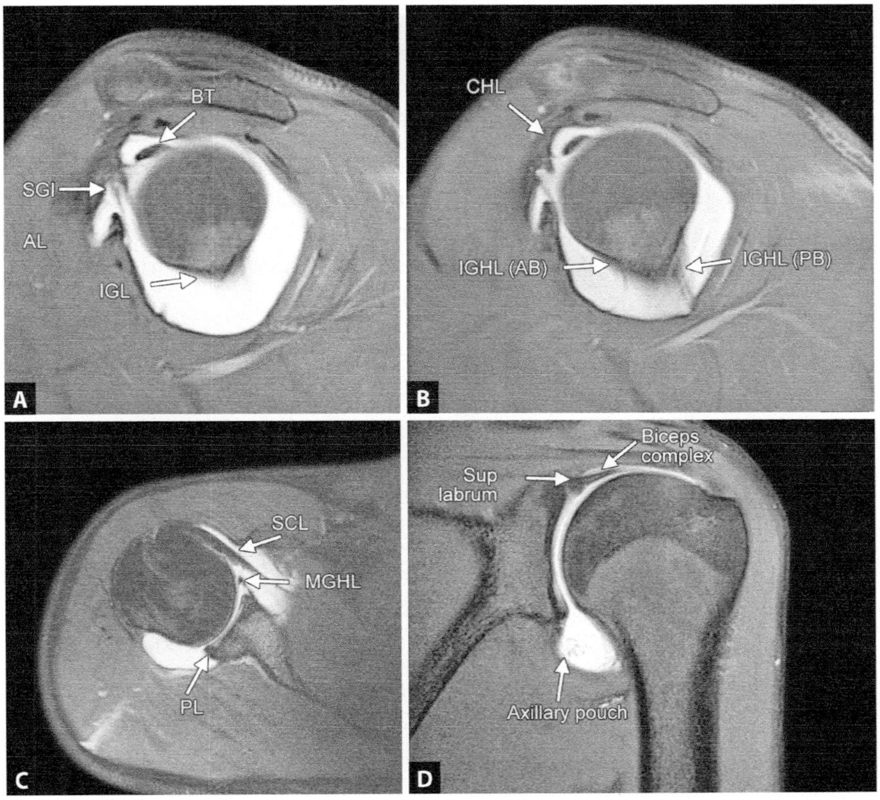

Figs. 4A to D: (A and B) Sagittal; (C) Axial; and (D) Coronal T1-weighted fat saturated arthrogram images show ligamentous anatomy. The superior glenohumeral ligament (SGHL) is seen coursing down from its coracoid attachment. Inferior glenohumeral ligament (IGHL) is seen with thick anterior and posterior bands outlining a distended axillary recess. The middle glenohumeral ligament (MGHL) is seen as a thin hypointense band beneath subscapularis tendon (SCT). The biceps-labral complex is firmly attached to the glenoid rim.

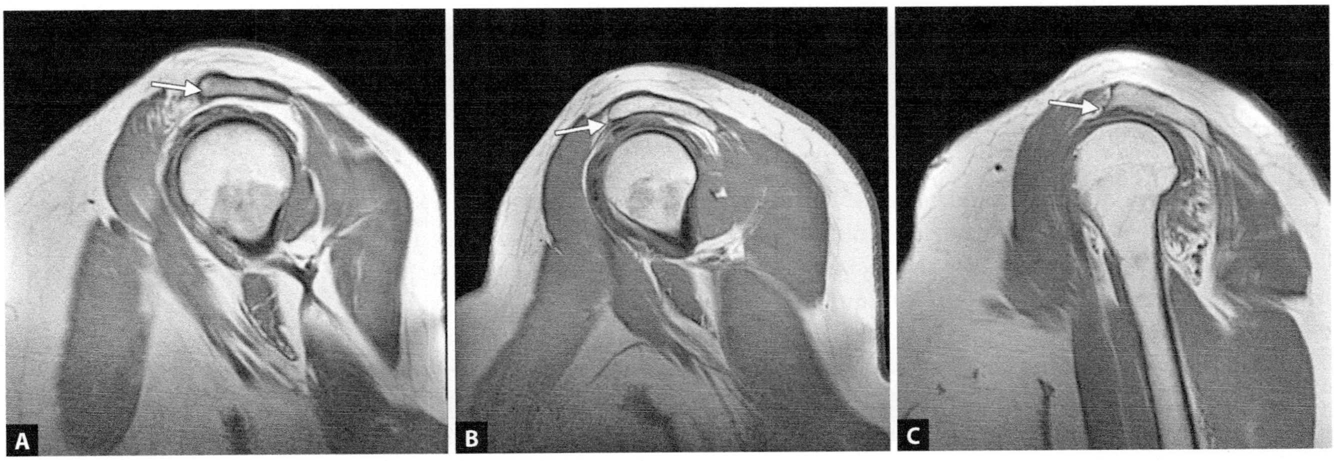

Figs. 5A to C: (A) Type I; (B) Type II; and (C) Type III acromion morphologies.

The subcoracoid impingement can be due to reduced distance between coracoid process and the medial aspect of humeral head leading to compression of SCT and biceps long head.

Secondary Extrinsic Impingement

Here the abnormality lies in the stability of the glenohumeral joint in the setting of a normal CCA. It usually occurs in young athletes involved in sports demanding overhead arm movements. Possible underlying defect of static stabilizers (glenohumeral ligaments) leads to overload on secondary stabilizers (cuff structures) and a reduced acromiohumeral gap.

Internal Impingement

It is due to contact between undersurface of rotator cuff and glenoid rim due to throwing with arm in abduction and maximal external rotation. Supraspinatus hypertrophy or an abnormality of the greater tuberosity may also be contributory factors.

ROTATOR CUFF TENDINOPATHY AND TEARS

Rotator cuff disease is one of the most common causes of shoulder pain and indication for MRI evaluation of shoulder. Multiple etiologies have been implicated in the development of degenerative changes (tendinopathy) in the rotator cuff tendons near greater tuberosity. Aforementioned rotator cuff impingement between CCA and humeral head is most often implicated. Acute and chronic trauma, sports, overuse, aging, collagen vascular, and metabolic diseases are also associated with rotator cuff tendinopathy and tears. Vascular insufficiency leading to degeneration in critical zone may also plays a role in rotator cuff tears (RCTs). Critical zone, approximately 1 cm from the insertion of the SST at the greater tuberosity, is the most susceptible area for tears.

Neer described three clinicopathologic stages of impingement.[14]

Stage I: There is reversible edema and hemorrhage within the distal SST usually in young patient (<25 years) and is managed conservatively.

Stage II: There is tendinitis and thickening with fibrosis. Bursal pathology aggravates the condition by compromising subacromial space. Patient are usually between 25 and 40 years of age. No radiographic changes are seen in stage I and II.

Stage III: These are characterized by partial or a full thickness tears of rotator cuff or biceps tendon usually seen in patients older than 40 years of age. Osseous changes in the form of degenerative changes at greater tuberosity and acromial osteophyte formation are seen on radiographs.

Impingement is a process of progressive wear and tear. MR interpretation in early stages is often equivocal. The injured tendon may appear thickened due to mucoid degeneration; however, histology of tendons of asymptomatic people also shows similar changes. The term "tendinosis or tendinopathy" is preferred over tendinitis as no inflammatory changes are seen within these tendons. In contrast to these intrasubstance changes of tendinosis, "tendon surface degeneration" is seen as irregularity of surface and may be indistinguishable from or coexist with "partial tears." There may also be associated features of bursal and peribursal inflammation.

Magnetic Resonance Appearance

Seeger[15] has classified impingement on coronal MR images into three types:

Type 1: Normal low-signal intensity on T1 and T2WI and normal morphology of the SST. Areas of increased signal intensity are noted on proton and GRE images.

Type 2: High-signal intensity of SST on T1WI. If T2WI also reveal high signal intensity, which is not involving the entire thickness, it may represent partial tear (bursal or articular surface or intra substance).

Type 3: High-signal intensity is found on T1 and T2WI traversing full thickness suggestive of complete RCT, with or without tendon retraction.

Carrino et al.[16] described more extensive MR grading for RCTs.

Grade 0 (normal): Uniform low-signal intensity of the tendons.

Grade I: Increased signal intensity in tendon, more obvious on T1WI and proton images but not seen or less obvious on T2WI **(Figs. 6A and B)**.

Grade II (tendinosis/tendinitis): Increased signal intensity on T2WI that does not involve articular or superior surface. The tendon may be thin, thick, or irregular, similar to Neer stage II **(Figs. 7A and B)**.

Grade III (degeneration): Increased signal intensity on T2WI in one or multiple areas but signal changes do not meet criteria for partial or complete tear.

Grade IV (partial tear): Increased signal intensity on T2WI that involve the inferior (articular) or superior (bursal) surface of the tendons **(Fig. 8)**.

Grade V: Full thickness tear with few spared fibers.

Grade VI: Full thickness tear without tendon retraction **(Fig. 9)**.

Grade VII: Full thickness tear with tendon retraction **(Fig. 10)**.

An increase in T2 signal intensity along with abnormality in tendon morphology increases the confidence level of diagnosing a tear. Partial tears are better shown on T2WI (with fat suppression), particularly in presence of joint effusion as a discontinuity or fraying of the tendon **(Fig. 8)**. Partial tears are classified as grade I, II, or III depending on involvement of less than 25%, 25–30%, or more than 50% of the tendon thickness.

Complete RCTs occur at sites of previous tendinopathy and can be diagnosed with greater confidence on MRI than the debatable early tendon pathology and partial tears. Full thickness tears can be classified as small (<1 cm or involvement of one tendon only) **(Fig. 11)**, medium (1–3 cm or involvement of two tendons), and massive (>3–5 cm or involvement of three or more tendons). Massive tears of the rotator cuff may also involve the subscapularis and biceps with or without dislocation **(Fig. 12)**. Both anteroposterior and mediolateral measurements of tears as well as quality of torn margins should be noted as these are important information from surgical point of view. Undersurface tears of posterior SST and IST, humeral head

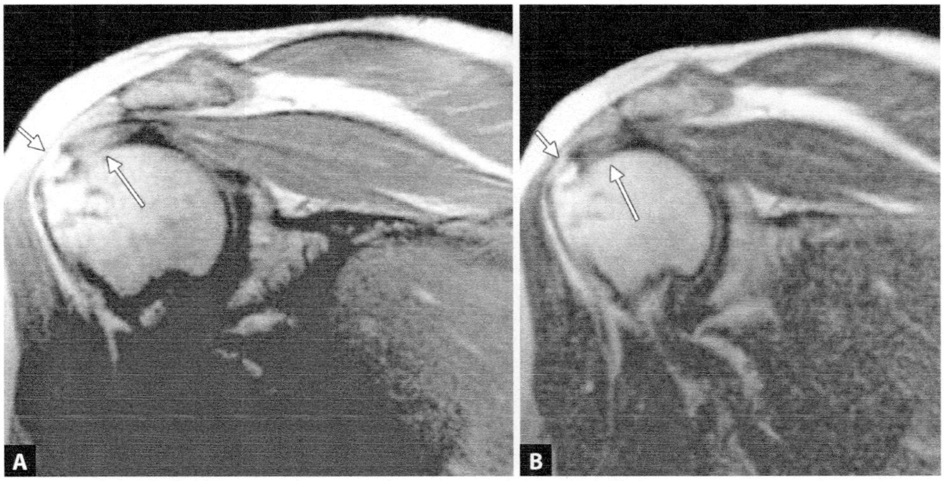

Figs. 6A and B: (A) Proton; and (B) T2 turbospin-echo (T2 TSE) coronal sections show increased signal within the supraspinatus tendon (SST) (A, long arrow); however, T2WI (B) shows less pronounced signal changes in the tendon suggesting tendinopathy. Partial retraction at the insertion site with cyst formation is also noted (short arrow).

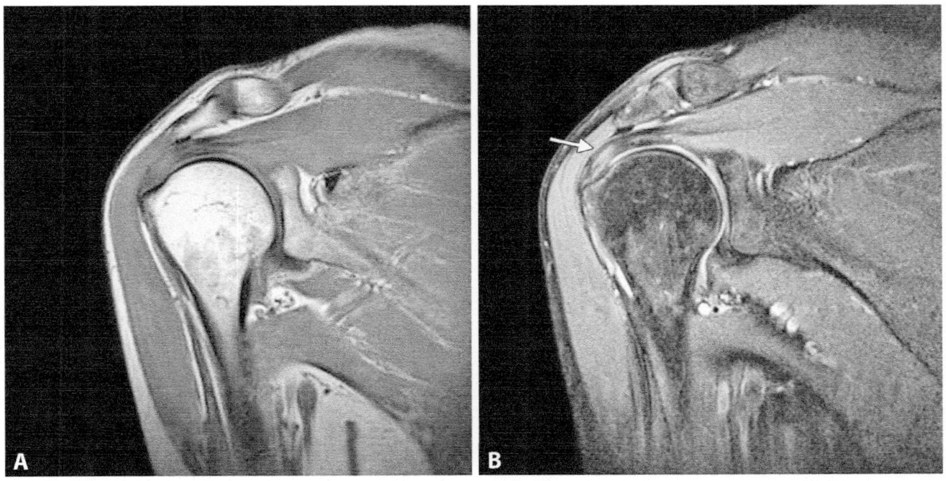

Figs. 7A and B: (A) T1; and (B) T2 fat saturated coronal sections show intrasubstance increased signal (tendinosis) in the supraspinatus tendon on both the images (arrow).

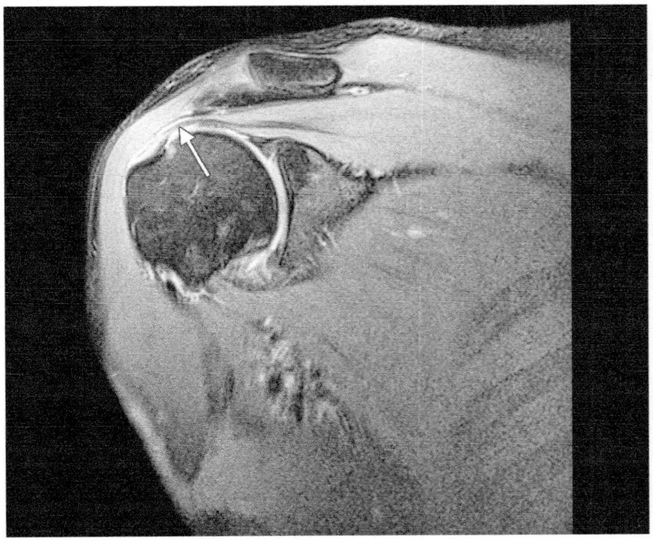

Fig. 8: Proton density (fat saturated) coronal section shows articular surface tear as a focus of bright signal area along the undersurface of the supraspinatus tendon (SST) (arrow).

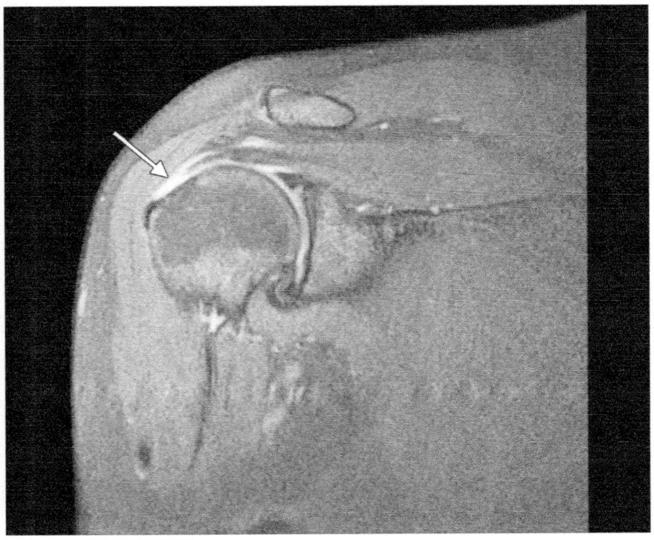

Fig. 9: Proton density (fat saturated) coronal section shows full thickness tear of supraspinatus tendon (SST) without retraction (arrow).

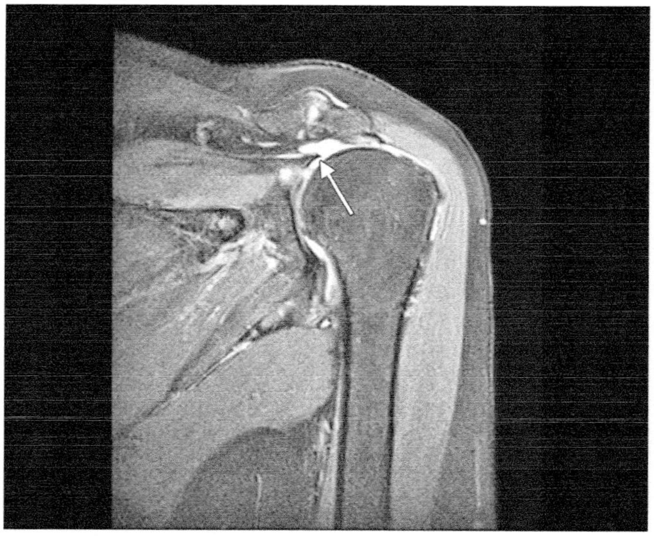

Fig. 10: Proton density (fat saturated) coronal section shows full thickness tear of supraspinatus tendon (SST) with retraction of fibers (arrow). Acromian osteophyte is also noted.

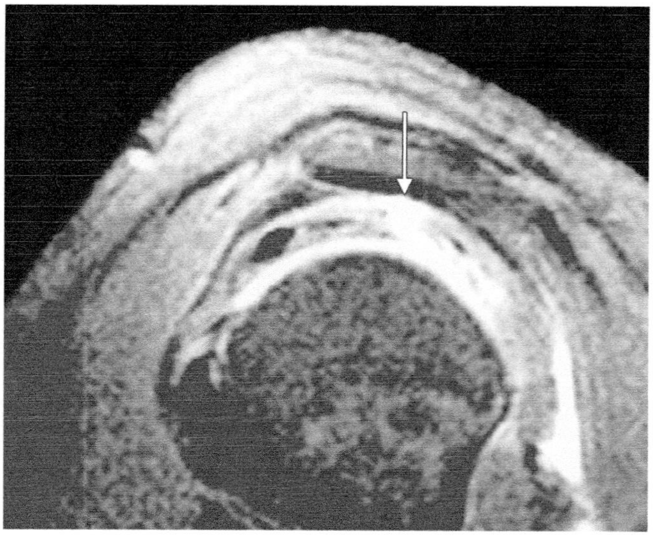

Fig. 11: Sagittal fat-suppressed T1 MR arthrographic image is showing tear of posterior supraspinatus tendon (SST) and possibly infraspinatus tendon (IST) (conjoint tendon) with a full thickness defect outlined by the contrast in posterior rotator interval (arrow).

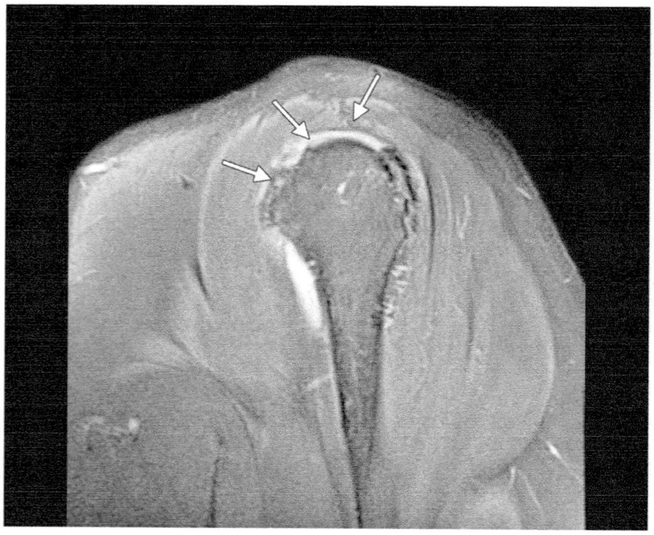

Fig. 12: Oblique sagittal proton density (fat saturated) section through the rotator cuff shows a massive tear involving subscapularis tendon (SCT), supraspinatus tendon (SST) as well as the infraspinatus tendon (IST) (from anterior to posterior-arrows) are seen as increased signal replacing normal low signal of the tendons.

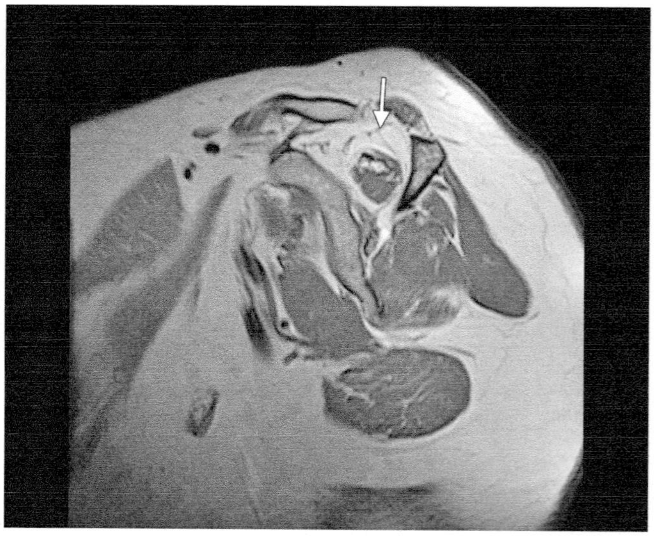

Fig. 13: T1 oblique sagittal section shows atrophy of the rotator cuff muscles and fatty changes are seen as T1 hyperintensity (arrow).

chondromalacia, and fraying of posterosuperior labrum are hallmarks of internal impingement syndrome seen in overhead throwers **(Fig. 11)**.

Sometimes tears may not show T2 hyperintensity due to granulation or fibrosis and appear to be normal. Although less specific, knowledge of secondary signs of RCT is useful in such difficult cases. MR may show fatty atrophy of muscle belly in complete tears as T1 hyperintensity and loss of volume **(Fig. 13)**. Humeral head may be apposed to the acromion in such chronic cases. Tendons may be completely nonvisualized due to musculotendinous retraction in complete tears. Tendon retraction, loss of peribursal/subdeltoid fat plane, and fluid in the subdeltoid subacromial bursa can be seen in 92% patients with complete RCT **(Figs. 14A and B)**.[17] However, bursal fluid can also be found in impingement (43%), labral abnormality (29%), bursitis (19%), tendinitis (14%), and even in asymptomatic people **(Fig. 15)**.[18] Joint effusion can be seen in both partial and complete tears. Marrow signal changes and cyst formation in the greater tuberosity

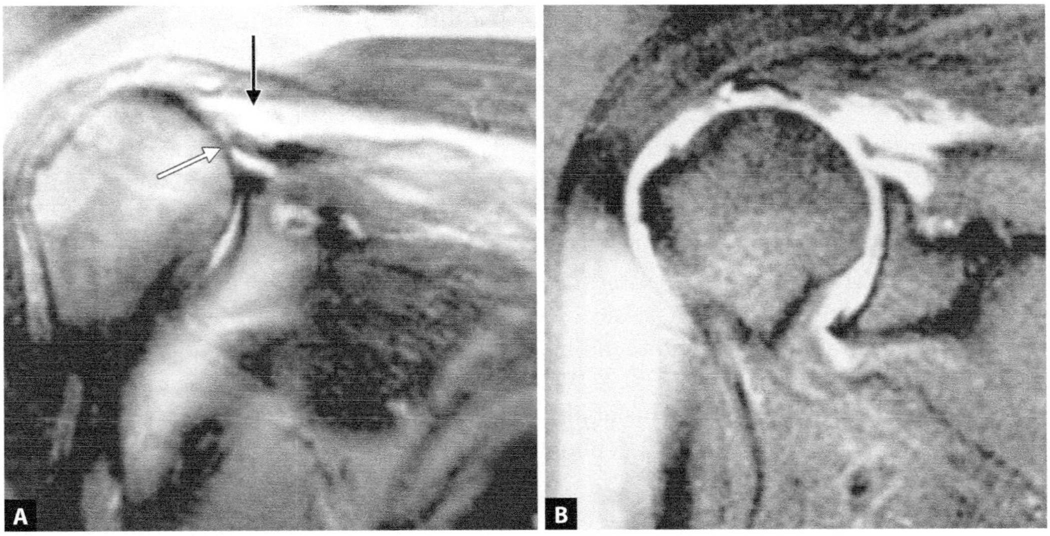

Figs. 14A and B: T2 turbospin-echo (T2 TSE) and arthrographic coronal sections show complete tear of SST (white arrow) with tendon retraction and fluid in the subacromial-subdeltoid bursa (SASDB) (black arrow) (A). There is free spillage of intraarticular contrast into the SASDB (B).

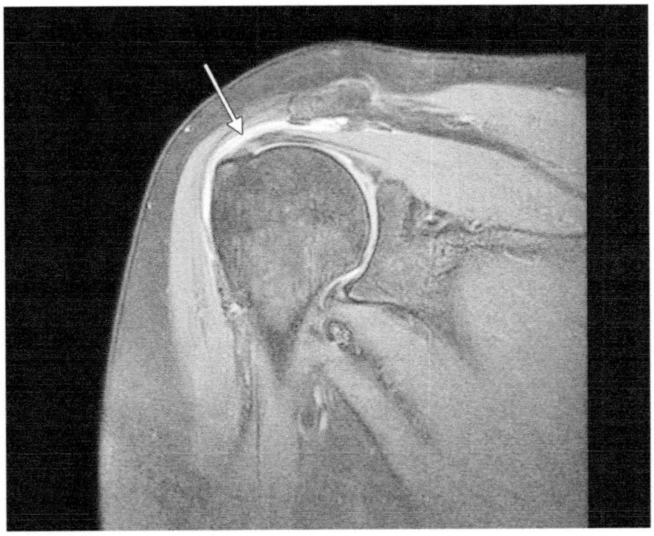

Fig. 15: Proton density (fat saturated) coronal section: The subacromial-subdeltoid bursa (SASDB) shows fluid (arrow) in absence of any visible rotator cuff tear.

on fat suppressed T2 WI and osseous changes like AC joint osteophytosis and subacromial spurs are secondary signs of cuff tendinopathy and indicate advanced disease **(Fig. 10)**. Artifactually increased signal may be noted within the tendons on proton images due to "magic angle effect" in areas where the tendon courses at 55° angle in relation to the magnetic field. Normal signal on T2WI differentiates this from actual tendinopathy.

According to Zlatkin and colleagues,[19] sensitivity and specificity of MR for imaging partial and full thickness tears are 91% and 88%, respectively, with 89% accuracy. MR arthrography though not used routinely is useful in difficult cases and is gaining in popularity **(Fig. 14B)**.[20] It is superior to conventional T2WI for evaluating partial tears particularly on the articular side and differentiating small complete tears (with fibrosis) from partial tears. It is also helpful for diagnosing associated instability and capsulolabral disorders.

Instability

Shoulder joint is one of the most mobile joints in the body. But this mobility comes at the expense of stability as the joint architecture, which allows maximum mobility, also predisposes it to dislocation.

Glenohumeral joint is relatively shallow with a large humeral head in comparison to glenoid fossa. The structures responsible for maintaining joint stability are dynamic stabilizers (rotator cuff) and static stabilizers (glenoid labrum, joint capsule, GHL and periarticular soft tissue) **(Fig. 4)**. Pathology of any of these structures can predispose to instability.

Anterior and posterior bands are thickenings of anterior and posterior margins of IGHL, which prevent anterior and posterior dislocation respectively. Most important static stabilizer of shoulder is anterior band of inferior GHL, which prevents anterior dislocation.[21]

For practical purpose, shoulder instability can be broadly classified into two types: (1) unidirectional traumatic instability and (2) multidirectional nontraumatic instability, former being more common.[22] As the name implies unidirectional traumatic instability follows trauma, is unidirectional, usually anterior and is unilateral. Anterior instability is often associated with anteroinferior labral tear with or without glenoid rim fracture (Bankart lesion). This condition usually requires surgery and has been given a name traumatic, unidirectional, Bankart, surgery

(TUBS).[22] MRI aids in planning surgical management in these patients as it can show associated capsulolabral-ligamentous defects, rotator cuff injury as well as osseous lesions.

Multidirectional nontraumatic instability is seen in young without history of trauma. It is often bilateral and invariably has an inferior component. These patients can voluntarily dislocate their shoulders. Basic pathology here seems to be capsular laxity which is difficult to assess by MRI. Treatment is usually conservative. These lesions are also named as AMBRI (atraumatic, multidirectional, bilateral, rehabilitation, inferior capsular shift).[22] As MR plays little role in evaluation of multidirectional instability, subsequent discussion will mainly focus on unidirectional instability (labral tears).

Imaging Techniques for Labral Tears

The shape of labrum varies from individual to individual (triangular, rounded, blunted, crescent shaped, etc). Most commonly, it is triangular anteriorly and rounded or triangular posteriorly **(Fig. 16)**. Few horizontal notches and vertical clefts along anterior aspect of labrum are considered normal. When seen posteriorly, these are considered tears.

Labral tear is seen as either complete absence of a portion of labrum, displacement of labrum from glenoid rim or linear area of increased signal intensity within the labrum on T2WI. Abnormal labral appearance in MRI is classified into four types as follows: Type 1—increased signal within the labrum not extending to the surface consistent with degeneration. Type 2—frayed appearance of labrum with normal signal. Type 3—increased signal within labrum extending to the surface consistent with tear and Type 4—combined features of Type 2 and Type 3. Type 2 to 4 labra are considered pathological. MR arthrography is the technique of choice for diagnosing labral pathology **(Fig. 17)**. Injected contrast distends the joint cavity and better delineates morphology of labrum and GHL. Contrast entering the labrum or tracking beneath the labrum to the external surface of joint also suggests tear **(Fig. 18)**. Positioning the arm is abduction and external rotation (ABER) has been shown to increase the sensitivity of MR arthrography.[23] This position puts tension on and improves evaluation of anterior band of IGHL and anterior inferior labrum.

Magnetic resonance arthrography has sensitivity of 91% and specificity of 93% for labral tears.[24] Conventional MRI, CT arthrography, and radiographic arthrography are alternative techniques for evaluation of labrum. Conventional MRI has shown variable accuracy with sensitivity ranging from 78 to 93% and specificity from 68 to 87%.[25,26] Relatively few studies have compared the accuracy of various techniques. However, one study by Chandnani et al.[27] compared CT arthrography, MR, and MR arthrography and showed MR arthrography to be the most sensitive modality among these (96%).

Magnetic Resonance Findings in Patients with Instability

Findings in anterior instability typically include anteroinferior labral tear with rupture of scapular periosteum (Bankart lesion), Bankart fracture (bony Bankart), and Hill Sach's lesion **(Figs. 17 and 19)**. When humeral head dislocates anteriorly, it can cause fracture

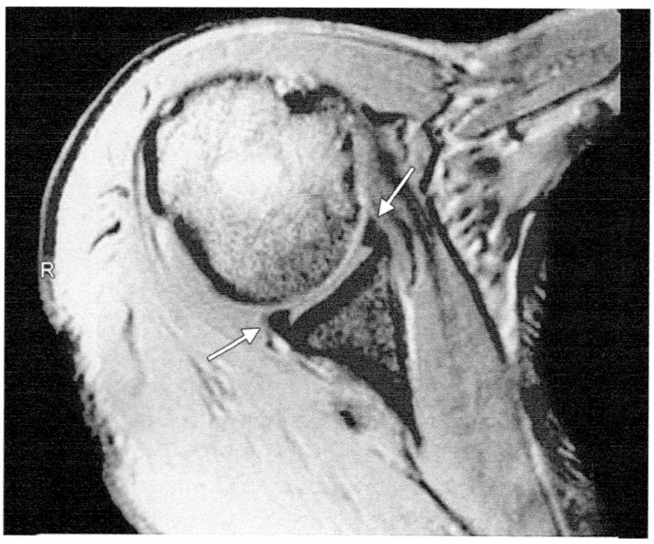

Fig. 16: Gradient-echo axial section shows normal anterior and posterior triangular labra undercut by a bright appearing articular cartilage (arrows).

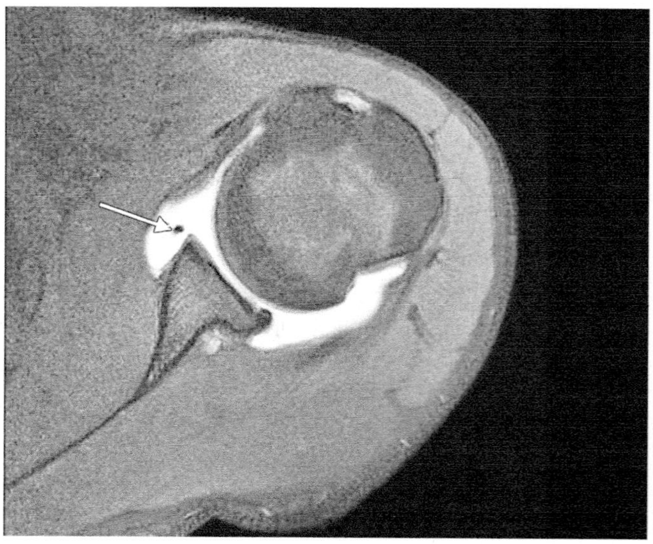

Fig. 17: T1 fat saturated arthrogram (axial section) at the inferior head level: Bankart lesion is seen as a separated anterior inferior labrum (arrow).

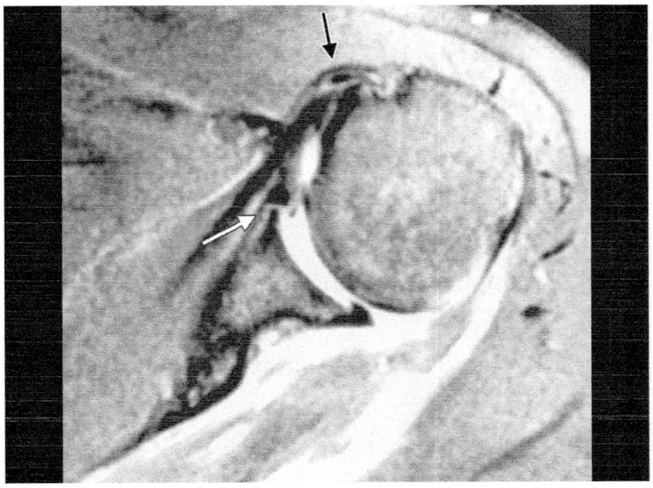

Fig.18: MR arthrogram shows a detached labrum with contrast outlining its base (white arrow). Partially sectioned middle glenohumeral ligament (MGHL) may at times mimic a labral fragment. Also note the medially dislocated biceps tendon from its groove and lying anterior to the subscapularis tendon (SCT) (black arrow).

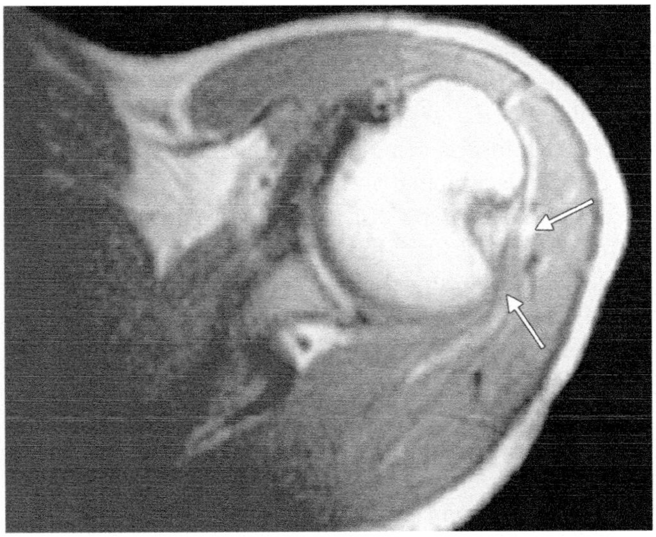

Fig. 19: T1 spin-echo axial section: There is a wedge-shaped defect at the posterosuperior aspect of the humeral head representing Hill-Sach's lesion (arrows) due to anterior dislocation of shoulder.

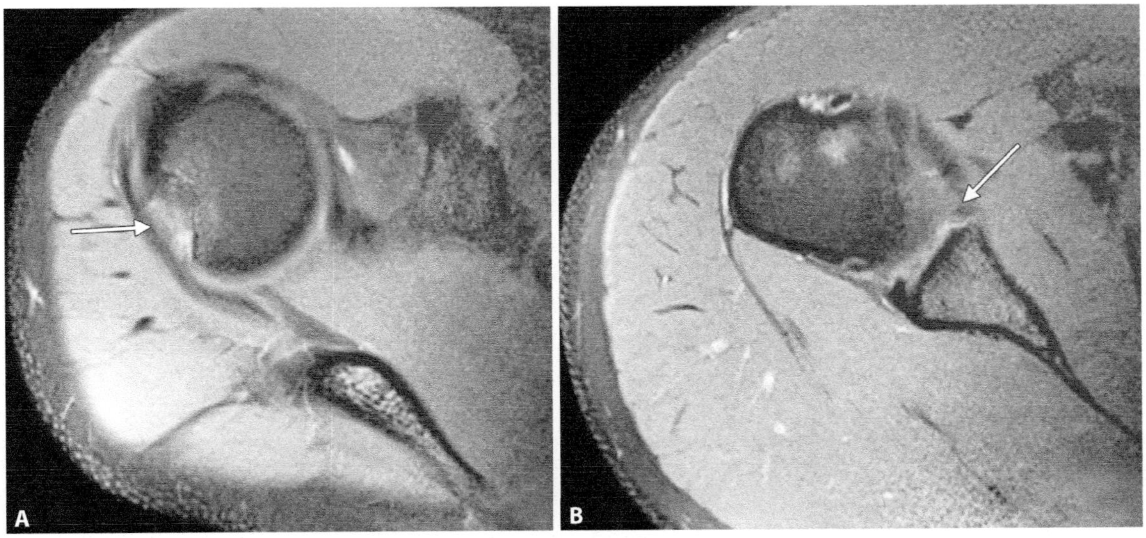

Figs. 20A and B: Proton density fat saturated axial sections (A and B) in another patient show typical Hill-Sach's defect in humeral head with anteroinferior glenoid injury (arrows).

of anterior glenoid rim (Bankart fracture) and can produce impaction fracture in superior posterolateral aspect of humeral head (Hill-Sach's lesion). On axial images, this is identified as a compression defect in the normally round posterolateral humeral head superior to the coracoid process (as opposed to normal defect of head below it)[28] **(Figs. 19 and 20)**. There may be associated marrow edema in recent injuries. Identification of these lesions is important as they predispose to recurrent dislocation with minimal trauma and may affect surgical planning.[29]

Some terms are used to describe Bankart variants. Glenolabral articular disruption (GLAD) lesions are described as tears of anteroinferior glenoid labrum with injury to glenoid articular cartilage. Scapular periosteum remains intact and holds labrum in place in GLAD. Loose bodies can occur in joint from detached avulsed articular cartilage fragment.[30] In ALPSA (anterior labroligamentous periosteal sleeve avulsion) lesion, there is tear of anterior labrum with periosteal stripping and displacement of labrum medially. Healing occurs typically with synovial fibrosis.[31] HAGL (humeral avulsion of GHL) lesions include detachment of capsule and IGHL from their anterior humeral attachment site. These lesions are uncommon cause of instability.[32] Perthe's lesion is described as an anterior labral tear having a scapular attachment with an intact periosteal sleeve[31] **(Fig. 21)**.

Three variations in anterior capsule insertion have been described.[33] Type I capsule inserts near the labrum, in type II, it inserts just medial to the labrum, and in type III, capsule is attached greater than 1 cm from the labral margin. Whether type III capsule predisposes to or is the result of anterior instability is not clear and debatable. However, a large capacious anterior pouch/subscapularis bursa is a frequent secondary finding in patients with recurrent anterior subluxation.

A close scrutiny of rotator cuff interval should also be done in all patients of clinical instability with RCT as capsule is weak in this area. The tear of the capsule may be isolated or associated with SST/SCT tears as well as biceps tendon dislocation.[34]

Superior labrum anterior to posterior (SLAP) lesions are important cause of traumatic instability. These lesions are typically seen in young people involved in sports activity requiring overhead movement of humeral head, like bowlers. They are believed to be caused by repetitive contact of humeral head with posterosuperior labrum. Consequently labrum becomes weak and tears away **(Fig. 22)**. Gradually tear progresses from posterior to anterior direction. The SLAP lesions were originally classified into four types by Snyder,[35] depending on the nature of labral injury and whether there is associated biceps tendon damage.

Type I: Fraying of glenoid labrum, but biceps tendon and labrum are not torn from glenoid (managed conservatively).

Type II: Stripping of labrum along with biceps tendon from glenoid (repaired surgically).

Type III: Bucket handle tear of labrum leaving biceps attachment to glenoid intact.

Type IV: Extension of bucket handle tear into biceps tendon.

This original classification was later expanded on the basis of arthroscopic findings however their clinical implication is questionable.

Type V: Bankart tear extending posterosuperiorly to biceps labral complex.

Type VI: Unstable flap or radial tear with separation of biceps from its anchor.

Type VII: Superior labral tear extending anteriorly beneath the middle GHL.

Type IX: Circumferential labral tear.

The SLAP lesions are associated with anterior instability and cuff tears. They are difficult to diagnose but important to identify as they respond well to arthroscopic repair.

Labral tears can be associated with labral cysts or ganglia which can cause compression neuropathy **(Fig. 23)**. These form because of one way valve mechanism leading to accumulation of joint fluid within them.

Anterior instability may also result from subscapularis injury. Subscapularis tears are seen after anterior dislocation over 40 years of age and after posterior dislocation at any age. Plain films and MRI may show lesser tuberosity fracture **(Fig. 24)**. Pfirrman et al.[36] graded subscapularis injury into four grades. Grade 0 tear is normal morphology. Grade I tear involves less than one-fourth and grade II tears involve greater than one fourth of subscapularis width. Grade III is complete detachment.

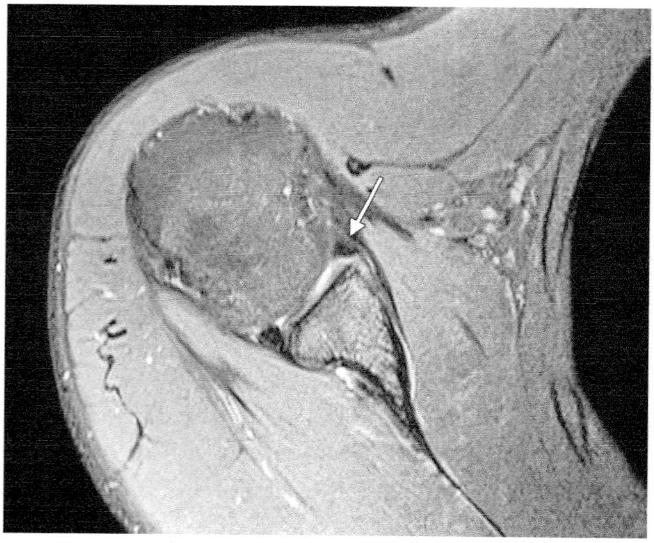

Fig. 21: Proton density fat saturated axial section showing avulsed labrum with a sleeve attached to the periosteum consistent with Perthe's variation of Bankart lesion (arrow).

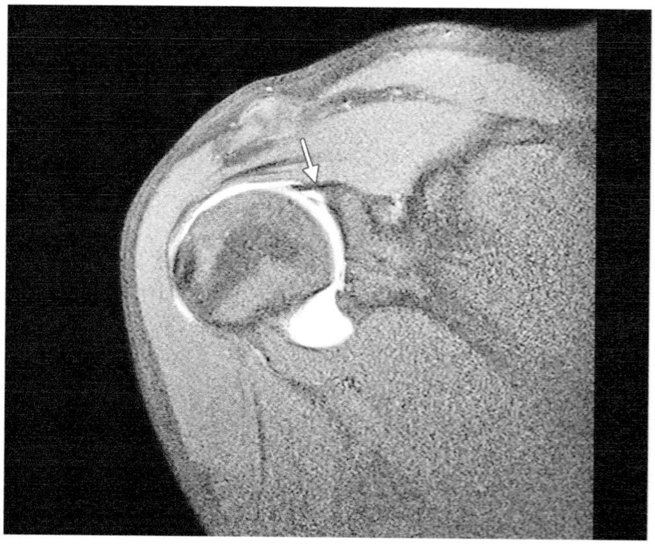

Fig. 22: T1 fat saturated arthrogram (coronal section) shows irregular shape tear with contrast filling in superior labrum suggestive of superior labrum anterior to posterior (SLAP) tear (arrow).

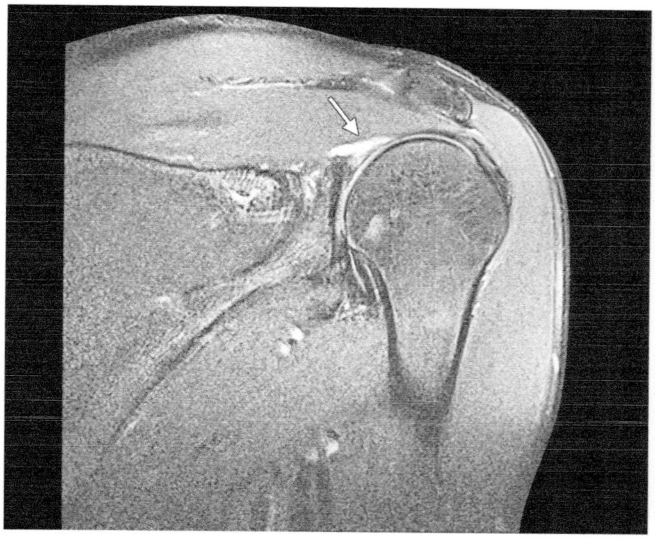

Fig. 23: Proton density fat sat coronal section shows superior labral tear with ganglion (arrow).

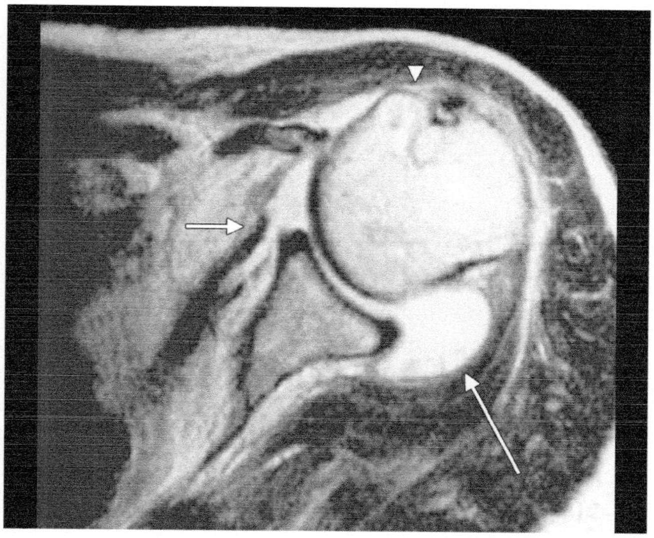

Fig. 24: T2 turbo spin-echo (T2 TSE) axial section shows a subscapularis tendon (SCT) tendon tear in a case of massive rotator cuff tear (RCT). The retracted tendon fibers (short arrow) and marrow edema at the lesser tuberosity (arrowhead) can be seen. A redundant posterior capsule indicates shoulder instability (long arrow).

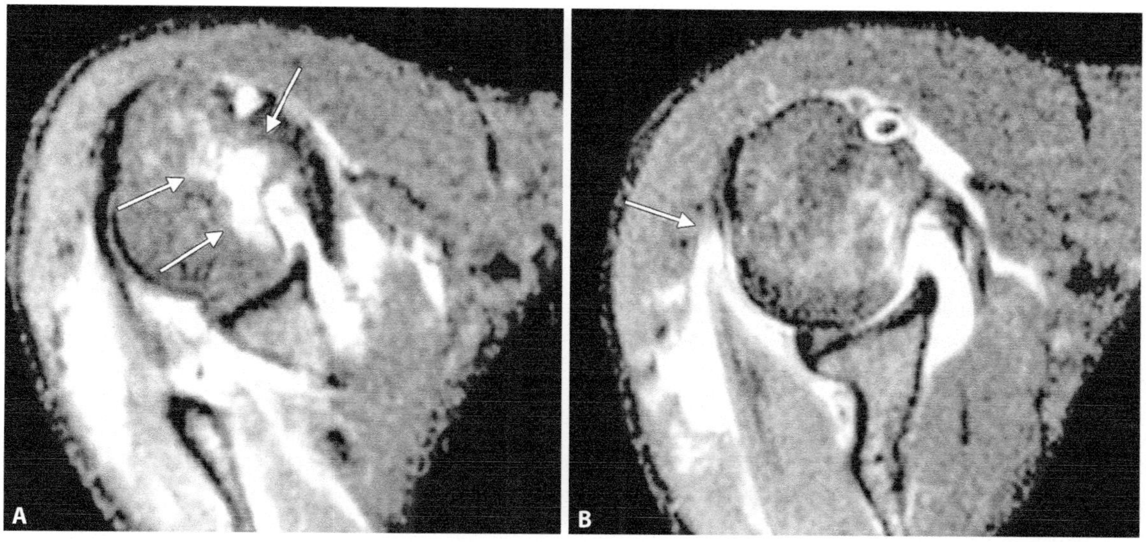

Figs. 25A and B: Turbo inversion recovery axial sections show classical anteromedial bony defect of reverse Hill-Sach's lesion due to posterior dislocation (A, arrows) and associated teres minor tendon tear (B, arrow). The posterior labrum is infolded and heterogeneous in signal.

Posterior instability is much less common than anterior (2–4%). It is usually a result of anterior direct blow on shoulder or seizures. Imaging findings in addition to subscapularis tears include teres minor injury, posterior labral and capsular tear and anteromedially located reverse Hill-Sach's lesion **(Figs. 25A and B)**.[37]

Pitfalls

Some anatomic variants that can mimic labral tear should be kept in mind while interpreting shoulder MR. The most significant normal variation is a deficient attachment of labrum in the anterosuperior quadrant of glenoid (sublabral foramen or recess). At superior portion of the labrum three types of attachments are seen.

Type I: Labrum firmly attached to glenoid rim.

Type II: A small recess is present between labrum and the cartilage.

Type III: A large sublabral recess is present.

Sublabral recess is seen in 30% of patients[38] and should be differentiated from an SLAP tear on MR arthrography by observing location and configuration of contrast. The SLAP tears are usually seen at or posterior to biceps tendon attachment while the recess is seen anterior to it. Contrast in sublabral recess is seen as a thin line with smooth margins that runs along the glenoid. Contrast in a tear has irregular margins, globular shape, and is seen to enter into labral substance.[39] Occasionally, contrast may be seen filling both sublabral recess and tear. This has been likened to a double chocolate or cream-filled cookie (Oreo sign).

A sublabral hole is seen in 17% normal people and is present at 2 O'clock position in pear-shaped glenoid cavities. Association of thick MGHL and an absent anterosuperior labrum has been termed as "Buford complex" and is also a normal variant.

The bright signal of hyaline cartilage between glenoid rim and labrum and the gap between MGHL and anterior glenoid can mimic tears of labrum. Following GHL on consecutive images can solve this problem.

ABNORMALITIES OF BICEPS TENDON

Bicipital Tendinopathy/Rupture

This usually occurs in middle aged or older patients with rotator cuff disease due to impingement of biceps tendon during flexion at shoulder joint beneath coracoacrominal ligament and anterior acromian.

This impingement may cause tendinopathy (or tenosynovitis) with flattening and thinning of tendon that may lead to complete rupture of the tendon **(Figs. 26A and B)**. Bicipital tendinopathy may also occur in patients with glenohumeral instability and attrition at the groove. Early bicipital tendinopathy often goes undetected on MR studies. MRI reveals increased signal intensity within the abnormal tendon.[40] "Magic angle effect" can also lead to fallacious increased signal intensity within the tendon.

Morphologic abnormalities such as fraying, flattening, and absence of tendon may sometime be identified. Disproportionate amount of fluid in bicipital tendon sheath as compared to the joint fluid may suggest bicipital abnormality, i.e., tenosynovitis.

Bicipital Tendon Dislocations

Bicipital tendon dislocation usually occurs with the chronic RCTs that have extended to involve the subscapularis tendons. The symptoms are usually masked by those of RCTs.

Some fibers of subscapularis along with deep fibers of coracohumeral and the superior GHL complex forms the pulley for biceps tendon and the bicipital groove is hooded by transverse humeral ligament. When all the three structures are disrupted, tendons of long head of biceps dislocates medially posterior to subscapularis tendon into the joint, where it may be mistaken for a detached anterior labrum. Rarely when subscapularis tendon remains intact, with the disruption of other two ligaments, biceps tendon displaces extra-articularly, anterior to SCM.[41] On axial MR images, bicipital groove is empty with medially dislocated tendon in cases of biceps dislocations **(Fig. 27)**.

NERVE ENTRAPMENT SYNDROMES

The following two nerve entrapment syndromes are uncommon but important causes of shoulder pain:

Quadrilateral Space Compression Syndrome

Quadrilateral space is bounded by teres minor superiorly, teres major inferiorly, shaft of humerus laterally, and long head of biceps medially. Axillary nerve and posterior humeral circumflex artery and vein pass through it.

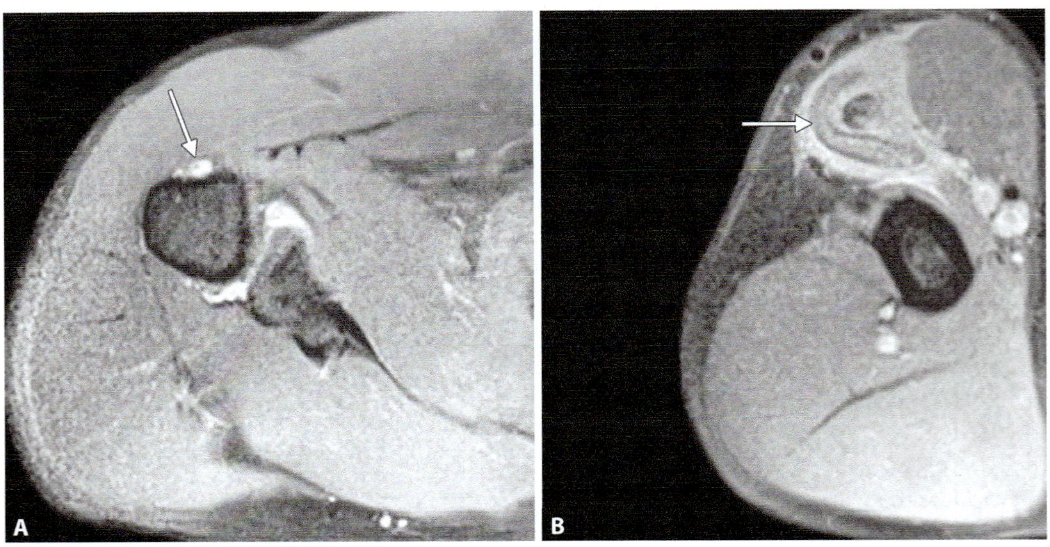

Figs. 26A and B: Proton density fat saturated axial section at the level of glenoid (A) shows empty bicipital groove suggestive of complete rupture of biceps tendon. Retracted biceps tendon (arrow) is seen in upper arm (B).

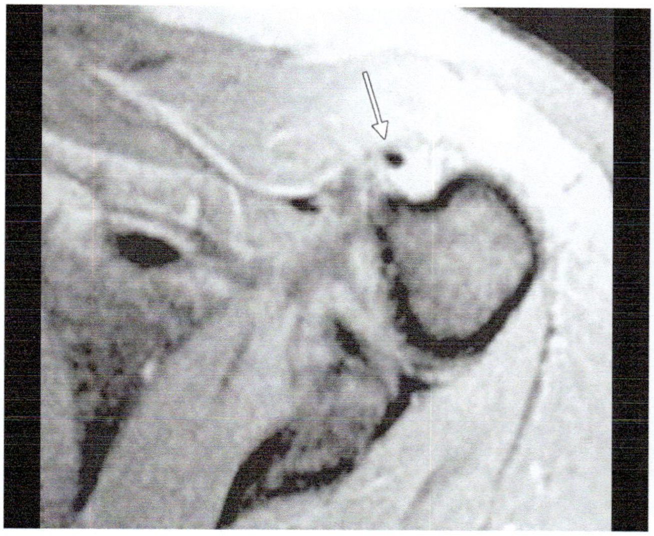

Fig. 27: Fat-suppressed T2 turbo spin-echo (T2 TSE) axial section: Biceps tendon is seen dislocated medially (arrow) with an empty bicipital groove.

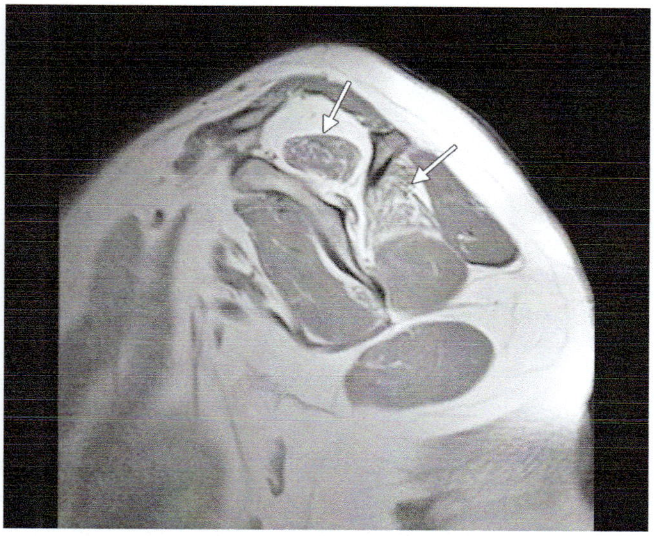

Fig. 28: T1 oblique sagittal section shows atrophy and fatty changes in supraspinatus and infraspinatus (arrows) secondary to impingement of suprascapular nerve.

Patients present with pain and paresthesia in axillary nerve distribution and muscle atrophy of teres minor and major muscles. MRI does not show actual entrapment but excludes other causes of shoulder pain and only shows atrophy of teres minor with major muscle.[42] MR angiography or DSA (digital subtraction angiography) may be helpful by showing occlusion of posterior circumflex humeral artery.

Suprascapular Nerve Entrapment

Suprascapular nerve passes through supraspinatus notch to enter supraspinatus fossa beneath supraspinatus muscles. Further posteriorly it passes through spinoglenoid notch to enter into the intraspinatus fossa. It supplies both supraspinatus as well as infraspinatus muscle. Compression of nerve at the level of suprascapular notch results in atrophy of both muscles **(Fig. 28)** and compression at the level of spinoglenoid notch results in atrophy of infraspinatus muscle only. Compression may be because of neoplasm, hematoma, or most commonly ganglion cyst. MR shows fatty replacement of involved muscle and soft tissue lesion responsible for compression.[43]

Ganglion cysts are either associated with labral tears or typically arise from a posterior capsular defect and present at spinoglenoid notch. They appear isointense to muscle on T1WI and hyperintense on T2WI. They are often septate and may show rim enhancement on gadolinium administration.

Adhesive Capsulitis

Adhesive capsulitis (frozen shoulder) is a clinical syndrome of pain and restricted joint movement secondary to thickening and contraction of the synovial sheath and joint capsule. It is most commonly seen in 40–60 years old females. It may be associated with trauma, osteoarthritis, or rheumatic disorders.

On MRI, abnormal soft tissue may be seen in the rotator cuff interval encasing SGHL or CHL and may extend to undersurface of the biceps anchor.

Joint capsule and synovial thickening of more than 4 mm at the level of axillary recess is a useful MR criterion to diagnose this condition[44] **(Figs. 29A and B)**. Postgadolinium enhancement of the rotator cuff interval or axillary recess may be present, increasing the diagnostic accuracy.

Magnetic resonance arthrography, though not preferred for diagnosis, reveals decreased joint volume (<10 cc), decreased fluid volume in biceps tendon sheath and axillary recess, corrugations of capsule with thickening, and rotator interval abnormality.

Calcific Tendinitis

Formation of calcific deposits in the tendon is a degenerative process. Calcification of rotator cuff most commonly occurs in supraspinatous tendon but can occur in other tendons.[45] The size of deposition may vary from few millimeter to several centimeter. MR examination shows linear or globular area of decreased signal in all pulse sequences; however, T2* GRE has more sensitivity and specificity to demonstrate hypointensity in the tendon **(Figs. 30A and B)**.

ARTHRITIS

The shoulder joint is frequently involved in osteoarthritis and other infective/inflammatory arthropathies. MRI can demonstrate early inflammatory soft tissue and osseous changes and can be used as a sensitive monitoring tool.

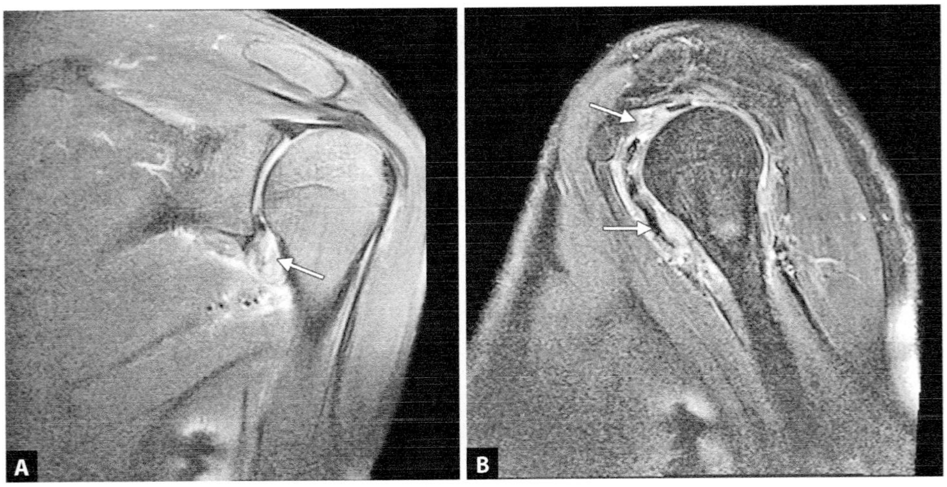

Figs. 29A and B: Proton density fat coronal section (A) and sagittal oblique (B): Thickened axillary pouch (arrows) with capsular edema and soft issue in rotator interval are indicative of adhesive capsulitis in a patient with frozen shoulder.

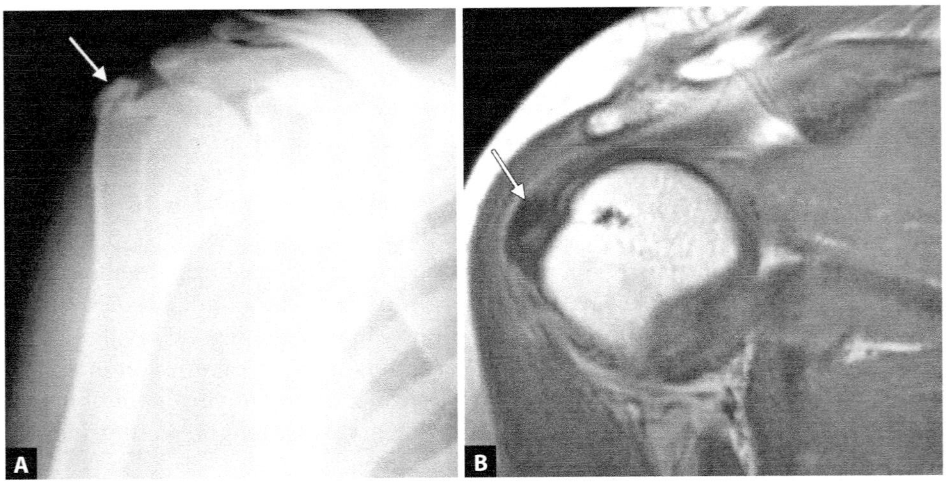

Figs. 30A and B: (A) Radiograph of shoulder shows globular calcification near greater tuberosity; (B) T1W coronal section shows globular area of hypointense signal (arrow) in the supraspinatus tendon suggestive of calcific tendinitis.

Osteoarthritis

Osteoarthritis of shoulder is characterized by chondral erosions, osteophyte formation, subchondral cyst, sclerosis, and synovitis.[46] Humeral head sclerosis and cartilage loss are usually central or superior in location. MRI is very good to identify cartilage thinning and loss. Subchondral cysts are seen in both humeral head and glenoid **(Fig. 31)**. Inferior capsule may be enlarged with contraction of anterior capsule. Loose bodies occur in glenohumeral joint and subacromial bursa which appear isointense to bone or hypointense on T2W images.

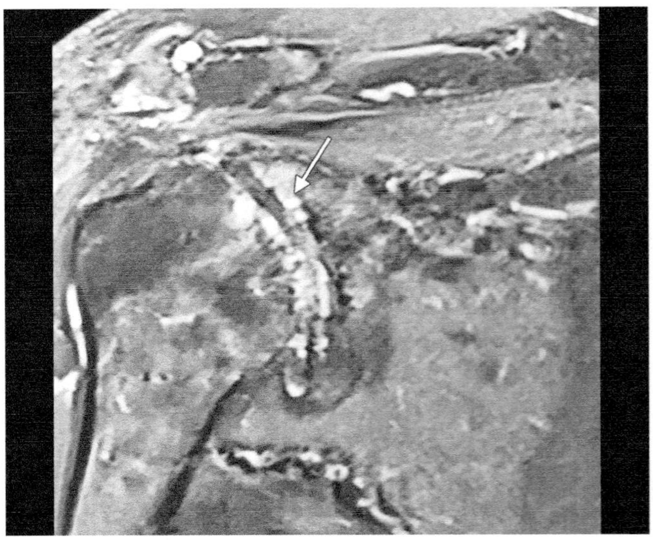

Fig. 31: T2 fat suppressed coronal section shows osteophytes, cartilage loss, and subchondral cysts which are typical findings of osteoarthritis.

Infective Arthritis

Septic arthritis is a clinical diagnosis relying on physical and laboratory parameters and microbiologic assessment of joint aspirate. Usually it affects older age group (average 65 years). The source of infection is either hematogenous or local. Immunocompromised status and pre-existing degenerative joint disease increases risk of septic arthritis. However, typical systemic and local symptoms may be absent in indolent infections like tuberculosis. Conventional radiographs may show associated osteoarthritis, osteomyelitis, or serve as a baseline study to monitor disease progression or response to treatment, but are insensitive to pick up early marrow or soft tissue changes. MR demonstrates these well along with bone changes; however, its specificity is low.[47]

Inflammation of synovial lining and joint effusion, the earliest pathologic changes, and associated bone marrow edema are seen well on fat-saturated T2WI and postcontrast T1WI **(Figs. 32A and B)**. Further progression of disease leads to cartilage destruction manifesting as joint space narrowing and marginal erosion of bare area. Subchondral bone changes in form of edema, subchondral cyst formation, and bone destruction follow when disease becomes subacute. Osteomyelitis, bone destruction, and joint ankylosis are features of chronic septic arthritis. RCTs can also be seen in subacute and chronic disease. MR cannot distinguish septic from nonseptic arthritis. Combination of bone erosions with marrow edema favors infectious etiology. Tuberculosis of shoulder joint is infrequent and has indolent clinical presentation. Patients usually presents with pain and restriction of movement for long duration. MRI is very useful to demonstrate synovial thickening, erosions, bone edema, and periarticular collections **(Figs. 33A and B)**.

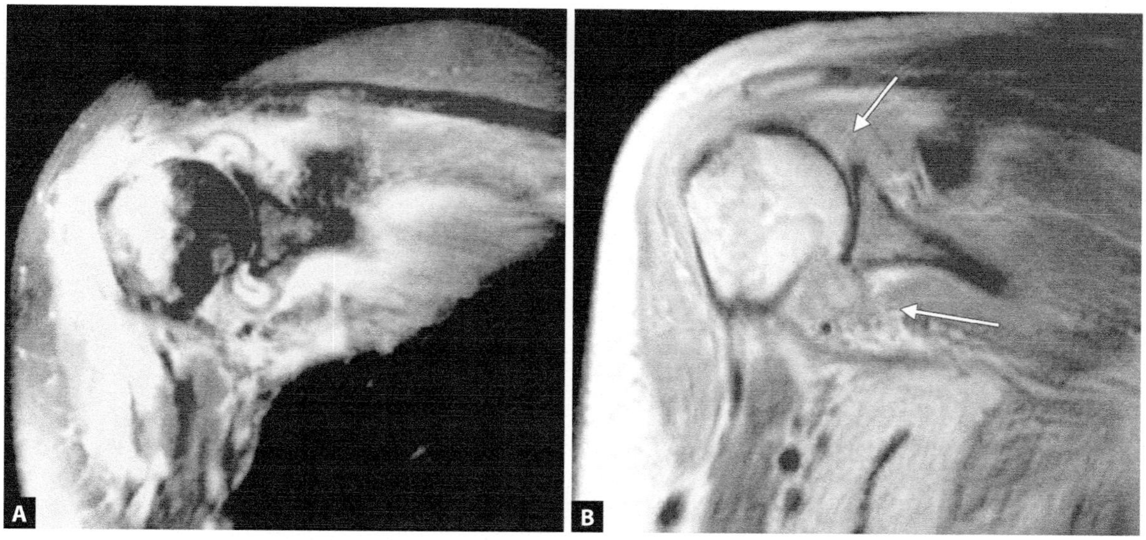

Figs. 32A and B: T2 turbo spin-echo (T2 TSE) fat-suppressed coronal section (A) reveals marked bone marrow and periarticular soft tissue edema and synovial thickening in a case of septic arthritis. T1 SE postcontrast (B) shows enhancement of the synovium and the periarticular tissue (arrows).

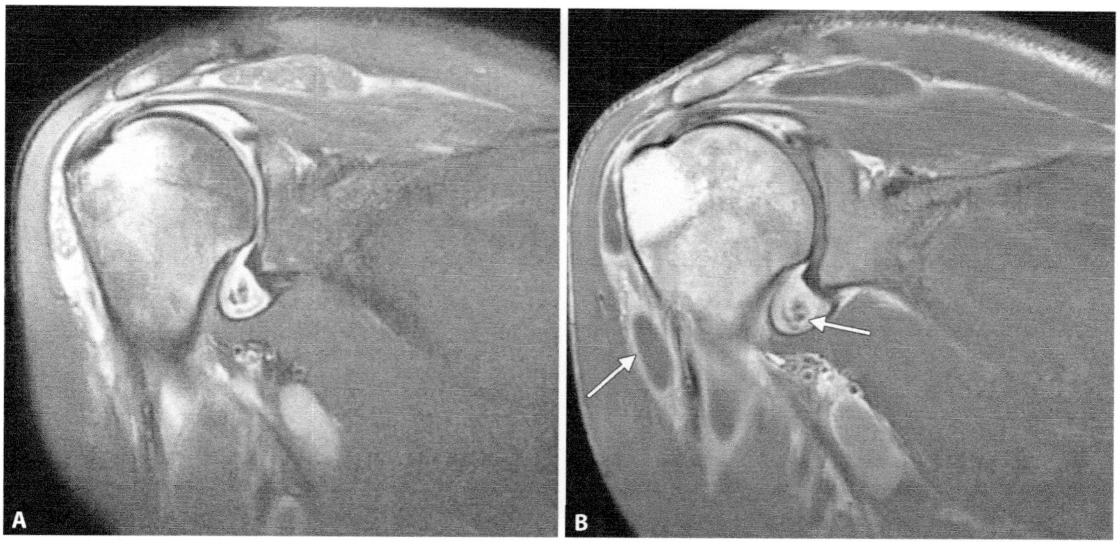

Figs. 33A and B: Tubercular arthritis: T2W fat saturated (A) and T1 fat saturated postcontrast coronal section (B) show joint effusion, synovial thickening, erosions, and periarticular collections.

Rheumatoid Arthritis

Rheumatoid arthritis (RA) is a chronic inflammatory joint disease, which involves synovial lining of joints. With disease progression there is involvement of articular cartilage, bone at joint margins, and periarticular soft tissue. Shoulder joint becomes involved later in the disease process. Proliferative synovitis involves glenohumeral joint, AC joint, and bursae around shoulder. Rotator cuff also becomes involved as disease progresses.

Magnetic resonance imaging is useful for detecting early changes of RA including synovitis, joint effusion, and marginal erosions. Marginal erosions are seen as low-signal areas on T1WI and variable signal intensity on T2WI. MRI may be superior to ultrasound, CT, or conventional radiographs for detecting marginal erosions.[48]

Cartilage destruction is difficult to evaluate with routine shoulder protocol including MR arthrography, as it is very thin. RCTs are commonly seen in RA due to destructive synovitis near greater tuberosity.

Presence, size, and extent of synovial cysts, clinically evident soft tissue swellings of subacromial, and subdeltoid bursitis and simultaneous arthritic involvement of AC joint, all well-known manifestations of RA can be well shown by MR.

AVASCULAR NECROSIS

It is associated with trauma, steroid use, sickle cell anemia, and alcoholism. It can be differentiated from osteoarthritis by signal abnormality confined to the humeral head and sparing of glenoid. The Neer classification for shoulder AVN is similar to Ficat classification for hip osteonecrosis.[49] MR may show focal subarticular dark signal, a dark line encircling normal marrow, or a double line sign early on and fragmentation and collapse of head later **(Fig. 34)**. Metadiaphyseal lesions may show classical serpiginous low-intensity line surrounding high-intensity center (in chronic infarcts) and high-intensity rim in more acute infarcts.

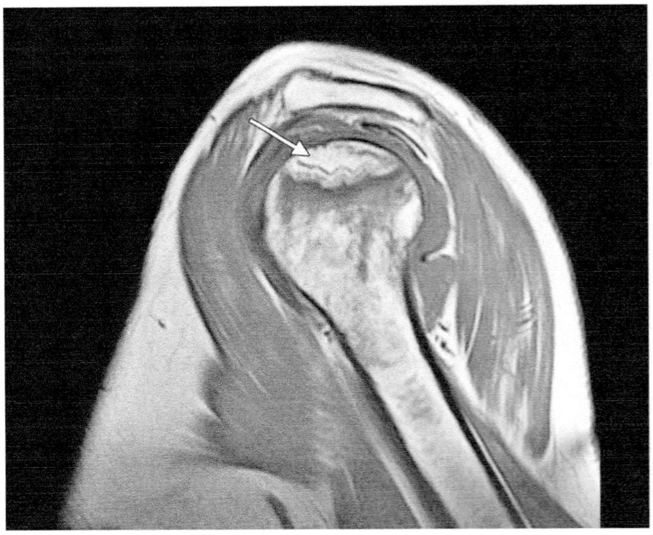

Fig. 34: T1 oblique sagittal section shows well-defined serpiginous area in humeral head suggestive of AVN (arrow).

NEOPLASMS

Magnetic resonance imaging is the imaging modality of choice for characterizing and staging both primary and secondary musculoskeletal neoplasms and tumor like lesions. MR shows joint involvement, soft tissue, and osseous components, involvement of neurovascular structures as well as helps in tissue characterization. T1WI (for marrow involvement), T2WI (for soft tissue extension), STIR, and postgadolinium fat-suppressed T1WI diagnose and stage tumors well. Metastatic disease is by far the most common malignant tumor around shoulder followed by myeloma, osteosarcoma, chondrosarcoma, and Ewing's sarcoma **(Figs. 35A and B)**.

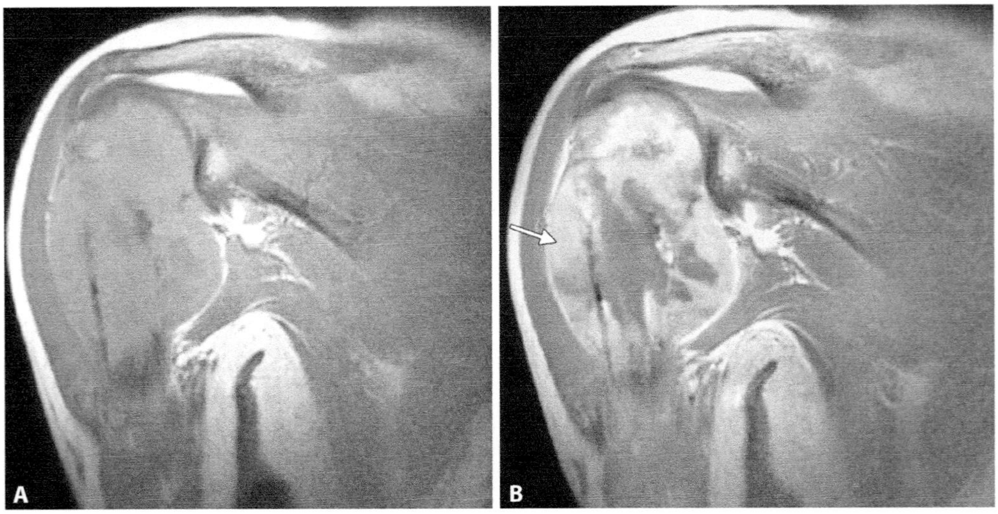

Figs. 35A and B: Ewing's sarcoma: T1W coronal (A) and postcontrast T1W, coronal section (B) shows malignant mass arising from metadiaphysis of right humerus associated with cortical destruction and adjacent soft tissue.

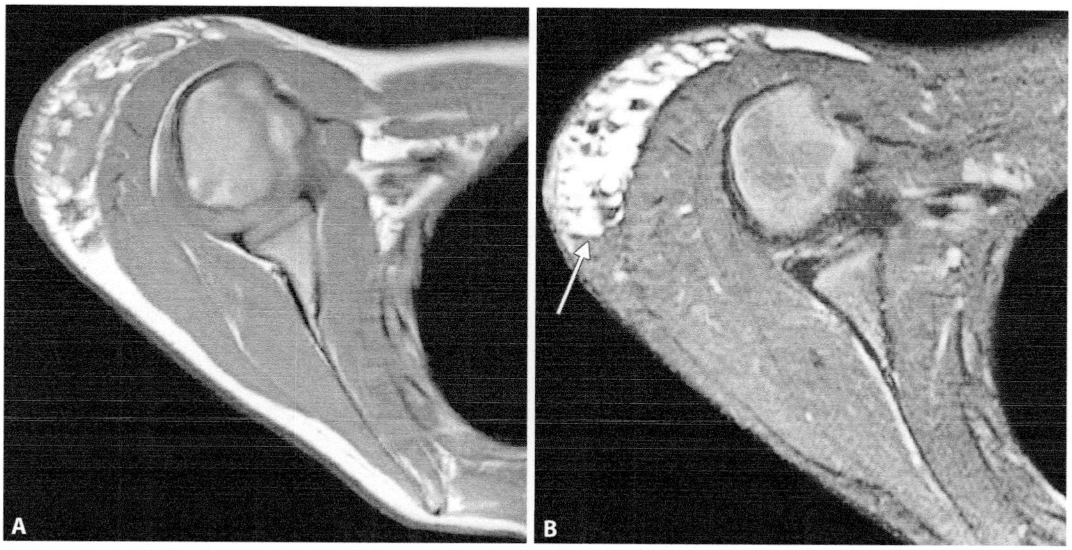

Figs. 36A and B: Soft tissue hemangioma: T1W axial (A) and T2W fat saturated axial section (B) of shoulder show altered signal soft tissue lesion superficial to deltoid muscle limited to subcutaneous tissue.

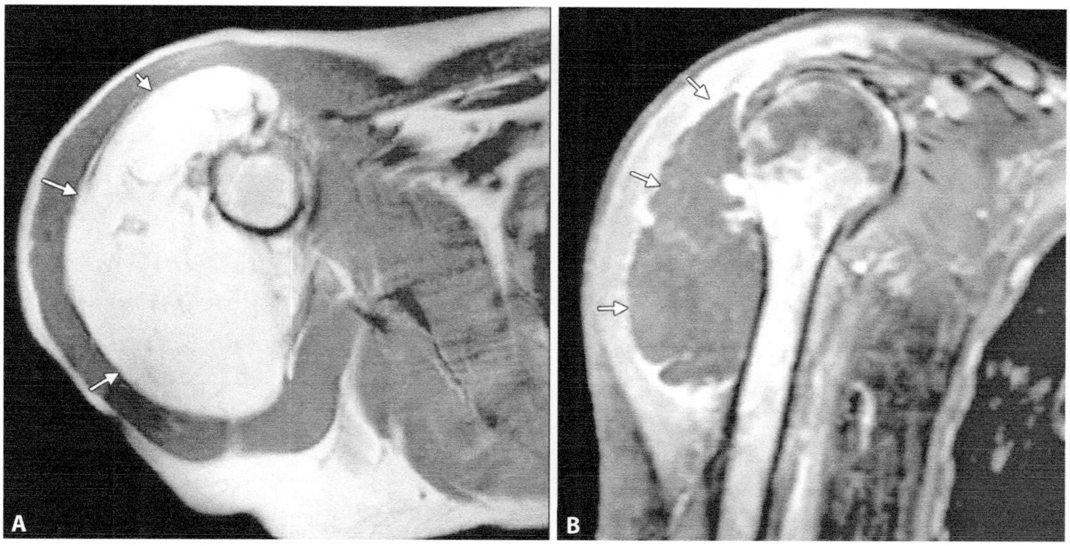

Figs. 37A and B: T1 axial section: A lipoma (arrows) in relation to the subacromial-subdeltoid bursa (SASDB) showing high-signal of fat (A). The inversion recovery image shows dark signal due to fat saturation (B).

Frequent benign lesions comprise osteochondroma, chondroma, chondroblastoma, and giant cell tumor. Common soft tissue lesions around the shoulder are hemangioma **(Figs. 36A and B)**, lipoma **(Figs. 37A and B)**, and extra-abdominal desmoid.[50]

ADVANCE MAGNETIC RESONANCE TECHNIQUES IN SHOULDER JOINT

The routine protocols used for MR examinations of shoulder are quite good to detect shoulder injuries and related pathologies; however, there has been advancement in MR techniques to answer some particular clinical queries.[51]

Axial 3D dual echo-time T1-weighted FLASH sequence: Assessment of bony injuries involving humeral head and glenoid are important for management of shoulder injuries. CT scan with 3D reconstructions provides details of bony injuries; however, it is associated with radiation exposure. 3D dual echo-time T1-weighted FLASH sequence can provide 3D reconstruction comparable to traditional CT.[52-53]

Oblique sagittal 3D volume-interpolated breathhold examination (VIBE): Rotator cuff tear may be associated with fatty degeneration of cuff muscle. The assement of fatty degeneration is important at it is important factor for outcome after rotator cuff repair. Goutallier classification system is established qualitative assessment method however recent studies have focused on the quantitative assessment of fat fractions to see relationship between muscular atrophy and fatty infiltration of the rotator cuff by using a 3D oblique sagittal volume-interpolated breathhold examination (VIBE) sequence with the 2-point Dixon method.[54-56]

Three-dimensional MRI reconstruction of the rotator cuff: 3D imaging can depict the exact shape of cuff tear which is useful for preoperative planning of these patients. Tendon tears can be classified as either longitudinal or crescent shaped. Longitudinal tears are those with length greater than its width. Crescent-shaped tears has more width then length. Longitudinal tear may be subdivided in U- or L-shaped tears.[57-58]

Radial MRI of the shoulder: There can be partial averaging of insertional fibers of rotator cuff with concealment of smaller tear. Radial MRI can improve the detection of small tear. Radial imaging has shown excellent promise in the evaluation of subtle RCTs, especially those involving the subscapularis tendon.[59]

Diffusion tensor imaging (DTI): It is an advanced method for quantify direction-dependent water diffusion. Rotator muscle fibers tracts are visualized by advanced postprocessing. As a functional MR technique, DTI may show muscle abnormalities before they become evident at conventional morphologic MR sequences.[60]

TEMPOROMANDIBULAR JOINT

INTRODUCTION

Temporomandibular joint (TMJ) dysfunction is a common condition that may affect up to 28% of the population.[61] The most common cause of TMJ dysfunction is internal derangement, which is defined as an abdominal relationship of the disc to the condyle. The TMJ dysfunction is best evaluated with MRI due to excellent demonstration of disc morphologic changes, disc displacement, and various other abnormalities of TMJ.[62]

MAGNETIC RESONANCE IMAGING TECHNIQUE

Magnetic resonance imaging of TMJ is performed by using the body coil as transmitter and dual surface coils as receiver (simultaneous examination of both sides is preferred as TMJ disorders often involve both sides). Axial plane is used for localization of condyle and planning of sagittal and coronal images. Sagittal images are obtained in both closed and open mouth positions, in a plane perpendicular to the horizontal long axes of mandibular condyles **(Fig. 38)**. Coronal images are acquired along the horizontal long axes of condyles in closed mouth position.

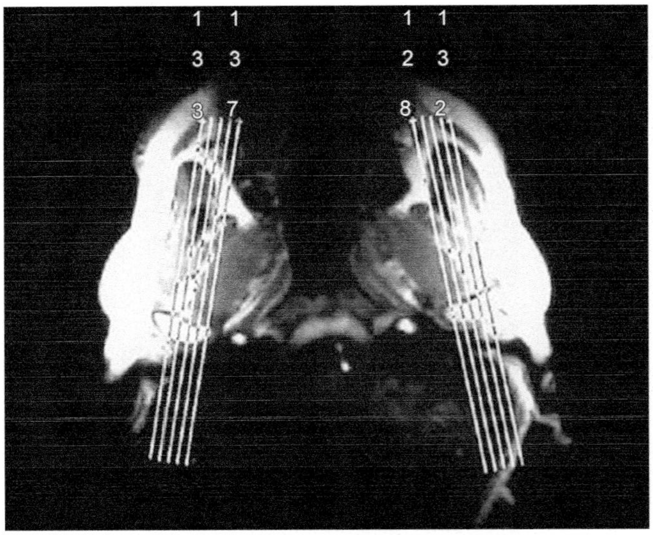

Fig. 38: For temporomandibular joint imaging, sagittal images are planned perpendicular to the horizontal axes of mandibular condyles on axial scout images as shown. The coronal images are planned perpendicular to the above prescribed sagittal plane.

Out of these sagittal plane is standard plane of imaging. The preferred sequences are T1 spin echo (shows fat as bright), T2 turbo spin echo (fluid sensitive), and proton density images. Functional joint dynamics at incremental mouth opening can be shown with small flip angle gradient echo imaging.

NORMAL ANATOMY AND MAGNETIC RESONANCE APPEARANCE (FIGS. 39 TO 42)

Temporomandibular joint is a diarthrodial synovial joint. Its articular surfaces are formed by articular eminence and anterior part of mandibular (glenoid) fossa superiorly and head of mandibular condyle inferiorly **(Figs. 39A and B)**. Articular surfaces are covered by a fibrocartilage. Mandibular condyles are elliptical in shape with their long axes converging posteriorly at around 15° **(Fig. 40C)**.[63] An intra-articular disc divides the joint into upper and lower compartments **(Figs. 39 and 40)**. The disc is composed of avascular fibrous connective tissue which merges with peripheral capsule. It is oval in shape, measuring approximately 18 mm in anteroposterior dimension and 20 mm in mediolateral extension. It is biconcave in sagittal plane and crescent shaped in coronal plane. Two localized thickenings are present in the disc, called anterior and posterior bands. Posterior band is thicker than the anterior band. Consequently, the disc is 2 mm thick in its anterior part, 1 mm centrally, and 3 mm in its posterior part.[54] Normally, in a closed mouth position, posterior band is located directly above the condyle, central thin zone between articular eminence and condyle and anterior band below articular eminence. Disc is attached posteriorly to temporal bone and posterior subcondylar area through a fibrofatty vascular connective

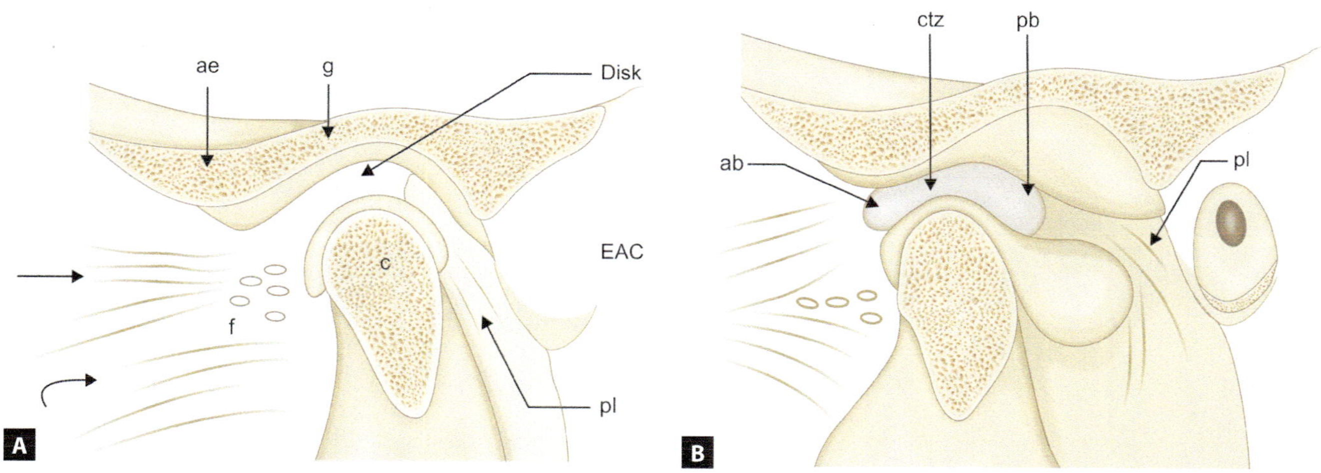

Figs. 39A and B: Diagrammatic representation of temporomandibular joint (TMJ) anatomy. (A) Close mouth position—oval disc lies between the condyle (c) and glenoid fossa (g). More anteriorly the articular eminence is seen (ae). The retrodiscal tissue (pl) acts as the posterior attachment. Bright lateral pterygoid fat plane (f), external auditory canal (EAC), superior (straight arrow) and inferior (curved arrow) bellies of lateral pterygoid muscles are also labeled; (B) Open mouth position—the condyle and the disc move anteriorly together to a position below the articular eminence with central thin zone interposed between the two. (ab: anterior band; ctz: central thin zone; pb: posterior band).

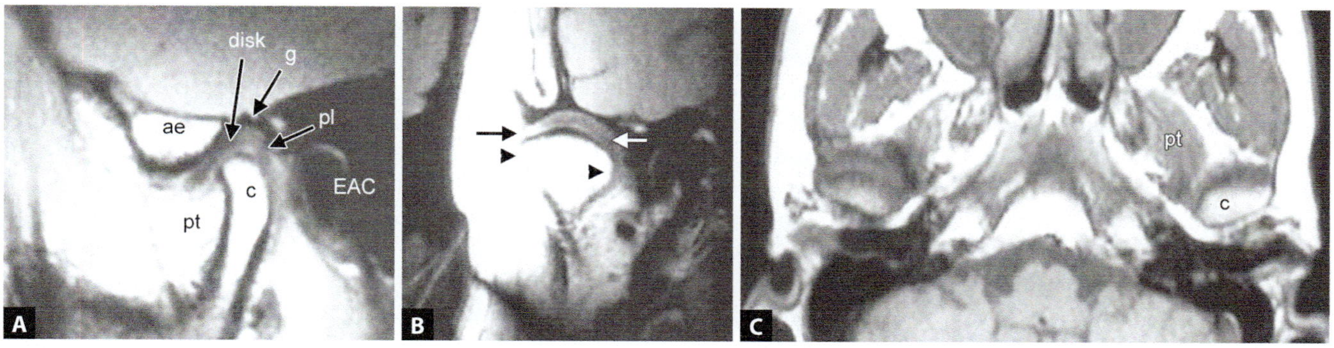

Figs. 40A to C: (A) Sagittal proton WI showing normal anatomy (compare with Fig. 2). The marrow in the condyle and articular eminence appears bright in signal. The articular margins of temporal bone are dark and well-defined. The disc shows intermediate signal; (B) Coronal proton WI: The crescent-shaped disc (white arrow), and lateral attachment of disc (black arrow) are seen. The lateral and medial poles of the condyle (arrow heads) can be seen with disc attaching just beneath them; (C) Axial anatomy T1WI: Elliptical condyles with posteriorly converging horizontal axes in relation to skull base. (c: condyle; pt: inferior belly of lateral pterygoid muscle)

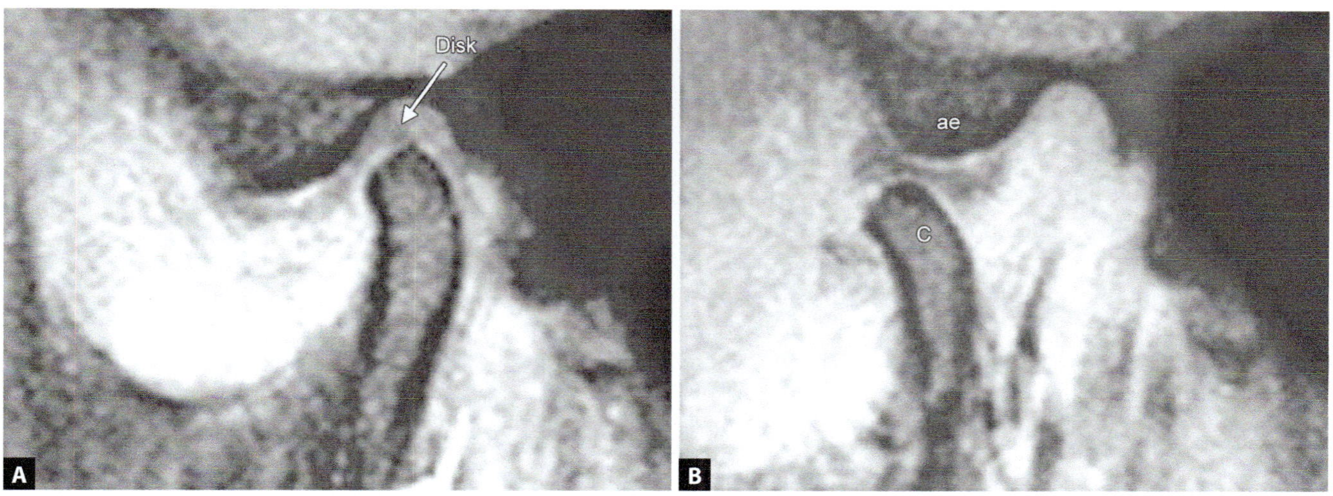

Figs. 41A and B: (A) Close mouth; and (B) Open mouth positions showing location of disc (arrow) in relation to the condyle. The posterior band lies just superior to condyle in (A) and the condyle lies opposite the articular eminence with interposed thin zone between them in open mouth position (B).

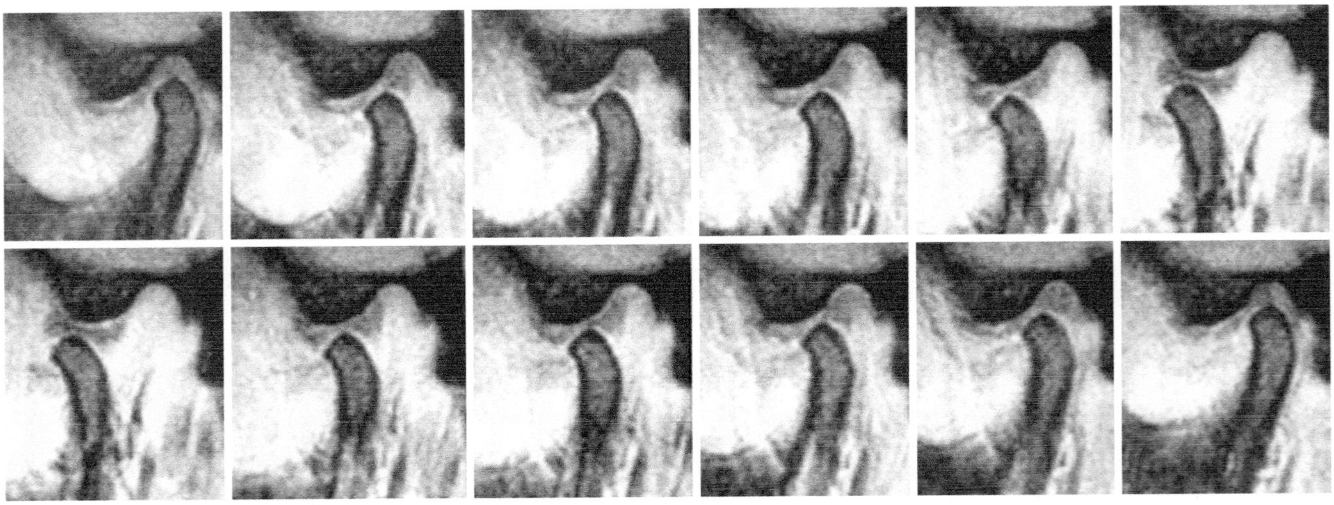

Fig. 42: Fast gradient echo serial sagittal sections showing condylar translation in the glenoid fossa and its constant relationship with the disc. (upper row—mouth opening and lower row—mouth closing). The posterior band at 12 O'clock position in the closed mouth position (first frame upper row). The head opposed to articular eminence with thin zone of disc interposed between the two (last frame upper row). Note expansion of the posterior soft tissues as mouth opens.

tissue called posterior attachment, retrodiscal tissue, or bilaminar zone through its superior and inferior lamina. This structure restrains its anterior movement. Joint is covered by a loose connective tissue capsule, attached superiorly to articular eminence and circumference of mandibular fossa and inferiorly to neck of condyle. The superior head of lateral pterygoid inserts on anterior capsule and adjacent condylar neck with its tendinous fibers directly attaching to the anterior band of the disc and helps in mouth opening. Medial pterygoid and temporalis muscles with their mandibular insertions also assist mandibular movements. Temporomandibular and sphenomandibular/stylomandibular ligaments reinforce the lateral and medioposterior capsule, respectively.

Normal Magnetic Resonance Appearance

The cortices of condyle and temporal component of the TMJ have smooth outline and low-signal intensity **(Fig. 40A)**. The articular covering and synovium show high-signal. Intra-articular disc shows low-signal intensity as it is composed of fibrous tissue; however, the posterior disc attachment has relatively high-signal intensity because of fatty tissue. The attachment of superior belly of lateral pterygoid to anteromedial disc and adjacent condyle can also be demonstrated as low-intensity structure. The medial pterygoid muscle lies inferiorly. The low-signal maxillary vessels can be seen between pterygoid muscles and mandibular condyle. The low-signal temporomandibular ligament can be seen as laterally supporting structures on coronal images **(Fig. 40B)**.

MOVEMENTS

The TMJ movements take place at both compartments. Translation occurs predominantly in the upper compartment and both rotation and translation in the lower compartment. During jaw opening, initially the condyles rotate in lower compartment followed by translatory movement in upper and subsequently in the lower joint compartment. During translation there is sliding movement of intraarticular disc along with condyle in relation to mandibular fossa. During all movements the central disc remains located between the condyle and the articular tubercle with anterior and posterior bands acting as functional guides. In contrast to the 12 O'clock location of posterior band in closed mouth position, in open mouth position the apex of the condyle lies opposite the articular eminence with interposed central thin zone between the two and there is marked expansion of the tissue in the region of posterior attachment **(Figs. 39 to 41)**. The disc does not move in the mediolateral direction unless these attachments are torn.

DISEASES OF TEMPOROMANDIBULAR JOINT

Temporomandibular joint disorders are more prevalent in young and middle age females. Patients with TMJ disorders present with complaints of myofacial pain syndrome (pain and muscle tenderness around the joint) and biomechanical dysfunction (clicking, crepitus, and limitation of jaw movements).

Internal Derangement

Internal derangement is defined as altered morphological and functional relationship between articular surface of the temporal bone, disc, and mandibular condyle.

Disc Displacements

This is the most common TMJ disorder.[65] Normally the posterior band is at 12 O'clock position in relation to mandibular condyle. Displacement is said to have occurred when this relationship is altered. Disc can displace in anterior, posterior, anteromedial, anterolateral, and sometimes purely in lateral and medial directions.[66] Anterior and posterior displacements are seen best in sagittal images. Lateral and medial displacements are best seen in coronal images.

Disc displacement is further categorized into "displacement without reduction" and "displacement with reduction." When an anteriorly displaced disc fails to return to normal position on jaw opening it is called displacement without reduction **(Figs. 43A and B)**. These patients can not open their mouths fully (closed lock jaw).[67] In displacement with reduction, displaced disc returns to normal position relative to condyle during jaw opening leading to reciprocal clicking[68] **(Figs. 44A and B)**.

Most common disc displacement is anterior however often it also has an anteromedial or anterolateral component **(Figs. 45A and B)**. Such displacements are also called rotational displacements. Further the disc displacement may be complete or partial when only the medial or lateral part of the disc is displaced. In pure medial and lateral disc displacements sagittal images will show no disc between condyle and mandibular fossa. Instead pulled up lateral or medial capsular tissue, respectively, will be seen, giving it an empty appearance (empty fossa sign).

Disc Deformity and Osteoarthritis

Internal derangements of TMJ are progressive disorders. The reducing disc leads to nonreducing disc in due course of time and a chronically displaced disc slowly gets deformed and later leads to osteoarthritis of the joint.[69] The above stages of displaced disc are also graded as acute (reducing disc with normal morphology), subacute (nonreducing disc with deformity), and chronic (adhesions, fibrosis, perforation, and degenerative joint disease).[70] Disc deformity is important to identify as it is treated with discectomy while disc repositioning is done for disc displacements.

Earliest MR findings of disc deformity is thickening of posterior band. As the disease progresses disc assumes rounded, biconvex, or sigmoid shaped instead of normal biconcave configuration. It may also show fissuring and surface irregularity. In some of the cases, the disc may show severely diminished volume.

Another tissue alteration seen in association with chronic disc displacement is formation of "pseudodisc." This appearance is because of fibrosis and anterior displacement of posterior attachment which comes to occupy the normal position of disc between condyle and mandibular fossa and simulates disc because of its low-signal intensity. Perforations are seen in 5–15% patients with disc displacement, more frequently at posterior disc attachment.[71] Secondary changes because of disc deformity include synovitis and joint effusion. It is best seen on T2 WI as increased signal intensity in upper, lower, or both compartments.

Marrow abnormality in form of marrow edema, osteonecrosis, or sclerosis in the condyle can be secondary to disc deformity **(Fig. 46)**. Normal marrow in condyle shows high signal intensity on both T1 and T2 WI. Marrow edema is seen as low-signal intensity on T1WI and high-signal intensity on T2WI. Osteonecrosis and sclerosis show low-signal intensity on T1WI and variable signal intensity on T2WI. Long-standing disc displacement without reduction can lead to osteoarthritis in TMJs. It is characterized by osteophyte formation with flattening and irregularity of articular surfaces **(Figs. 47A and B)**.

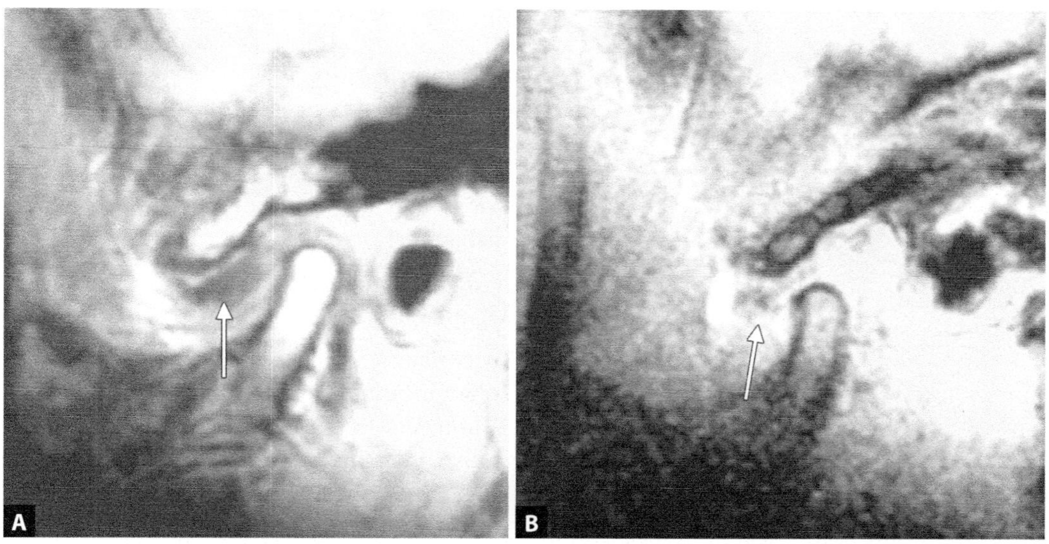

Figs. 43A and B: Nonreducing disc. Sagittal section (A) closed mouth and (B) open mouth. The nonreducing anteriorly displaced disc is shown (arrows).

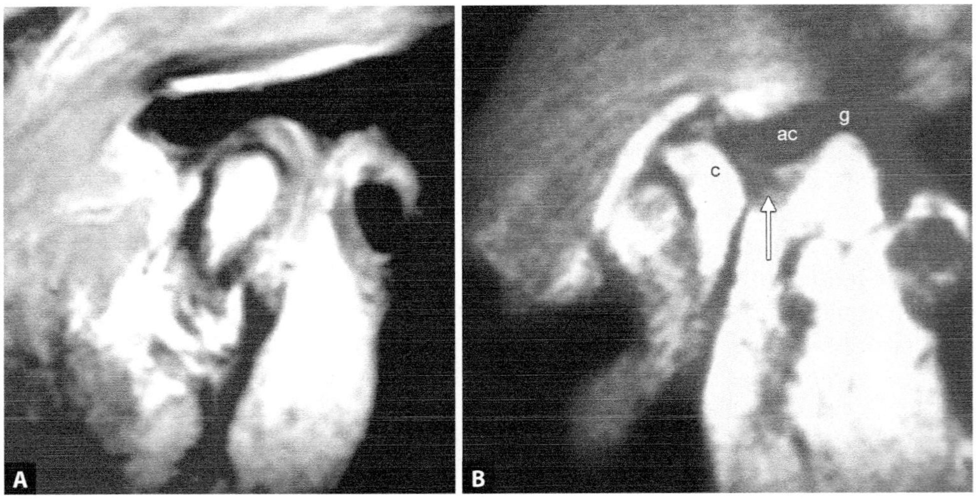

Figs. 44A and B: Reducing disc. Sagittal section (A) closed mouth and (B) open mouth. (A) There is mild anterior displacement of the disc; (B) Dislocation of condyle into infratemporal fossa anterior to the articular eminence. The eminence and the reduced disc (arrow) prevents condyle from returning to the glenoid fossa.

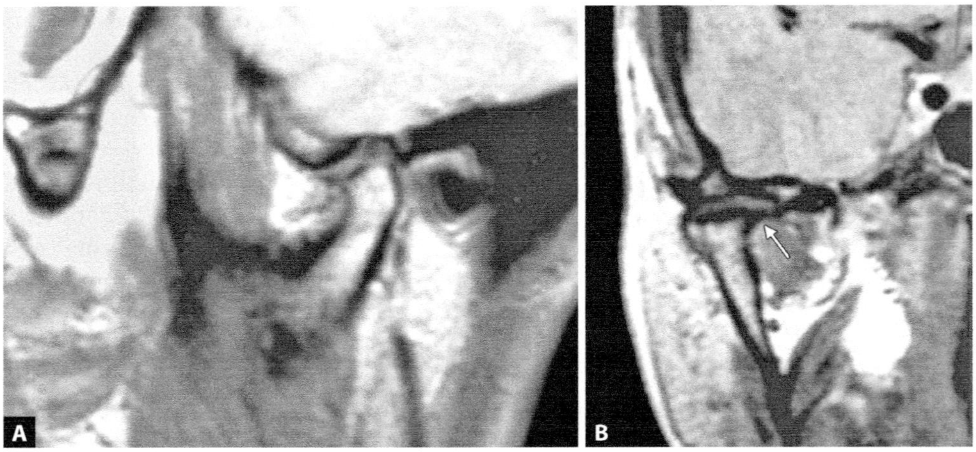

Figs. 45A and B: (A) Proton weighted sagittal section: The disc is not well seen in the glenoid fossa; (B) Coronal section: The disc is anteromedially displaced (arrow).

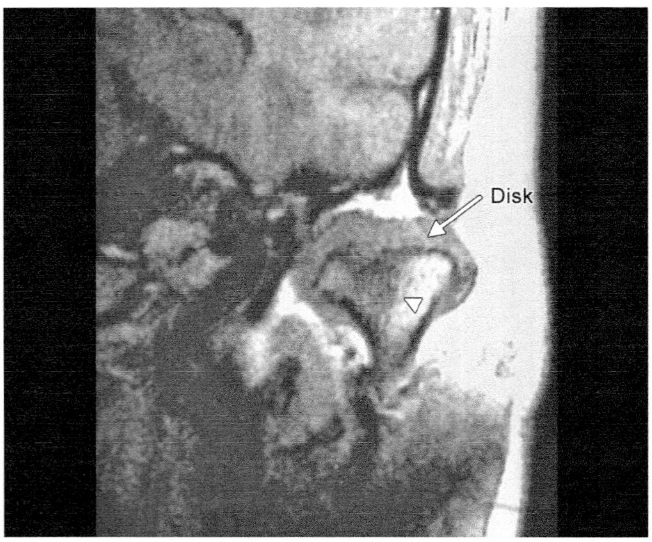

Fig. 46: Coronal T1WI: Low-intensity area in the medial part of the condyle (arrowhead) in case of displaced disc (arrow) likely representing a focus of avascular necrosis.

Stuck Disc

Upper compartment permits translational movements only, in which the disc slides or translates relative to the mandibular fossa. This movement is important in later part of jaw opening. In pathology of upper compartment, this movement gets blocked, consequently the patients is not able to open his mouth fully. This can cause pain and discomfort.

Open Lock Jaw

In contrast to "closed lock state" described above, in "open lock jaw," after wide opening of the mouth patient is not able to close mouth temporarily or permanently due to the dislocation of condyles in infratemporal fossa anterior to articular eminence. The latter prevents the condyle from returning back into glenoid fossa. On the other hand, a reducing disc may do the same **(Figs. 44A and B)**.

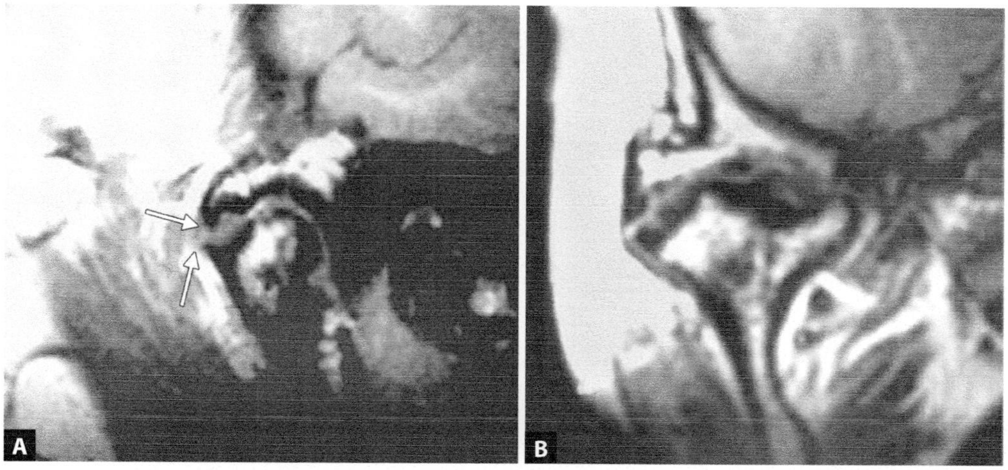

Figs. 47A and B: Sagittal (A) and coronal (B) T1-weighted sections: Articular surface irregularity, subchondral sclerosis, and osteophytes (arrows) along anterior glenoid rim and condyle in a case with osteoarthritis of TMJ.

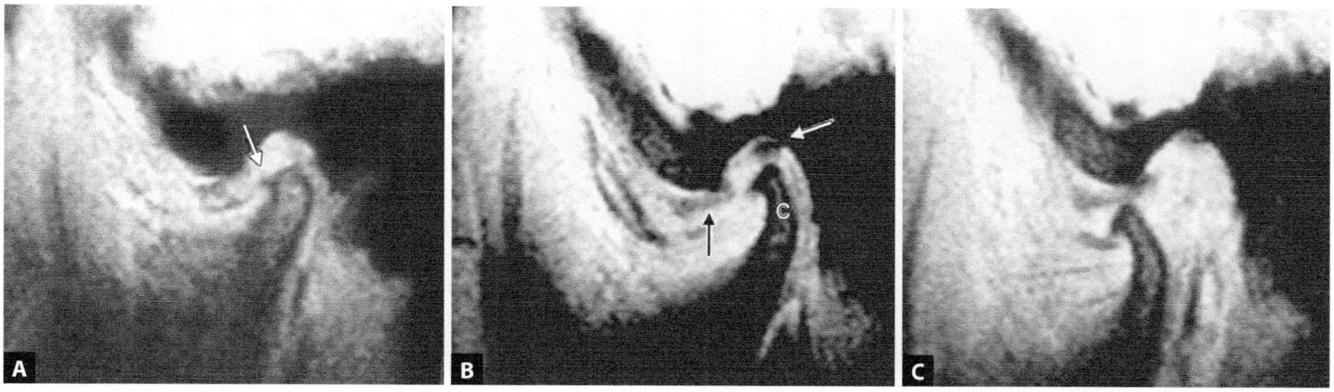

Figs. 48A to C: Mandibular asymmetry due to disc dislocation. (A) Right side—closed mouth; (B) Left side—closed mouth; (C) Left side—open mouth. The left condyle is hypoplastic (B). There is anterior dislocation of the disc on this side (black arrow) with fibrosis of posterior attachment (white arrow). The disc is nonreducing (C). The right-sided disc also shows features of degeneration (arrow—A).

Further indications of imaging of TMJ are demonstration of loose bodies, postoperative evaluation, mandibular asymmetry, trauma, infective/noninfective arthritis, and neoplasia.

Osteonecrosis and Osteochondritis Dissecans

Low-signal areas on T1WI within the marrow of mandibular condyle may represent above two conditions. Increased signal on T2 WI may indicate presence of edema and may be a precursor of osteonecrosis. The probable precipitating factors are local trauma and disc displacement[72] **(Fig. 46)**. Loose bodies may be seen within the joint in osteochondritis dissecans as hypointense structures.

POSTOPERATIVE IMAGING

Magnetic resonance is valuable in demonstrating joint mobility and postoperative adhesions/fibrosis after disc repositioning surgery and discectomy and also for evaluation of alloplastic implants. Contrast administration may be useful in postoperative evaluations of the joint.

EVALUATION OF MANDIBULAR ASYMMETRY

This is multifactorial and could be due to trauma or internal derangement. Unilateral condylar hyperplasia on long side may be seen in these patients.[73] In children with facial asymmetry, decreased condylar growth, or degenerative joint changes on short side may be demonstrated in response to displaced disc[74] **(Figs. 48A to C)**.

INFECTIONS AND ARTHRITIDES

Infections of TMJ are rare and seen postoperatively or through spread from adjacent structures, i.e., ear cavity.[75] Fluid sensitive sequences (T2 TSE) and postcontrast imaging provide valuable information in infections. TMJ is involved in 50% of patients with RA, ankylosing spondylitis, psoriatic arthritis, and pseudogout. MRI shows soft tissue involvement, erosions, and synovial proliferation.[76]

TUMORS AND TUMOR-LIKE CONDITIONS

Tumors of TMJ region are uncommon and more than two-thirds are benign.[77] Synovial chondromatosis

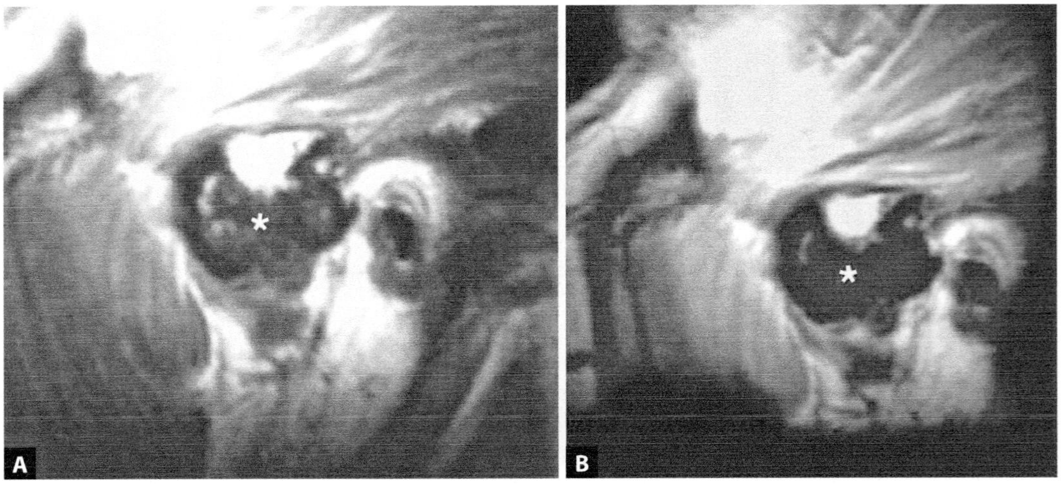

Figs. 49A and B: T1WI (A) and T2WI (B) show a densely sclerotic lesion in the articular eminence (asterix) suggestive of osteoma.

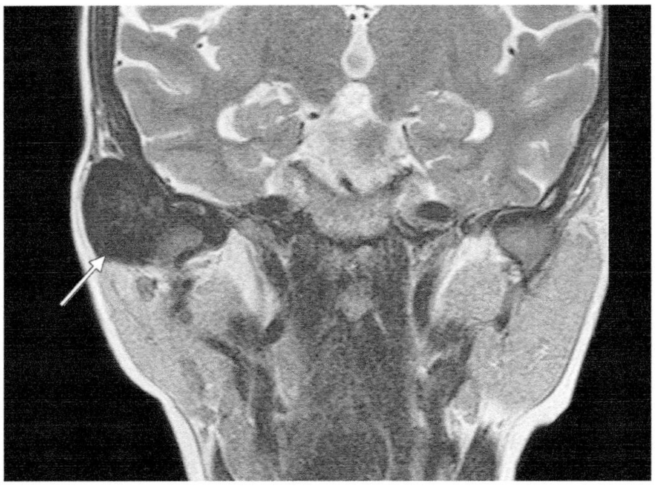

Fig. 50: T2W coronal section shows lobulated hypointense mass in right temporomandibular joint with widened joint space (arrow) suggestive of pigmented villonodular synovitis (PVNS).

has been reported in TMJ,[78,79] and MR may show joint expansion, synovial thickening with low-intensity foci within it. Osteochondroma is also a common tumor of the mandibular condyle and needs to be differentiated from osteoma and hypertrophic condylar changes **(Figs. 49A and B)**. Pigmented villonodular synovitis is uncommon but reported in TMJ. MR features include synovial thickening/mass with hypointensities on both TI and T2W images **(Fig. 50)**.[80] Meta-static diseases from a remote site (mostly adenocarcinoma from breast) can present around the TMJ in less than 1% cases. Synovial cysts, aneurysmal bone cyst, eosinophilic granuloma, chondrosarcoma, and lymphoma are reported in TMJ or mandibular condyle.[81-82]

REFERENCES

1. Stoller DW, wolf EM, LI AE, Nottage WM, Tirman FJP. The shoulder. In: Stoller DW (Eds). Magnetic Resonance Imaging in Orthopaedics and Sports Medicine, 3rd edition. Philadelphia: Lippincott, Williams and Wilkins; 2007. p. 1131.
2. Mack LA, Matsen FA III, Kilcoyne RF, Davies PK, Sickler ME. US evaluation of rotator cuff. Radiology. 1985;157:205-9.
3. Middleton WD, Edelstein G, Reinus WR, Melson GL, Totty WG, Murphy WA. Sonographic detection of rotator cuff tears. Am J Roentgenol. 1985;144:349-53.
4. Van Holsbeeck M, Strouse PJ. Sonography of the shoulder: Evaluation of the subacromial subdeltoid bursa. AJR Am J Roentgenol. 1993;160:561-4.
5. Martinoli C, Bianchi S, Prato N, Pugliese F, Zamorani MP, Valle M, et al. US of the shoulder: Nonrotator cuff disorders. Radiographics. 2003;23:381-401.
6. Berquist TH. MRI of the Musculoskeletal System, 3rd edition. New York: Raven Press; 1990. pp. 517-607.
7. Cook TS, Stein JM, Simonson S, Kim W. Normal and variant anatomy of the shoulder on MRI. Magn Reson Imaging Clin N Am. 2011;19:595-608.
8. Chung CB, Dwek JR, Feng S, Resnick D. MR arthrography of the glenohumeral joint: A tailored approach. Am J Roentgenol. 2001;177:217-19.
9. Chung CB, Corrente L, Resnick D. MR arthrography of the shoulder joint. MRI Clinics North Am. 2004;12:217-9.
10. Rudez J, Zanetti M. Normal anatomy, variants and pitfalls on shoulder MRI. Eur J Radiol. 2008;68:25-35.
11. Gumina S, Postacchini F, Orsina L, Cinotti G. The morphometry of the coracoid process - its aetiologic role in subcoracoid impingement syndrome. Int Orthop. 1999;23:198-201.
12. Prescher A, Klompen T. The glenoid notch and its relation to the shape of glenoid cavity of the scapula. J Anat. 1997;190:457-60.
13. Bigliani LU, Morrison DS, April EW. Morphology of acromion and its relationship to rotator cuff tears. Orthop Trans. 1986;10:228.
14. Neer CS. Anterior acromioplasty for the chronic impingement syndrome: A preliminary report. J Bone Joint Surg (Am). 1972;54:41-50.

15. Seeger LL, Gold RH, Bassett LW, Ellman H. Shoulder impingement syndrome: MR findings in 53 shoulders. AJR Am J Roentgenol. 1988;150:343-7.
16. Carrino JA, McCauley TR, Katz LD, Smith RC, Lange RC. Rotator cuff: Evaluation with fast spin echo versus conventional spin echo imaging. Radiology. 1997;202:533-9.
17. Zlatkin MB, Reicher MA, Kellerhouse ME, McDade W, Vetter L, Resnick D. The painful shoulder: MR imaging of the glenohumeral joint. J Comput Assist Tomogr. 1988;12:995-1001.
18. Mirowitz SA. Normal rotator cuff: MR imaging with conventional and fat suppression techniques. Radiology. 1991;180:735-40.
19. Zlatkin MB, Iannotti JP, Roberts MC, Esterhai JL, Dalinka MK, Kressel HY, et al. Rotator cuff tears: Diagnostic performance of MR imaging: Comparison with arthrography and correlation with surgery. Radiology. 1989;172:223-9.
20. Hoddler J, Kursunoglu-Brahme S, Syndler SJ, Cervilla V, Karzel RP, Schweitzer ME, et al. Rotator cuff disease: Assessment with MR arthrography versus standard MR imaging in 36 patients with arthroscopic confirmation. Radiology. 1992;182:431-3.
21. Turkel SJ, Panio MW, Marshal JL, Girgis FG. Stabilizing mechanisms preventing anterior dislocation of the glenohumeral joint. J Bone Joint Surg Am. 1981;63:1208-17.
22. Cleeman E, Flatow EL. Shoulder dislocations in the young patient. Orthop Clin North Am. 2000;3:217-29.
23. Kwak SM, Brown RR, Trudell D, Resnick D. Glenohumeral joint: Comparison of shoulder positions at MR arthrography. Radiology. 1998;208:375-80.
24. Palmer WE, Caslowitz PL. Anterior shoulder instability: Diagnostic criteria determined from prospective analysis of 121 MR arthrograms. Radiology. 1995;197:819-25.
25. Garneau RA, Renfrew DL, Moore TE, el-Khoury GY, Nepola JV, Lemke JH. Glenoid labrum: Evaluation with MR imaging. Radiology. 1991;179:519-22.
26. Legan JM, Burkhard TK, Goff WB II, Balsara ZN, Martinez AJ, Burks DD, et al. Tears of the glenoid labrum: MR imaging of 88 arthroscopically confirmed cases. Radiology. 1991;179:241-6.
27. Chandnani VP, Yeager TD, De Berardino T, Christensen K, Gagliardi JA, Heitz DR, et al. Glenoid labral tears: Prospective evaluation with MR imaging, MR arthrography and CT arthrography. Am J Roentgenol. 1993;161:1229-53.
28. Richards RD, Sartoris DJ, Pathria MN, Resnick D. Hill Sach's lesion and normal humeral groove: MR imaging features allowing their differentiation. Radiology. 1994;190:665-8.
29. Sugaya H, Moriishi J, Dohi M, Kon Y, Tsuchiya A. Glenoid rim morphology in recurrent anterior glenohumeral instability. J Bone Joint Surg Am. 2003;85:878-84.
30. Sanders TG, Tirman PF, Linares R, Feller JF, Richardson R. The glenolabral articular disruption lesion: MR arthrography with arthroscopic correlation. Am J Roentgenol. 1999;172:171-5.
31. Levine WN, Flatow EL. The pathophysiology of shoulder instability. Am J Sports Med. 2000;28:910-7.
32. Bui-Mansfield LT, Taylor DC, Uhorchak JM, Tenuta JJ. Humeral avulsions of the glenohumeral ligament: Imaging features and a review of the literature. AJR Am J Roentgenol. 2002;179:649-55.
33. Mosley HF, Overgaard B. The anterior capsular mechanism in recurrent anterior dislocation of the shoulder morphological and clinical studies with special reference to glenoid labrum and the glenohumeral ligaments. J Bone Joint Surg. 1962;44:913-27.
34. Bigoni JB, Christine B, Chung MD. MR imaging of the rotator cuff interval. Magn Reson Imaging Clin North Am. 2004;12:61-73.
35. Snyder Sj, Karzel RP, Del Pizzo, Ferkel RD, Friedman MJ. SLAP lesions of the shoulder. Arthroscopy. 1990;6:274-9.
36. Pfirrman CWA, Zannette M, Weishaupt D, Gerber C, Hodler J. Subscapularis tendon tears: Detection and grading at MR arthrography. Radiology. 1999;213:709-14.
37. Tung GA, Hou DD. MR arthrography of the posterior labrocapsular complex: Relationship with glenohumeral joint alignment and clinical posterior instability. Am J Roentgenol. 2003;180:369-75.
38. Stoller W. MR arthrography of the glenohumeral joint. Radiolol Clin North Am. 1997;35:97-116.
39. Jee WH, McCauley TR, Kalz LD, Matheny JM, Ruwe PA, Daigneault JP. Superior labral anterior posterior (SLAP) lesions of the glenoid labrum: Reliability and accuracy of MR arthrography for diagnosis. Radiology. 2001;218:127-32.
40. Erickson SJ, Fitzgerald SW, Quinn SF, Carrera GF, Black KP, Lawson TL. Long bicipital tendon of the shoulder: Normal anatomy and pathologic findings on MR imaging. Am J Roentgenol. 1992;158:1091-6.
41. Bennet WF. Visualisation of the anatomy of the rotator interval and bicipital sheath. Arthroscopy. 2001;17:107-11.
42. Linker CS, Helms CA, Fritz RC. Quadrilateral space syndrome: Findings at MR imaging. Radiology. 1993;188:675-6.
43. Fritz RC, Helms CA, Steinback LS, Genant HK. Suprascapular nerve entrapment: Evaluation with MR imaging. Radiology. 1992;183:437.
44. Emig EW, Schweitzer ME, Karasick D, Lubowitz J. Adhesive capsulitis of the shoulder: MR diagnosis. Am J Roentgenol. 1995;164:1457-9.
45. Rockwood C, Uhthoff HK, Dervin G, et al. Calcifying tendinitis. In: Rockwood C, Matsen III F, Wirth M, Lippt S (Eds). The Shoulder, 3rd edition. Philadelphia: Saunders; 2004. p. 1033.
46. Lee E, Flatow, E. The shoulder and arm. In: Weinstein S, Buckwalter J (Eds). Turek' Orthopedics, 6th edition. Philadelphia: Lippinkot Williams and Wilkins; 2005. p. 345.
47. Learch TJ, Farooki S. Magnetic resonance imaging of septic arthritis. Clin Imaging. 2000;24:336-42.
48. Alasaarela E, Suramo I, Tervonen O, Lähde S, Takalo R, Hakala M. Evaluation of humeral head erosions in rheumatoid arthritis: A comparison of ultrasonography, magnetic resonance imaging, computed tomography and plain radiography. Br J Rheumatol. 1998;37:1152-6.
49. Neer CS. Shoulder Reconstruction. Philadelphia: WB Saunders; 1990. p. 194.
50. Enzinger FM, Weiss SW. Soft Tissue Tumors. St. Louis, MO: CV Mosby; 1983.

51. Gottsegen CJ, Merkle AN, Bencardino JT, Gyftopoulos S. Advanced MRI techniques of the shoulder joint: Current applications in clinical practice. Am J Roentgenol. 2017;209(3):544-551.
52. Gyftopoulos S, Yemin A, Mulholland T, Bloom M, Storey P, Geppert C, et al. 3DMR osseous reconstruction of the shoulder using a gradient-echo based two-point Dixon reconstruction: A feasibility study. Skeletal Radiol. 2013;42:347-352
53. Gyftopoulos S1, Beltran LS, Yemin A, Strauss E, Meislin R, Jazrawi L, et al. Use of 3D MR reconstructions in the evaluation of glenoid bone loss: A clinical study. Skeletal Radiol. 2014;43:213-8.
54. Schiefer M, Mendonca R, Maganini MM, Fontenelle C, Pires Carvalho AC, Almeida M, et al. Intraobserver and interobserver agreement of Goutallier classification applied to magnetic resonance images. J Shoulder Elbow Surg. 2015;24:1314-21.
55. Lee YH, Kim S, Lim D, Song H, Suh J. MR quantification of the fatty fraction from T2*-corrected Dixon fat/water separation volume-interpolated breathhold examination (VIBE) in the assessment of muscle atrophy in rotator cuff tears. Acad Radiol. 2015;22:909-91.
56. Nozaki T, Tasaki A, Horiuchi S, Osakabe C, Ohde S, Saida Y, et al. Quantification of fatty degeneration within the supraspinatus muscle by using a 2-point Dixon method on 3-TMRI. Am J Roentgenol. 2015;205:116-22.
57. Burkhart SS, Danaceau SM, Pearce CE. Arthroscopic rotator cuff repair: Analysis of results by tear size and by repair technique—margin convergence versus direct tendon to bone repair. Arthroscopy. 2001;17:905-12.
58. Davidson JF, Burkhart SS, Richards DP, Campbell SE. Use of pre-operative magnetic resonance imaging to predict rotator cuff tear pattern and method of repair. Arthroscopy. 2005;21:1428.
59. Furukawa R, Morihara T, Arai Y, Ito H2, Kida Y1, Sukenari T, et al. Diagnostic accuracy of magnetic resonance imaging for subscapularis tendon tears using radial-slice magnetic resonance images. J Shoulder Elbow Surg. 2014;23:e283-e290.
60. Budzik JF, Balbi V, Verclytte S, Pansini V, Le Thuc V, Cotten A. Diffusion tensor imaging in musculoskeletal disorders. Radiographics. 2014;34:E56-72.
61. Guralnick W, Kaban LB, Merrill RG. Temporomandibular joints afflictions. N Engl J Med. 1978;299:123-9.
62. Tomas X, Pomes J, Berenguer J, Quinto L, Nicolau C, Mercader JM, et al. MR imaging of temporomandibular joint dysfunction: A pictorial review. Radiographics. 2006;26:765-81.
63. Yale SH. Radiographic evaluation of the temporomandibular joint. J Am Dent Assoc. 1969;79:102-7.
64. Hansson T, Nordström B. Thickness of soft tissue layers and articular disc in the temporomandibular joint. Acta Odontol Scand. 1977;35:77-83.
65. Paesani D, Westesson PL, Hatala M, Tallents RH, Kurita K. Prevalence of internal derangement in patients with craniomandibular disorders. Am J Orthod Dentofacial Orthop. 1992;101:41-7.
66. Katzberg RW, Westesson PL, Tallents RH, Anderson R, Kurita K, Manzione JV Jr, et al. Temporomandibular joint: MR assessment of rotational and sideways disc displacements. Radiology. 1988;169:741-8.
67. Wikes CH. Arthrography of the temporomandibular joint in patients with temporomandibular joint pain dysfunction syndrome. Minn Med. 1978;39:319-23.
68. Farrar WB. Characteristics of the condylar path in internal derangement of the TMJ. J Prosthet Dent. 1978;39:319-23.
69. Wikes CH. Internal derangement of the temporomandibular joint: Pathological variations. Arch Otolaryng Head Neck Surg. 1989;115:469-77.
70. Hasso AN, Christiansen EL, Alder ME. The temporomandibular joint. Radiol Clin North Am. 1989;27:301.
71. Westesson PL, Bronstein SL, Leidberg JL. Internal derangement of the temporomandibular joint: Morphological description with correlation to joint function. Oral Surg Oral Med Oral Path. 1985;59:323-31.
72. Schellhas KP, Wikes CH, Fritts HM, Omlie MR, Lagrotteria LB. MR of osteochondritis dissecans and avascular necrosis of the mandibular condyle. AJNR. 1989;10:3-12.
73. Jonck LM. Facial asymmetry and condylar hyperplasia. Oral Surg Oral Med Oral Pathol. 1975;40:567-73.
74. Katzberg RW, Tallents RH, Hayakawa K, Miller TL, Goske MJ, Wood BP. Internal derangements of the temporomandibular joint: Findings in paediatric age group. Radiology. 1985;154:125-7.
75. Thomson HG. Septic arthritis of the temporomandibular joint complicating otitis externa. J Otolaryngol Otol. 1989;103:319-21.
76. Smith HJ, Larheim TA, Aspestrand F. Rheumatic and non-rheumatic disease in the temporomandibular joint: Gadolinium enhanced MR imaging. Radiology. 1992;185:229-34.
77. Poveda-Roda R, Bagán JV, Sanchis JM, Margaix M. Pseudotumors and tumors of the temporomandibular joint: A review. Med Oral Patol Oral Cir Bucal. 2013;18:e392-e402.
78. Heffez LB. Imaging of internal derangements and synovial chondromatosis of the temporomandibular joint. Radiol Clin North Am. 1993;31:149-62.
79. Benslama L, Schouman T, Toure S, Chardain J, Goudot P. Synovial chondromatosis of the temporomandibular joint: Report and analysis of 12 cases. J Stomatol Oral Maxillofac Surg. 2019;120(5):476-9.
80. Bravo SM, Winalski CS, Weissman BN. Pigmented villonodular synovitis. Radiol Clin North Am. 1996;34: 311-26.
81. Rai KK, Dharmendrashinh R, Shiva Kumar HR. Aneurysmal bone cyst: A lesion of the mandibular condyle. J Maxillofac OralSurg. 2012;11:238-42.
82. Giorgione C, Passali FM, Varakliotis T, Sibilia M, Ottaviani F. Temporo-mandibular joint chondrosarcoma: Case report and review of the literature. Acta Otorhinolaryngol Ital. 2015;35(3):208-11.

CHAPTER

17

Magnetic Resonance Imaging of Wrist

Anindita Sinha, Harish Bhujade, Mahesh Prakash

INTRODUCTION

Wrist is composed of complex joint formed by small bones, ligaments, tendons, and cartilage. Magnetic resonance imaging (MRI) is an important diagnostic tool in evaluation of common wrist disorders and ligamentous injuries. For accurate diagnosis of various pathologies of wrist, it is important to know detailed anatomy of wrist.

BONES AND JOINTS

Wrist is formed by distal radius and ulna, eight carpal bones and bases of metacarpals. The proximal row is formed by scaphoid, lunate, triquetrum, and pisiform; the distal row is formed by trapezium, trapezoid, capitate, and hamate (from lateral to medial). The distal ends of radius and ulna form the distal radioulnar joint (DRUJ). The radius has a triangular articular surface for the scaphoid and a quadrilateral articular surface for the lunate at its distal end to form the radiocarpal joint.

The two rows of carpal bones form *Gilula's arc*, which comprised of Arc I along the proximal surfaces of proximal carpal bones (scaphoid, lunate, and triquetral), Arc II along the distal surfaces of these proximal carpal bones, and Arc III along the proximal surfaces of capitate and hamate **(Fig. 1)**.[1]

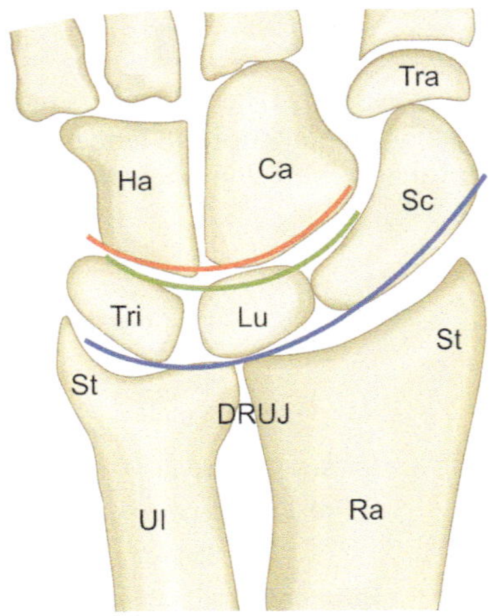

Fig. 1: Bones of the wrist with carpal bones forming the three arcs of Gilula. Proximal row (blue) is formed by the proximal articulating surfaces of scaphoid (Sc), lunate (Lu), and triquetral (Tri). The II arc (green) is formed by the distal articulating surfaces of the proximal carpal bones. The III arc (red) is formed by the proximal articulating surface of capitate (Ca) and hamate (Ha). The radius (Ra), ulna (Ul), and the styloid processes (St) and the distal radioulnar joint (DRUJ) are shown. Note the neutral ulnar variance.

Ulnar Variance or Hulten Variance

It is the difference in lengths of articular surfaces of distal ends of radius and ulna.[2] This can be neutral when both articular surfaces are at the same level, negative (ulnar articular surface >2 mm proximal to the radial articular surface), and positive (ulnar articular surface >2 mm distal to radial articular surface) **(Figs. 2A to C)**.

Ligaments of Wrist

For convenience, the wrist ligaments are grouped into intrinsic ligaments, extrinsic ligaments, and ligaments of thumb.

Intrinsic ligaments attach only to carpal bones and include scapholunate ligament, lunotriquetral ligament, and triangular fibrocartilage complex (TFCC) **(Fig. 3)**.

Extrinsic ligaments attach to other structures besides carpal bones. These are further divided into volar extrinsic and dorsal extrinsic ligaments.

- *Volar extrinsic ligaments* consist of volar radio-scaphocapitate, volar radiotriquetral, volar ulnolunate, volar ulnotriquetral, and volar radioulnar ligaments.
- *Dorsal extrinsic ligaments* consist of dorsal intercarpal, dorsal radiotriquetral, and dorsal radioulnar ligaments.

Scapholunate Ligament (Fig. 3)

Scapholunate ligament is a U-shaped ligament and has three components—Volar, dorsal, and interosseous.[3] The volar component, which courses obliquely, is thinner (1 mm in thickness) and weaker. The dorsal component is the thickest component (3 mm). The volar and dorsal components are best seen on axial images, appearing as band-like structures, the dorsal showing

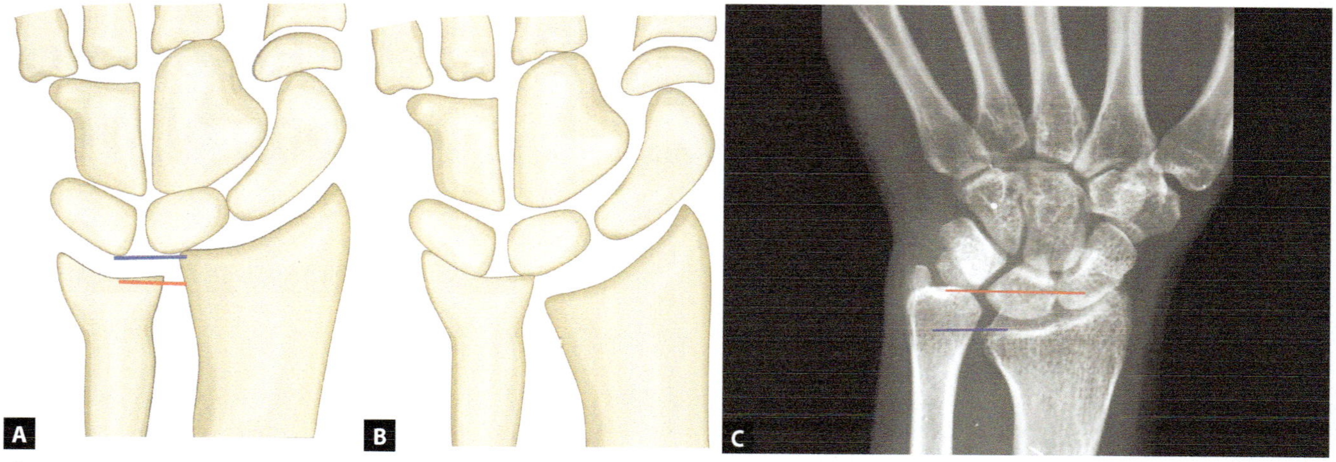

Figs. 2A to C: Ulnar variance. Ulnar variance is measured as the distance between two lines, one drawn tangential to the lunate fossa of radius (blue line) and another drawn tangential to the ulnar articular surface of ulna. (A) Negative ulnar variance with a short ulna; (B) Positive ulnar variance with ulna longer than the distal radius; (C) Radiograph of the wrist showing positive ulnar variance.

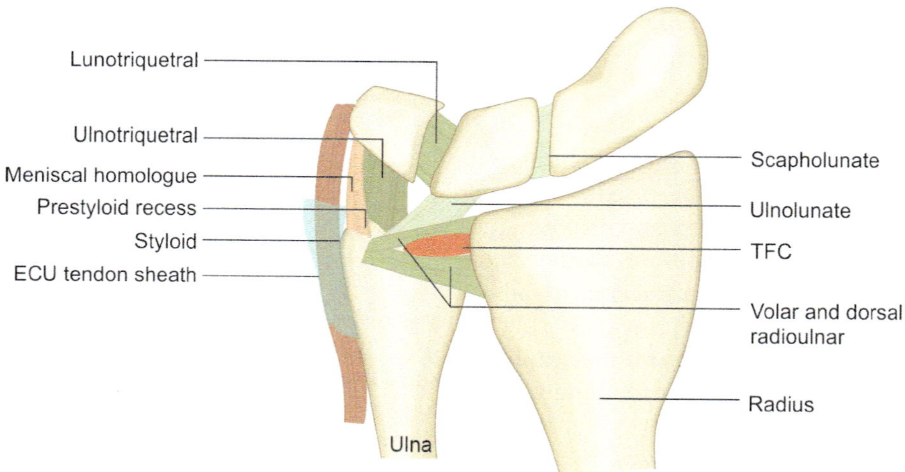

Fig. 3: Components of triangular fibrocartilage complex. The triangular articular disc (TFC disc proper), the volar, and dorsal radioulnar ligaments, the ulnolunate ligament, the ulnotriquetral ligament, the ulnar collateral ligament, the meniscus homologue, and part of the sheath of the extensor carpi ulnaris tendon. The scapholunate and lunotriquetral ligaments are also shown. (ECU: extensor carpi ulnaris; TFC: triangular fibrocartilage).

homogeneous-signal intensity and the volar showing heterogeneous-signal intensity. The interosseous component is best viewed on coronal sections. It appears band-like at its dorsal aspect, triangular at its central aspect, and trapezoidal at its volar aspect.

Lunotriquetral Ligament (Fig. 3)

Lunotriquetral ligament appears V-shaped and has volar, dorsal, and proximal components. The dorsal component is important for carpal stability and resistance to rotation.[3] The volar and dorsal components appear band-like on axial images.

Triangular Fibrocartilage Complex (Fig. 3)

Triangular fibrocartilage complex lies between the distal end of ulna and proximal carpal bones (lunate and triquetral). It consists of a triangular articular disc [triangular fibrocartilage (TFC) disc proper], dorsal radioulnar ligament, volar radioulnar ligament, ulnolunate ligament, ulnotriquetral ligament, ulnar collateral ligament, meniscus homologue, and part of the sheath of the extensor carpi ulnaris (ECU) tendon. The appearance of TFCC varies with ulnar variance. It is thicker and short with negative ulnar variance and thin and stretched with positive ulnar variance.

Triangular fibrocartilage disc appears as an asymmetric bowtie structure, which is best seen on coronal sections as a low-signal intensity structure on all pulse sequences. The triangular ligament has two bands, which attach the disc proper to the tip and fovea of the styloid process of ulna **(Figs. 4A to C)**. The vascularized tissue between the two bands is called the ligamentum subcruentum. TFC is supplied by the palmar and dorsal branches of

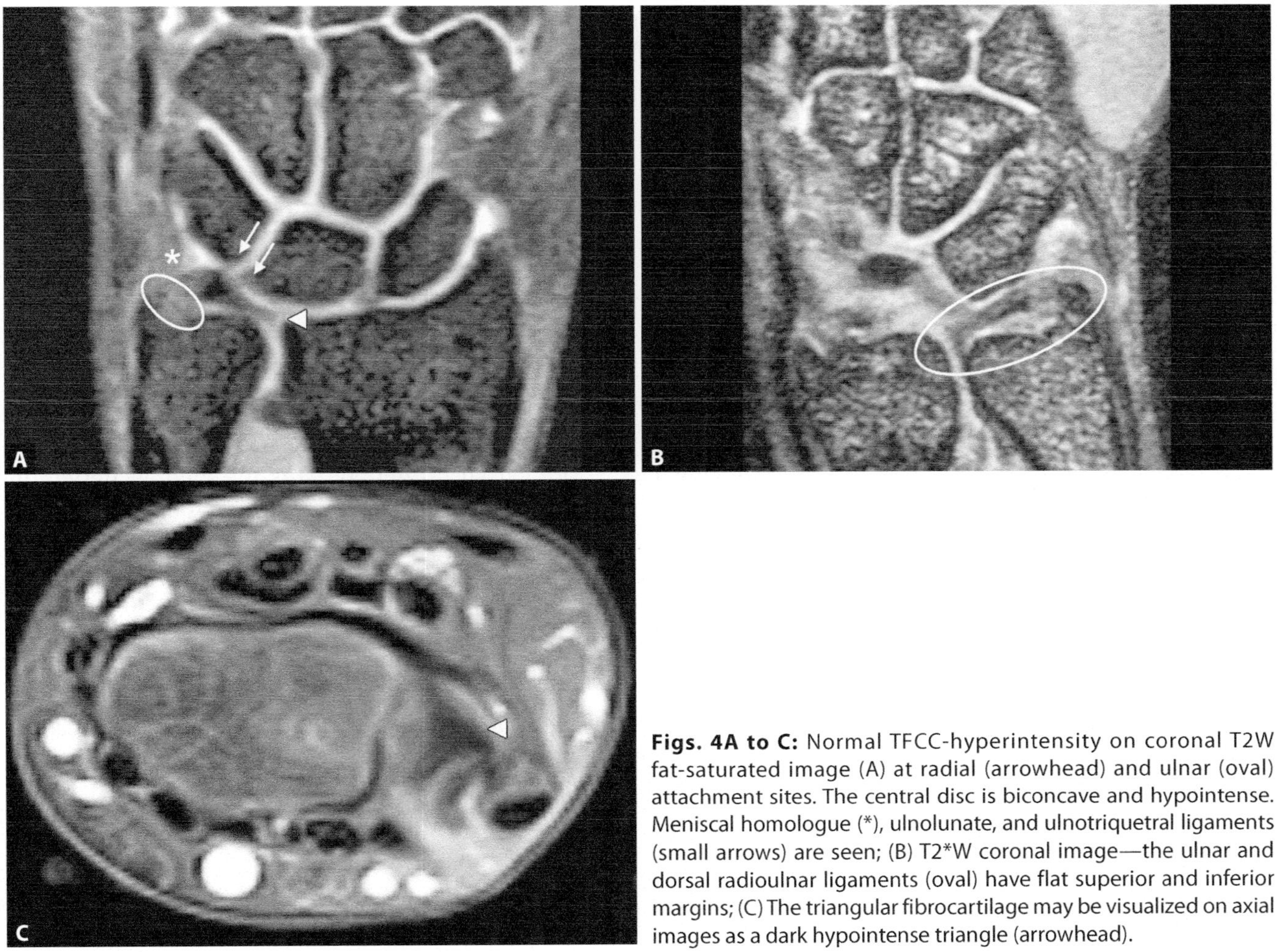

Figs. 4A to C: Normal TFCC-hyperintensity on coronal T2W fat-saturated image (A) at radial (arrowhead) and ulnar (oval) attachment sites. The central disc is biconcave and hypointense. Meniscal homologue (*), ulnolunate, and ulnotriquetral ligaments (small arrows) are seen; (B) T2*W coronal image—the ulnar and dorsal radioulnar ligaments (oval) have flat superior and inferior margins; (C) The triangular fibrocartilage may be visualized on axial images as a dark hypointense triangle (arrowhead).

the anterior interosseous artery and branch of the ulnar artery. The central and radial part of TFC is avascular while the periphery is vascularized. The tears of the vascularized part of TFC get healed while those of the central and radial part do not heal.[3]

The meniscal homologue appears as a triangular fat intensity structure between the ulnar styloid and triquetrum. It joins the ECU tendon sheath and joint capsule to form a ligamentous stabilizer.[4]

The radioulnar ligaments (dorsal and volar) are the main stabilizers of the wrist and DRUJ. It has superficial and deep fibers, both arising from the ulnar side of the distal radius at the sigmoid notch. The deep fibers insert on the fovea of the styloid process of ulna and are most important for joint stability, and the superficial fibers attach to the tip of the ulnar styloid.[5]

The volar ulnolunate ligament arises from the volar radioulnar ligament. It attaches distally to the lunate, parallel to the long axis of the wrist and forearm. Some of its fibers also attaches to the lunotriquetral ligament. The volar ulnotriquetral ligament also arises at the volar radioulnar ligament, medial to the volar ulnolunate ligament. This ligament then broadens and attaches on the triquetrum. Both these volar ligaments can be best seen on coronal images. The volar radioscaphocapitate ligament arises from the radial styloid and courses distally and medially to the capitate. Few of its fibers attach to the waist of scaphoid.

The volar radiolunate ligament also arises from the radial styloid, adjacent to the radioscaphocapitate ligament origin. The volar radiolunate ligament extends obliquely to attach on the lunate.

The dorsal radiotriquetral ligament arises from the dorsal styloid process of radius and attaches to the dorsal tubercle of the triquetrum. It courses in an oblique fashion, attaching and crossing the medial aspect of the lunate. The dorsal intercarpal ligament spans from the dorsal tubercle of the triquetrum to the dorsal groove of the scaphoid. The dorsal radiotriquetral and dorsal intercarpal ligaments are best evaluated on coronal images.[3]

Extensor Compartment (Fig. 5)

The extensor retinaculum stretches between the ulnar styloid process, the medial margin of pisiform and triquetrum, and the lateral radius margin. From the radial

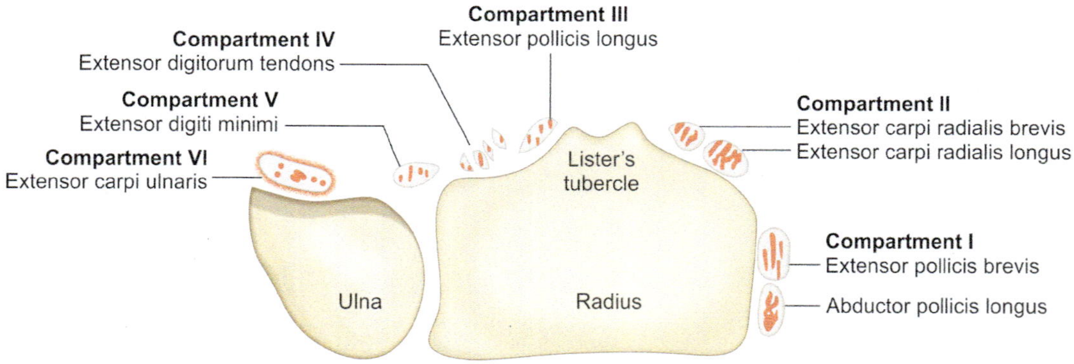

Fig. 5: From the radial to the ulnar side, the extensor tendons are arranged under the extensor retinaculum into six extensor compartments. Lister's tubercle is a landmark dividing compartments II and III.

to the ulnar side, the extensor tendons are arranged under the extensor retinaculum into six extensor compartments. The extensor tendons are best evaluated on axial images.

1. *Compartment I:* The abductor pollicis longus (APL) and extensor pollicis brevis (EPB) tendons
2. *Compartment II:* The extensor carpi radialis longus and brevis tendons
3. *Compartment III:* The extensor pollicis longus (EPL) tendon
4. *Compartment IV:* The extensor digitorum and indices tendons
5. *Compartment V:* The extensor digiti minimi tendon
6. *Compartment VI:* The ECU tendon.

Flexor Compartment (Figs. 6A to C)

A total of nine tendons traverse the carpal tunnel passing under the flexor retinaculum, which includes the four deep flexor digitorum profundus (FDP) tendons, the four superficial flexor digitorum superficialis (FDS) tendons, and the single flexor pollicis longus (FPL) tendon.

- *Guyon's canal* is a small anatomic space containing the ulnar nerve.
- *The medial border:* Pisiform bone and the hook of the hamate
- *The roof:* The palmar carpal ligament, palmar fascia, and palmaris brevis muscle
- *The floor:* FDP tendons, transverse carpal ligament (flexor retinaculum), pisohamate and pisometacarpal ligaments, and opponens digiti minimi muscle
- *Contents:* Ulnar nerve and vessels.

Carpal Tunnel (Figs. 6A to C)

Carpal tunnel is formed on the volar aspect of the wrist joint by the flexor retinaculum (transverse carpal ligament) forming the fibrous roof. The floor is formed by the carpal bones. The flexor retinaculum attaches to the scaphoid proximally on the radial side and tubercle of trapezium distally. The retinaculum attaches to the pisiform proximally and hook of hamate distally on the ulnar side.

The carpal tunnel contains the median nerve, the flexor tendons (four each of FDS and FDP surrounded by a single synovial sheath), and the FPL in a separate synovial sheath.

IMAGING TECHNIQUE OF WRIST

Magnetic Resonance Imaging

The wrist can be imaged at 1.5 Tesla. The 3 Tesla scanner is preferable for high-resolution imaging of the small intrinsic ligamentous structures of the wrist.[6]

Positioning

Patients can be placed in prone position with arms outstretched above the level of head (Superman position).

Patients unable to stay in this position can stay in supine position with hand beside the body. In this position, a single hand and wrist can be imaged by a phased array coil; however, image quality including fat suppression may be suboptimal due to distance of wrist and hand from the isocenter of the magnet. Additional manual shimming and use of fat suppression techniques such as IDEAL (iterative decomposition of water and fat with echo asymmetry and least-squares estimation) can overcome these problems.[6]

Coil

A dedicated 8–16-channel wrist (surface) coil is ideal for wrist. Small flex or loop coils can be used for cases where only a small field of view is needed for imaging of a dedicated structure. These coils can be closely wrapped around the anatomical part to be imaged.

The suggested protocol is given in **Table 1**.

Sequences are given in **Table 2**.

The three-dimensional fast spin-echo (3D FSE) isotropic sequences are better than GRE for cartilage, ligament, and osseous evaluation. These techniques can be quickened by parallel imaging, driven equilibrium techniques, compressed SENSE, or variable flip angles of the radiofrequency (RF) refocusing pulse [e.g., SPACE

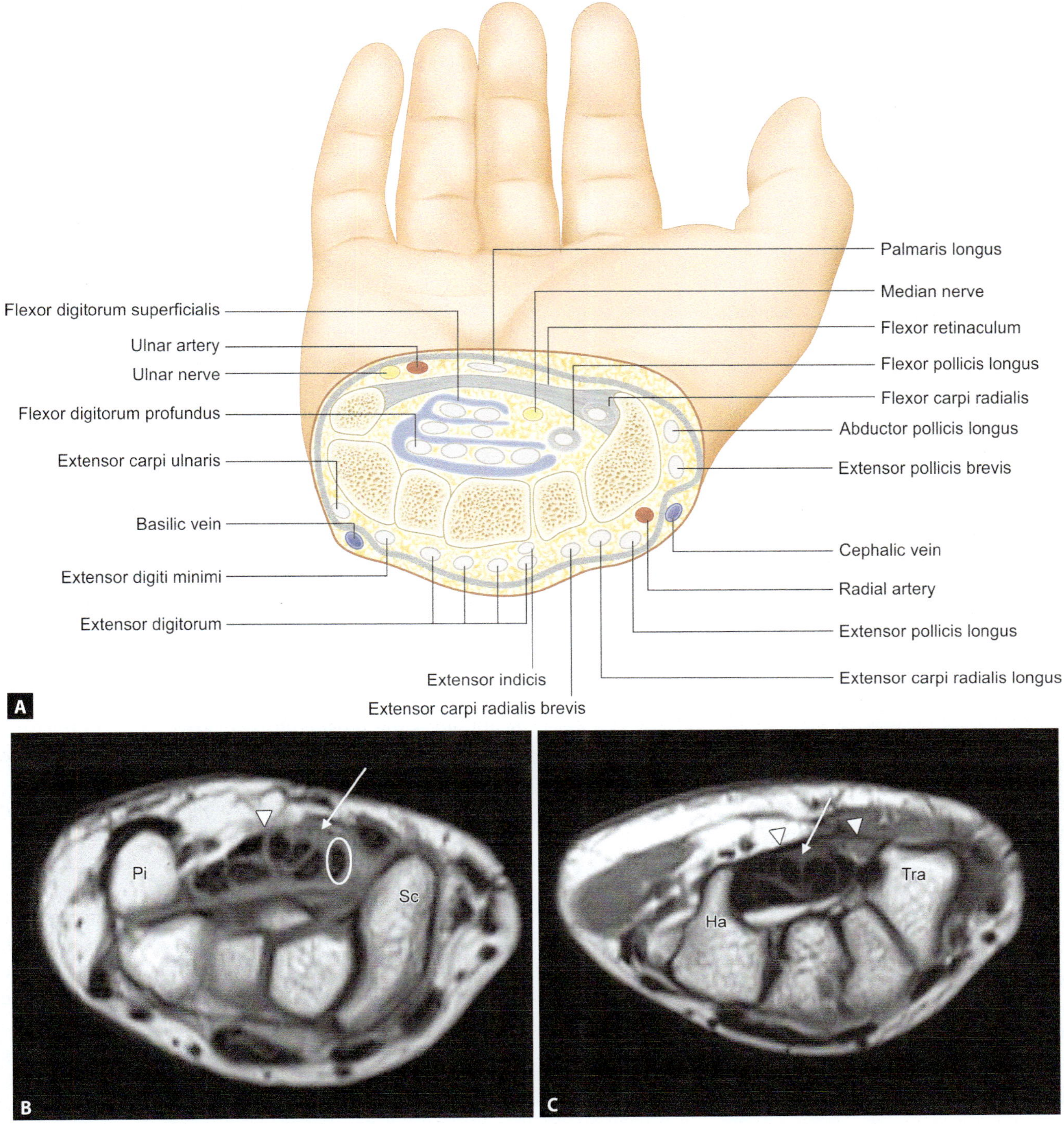

Figs. 6A to C: (A) Carpal tunnel and Guyon's canal. Normal magnetic resonance (MR) anatomy of the carpal tunnel; Axial T1W MR images at the level of pisiform (B) and at the level of hook of hamate (C) show the fibro-osseous carpal tunnel bounded by the carpal bones posteriorly, by the pisiform and hook of hamate on the ulnar side, and the scaphoid and tubercle of trapezium on the radial side. Superiorly, the hypointense linear flat flexor retinaculum (arrowheads) forms the roof of the carpal tunnel. The hypointense flexor digitorum superficialis and profundus tendons and the fasciculated speckled median nerve (arrow) are seen traversing the tunnel. The tendon of flexor pollicis longus (oval) is deep to the median nerve.

(Sampling Perfection with Application optimized Contrasts using different flip angle Evolution), CUBE, VISTA (volume isotropic turbo spin-echo acquisition) are techniques in various scanners].[7]

Cartilage Imaging

Cartilage imaging has the potential of early detection of degenerative changes and tears of TFCC and articular cartilage of carpal bones. Preliminary studies have

Table 1: MRI protocol planning routine imaging of the wrist.

FOV	8–10 cm
Matrix	416 × 192, 224 × 224 (for 3D sequences)
Slice thickness	2–2.5 mm with no interslice gap
Imaging plane	Axial scout-to-plan coronal (coronal should be the first sequence)
Coronal	Coronal-parallel to ulnar and radial styloid process [coverage from bases of metacarpals to distal radioulnar joint (DRUJ)]
Axial	Coronal scout-to-plan axial
	Axial images should include carpometacarpal joints and DRUJ
Sagittal	Use axial images to plan
	Sagittal images should be perpendicular to volar tips of the scaphoid tubercle and pisiform

(FOV: field of view)

Table 2: MRI sequences.

Coronal	• T2 FS • T1 • PD FS* (keep TE at 40, not less for PD sequences)
Axial	• T2 FS • T1
Sagittal	PD FS
Coronal 3D isotropic sequence[7]	T2 *GRE, 3D volumetric FSE PD FS turbo spin echo with <1 mm slice thickness

*Keep TE at 40, not less for PD sequences.
(FS: fat-saturated; FSE: fast spin-echo; GRE: gradient recalled-echo; PD: proton density; TE: echo time)

suggested changes in T1rho (T1ρ) and T2 relaxation times in torn ligaments and in degenerative and inflammatory conditions, as well as changes in response to different medications in inflammatory arthritis.[8,9]

Magnetic Resonance Arthrography of Wrist

Magnetic resonance arthrography of wrist can be single-compartmental (most commonly radiocarpal), two-compartmental, or rarely three-compartmental (radiocarpal, DRUJ, and midcarpal) arthrography. The fluoroscopic guidance is used for injections into the joint. The dorsal approach is commonly used for radiocarpal injections. The lateral approach can be used for radiocarpal injections.[10] The radiocarpal joint is visualized, and skin surface is marked at the level of the midscaphoid. Local anesthesia is given with a 22–26 gauge, hypodermic needle on the dorsum of the wrist. 3–5 mL of 1:1 contrast media (diluted iodinated contrast and gadolinium) is injected till the resistance is felt under fluoroscopic/cine guidance after advancing the needle into radiocarpal joint.

The dorsal approach can also be used for midcarpal and DRUJ injections. For midcarpal injections, the needle is advanced into the central part of the junction of the hamate, lunate, capitate, and triquetrum. For DRUJ injection, the needle extends to the radial aspect of the ulnar head.[11]

Indications for MR arthrography include peripheral TFC tears, undersurface TFCC tears as well as for evaluation of the postoperative TFCC where the injection site should be DRUJ. MR arthrography also increases diagnostic confidence in detecting tears of scapholunate and lunotriquetral ligaments.[12]

The contraindications for wrist injections include local skin infections. Pain and swelling may be seen after the injections, which is likely due to overdistension of joints.

Magnetic resonance arthrography is performed after the injections on 1.5 T or higher tesla machine. The position of patient is like conventional MR wrist (superman position). Fat-suppressed (FS) T1 fast spin-echo sequences in axial, coronal, and sagittal planes are acquired with 2 mm slice thickness. Additional sequences, T2 fat-saturated coronal and T1 coronal can be taken.[13]

Scaphoid Fracture

Scaphoid is the most common carpal bone to fracture; 70% of the fractures around the carpal bones are scaphoid fractures.

The mechanism of injury is a fall on the outstretched hand with pain in the anatomical snuffbox.

Fractures through the waist of scaphoid are most common.

Fractures through tubercle of scaphoid and incomplete scaphoid waist fractures are stable. Fractures through proximal pole, fracture dislocations, distal pole oblique fractures, and complete fractures through waist are unstable fractures (Herbert classification) **(Figs. 7A to C)**.

The Russe classification divides the fractures according to the orientation of the fracture line—horizontal oblique, vertical oblique, and transverse. The vertical oblique orientation has the most propensity to displace.[14]

However, none of the classifications can predict nonunion.

Clinical symptoms: May be minimal with very little restriction of movement, leading to delay in diagnosis as fractures may be radiologically occult.

Radiographs should be obtained in posterior-anterior and lateral views, hand in 45° ulnar deviation and pronation and an oblique view in 45–60° pronation.

Radiologically occult fractures may be evident on computed tomography (CT) or MRI. About 80% of scaphoid is covered by articular cartilage, and the space

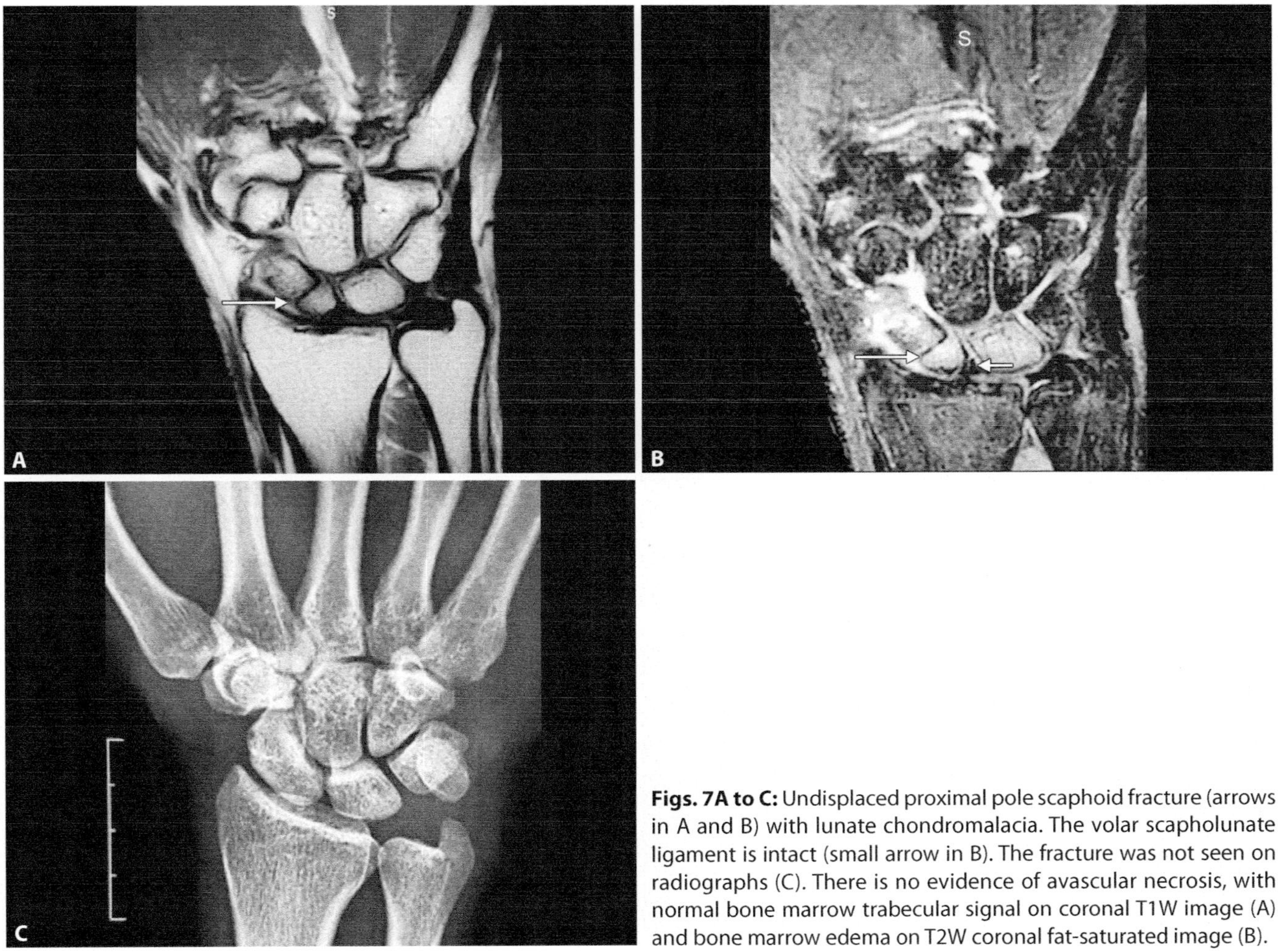

Figs. 7A to C: Undisplaced proximal pole scaphoid fracture (arrows in A and B) with lunate chondromalacia. The volar scapholunate ligament is intact (small arrow in B). The fracture was not seen on radiographs (C). There is no evidence of avascular necrosis, with normal bone marrow trabecular signal on coronal T1W image (A) and bone marrow edema on T2W coronal fat-saturated image (B).

left for blood supply from the recurrent radial artery branch is minimal. The neglected fractures are at a risk of nonunion due to tenuous blood supply of the scaphoid from the dorsal branch of the radial artery, which enters distal to the waist.[15]

Stable scaphoid fractures are treated conservatively by casts. Delayed union can occur even in stable fractures, which is evident as a persistently visible fracture line 16 weeks after fracture.[16]

Magnetic Resonance Imaging of Scaphoid Injuries

Chronic scaphoid delayed union or nonunion results in sclerosis in radiographs or CT. However, sclerosis does not imply avascular necrosis.

Presence of sclerosis and fluid in the cleft of the fracture fragment are signs of nonunion on MRI **(Figs. 8A to C)**. MRI is superior to CT or bone scintigraphy in detecting possible avascular necrosis due to its superior resolution.

The proximal pole is prone to avascular necrosis in scaphoid waist fractures due to blood supply from the distal pole traversing through the waist to reach the proximal pole.

Magnetic resonance appearance of hypointensity of >50% of the proximal pole on both T1-weighted (T1W) and T2-weighted (T2W) images suggests avascular necrosis.[17]

However, sensitivity and specificity of noncontrast-enhanced MRI is low in detecting avascular necrosis due to a common finding of a heterogeneous signal on T2W images, and hypointensity on both T1W and T2W images also found in ischemic bone (**Figs. 9A to C**).

Hyperintensity on T2W images may also be present in avascular necrosis and hypointensity is seen in only 50% of the cases.[18]

Contrast-enhanced MRI is necessary to distinguish between ischemic and necrotic bone. Complete lack of enhancement on postcontrast fat-saturated T1W images suggests severe ischemia or avascular necrosis.[19]

However, some patients have increased enhancement of the proximal pole on postcontrast images, possibly due to ingrowth of fibrovascular tissue or diffusion of contrast into necrotic bone from the surrounding tissue.[20]

Diagnostic algorithm: Recent recommendations in imaging of scaphoid fractures suggest that CT be

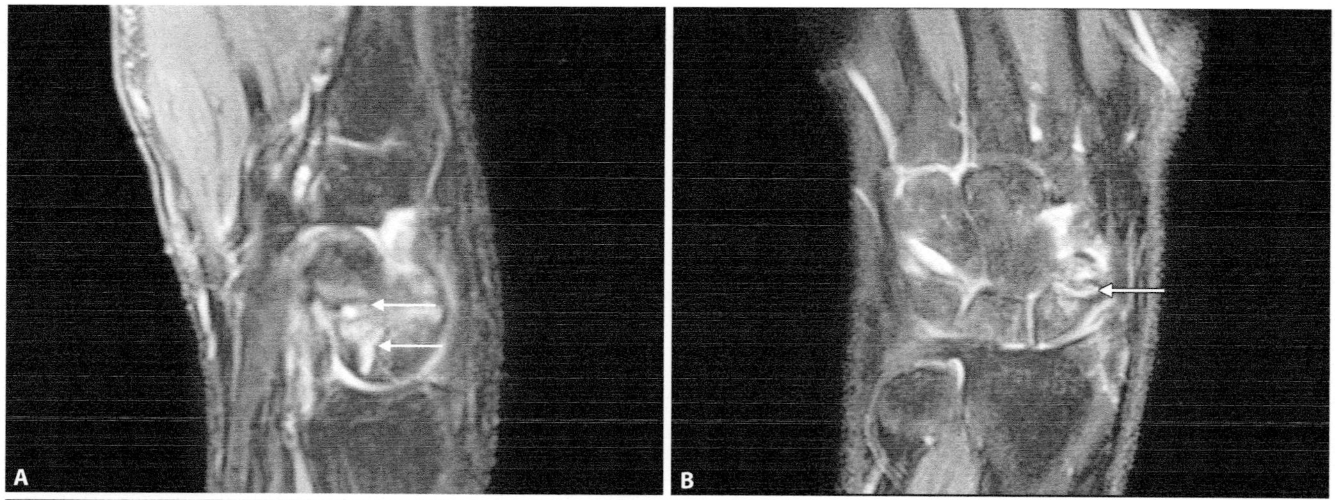

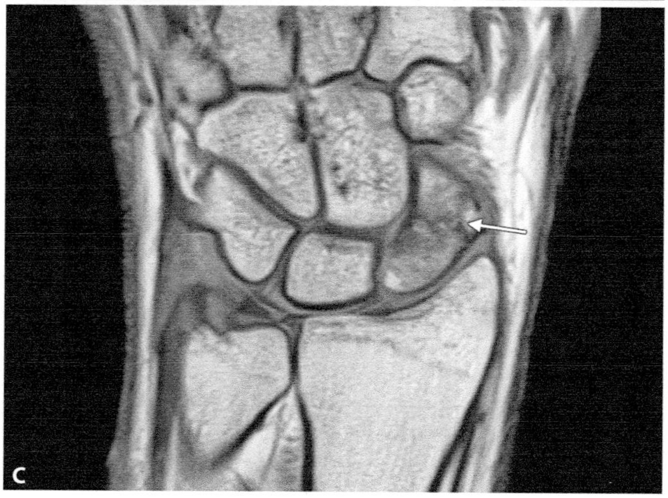

Figs. 8A to C: Scaphoid nonunion 2 months after trauma. (A) Sagittal; and (B) Coronal T2W fat-saturated images show a fluid-filled gap between the fractures through the waist of scaphoid (arrows); (C) A hypointense line is visible on coronal T1W image (arrow).

acquired/reformatted in sagittal-oblique and coronal-oblique planes in cases of normal or equivocal radiographs. CT is better in demonstrating a fracture pattern including fracture orientation and dislocation or fragmentation. However, CT is inferior to MRI in detecting microtrabecular fracture and nondisplaced fractures. MRI is useful in detecting all scaphoid fractures, and additional sequences should be acquired in sagittal-oblique and coronal-oblique planes along long axes of scaphoid. However, diagnostic confusion may persist in cases of bone marrow edema (bone contusion) and nondisplaced fracture.[21]

Fractures of Other Carpal Bones

Fractures of other bones are uncommon. Hook of hamate fractures also occurs due to a fall on the outstretched hand and can occur due to avulsion at the flexor retinaculum attachment site.[15] Hook of hamate fractures can be easily missed on radiographs, where absence of visibility of hook of hamate can be the only sign on routine posteroanterior (PA) views. Ulnar styloid fractures can lead to DRUJ instability, when associated with the base of styloid fractures which disrupt the TFCC. Pisiform is also prone to fractures due to its superficial location and can be detected on routine radiographic views or carpal tunnel view; undiagnosed pisiform fractures lead to pisotriquetral chondromalacia, intra-articular loose bodies, and ulnar nerve impingement.[22]

Kienböck's Disease

Kienböck's disease is referred to avascular necrosis of the lunate bone. It was first described by the Austrian radiologist Robert Kienböck's in 1910.[23]

The etiology of Kienböck's disease is multifactorial. Predisposing factors include trauma, disruption of venous outflow and local vascular anatomy, ulnar variance, metabolic factors, and repetitive mechanical load. A negative ulnar variance has been found in 78% of cases.[24] Type II lunate with an articulating facet with the hamate also shows higher risk of Kienböck's disease **(Figs. 10A and B)**.[25]

The terminal arterial branches without sufficient collateral vessels and cases with a single palmar vessel are more prone to Kienböck's disease **(Table 3)**.

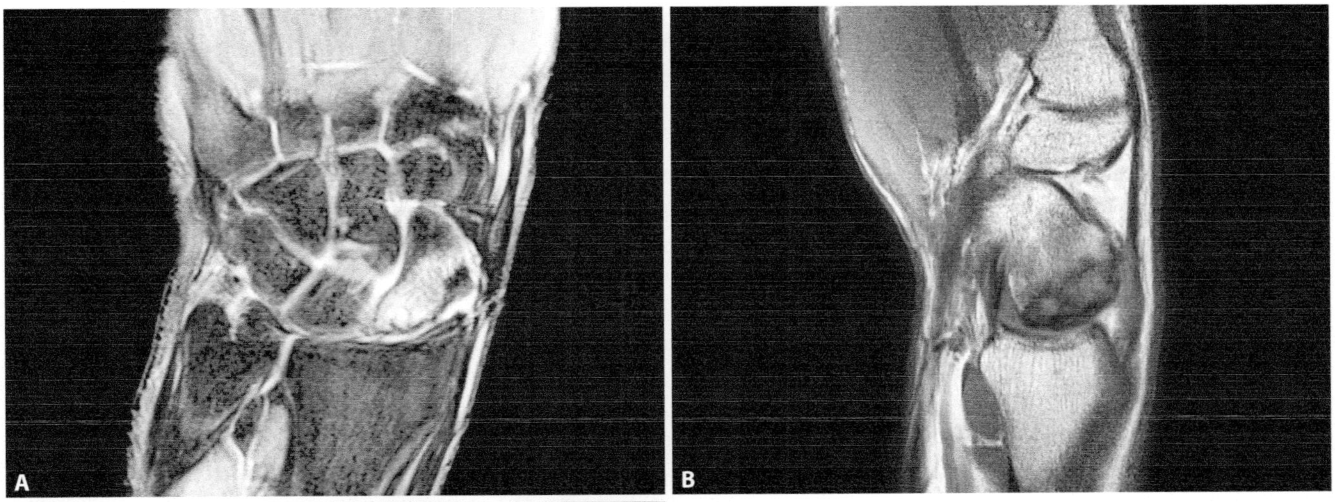

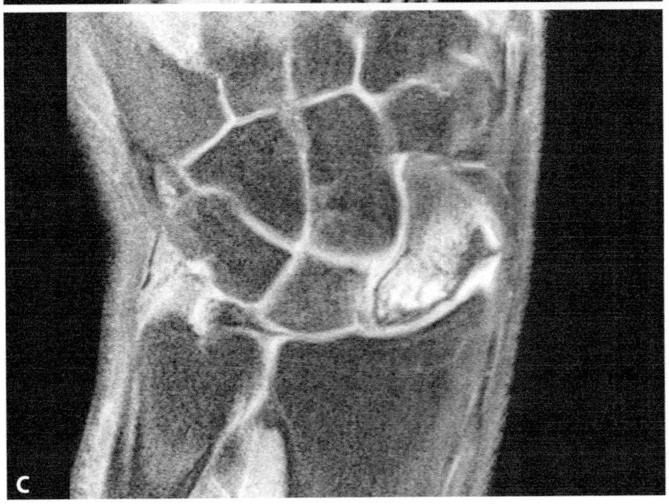

Figs. 9A to C: Scaphoid proximal pole cystic change with bone marrow edema sparing distal pole on proton density (PD)-weighted fat-saturated coronal image (A) with hypointensity of proximal pole on sagittal T1W image (B). However, homogeneous enhancement is seen on postcontrast image (C), suggesting lack of avascular necrosis.

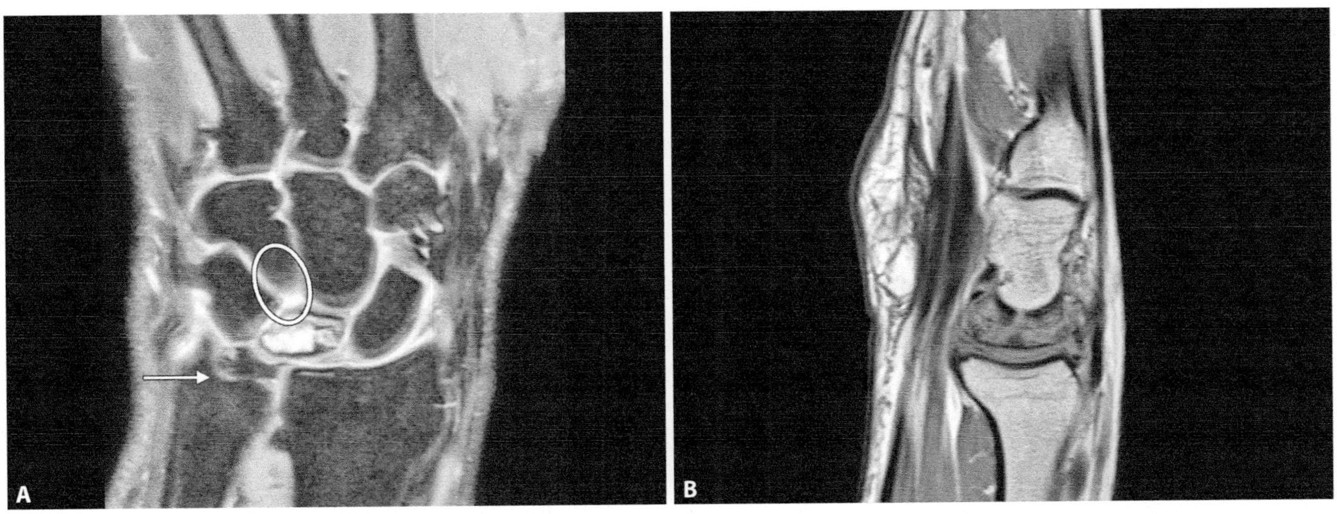

Figs. 10A and B: Kienböck's disease with negative ulnar variance with flattened type II lunate. Proton density fat-saturated coronal image (A) shows flattened lunate bone with hyperintensity on fat-saturated images involving the entire lunate (A) and hypointensity of the lunate on the T1W image (B). The lunate has a facet for articulation with hamate (oval in A). The articular surface of distal ulna is proximal to that of the radius (negative ulnar variance) (arrow in A), another predisposing factor for Kienböck's disease.

The onset of disease is seen between the ages of 20 and 40 years with a 2:1 ratio of men to women. It commonly affects the dominant wrist, but bilateral disease can be seen. The clinical onset can be abrupt or insidious and patients can also remain asymptomatic in the precollapse stage.[26]

Table 3: Lichtman staging of Kienböck's disease.[28]

Stages	*Radiographic and CT findings*	*MRI findings*
I	Normal morphologic findings	• Morphologic preservation • Edema pattern in bone marrow
II	• Normal morphologic findings • Sclerosis in bone marrow	• Morphologic preservation • Signal intensity low on T1W images, variable on T2W images
IIIA	• Collapse of lunate bone • Radioscaphoid angle <60°	• Morphologic collapse of lunate bone • Signal intensity low on T1W images, variable on T2W images
IIIB	• Collapse of lunate bone • Radioscaphoid angle >60°	• Morphologic collapse of lunate bone • Signal intensity low on T1W images, variable on T2W images
IIIC	• Collapse of lunate bone • Coronal lunate fracture (chronic)	• Morphologic collapse of lunate bone • Signal intensity low on T1W images, variable on T2W images Coronal lunate fracture (chronic)
IV	Radiocarpal or midcarpal degenerative arthritis	• Radiocarpal or midcarpal degenerative arthritis • Signal intensity low on T1W images, variable on T2W images

Patients present with dorsally located central wrist pain with dorsal tenderness around the lunate, swelling, reduced wrist motion, and grip after acute or repetitive trauma.[27]

Contrast-enhanced MRI helps in differentiation between bone marrow edema and partial or complete necrosis. Enhancement is homogeneous in non-necrotic edematous bone. Partial necrosis shows a heterogeneous enhancement pattern and complete necrosis shows absence of enhancement.[28]

The Lichtman classification may help in treatment decision-making. Options include nonoperative management in early stage disease (stages I to IIIA) to vascularized grafting, proximal row carpectomy, or arthrodesis in late stages (stages IIIB to IV). However, treatment remains controversial and may not alter the natural history of the disease.[29]

Triangular Fibrocartilage Complex Lesions

Triangular fibrocartilage is a hypointense, biconcave, or bow-tie shaped on coronal sections, discoid or biconcave on sagittal, and triangular on axial sections[30] **(Figs. 11A to C)**. The volar and dorsal radioulnar ligaments of the TFCC have parallel upper and lower margins **(Figs. 12A and B)**.

At the radial attachment, minimal hyperintensity due to hyaline cartilage may be seen and may be mistaken for a tear.[30]

At the ulnar attachment, there are two laminae, one from the styloid process of ulna and one from fovea which are striated but hypointense. Intervening ligamentum subcruentum may appear hyperintense normally.

Triangular fibrocartilage complex lesions can occur due to trauma or repetitive overuse. The Palmer classification divides TFCC injuries into two classes—traumatic (Class I) and degenerative (Class II) **(Table 4)**.[22]

However, the Palmer classification does not classify tears of volar or dorsal radioulnar ligaments or subclassify type IB ulnar avulsions further into distal (styloid) avulsions or proximal (foveal) avulsions, which have prognostic and therapeutic significance, since the foveal attachment damage is more disabling and styloid avulsion fractures associated with distal lamina tears can cause instability. Combinations of different tears and partial tears are also common and have not been classified.[31]

Type IA tears are central perforations of the TFC, often found in asymptomatic individuals and do not result in any dysfunction of the DRUJ. Central perforations are seen as fluid-signal intensity or contour irregularity within the central or paracentral portion of the triangular fibrocartilage proper and may be partial-thickness tear of either the proximal or the distal (less common) articular surface. Type IA tears are in the avascular zone and cannot be surgically repaired **(Figs. 13A and B)**.

Type IB tears near the ulnar attachment are difficult to diagnose on MRI; features of ulnar-sided synovitis and focal fluid on the ulnar side are clues to diagnosis. Ulnar-sided tears and type IC tears are vascular and respond well to interventions.[31] MR arthrography with DRUJ injections have better sensitivity in detecting type IA and IB lesions **(Figs. 14A and B)**.

Type IC tears appear as thickening with edema within the ligament on long TE sequences.[31] Type ID tears near the radial attachment can be associated with radial avulsion fractures of sigmoid notch.

Degenerative Tears

Triangular fibrocartilage complex degeneration manifests as intrasubstance hyperintensity not communicating

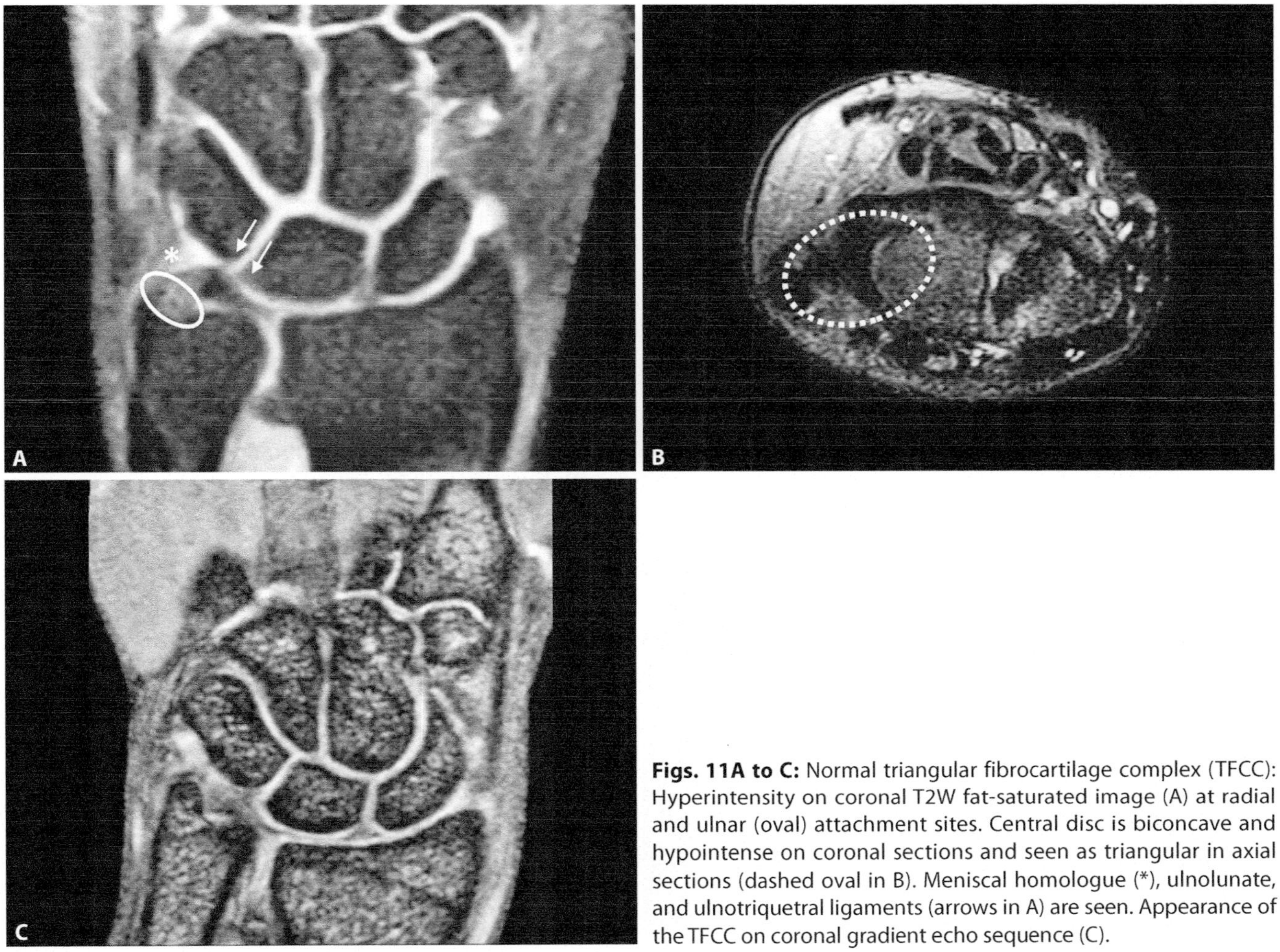

Figs. 11A to C: Normal triangular fibrocartilage complex (TFCC): Hyperintensity on coronal T2W fat-saturated image (A) at radial and ulnar (oval) attachment sites. Central disc is biconcave and hypointense on coronal sections and seen as triangular in axial sections (dashed oval in B). Meniscal homologue (*), ulnolunate, and ulnotriquetral ligaments (arrows in A) are seen. Appearance of the TFCC on coronal gradient echo sequence (C).

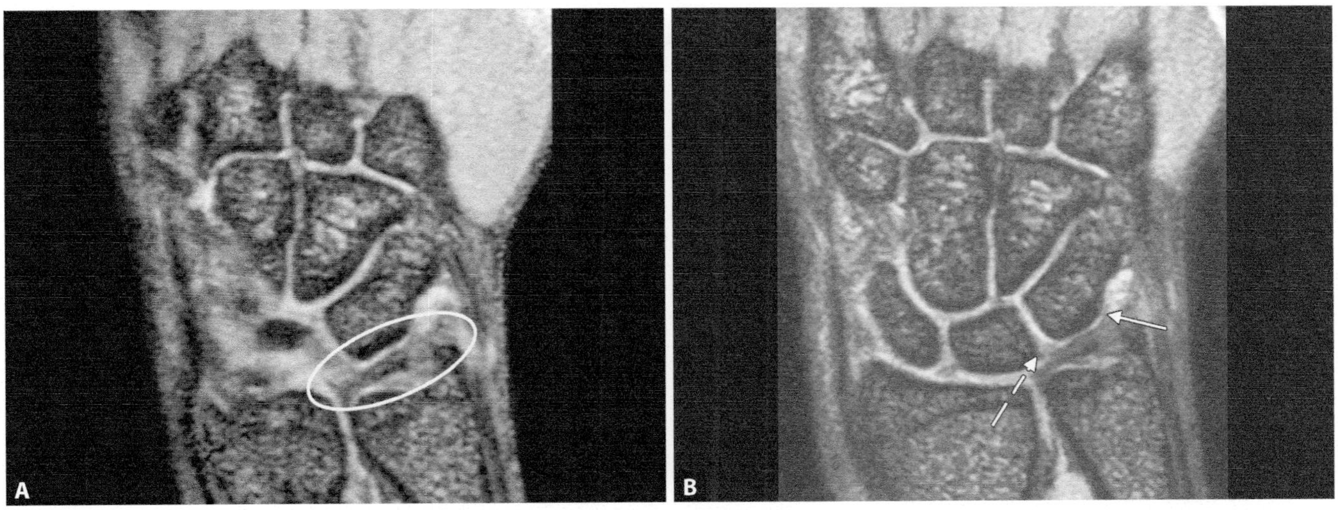

Figs. 12A and B: (A) Dorsal radioulnar ligament (oval) which has horizontal superior and inferior margins unlike the biconcave triangular fibrocartilage articular disc proper; (B) Ulnolunate (dashed arrow) and ulnotriquetral ligaments (arrow).

with the articular surface. The disc may appear diffusely thinned in degenerative tears. Degenerative tears are common with aging and rarely seen before 30 years and are associated with positive ulnar variance and ulnar impaction with chondromalacia of lunate or degenerative subchondral cysts.[31]

Table 4: Classification of triangular fibrocartilage complex (TFCC) tears.

Class I tears (traumatic)	
IA	Central perforations
IB	Ulnar avulsion with or without distal ulnar fracture
IC	Distal avulsion at carpal attachment
ID	Radial avulsion with or without sigmoid notch fracture
Class II tears (degenerative)	
IIA	TFCC wear
IIB	TFCC wear with lunate and/or ulnar chondromalacia
IIC	TFCC perforation with lunate and/or ulnar chondromalacia
IID	C and lunotriquetral ligament perforation
IIE	D and ulnocarpal arthritis

Three-dimensional Imaging

Three-dimensional isotropic imaging is specifically useful for evaluating the TFCC since in the imaging position, the TFCC is not orthogonal to the coronal plane but oblique to it, resulting in false-positive diagnosis of tears as the entire ligament may not be visualized in one section due to its obliquity. 3D sequences with a section thickness of 1 mm or less with no interslice gap can be reconstructed with multiplanar reconstructions for better evaluation of the TFCC. Punctate hypointensity on 3D gradient echo sequences is an early sign of degeneration.[32]

Radioulnar Ligament Lesions

Injuries of dorsal and volar radioulnar ligaments result in DRUJ dysfunction with ulnar-sided wrist pain.

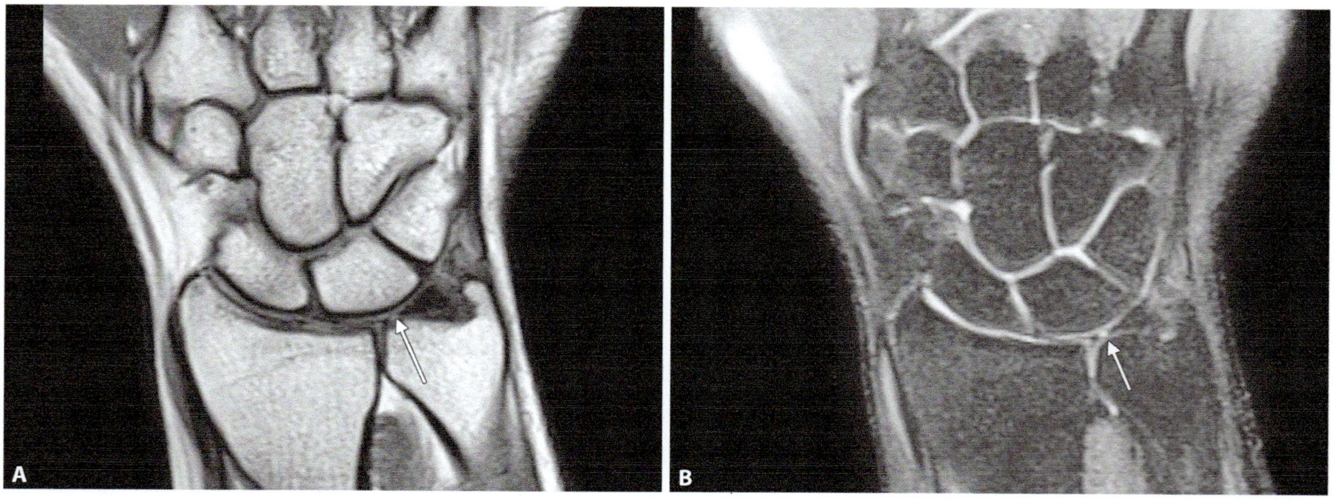

Figs. 13A and B: Central triangular fibrocartilage complex (TFCC) tear. Coronal PD weighted (A) and T2W fat saturated (B) images show a central perforation of the TFCC (arrow), with fluid signal within the central portion of the disc. These tears are often asymptomatic.

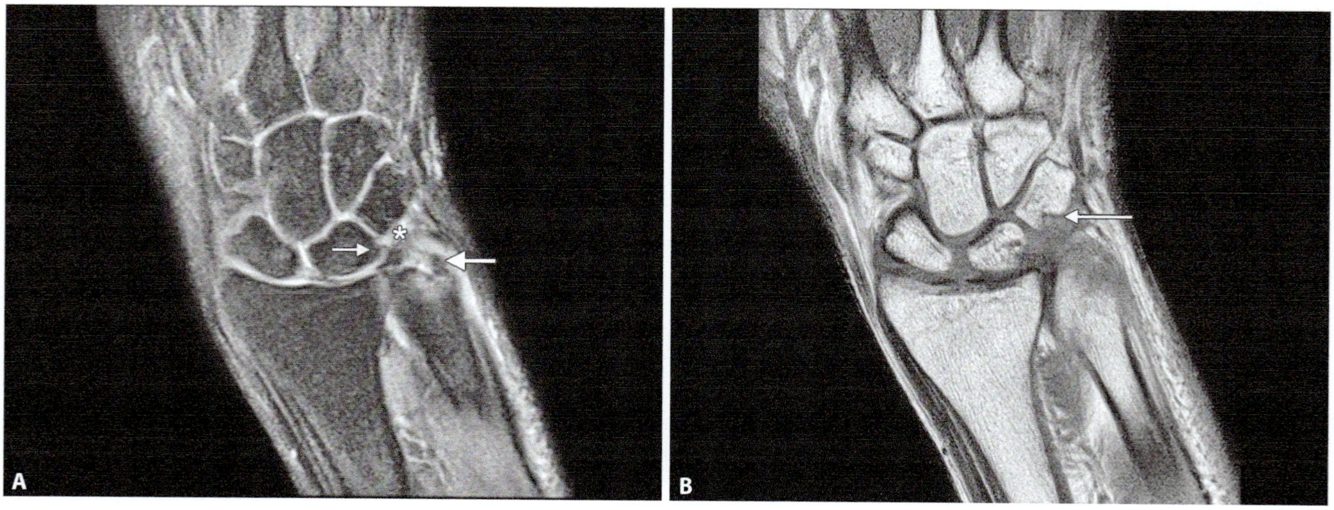

Figs. 14A and B: (A) PD-weighted fat-saturated coronal MRI reveals fracture of base of ulnar styloid (thick arrow) with thickened and hyperintense proximal and distal lamina of TFC (thick arrow). The ulnolunate ligament is hypointense (thin arrow). Hyperintensity and thickening of ulnotriquetral ligament is seen (*); (B) Coronal T1W image shows osteochondral impaction injury at the proximal radial side of triquetrum (arrow) at the ulnolunate ligament attachment site.

The dorsal and volar radioulnar ligaments have flat superior and inferior margins unlike the biconcave margins of the TFC and are hypointense on all pulse sequences, but mildly more hyperintense than the TFC proper.

Disruptions of the radioulnar ligaments should be carefully evaluated on the peripheral MRI sections. The ulna commonly subluxates dorsally relative to the sigmoid notch due to tear of the dorsal radioulnar ligament with loss of concentric relation between sigmoid notch of radius and ulnar head **(Figs. 15A to C)**.[30]

Ulnar Impaction Syndrome (Ulnocarpal Abutment)

This is a common cause of ulnar-sided wrist pain and is occasionally associated with positive ulnar variance causing excessive load on the ulnar side of the wrist with ulnar impaction on the TFCC and ulnar-sided carpal bones. The condition can also be seen in neutral or negative ulnar variance.[22]

Radiography with forearm in pronation with hand gripped may show the actual increase in positive ulnar variance and impaction. Foreshortened radius may also be found postsurgically, post-traumatically in malunited foreshortened radius, due to premature physeal fusion of the distal radius (congenitally or in post-traumatic cases in skeletally immature patients).[2,22]

Magnetic resonance imaging is useful in detecting early changes since radiographic findings may be subtle or normal even in advanced disease. MRI shows the ulnar-sided degenerative changes involving ulnar-sided carpal bones (ulnar side of lunate, triquetrum) and ulnar head. Cartilage thinning, subchondral cysts, marrow edema, and sclerosis along the ulnar aspect of the lunate and/or triquetrum may be seen **(Figs. 16A and B)**.[22] Degenerative changes in the thinned-out TFCC are also seen. Advanced cases lead to ulnocarpal joint arthritis.

Ulnar Styloid Impaction Syndrome

This causes ulnar-sided wrist pain due to impaction between a long styloid process of ulna (>6 mm) and a nonunited styloid process fracture fragment and the triquetral bone.

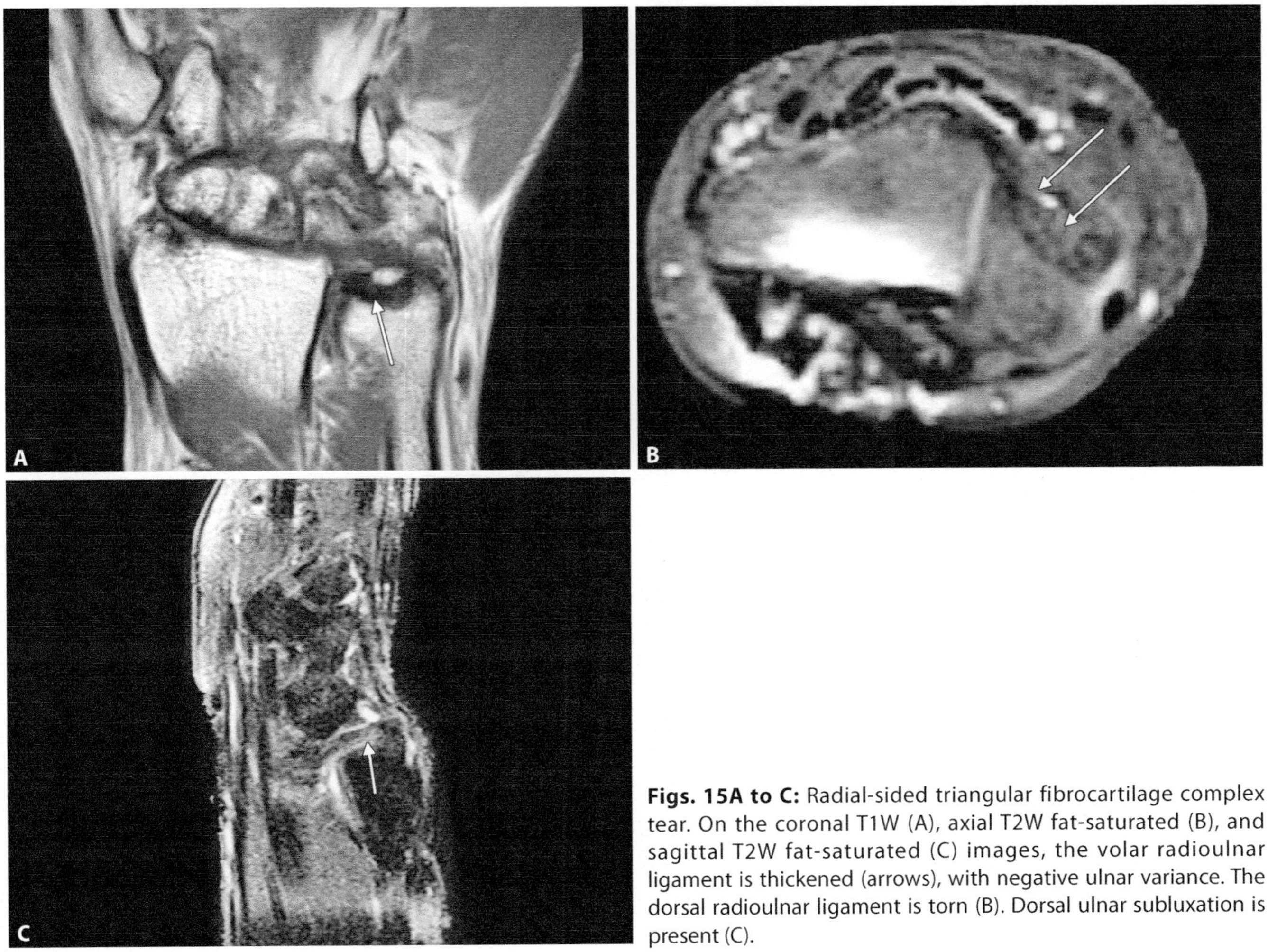

Figs. 15A to C: Radial-sided triangular fibrocartilage complex tear. On the coronal T1W (A), axial T2W fat-saturated (B), and sagittal T2W fat-saturated (C) images, the volar radioulnar ligament is thickened (arrows), with negative ulnar variance. The dorsal radioulnar ligament is torn (B). Dorsal ulnar subluxation is present (C).

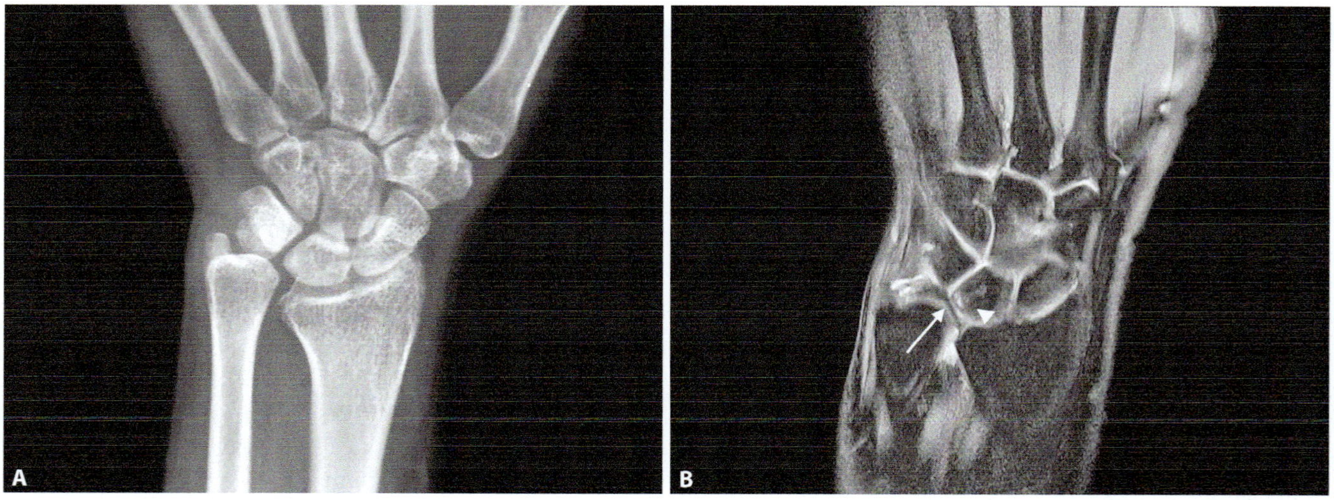

Figs. 16A and B: Ulnocarpal abutment. (A) Radiograph; and (B) Coronal T2W fat-saturated image. Positive ulnar variance with thinned-out TFC and chondromalacia along the ulnar aspect of the lunate (arrowhead).

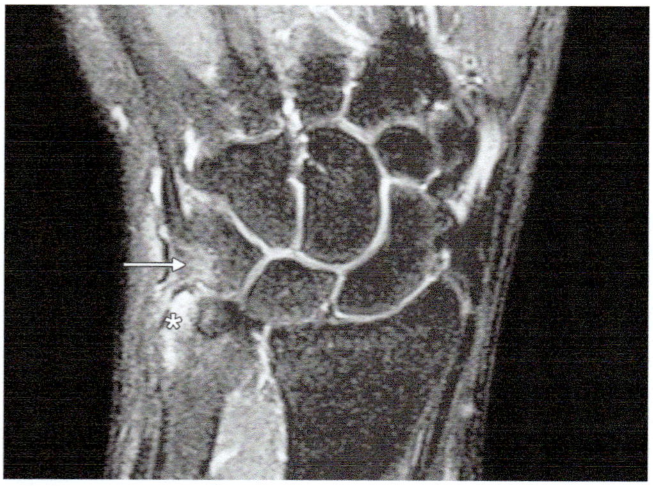

Fig. 17: Coronal T2W fat-saturated image shows ulnar styloid impaction with edema of the ulnar styloid process (*) and ulnar aspect of triquetrum (arrow).

Magnetic resonance imaging findings: Degenerative changes are noted in a long or curved ulnar styloid process and in triquetrum with bone marrow edema, cartilage changes, subchondral cysts, and sclerosis along the styloid process and triquetrum **(Fig. 17)**.[22]

Ulnar Impingement Syndrome

In this condition, a shortened ulna, which lies proximal to the sigmoid notch, impinges against the radius. MRI shows a foreshortened ulna with bone marrow edema at the level of impingement on the radius proximal to sigmoid notch. Later stages show sclerosis, scalloping along the ulnar margin of distal radius, and degenerative changes with osteophytes.[22]

Hamatolunate Impingement

Hamatolunate impingement occurs due to a type II lunate where there is an additional facet on the distal articular surface of the lunate where the hamate and lunate articulate. Impingement at this articulation can cause chondromalacia and pain.[33]

Table 5: Classification of carpal instability.

Nomenclature	*Area of abnormality*
Carpal instability dissociative (CID)	Between the proximal row (most common) and distal row of carpal bones in the same row
Carpal instability nondissociative (CIND)	Between radiocarpal and midcarpal rows
Carpal instability complex	Combination of the above two
Adaptive carpus	Due to abnormality proximal or distal to carpal rows

Carpal Instability

Carpal instability is defined as the inability to bear physiological load.

Carpal instabilities are most commonly caused by injuries to the intrinsic ligaments of the wrist, though inflammatory and congenital conditions can also lead to instability. Based on the type of injury, carpal instability is classified into four types according to the Mayo classification **(Table 5)**.

Carpal Instability Dissociative

Scapholunate instabilities are the most common carpal instabilities, and the scapholunate and lunotriquetral ligament injuries are the most common causes of dissociative carpal instability. Scaphoid fractures, Kienböck's disease, and rheumatoid arthritis (RA) also cause scapholunate instability.[34]

Scapholunate ligament injury: Scapholunate ligament injuries are associated with radial-sided wrist pain and popping or clicking on physiological loading of the wrist joint. Scapholunate ligament injury can result in scapholunate dissociation, scapholunate advanced collapse (SLAC), and scaphoid nonunion advanced collapse (SNAC).[35]

The scapholunate ligament has three components—dorsal, interosseous, and volar. The dorsal component is most important for maintaining stability. The dorsal intercarpal ligaments also act as secondary stabilizers.[36]

Scapholunate dissociation causes widening of the scapholunate interval to >3 mm on radiographs. This is known as Terry Thomas sign. However, routine radiographs may be normal even in complete scapholunate ligament tears and stress radiographs may be required with clenched fist views or wrist in ulnar and radial deviation. MRI or MR arthrography can demonstrate the ligament tear.

Scapholunate ligament injuries cause a pattern of injury known as dorsal intercalated segment instability (DISI) with a dorsal tilt of the concave distal articular surface of the lunate and volar tilt of the scaphoid with an increase in the scapholunate angle (>60°). These injuries occur due to damage to scapholunate ligament along with secondary stabilizers such as radioscaphocapitate and scaphocapitate ligaments.[34,35]

Further progression leads to degenerative changes in the radioscaphoid articulation and ultimately carpal collapse **(Figs. 18A to C)**. Nontraumatic scapholunate dissociation and SLAC are seen in patients with calcium pyrophosphate deposition disease.

On MRI, partial tears may appear as an elongated or a focally thin ligament or a focal area of high-signal intensity. Complete tears appear as a complete discontinuity.[12] Double-compartment MR arthrography can demonstrate tears with greater sensitivity and specificity.[12,37]

Lunotriquetral ligament injury: The lunotriquetral ligament, like the scapholunate ligament, has three components (dorsal, interosseous, and volar) and plays an important role in maintaining stability of the proximal carpal row. The volar component of the lunotriquetral ligament is the strongest. Lunotriquetral ligament injuries present with ulnar-sided wrist pain.

Lunotriquetral ligament injury along with injury of the secondary stabilizers (dorsal radiotriquetral and dorsal scaphotriquetral ligaments) leads to volar intercalated segment instability (VISI). The lunate rotates in a volar direction.[38]

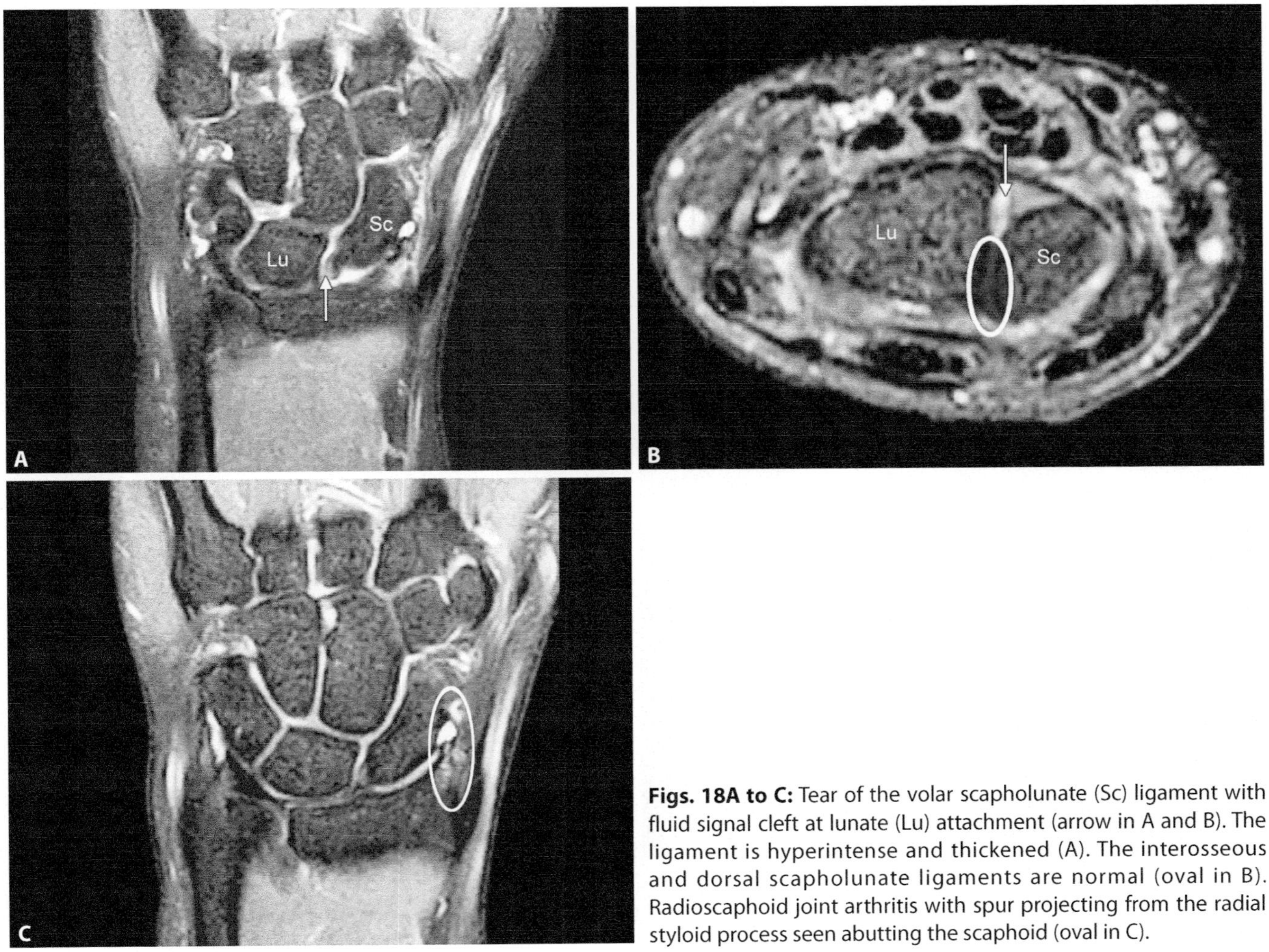

Figs. 18A to C: Tear of the volar scapholunate (Sc) ligament with fluid signal cleft at lunate (Lu) attachment (arrow in A and B). The ligament is hyperintense and thickened (A). The interosseous and dorsal scapholunate ligaments are normal (oval in B). Radioscaphoid joint arthritis with spur projecting from the radial styloid process seen abutting the scaphoid (oval in C).

The lunotriquetral ligament is triangular or linear. The tears of this ligament are not easily detected on MRI, and MR arthrography has greater sensitivity in detecting tears. Widening of the lunotriquetral interval is rarely seen, unlike scapholunate ligament tears.[12]

Distal Radioulnar Joint

The distal radius, ulna, TFCC, and joint capsule form the DRUJ. The head of ulna forms a pivot joint after it articulates with the sigmoid notch on the ulnar aspect of the distal radius. Forearm movement of pronation and supination occur at the DRUJ, which also plays an important role in stabilization of the forearm. The foveal attachment of the radioulnar ligaments of the TFCC and the ulnotriquetral ligament also have a role in maintaining stability. Distal radial fractures are also associated with DRUJ injuries, which often go unrecognized.[39]

The clinical features of DRUJ instability include pain or audible clicking on pronation/supination or restricted movement. The empty groove of extensor carpi ulnaris can be palpated. The ulna which subluxates dorsally can also be palpated.[39]

Associated osseous injuries—Colles', Smith's (reverse Colles, fracture), Essex-Lopresti, Galeazzi, Chauffeur's, and Barton's fractures—can be associated with DRUJ instability. DRUJ instability causes ulnar-sided pain and early onset of degenerative arthritis in patients with distal radial fractures.[13,39]

Radiography is the primary investigation of choice and in a well-positioned lateral radiograph, the ulnar anterior and posterior margins overlap with the radius. However, positioning may be difficult and subtle subluxations may be missed.

The CT and MRI are useful for detecting the congruence of the DRUJ on axial images. In addition to ligamentous and osseous injuries, entrapment of ECU may also be detected, which may result in failure of closed reduction in certain osseous injuries such as Barton's fracture.[40]

Post-traumatic fractures of ulnar styloid, especially base of ulnar styloid, are also associated with DRUJ instability due to concomitant injury to foveal attachment of TFCC. Chronic unstable styloid fractures or malunited ulnar styloid fractures also results in repetitive trauma and dislocation or tears of ECU. Post-traumatic distal radial fractures and physeal fusion can lead to positive ulnar variance and DRUJ instability due to TFCC tears.[39]

Tendon Disorders

Tendons have low-signal intensity on all pulse sequences due to a parallel arrangement of fibers with low water content. APL can have a normally striated appearance due to multiple tendon slips with interspersed fat. Magic angle artifact can cause artifactual intermediate-signal intensity, especially in the FPL and ECU.[41]

De Quervain's Tenosynovitis

De Quervain's tenosynovitis affects the first extensor compartment containing the APL and EPB. This is commonly seen in middle-aged females and can be bilateral in 30%.[41] It is also common in the peripartum period.[33] Positive Finkelstein's test with pain on ulnar deviation of the thumb is diagnostic.

The MRI findings include tendon thickening, fluid around the tendon sheath, and surrounding edema. A septum may be found between the tendon sheaths **(Figs. 19A and B)**. Ultrasound is an alternative tool to MRI to look for septum between the two tendons.

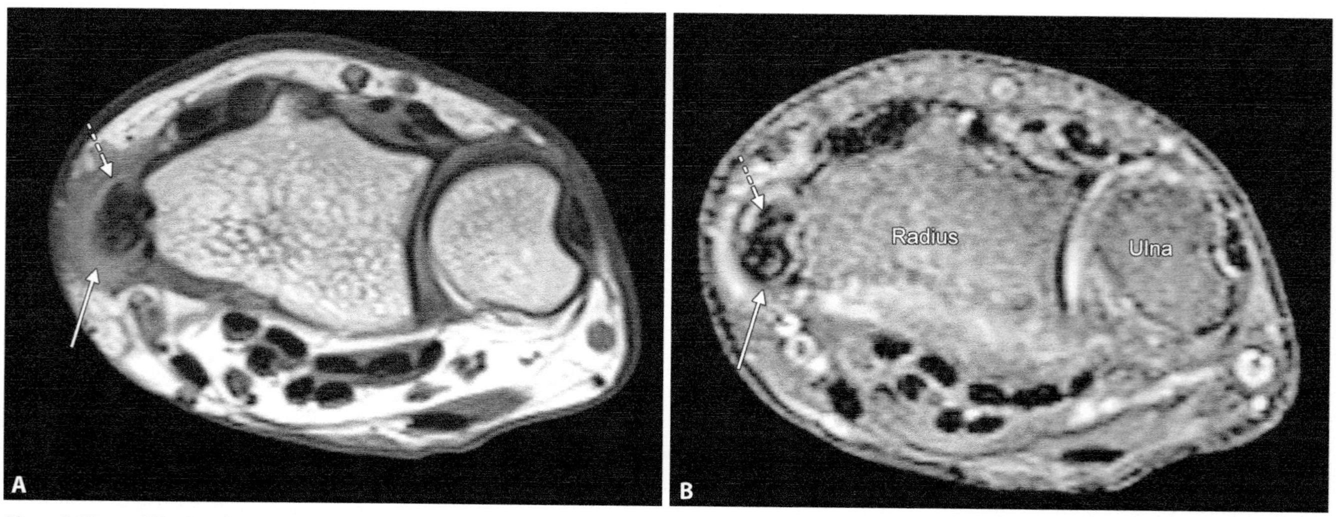

Figs. 19A and B: De Quervain's tenosynovitis. (A) Axial T1W and (B) T2W fat-saturated images show thickening and intratendinous intermediate signal of abductor pollicis longus (arrow) and extensor pollicis brevis (dashed arrow). Fluid seen surrounding the tendons and mild surrounding soft tissue edema are also present.

Intersection Syndrome

The first compartment tendons of APL and brevis cross from ulnar to radial side over the second compartment extensor tendons of extensor carpi radialis longus and brevis. Overuse or repeated friction at this intersection 3–4 cm proximal to Lister's tubercle of the radius causes tenosynovitis of the second compartment with pain in the distal forearm. The site of pain is proximal to the site of pain in de Quervain's tenosynovitis, at the site of intersection. Overhead racket players and weight-lifters are prone to this overuse injury.

Distal Intersection Syndrome

This is a rare cause of pain on the dorsal side of the wrist over Lister's tubercle at the point of crossing of the third compartment tendon of extensor pollicis longus (EPL) over the second compartment tendons of extensor carpi radialis brevis and longus.

Extensor Carpi Ulnaris Tenosynovitis

Extensor carpi ulnaris tenosynovitis is common and seen most commonly in patients with RA and in patients with subluxation of the ECU due to DRUJ instability, which may be postinflammatory or post-traumatic **(Figs. 20A and B)**.

Flexor Tenosynovitis

Flexor tenosynovitis occurs commonly in patients with RA or tubercular arthritis, both of which can lead to synovial thickening and intrasynovial rice bodies. Distension of the common flexor tendon sheath can present as carpal tunnel syndrome (CTS) **(Figs. 21A and B)**.

Carpal Tunnel Syndrome

Carpal tunnel syndrome accounts for approximately 90% of all entrapment neuropathies and is caused by compression of the median nerve at the carpal tunnel in the volar aspect of the wrist. Patients present with complaints of pain, numbness, or tingling feeling in the hands in the median nerve distribution.[42] Nerve conduction studies remain the gold standard for diagnosing and grading CTS, but provide limited information about the exact location, extent, and possible cause of nerve entrapment and is also uncomfortable for the patient.[43] Magnetic resonance neurography (MRN) is a specific MR technique to enhance the peripheral nerve visualization with the help of high-resolution and high-contrast pulse sequences. MRI has the advantage of excellent soft-tissue resolution, the capacity to delineate the site of nerve injury, and to demonstrate the secondary causes of CTS.[44]

Magnetic resonance neurography sequences recommended include axial T1W pulse sequence, axial FS pulse sequence, preferably T2-spectral adiabatic inversion recovery (SPAIR) sequence, coronal proton density sequence, and 3D nerve imaging.[45] The advantage of the 3D isotropic technique lies in the ability to allow thinner slices and multiplanar reconstructions derived from isotropic voxels for clear display of nerves along the long axis. A diffusion-based 3D reversed fast imaging with steady-state free precession (3D PSIF) is another sequence which can be used to cause vascular signal suppression in peripheral nerves creating nerve specific images.[44,45] Diffusion tensor imaging can also be performed as a problem-solving tool for quantification of the fractional anisotropy (FA). Axial T2 SPAIR sequence is adequate for assessing the median nerve; T2 fat-suppressed 3D PSIF sequence is useful to delineate the margins and course of the median nerve.[46]

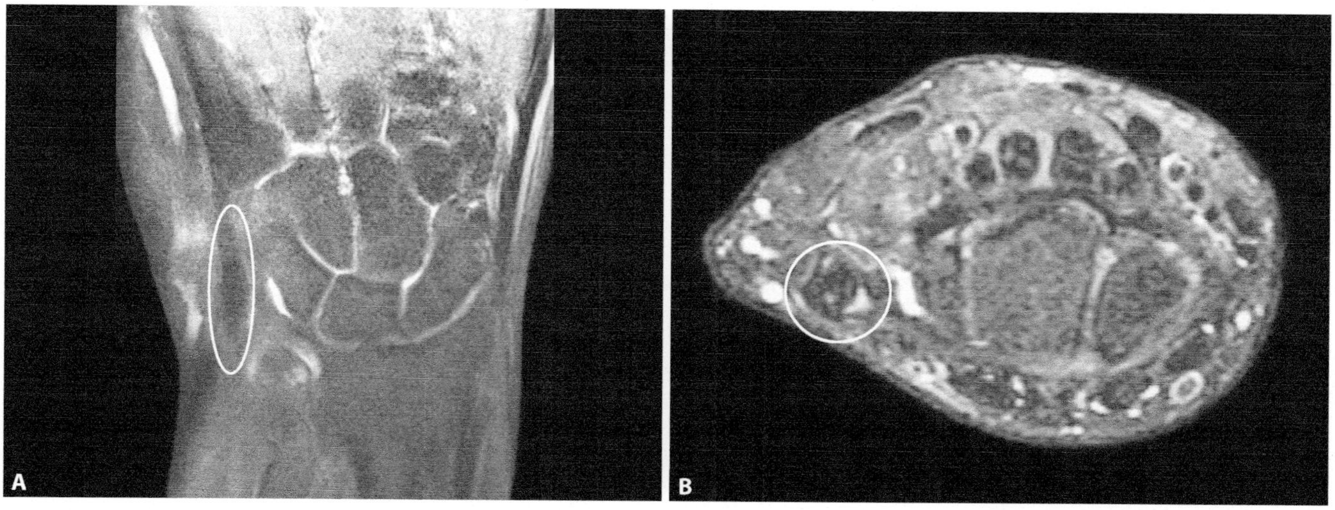

Figs. 20A and B: Flexor carpi ulnaris tendinopathy in a patient with ulnar wrist pain. Coronal PD-weighted fat-saturated images show a focal thickening of flexor carpi ulnaris with mild fluid (ovals in A and B). Fluid is also seen in the adjacent distal radioulnar joint.

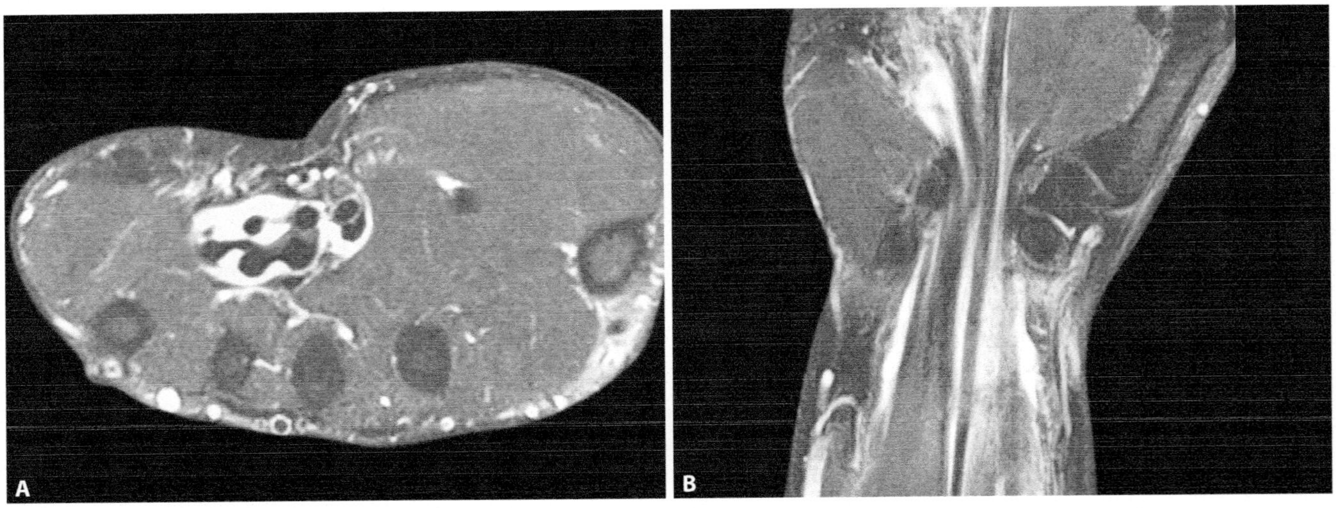

Figs. 21A and B: Flexor tenosynovitis. Fluid is seen around the flexor tendons in the axial (A) and coronal (B) T2W fat-saturated sequences.

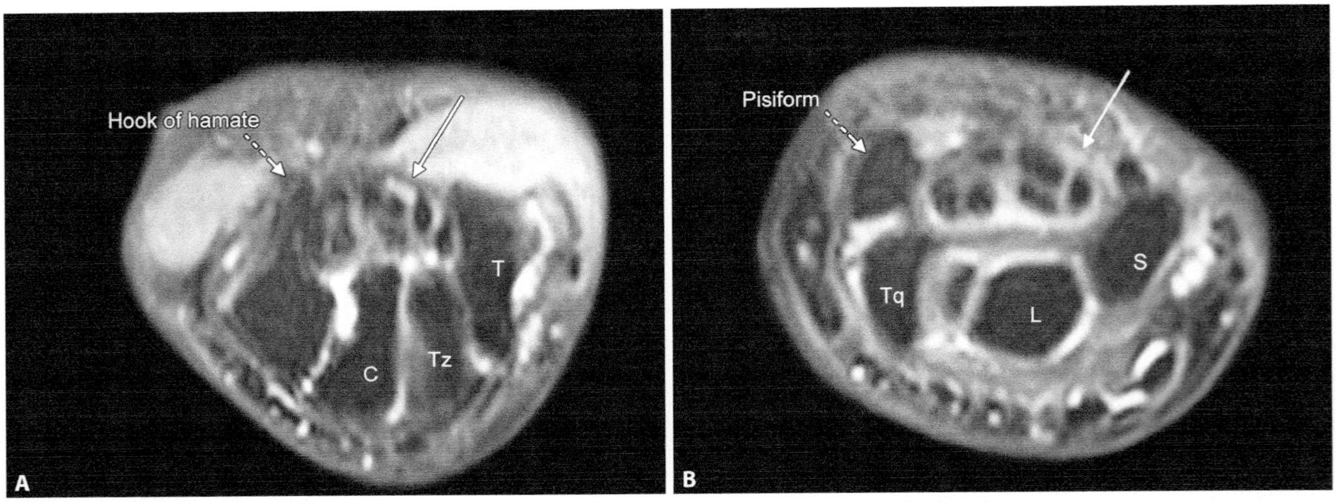

Figs. 22A and B: Normal median nerve on MRI. Axial T2 SPAIR images at the (A) hamate hook level (dashed arrow in A), (B) level of pisiform bone (dashed arrow in B) depicting normal size and signal intensity of the median nerve (arrow) at the CT in the right wrist of a patient in the control group. (C: capitate, L: lunate; R: radius; S: scaphoid; T: trapezium; Tq: triquetrum; Tz: trapezoid; U: ulna; SPAIR: spectral adiabatic inversion recovery)

Cross-sectional area (CA) of the median nerve is the most well-studied parameter, with measurement just proximal to the tunnel or at the site of the most marked swelling of the nerve being the most useful.[47-50] A cutoff value of CA of >0.165 cm^2, 1 cm proximal to the pisiform, had the highest sensitivity of 91.1% and specificity of 87.5% **(Figs. 22A and B).**[46] Koh et al. found a value of 0.143 cm^2 at the same level to give a sensitivity of 76.2% and specificity of 73.8%.[47] Klauser et al. found a cutoff value of 0.575 for FA to have sensitivity and specificity of 73.9% and 80%, respectively, and a maximum CA value of 0.17 cm^2 to have a sensitivity of 93.3% and specificity of 93.3%.[51]

Median nerve signal intensity on MRI relative to the hypothenar muscle is significantly different between patient and control group **(Figs. 23A and B).**[47,52] Retinacular bowing of >0.122 cm has a sensitivity and specificity of 60.0% and 65.6%, respectively.[46] Associated findings of extraosseous ganglion cysts and flexor tenosynovitis may be found.

Guyon's Canal Syndrome

Guyon's canal syndrome is a rare ulnar neuropathy. The ulnar nerve while traversing through the narrow Guyon's canal in the wrist can be compressed by ganglion cysts. Repetitive trauma can cause ulnar artery thrombosis or aneurysm, a condition known as hypothenar hammer syndrome.[53]

Wartenberg's Syndrome

Wartenberg's syndrome is pain or paresthesia along the radial aspect of dorsal forearm and over dorsal thumb and

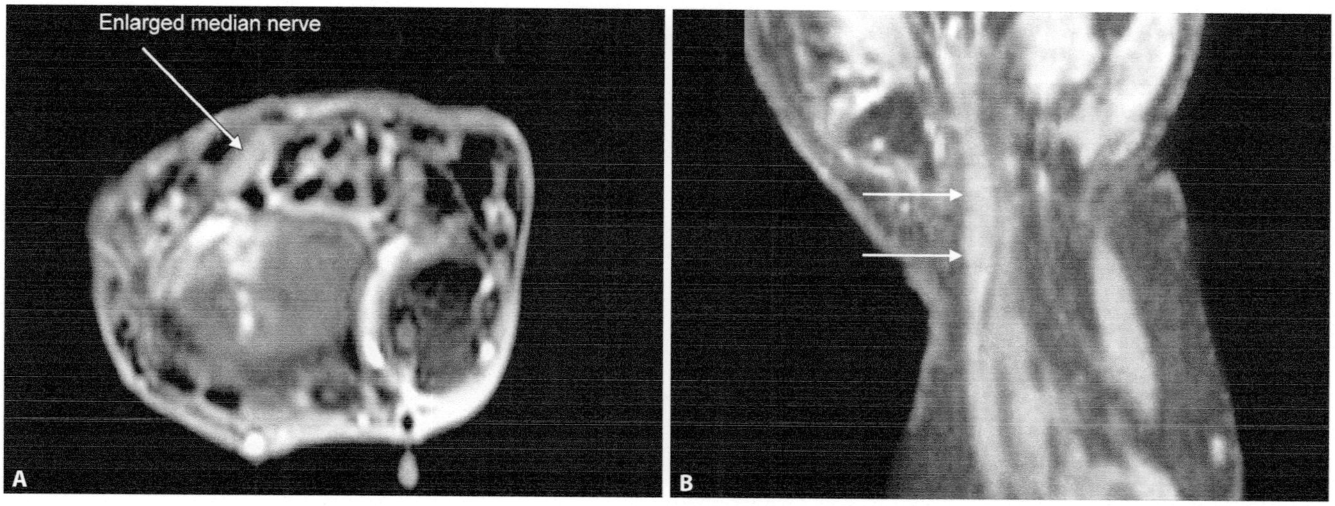

Figs. 23A and B: (A) T2 SPAIR axial image showing enlarged median nerve; (B) 3D PSIF curved reformatted image showing focal thickening of the median nerve just proximal and at the carpal tunnel in a patient with severe carpal tunnel syndrome (CTS) on nerve conduction studies.

index finger due to injury or compression of the superficial radial nerve, which emerges and courses between the brachioradialis and extensor carpi radialis longus tendon.

Inflammatory Arthritis

Rheumatoid Arthritis

Changes of RA can be detected early before radiographic evidence of the disease by both ultrasound and MRI, as early as 4 months from clinical onset. Synovitis, erosions, and tenosynovitis can be detected by both modalities. However, MRI can also reveal bone marrow edema, which is a precursor of erosions[54] **(Figs. 24A to C)**.

Contrast-enhanced MRI can differentiate between synovitis, which enhances, and effusion, which is nonenhancing. However, in late acquisitions, gadolinium can diffuse into the synovial fluid and this occurs more rapidly in small joint.[55] Dynamic gadolinium-enhanced MRI can quantify the degree of synovial enhancement. The extent of erosions and bone marrow edema on MRI can also be used for longitudinal follow-up and assessment of response.

Synovitis, erosions, and bone marrow edema can be graded with scores of 0–3 according to the Outcome Measures in Rheumatology Clinical Trials (OMERACT) and European League Against Rheumatism (EULAR) Rheumatoid Arthritis Magnetic Resonance Imaging Score (RAMRIS) system.[56]

Seronegative Spondyloarthropathies

Magnetic resonance imaging is sensitive in diagnosing erosions, edema, and synovitis but not specific. Similar findings can be detected in other causes of inflammatory arthritis including seronegative spondyloarthropathies such as psoriatic arthritis and Reiter's disease. Involvement of the axial skeleton and enthesitis helps in differentiating between RA and seronegative arthropathies.[54]

Infections

Infectious Tenosynovitis

Acute suppurative tenosynovitis is bacterial and commonly spreads from the adjacent soft-tissue infections after a penetrating injury. Fluid or pus within the tendon sheath along with heterogeneous tendon thickening may be found. In chronic tenosynovitis due to tubercular infections, intrasynovial hypointense rice bodies may be found **(Fig. 25)**.[57]

Palmar Space Infections

There are many potential spaces in the wrist joint and hand—thenar space, midpalmar space, hypothenar space, and space of Parona (between the pronator quadratus and the FDP tendon). The radial bursa, which is a sheath covering FPL, and ulnar bursa, which is a continuation of the flexor tendon sheath of the little finger, communicate with the space of Parona.[58] Infections in these spaces can occur after penetrating injury or rupture of the radial or ulnar bursa into space of Parona.

Chronic Infectious Arthritis

Tubercular arthritis can present with heterogeneous synovial thickening, erosions, and tenosynovitis. Sinus tracks and ulcers or abscesses or periarticular soft-tissue nodules or masses may also be seen and should raise the suspicion of atypical bacterial or fungal infections.[58]

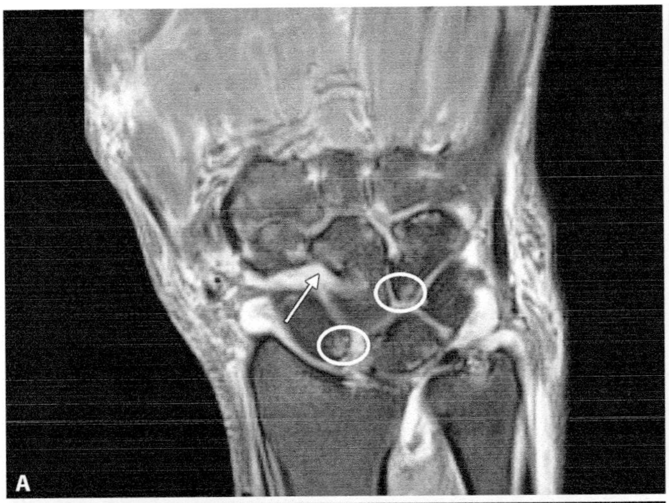
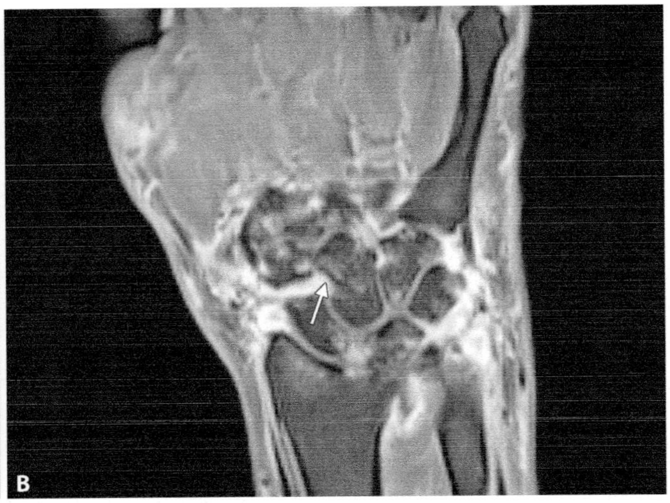
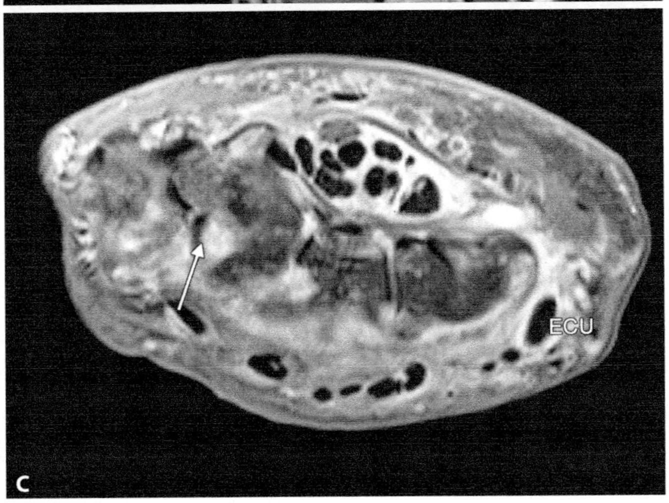

Figs. 24A to C: Coronal T2W (A), postcontrast coronal T1W (B) and postcontrast axial T1W (C) fat-saturated images show erosion in capitate (small arrow) and bone marrow edema (oval) in the carpal bones. Synovitis is seen in the distal radioulnar, radiocarpal, ulnocarpal, and intercarpal joints along with tenosynovitis of flexor tendons and extensor carpi ulnaris (ECU). Erosions must be seen in two planes.

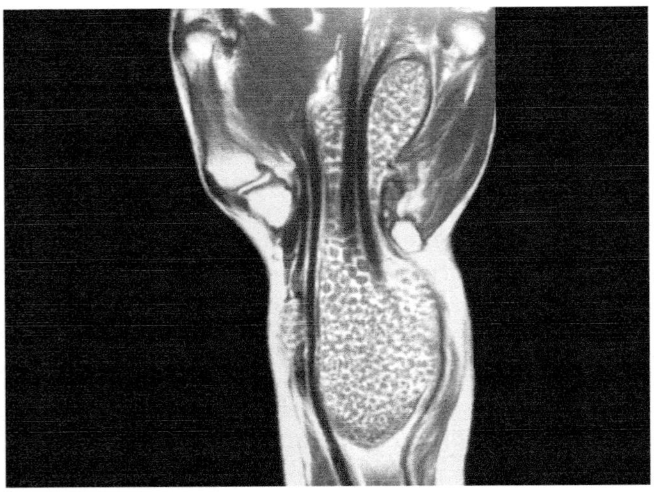

Fig. 25: Intrasynovial hypointense rice bodies in the common flexor tendon sheath on a coronal T2W image. Rice bodies can also be seen in inflammatory arthritis like rheumatoid arthritis.

Degenerative Arthritis

Wrist osteoarthritis (OA) occurs most commonly as post-traumatic sequelae after SLAC or scaphoid nonunion advanced collapse which progresses from radiocarpal arthritis to midcarpal arthritis, involving scaphocapitate and capitolunate joints. Patients with inflammatory arthritis and pyrophosphate deposition disease also develop OA. Idiopathic OA may also develop and in some studies, idiopathic OA is more common than post-traumatic arthritis of the wrist.

Radiographs show osteophytes, subchondral sclerosis and cysts, joint space narrowing, and marginal erosions (in erosive OA). Although scoring systems for hand and wrist OA on radiographs exist (Kellgren-Lawrence Scale), there is poor correlation between clinical severity and radiographic findings.[59]

The MRI is more reliable and sensitive in detecting radiocarpal arthritis, especially radiolunate arthritis, which has implications in deciding the arthrodesis procedure **(Figs. 26A to C)**.[60]

Tumors

Tumors include ganglion, intraosseous synovial cyst/ganglion/soft-tissue giant cell tumor (GCT) of the tendon sheath (GCTTS) and tumors like neurofibromas and schwannomas.

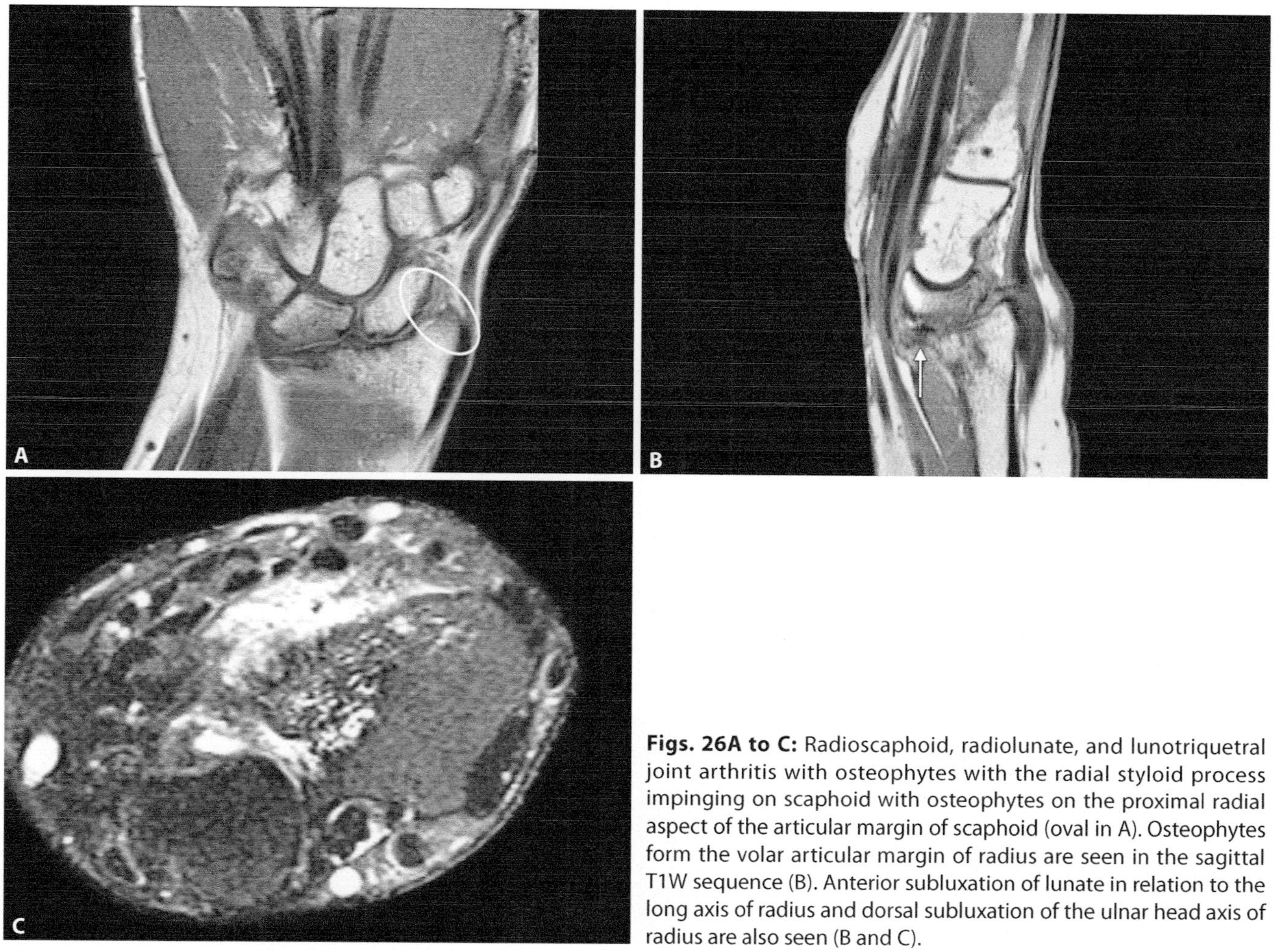

Figs. 26A to C: Radioscaphoid, radiolunate, and lunotriquetral joint arthritis with osteophytes with the radial styloid process impinging on scaphoid with osteophytes on the proximal radial aspect of the articular margin of scaphoid (oval in A). Osteophytes form the volar articular margin of radius are seen in the sagittal T1W sequence (B). Anterior subluxation of lunate in relation to the long axis of radius and dorsal subluxation of the ulnar head axis of radius are also seen (B and C).

Soft Tissue Tumors

The common soft tissue tumors in the wrist joint are cystic, and ganglion cyst is the most common soft tissue tumor commonly seen. Ganglion cysts or synovial cysts are associated with ligamentous injury or degenerative conditions where increased intra-articular pressure causes extrusion of joint fluid, or there is mucoid degeneration of the collagenous tissue. On imaging, a small communication may be visible with the joint space, most commonly on the dorsal radial aspect of the wrist. An uncomplicated cyst appears isointense on T1W image and hyperintense on T2W image **(Figs. 27A and B)**. However, a hemorrhagic or ruptured cyst may have internal debris and content and mimic a neoplasm. On contrast enhancement, peripheral enhancement can be noted in a ganglion cyst and is helpful in differentiating it from a solid neoplasm.[61,62]

Benign soft tissue tumors are more common than malignant tumors. Soft tissue tumors commonly seen in the wrist joint are lipomas, vascular malformations **(Figs. 28A to C)**, GCTTS, neurogenic tumors, and lipofibromatous hamartoma of the median nerve **(Figs. 29A and B)**.

Giant cell tumor of the tendon sheath, also known as pigmented villonodular synovitis, presents as a firm multinodular nontender mass. It is the second most common tumor after ganglion cysts. Long-standing tumors can cause pressure erosion over bone. They appear as hypointense on both T1W and T2W imaging, and can also be located along the carpal bones.[63] GCTTS can be classified as type I with a single round or multilobulated tumor and type II where there are two or more distinct tumors which are not joined.[64] These tumors have a high recurrence rate if they are not completely excised or in type II tumors[63] **(Figs. 30A to C)**.

Among the malignant tumors, epithelioid sarcoma, synovial sarcomas, and malignant peripheral nerve sheath tumors are common in adults and rhabdomyosarcomas in pediatric population.

Osseous Lesions

Intraosseous ganglion is a very common cystic lesion of the hand and wrist, in a carpal bone.[62]

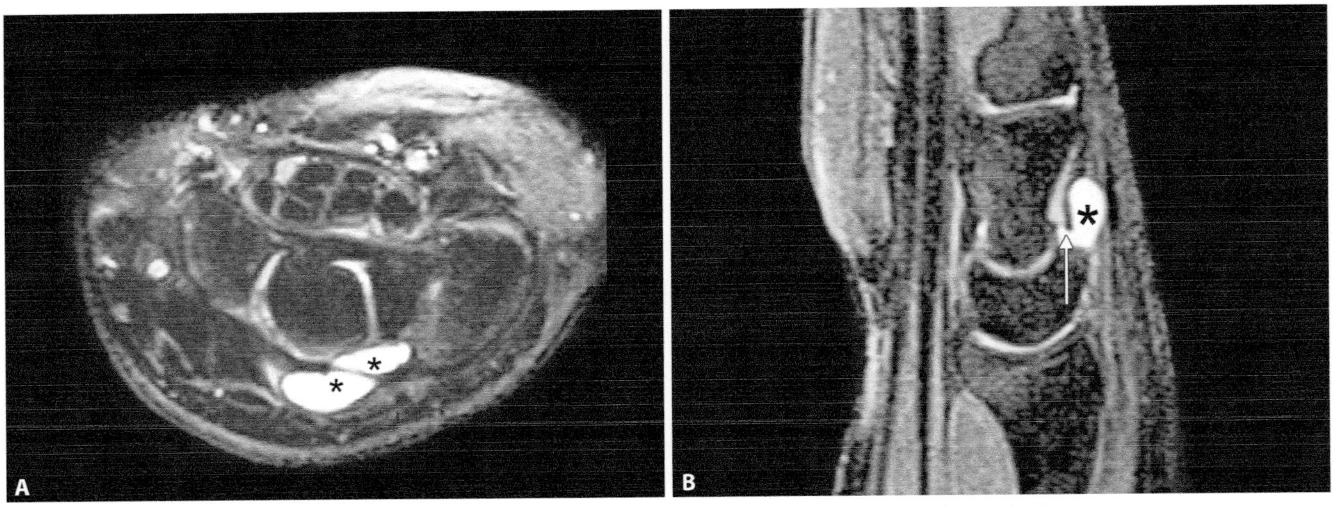

Figs. 27A and B: Ganglion. A lobulated hyperintense lesion (*) seen in the dorsal wrist with a small beak-like extension (arrow in B) from the capitolunate joint.

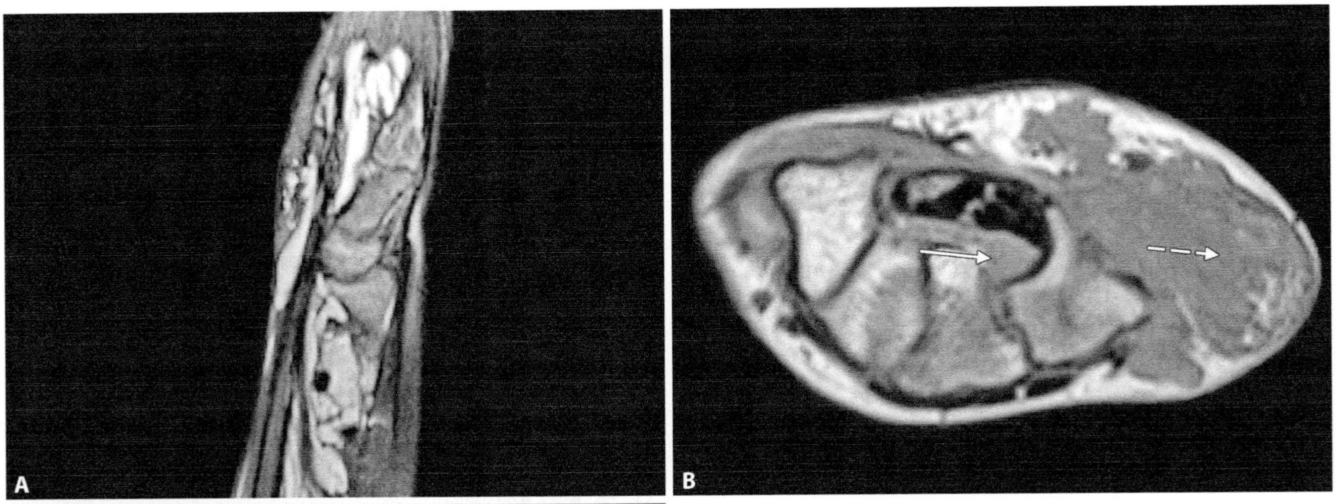

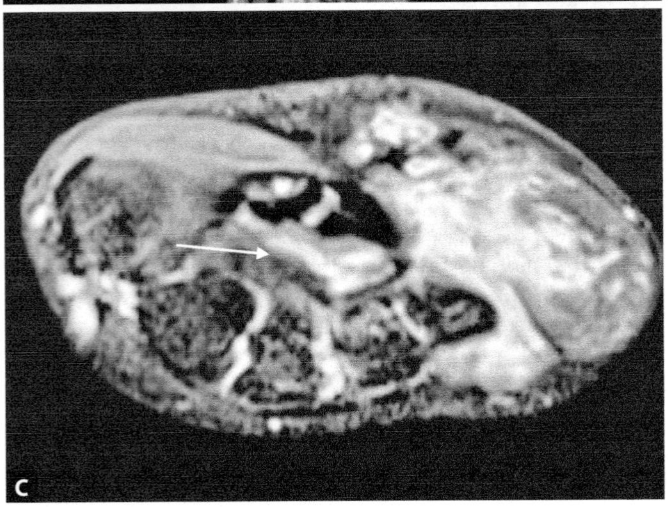

Figs. 28A to C: (A) Sagittal T2W fat-saturated image shows an infiltrative hyperintense lobulated mass with thin septae and hyperintense foci extending along the flexor tendons on the volar aspect of wrist; (B and C) On axial T1W and postcontrast T1W fat-saturated images, the extension into carpal tunnel (arrow) and interspersed fat (dashed arrow) are seen in this low-flow vascular malformation.

Benign bone tumors are far more common than malignant lesions. Enchondromas, GCTs, giant cell reparative granulomas, osteoid osteomas, and aneurysmal bone cysts are found in the metacarpals and phalanges and rarely in the carpal bones. Lymphomas, eosinophilic granulomas, chondrosarcomas, and osteosarcomas and rarely Ewing's sarcoma can affect the hand and wrist.

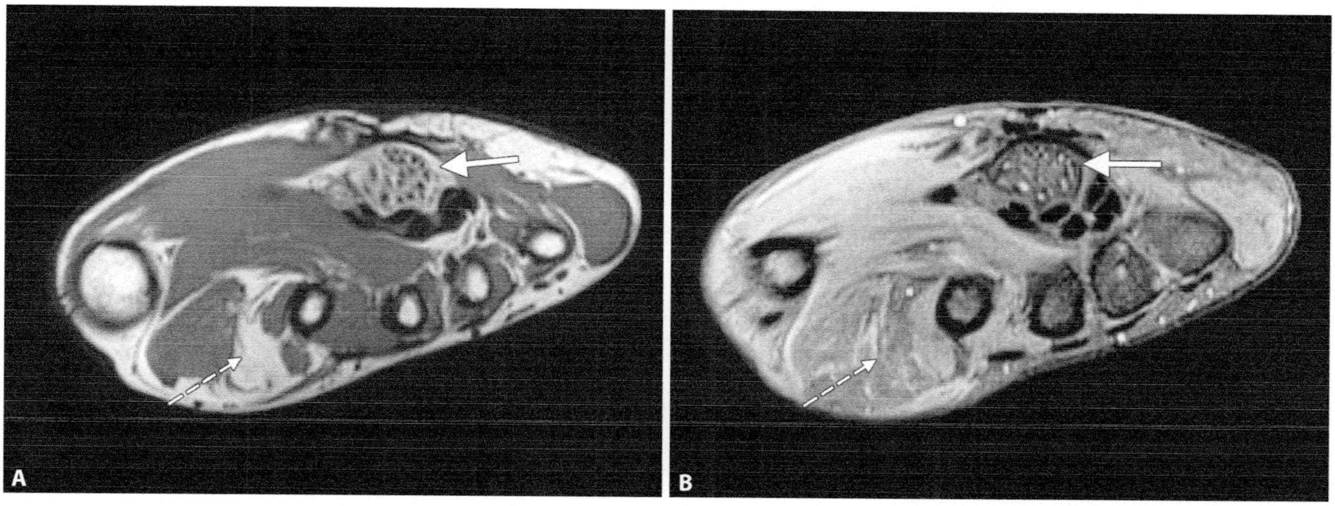

Figs. 29A and B: Fibrolipomatous hamartoma of the median nerve. The median nerve is thickened with a stippled appearance (arrow) with separation of the enlarged fascicles by fat, which is suppressed on the PD-weighted fat-saturated images. The digital branch of the median nerve is also involved (dashed arrow).

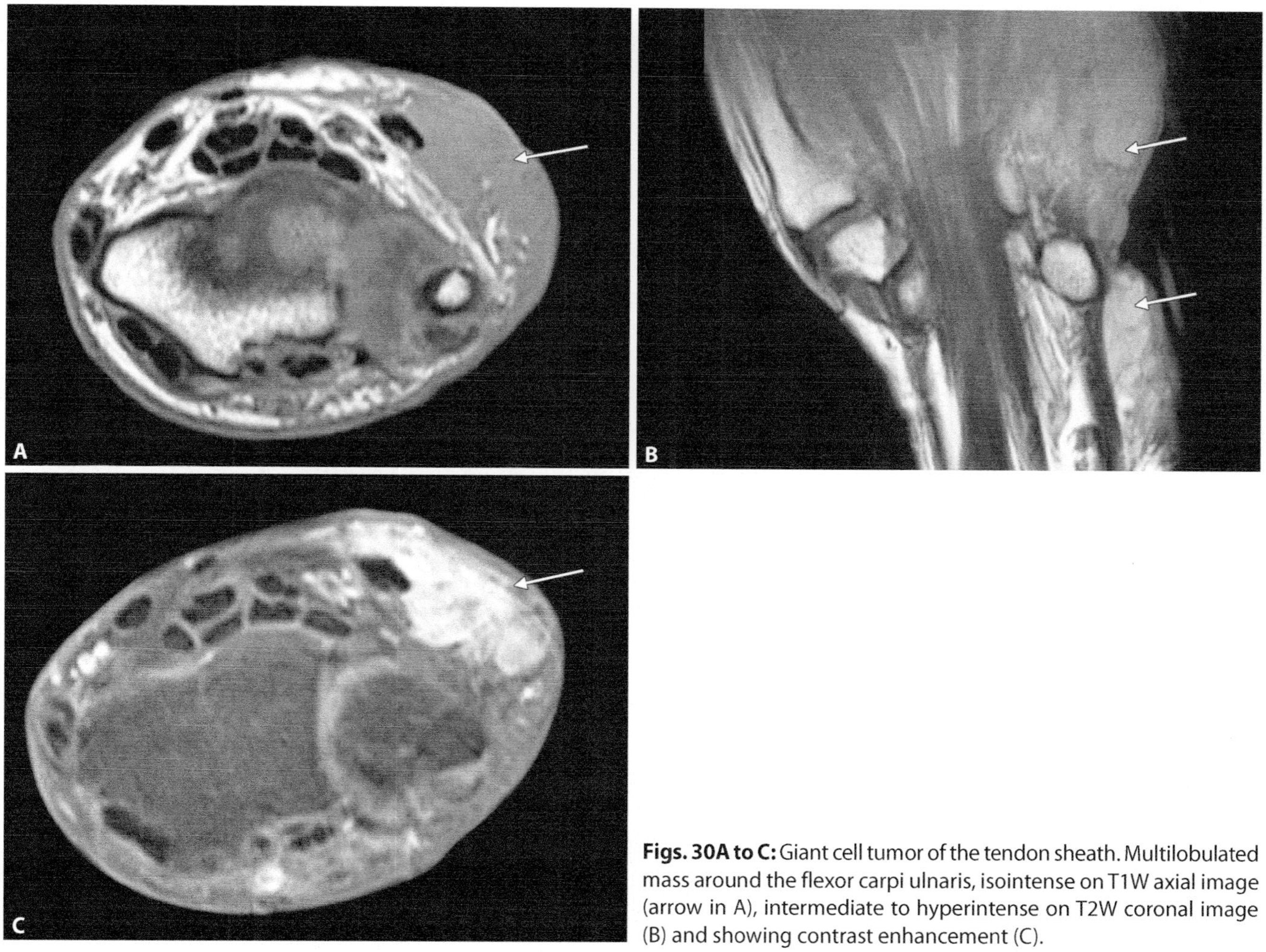

Figs. 30A to C: Giant cell tumor of the tendon sheath. Multilobulated mass around the flexor carpi ulnaris, isointense on T1W axial image (arrow in A), intermediate to hyperintense on T2W coronal image (B) and showing contrast enhancement (C).

Ulnar-sided Wrist Pain

The causes of ulnar-sided wrist pain are given in **Table 6**.

Radial-sided Wrist Pain

The causes of ulnar-sided wrist pain are given in **Table 7**.

Table 6: Causes of ulnar-sided wrist pain.[2,22]

Ligamentous injuries	• Triangular fibrocartilage complex (TFCC) lesions
Impaction syndromes	• Ulnar impaction syndrome • Ulnar impingement syndrome • Ulnar styloid impaction syndrome • Hamatolunate impingement syndrome
Osseous injuries	• Kienböck's disease • Ulnar styloid fracture • Hamate fracture • Pisiform fracture • Base of fifth metacarpal fracture
Joint disorders	• Carpal instability • Distal radioulnar joint disorders
Tendon disorders	• Extensor carpi ulnaris disorder • Flexor carpi ulnaris tendinitis
Nerve impingement	• Guyon's canal syndrome

Table 7: Causes of radial-sided wrist pain.

Ligamentous injuries	• Scapholunate ligament injury
Osseous injuries	• Scaphoid fracture and avascular necrosis (AVN) of scaphoid
Joint disorders	• Scapholunate advanced collapse and scaphoid nonunion advanced collapse • Trapeziometacarpal joint arthritis
Tendon disorders	• De Quervain's tenosynovitis • Intersection syndromes (between I and II compartments proximal and II and III compartments distal to Lister's tubercle) • Flexor carpi radialis tenosynovitis
Nerve impingement	• Wartenberg's syndrome

REFERENCES

1. Mann FA, Gilula LA. Post-traumatic wrist pain and instability: a radiographic approach to diagnosis. In: Lichtman DM, Alexander AH (Eds). The Wrist and Its Disorders, 2nd edition. Philadelphia PA: Saunders; 1997. pp. 91-108.
2. Cerezal L, Del piñal F, Abascal F, García-Valtuille R, Pereda T, Canga A. Imaging findings in ulnar-sided wrist impaction syndromes. Radiographics. 2002;22 (1):105-21.
3. Bateni CP, Bartolotta RJ, Richardson ML, Mulcahy H, Allan CH. Imaging key wrist ligaments: what the surgeon needs the radiologist to know. Am J Roentgenol. 2013;200(5):1089-95.
4. Buck FM, Gheno R, Nico MA, Haghighi P, Trudell DJ, Resnick D. Ulnomeniscal homologue of the wrist: correlation of anatomic and MR imaging findings. Radiology. 2009;253(3):771-9.
5. Haugstvedt JR, Berger RA, Nakamura T, Neale P, Berglund L, An KN. Relative contributions of the ulnar attachments of the triangular fibrocartilage complex to the dynamic stability of the distal radioulnar joint. J Hand Surg Am. 2006; 31(3):445-51.
6. Johnson D, Stevens KJ, Riley G, Shapiro L, Yoshioka H, Gold GE. Approach to MR imaging of the elbow and wrist: technical aspects and innovation. Magn Reson Imaging Clin N Am. 2015;23(3):355-66.
7. Chang AL, Yu HJ, von Borstel D, Nozaki T, Horiuchi S, Terada Y, et al. Advanced imaging techniques of the Wrist. Am J Roentgenol. 2017;209(3):497-510.
8. Akella SV, Regatte RR, Borthakur A, Kneeland JB, Leigh JS, Reddy R. T1rho MR imaging of the human wrist in vivo. Acad Radiol. 2003;10(6):614-9.
9. Ku E, Pedoia V, Tanaka M, Heilmeier U, Imboden J, Graf J, et al. Evaluating radiocarpal cartilage matrix changes 3-months after anti-TNF treatment for rheumatoid arthritis using MR T1ρ imaging. J Magn Reson Imaging. 2017;45(5):1514-22.
10. Medverd JR, Pugsley JM, Harley JD, Bhargava P. Lateral approach for radiocarpal wrist arthrography. Am J Roentgenol. 2011;196(1):W58-60.
11. Limarzi GM, O'Dell MC, Scherer K, Pettis C, Wasyliw CW, Bancroft LW. Magnetic resonance arthrography of the wrist and elbow. Magn Reson Imaging Clin N Am. 2015;23(03):441-55.
12. Cerezal L, Abascal F, Garcia-Valtuille R, del Pinal F. Wrist MR arthrography: how, why, when? Radiol Clin N Am. 2005;43(4):709-31.
13. Squires JH, England E, Mehta K, Wissman RD. The role of imaging in diagnosing diseases of the distal radioulnar joint, triangular fibrocartilage complex, and distal ulna. Am J Roentgenol. 2014;203(1):146-53.
14. Ten Berg PW, Drijkoningen T, Strackee SD, Buijze GA. Classifications of acute scaphoid fractures: a systematic literature review. J Wrist Surg. 2016;5(2):152-9.
15. Cockenpot E, Lefebvre G, Demondion X, Chantelot C, Cotten A. Imaging of sports-related hand and wrist injuries: sports imaging series. Radiology. 2016;279(3):674-92.
16. Amadio PC, Berquist TH, Smith DK, Ilstrup DM, Cooney WP 3rd, Linscheid RL. Scaphoid malunion. J Hand Surg [Am]. 1989;14(4):679-87.
17. Trumble TE, Irving J. Histologic and magnetic resonance imaging correlations in Kienböck's disease. J Hand Surg Am. 1990;15(6):879-84.
18. Desser TS, McCarthy S, Trumble T. Scaphoid fractures and Kienböck's disease of the lunate: MR imaging with histopathologic correlation. Magn Reson Imaging. 1990;8(4):357-61.
19. Cerezal L, Abascal F, Canga A, García-Valtuille R, Bustamante M, del Piñal F. Usefulness of gadolinium-enhanced MR imaging in the evaluation of the vascularity of scaphoid nonunions. Am J Roentgenol. 2000;174(1):141-9.
20. Anderson SE, Steinbach LS, Tschering-Vogel D, Martin M, Nagy L. MR imaging of avascular scaphoid nonunion before and after vascularized bone grafting. Skeletal Radiol. 2005;34(6):314-20.
21. Schmitt R, Rosenthal H. Imaging of scaphoid fractures according to the New S3 guidelines. Fortschr Röntgenstr. 2016;188(5):459-69.

22. Watanabe A, Souza F, Vezeridis PS, Blazar P, Yoshioka H. Ulnar-sided wrist pain. II. Clinical imaging and treatment. Skeletal Radiol. 2010;39(9):837-57.
23. Kienböck R. Über traumatische malazie des mondbeins und ihre folgezustände: entartungsformen und kompressionsfrakturen. Fortschr Geb Roentgenstrahlen. 1910;16:77-103.
24. Hulten O. Über anatomische variationen der handgelenkknochen. Acta Radiol. 1928;9:155-68.
25. Antuña Zapico JM. Malacia del semilunar. Vall-adolid, Spain: University of Valladolid; 1966.
26. van Leeuwen WF, Janssen SJ, ter Meulen DP, Ring D. What is the radiographic prevalence of incidental Kienböck disease? Clin Orthop Relat Res. 2016;474(3):808-13.
27. Stoller DW. Magnetic Resonance Imaging in Orthopaedics and Sports Medicine, 3rd edition. Baltimore, MD: Lippincott Williams & Wilkins; 2007
28. Arnaiz J, Piedra T, Cerezal L, Ward J, Thompson A, Vidal JA, et al. Imaging of Kienböck disease. Am J Roentgenol. 2014;203(1):131-9.
29. Kennedy C, Abrams R. Lichtman classification for Kienbock disease. Clin Orthop Relat Res. 2019;477(6):1516-20.
30. Helms C, Major N, Anderson M, Kaplan PE, Dussault R (Eds). Musculoskeletal MRI, 2nd edition. Philadelphia: Saunders; 2009. pp. 252-9.
31. Ng AW, Griffith JF, Fung CS, Lee RK, Tong CS, Wong CW. MR imaging of the traumatic triangular fibrocartilaginous complex tear. Quant Imaging Med Surg. 2017;7(4):443-60.
32. Bae WC, Ruangchaijatuporn T, Chang EY, Biswas R, Du J, Statum S, et al. MR morphology of triangular fibrocartilage complex: correlation with quantitative MR and biomechanical properties. Skeletal Radiol. 2016;45(4): 447-54.
33. Moser TP, Martinez AP, Andoulsi S, Jeantroux J, Cardinal E. Radiographic/MR imaging correlation of the wrist. Magn Reson Imaging Clin N Am. 2019;27:601-23.
34. Kani KK, Mulcahy H, Chew FS. Understanding carpal instability: a radiographic perspective. Skeletal Radiol. 2016;45(8):1031-43.
35. Treiman ML, Strle NA, Matthews CR, von Borstel D. Carpal instability: clarification of the most common etiologies and imaging findings. J Am Osteopath Coll Radiol. 2019;8(4):5-10.
36. Shahabpour M, Staelens B, Van Overstraeten L, De Maeseneer M, Boulet C, De Mey J, et al. Advanced imaging of the scapholunate ligamentous complex. Skeletal Radiol. 2015;44 (12):1709-25.
37. Schmitt R, Christopoulos G, Meier R, Coblenz G, Fröhner S, Lanz U, et al. Direct MR arthrography of the wrist in comparison with arthroscopy: a prospective study on 125 patients. Rofo Fortschr Geb Rontgenstr Neuen Bildgeb Verfahr. 2003;175(7):911-9.
38. Lee DJ, Elfar JC. Carpal ligament injuries, pathomechanics, and classification. Hand Clin. 2015;31(3):389-98.
39. Mespreuve M, Vanhoenacke F, Verstraete K. Imaging findings of the distal radio-ulnar joint in trauma. J Belgian Soc Radiol. 2015;99(1):1-20.
40. Amrami KK, Moran SL, Berger RA, Ehman EC, Felmlee JP. Imaging the distal radioulnar joint. Hand Clin. 2010;26(4):467-75.
41. Bencardino JT. MR imaging of tendon lesions of the hand and wrist. Magn Reson Imaging Clin N Am. 2004;12 (2):333-47.
42. Ghasemi-Rad M, Nosair E, Vegh A, Mohammadi A, Akkad A, Lesha E, et al. A handy review of carpal tunnel syndrome: from anatomy to diagnosis and treatment. World J Radiol. 2014;6(6):284-300.
43. Filler AG, Kliot M, Howe FA, Hayes CE, Saunders DE, Goodkin R, et al. Application of magnetic resonance neurography in the evaluation of patients with peripheral nerve pathology. J Neurosurg. 1996;85(2):299-309.
44. Chhabra A, Lee PP, Bizzell C, Soldatos T. 3 Tesla MR neurography—technique, interpretation, and pitfalls. Skeletal Radiol. 2011;40(10):1249-60.
45. Chhabra A, Flammang A, Padua A Jr. Carrino JA, Andreisek G. Magnetic resonance neurography: technical considerations. Neuroimaging Clin N Am. 2014;24(1): 67-78.
46. Bagga B, Sinha A, Khandelwal N, Modi M, Ahuja CK, Sharma R. Comparison of magnetic resonance imaging and ultrasonography in diagnosing and grading carpal tunnel syndrome: a prospective study. Curr Prob Diagn Radiol. 2020;49(2):102-15.
47. Koh SH, Kwon BC, Park C, Hwang SY, Lee JW, Kim SS. A comparison of the performance of anatomical MRI and DTI in diagnosing carpal tunnel syndrome. Eur J Radiol. 2014;83(11):2065-73.
48. Uchiyama S, Itsubo T, Yasutomi T, Nakagawa H, Kamimura M, Kato H. Quantitative MRI of the wrist and nerve conduction studies in patients with idiopathic carpal tunnel syndrome. J Neurol Neurosurg Psychiatry. 2005;76(8):1103-8.
49. Britz GW, Haynor DR, Kuntz C, Goodkin R, Gitter A, Kliot M. Carpal tunnel syndrome: correlation of magnetic resonance imaging, clinical, electrodiagnostic, and intraoperative findings. Neurosurgery. 1995;37(6):1097-103.
50. Monagle K, Dai G, Chu A, Burnham RS, Snyder RE. Quantitative MR imaging of carpal tunnel syndrome. Am J Roentgenol. 1999;172(6):1581-6.
51. Klauser AS, Abd Ellah M, Kremser C, Taljanovic M, Schmidle G, Gabl M, et al. Carpal tunnel syndrome assessment with diffusion tensor imaging: value of fractional anisotropy and apparent diffusion coefficient. Eur Radiol. 2018;28(3):1111-7.
52. Radack DM, Schweitzer ME, Taras J. Carpal tunnel syndrome: are the MR findings a result of population selection bias? Am J Roentgenol. 1997;169(6):1649-53.
53. Hui-Chou HG, McClinton MA. Current options for treatment of hypothenar hammer syndrome. Hand Clin. 2015;31(1):53-62.
54. Jbara, M, Patnana M, Kazmi F, Beltran J. MR imaging: arthropathies and infectious conditions of the elbow, wrist, and hand. Magn Reson Imaging Clin N Am. 2004;12:361-79.
55. McQueen FM. Magnetic resonance imaging in early inflammatory arthritis: what is its role? Rheumatology. 2000;39(7):700-6.

56. Ejbjerg B, McQueen F, Lassere ME, Haavardsholm P, Conaghan P, O'Connor P, et al. The EULAR-OMERACT rheumatoid arthritis MRI reference image atlas: the wrist joint. Ann Rheum Dis. 2005;64:i23-i47.
57. Plotkin B, Srihari SC, Srinath SC, Motamedi K. MR imaging and US of the WRIST Tendons. Radiographics. 2016;36(6):1688-700.
58. Patel DB, Emmanuel NB, Stevanovic MV, Matsuk GR, Gottsegen CJ, Forrester DM, et al. Hand infections: anatomy, types and spread of infection, imaging findings, and treatment options. Radiographics. 2014;34(7): 1968-86.
59. Haugen IK, Bøyesen P. Imaging modalities in hand osteoarthritis—status and perspectives of conventional radiography, magnetic resonance imaging, and ultrasonography. Arthritis Res Ther. 2011;13:248.
60. Li AE, Lee SK, Rancy SK, Burge AJ, Potter HG, Wolfe SW. Comparison of magnetic resonance imaging and radiographs for evaluation of carpal osteoarthritis. J Wrist Surg. 2017;6(2):120-5.
61. Vanhoenacker FM, Eyselbergs M, Van Hul E, Van Dyck P, De Schepper AM. Pseudotumoural soft tissue lesions of the hand and wrist: a pictorial review. Insights Imag. 2011;2(3):319-33.
62. Plate AM, Lee SJ, Steiner G, Posner MA. Tumor-like lesions and benign tumors of the hand and wrist. J Am Acad Orthop Surg. 2003;11(2):129-41.
63. Di Grazia S, Succi G, Fragetta F, Perrotta RE. Giant cell tumor of tendon sheath: study of 64 cases and review of literature. G Chir. 2013;3(5-6):149-52.
64. Al-Qattan M. Giant cell tumors of tendon sheath: classification and recurrence rate. J Hand Surg Br. 2001;26(1):72-5.

CHAPTER

18

Magnetic Resonance Imaging of the Hip and Pelvis

Anjali Prakash, Alpana Manchanda, Rashmi Dixit

INTRODUCTION

The hip joint is a primary weight-bearing joint. The pelvis transmits the weight of the body to both the feet and at the same time allows extensive movement of the hip. Pain in the hip is one of the most common orthopedic complaints which has a broad differential diagnosis and includes both intra and extra-articular causes.

Conventional radiography is used as a first-line tool in trauma, arthritis, and suspected tumors; however, it is insensitive to early osseous changes and may depict only advanced stage of the disease where treatment options are limited to hip replacement. It is also unable to detect soft tissue injury, cartilage, and labral pathology. Magnetic resonance imaging (MRI) has become the imaging study of choice for diagnosing most hip disorders.

NORMAL ANATOMY

The pelvis is a complex structure composed of an osseous ring formed by the innominate bones and the sacrum with numerous muscles attached for support and ambulation. The sacroiliac joints allow little movement and the articulating surfaces serve to transmit weight. These surfaces are covered by hyaline cartilage and bound together by strong ligaments—the interosseous anteriorly and by the sacroiliac ligaments posteriorly.

The hip is a ball and socket joint formed by the articulation of the spherical femoral head with the acetabulum. The acetabulum covers 40% of the femoral head and is formed by the ilium, ischium, and the pubis. In infants, the acetabulum is united by a Y-shaped cartilage. The acetabulum is tilted anteriorly, making hip flexion easier than extension. The concave shape of the acetabulum adds to stability of the joint. The semilunar surface of the acetabulum is covered by hyaline cartilage shaped like an inverted horseshoe. It contains nonarticulating central depression, the acetabular fossa. The depth of the acetabulum is increased by the fibrocartilaginous labrum that surrounds it.

The femoral head is almost completely covered by hyaline cartilage sparing only the depression of the acetabular fovea where the ligamentum teres attaches. The ligamentum teres carries an artery which supplies blood to the femoral head in children and involutes with age.

The trochanters are apophysis which add to the width of the bone. There are four distinct facets in the greater trochanter of the hip three of which have corresponding tendon attachment sites. The tendons of the gluteus medius and minimus, the obturator internus and externus, and piriformis muscle attach to the greater trochanter. The facets of the greater trochanter have bursae that are intimately associated with them. These include the subgluteus minimus and medius bursae, these bursae lay beneath the gluteus minimus and medius tendon osseous attachment sites, respectively. In addition, there is a subgluteus maximus bursa, the largest of the three. The iliopsoas tendon inserts at the lesser trochanter **(Figs. 1 and 2)**.

Similarly, the attachment sites of the proximal hamstring tendons correspond to changes in osseous contour. The proximal hamstring attachment complex is composed of the semimembranosus, semitendinosus, and biceps femoris tendons. All three, except for the short head of the biceps femoris, arise from the posterolateral ischial tuberosity, lateral and inferomedial facets. The semimembranosus tendon originates from the superolateral facet while the semitendinosus and long head of the biceps femoris form a conjoint tendon that attaches to the inferomedial facet. Rarely, the conjoint tendon is absent and the two tendons arise separately. The coronal plane on MR imaging is superior in visualization of the proximal hamstring attachment to these facets. In the transverse plane, the semimembranosus tendon can be found anterolaterally to the conjoint tendon. More distally, the tendon runs more medial and anterior to the other two hamstring tendons.

The trabecular pattern within the femoral head and neck is reinforced by two regions of increased trabeculation corresponding to areas of relative increase in stress. The largest of these areas runs from the apex of the femoral head inferolaterally crossing the physeal plate to the medial femoral neck. This region is referred to as primary weight-bearing trabecula. Primary weight-bearing

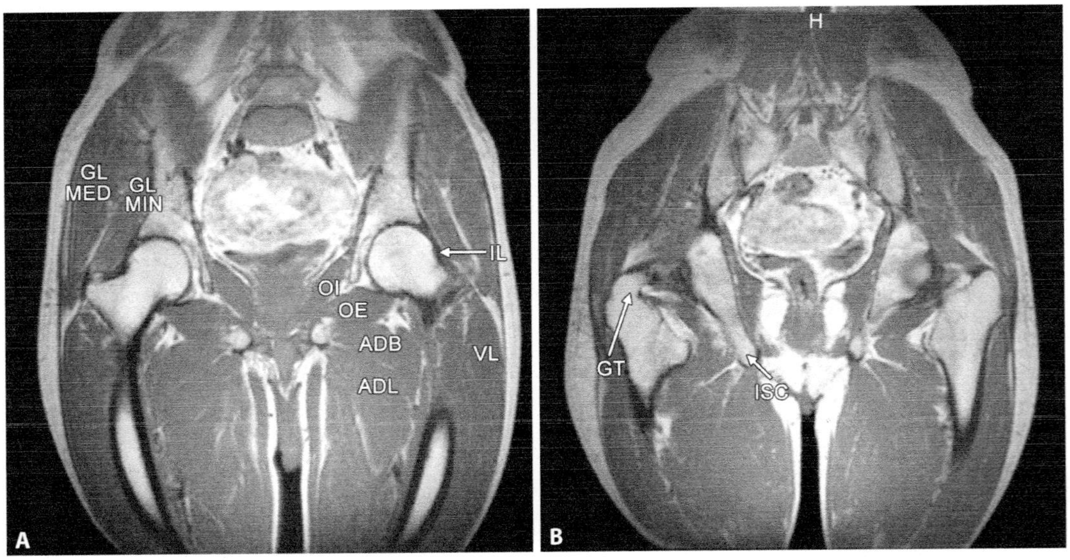

Figs. 1A and B: T1-weighted coronal image of both hips anterior (A) to posterior (B) depicting normal anatomy. (ADB: adductor brevis; ADL: adductor longus; GL MED: gluteus medius; GL MIN: gluteus minimus; GT: greater trochanter; IL: iliofemoral ligament; ISC: ischium; OE: obturator externus; OI: obturator internus; VL: vastus lateralis)

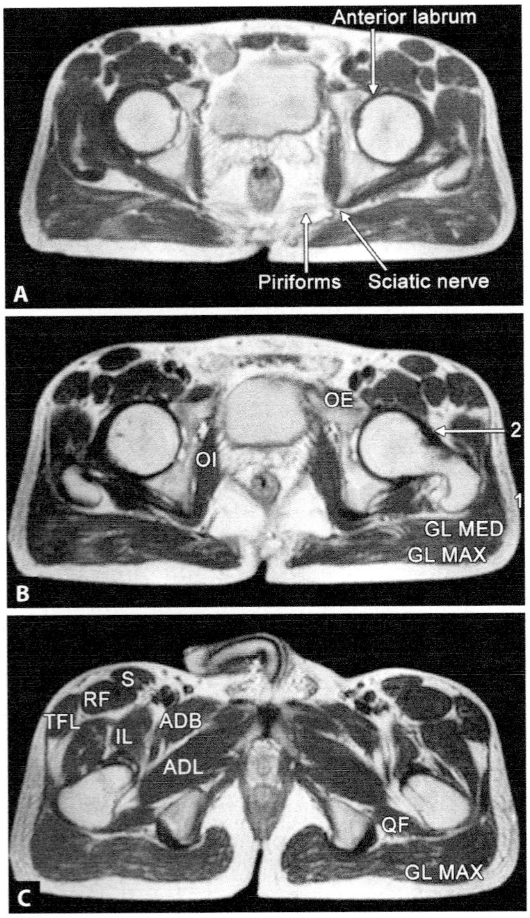

Figs. 2A to C: T1-weighted axial image of both hips depicting normal anatomy superior to inferior. Arrow marked 2-iliofemoral ligament (anterior fold of the hip capsule).
(ADB: adductor brevis; ADL: adductor lingus; GL MAX: gluteus maximus; GL MED: gluteus medius; IL: iliopsoas muscle; OE: obturator externus; OI: obturator internus; QF: quadratus femoris; RF: rectus femoris; S: sartorius; TFL: tensor fascia lata)

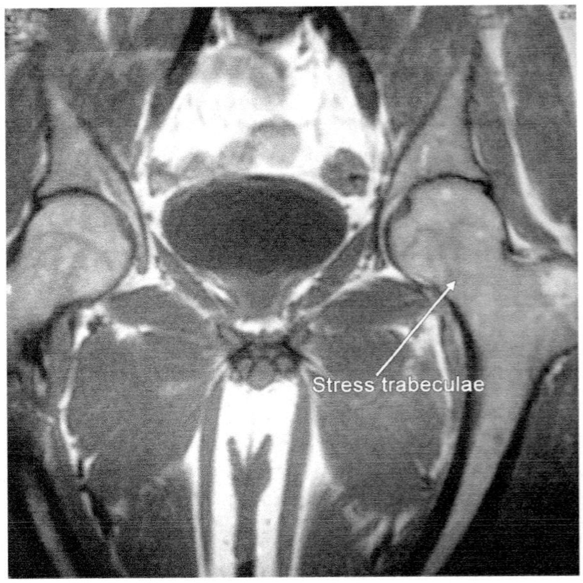

Fig. 3: T1-weighted coronal image of both hips—stress trabeculae seen as fan-shaped region of hypointensity in the femoral neck.

trabeculae produce a fan-shaped area of lower signal within the femoral head and neck, produced by increased concentration of calcium relative to fat. A second area of trabecular prominence runs from the inferomedial femoral head laterally and across the neck toward the greater trochanter **(Fig. 3)**.

MAGNETIC RESONANCE IMAGING TECHNIQUE

Conventional Magnetic Resonance Imaging

The technique for performing MRI of the hip is designed to image the entire pelvis and both hips. Hip MRI is best performed on a 1.5 or 3 Tesla magnet. The patient is placed in a supine position as straight as possible with the toes taped together to maintain slight internal rotation of the hip and to immobilize. A multichannel body coil with a large field of view is used to get an overview of the entire pelvis.[1]

Magnetic resonance examination of the hip begins with a triplane localization which is a low resolution gradient recalled echo imaging technique. This allows accurate positioning. Imaging is done in three standard planes **(Figs. 4A to C)**. Coronal images should cover the insertion of the adductor tendons and the iliopsoas. An axial whole pelvis sequence should extend from the level of sacroiliac joints to the level of insertion of iliopsoas at the lesser trochanter. Sagittal images must include from the medial acetabular wall to the greater trochanter. Images in axial oblique plane to look for abnormal femoral head-neck offset are also obtained. The axial oblique plane is obtained by using a coronal localizer and angling the slices parallel to the femoral neck **(Figs. 5A and B)**.

Standard hip MR protocol **(Table 1)** consists of anatomical sequences such as nonfat saturated T1W TSE. Fluid sensitive sequences such as T2W FSE with fat saturation and short tau inversion recovery (STIR in coronal plane) are also obtained. Postcontrast fat saturated T1W images are obtained as a routine in suspected cases of tumor and infection.

This is followed by a tailored high-resolution protocol for the area of interest. There is no true hip coil and hip imaging is best performed with a shoulder coil or a small field of view surface coil. The hip is centered in the magnetic field. Specific protocols for deep gluteal syndrome, adductor tendinitis, gluteal tendons, rectus femoris, and athletic pubalgia can be used based on patient symptomatology and clinical findings.

Radial Imaging

The nearly spherical femoral head, anteverted orientation, and anatomically abducted hip joint make imaging of the hip in conventional planes a challenge due to volume

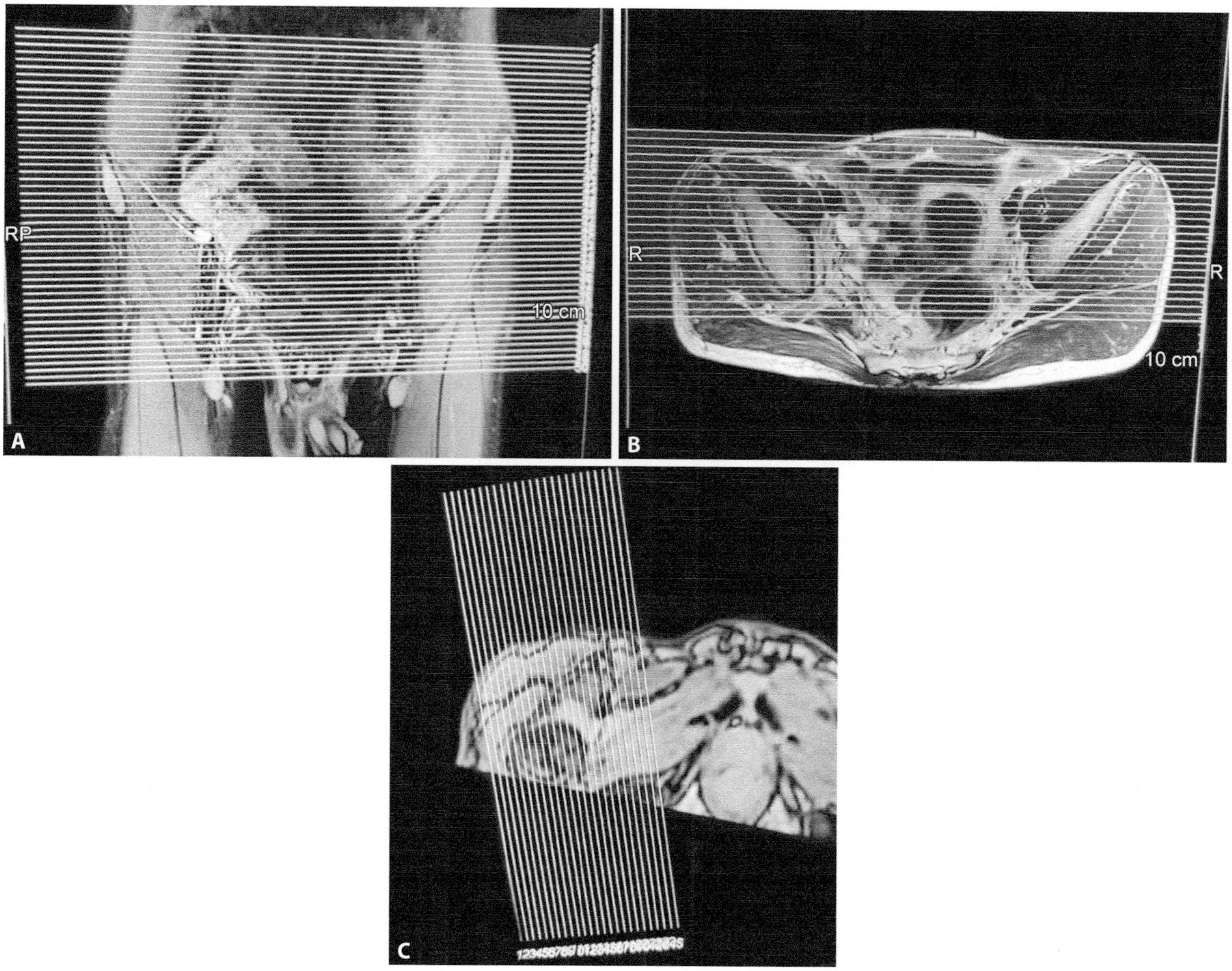

Figs. 4A to C: Triplane localizer on which planning is done for MR pelvis and hip.

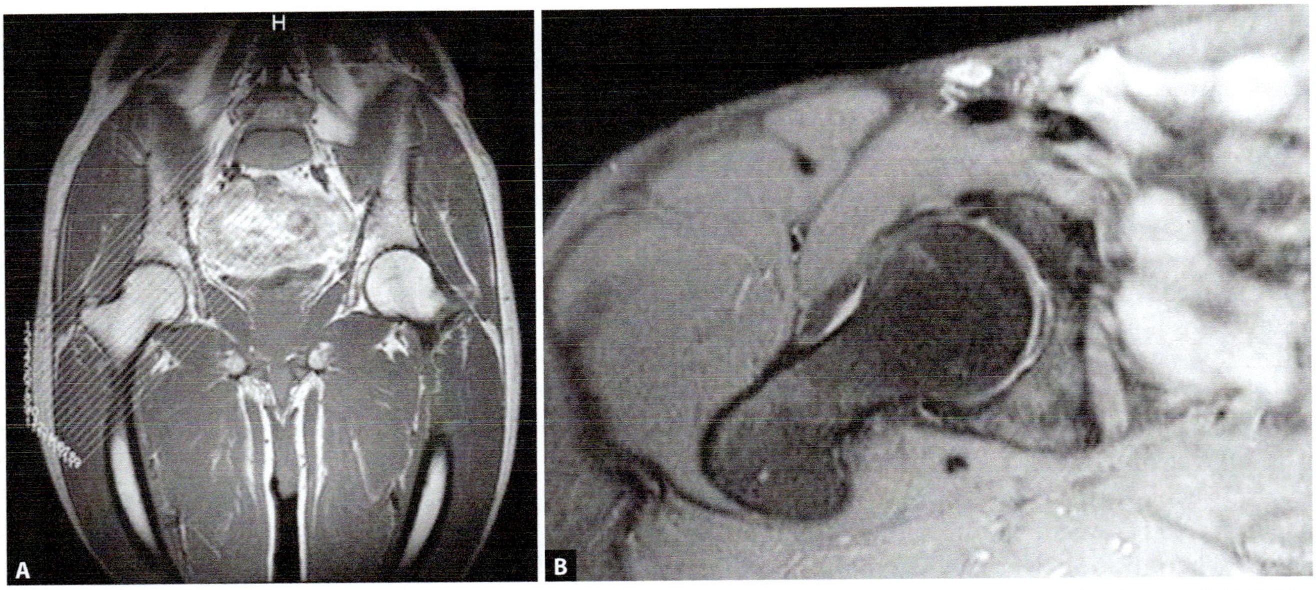

Figs. 5A and B: (A) T1-weighted coronal image, used as localizer to obtain axial-oblique proton density-weighted image (PDWI) (B).

Table 1: Magnetic resonance protocol for routine examination of hip.

Sequence	*FOV (mm)*	*Matrix*	*TR (ms)*	*TE (ms)*	*TI (ms)*	*Bandwidth (kHz)*	*Echo train length*
Coronal STIR (pelvis)	360	320 × 192	4,060	48	200	200	7
Axial PD FSE	200	256 × 256	2,730	9	-	300	5
Coronal T1 FSE	200	384 × 307	650	15	-	303	5
Coronal T2 FSE FS	200	256 × 256	3,070	60	-	250	11
Sagittal PD FSE	200	384 × 307	3,500	43	-	303	7
Oblique axial PD FSE FS	160	384 × 257	3,640	48	-	303	5
Axial T2 FSE FS	200	256 × 154	4,000	69	-	250	11

(FS: fat saturation; FSE: fast spin echo; PD: proton density image; STIR: short tau inversion recovery)

averaging. The regions most affected are the anterior and posterosuperior regions of the hip joint in the axial plane and the superior part in the sagittal plane. Labral and cartilage pathology in these regions may be masked.

Radial imaging plane is perpendicular to the curved surfaces of the joint with the imaging plane going through the center of the joint or along the radius of the sphere. This provides a cross section of the cartilage and labrum. Radial sections are obtained in the plane of the acetabular opening and are planned on the enface view of the acetabulum **(Fig. 6)**. Acquisition of the enface view requires the use of a double oblique orientation. Two localizers are obtained—first is axial oblique, second is the coronal localizer. Plane of section is adjusted to go through the edge of the acetabular rim on both localizer images. Sections are obtained with a spectral presaturation attenuated inversion recovery with proton density weighting. Each section provides information about diametrically opposite positions in the joint.[2,3]

Magnetic Resonance Arthrography

Direct magnetic resonance arthrography (MRA) is the mainstay in hip imaging to detect labral and chondral pathology. It is the current gold standard for detection of intra-articular lesions.[4] Injection of gadolinium into the joint distends it and increases the intra-articular pressure forcing contrast into cartilage and labral tears and detachments. Recent studies have suggested that due to a higher signal-noise ratio (SNR), noncontrast MRI imaging at 3T MRI could replace direct MR arthrography at 1.5T MRI.[5]

Direct MR arthrography of the hip consists of two steps. Initially, the joint injection is performed in the fluoroscopic suite. After instillation of iodinated contrast material to document the intra-articular position of the needle, 10 mL of 1:200 dilution of gadolinium contrast is injected into the joint. The second step is the actual MR imaging in the MR suite. MR arthrogram protocol is given in **Table 2**. Concurrent injection of local anesthetic into

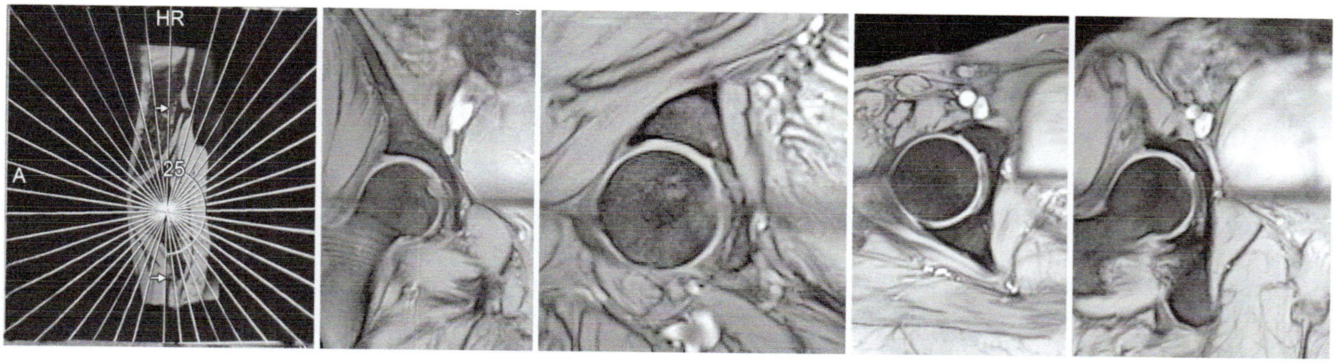

Fig. 6: Radial sections obtained around the enface view of acetabulum.

Table 2: Magnetic resonance arthrogram protocol.

			Routine hip MR arthrogram protocol			
Sequence	*FOV (mm)*	*Matrix*	*TR (ms)*	*TE (ms)*	*Bandwidth (kHz)*	*Echo train length*
Coronal T1 FSE	160	448 × 269	610	15	302	3
Coronal T1 FSE FS	160	384 × 230	570	15	237	3
Oblique axial T1 FSE	160	384 × 230	650	14	237	3
Axial T2 FSE FS	160	384 × 230	3,500	82	237	11
Coronal T2 FSE FS	160	384 × 230	3,960	82	210	11
Sagittal T1 FSE FS	160	448 × 318	640	13	211	3

(FS: fat saturation; FSE: fast spin echo; STIR: short tau inversion recovery)

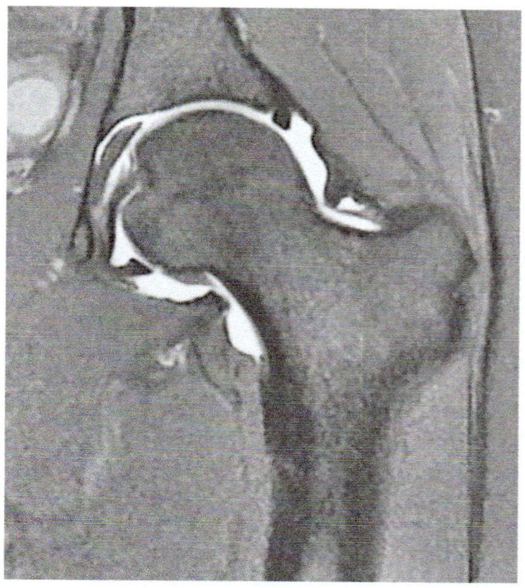

Fig. 7: MR arthrogram-contrast injected directly into the joint. Labrum appreciated as low signal triangular structure.

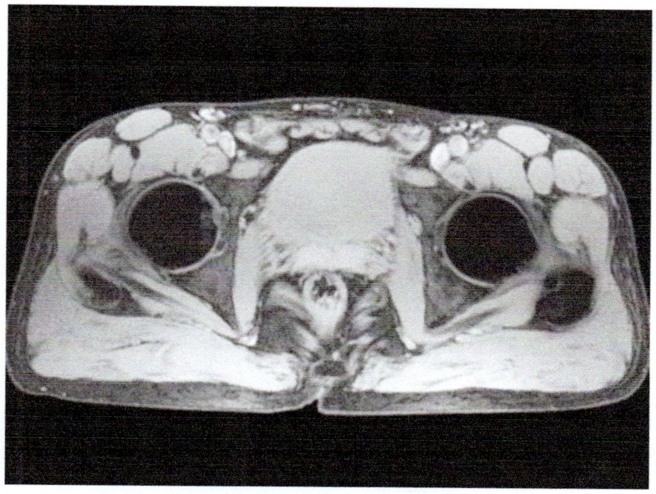

Fig. 8: Indirect MR arthrogram—diffuse enhancement seen within the joint.

the joint and performing provocative maneuvers can help correlate symptoms to pathology **(Fig. 7)**.

Indirect MRA is an alternate technique that is performed after intravenous injection of gadolinium. The contrast eventually enters the joint by diffusion and bulk flow from the synovium producing an arthrogram-like effect. Imaging is done 30 minutes after the injection. Exercise after injection helps to promote contrast accumulation into the joint **(Fig. 8)**. This technique can be helpful in certain select patients. High sensitivity and specificity for this technique performed at 3T MRI has been found for labral pathology with lower accuracy for acetabular and femoral head cartilage lesions.

Indirect MRA suffers from several drawbacks, as there is no increase in intra-articular pressure, some labral tears may not be detected. Presence of contrast in multiple compartments in the joint does not imply abnormal communication as it would in direct MRA.[6,7]

MAGNETIC RESONANCE APPEARANCES OF NORMAL HIP

The appearance of the hip on MRI varies depending on the type of sequence and the skeletal maturity of the patient. Cortical bone produces a thin sharply defined black line. Thicker cortex is noted in the femoral diaphysis. Higher signal is always present within the medullary cavity of both the femoral head and acetabulum. In the adult, the epiphysis is filled completely with fatty marrow that is high in signal on all sequences, except STIR and fat saturation techniques, in which the epiphysis becomes dark. The nonossified epiphyseal cartilage of the child is homogeneous and moderately high in signal. Maturation replaces the cartilage with larger amounts of fatty marrow within the bony epiphysis **(Figs. 9 and 10)**.

The immature metaphysis contains hematopoietic marrow and is intermediate in signal on all sequences. The adult metaphysis contains a mix of fatty and

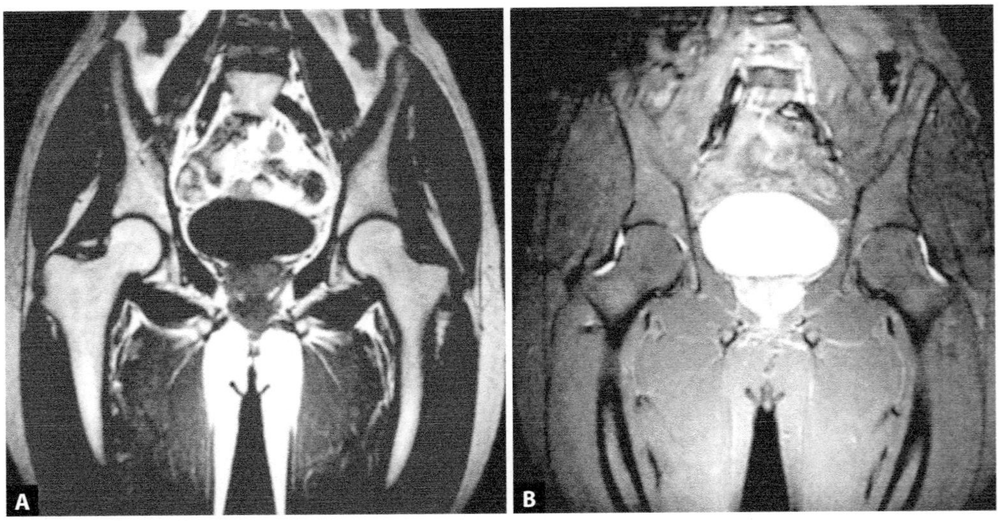

Figs. 9A and B: (A) T1-weighted coronal image of bilateral hips and pelvis; and (B) Short tau inversion recovery (STIR) coronal image showing fatty marrow of the femoral head, which is suppressed on STIR. Cortical outline is sharply defined and black on both sequences—normal appearance.

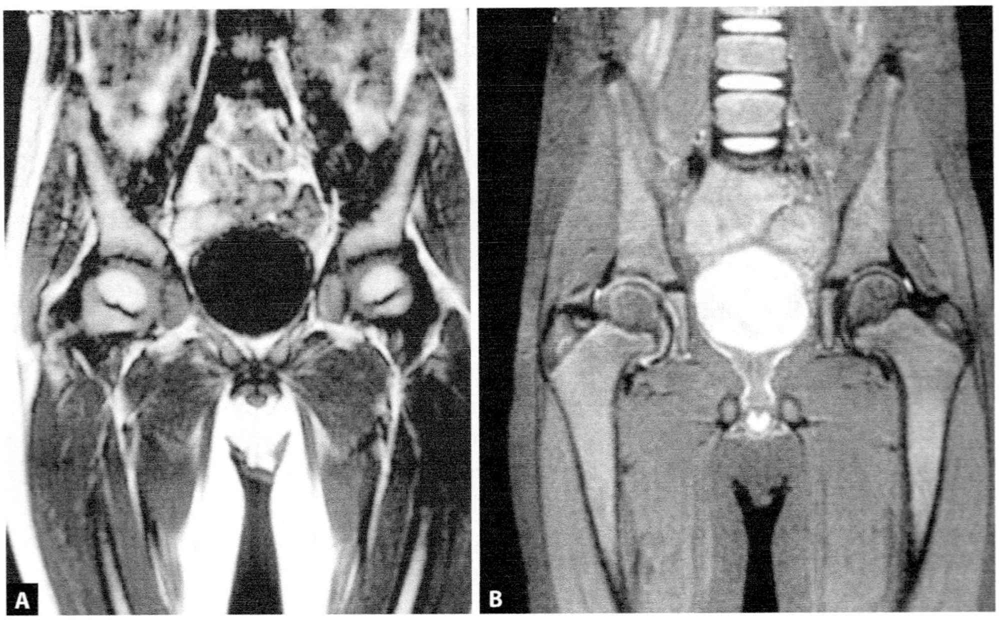

Figs. 10A and B: (A) T1-weighted coronal image; and (B) Short tau inversion recovery (STIR) coronal image shows moderately high signal in the epiphyseal cartilage with ossifying femoral head exhibiting fatty marrow in a child.

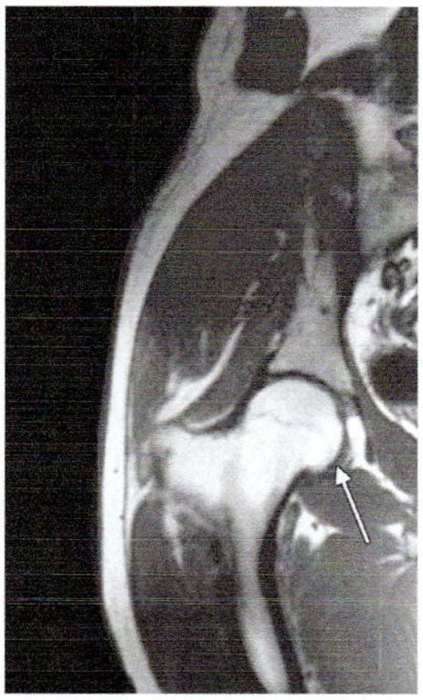

Fig. 11: T1-weighted coronal image of the right hip showing normal physeal scar seen as a thin hypointense line separating epiphysis from metaphysis.

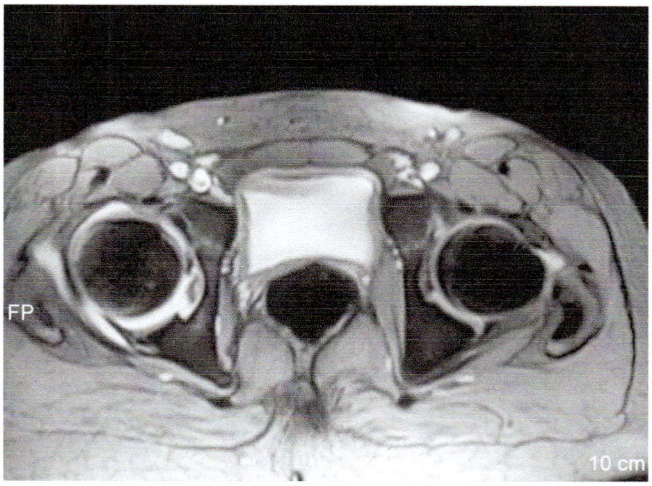

Fig. 12: T2-weighted fat-saturated fast spin-echo (FSE)—axial scan depicts normal hypointense labrum and intermediate signal articular cartilage.

hematopoietic marrow that is lower in signal than the epiphysis and is often heterogenous. Hematopoietic marrow dominates in younger patients and fatty marrow in older patients. This may be due to decreased blood supply of the marrow with age and a change from the sinusoidal blood flow of hematopoietic marrow to the more sparse capillary flow in fatty marrow. The physeal scar separating the epiphysis from the metaphysis is seen on all MR examinations of the hip **(Fig. 11)**. The inability to identify some part of the physeal scar indicates an examination of inadequate quality. The physeal scar, best seen on T1W images is seen as a thin black line on all sequences.

Labrum is seen as a triangular structure, hypointense on all sequences. The articular cartilage of the femoral head and acetabulum produces a thin, smooth uniform intermediate signal, the signal being higher on STIR, gradient, and fat saturation sequences **(Fig. 12)**.

The structures to be evaluated on a hip MRI are given in **Box 1**.

Box 1: Structures to evaluate in different planes.

- *Coronal:*
  - *Osseous structures:*
    - Acetabulum
    - Femoral head, neck
    - Greater, lesser trochanter
    - Sacrum
    - Ilium
    - Sacroiliac joints
  - *Muscles:*
    - Gluteal muscles
    - Adductors
    - Abductors
    - Hamstrings
    - Quadriceps
  - *Labrum*
  - *Pulvinar*
- *Axial:*
  - *Osseous structures:*
    - Femoral head, neck
    - Greater, lesser trochanter
    - Sacrum
    - Sacroiliac joints
    - Acetabulum
  - *Muscles:*
    - Gluteus maximus, medius, and minimus
    - Sartorius, rectus femoris
    - Gracilis, pectineus, adductor longus, brevis, and magnus
    - Tensor fascia lata
    - Piriformis
    - Obturator internus, externus
    - Gemelli superior and inferior
    - Quadratus femoris
  - *Labrum*
  - *Pulvinar*
- *Sagittal*
  - *Osseous structures*
    - Femoral head
- *Labrum*

Pathological Conditions of the Hip

Avascular Necrosis

Osteonecrosis (ON) **(Box 2)** refers to bone death secondary to interruption of the blood supply. The term avascular necrosis (AVN) describes the occurrence of ON in the epiphysis or subarticular bone and the term bone infarction to ischemia occurring at metadiaphyseal sites.

Etiopathogenesis: Avascular necrosis has a varied etiology, the most common causes being idiopathic, trauma, use of corticosteroids and alcoholism.[8,9]

In the hip, AVN occurs as a complication of displaced femoral neck fracture or hip dislocation. The risk of AVN is related to the degree of fracture displacement and a delay in reduction. Blood supply to the femoral head is

Box 2: Causes of osteonecrosis.

- Trauma
- Corticosteroids (exogenous and endogenous)
- Idiopathic
- Sickle cell anemia
- Collagen vascular disease
- Alcoholism
- Pancreatitis
- Renal transplantation
- Drug therapy [immunosuppressive, cytotoxic therapy bisphosphonates (jaw)]
- Pregnancy
- Radiation therapy
- Occlusive vascular disease (thromboembolic disease and arteriosclerosis)
- Infection (including immunodeficiency virus)
- Leukemia/lymphoma
- Vasculitis
- Diabetes
- Dysbaric conditions (caisson disease)
- Hemophilia
- Gout
- Thermal injury (burn, frostbite)
- Gaucher disease
- Langerhans cell histiocytosis
- Neuropathic arthropathy
- Polycythemia vera
- Multiple epiphyseal dysplasia

derived primarily from the medial circumflex artery. The medial and lateral circumflex artery sends branches with the capsular reflections (retinacula) of the hip joint to the femoral head. These branches are oriented along the long axis of the femoral head. Consequently, a subcapital fracture or a fracture of the femoral neck traverses these branches, which renders the head susceptible to ischemic necrosis. In some individuals, blood supply to the femoral head reaches via the foveal artery, which runs in the ligamentum teres. This artery may also be disrupted in the setting of trauma. Traumatic AVN is typically unilateral.

The pathogenesis of corticosteroid-induced ON is due to fatty embolization with osteoporosis-induced microfractures and increased blood viscosity. Long duration of steroid therapy, high and divided doses increases the likelihood of ON.

The first phase is interruption of blood supply. This leads to cell death and loss of cellular metabolic activity. Bone marrow is composed of three separate cell types—hematopoietic cells, osteocytes, and marrow fat cells. When these cells are exposed to an ischemic insult, they die at a different rate. Hematopoietic cells tend to die within 6–12 hours after insult, whereas osteocytes live up to 12–48 hours after blood flow is interrupted while fat cells live up to 5 days after the ischemic insult.

The second pathological phase of AVN is characterized by a rim of hyperemia surrounding the infarcted marrow. This marks an attempt to wall off and repair the ON area. Centripetal neovascularization of the necrotic zone characterizes the third pathological phase. This reactive interface is an attempt to repair the necrotic area and is called the *creeping zone of substitution.* The dead bone is resorbed and trabecular structure gets weakened. This initiates early fracture of the overlying cartilage with cleavage of the subchondral fracture plane and has a crescentic appearance in the femoral head. During this time, the weakened articular surface collapses with consequent joint space narrowing and degenerative arthritis.

Clinical features: The condition is seen mainly in young men in the third to fourth decade and is bilateral in up to 72% of cases. There are no specific symptoms. Patients may present with intermittent groin pain of gradual onset that is present at rest, exacerbated by weight bearing and it may radiate to the knee or buttocks. Movement of hip is associated with pain particularly on internal rotation. AVN does not always produce pain. Hips with stage I, II disease may be completely asymptomatic. Initially the pain is due to increased intramedullary pressure due to marrow edema.

Imaging

Plain radiographs are used in the initial workup of clinically suspected AVN; an anteroposterior (AP) and frog leg lateral projection should be obtained (this increases the likelihood of detecting a subchondral fracture.

Early changes of AVN may take several months to appear on radiographs; hence, they are insensitive for early disease detection. In late stages, the appearances are characteristic, if the radiographs are positive for advanced disease, further imaging is unnecessary except in the determination of clinically occult contralateral disease in patients at risk for AVN. A negative radiographic examination requires additional imaging. At the initial stages, plain radiograph may show nonspecific patchy areas of sclerosis and lucency. The earliest manifestation of advanced disease seen on radiographs is the *crescent* like subchondral fracture which will eventually lead to articular collapse followed by osteoarthritis.[10]

Radionuclide imaging for AVN is performed with a bone-seeking agent ^{99m}Tc-methylene diphosphonate (^{99m}Tc MDP) or marrow-seeking agent such as ^{99m}Tc sulfur colloid. Early in the course of disease, a cold photopenic zone may be observed in the anterosuperior part of the femoral head, which is virtually pathognomic for AVN. Later the reactive hyperemia and reparative response may result in a doughnut sign. Between the two phases is a window where bone scan may be normal.[11,12]

Computed tomography is not indicated for early detection, as it is less sensitive to MR and scintigraphy.

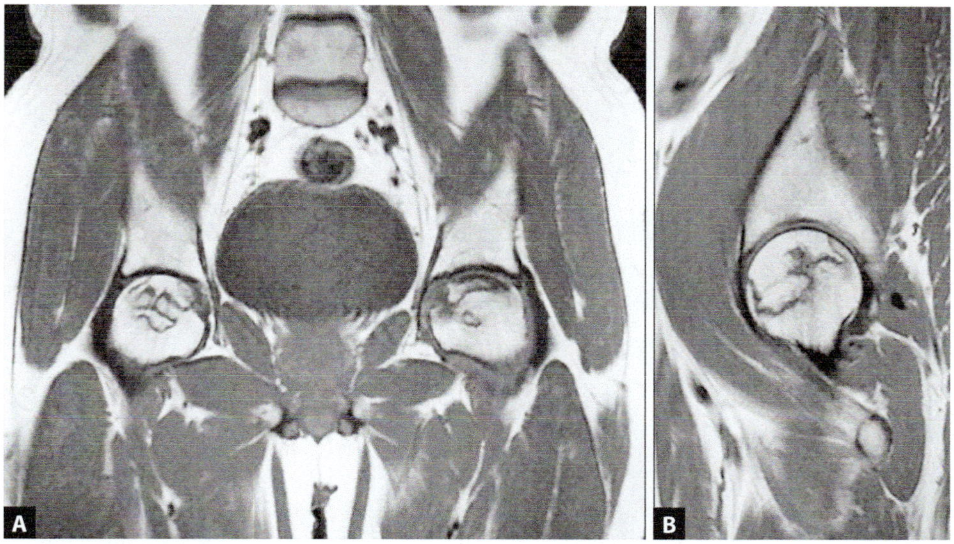

Figs. 13A and B: (A) T1-weighted (T1W) axial image of both hips; (B) T1W sagittal image of right hip showing characteristic serpiginous area of altered signal intensity of the anterosuperior part of the femoral head—avascular necrosis.

Alteration of the normal asterisk of the femoral head (condensation of compressive and tensile trabeculae) is seen in early stages. Later changes include serpentine sclerotic margins. Multidetector row computed tomography (MDCT) is useful in providing information on the location of articular collapse and extent of the epiphyseal ON. CT is required in surgical planning for rotational arthroplasty.[10]

Magnetic resonance imaging is the most sensitive and specific modality for the identification of ON with reported 97–100% accuracy.[9,10] MR imaging findings were reported to appear within a week of vascular insult in animal models.[13]

The most common MR appearance of AVN is that of a circumscribed subchondral geographic area of yellow marrow surrounded by a low signal intensity rim on all pulse sequences in the anterosuperior portion of the femoral head. This site represents the most peripheral site in the intraosseous circulation of the proximal femur and correlates histologically with the reactive interface between viable and nonviable bone **(Figs. 13A and B)**. The yellow marrow signal intensity is maintained because viable and nonviable fat have similar MR appearance. The rim of sclerosis is cresenteric/band like/rings like or wedge shaped.[14]

Another sign, seen on T2W images, in patients who have AVN is the "double line" sign.[11] This consists of an outer low intensity rim and an inner high intensity band on T2W images **(Fig. 14)** and has been described in up to 80% of cases. The high intensity component of this sign is believed to represent a zone of hyperemia and granulation tissue at the reactive interface between viable and nonviable bone. This sign was introduced by Mitchell and was considered as pathognomonic for AVN.

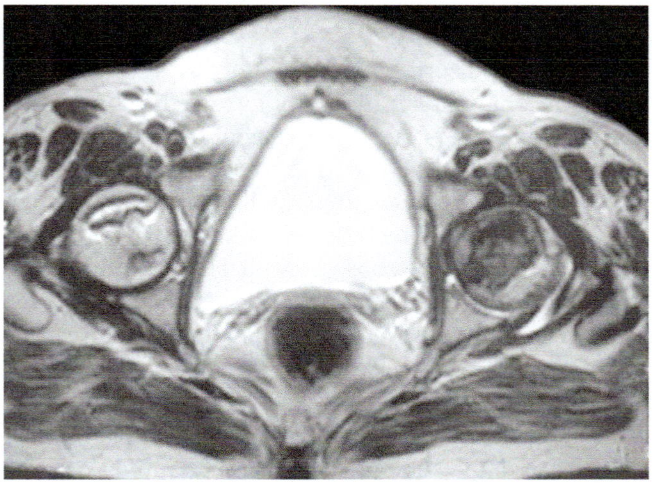

Fig. 14: T2-weighted axial image of both hips showing the "Double line" sign—outer hypointense and inner hyperintense rim—avascular necrosis.

It has been noted that transposition of the frequency and phase encoding axis results in the reversal of the positions of the bright and dark rims, suggesting the possibility of a chemical shift artifact as the etiology behind this sign. The artifactual nature of the double line sign does not reduce its diagnostic value for the diagnosis of AVN when conventional T2W SE or nonfat suppressed turbo spin echo sequences are applied. The newer high field scanners do not show this sign as spectral presaturation is applied with T2WFSE/TSE sequences.[15,16]

The MR signal intensity in the area of ON may show signal other than fat. Mitchell proposed a classification system based on the appearance of the center region signal, bounded by a low signal rim on T1 and T2W images.[11] Class A lesions have fat-like signal, class B has signal similar to subacute blood, Class C has fluid signal

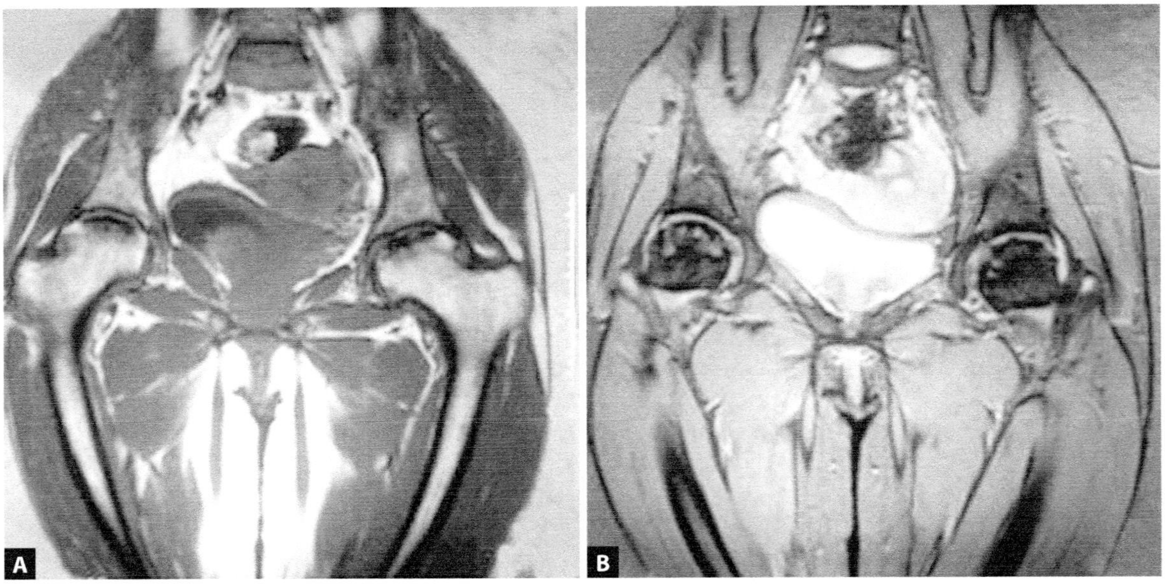

Figs. 15A and B: (A) T1-weighted coronal; and (B) Short tau inversion recovery (STIR) coronal depict insufficiency fracture of osteoporosis as irregular, discontinuous low signal intensity lines.

while low signal corresponding to fibrosis is seen in Class D lesions. This classification is not widely used as it does not correlate with radiographic staging and prognosis.

Subchondral fractures may occur in AVN. These are seen as low signal intensity lines on T1-weighted MR images and can be differentiated from subchondral insufficiency fractures based on the shape of the lesion. In AVN, the low signal band is smooth, concave to the articular surface and circumscribes the entire necrotic segment, whereas in insufficiency fractures, the low signal intensity band is irregular, discontinuous, and convex to the articular surface **(Figs. 15A and B)**. Unlike in most cases of AVN, the subchondral fragment and distal bone are edematous because both fragments are viable.[17,18]

Joint effusion is seen in 58–72% of patients and is due to associated synovitis **(Fig. 16)**.[19] This is often associated with bone marrow edema (BME) and is considered to be a cause of pain. BME may be seen in up to 30–59% of patients with AVN **(Figs. 17A and B)**. It is located within the femoral head, neck, and intertrochanteric region, as a reaction to subchondral fracture and blockage of venous drainage. BME is never found in the early stages of AVN as earlier thought. It develops after the onset of pain, typically in advanced disease, correlates with necrotic volume and articular collapse. Presence of BME is a poor prognostic indicator associated with failure of core decompression, failure of vascularized bone grafting.[19]

The use of contrast-enhanced MR is not necessary for the diagnosis or assessment in most cases. Lack of enhancement of the necrotic part with a peripheral rim of enhancement is seen **(Figs. 18A and B)**. Dynamic contrast-enhanced MR shows increased peak enhancement and delayed time to peak enhancement. Use of contrast-enhanced MR to predict risk of development of AVN post femoral neck fractures has also been studied.[20,21]

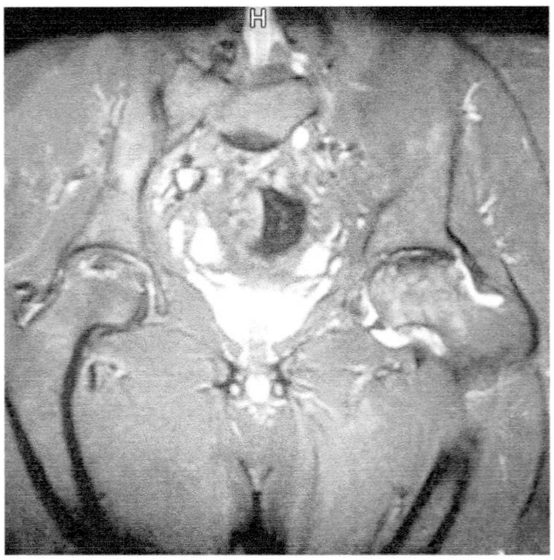

Fig. 16: Short tau inversion recovery (STIR) coronal image of both hips showing joint effusion on the left side with bilateral avascular necrosis.

Use of advanced MR techniques such as diffusion-weighted imaging,[22] perfusion weighted imaging, T2 mapping, and magnetic resonance spectroscopy are being researched to increase the accuracy of MRI in AVN. The ADC values in hip AVN are significantly higher than normal marrow but diffusion weighted MRI fails to distinguish between different stages of AVN **(Box 3)**. Preliminary studies have shown that proton MR spectroscopy can detect changes in the lipid/water spectra of patients with AVN before any morphological changes are evident.[23]

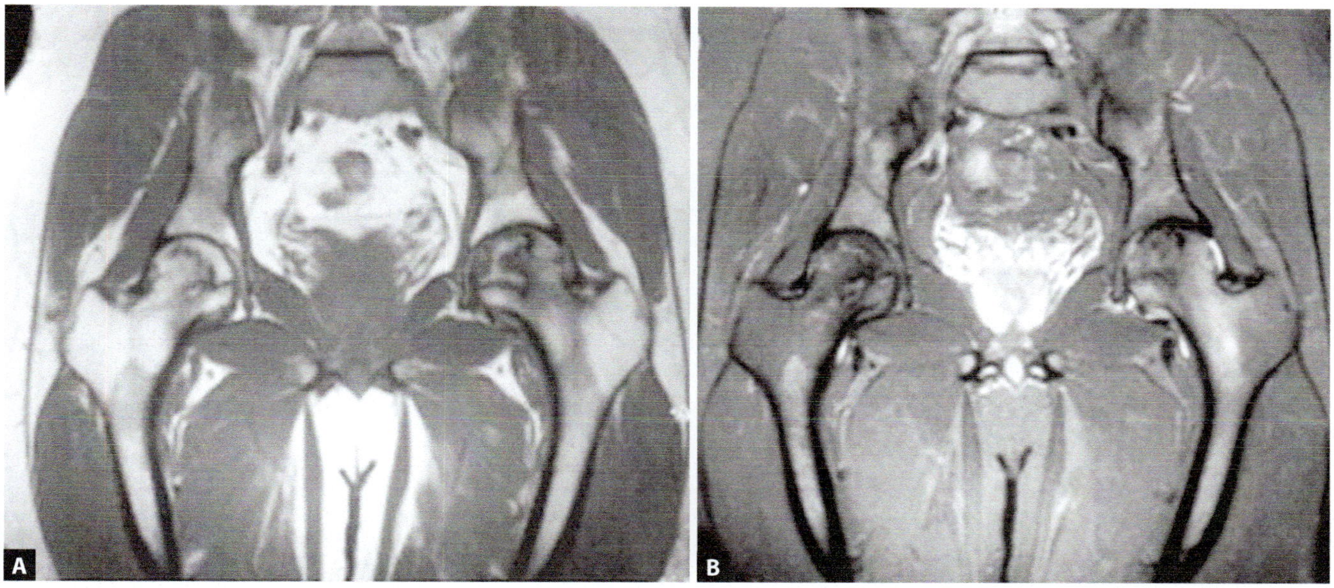

Figs. 17A and B: (A) T1-weighted coronal; and (B) Short tau inversion recovery (STIR) coronal images of both hips, showing increase in intertrochanteric fatty marrow on the right side with marrow edema on the left side with bilateral avascular necrosis.

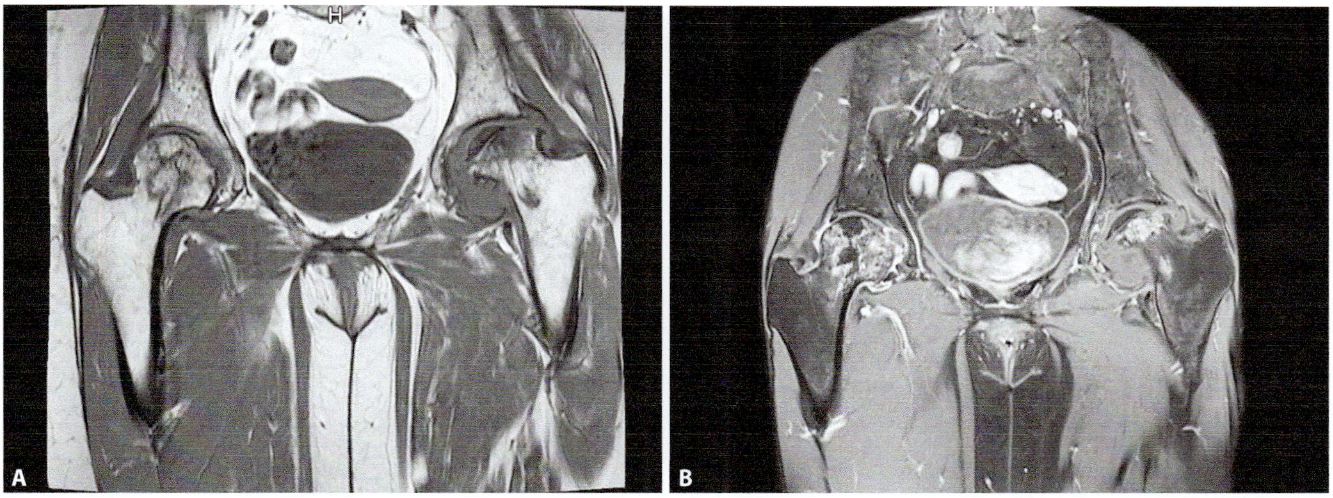

Figs. 18A and B: Bilateral avascular necrosis. (A) T1-weighted coronal; and (B) T1-weighted coronal fat suppressed, postgadolinium image of both hips showing necrotic nonenhancing areas with enhancing viable interface.

Box 3: Avascular necrosis: Magnetic resonance imaging.

- Anterior femoral head affected first
- 10 O'clock–2 O'clock position on coronal images
- Diffuse bone marrow edema
- Focal serpiginous low signal line
- Double line sign
- Focal subchondral low signal lesion on T1 with variable signal on T2

Staging

Various staging systems have been developed for the assessment of femoral head ON. These are the Ficat and Arlet, Steinberg **(Table 3)** and the association research circulation osseous (ARCO). All systems progress from radiologically occult disease to imaging findings consistent with femoral head collapse and degenerative arthritis**.**

Ficat and Arlet devised a staging system for hip AVN, based on clinical and plain radiographic findings.[24]

- *Stage 0*: Represents biopsy proven AVN in asymptomatic patients with normal radiographs and bone scan.
- *Stage 1*: Patients may have normal radiographs, abnormal bone scans and is associated with hip pain and decreased range of motion.
- *Stage 2*: Femoral head osteoporosis with areas of cystic lucency and sclerosis.
- *Stage 3*: There is subchondral collapse (crescent sign) of the femoral head with preservation of joint space.

Table 3: Steinberg classification of avascular necrosis (AVN).[25]

Stage	*Clinical features*	*Radiologic findings*	*Histologic findings*
0	No symptoms	Normal radiographs and MR images	ON present
I	Presence or absence of symptoms	Normal radiographs Abnormal MR images	ON present
II	Symptoms present	Radiographs with trabecular bone changes without subchondral bone changes and preserved joint spaces Diagnostic MR images	ON present
III	Symptoms present	Variable trabecular bone changes with subchondral bone fracture (crescent sign and/or subchondral bone collapse) Preserved femoral head shape and hip joint space	ON present
IV	Symptoms present	Altered shape of femoral head with variable joint space	ON present

Table 4: ARCO staging system for avascular necrosis (AVN).

Stage	*Clinical features*	*Radiologic findings*	*Histologic findings*
0	No symptoms	Normal radiographs and MR images	ON present
I	Presence or absence of symptoms	• Normal radiographs • Abnormal MR images	ON present
II	Symptoms present	• Radiographs with trabecular bone changes without subchondral bone changes and preserved joint spaces • Diagnostic MR images	ON present
III	Symptoms present	• Variable trabecular bone changes with subchondral bone fracture (crescent sign and/or subchondral bone collapse) • Preserved femoral head shape and hip joint space	ON present
IV	Symptoms present	Altered shape of femoral head with variable joint space	ON present

- *Stage 4*: There is frank cortical collapse of the femoral head.
- *Stage 5*: Superimposed degenerative joint disease.

Magnetic resonance is an integral part of several staging systems. The most critical part in all systems is the loss of spherical contour of the femoral head; MRI is to be used in precollapse stages of AVN.

The Toulouse, France-based Association *Internationale de Recherche sur la Circulation Osseuse (the association research circulation osseous)*[26] has proposed a more comprehensive staging system (*ARCO Classification,* **Table 4**).

MAGNETIC RESONANCE IMAGING AND PROGNOSTIC INDICATORS

A normal MR image is a good predictor of disease absence and is rare in case of biopsy proven disease. The natural history of AVN is typically of progression, though the rate of progression is unpredictable. The lesions themselves do not increase in size and small lesions remain stable. The larger the area involved, the more likely it is to collapse. As the lateral weight-bearing portion gets involved, the likelihood of collapse increases. In case of chronic renal failure, MRI positive asymptomatic, radiographically occult lesions have been seen to disappear without therapy.

When AVN is present, the percentage of weight bearing surface that is involved by the AVN lesion is the most reliable factor in predicting outcome. The size of the necrosis is important in predicting whether a fracture and further joint destruction will occur. Methods of quantification vary from the simple to the sophisticated, requiring advanced software. The extent of femoral head involvement has been estimated with MR imaging as percentage of the weight-bearing area, index of necrotic extent, and absolute necrotic volume. The extent and location of the necrotic fragment can be assessed using coronal MR images. The femoral head is viewed as a circle. If the necrotic fragment involves less than 25% of the diameter of the circle, there is less likelihood of lesion progressing to collapse. The location of the lesion is also important to determine future deterioration. The weight-bearing surface of the femoral head is defined as a segment extending from the medial aspect of the acetabulum to the lateral aspect of the acetabular roof. If more than 2/3rd of the weight-bearing surface is involved, there is

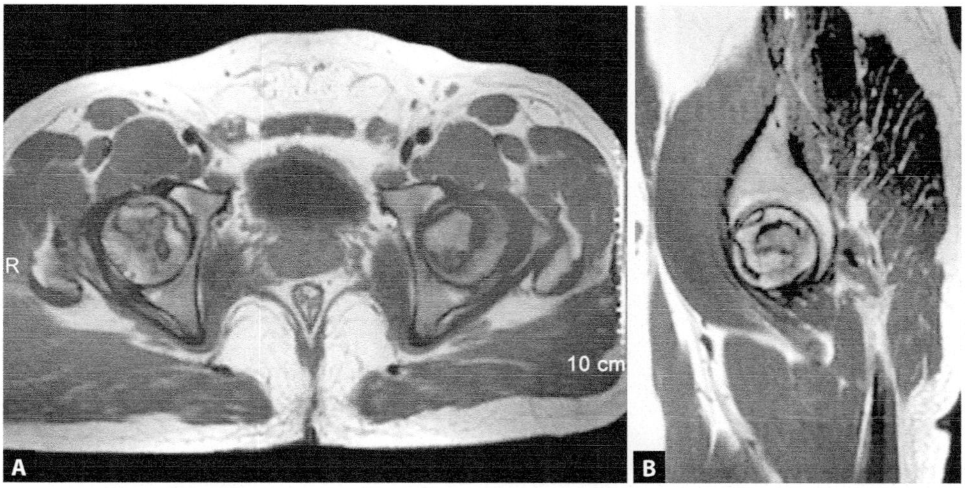

Figs. 19A and B: (A) T1-weighted axial image (T1W) of bilateral hips; and (B) T1W sagittal image of right hip shows bilateral avascular necrosis with >30% involvement of femoral head; the lesion is seen to cross the 12 O'clock position with an increased likelihood of collapse on the right side.

74% chance of collapse of the femoral head. Sagittal MR imaging can also be used to assess the extent and location of the necrotic fragment. If the reactive interface crosses the zenith (12 O'clock position), there is an 82% chance of collapse **(Figs. 19A and B)**.[27-29]

Two high-risk markers of disease may be observed in patients who have clinically suspected AVN. These are an early conversion from hematopoietic to fatty marrow and a dense intact physeal scar. The presence of either of these findings and the absence of definite disease warrants a follow-up in patients with risk factors for AVN and hip pain.[30,31]

Treatment

Patients, whose disease is discovered prior to articular collapse, are candidates for a host of operative and nonoperative interventions aimed at preserving the femoral head. These include administration of bisphosphonates, core decompression, nonvascularized and vascularized bone grafting, porus tantalum implant, mesenchymal stem cells, rotational osteotomy, etc. Hip arthroplasty is performed in cases of femoral head collapse and intractable pain. The results of hip replacement in patients with AVN are poorer than those of age-related controls.

Monitoring of Treatment

The MR features indicating normal incorporation of the graft includes enhancement surrounding the graft, revascularization of the previously necrotic area, reduction in BME, and an increase in signal of the necrotic bone. Dynamic CEMRI shows vascular ingrowth at 1–7 months postsurgery.

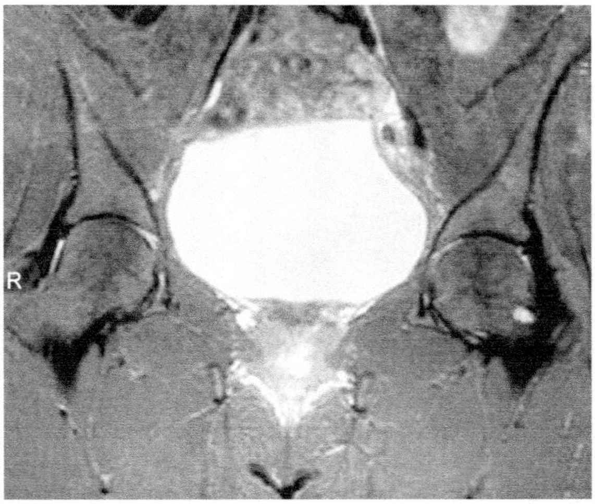

Fig. 20: T2-weighted fat suppressed coronal image of both hips shows herniation pit in the characteristic location on the left side.

Pitfalls in Diagnosis[1]

- Occasionally normal red marrow can be present in the femoral head, leading to a misinterpretation.
- Synovial herniation pit, which represents a tiny defect in the bone that allows joint fluid to fill this space, can be erroneously identified as an area of AVN **(Fig. 20)**.
- Subchondral bone cysts resulting from degenerative joint disease of the hip may appear similar to AVN but the low signal margins of the cyst are smooth and regular, rather than serpiginous as with AVN **(Figs. 21A and B)**.
- Fovea centralis, a normal anatomic finding, can be diagnosed as a site of AVN **(Fig. 22)**.

Minimal Avascular Necrosis

This entity is seen as a small and eccentrically located focal lesion at the femoral head, believed to be as a

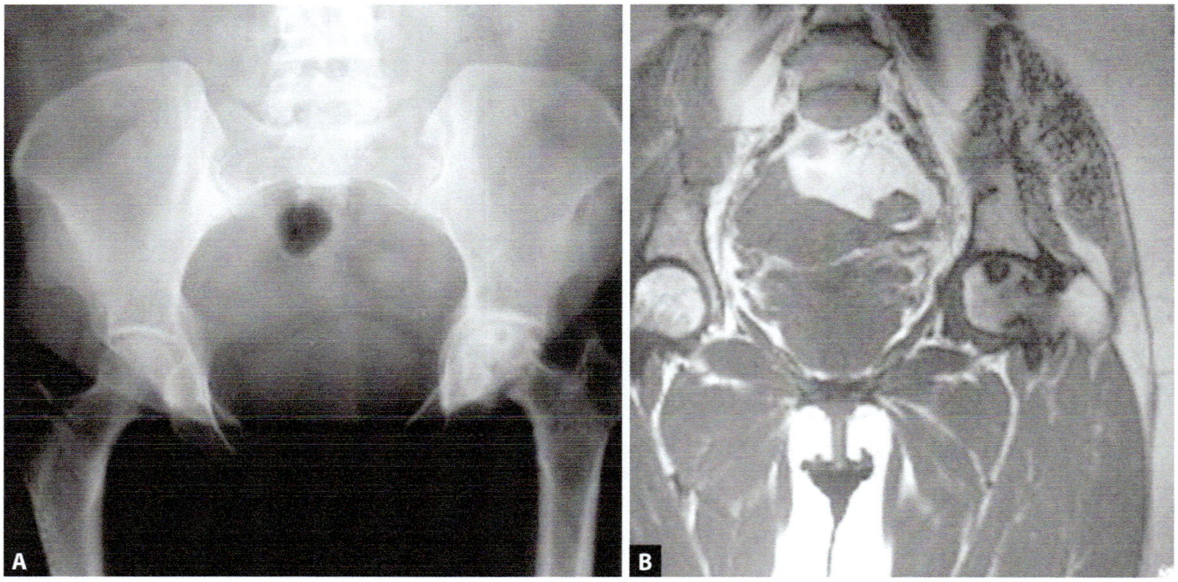

Figs. 21A and B: X-ray pelvis and both hips—(A) AP view shows decreased joint space on the left with subchondral cystic changes and osteophytes; (B) T1-weighted coronal image of both hips depicting subchondral cyst with osteophytes—degenerative changes.

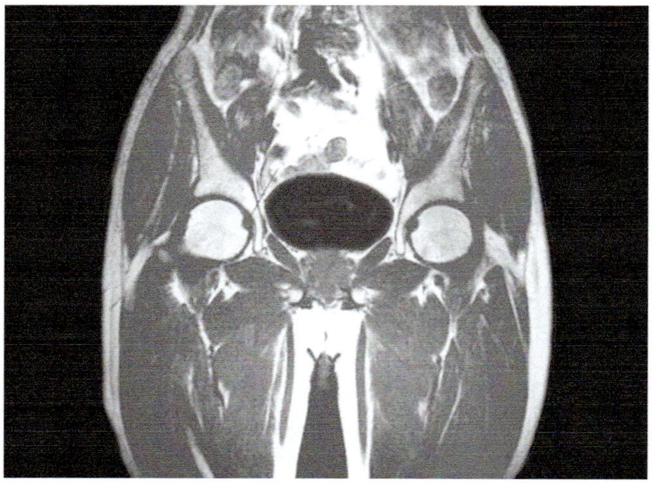

Fig. 22: T1-weighted coronal image of both hips—normal fovea central is seen on both sides.

result of single episode of infarction rather than recurrent ischemia. This does not lead to articular collapse. Differential diagnosis includes bone tumors and synovial herniation pits.[32]

ACUTE BONE MARROW EDEMA SYNDROME

The term "acute BME syndrome" refers to two clinical entities—transient osteoporosis of the hip and regional migratory osteoporosis. Both conditions present with pain of acute onset in middle-aged men and women in the peripartum period. The symptoms gradually resolve with conservative treatment. BME is noted on MR in both conditions.[33,34]

Box 4: Transient osteoporosis of the hip.

- Middle-aged men
- Pregnant women
- Male:female 3:1
- No history of trauma
- Low T1, high T2 signal femoral head to intertrochanteric line
- Spontaneous resolution (6–8 months)
- Differential diagnosis—AVN, osteoid osteoma, septic hip

The pathophysiology of the BME remains unknown. Links with ischemia, fractures, neurogenic compression, intraosseous thrombosis, and reflex sympathetic dystrophy syndrome have been suggested. The appearance of BME is nonspecific and probably results from different causes.

Transient osteoporosis of the hip (TOH) ***(Box 4)*** was first described by Curtiss and Kincaid in pregnant women during third trimester since then most cases have been observed in middle-aged men.[35] TOH has a predilection for hip, though similar changes may be seen in knee, ankle, and foot.

Generally, only one hip is involved. Unilateral hip pain begins spontaneously without history of trauma, may be rapid or gradual in onset, and is aggravated by weight bearing. After a plateau phase, pain progressively decreases until complete regression by 6–12 months after the onset without residual sequelae.

Regional migratory osteoporosis presents as migratory arthralgia of the weight-bearing joints of the appendicular skeleton. Migration follows a predicted pattern of proximal to peripheral location and time of symptom occurrence from 4 to 12 months.[36]

Imaging

Initial radiographs are normal but marked osteoporosis of the femoral head with preserved joint space is seen on radiographs obtained several weeks (at least 5 weeks) after the onset of symptoms. The bone resorption can be so intense that the subchondral bone plate becomes indistinguishable on conventional radiographs. Follow-up radiographs demonstrate a return to a normal appearance. Radionuclide studies with bone-seeking agents reveal abnormal accumulation. The severity of osteopenia does not correlate with the extent of marrow edema

Magnetic resonance imaging shows extensive BME of the proximal femur within 48 hours of the onset of symptoms. It appears moderately hypointense on T1-weighted images and intermediate to high on T2-weighted images. Edema may spare the inferomedial part of the femoral head and the greater trochanter called the "sparing sign." This is noted in a majority of patients, however, the specificity of this sign is not yet known. Edema may extend into the femoral neck. The lesion lacks definite margins and the transition zone between the lesion and the adjacent marrow is large. The lesion is homogeneous in signal, without obvious focal round or lobulated changes and without residual intralesional fatty areas **(Figs. 23A to C)**. After intravenous contrast injection, homogeneous and moderate to marked enhancement is seen. Moderate joint effusion is usually present and surrounding soft tissue edema.[37,38]

Small subchondral areas of low signal intensity (on T2W or T1W postcontrast) are seen in 30% of patients with BME syndrome. Subchondral low signal lesions that were <4 mm thick or 12.5 mm long returned to normal as opposed to those that were larger and continued on to collapse, representing progression to AVN. In transient osteoporosis, diffuse homogenous enhancement is seen in contradistinction to AVN where enhancement is heterogeneous with avascular foci of low signal. Dynamic contrast-enhanced MR shows distinct patterns, with transient bone marrow edema showing a subchondral spot of marked hyperfusion while ON showing high flow surrounding a subchondral area without detectable flow.

Bone marrow edema is a frequent MR imaging finding that is seen in a spectrum of hip conditions with wide variability in terms of prognosis and treatment options. Knowledge of various patterns of BME along with laboratory and clinical data is helpful in narrowing the differential **(Table 5)**.[39]

Analysis of the T1-weighted SE images is mandatory to differentiate a true "bone marrow edema syndrome" from other lesions in which marrow edema can also be a predominant feature like tumors, infection, cysts and systemic ON. After confirmation of the BME on T1-weighted SE images, high-resolution T2-weighted SE sequences are useful to assess (1) the articular cartilage, (2) the subchondral bone plate, and (3) the subchondral marrow.

If the articular cartilage is abnormal, the lesion is clinically irreversible (osteoarthritis or ON); if the subchondral bone plate is interrupted and the epiphysis lacks sphericity, the lesion is irreversible; if a fluid-like signal intensity plane is visible underneath the epiphyseal contour (cleft fracture), the lesion is irreversible.

After exclusion of a cartilage lesion and obvious fracture of the subchondral bone plate, detection and quantitative assessment of possible focal subchondral changes (low signal intensity subchondral area on T2- or enhanced T1-weighted SE images) are done. The lack of any additional focal changes in the subchondral edematous marrow area indicates a favorable prognosis, i.e., spontaneous resolution of the lesions and symptoms. The presence of a crescent-shaped low signal intensity area in the subchondral region with a thickness equal or superior to 4 mm on T2-weighted images suggests an irreversible lesion. In some situations, the prognosis

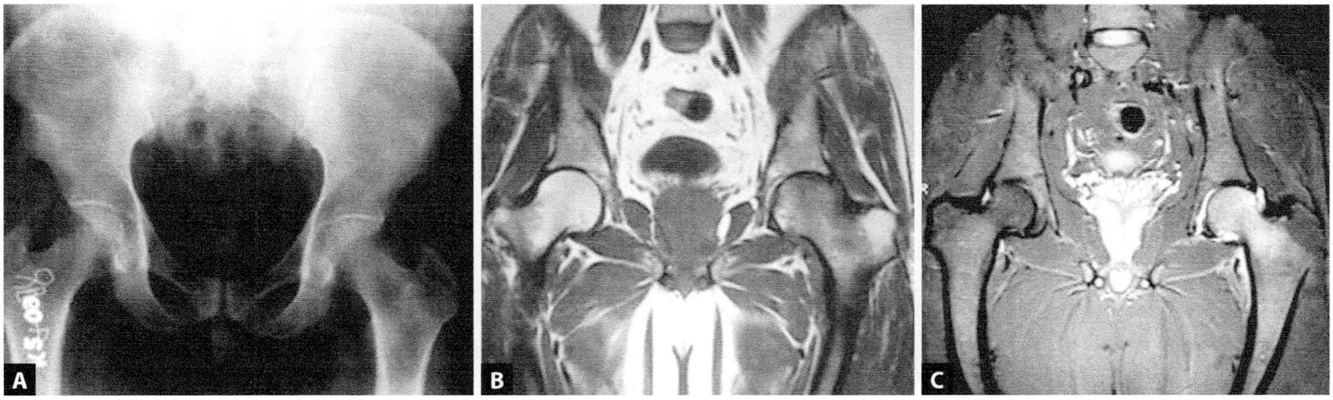

Figs. 23A to C: (A) X-ray pelvis and both hips of a patient with hip pain shows no abnormality; (B) T1-weighted coronal image; (C) Short tau inversion recovery (STIR) coronal image of the same patient show homogeneous area of altered signal intensity seen as hypointense on T1-weighted and bright on STIR images involving the left femoral head, extending to intertrochanteric region—bone marrow edema.

Table 5: Various causes of bone marrow edema and their differentiation.

	Avascular necrosis	*Transient osteoporosis of hip*	*Regional migratory osteoporosis*
Patients age	3rd–4th decade	4th–6th decade	4th–6th decade
Patients sex predominance	Males	Males Females (3rd trimester of pregnancy/postpartum)	Males
Onset of symptoms	Subacute	Acute	Acute
Most common location	Hip	Hip	Weight-bearing joints of appendicular skeleton
Migration	-	-	Yes; typically within 4–12 months from initial involvement
Plain radiographs	Normal in early stage lucency and surrounding sclerosis Subchondral fracture (crescent sign) Articular collapse osteoarthritis	osteopenia	osteopenia
MR imaging	Band-like lesion Double-line sign Crescent sign (subchondral fracture) BME (late stages following articular collapse)	BME (initial stages) With or without subchondral fracture, Not progressing to collapse	BME (initial stages) With or without subchondral fracture not progressing to collapse
Main associations	Corticosteroids Alcohol consumptions Idiopathic Trauma Hematologic diseases Irradiations	Osteopenia Osteoporosis Pregnancy	Osteopenia Osteoporosis Pregnancy
Treatment	Medical Surgical (core decompression Vascularized grafting, total arthroplasty)	Weight-bearing restriction Analgesics	Weight-bearing restriction Analgesics

remains uncertain and follow-up MR studies obtained 3 months later represent a valid alternative to further evaluate the femoral head lesion.

Labrum

The labrum is present in approximately three-fourths of the circumference of the acetabulum and absent along its inferior aspect. It is innervated by nerves that play a role in proprioception and pain production. The normal labrum has low signal on all imaging sequences and appears as a triangular structure attached to the acetabulum on all imaging planes **(Box 5)**.

Labral tears occur due to acute injury, impingement or developmental dysplasia. Patient has pain, clicking and restricted motion. MR arthrography is the recommended imaging technique for the labrum.

The shape of the acetabular labrum shows a tendency to become rounded and irregular with age. When degeneration is present, the labrum shows globular foci of increased signal intensity on the T2 and proton density weighted images frequently associated with a volume increase of the labrum. A labral tear is established when contrast material can be seen traversing or undercutting the labrum. Displacement of the labrum or the presence of a para-labral cyst can increase diagnostic confidence. Since most labral tears occur in the anterior/superior labrum, oblique coronal, oblique axial, and sagittal planes are most useful in detection. In Asian population, the labral tear is most commonly posterior in location.

Box 5: Labrum.

- *Normal*
  - Triangular, low signal on all sequences
  - Best seen with use of surface coil and MR arthrography
- *Abnormal*
  - Complaints of clicking, pain ± decreased range of motion
  - High signal in or through labrum
  - Deformed contour
  - Detached from acetabulum

An absent labral segment at MR arthrography should always been considered abnormal in patients with symptoms suggesting a pathologic labral condition. A normal cleft along the anteroinferior and posteroinferior labrum near its junction, with the transverse ligament, which spans the inferior aspect of the acetabulum along the acetabular notch, is seen. The presence of gadolinium in this cleft should not be misinterpreted as a labral tear. In addition, there is a normal recess superficial to the superior labrum and as gadolinium enters this recess, the appearance can mimic a labral tear. The iliopsoas tendon crosses anterior to the labrum and is potential mimic of a tear.[40]

FEMOROACETABULAR IMPINGEMENT

Femoroacetabular impingement (FAI) is a recently recognized cause of hip pain in all age groups and a proposed mechanism in the development of early osteoarthritis. FAI occurs due to an abnormal relationship between the femur, typically the junction between the anterior/superior femoral head and neck, and the acetabular rim. Repetitive contacts between the two may instigate chondral lesions and labral tears leading to early degenerative disease. A number of predisposing conditions have been described with deformities of the femur and/or the acetabulum which result in abnormal contact between these two structures, such as Legg-Calve-Perthes, slipped capital femoral epiphysis, coxa magna, hip dysplasia, and fractures of the femoral neck are known to predispose to FAI. However, a subset of patients who have no history of developmental or acquired disease of the hip joint may also be predisposed to FAI. Clinically, FAI is characterized by anterior inguinal pain and decreased range of motion with flexion, adduction, and internal rotation.[41-44]

Classically, two types of FAI have been described. The first has been labeled cam impingement and is most often seen in young athletic males. The second is pincer impingement and is more common in middle-aged and older females.

Cam Impingement

In cam type impingement of the hip, the predominant abnormality is in the contour of the anterior/superior femoral head-neck junction with a normal morphology of the acetabulum. Normally, the anterior/superior femoral head-neck junction has a concave configuration. However, this junction is either flattened or convex in cam type impingement. In addition, the femoral head may become somewhat aspherical due to this morphologic abnormality. During forceful motion, especially flexion, the nonspherical portion of the femoral head is squeezed under the acetabular rim. This abnormal contact results in damage predominately to the acetabular cartilage in a rather constant location along the anterosuperior acetabular rim. Chondral abrasion or avulsion in turn

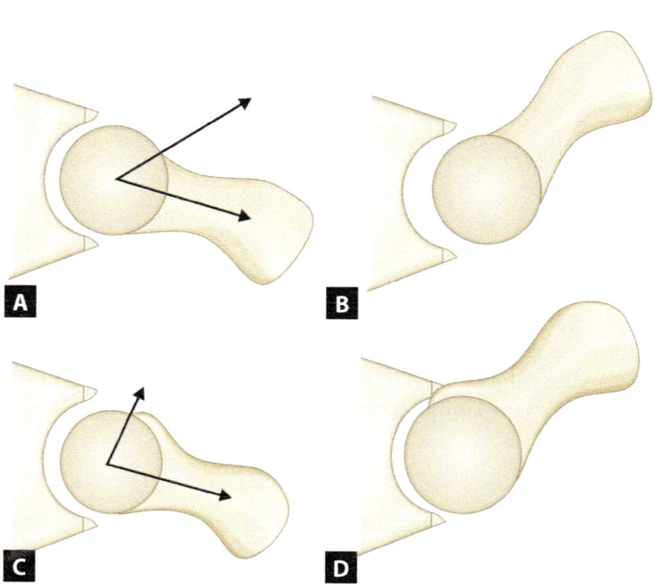

Figs. 24A to D: Schematic diagram through the femoral neck in the axial-oblique plane (A) alpha angle is measured, the normal angle = 42°; (B) A normal femoral head/neck junction allows clearance of the acetabular labrum during flexion of the hip; (C) Abnormal head/neck offset with an alpha angle greater than 55°; and (D) This creates an abnormal contact on the acetabular labrum during hip flexion cam impingement.

leads to a tear or detachment of the acetabular labrum **(Figs. 24A to D)**. Repetitive osseous impingement can then result in osteophyte formation on the anterior femoral neck, further exacerbating the problem.[45,46]

Pincer Impingement

In pincer type impingement, the predominant abnormality is with the morphology of the acetabulum with a relatively normal contour of the proximal femur. Abnormalities in acetabular morphology include acetabular retroversion, anterior and/or lateral over-coverage, and protrusio acetabulae. All these conditions increase either the relative depth of the acetabulum or the circumferential overcoverage of the femoral head. Continued impact of the relatively normal femoral neck against the acetabular rim leads to pincer abutment and lesions in the acetabular rim **(Figs. 25A and B)**. The first lesion to appear is degeneration of the labrum with formation of an intrasubstance cyst or ossification of the rim responsible for additional deepening of the acetabulum and worsening of the overcoverage. The repetitive abutments occur more often anteriorly and can result in chondral injury in the conter-coup region of the posteroinferior acetabulum. Acetabular cartilage lesions are typically limited to a small region on the acetabular rim. In contrast, cam impingement is characterized by deeper cartilage lesions (some of which are very large flaps) and more extensive labral tears.

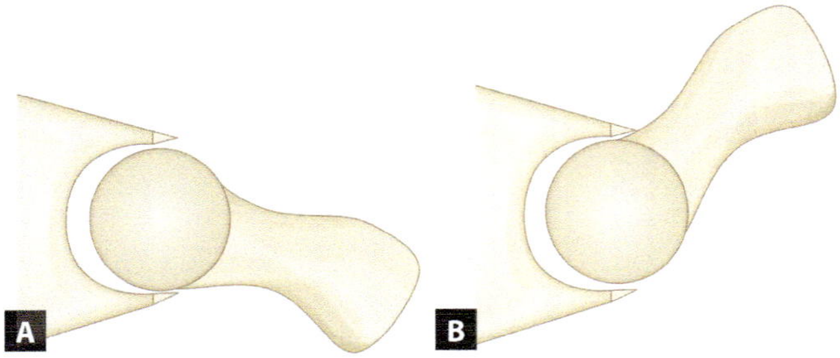

Figs. 25A and B: Schematic diagram through the femoral neck in the axial-oblique plane. Redundant acetabulum with over coverage of the femoral head (A), which causes abnormal linear contact with the labrum during flexion (B) Pincer impingement.

Box 6: Cam morphology.

- Asphericity of the femoral head
- Abnormal waisting at the FHNJ
- Femoral head-neck offset <10 mm
- Femoral head-neck offset to femoral head diameter ratio <0.17
- Alpha angle >55°

(FHNJ: femoral head neck junction)

Imaging

Femoroacetabular impingement is assessed with radiography and MR arthrography. Radiography depicts osseous abnormalities while MR imaging allows multiplanar visualization of the same and stages soft tissue.

Radiography in Femoroacetabular Impingement

High quality radiography in AP projection without rotation or tilt is mandatory for assessment of FAI. Centering of the radiograph has to be the patient's midline and not the hip. The patient position should be upright for the AP projection. A lateral view—frog leg lateral is also required. Suboptimal radiographs may overestimate, underestimate or falsely diagnose FAI. Comprehensive radiographic assessment is done following a suggested checklist.[47,48]

Radiographs in patients with impingement may initially appear normal because the abnormalities can be subtle.

Cam—on an AP view of the hip, the normal concavity along the lateral aspect of the femoral head-neck junction becomes flattened or slightly convex. This abnormal waisting at femoral head-neck junction has been referred to as the pistol-grip deformity or an abnormal epiphyseal extension. Loss of the normal concavity along the anterior femoral head-neck junction can also be appreciated on a true lateral view. Qualitative assessment is performed by approximating the femoral head with a circle; no bone should extend beyond this circle in normal morphology. Femoral head neck offset (FHNO) is assessed on lateral view with FHNO <10 mm indicating Cam morphology **(Box 6)**.

Pincer impingement—assessment of pincer morphology begins with qualitative assessment of global acetabular depth.

Coxa profunda occurs when the medial border of the acetabular fossa contacts or is medial to the ilioischial line **(Fig. 26A)**.

Coxa protrusio occurs when the medial border of the femoral head contacts or is medial to the ilioischial line **(Fig. 26B)**.

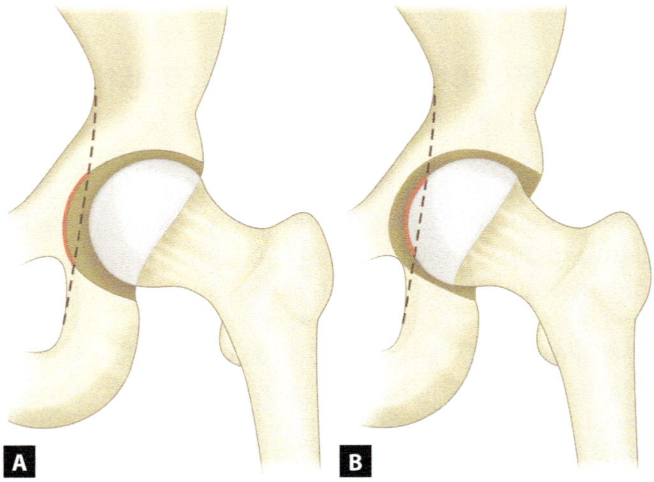

Figs. 26A and B: Schematic diagram depicting (A) Coxa profunda—the medial border of the acetabular fossa contacts or is medial to the ilioischial line; and (B) Coxa protrusio—the medial border of the femoral head contacts or is medial to the ilioischial line.

Various signs for retroversion of the acetabulum have been described **(Figs. 27A to C)**.

- *Crossover sign*: The anterior rim of the acetabular fossa normally is medial to the posterior rim. If the anterior rim extends lateral to the posterior rim in the superior part, a crossover sign is present.
- *Posterior wall sign*: The posterior rim should cross at or near the femoral head center. If posterior rim is lateral then posterior wall over coverage is said to be present. A deficient posterior wall is present if the posterior rim is medial.
- *Ischial spine sign*: The ischial spine is normally largely obscured by the medial acetabulum. Visualization of prominent ischial spine is seen in acetabular retroversion.

Care must be taken as slight craniocaudal or transverse angulation can either mimic or obscure true retroversion of the acetabulum.[49]

Global acetabular overcoverage can also be assessed by measuring the center edge angle (normal = 25 acetabular overcoverage = 39°) and acetabular index (normal-2–10°).

An association between an os acetabuli and hip impingement has also been suggested. Some believe that this heterotopic bone formation on the acetabular

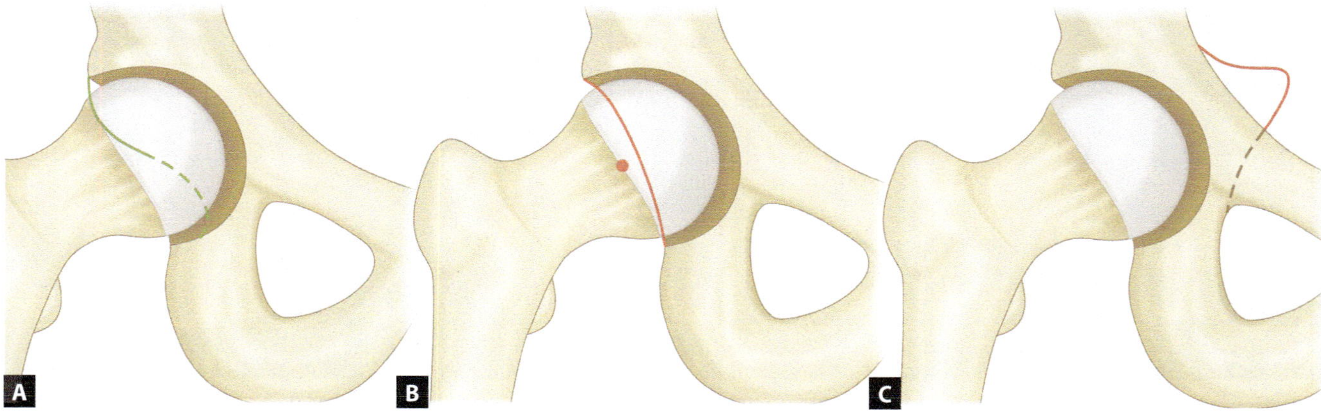

Figs. 27A to C: Schematic diagram of signs of acetabular retroversion—(A) Crossover sign; (B) Posterior wall sign; (C) Ischial spine sign.

rim is due to abnormal contact with the femur. The mineralization may be seen in the soft tissues or in the labrum. There is a high prevalence of herniation pits in patients with FAI.

Magnetic Resonance Imaging

Apart from routine imaging of the hip to be assessed and a survey of the entire pelvis, sequences **(Table 6)** to look specifically for FAI are obtained. MR arthrography is usually done and can be done using leg traction to break the seal effect of labrum with potential improvement in visualization of cartilage injury.

The same morphologic osseous abnormalities as seen on radiography are seen at MR imaging. Epiphyseal extension is best seen on coronal sequences as they most closely approximate the AP view of the hip. The abnormal femoral head-neck offset on the anterior/superior head-neck junction is often best seen on oblique (oblique axial or oblique sagittal) images that parallel the femoral neck to measure the sphericity of the femoral head as well as the abnormal offset at the femoral head-neck junction.

Quantitative measurement is done by measuring the alpha angle. The alpha angle is measured on an oblique image through the center of the femoral neck. A line is drawn along the long axis of the femoral neck bisecting a circle which outlines the femoral head. A second line is then drawn from the center of the circle to the point at which the femoral head or neck protrudes beyond the confines of the circle anteriorly. The angle formed by these two lines comprises the alpha angle. An alpha angle >50° is abnormal although using a threshold of 55° may be more specific to impingement. The alpha angle will be greater in many causes of impingement due to an abnormality of the shape of the femoral head-neck junction such as a wide femoral neck, osteophytes or posterior displacement of the femoral head **(Figs. 28A to C)**.[50]

Magnetic resonance arthrography helps visualize the cartilage and labral lesions that are often associated with FAI **(Fig. 29 and Box 7)**.

Table 6: Magnetic resonance imaging (MRI) sequences for suspected femoroacetabular impingement.

Axial oblique (Swiss axial)	Obtained parallel to the femoral neck Allows better visualizations of the anterior and posterior labrum with decreased geometric distortions
Radial imaging	Images are perpendicular to a double-oblique en face view of the acetabulum. Minimizes geometric distortion and partial volume average effects inherent when imaging spherical structures using routine anatomic planes
3D GRE	Obtained with 1.5 mm isotropic voxels Allows multiplanar assessment of osseous morphology
SS-FSE of knee and hip	To assess for femoral torsion

A triad of MR arthrographic findings has been described in patients with cam type FAI. The triad consists of an abnormally increased alpha angle, an anterior/superior acetabular cartilage lesion, and an anterior/superior acetabular labral tear.[51-54]

Femoroacetabular impingement is often bilateral but one hip may be asymptomatic, therefore both hips must be assessed. A large number of patients with cam FAI have an associated acetabular deformity (Pincer) **(Table 7)**.

Role of preventive treatment in asymptomatic patients with FAI morphology is unclear. Symptomatic patients, however, benefit from early noninvasive and surgical interventions.

Herniation Pits

Conversion defects (herniation pits) result from an abrasive effect of the anterior hip capsule in an area of the anterosuperior subcapital region of the femoral neck. This phenomenon is common, affecting 4–5% of adults and occurs in an area where there are normal cortical defects. The medullary canal is exposed to erosion from

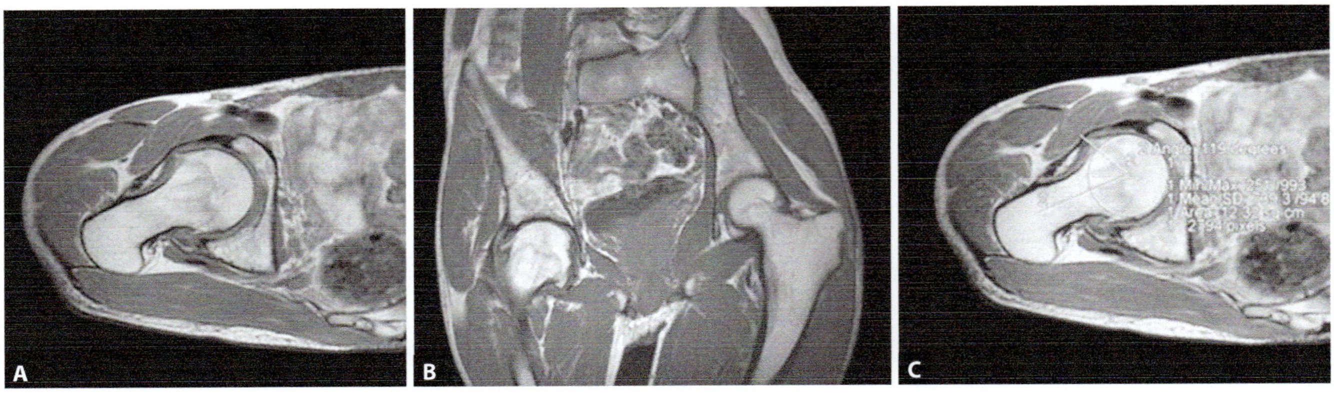

Figs. 28A to C: Abnormal head/neck offset in the right hip of a young adult, appreciated on the axial oblique image (A), with degenerative changes seen on T1-weighted coronal image (B), alpha angle measures 119° (C).

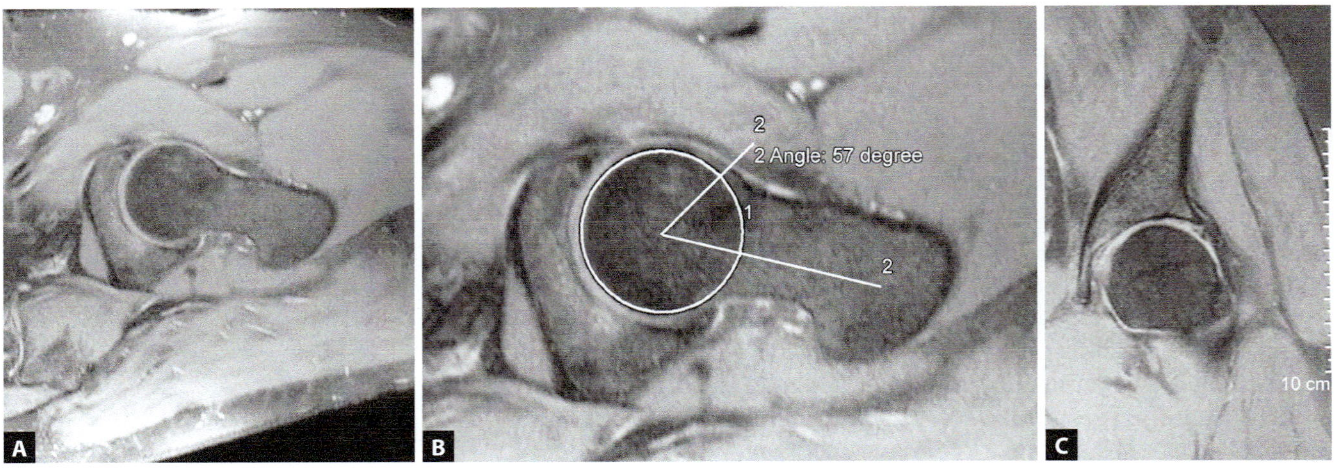

Figs. 29A to C: Indirect MR arthrogram shows abnormal femoral head neck offset in axial oblique image (A), increased alpha angle (B) and an anterior labral tear seen on coronal image (C).

Box 7: Magnetic resonance (MR)/magnetic resonance arthrography (MRA) checklist in the assessment of femoroacetabular impingement.

- Presence and character of acetabular over-coverage of the femoral head
- Femoral head asphericity or morphologic alterations of the femoral head neck junction
- Articular cartilage injury
- Acetabular labral injury
- Additional injuries to the soft tissues about the hip
- Presence of osteoarthritis
- Bone marrow abnormalities

Table 7: Pincer morphology.

Global acetabular over-coverage	*Acetabular retroversion*
• Negative acetabular depth (femoral head center medial to line connecting anterior and posterior acetabular rims) • Center-edge angle > 39°	Negative cranial or equatorial acetabular version

the overlying soft tissue and synovium, which create a subcortical pit. Previously considered an incidental finding, these are now considered as potential imaging indicators for FAI.

On MR images, herniation pits show marrow replacement in the subcapital region with a rim of low signal on all pulse sequences corresponding to an area of sclerosis. Internally, the lesions are composed primarily of fibrocartilaginous tissue and fluid components. Lesions show a low to intermediate signal intensity on T1 and are of variable signal intensity on T2WI; those with fibrous component being low and those with fluid being hyperintense on T2WI **(Figs. 30A and B).**[55]

HIP TRAUMA

Hip fractures are seen with increasing frequency in older population due to falls and in younger population with high impact motor vehicle accidents. Fractures of the pelvis, hip, and proximal femur are usually identified at radiography. CT adds substantially in further evaluation

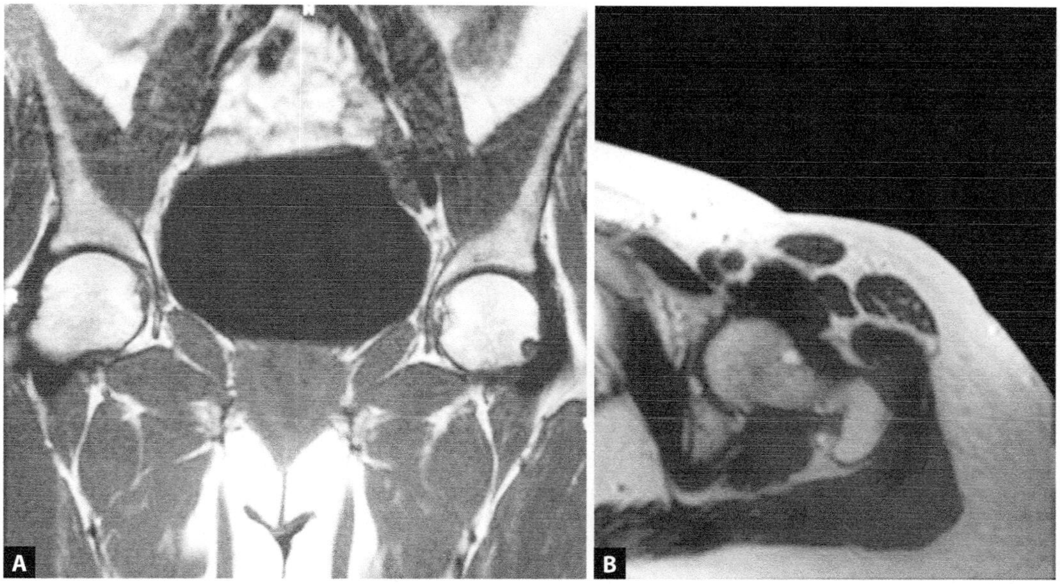

Figs. 30A and B: Herniation pit seen as a smooth well-marginated lesion in anterosuperior aspect of left femoral head with fluid characteristics on (A) T1-weighted coronal image; and (B) T2-weighted axial image of both hips.

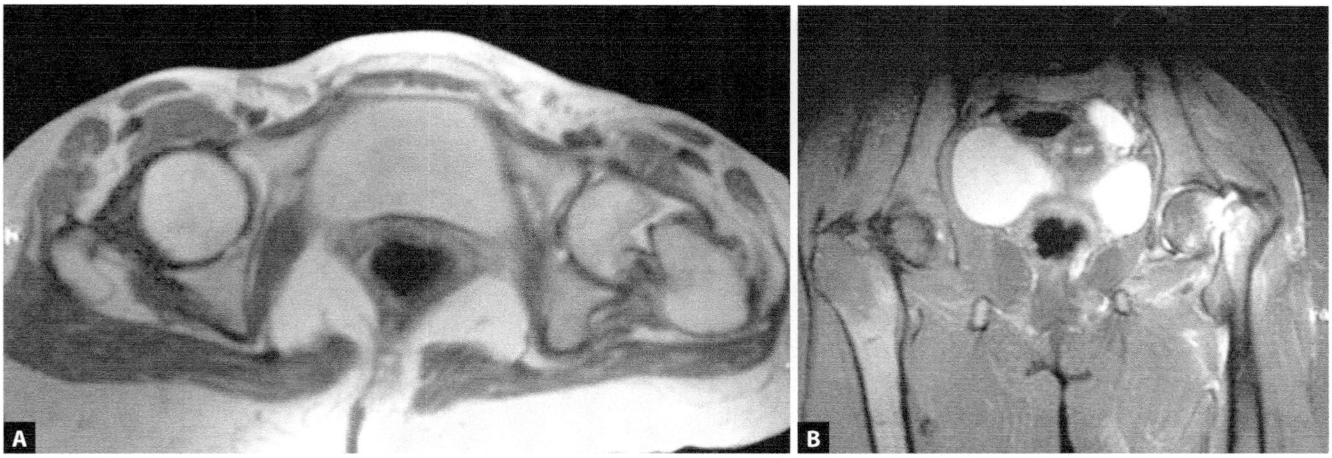

Figs. 31A and B: Fracture neck left femur. (A) T2-weighted axial; and (B) Short tau inversion recovery (STIR) coronal images of both hips show marrow edema and fluid at the fracture site.

of complex pelvic fractures. MR imaging adds another dimension to the study of hip trauma as immediate changes in the appearance of marrow are identified on MR **(Figs. 31A and B)**. Thus, it is useful in nondisplaced fractures, stress fractures, insufficiency fractures, and fractures in axial plane that cannot be identified on CT.

Magnetic resonance imaging is the method of choice in detecting 2–10% occult fractures of the hip.[56] Additional information about soft tissue pathology is provided by MRI specifically in fractures of the greater trochanters. All avulsion fractures of the greater or lesser fractures of the adults without history of significant trauma necessitate investigation for potential metastatic disease.

A low signal intensity linear or curvilinear line with surrounding BME on T1W images is seen in fractures. It is best appreciated in coronal plane. This single sequence is considered sufficient for the diagnosis of occult fracture of the hip. Contrast-enhanced MR perfusion of the femoral head may be useful to assess femoral head perfusion after femoral neck fracture to aid the clinician in deciding between joint preserving surgery and hip arthroplasty.[57,58]

Stress Fractures

Stress fractures can be further divided into fatigue and insufficiency fractures.

Fatigue fractures occur commonly in pelvis and hips. Fatigue fractures result from increased or abnormal stress applied to normal bone. MRI is sensitive and specific because it shows the fracture line as a linear low signal band/line on both T1W andT2W images with surrounding

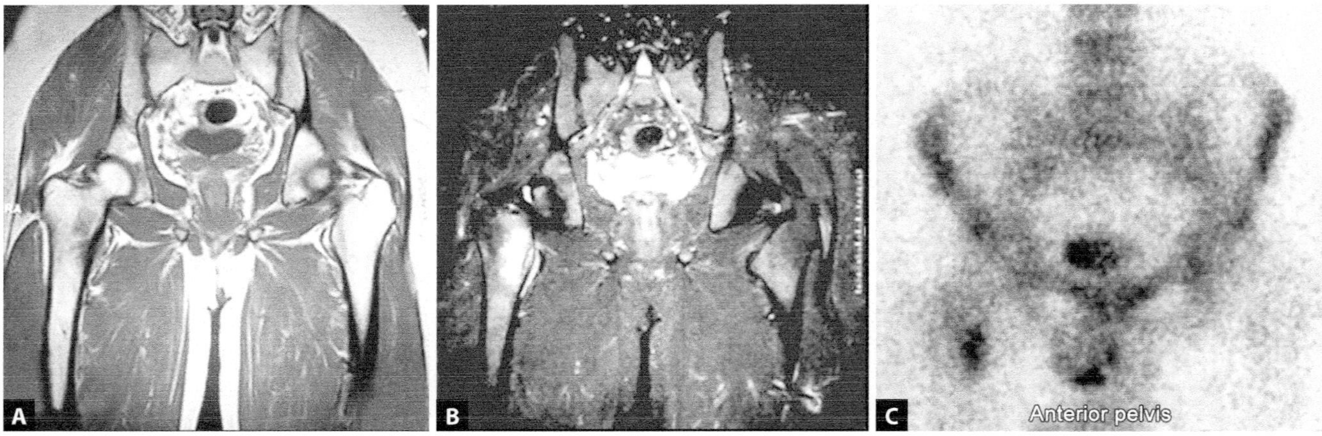

Figs. 32A to C: T1-weighted (T1W) coronal image of both hips (A) and short tau inversion recovery (STIR) coronal image of both hips (B), showing an area of edema on the compressive medial surface of the right femur (hypo on T1W image and hyper on STIR) with associated soft tissue swelling and corresponding hot spot on the bone scan; (C) Stress reaction.

marrow edema. Increased signal may be seen within the fracture site on fluid sensitive sequences because of hemorrhage within the fracture site. The signal alterations related with stress injury resolve by 6–12 weeks. Stress reactions occur along the medial aspect of the femoral neck (compressive surface) or superior surface (tensile surface). Additional locations include pubic rami and sacrum **(Figs. 32A to C).**[59]

In the pelvis, fatigue fractures are seen in the sacrum. These are frequently bilateral in the supra-acetabular region of ilium.

Insufficiency fractures occur from normal strain on a bone weakened by osteoporosis, osteomalacia, steroids, rheumatoid arthritis (RA), etc. In a clinical setting of osteoporosis and a painful hip, even in absence of trauma an occult fracture may be present. A limited MRI examination consisting of coronal and axial images of the entire pelvis using T1 and fat suppressed T2W sequences can be used. MR demonstrates low signal fracture line surrounded by marrow edema. Multiple fractures coexist. The most common locations for insufficiency fractures of hip and pelvis are subcapital, intertrochanteric, sacral, supra-acetabular, pubic bones, and pubic rami.

Salter Fracture

Traumatic epiphyseal slip can occur in skeletally immature individuals in setting of infant abuse or birth trauma. A fast spin echo T2W sequence with fat suppression and STIR imaging shows edema and the hemorrhage through the physis and is diagnostic of shear injury.

Traumatic Musculotendinous Injury

Musculotendinous injuries are among the most common form of sport-related injury to the pelvis and hip. The pelvic ring and proximal femur are the sites of origin or insertion for several major muscle groups including the abdominal, gluteal, adductors, hamstrings, and iliopsoas muscles. The injuries occur as a result of blunt direct trauma or secondary to indirect trauma from excessive tension or forceful contraction. The injuries can be categorized based on the mechanism of trauma and the site of involvement. These include tendinous avulsion injury, muscle contusion, and myotendinous strain.[60-62]

Avulsion Injury

Acute avulsion injury at the tendinous insertion site results from forceful eccentric muscle contraction or passive lengthening. It is manifested on MR as a hematoma and periosteal stripping at the tendinous attachment site. Waviness and retraction of the torn end of the tendon along with a fragment of bone or cartilage may be present. Avulsion injuries about the hip joint occur primarily at six sites.

- Ischial tuberosity
- Anterosuperior iliac spine
- Anteroinferior iliac spine
- Lesser trochanter
- Greater trochanter
- Pubic bone.

Nondisplaced bony avulsions appear on T1W images as curved sharply marginated bone fragment adjacent to the apophysis from which it has originated. Increased distance between a displaced fragment and the parent bone is a poor prognostic indicator and may lead to fibrous union and disability.

Muscle Contusions

These are secondary to direct trauma usually by a blunt object. They often occur deep in the muscle belly and tend to be less symptomatic than strains because the latter are commonly localized in the superficial muscle layers. Common sites of muscle contusion about the hip joint

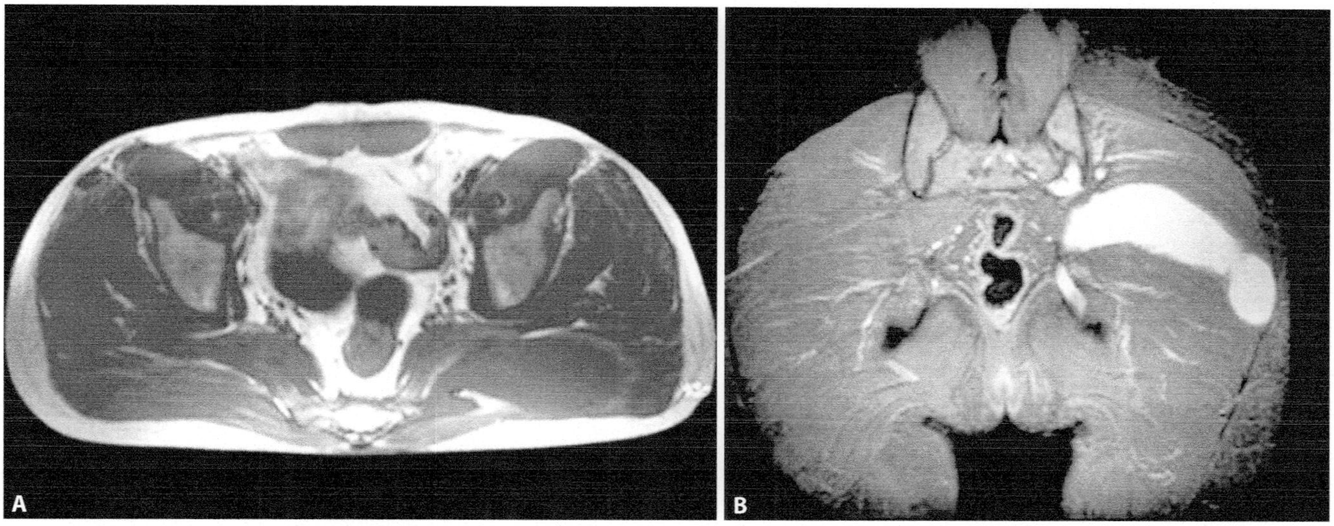

Figs. 33A and B: (A) T1-weighted axial image; and (B) Short tau inversion recovery (STIR) coronal image of the pelvis shows well-marginated area of altered signal in the gluteus maximus suggestive of a tear.

include the gluteal region and proximal thigh. Muscle contusions are seen in MR examinations of clinically suspected hip fractures and negative radiographs.

The MR imaging appearance varies according to the severity of the lesion. Diffuse edematous changes of the muscle are manifested by a feathery MR imaging appearance on STIR and T2W images along with an increased muscle girth. Intramuscular hemorrhages may develop with more severe trauma.

Muscle Strain—Myotendinous Strain

Strain injuries affect the myotendinous junction, the weakest point of the musculotendinous unit. The most common strained muscles about the hip joint are the rectus femoris and the hamstrings. In the first-degree strains implying minor degrees of fiber disruption, there is interstitial edema and hemorrhage at the myotendinous junction extending into the fascicles producing a feathery pattern. Partial tears without retraction characterize the second-degree tears. Hematoma and perifascial fluid collections may also be seen. Third-degree tears refer to complete rupture of the myotendinous unit. MRI is used for preoperative assessment of the extent of retraction.

Gluteus Medius Tendon Tear—Greater Trochanteric Pain Syndrome

The rotator cuff lesions of the hip involve tears of the abductor musculature, namely the gluteus medius and minimus. Proposed causes include friction of the iliotibial band with the underlying tendons, abnormal gait leading to altered biomechanics, repetitive stress in runners, and trauma. It more commonly affects middle-aged to elderly women who complain of chronic pain around hip or groin region, mimicking intra-articular hip pathology. It is also seen in recreational runners and participants of step aerobics. The most common symptom is lateral hip pain which has a broad differential diagnosis including entities such as bursitis, tendonitis, muscle insufficiency fractures, nerve entrapment, muscle strain, and bursitis **(Figs. 33A and B)**. Small focal tears are more common than diffuse avulsions. Various MR findings such as increased T2 signal superior to the greater trochanter and atrophy of the gluteal muscles may be seen.[63]

Morel-Lavallée Lesion

It is a post-traumatic encapsulated fluid collection between the superficial and deep layers of the fascia in the lateral thigh, in the trochanteric region adjacent to fascia lata. It is distinct from trochanteric bursitis. Vessels perforating the facial layers get damaged due to compression in closed space or due to shear forces and leak into this space. It does not resolve spontaneously and requires surgical drainage. If chronic, it may mimic a soft tissue sarcoma.

Snapping Hip Syndrome

A cause of hip pain in athletes in high energy sports like soccer; this is due to sudden movements of the iliopsoas tendon over the iliopectineal eminence, the femoral head or a paralabral cyst. It can be associated with iliopsoas tendinopathy and iliopsoas bursitis. Thickened iliopsoas tendon with increased signal on fluid sensitive sequences is seen. Iliopsoas tendon tears at its tendinous part while the muscular insertion into the iliacus remains intact.[64]

ATHLETIC PUBALGIA

Athletic pubalgia was formerly called as "sports hernia." It is seen as groin injury in professional soccer players. Pubalgia is caused by injuries to the rectus abdominis

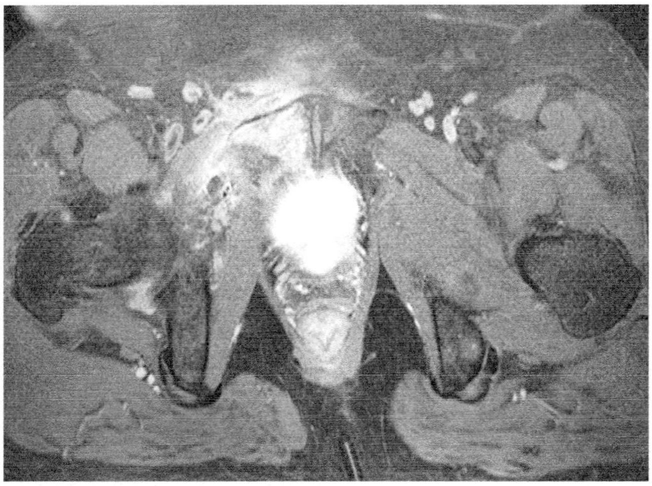

Fig. 34: T2-weighted fat-saturated fast spin-echo (FSE)—marrow edema right pubic bone with soft tissue edema in a case of pubalgia.

insertion, origin of the hip adductors tendons, and the pubic symphysis. Tears of the aponeurosis connecting the rectus abdominis muscle and the adductor longus muscle can be detected as fluid-like areas underneath the aponeurosis. Sagittal and oblique coronal planes that are perpendicular to the aponeurosis and a small field of view are recommended for imaging. Separation of the aponeurotic plate from the underlying pubic bone causes a fluid filled cleft. Tendon avulsion from the parent bone may be seen. Signal changes are seen in the involved muscles **(Fig. 34)**. Osteitis pubis may be noted in chronic changes.[65,66]

ARTHRITIS

Arthropathies commonly affect the following joints of the pelvis: The sacroiliac joint, the hips, and to a lesser extent of the symphysis pubis. Primary and secondary arthritis are common, RA can affect the hip in a small percentage, often bilaterally symmetrically with axial joint space narrowing. Hip involvement in ankylosing spondylitis is seen in 24–36% of patients. Calcium pyrophosphate dihydrate deposition (CPPD) disease and occasionally gout also involve the hip. The hip is a preferred site for several unusual articular diseases including pigmented villonodular synovitis (PVNS) and primary synovial chondromatosis.

Radiography remains the primary modality by which arthropathy of the hip is evaluated. With the advent of aggressive and advanced treatment options, MRI can demonstrate extent of synovial hypertrophy (pannus) that is common to all inflammatory arthritis but not evident on radiographs. Pannus shows low signal on T1 and high signal intensity on T2 images. It may be difficult to differentiate from synovial fluid. Pannus shows slightly higher signal intensity on short TR images and has more heterogenous and mildly lower signal intensity on long TR images. Pannus and synovitis enhance more dramatically and diffusely compared to synovial fluid which enhances only peripherally. Fibrotic component of pannus may be of low SI on T2W images. These are often more prominent in seronegative spondyloarthropathy and reflect inactive disease or therapeutic effect.

Magnetic resonance imaging also depicts the degree of bone erosion and cartilage thinning. MRI can be used to monitor therapy by quantitating the volume of pannus.

Rheumatoid arthritis: BME is seen as an early marker in patients with RA. It correlates with the presence of acute phase reactants in the blood. Seen in subchondral regions or with bone erosions, BME is a marker of synovitis and subsequent erosive damage which may occur after a lag of almost a year. Intense contrast enhancement, effusions, and erosions (seen as sharply marginated juxta-articular enhancing lesions) are other features on MRI.[67,68]

Pigmented villonodular synovitis (PVNS) is an uncommon disorder characterized by synovial proliferation with hemosiderin deposition in the involved synovial tissue. Pressure erosions of bone by the synovial masses may occur. Pigmented villonodular synovitis occurs most commonly in 2nd and 5th decade and is usually monoarticular. The knee is the most often involved joint but it can also occur in the hip.

Magnetic resonance imaging: Hemosiderin deposition is pathognomic of the condition and is seen as large globular areas of low signal intensity on all imaging sequences with blooming on gradient echo imaging. Pigmented villonodular synovitis is characterized by low signal intensity on T1W and T2W images distinguishing it from almost all tumors and inflammatory conditions, which have high signal on T2W images.[69]

Primary synovial chondromatosis: This results from metaplastic proliferation of synovium with formation of multiple cartilaginous or osseous loose bodies. It is not associated with degenerative change until later in the course of disease. On conventional radiography, it is not possible to differentiate it from PVNS.

Magnetic resonance imaging: MRI makes the differentiation possible as synovial chondromatosis follows the signal characteristics of cartilage. Cartilaginous loose bodies are low in signal on T1 and higher in signal on T2 images. Ossified loose bodies may be diffusely dense and sclerotic (low signal on all pulse sequences) or may have low signal cortical margin with a fatty center (chewy nougat).[70]

Amyloid arthropathy is a rare entity and typically presents in patients of renal failure with clinical features similar to RA. There may be erosions within acetabulum and femoral head and neck that show low signal on T1 and low to intermediate signal on T2 images. History and absence of hemosiderin, allows it to be differentiated from PVNS.

SACROILIITIS

This is a nonspecific term suggesting an inflammatory process involving the sacroiliac joints. A variety of disease process affect this joint including HLA-B27 spondyloarthropathies such as ankylosing spondylitis, psoriasis, and Reiter's syndrome. Other common conditions that affect these joints include osteoarthritis, gout, RA, and infection including tuberculosis.

In contrast to the hip, conventional radiography of the sacroiliac joints is often difficult even with specialized projections. The complex shape of the sacrum and iliac bones, curved nature of SI joints, and the overlapping bowel gases make the assessment suboptimal with early changes being difficult to interpret.

Magnetic resonance imaging is an accurate method for assessing early sacroiliac joint disease. The advantages of MR evaluation are direct visualization of cartilage, imaging in the oblique coronal plane for evaluation of synovial compartment, and lack of ionizing radiation as most patients of sacroiliitis are young and of reproductive age group. It is more sensitive than CT in detecting cartilage loss, edema, and small erosions.

The normal sacroiliac joint is well depicted with MR imaging. It clearly distinguishes the synovial and ligamentous compartments of the sacroiliac joint. The ligamentous part of the joint is posterior and obliquely oriented and contains adipose tissue with focal areas of low signal intensity representing loose connective tissue and the interosseous sacroiliac ligaments. The synovial compartment of the sacroiliac joint is anterior and more vertically oriented corresponding to the inferior one-half to two-thirds on plain radiographs MR imaging allows identification of the hyaline cartilage in the synovial compartment as a thin zone of intermediate signal, the maximum thickness of the cartilage is 5 mm. The iliac and sacral cortices are seen as areas of low signal intensity on either side of the cartilage **(Fig. 35)**. The most characteristic finding of sacroiliitis at MR imaging is loss of the normal thin band of intermediate signal intensity representing cartilage on T1W images. Altered signal intensity in the sacral and iliac cortices with adjacent marginal irregularity and deeper defects in the juxtaposed marrow are seen on T1W images. Erosions are more prominent anteroinferiorly and on the iliac side of the synovial compartment where cartilage is thinned and subchondral bone is not well protected. Area of increased signal is seen on T2 images in the synovial compartment.

The use of dynamic gadolinium-enhanced MR imaging has shown to be more sensitive than conventional MR imaging. Rapid (>90%) increase in signal intensity of articular and periarticular region represents active sacroiliitis. Intra-articular enhancement is noted in patients with active sacroiliitis. The fluid within the joint space does not enhance whereas the inflammatory reaction (phlegmon) may enhance **(Figs. 36 and 37)**.[71,72]

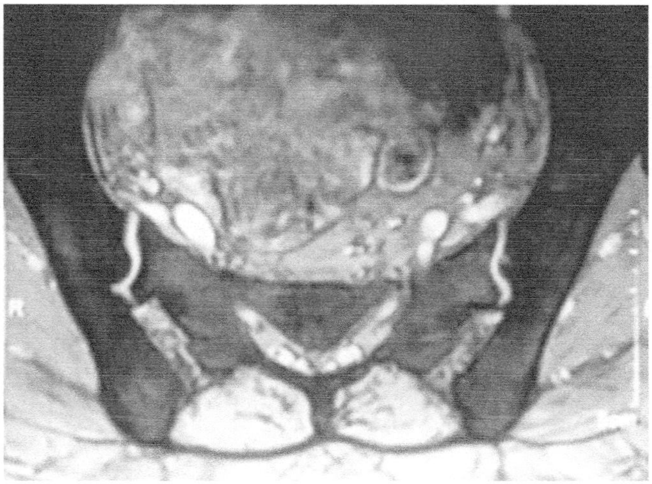

Fig. 35: Gradient T2-weighted axial image shows vertical anterior synovial part of the joint and posterior obliquely oriented ligamentous part—normal sacroiliac joint.

The cause of sacroiliitis cannot be distinguished with MR imaging. The asymmetry of appearance aids the differential diagnosis, as ankylosing spondylitis is generally bilateral and symmetric. Unilateral disease with prominent edema in the soft tissue and marrow adjacent to the joint suggests infection.

INFECTION

The MRI protocol for diagnosis of soft tissue infections and osteomyelitis differs from the routine protocol. Additional imaging sequences using fat suppressed T1 FSE sequences pre- and post-IV gadolinium are performed to enable the diagnosis of sinus tracts and abscesses. The presence of BME and enhancement on MR images is very sensitive for osteomyelitis and the absence of these findings excludes the presence of acute osteomyelitis. The distinction between para-articular cellulitis and osteomyelitis can be made with MR imaging, which is also useful in defining the extent of osteomyelitis before surgery.[73]

Soft tissue infection about the hips can involve the joint or surrounding muscles. Hip joint infection is common in infancy and childhood. MRI shows early cartilage destruction. Any case of monoarticular arthritis should be considered infectious unless proved otherwise.

Tubercular arthritis: Articular manifestations of musculoskeletal TB are second to spinal disease in frequency of presentation. The most commonly involved are the hip and knee followed by the sacroiliac joint, shoulder, elbow, and ankle. Magnetic resonance demonstrates synovitis and joint effusion. Indolent infections such as tuberculosis result in prominent synovitis and MRI can then simulate a noninfectious inflammatory arthritis.

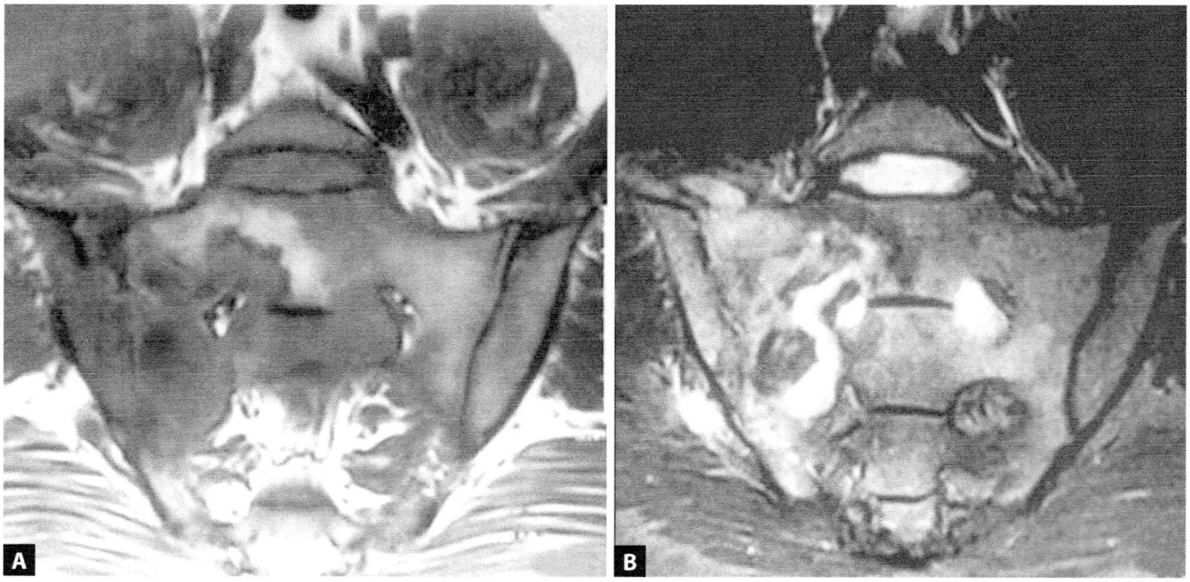

Figs. 36A and B: (A) T1-weighted coronal image of both sacroiliac joints; and (B) T2-weighted coronal image show altered signal in the right sacral ala and iliac blade, with articular erosion and decreased joint space—right sacroiliitis.

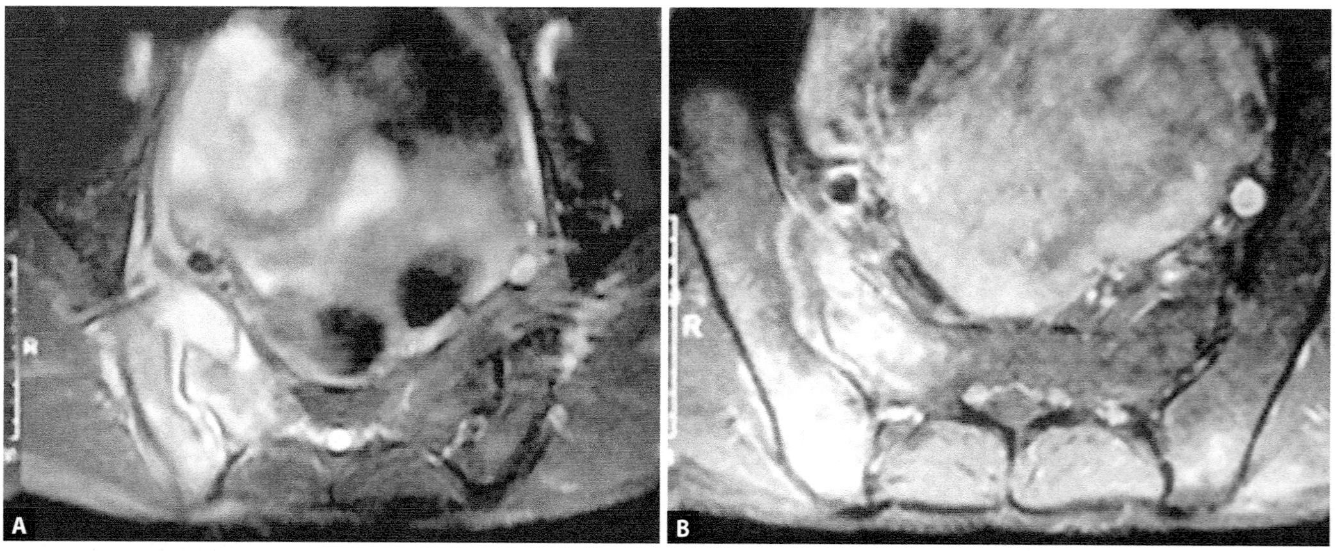

Figs. 37A and B: (A) T2-weighted axial; and (B) Short tau inversion recovery (STIR) axial image of both sacroiliac joints showing altered signal in right sacroiliac joint with widened joint space and periarticular collection—tubercular sacroiliitis.

MRI may demonstrate intraosseous involvement earlier than with other modalities **(Figs. 38A and B)**. Tuberculosis of the joints is discussed in detail elsewhere in the book.

BURSAE

There are several bursae in the hip region, which can get inflamed. *The iliopsoas bursa* is the largest bursa in the body and communicates with the hip joint in 15% of population. The iliopsoas bursa is located anterior to the hip joint and adjacent to femoral vessels. It lies between the psoas muscle and the anteromedial surface of the hip joint. The bursa measures 3–7 cm in length and is 2–4 cm in width. It gets distended in inflammatory, infective or degenerative disease. Patient may have groin pain and a palpable mass. It is not seen unless distended with fluid. Postcontrast scanning delineates the bursa better as the lining of the bursa enhances and the fluid does not. Asymptomatic bursal fluid may occur in the presence of joint effusion due to communication with the joint.

Greater trochanteric bursitis is another cause of hip pain, with patient localizing the pain to lateral aspect of the hip; this results from repetitive hip flexion. The findings on MR consist of no perceptible abnormality on T1W images. On T2 images, there is increased signal paralleling the greater trochanter. Instead of a well-defined fluid collection, a focus of interdigitating high signal may

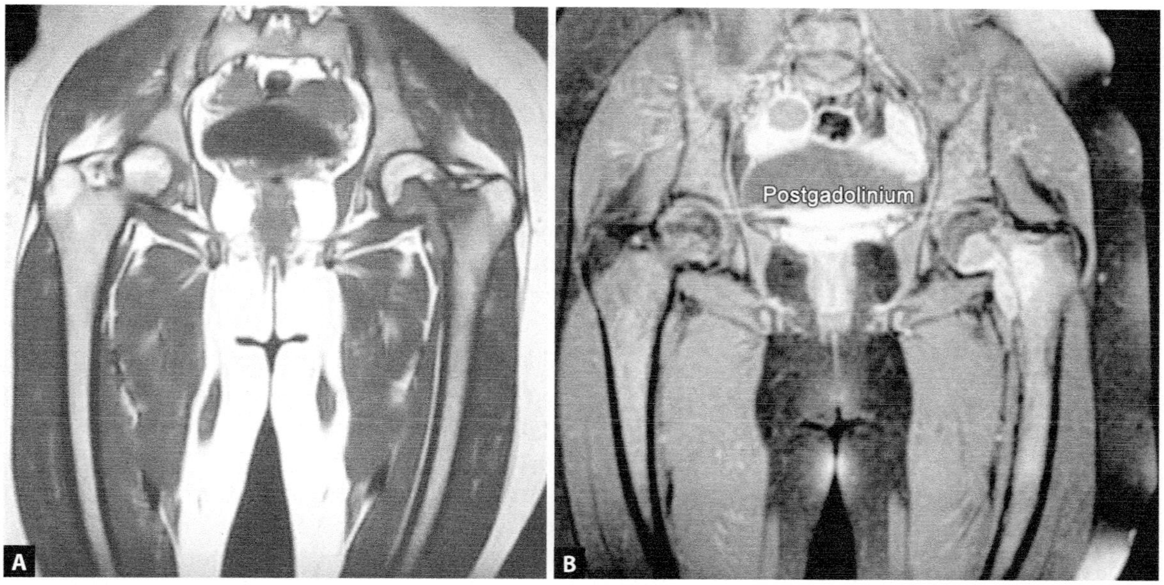

Figs. 38A and B: (A) T1-weighted (T1W) coronal image of the pelvis; and (B) T1W coronal postgadolinium image show an area of cortical erosion in the femoral neck with associated marrow edema—tubercular arthritis.

be seen around the tendons of the greater trochanter. Clinically, it may not be possible to differentiate bursitis from gluteus medius/minimus tears.

NERVES

The largest nerve adjacent to the hip joint is the sciatic nerve. It is located immediately posterior to the posterior column of the acetabulum and lateral to the L4-S3 nerve roots. The nerve exits the infrapiriformis portion of the greater sciatic foramen and courses between the ischial tuberosity and greater trochanter surrounded by fat. It is located between quadratus femoris muscle anteriorly and gluteus maximus posteriorly. On MRI, the sciatic nerve is identified as intermediate signal intensity stippled structure surrounded by fat just lateral to the ischial tuberosity on axial images. MR neurography depicts the sciatic nerve in detail **(Fig. 39)**.[74]

The sciatic nerve can be compressed by a nearby mass or may be traumatized by a direct blow resulting in swelling of the nerve with an increased signal on T2W images.

Magnetic resonance imaging of acetabular fractures can be used to detect subclinical injury to the sciatic nerve. The injured nerve shows perineural or intraneural enhancement. Preoperative detection of such abnormalities warrants intraoperative monitoring as these patients would be at risk for further (iatrogenic) nerve injury. Compared with neurological examinations and somatosensory-evoked potential (SEP) monitoring, MR may be a more sensitive indicator of sciatic nerve trauma.[75]

Fibrolipomatous hamartoma may be seen in relation to the sciatic nerve in which fascicles of the nerve are surrounded by fat.

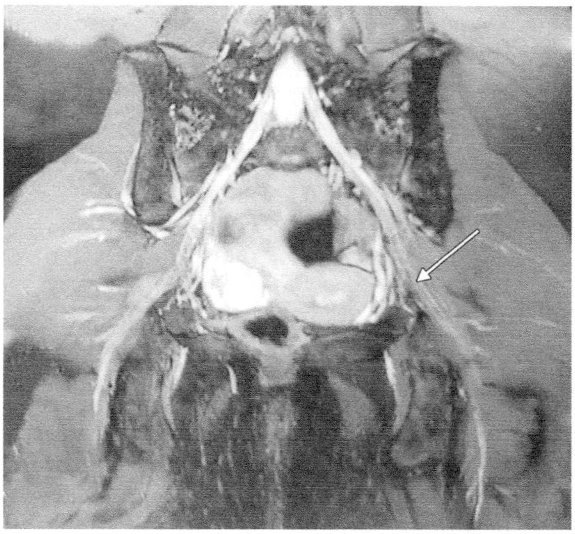

Fig. 39: MR neurography—maximum intensity projection (MIP) image depicting the sciatic nerve on both sides (marked with arrow on the left).

PIRIFORMIS SYNDROME

The sciatic nerve exits the pelvis at the greater sciatic notch and is located immediately anterior to the piriformis muscle. The sciatic nerve can split through piriformis and a portion of the nerve can be superficial to the piriformis muscle. Due to this variation in location of the sciatic nerve, compression, hypertrophy or injury to the piriformis muscle can cause irritation to the sciatic nerve, mimicking radicular symptoms of disc disease.

Magnetic resonance imaging may show asymmetry in size of one piriformis compared to opposite side. In case of trauma, high signal may be noted.

MAGNETIC RESONANCE IMAGING IN POSTARTHROPLASTY HIP

Complications of hip replacement procedures can be hardware failure, periprosthetic fractures, implant loosening, infections, and adverse tissue reactions. Tendinopathy, heterotopic ossification, neuropathy, and component-induced synovitis are other complications. MR plays an important role in the diagnosis and grading of adverse tissue reactions because of poor sensitivity of radiography and CT.

Imaging of the hip after total hip arthroplasty was a challenge due to susceptibility artifacts. With pulse modifications designed to reduce artifacts, better hardware, MRI is now being used to detect postoperative complications. MRI protocols to image implants include use of sequences with high spatial resolution, smaller fields of view, and higher imaging matrices. A lower strength magnet (1.5T instead of 3T),with stronger gradients, use of Spin echo instead of gradient echo sequences, increasing receiver bandwidth, and use of STIR (instead of frequency selective fat suppression) for a more uniform fat saturation are other steps to reduce susceptibility. Newer techniques such as slice encoding for metal artifact correction (SEMAC), multiacquistion variable resonance image combination (MAVRIC), and view angle tilting are now available which have improved imaging around prosthesis.[76,77]

Initially metal on metal (MOM) arthroplasties were done which were replaced by metal on polymer (MOP) implants due to high incidence of aseptic loosening in the former. MOP arthroplasties have metallic femoral head prosthesis and a polyethylene liner within the prosthetic acetabular cup. Aseptic loosening and shedding of polyethylene fragments from this led to periprosthetic loosening and aseptic loosening (particle disease) of second-generation MOM implants constructed from chromium cobalt and molybdenum alloy were introduced in the late 1990s. These are now known to have complications like adverse reaction to metal debris (ARMD) due to reaction to shed metallic microparticles. Granulomatous inflammation and aseptic lymphocytic vacuities associated lesions (ALVAL) have also been documented. Clinical long-term follow-up and monitoring of cobalt and chromium levels are used to detect ARMD.[78]

Direct visualization by MRI is the least invasive technique to determine the occurrence of ARMD. Periprosthetic collections are seen in both types of implant. They may have signal like simple fluid, others have more ill-defined solid debris with thicker, irregular pseudocapsule, appreciated on fluid sensitive sequences. MRI plays a significant role in the assessment of soft tissues adjacent to the prosthesis and can detect insertional tears of gluteal tendons, muscle edema/atrophy, and periprosthetic marrow edema. Metallosis is noted as a low signal intensity halo around the prosthesis on all sequences.

Trochanteric bursitis, avulsion of the gluteus tendons, and short external rotators can be identified on MRI.

HIP AND PELVIS-BONE TUMORS

Any bone tumor or tumors-like lesion can occur in and round the hip and pelvis, but there are certain tumors that are preferentially seen in this region **(Box 8)**.

The pelvis and proximal femur contain hematopoietic red bone marrow that persists throughout life and a mix of red and yellow marrow is seen in adults. Both the apophysis and epiphysis should have yellow marrow. Fat marrow can convert to red marrow in times of increased physiological demands. Variations in the red marrow pattern are a source of diagnostic errors. Normal red marrow has serpiginous margins which do not disrupt normal anatomical barriers and appear iso to hyperintense to skeletal muscles on T1W images after neonatal period.

Most bone tumors in the pelvis are malignant and most tumors in proximal femur are benign in the adults. Metastasis and multiple myeloma are very common in the pelvis in patients >40 years of age and must be excluded in patients presenting with a lytic/blastic lesion in the pelvis. The most common primary malignant bone tumors of the pelvis are chondrosarcoma **(Figs. 40A to C)**, followed by Ewing's sarcoma and the osteosarcoma.[79] Same are also seen in proximal femur (chondrosarcoma being the most common followed by osteosarcoma and Ewing's sarcoma). The most common primary benign tumors in pelvis are osteochondroma, giant cell tumors, and Langerhans cell histiocytosis, and in the proximal femur are fibrous dysplasia, solitary bone cyst, and osteoid osteoma.

Transarticular spread across joints—sacroiliac, symphysis pubis, and a hip via ligamentum teres is mostly seen with aggressive lesions such as chondrosarcoma, osteosarcoma, metastasis, and giant cell tumor.

Bone islands (enostosis) are common incidental and asymptomatic findings with pelvis and sacrum being common sites. Suspicion of metastasis may be raised in

Box 8: Common bone tumors of the hip and pelvis.

- *Benign*
  - Osteochondroma
  - Enchondroma
  - Chondroblastoma
  - Giant cell tumor
  - Osteoid osteoma
  - Geode
- *Malignant*
  - Metastasis
  - Chondrosarcoma
  - Ewings sarcoma
  - Plasmacytoma

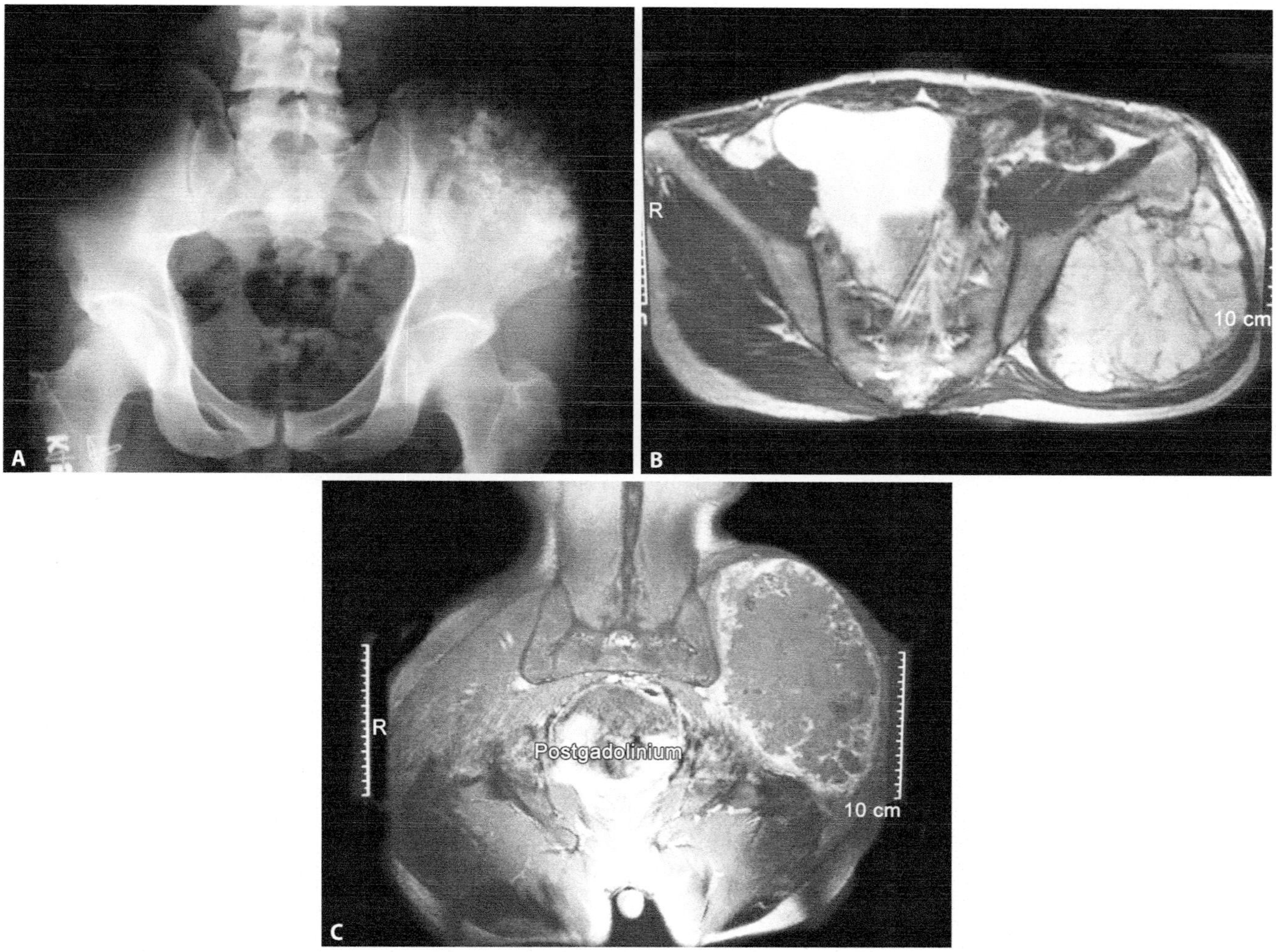

Figs. 40A and C: (A) X-ray pelvis radiograph shows a large mass with typical chondroid calcification in relation to left iliac blade; (B) T2 hyperintensity seen on axial MR image; (C) Rings and arc pattern of enhancement in postgadolinium coronal image—chondrosarcoma.

patients with a known malignancy. Clinical correlation, metabolic profile, and review with previous imaging are required to reach a diagnosis.

CONCLUSION

Magnetic resonance imaging is the diagnostic modality of choice for most disorders of the hip and pelvis in evaluating cases with radiographic findings that are inconclusive or do not explain the patient's complaints. In the evaluation of hip and pelvis, MRI is often the problem solving technique bypassing bone scintigraphy and CT. With MRI, one can stage the pathology of the hip and pelvis to prognosticate and influence therapeutic decisions.

REFERENCES

1. Hips and pelvis. In: Helms C, Major N, Anderson MW, Kaplan P, Dussault R (Eds). Musculoskeletal MRI, 2nd edition. Philadelphia: WB Saunders; 2009. pp. 324-51.
2. Sutter R, Zanetti M, Pfirrmann CWA. New developments in hip imaging. Radiology. 2012;264(03):651-67.
3. Petchprapa CN, Dunham KS, Lattanzi R, et al. Demystifying radial imaging of the hip. Radiographics. 2013;33:E97-112.
4. Llopis E, Fernandez E, Cerezal L. MR and CT arthrography of the hip. Semin Musculoskelet Radiol. 2012;16(01):42-56.
5. Crespo-Rodríguez AM, De Lucas-Villarrubia JC, Pastrana-Ledesma M. The diagnostic performance of non-contrast 3-Tesla magnetic resonance imaging (3-T MRI) versus 1.5-Tesla magnetic resonance arthrography (1.5-T MRA) in femoro-acetabular impingement. Eur J Radiol. 2017;88:109-16.
6. Morrison WB. Indirect MR arthrography: concepts and controversies. Semin Musculoskelet Radiol. 2005;9:125-34.
7. Zlatkin MB, Pevsner D, Sanders TG, Hancock CR, Ceballos CE, Herrera MF. Acetabular labral tears and cartilage lesions of the hip: indirect MR arthrographic correlation with arthroscopy–a preliminary study. Am J Roentgenol. 2010;194:709-14.
8. Hungerford DS, Zizic TM. Pathogenesis of ischemic necrosis of the femoral head. Hip; 1983. pp. 249-62.
9. Malizos KN, Karantanas AH, Varitimidis SE, Dailiana ZH, Bargiotas K, Maris T. Osteonecrosis of the femoral head: Etiology, imaging and treatment. Eur J Radiol. 2009;63:16-28.

10. Murphey MD, Foreman KL, Klassen-Fischer MK, Fox MG, Chung EM, Kransdorf MJ. From the radiologic pathology archives imaging of osteonecrosis: Radiologic-pathologic correlation. Radiographics. 2014;34(04):1003-28.
11. Mitchell DG, Rao VM, Dalinka MK, Spritzer CE, Alavi A, Steinberg ME, et al. Femoral head avascular necrosis: Correlation of MR imaging, radiographic staging, radionuclide imaging and clinical findings. Radiology. 1987;162(3):709-15.
12. Beltran J, Herman LJ, Burk JM, Zuelzer WA, Clark RN, Lucas JG, et al. Femoral head avascular necrosis: MR imaging with clinical pathological and radionuclide correlation. Radiology. 1988;166:215.
13. Nadel DN, Debatin JT, Richardson LW. Detection of acute avascular necrosis of the femoral head in dogs: Dynamic contrast enhanced MR imaging vs spin echo and STIR sequences. Am J Roentgenol. 1992;159:1255.
14. Karantanas AH, Drakonaki EE. The role of MR imaging in vascular necrosis of the femoral head. Semin Musculoskelet Radiol. 2011;15:281-300.
15. Duda SH, Laniado M, Schick F, Claussen CD. The Double line sign of osteonecrosis: Evaluation on chemical shift MR images. Eur J Radiol. 1993;16(3):233-8.
16. Omar I, Blount J. Magnetic Resonance Imaging of the hip. Top Magn Reson Imaging. 2015;24:165-87.
17. Ikemura S, Yamamota T, Motomura G, Nakashima Y, Mawatari T, Iwamoto Y. MRI evaluation of collapsed femoral head in patients 60 years old or older: Differentiation of subchondral insufficiency fracture from osteonecrosis of the femoral head. Am J Roentgenol. 2010;195(1):W63-8.
18. Yeh LR, Chen CK, Huang YL, Pan HB, Yang CF. Diagnostic Performance of MR imaging in the assessment of subchondral fractures in avascular necrosis of the femoral head. Skeletal Radiol. 2009;38(06):559-64.
19. Huang GH, Chan WP, Chang YC, Chang CY, Chen CY, Yu JS. MR imaging of bone marrow edema and joint effusion in patients with osteonecrosis of the femoral head: relationship to pain. Am J Roentgenol. 2003;181:545-9.
20. Vande Berg B, Malghem J, Labaisse MA, Noel H, Maldague B. Avascular necrosis of the hip. Comparison of contrast enhanced and nonenhanced MR imaging with histological correlation. Radiology. 1992;182:445-50.
21. Chan WP, Liu YJ, Huang GS, Lin MF, Huang S, Chang YC, et al. Relationship of the idiopathic osteonecrosis of the femoral head to perfusion changes in the proximal femur by dynamic contrast enhanced MRI. Am J Roentgenol. 2011;196:637-43.
22. Oner AY, Aggunlu L, Akpek S, Celik A, Le Roux P, Tali T, et al. Staging of hip avascular necrosis: Is there a need for DWI? Acta Radiol. 2001;52:111-4.
23. Hou CH, Shih TT, Liu CY, Li YD, Enright T. Proton MR spectroscopy of the femoral head-evaluation of patients at risk for vascular necrosis. J Magn Reson Imaging. 2006;24(2):409-17.
24. Arlet J, Ficat RP. [Diagnosis of primary femur head osteonecrosis at stage 1 (preradiologic stage)]. Rev Chir Orthop Reparatrice Appar Mot. 1968;54(7):637-48.
25. Steinberg ME, Hayken GD, Steinberg DR. A quantitative system for staging avascular necrosis. J Bone Joint Surg Br. 1995;77(1):34-41.
26. Association for Research on Osseous Circulation. Committee on Terminology and Classification. ARCO News. 1992;4:41-6.
27. Shimizu K, Moriya H, Akita T, et al. Prediction of collapse with magnetic resonance imaging of avascular necrosis of the femoral head. J Bone Joint Surg. 1994;76A:215-21
28. Bradway JK, Morrey BF. The natural history of the silent hip in bilateral atraumatic osteonecrosis. J Arthroplasty. 1993;8(4):383-7.
29. Hu LB, Huang ZG, Wei HY, Wang W, Ren A, Xu YY. Osteonecrosis of the femoral head: Using CT, MRI and gross specimen to characterize the location, shape and size of the lesion. Br J Radiol. 2015;88(1046):20140508
30. Mitchell DG, Rao UM, Dalinka MK, Spritzer CE, Axel L, Gefter W, et al. Hematopoietic and fatty bone marrow distribution in the normal and ischemic hip: New observations with 1.5T MR imaging. Radiology. 1986;161(1):199-202.
31. Jiang CC, Shih TT. Epiphyseal scar of the femoral head: Risk factor of osteonecrosis. Ra diology. 1994;191(2):409-12.
32. Coleman BG, Kressel HY, Dalinka MK, Scheibler ML, Burk DL, Cohen EK. Radiographically negative avascular necrosis detection with MR imaging. Radiology. 1988;168:525-8.
33. Vande Berg BC, Lecovet FE, Koutaissoff S. Bone marrow edema of the femoral head and transient osteoporosis of the hip. Eur J Radiol. 2008;67:68-77.
34. Kaplan SS, Stegman CJ. Transient osteoporosis of the hip. J Bone Joint Surg Am. 1985;67A:490-2.
35. Curtiss PH, Kincaid WE. Transitory demineralisation of the hip in pregnancy. J Bone Surg Am. 41A:1237-1333.
36. Uzun M, Ayhan E, Beksac B, Karaman O. Regional migratory osteoporosis and transient osteoporosis of the hip: Are they all the same? Clin Rheumatol. 2013;32(6):919-23.
37. Vande Berg BE, Malghem JJ, Labaisse MA, Noel HM, Maldague BE. MR imaging of avascular necrosis and transient marrow edema of the femoral head. Radiographics. 1993;13(3):501-20.
38. Klontzas ME, Vassalou EE, Zibis AH, Bintoudi AS, Karantanas AH. MR imaging of transient osteoporosis of the hip: an update on 155 hip joints. Eur J Radiol. 2015;84(3):431-43.
39. Klontzas ME, Zibis AH, Vassalou EE, Karantanas AH. MRI of the hip: current concepts on bone marrow oedema. Hip Int. 2017;27(4):329-35.
40. Naraghi A, White LM. MRI of labral and chondral lesions of the hip. Am J Roentgenol. 2015;205:479-90.
41. Kassarjian A, Brisson M, Palmer WE. Femoroacetabular impingement. Eur J Radiol. 2007;63:29-35.
42. Anderson SE, Siebenrock KA, Tannast M. Femoroacetabular impingement: evidence of an established hip abnormality. Radiology. 2010;257(1):8-13.
43. Ganz R, Parvizi J, Beck M, Leuing M, Notzli H, Siebenrock KA. Femoroacetabular impingement: A cause of osteoarthritis of the hip. Clin Orthop Relat Res. 2003;417:112-20.
44. Amanatullah DF, Antkowiak T, Pillay K, Patel J, Refaat M, Toupadakis CA, et al. Femoroacetabular impingement: Current concepts in diagnosis and treatment. Orthopedics. 2015;38:185-99.
45. Siebenrock KA, Wahab KH, Werlen S, Kalhor M, Leunig M, Ganz R. Abnormal extension of the femoral head epiphysis

as a cause of cam impingement. Clin Orthop Relat Res. 2004;418:54-60.
46. Notzli HP, Wyss TF, Stoecklin CH, Schmid MR, Treiber K, Hodler J. The contour of the femoral head-neck junction as a predictor for the risk of anterior impingement. J Bone Joint Surg Br. 2002;84:556-60.
47. Ghaffari A, Davis I, Storey T, Moser M. Current concepts of femoroacetabular impingement. Radiol Clin North Am. 2018;56(6):965-82.
48. Sutter R, Pfirrmann CWA. Update on femoroacetabular impingement: What is new, and how should we assess it? Semin Musculoskelet Radiol. 2017;21(5):518-28.
49. Siebenrock KA, Kalbermatten DF, Ganz R. Effect of pelvic tilt on acetabular retroversion: A study of pelvis from cadavers. Clin Orthop Relat Res. 2003;407:241-8.
50. Ito K, Minka A, Leunig M, Werlen S, Ganz R. Femoroacetabular impingement and the cam effect: An MRI based quantitative anatomical study of the femoral head-neck offset. J Bone Joint Surg Br. 2001;83:171-6.
51. Schmaranzer F, Lerch TD, Strasser U, Vavron P, Schmaranzer E, Tannast M. Usefulness of MR arthrography of the hip with and without leg traction in detection of intra-articular bodies. Acad Radiol. 2019;26(9):e252-e259.
52. Pfirrmann CWA, Mengiardi B, Dora C, Kalberer F, Zanetti M, Hodler J. Cam and pincer femoroacetabular impingement: Characteristic MR arthrographic findings in 50 patients. Radiology. 2006;240(3):778-85.
53. Li AE, Jawetz ST, Greditzer HG 4th, Burge AJ, Nawabi DH, Potter HG. MRI for the preoperative evaluation of femoroacetabular impingement. Insights Imaging. 2016;7(2):187-98.
54. Kassarjian A, Yoon LS, Belzile E, Connolly SA, Millis MB, Palmer WE. Triad of arthrographic findings in patients with cam type femoroacetabular impingement. Radiology. 2005;236:588-92.
55. Nokis SR, Vogler JB, Spritzer CE, Martinez S, Herfkens RJ. Herniation pits of the femoral neck: Appearance at MR imaging. Radiology. 1989;172(1):231-4.
56. Rehman H, Clement RG, Perks F, White TO. Imaging of occult hip fractures: CT or MRI? Injury. 2016;47(6):1297-1301.
57. Nachtrab O, Cassar-Pullicino VN, Lalam R, Tins B, Tyrrell PN, Singh J. Role of MRI in hip fractures, including stress fractures, occult fractures, avulsion fractures. Eur J Radiol. 2012;81(12):3813-23.
58. Lang P, Mauz M, Schörner W, Schwetlick G, Henkes H, Berthezene Y, et al. Acute fracture of the femoral neck: Assessment of femoral head perfusion with gadopentetate Dimeglumine—Enhanced MR imaging. Am J Roentgenol. 1993;160(2):335-41.
59. Steele CE, Cochran G, Renninger C, Deafenbaugh B, Kuhn KM. Femoral neck stress fractures: MRI risk factors for progression. J Bone Joint Surg Am. 2018;100(17):1496-502.
60. Kassarjian A, Rodrigo RM, Santisteban JM. Current concepts in MRI of rectus femoris musculotendinous (myotendinous) and myofascial injuries in elite athletes. Eur J Radiol. 2012;81(12):3763-71.
61. Bencardino JT, Palmer WE. Imaging of hip disorders in athletes. Radiol Clin North Am. 2002;40(2):267-87.
62. Boutin RD, Newman JS. MR imaging of sports-related hip disorders. Magn Reson Imaging Clin N Am. 2003; 11(2):255-81.
63. Kingzett-Taylor A, Tirman PF, Feller J, McGann W, Prieto V, Wischer T, et al. Tendinosis and tears of gluteus medius and maximus muscles as a cause of hip pain: MR imaging findings. Am J Roentgenol. 1999;173(4):1123-6.
64. Lee KS, Rosas HG, Phancao JP. Snapping hip: Imaging and treatment. Semin Musculoskelet Radiol. 2013;17(3):286-94.
65. Mullens FE, Zoga AC, Morrison WB, Meyers WC. Review of MRI technique and imaging findings in athletic pubalgia and the "sports hernia.". Eur J Radiol. 2012;81(12):3780-92.
66. Agten CA, Sutter R, Buck FM, Pfirrmann CWA. Hip imaging in athletes: Sports imaging series. Radiology. 2016;280(2):351-69.
67. Narváez JA, Narváez J, De Lama E, De Albert M. MR imaging of early rheumatoid arthritis. Radiographics. 2010;30(1):143-63; discussion 163-5.
68. Hetland ML, Ejbjerg B, Hørslev-Petersen K, Jacobsen S, Vestergaard A, Jurik AG, et al. MRI bone oedema is the strongest predictor of subsequent radiographic progression in early rheumatoid arthritis. Results from a 2-year randomised controlled trial (CIMESTRA). Ann Rheum Dis. 2009;68:384-90.
69. Flandry F, Hughston J, McCann S, Kurtz DM. Diagnostic features of diffuse pigmented villonodular synovitis of the knee. Clin Orthop. 1994;298:212-20.
70. Hermann G, Abdelwahab IF, Klein M, Kenan S, Lewis M. Synovial chondromatosis. Skeletal Radiol. 1995;24:298-300.
71. Murphey MD, Wetzel LH, Bramble JM, Levine E, Simpson KM, Lindsley HB. Sacroiliitis: MR imaging findings. Radiology. 1991;180:239-44.
72. Bollow M, Braun J, Hamm B, Eggens U, Schilling A, König H, et al. Early sacroiliitis in patients with spondyloarthropathy: Evaluation with dynamic gadolinium enhanced MR imaging. Radiology. 1995;194:529-36.
73. Maj L, Gombar Y III, Morrison WB. MR imaging of hip infection and inflammation. Magn Reson Imaging Clin N Am. 2013;21(01):127-39.
74. Chhabra A, Chalian M, Soldatos T, Andreisek G, Faridian-Aragh N, Williams E, et al. 3-T high-resolution MR neurography of sciatic neuropathy. AJR Am J Roentgenol 2012;198(4):W357-64.
75. Potter HG, Montgomery KD, Heise CW, Helfet DL. MR imaging of acetabular fractures: Value in detecting femoral head injury, intra-articular fragments and sciatic nerve injury. Am J Roentgenol. 1994;163(4):881-6.
76. Berkowitz JL, Potter HG. Advanced MRI techniques for the hip joint: focus on the postoperative hip. Am J Roentgenol. 2017;209(3):534-43.
77. Fritz J, Lurie B, Miller TT, Potter HG. MR imaging of hip arthroplasty implants. Radiographics. 2014;34(4):E106-32.
78. Müller GM, Lundin B, von Schewelov T, Müller MF, Ekberg O, Månsson S. Evaluation of metal artifacts in clinical MR images of patients with total hip arthroplasty using different metal artifact-reducing sequences. Skeletal Radiol. 2015;44(3):353-9.
79. Afonso PD, Weber MA, Issac A, Bloem JL. Hip and pelvis bone tumours: Can you make it simple. Semin Musculoskelet Radiol. 2019;23:e37-e57.

CHAPTER

19

Magnetic Resonance Imaging of the Knee

Sapna Singh, Anjali Prakash, Gaurav Shanker Pradhan

INTRODUCTION

The knee is one of the important weight bearing (WB) joints capable of performing complex and extensive movements. It is therefore most frequently affected by traumatic and degenerative conditions.

Since its inception, magnetic resonance imaging (MRI) has been found to be a very informative imaging method widely accepted by the orthopedic community for evaluating the knee joint. MRI has reduced the number of diagnostic arthroscopies and has enabled selection of patients for therapy-oriented arthroscopy.[1,2] Soft tissue discrimination with MRI is excellent and differentiation can be made between cortex, marrow, ligaments, tendons, muscles, synovium, vascular, and cartilage elements.[3] This differentiation is not possible with conventional radiographic techniques. Additional advantages of MRI are its multiplanar and thin section capabilities and the ability to evaluate subchondral bone and marrow. MR is the recommended imaging modality over CT for the evaluation of bone contusions and occult knee fractures including the tibial plateau fractures. It has supplanted nuclear scintigraphy in the characterization of osteonecrosis and can be used to assess the integrity of overlying articular cartilage surfaces. Kinematic and dynamic MR techniques provide an improved perspective for assessing the biomechanics of the patellofemoral joint and the normal functions of the ligamentous structures of the knee.

3 Tesla (3T) MRI has revolutionized musculoskeletal imaging. The gain in the signal-to-noise ratio (SNR) improves image quality with increased signal and higher spatial resolution leading to an improved diagnostic accuracy. The ligamentous and cartilaginous structures are elucidated in better details on a 3T MR scanner. The smaller structures such as the posterolateral corner (PLC) are also assessed better.

IMAGING PROTOCOLS/TECHNICAL FACTORS

An ideal MR technique should yield images of the osseous and soft tissue structures of the knee with good contrast and spatial resolution in a reasonable time to maximize patient acceptability. The use of a dedicated knee coil is mandatory for a quality study because it improves the SNR. Using a small field of view (FOV) in the range of 10–14 cm greatly improves spatial resolution and facilitates optimal assessment of the small anatomical structures of the knee. A matrix of 256 × 256 is usually standard.

Patient Positioning

The patient is placed supine, feet first with the leg in full extension. The knee is placed in 10–15° of external rotation to realign the anterior cruciate ligament (ACL) parallel with the sagittal imaging plane. This is typically the position of the knee in the relaxed state and no effort at externally rotating the knee needs to be made in the majority of patients. The knee is placed in a dedicated knee coil to produce a uniform signal intensity across the image and foam pads are used to immobilize the knee within the center of the coil. Only one knee can be imaged at a time.

Slice Thickness

Four millimeter sections are used for axial, coronal, and sagittal images of the knee.[4] When needed, submillimeter resolution can be obtained with three-dimensional Fourier transformation (3D FT) volume protocols. In children, 3 mm slices allow optimal medial to lateral joint coverage in the sagittal plane and anterior to posterior coverage in the coronal plane.

Imaging Planes and Pulse Sequences

Acquisition of images in three orthogonal planes is helpful in defining and characterizing abnormalities.[4,5] An axial acquisition through the patellofemoral joint is used as the initial localizer for subsequent sagittal and coronal plane images. Menisci and cruciate ligaments are best evaluated on sagittal images with coronal views for secondary visualization and confirmation of pathology. The medial and lateral collateral ligaments are best displayed on coronal images. The articular cartilage surfaces of medial and lateral compartments are assessed in both coronal and sagittal planes. The patellofemoral joint including patellar facet and trochlear groove is best seen on axial images.

Standard MR Pulse Sequences

Short echo time (TE) conventional spin echo (CSE) images generally provide the best contrast for anatomical evaluation. The more rapidly acquired, fast spin echo (FSE) pulse sequences with short echo train length provide high SNR, excellent soft tissue contrast, high in-plane spatial resolution, and shorter scan times compared to CSE sequences. Short tau inversion recovery (STIR) and fat-saturated FSE pulse sequences are best for the evaluation of bone contusions and other marrow abnormalities. A knee protocol that works well includes FSE proton density (PD) and T2-weighted (T2W) sequence in the sagittal plane, a STIR sequence in the coronal plane, T1-weighted (T1W) coronal images, T2W axial images, and a sequence for articular cartilage.

Isotropic 3D Fast Spin Echo Acquisition

Many 3D techniques with gradient echo (GRE) based and fat suppressed (FSE) based sequences are available which have been discussed in detail in the section on articular cartilage. These sequences provide thinner sections and reduce partial volume averaging excellent for the depiction of subtle cartilaginous defects.

Metallic Artifact Reduction Sequences (MARS)

The metallic susceptibility artifacts cause both through plane and in plane distortions which can be corrected by view angle tilting (VAT), slice-encoding for metal artifact correction (SEMAC), and multiple-acquisition with variable resonance image combination (MAVRIC) sequences.[6]

Intravenous gadolinium is useful in assessment of inflammatory arthritides as it causes enhancement of the pannus. The biomechanics of patellar tracking can be assessed with kinematic technique with a cine loop display of acquired images.

MR EVALUATION OF THE KNEE

The structures that are studied can be broadly categorized as:

- Menisci
- Central structures of the knee [ACL, posterior cruciate ligament (PCL)]
- Medial structure of the knee [medial collateral ligament (MCL)]
- Corner based anatomy [PLC, posteromedial corner (PMC), anterolateral corner (ALC), anteromedial corner (AMC) or the extensor mechanism of the knee]
- Patellofemoral joint and MR kinematics
- Articular cartilage
- Synovium
- Bone marrow
- Subchondral bone

MENISCI

Magnetic resonance imaging is the modality of choice for evaluating a patient with suspected meniscal pathology. By displaying the morphology of meniscal tear, MR provides valuable information for determining the need for operative intervention and predicting the feasibility of meniscal repair.

Microanatomy of the Menisci

The menisci are predominantly made up of type I collagen arranged into bundles. Most of the bundles course circumferentially parallel to the long axis of the meniscus. A smaller number of fibers are oriented in a radial fashion functioning as stabilizing tie fibers. With axial loading of the joint, the circumferential orientation of most of the collagen bundles allows for meniscal deformation, the development of "hoop stresses", and a relatively even distribution of the load across the joint surfaces. Up to one-third of the peripheral meniscus is vascularized and innervated (the "red zone") whereas the remaining inner two-thirds or more is strictly fibrocartilaginous (the "white zone").[7,8]

Macroanatomy and MRI Appearance

The menisci are C-shaped structures that are conventionally described as having three segments **(Figs. 1A to C)**:

1. Anterior horn
2. Body
3. Posterior horn

Each meniscus measures approximately 5 mm in height along its periphery and tapers to a thin inner edge and hence shows a triangular shape when cut in cross section **(Fig. 2)**. The upper margin is called the superior articular surface whereas the lower margin is called the inferior articular surface. The superior articular surface is completely visible to the arthroscopist, the inferior to some extent, while the outer nonarticular capsular surface is not seen.

The menisci demonstrate diffusely low signal on all MRI pulse sequences because of their fibrocartilaginous nature. Meniscal pathology is best demonstrated on sequences that use a short TE (<20 ms), i.e., T1W, PD, and gradient echo images. If a FSE technique is used, the echo train length should be kept below 4–5 and the interecho space minimized to reduce the blurring effect inherent to this technique that can obscure a meniscal tear.[9,10] The menisci can also be evaluated by 3D volumetric acquisitions and radial imaging. Radial imaging in which multiple planes are rotated from the center of each meniscus or center of tibia can section portions of both the medial and lateral meniscus in views similar to conventional arthrogram.

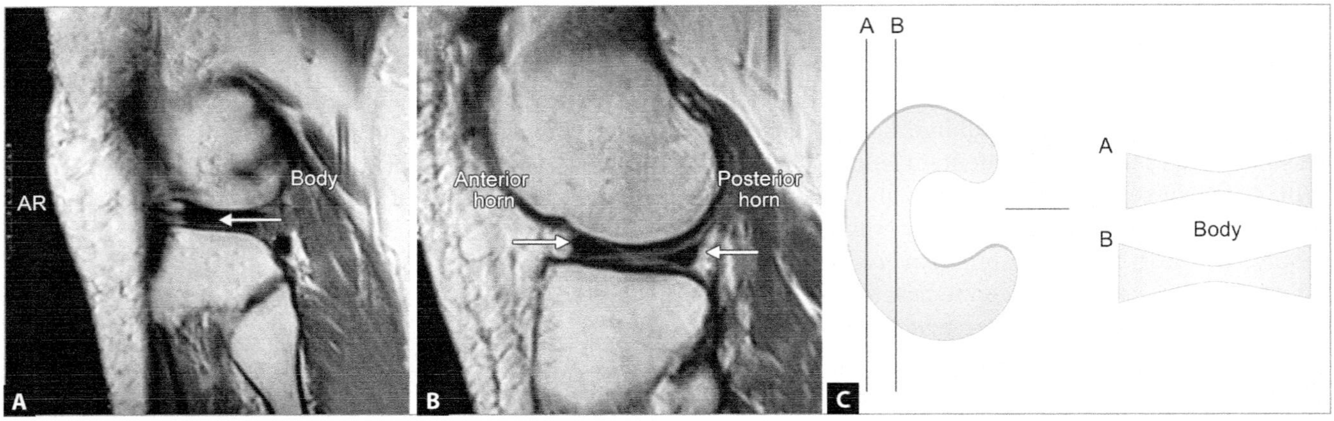

Figs. 1A to C: Sagittal T2W MR images of the knee showing a bow-tie configuration of the body of the lateral meniscus (A) and the symmetric equal size anterior and posterior horns (B). (C) Schematic diagram of the body of the meniscus seen as a bow-tie. Normal diffuse low-signal intensity of the meniscus is seen throughout—normal lateral meniscus.

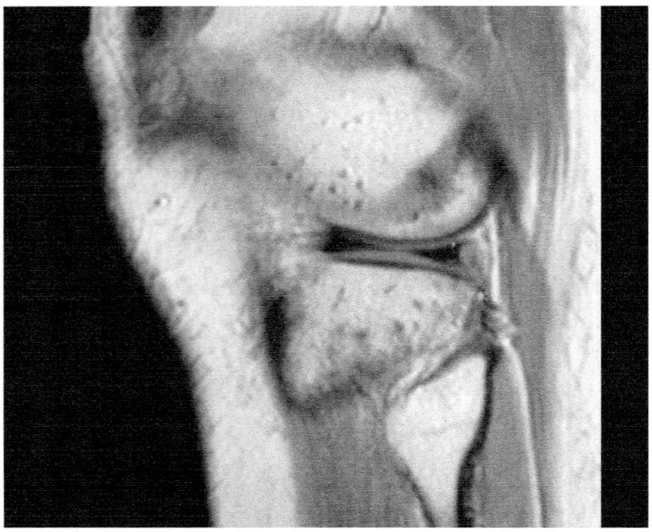

Fig. 2: Sagittal proton density MR image through the lateral meniscus showing the normal triangular shape of the meniscus thick peripherally and tapering to a thin inner edge. The normal meniscus measures 3–5 mm in height along its periphery.

Medial Meniscus

The semicircular medial meniscus has a wide posterior horn, narrows anteriorly, and has a more open C-shaped configuration than the more circular lateral meniscus. The anterior horn is roughly one-third to one-half as large as the posterior horn on sagittal images. The body of the meniscus is seen as a bow tie-shaped structure on the two most peripheral sagittal slices through the meniscus when 3- or 4-mm thick slices are obtained.[11]

The medial meniscus is attached to the joint capsule along its entire peripheral circumference. It is attached to medial femoral condyle and tibial plateau by the coronary ligament [deep fibers of medial collateral ligament (MCL)]. The less mobile medial meniscus attachment to the deep layer of the MCL and the capsule makes the medial meniscus more susceptible to injury.

Lateral Meniscus

The lateral meniscus forms a tight C-shape (more circular than the medial meniscus) and is symmetric in width from anterior to posterior. The lateral meniscus is relatively mobile, it is more loosely attached to the joint capsule especially along its posterolateral aspect where the popliteus tendon courses through its intra-articular tunnel. There is no direct attachment of the lateral meniscus to the fibular collateral ligament or lateral collateral ligament. The meniscofemoral ligaments course from the posterior horn of the lateral meniscus, along either side of PCL, to attach to the inner margin of the medial femoral condyle. The ligament of Humphry courses anterior to PCL whereas the ligament of Wrisberg passes posterior to it. One of these two limbs is present in approximately 70% of the knees, both are present in only 6%.[6]

Anatomic Variants

Discoid Meniscus

A discoid meniscus is a dysplastic meniscus in which the meniscus is disc-shaped rather than C-shaped. The lateral meniscus is most commonly affected with a reported incidence of around 3%. Often a discoid meniscus is enlarged and affects the anterior or posterior horns of the meniscus asymmetrically. On sagittal images using 4–5 mm slice thickness, a discoid meniscus exhibits a continuous or bow tie appearance on three or more consecutive images (**Figs. 3A to C**). Central tapering seen in normal menisci is lost in discoid fibrocartilage. Coronal images show the extension of the discoid meniscus apex toward or into the intercondylar notch and can be diagnosed when the body of the meniscus is more than 15 mm on a midline coronal image. Although often encountered incidentally, discoid menisci are more prone to undergo cystic degeneration with subsequent tears and multiple tears within the same meniscus are not uncommon.[12]

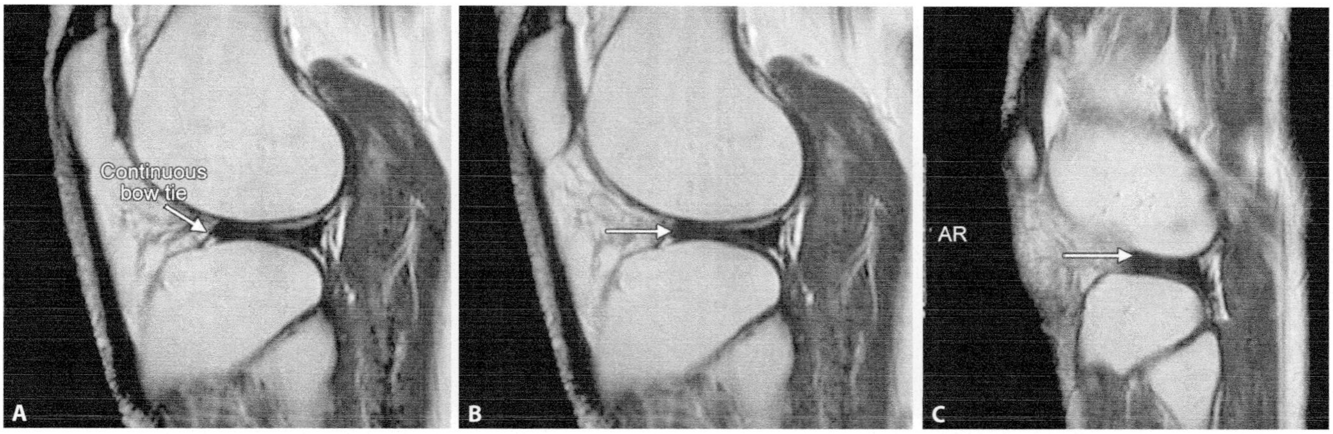

Figs. 3A to C: Consecutive 4 mm T2W sagittal MR images through the lateral meniscus showing a continuous bow-tie appearance on three sections—discoid meniscus.

Meniscus Flounce (Buckled Meniscus)

Occasionally, the medial meniscus demonstrates an undulating or buckled appearance on sagittal MR images. This redundancy is a normal variant that is related, at least in part, to knee position. Close inspection of the meniscus is needed however because a meniscal tear may occasionally result in a similar appearance.[13]

Meniscal Ossicle

This is an embryologic variant or sequelae of prior trauma. It is a small focus of ossification within the meniscus and usually involves the posterior horn of the medial meniscus.[14] Although mostly asymptomatic, a meniscal ossicle may cause mechanical symptoms or pain and can be mistaken for a loose body on radiographs or MRI.

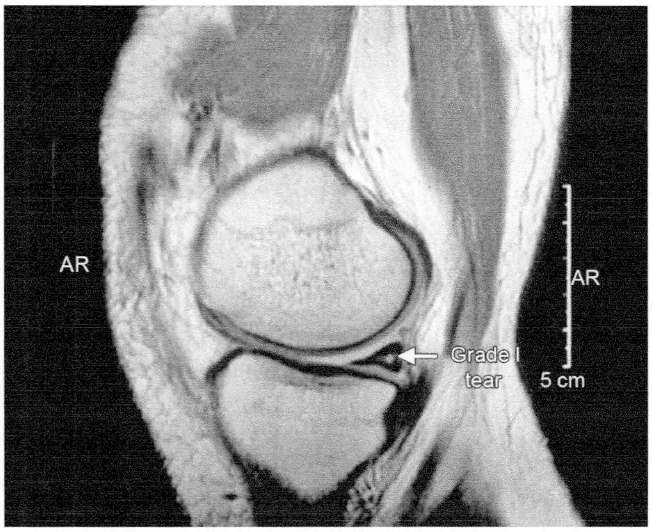

Fig. 4: Proton density sagittal MR image showing intrasubstance focal/globular increased signal within the posterior horn of the medial meniscus—Grade I meniscal signal.

Abnormal Meniscus

Meniscal Degenerations and Tears

The rotation of femur against a fixed tibia during flexion and extension places the menisci at risk for injury. Degeneration and tears of the meniscus demonstrate increased signal attributed to the imbibed synovial fluid.

MR Grading of Meniscal Tears

The MRI diagnosis of a meniscal tear is based on the alteration of intrameniscal signal characteristics. An MRI grading system divides increased intrameniscal signal into three grades according to their configuration and relation to articular surface.[15]

Grade I: In grade I, a nonarticular focal or globular intrasubstance increased signal is seen **(Fig. 4)**. Histologically, grade I signal intensity correlates with foci of early mucinous degeneration and chondrocyte deficient or hypocellular regions. Grade I signal intensity may be observed in asymptomatic athletes and normal volunteers and is not clinically significant.[16]

Grade II: In grade II, a linear intrasubstance horizontal increased signal extends from the capsular periphery of the meniscus. However, it does not involve an articular meniscal surface **(Figs. 5A and B)**. Areas and bands of mucinous degeneration are more extensive in grade II than in grade I.

Grade III: The increased signal intensity of the meniscus extends to at least one of the two articular surfaces **(Figs. 6A and B)**.

Abnormal Morphology

In addition to abnormal signal intensity, the morphology, i.e., size and shape of the meniscus should be assessed when evaluating meniscal lesions. The normal meniscus measures 3–5 mm in height. The medial meniscus varies in width from 6 mm at the anterior horn to 12 mm at the posterior horn. The lateral meniscus is approximately

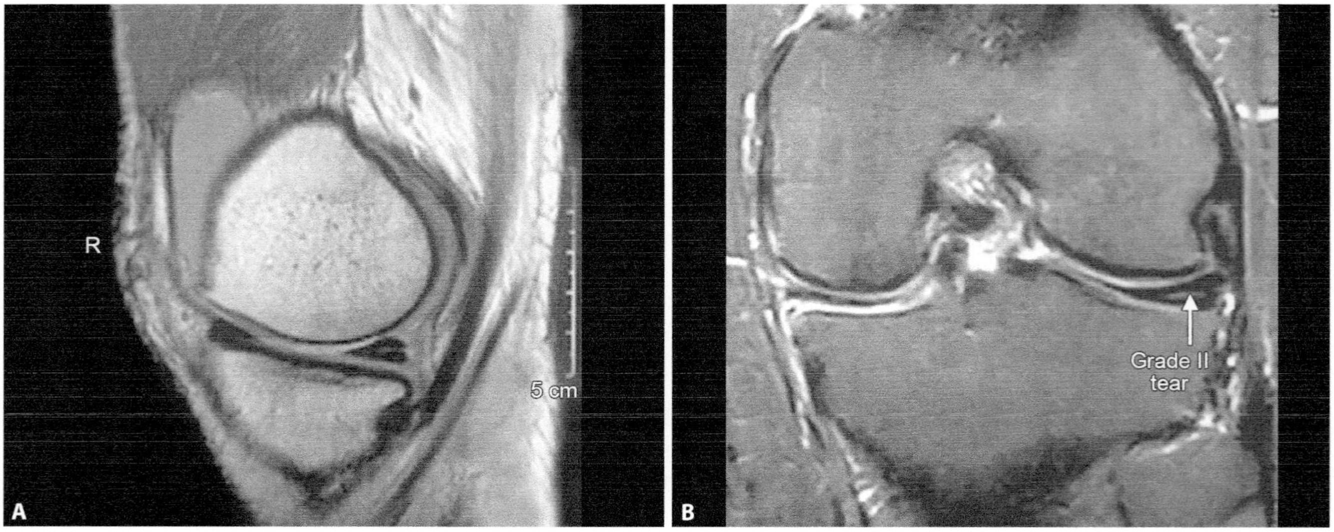

Figs. 5A and B: (A) T2W sagittal MR; and (B) STIR coronal images showing a horizontal, linear intrasubstance increased signal extending from the capsular periphery of the meniscus but not involving an articular meniscal surface—Grade II meniscal signal.

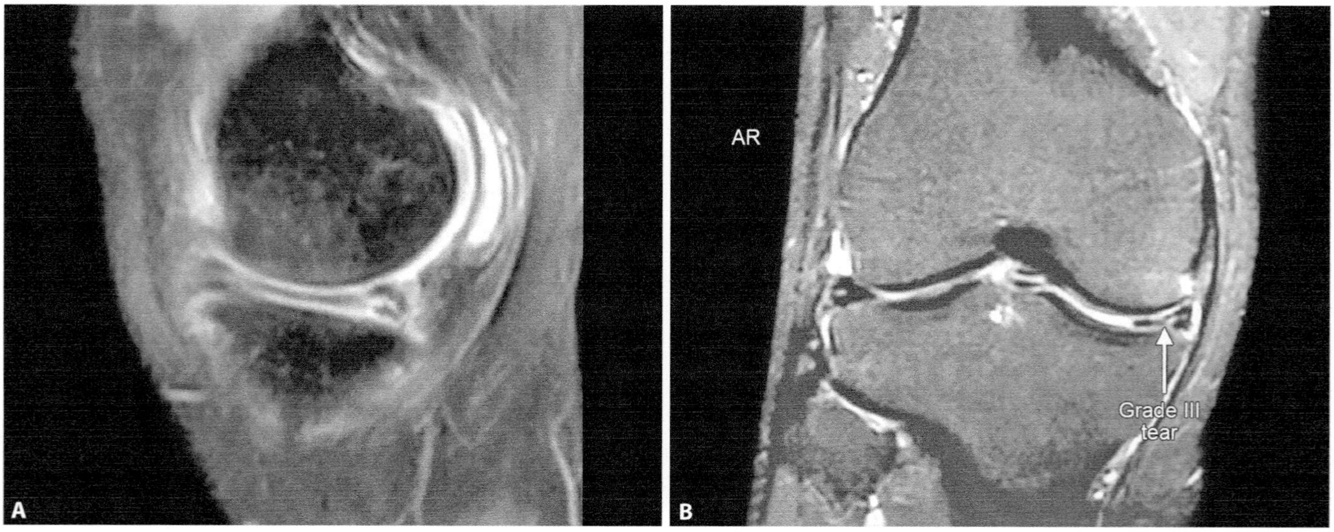

Figs. 6A and B: T2W fat suppressed sagittal (A) and (B) STIR coronal MR images showing increased signal intensity within the meniscus communicating or extending to the inferior articular surface—Grade III meniscal signal.

10 mm in width throughout its length. Irregularity of the meniscal margin, a focal defect in one of its articular surfaces or an abnormally small meniscal segment, may be indicative of a tear **(Figs. 7A and B)**. Focal step such as contour deformities and wedge defects in the contour of the articular surface "Notch sign" may be the only sign present in some tears.[17] If a smaller than normal meniscal segment is observed, a thorough search should be performed to identify a displaced fragment.

"Two-slice-touch" rule: Meniscal distortion in the absence of prior surgery and intrasubstance signal intensity extending to the articular surface, if seen on two or more consecutive images, is called the two-slice-touch rule. The positive predictive value of this sign is 94% in the medial meniscus and 96% in the lateral meniscus and should be reported as a meniscal tear.[18]

Classification of Meniscal Tears

Meniscal tears are divided into two basic types—vertical and horizontal. Vertical tears are often of a traumatic origin whereas horizontal tears are usually secondary to meniscal degeneration.

Vertical Tears

Vertical tears are further subdivided into radial (perpendicular to the long axis of the meniscus) and longitudinal (parallel to the long axis) varieties **(Fig. 8)**.

Horizontal Tears

A horizontal or oblique tear extends through the meniscus along a plane parallel to the tibial plateau, separating the meniscus into superior and inferior fragments **(Fig. 9)**.

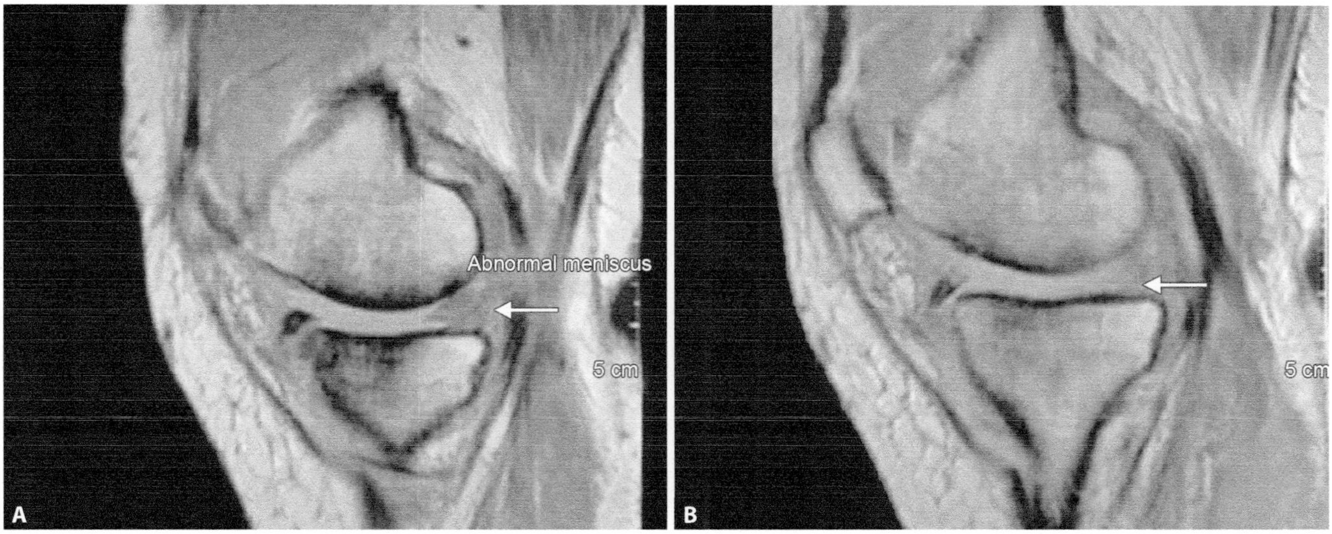

Figs. 7A and B: Consecutive proton density sagittal MR images of the knee showing irregularity and abnormally small posterior horn of the medial meniscus suggestive of a tear.

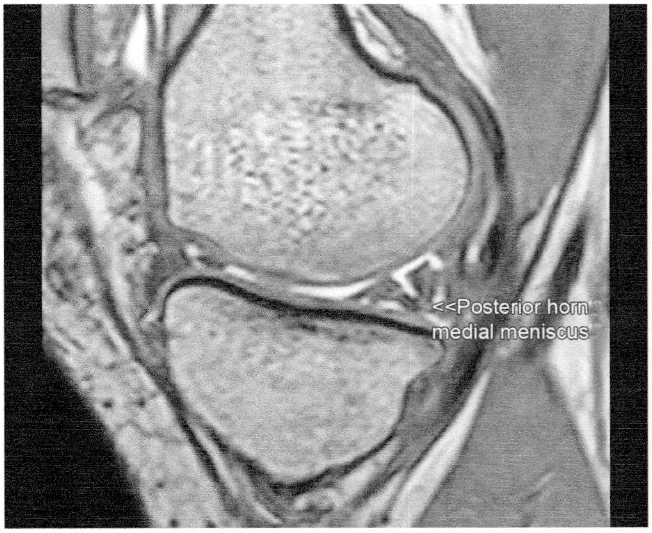

Fig. 8: Double echo steady state (DESS) sequence sagittal MR image showing a vertical longitudinal tear of the posterior horn of the medial meniscus seen as a vertically oriented linear focus of abnormal signal intensity within the substance of the meniscus along its long axis.

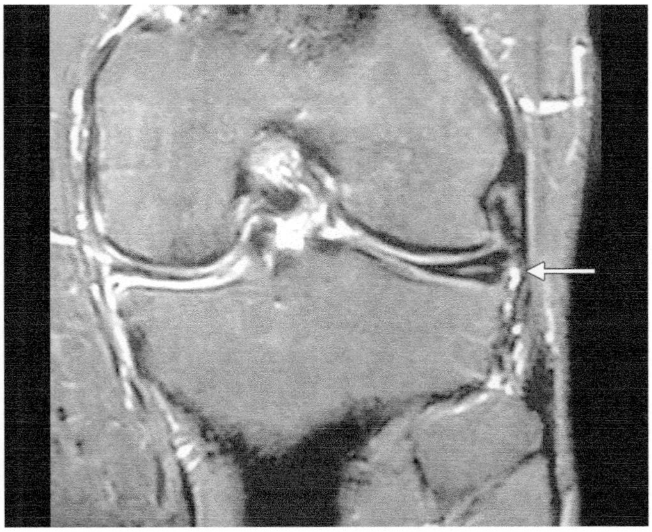

Fig. 9: STIR coronal MR image showing a horizontal tear in the body of the lateral meniscus.

Also called a horizontal cleavage tear, this is the most common type of tear to be associated with a meniscal cyst.[19] The cyst occurs as a result of fluid extending through the tear by a ball valve effect and collecting either within the meniscus (intrameniscal cyst) **(Figs. 10A and B)** or at the meniscocapsular junction (parameniscal cyst) **(Figs. 11A and B)**. If a cyst is seen along the meniscocapsular junction, an underlying meniscal tear should be excluded because the cysts tend to recur after resection if the underlying tear is not repaired. There are three criteria for the diagnosis of a meniscal cyst:

1. A tear which is horizontal in morphology
2. Accumulation of fluid seen as high-signal intensity on T2W images
3. Flat lining against the outer margin of the meniscus.

A meniscal cyst does not communicate with the joint space and is hence not opacified by contrast on MR arthrography.

Radial/Free Edge Tears

Radial tears extend perpendicular to the long axis of the meniscus. These range from a small injury along its free edge to a large tear extending through its entire circumference. MR images obtained perpendicular to the orientation of a radial tear demonstrate the tear as a small gap or cleft in the meniscus *(cleft sign)* which can sometimes be observed to move across the meniscus on successive images *(marching cleft sign)*.[20] If the orientation of the imaging plane is in the same direction as a full-thickness radial tear, a section through the same plane of the tear will demonstrate an absent meniscus or high-signal intensity resulting in the so called *ghost sign*. A partial-thickness

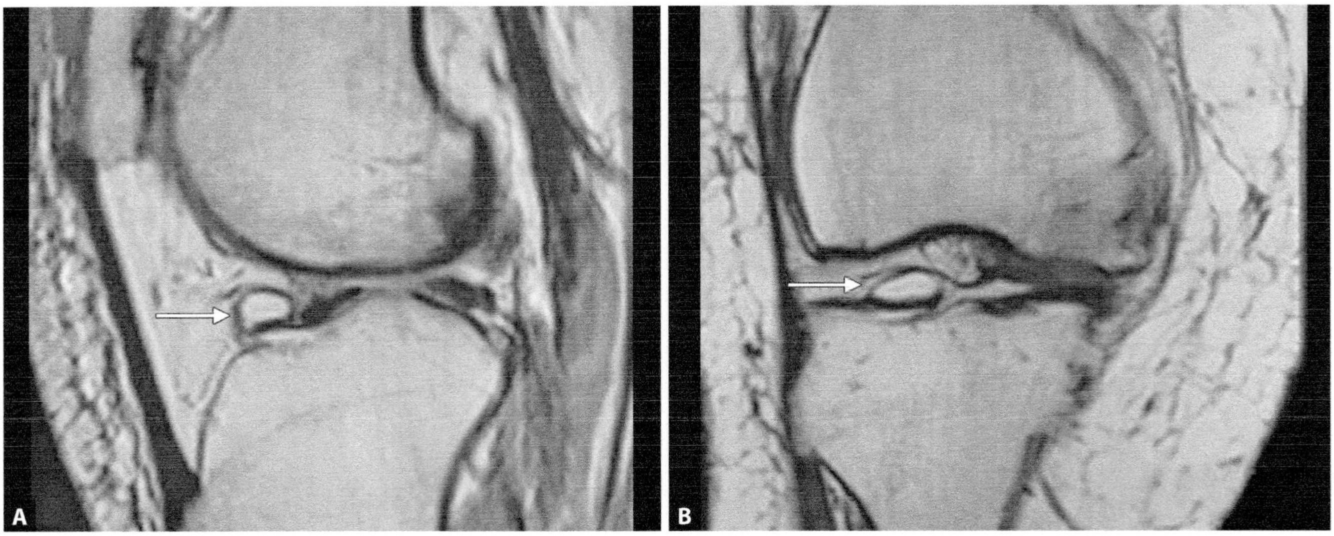

Figs. 10A and B: Sagittal and coronal MR images showing a meniscal cyst giving a slightly swollen appearance to the meniscus.

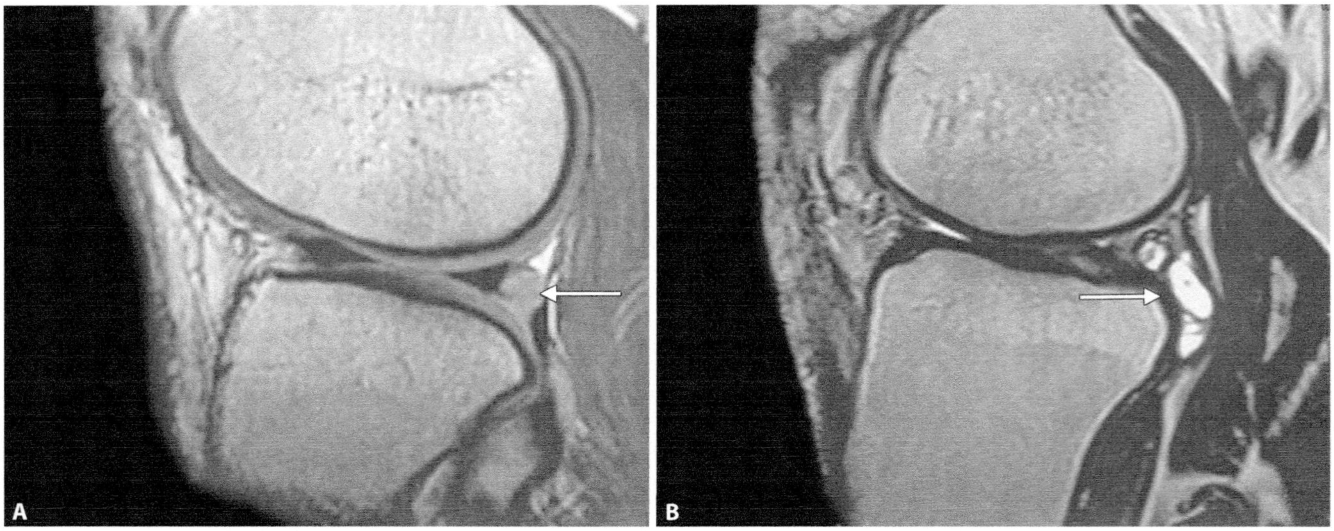

Figs. 11A and B: (A) Sagittal proton density; and (B) T2W MR images showing a fluid signal intensity structure at the meniscocapsular junction—parameniscal cyst.

radial tear will demonstrate blunting or abrupt truncation of the apex of the meniscus *(truncated triangle sign)*. A full-thickness radial tear severely compromises meniscal function by disrupting the critical circumferential collagen bundles such that the meniscus can no longer develop the "hoop stresses" necessary to disperse an axial load.[21] The middle third of the lateral meniscus is a common location for radial tears, probably because of its more circular shape and decreased radius of curvature, its increased mobility, and excessive loading during valgus stress.

Root tears: Root tears are full-thickness radial tears at the central tibial attachments of the menisci. Root tears should be suspected in cases of peripheral subluxation of the involved meniscus.[22] On posterior coronal MR images, abrupt loss or blunting of the normal meniscotibial attachment and foreshortening of the meniscus toward the posterior aspect of the intercondylar notch are seen.

Longitudinal Tears

Vertical longitudinal tears make up the common bucket handle tear that occurs in about 10% of meniscal tears. The normal meniscus has a body width of about 9 mm which is seen on sagittal images as a single slab of meniscal tissue that has a shape similar to a bow tie. When the inner edge of the meniscus displaces, a bucket handle tear is easily diagnosed by noting only one instead of the normal two body segments present on the outermost sagittal images through the meniscus. This is called the "absent bow tie sign"[10] and may be the only indication of a bucket handle tear. The anterior and posterior cruciate ligaments are the only two structures seen in the intercondylar fossa in a normal knee. A structure, in addition to these two, in the intercondylar fossa, is abnormal and is most likely to be a displaced meniscal fragment. A displaced meniscal fragment, usually, but not always, can be found especially in the intercondylar notch and a careful inspection for a fragment should always be made when only one body segment is seen on the sagittal images **(Fig. 12)**.[23,24] The displaced meniscal fragment can lie in front of the PCL which is called a "double PCL sign" **(Figs. 13A to C)**. The displaced fragment may also flip over the anterior horn of the affected meniscus which is called an "anterior flipped meniscus sign". On coronal images, a truncated appearance of the meniscus may be seen **(Figs. 14A to C)**.

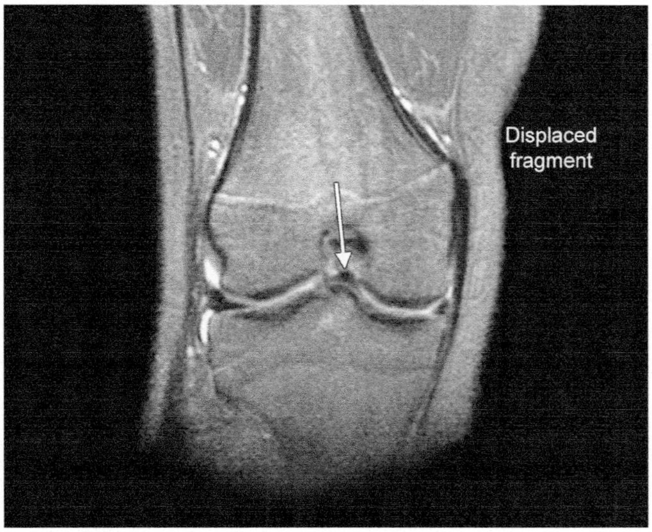

Fig. 12: STIR coronal MR image showing the displaced fragment lying within the intercondylar notch—bucket handle tear of the medial meniscus.

A new sign has been described recently for the diagnosis of bucket handle tears called the "V sign". The V sign is seen on the axial images and is seen at the junction of the displaced fragment and the meniscus, which is in place. The acute angle created accounts for the appearance as an inverted V. The V sign, when seen on axial images, is highly suggestive of a bucket handle tear.[25]

Peripheral Tear

If a tear is confined to the outer one-third of the meniscus, it is described as a peripheral tear because this changes the therapeutic plan for the patient. Except for the peripheral 10–25% of the meniscus which is supplied by the perimeniscal capillary plexus, the meniscus in adults is relatively avascular. Because of the rich vascularity in peripheral portion of the meniscus (red zone), this type of tear is more likely to heal with conservative therapy or operative repair, whereas tears confined to the inner white zone of the meniscus (avascular) have to be debrided or resected.[26]

Complex Tear

A combination of horizontal, longitudinal, and radial components constitutes a complex tear. The tear extends in more than one plane and the meniscus appears fragmented.[27]

Meniscocapsular Separation

A meniscocapsular separation refers to an injury in which the meniscus separates from the adjacent capsule. This can lead to meniscal instability if unrecognized and is most commonly seen along the medial meniscus, which is more tightly adherent to the joint capsule. It can also occur along

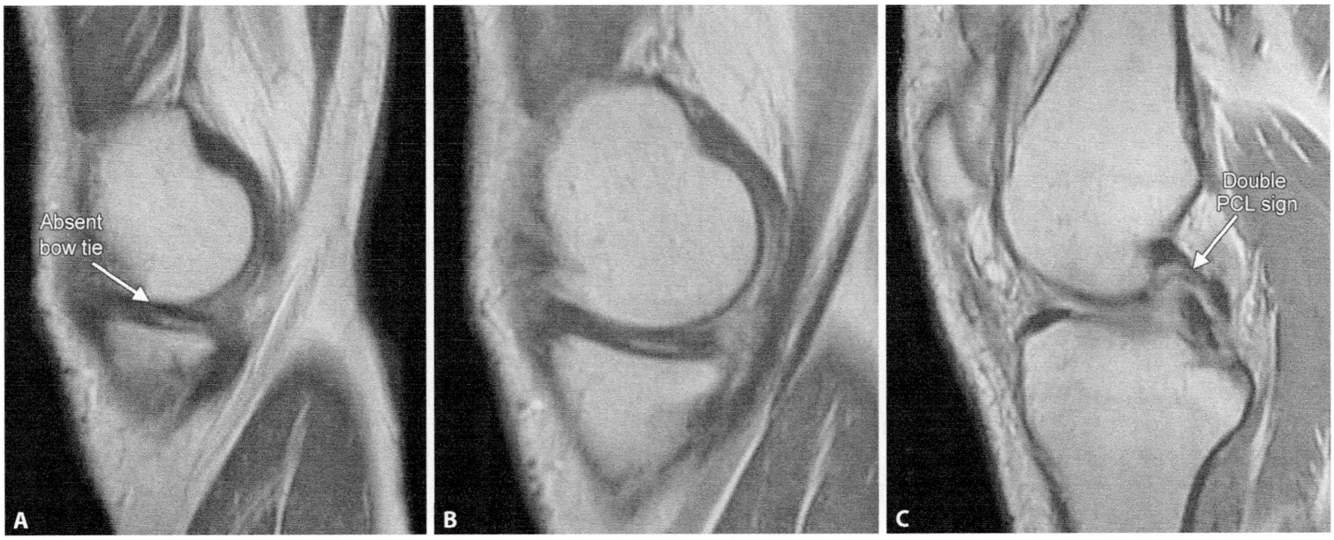

Figs. 13A to C: T2W sagittal MR images showing absent bow tie sign (A and B) and a displaced meniscal fragment beneath the posterior cruciate ligament (PCL) designated as a double PCL sign (C)—bucket handle tear of the medial meniscus.

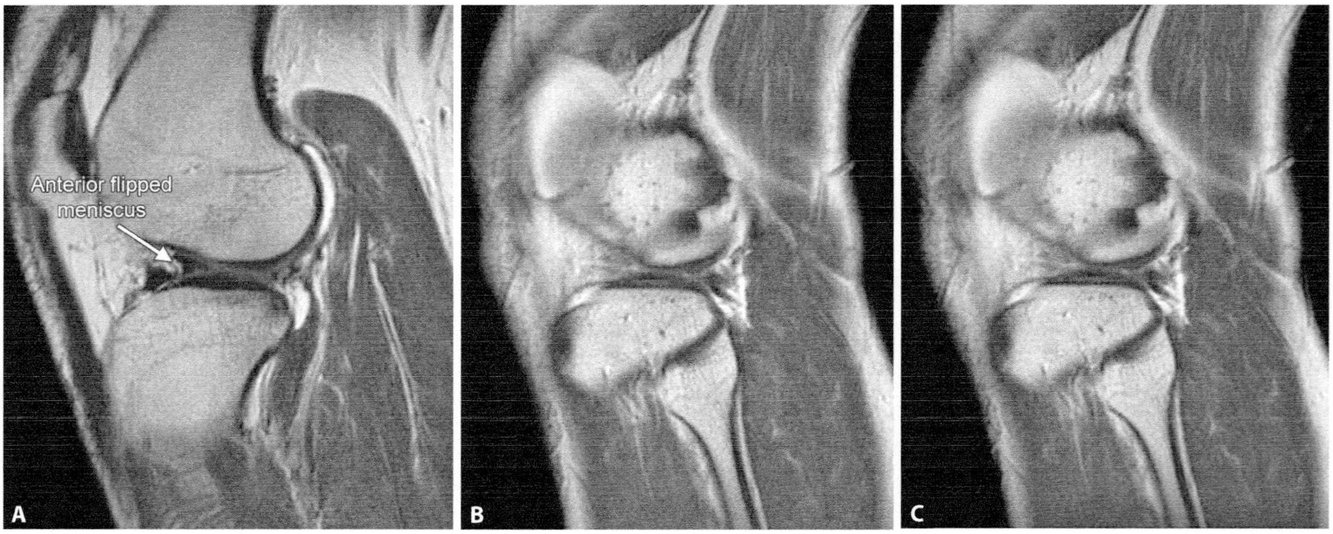

Figs. 14A to C: T2W sagittal MR images showing the displaced fragment flip over the anterior horn of the lateral meniscus (A) with an absent bow-tie sign (B and C)—bucket handle tear of the lateral meniscus.

the PLC of the joint where the lateral meniscus is attached by the popliteal meniscal fascicles. This injury is diagnosed when true fluid signal intensity is seen interposed between the meniscus and adjacent capsule or when the popliteal meniscal fascicles are disrupted.

Indirect Signs of the Meniscal Tear

There are some indirect signs that suggest a meniscal tear.[27]

Parameniscal Cysts

A parameniscal cyst when present suggests a horizontal tear of the meniscus. These represent the peripheral escape of joint fluid through a meniscal tear. Parameniscal cysts are differentiated from bursae and ganglion cysts owing to their intimate contact with a meniscus either directly or via a fluid track.

Meniscal Extrusion

It is said to be present when the peripheral margin of the meniscus extends 3 mm or more beyond the tibial plateau edge. There is a close association between meniscal extrusion and root tears.

Subchondral Marrow Edema

Linear subchondral bone marrow edema adjacent to the meniscal attachment site less than 5 mm deep and paralleling the articular surface can be seen with 90% of lateral meniscus tears and 60% of medial meniscus tears.[28] Contusions/bone bruises in the posterior medial tibial plateau have an associated tear of the posterior horn of the medial meniscus.

Imaging Challenges

Although MRI is extremely accurate in diagnosing meniscal pathology, there are numerous imaging pitfalls and artifacts that may simulate a tear and lead to an erroneous diagnosis. These are especially common in the posterior horn of the lateral meniscus.

Potential Pitfalls

Transverse Intrameniscal Ligament

On sagittal scans, the attachment of the transverse ligament to the anterior horn of the medial or lateral meniscus may be mistaken for a tear. This pitfall is avoided by following the meniscal fragment on successive sagittal scans, recognizing that it is contiguous with the normal ligament coursing across the infrapatellar fat.

Meniscofemoral Ligaments

Similarly, the attachment of the meniscofemoral ligaments of Humphry or Wrisberg to the posterior horn of the lateral meniscus may be mistaken for a tear on sagittal scans. Again, examination of sequential sagittal or appropriate coronal scans should allow for accurate diagnosis.[29]

Popliteus Tendon

There is usually at least a small amount of fluid within the popliteus tendon sheath that can be mistaken for a tear at the junction of the posterior horn and body of the lateral meniscus on sagittal or coronal scans.[30]

Magic Angle Effect

The posterior horn of the lateral meniscus courses slightly upward as it extends into the posterior intercondylar notch. As a result, artifactually increased signal may be seen within the meniscus on short TE sequences because of the magic angle artifact. This is due to the magic angle phenomenon caused by 55° orientation of this meniscus with respect to the static magnetic field. The signal, however, is often of a rather diffuse nature and disappears on long TE images (>40 ms).[31]

Pulsation Artifact from the Popliteal Artery

Phase artifacts propagating from the popliteal artery may mimic a tear in the posterior horn of the lateral meniscus on sagittal scans. Misdiagnosis can be avoided by recognizing the alternating lines of increased and decreased signal propagating across the entire image at that level.

Surgical Considerations in Meniscal Tear

When faced with a meniscal tear, the surgeon has three options—(1) leave the tear alone, (2) attempt a primary meniscal repair, and (3) perform a partial or complete meniscectomy. The paramount goal is to preserve as much meniscal tissue as possible to lessen the probability of developing osteoarthritis (OA).[32] Several features have been shown to be correlated with a higher probability of a successful meniscal repair and these features should be included in the MRI report by the radiologist.

Tear Location

The most important factor in predicting the success of a meniscal repair is where the tear is located in the meniscus, e.g., a tear in the periphery of the meniscus (within 3 mm of its capsular surface) has the highest probability for healing because of the excellent vascularity in that region.[26]

Blind spots for the arthroscopist include the anterior horn of each meniscus, the extreme inner portion of the posterior horn of the medial meniscus, and the undersurface of both menisci. It is also important to describe any meniscal tissue that has become displaced into a para-articular "gutter" so that the arthroscopist is able to probe for and resect the fragment, which might otherwise be missed.

Tear Morphology and Length

Vertical longitudinal tears have the best prognosis for healing because they do not disrupt the circumferential collagen bundles that are important for maintaining normal meniscal function.

Small partial tears (involving less than half the height of the meniscus) and radial tears measuring less than 5 mm in length also have a higher rate of healing than do larger tears.[26,33] A radial tear extending through the meniscus to the capsule is essentially unrepairable because of the complete disruption of the circumferential collagen bundles. Most horizontal tears are also not amenable to repair and the surgeon typically resects either the superior or inferior flap, leaving the other *in situ*.

Accuracy of MR in the Diagnosis of the Meniscal Tears

The accuracy of MR imaging of meniscal tears is greater than 90% in most series and the negative predictive value approaches 100%.[34,35] An additional advantage of MRI is the ability to evaluate extra-articular cause of knee pain masquerading as meniscal disease.

CENTRAL STRUCTURES OF THE KNEE

Anterior Cruciate Ligament

Anatomy

The ACL provides central support of the knee joint, contributing the most significant stabilizing mechanism against excessive anterior translation of the tibia. The ACL is a fan-shaped structure, with a tightly bound femoral attachment that expands broadly at the tibial attachment. The ACL is 11 mm wide and 31–38 mm long. The individual fascicles of the ACL are divided into two longitudinal fiber bundles, the longer and stronger anteromedial bundle (AMB) and the shorter posterolateral bundle (PLB).[36]

MR Appearance

T2W sagittal 3–4 mm thickness images are recommended for evaluating the ACL. It is also well-visualized on the axial and coronal images. The normal ACL has straight, taut fibers that run parallel to the roof of the intercondylar notch **(Figs. 15A and B)**. It typically has a striated appearance with some high signal within it especially at its insertion on the tibia.

ACL Tears

The most common mechanism of ACL tear is external rotation of femur on a fixed tibia combined with valgus force (i.e., twisting injury).

On MRI, an ACL tear is diagnosed by alterations in signal intensity, morphology, and the course of the ligament. An increased signal intensity within the ACL on PD and T2W images indicates an acute or subacute injury. A cloud-like amorphous mass of increased signal intensity may be evident within the ligament reflecting edema or hemorrhage **(Figs. 16A and B)**.

A complete ACL tear can be diagnosed when the ligament is either absent ("empty notch sign" in coronal images) **(Figs. 17A and B)** or discontinuous. An irregular or wavy contour and disruption of fibers also suggests a complete tear.[37]

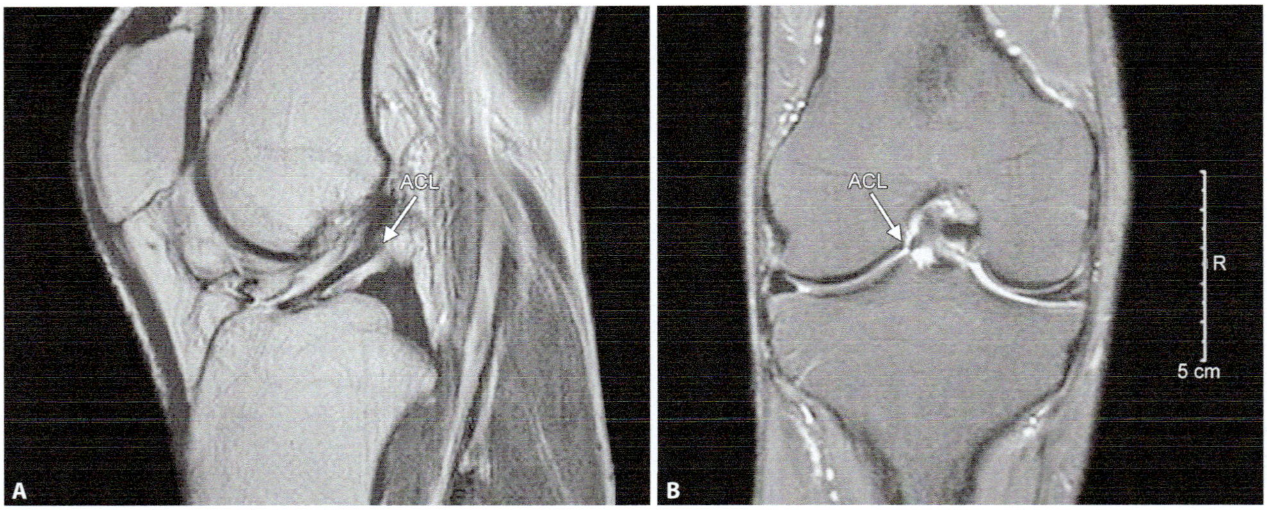

Figs. 15A and B: (A) T2W sagittal MR image of the knee depicting the normal anterior cruciate ligament (ACL) with straight, taut fibers that run parallel to the roof of the intercondylar notch; (B) STIR coronal MR image showing the ACL as a triangular structure within the notch.

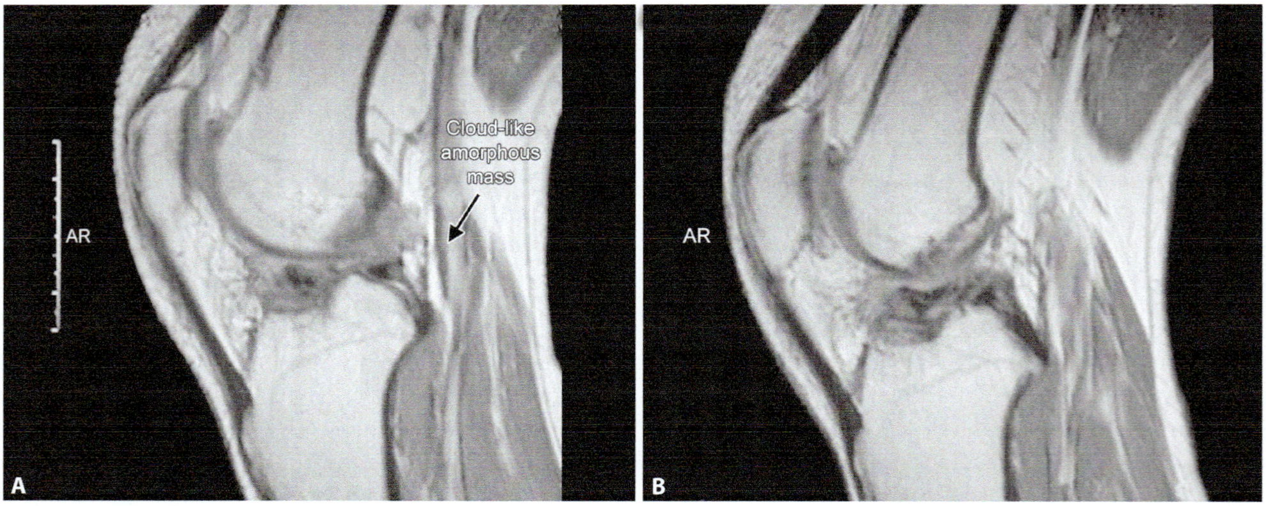

Figs. 16A and B: T2W sagittal MR images of the knee showing complete disruption of anterior cruciate ligament (ACL) fibers with a cloud-like amorphous mass of increased signal intensity in the region of ACL reflecting edema and hemorrhage—complete ACL tear.

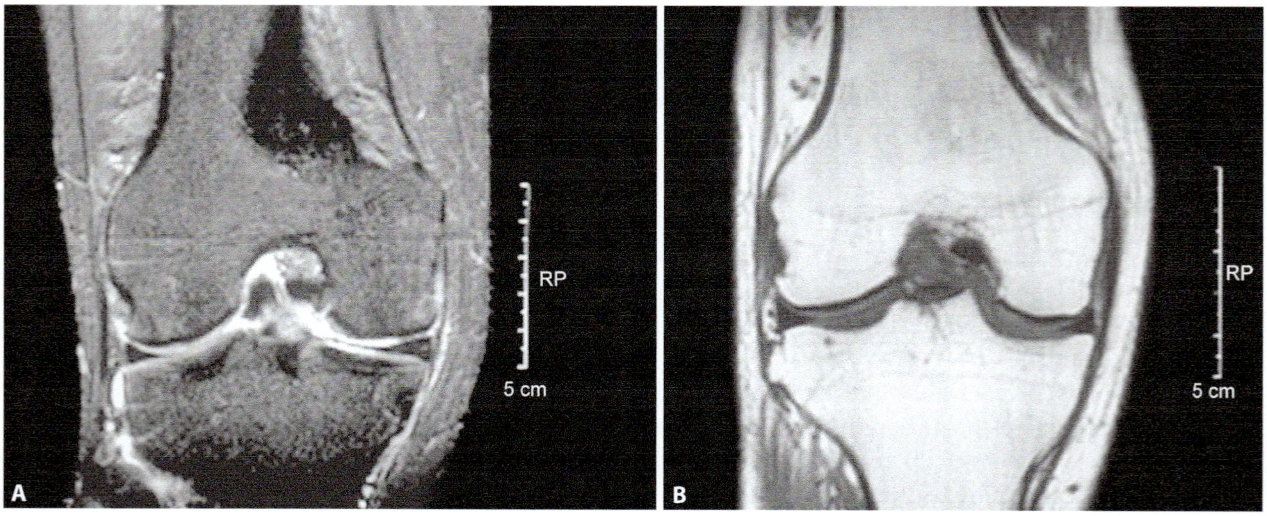

Figs. 17A and B: (A) STIR coronal image of the knee showing normal anterior cruciate ligament (ACL) and posterior cruciate ligament (PCL) in the intercondylar notch; (B) T1W coronal image shows the ACL to be absent (empty notch sign) in a case of ACL tear.

Indirect signs of ACL tear include:

- Buckling (abnormal high arc) of the PCL giving rise to a "question mark" configuration **(Fig. 18)**.
- Undulation and redundancy of the patellar tendon.
- *Uncovered lateral meniscus sign*: This sign is positive if a vertical line drawn tangentially to the most posterior margin of the lateral tibial plateau intersects any part of the posterior horn of the lateral meniscus. A positive uncovered lateral meniscus sign indicates that the lateral meniscus does not subluxate anteriorly with the tibia in an ACL injury.

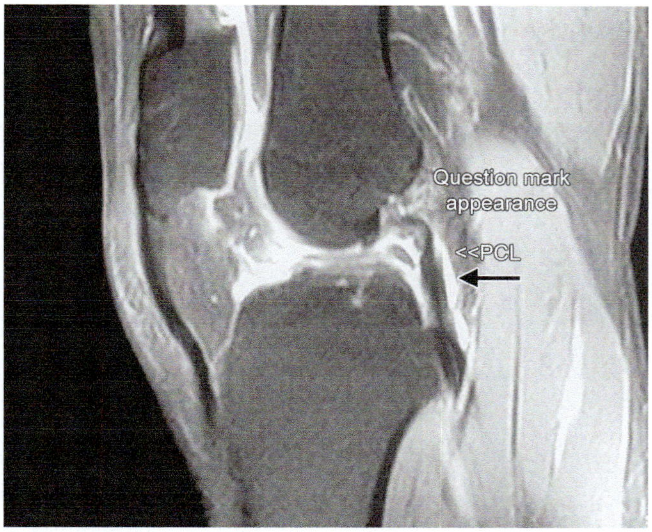

Fig. 18: T2W fat suppressed sagittal image of knee showing abnormal high arc (buckling) of the posterior cruciate ligament (PCL) giving rise to a "question mark" configuration—indirect sign of anterior cruciate ligament tear.

- Anterior tibial subluxation larger than 5 mm with respect to femur is a very sensitive and specific sign of complete ACL tear. If the distance between two parallel lines drawn tangential to the posterior lateral femoral condyle and posterior lateral tibial plateau is more than 5 mm, it is a sensitive ancillary sign of complete ACL tear **(Figs. 19A and B)**. This sign offers improved discrimination of complete from partial tears which is clinically important since the presence of partial tear is not considered an indication for surgical reconstruction.[38]
- Lateral notch sign in which the deep lateral femoral notch exceeds 2 mm in depth.
- Bone bruises/contusions in the midportion of the lateral femoral condyle and posterior portion of the lateral tibial plateau.[39,40] These so-called kissing contusions are representative of edema and hemorrhage caused by impaction trabecular microfractures that occur when the ACL ruptures **(Figs. 20A to C)**.
- Avulsion fracture of the lateral tibial rim (Segond fracture) is also suggestive of ACL tear.
- Joint effusion/hemarthrosis is a common finding associated with ACL injuries **(Fig. 20C)**.[41]
- A tibial spine avulsion is an uncommon but specific finding for ACL injury. Chronic tears of ACL may present with slumping of the distal fragment over the tibial indicating increased laxity of the ligament which may also be attenuated. In chronic tears, edema and synovitis are usually not present. MR also has an important role in defining partial tears of the ACL because these injuries are difficult to differentiate from complete ACL tears clinically. The detection of a discrete area or focus of increased signal intensity

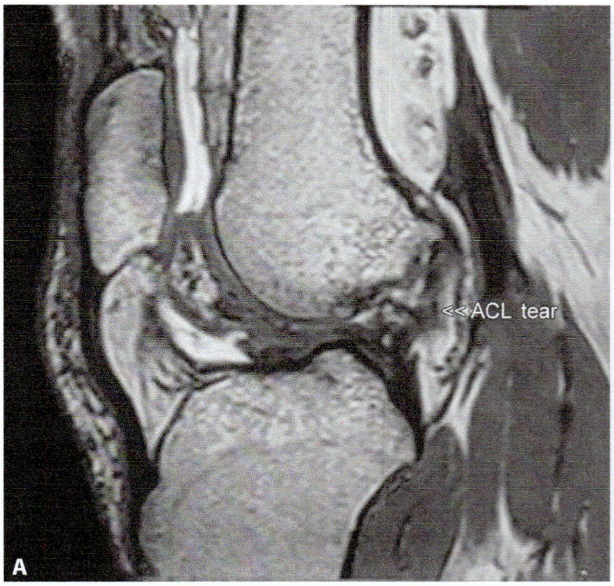

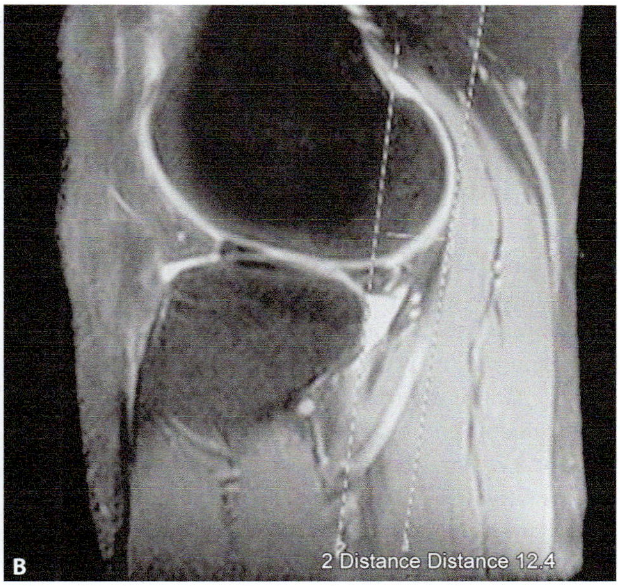

Figs. 19A and B: (A) Double echo steady state sagittal; and (B) T2W fat suppressed sagittal MR images of the knee showing cloud-like amorphous mass of increased signal in the region of anterior cruciate ligament (ACL) with anterior tibial translation larger than 5 mm with respect to femur—indirect sign of complete ACL tear.

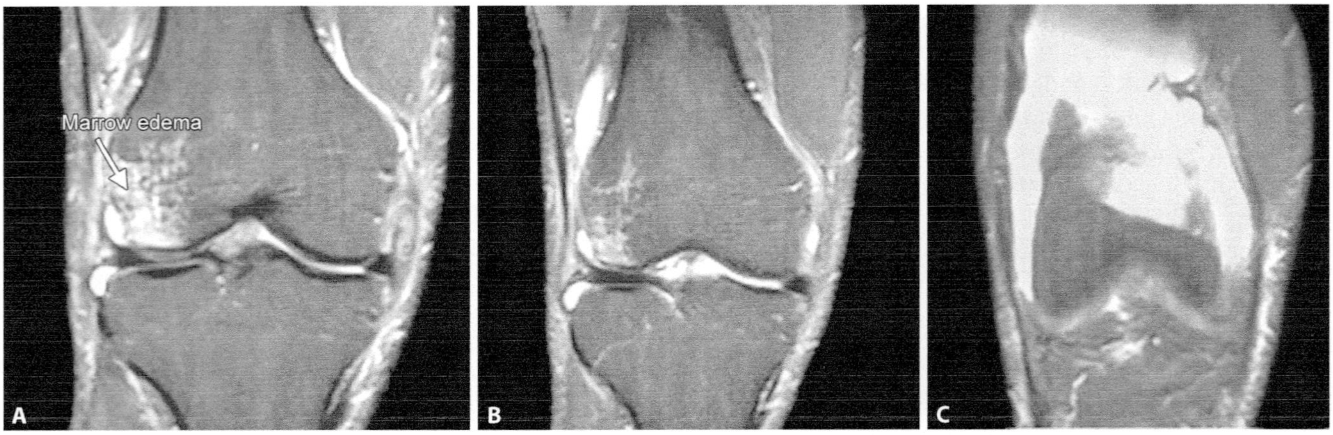

Figs. 20A to C: STIR coronal MR images of the knee showing marrow edema in the lateral femoral condyle and suprapatellar joint effusion—indirect signs of anterior cruciate ligament tear.

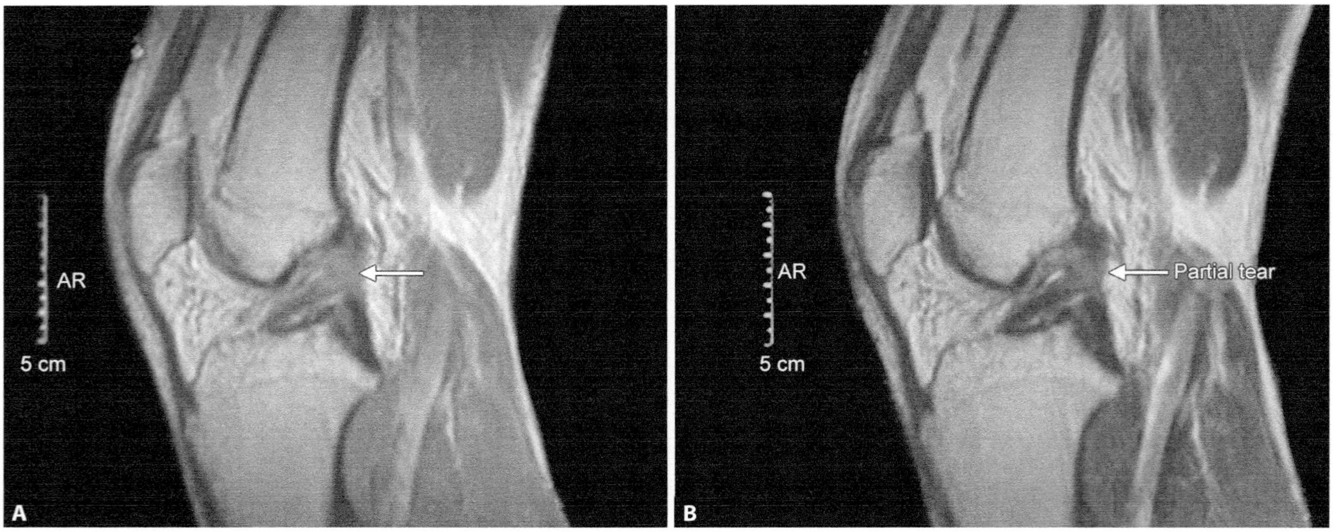

Figs. 21A and B: (A) Proton density; and (B) T2W sagittal MR images showing a discrete area of increased signal intensity within the substance of the anterior cruciate ligament (ACL), the ligament appearing intact—partial tear of ACL.

within the substance of the ACL is consistent with a diagnosis of partial tear **(Figs. 21A and B)**. In partial tear, although the bulk of the ligament appears to be intact with a relatively normal axis, there may be localized angulation of the ligament at the site of fiber disruption. False-negative diagnosis may result from the formation of scar tissue with adherence of ACL to the postcruciate ligament simulating a normal course and signal of the ACL. A partial volume averaging with the lateral femoral condyle and periligamentous or intraligamentous fat should be differentiated from partial ACL tears to avoid false positive diagnosis. A false positive diagnosis may also be seen in mucoid degeneration and ganglion cyst of the ACL. However, the ligament in these cases has a striated appearance on T2W images with interspersed intact ligamentous fibers resembling a "celery stalk".[42] Often an intraosseous ganglion cyst is seen at the tibial insertion of the ACL. Typically, there is no previous history of trauma.

O'Donoghue triad: A triad of ACL injury associated with MCL disruption and medial meniscus tear is known as O'Donoghue triad **(Figs. 22A to C)**.

Accuracy of MR in ACL tears: Accuracy of MRI for tears of the ACL is extremely high approaching 95–100% in almost all reported series.[4]

Posterior Cruciate Ligament

Anatomy

The PCL originates in the lateral aspect of the medial femoral condyle, crosses the ACL, and attaches to the posterior intercondylar fossa of tibia.[43] It averages 38 mm in length and 13 mm in width at its midportion. The PCL

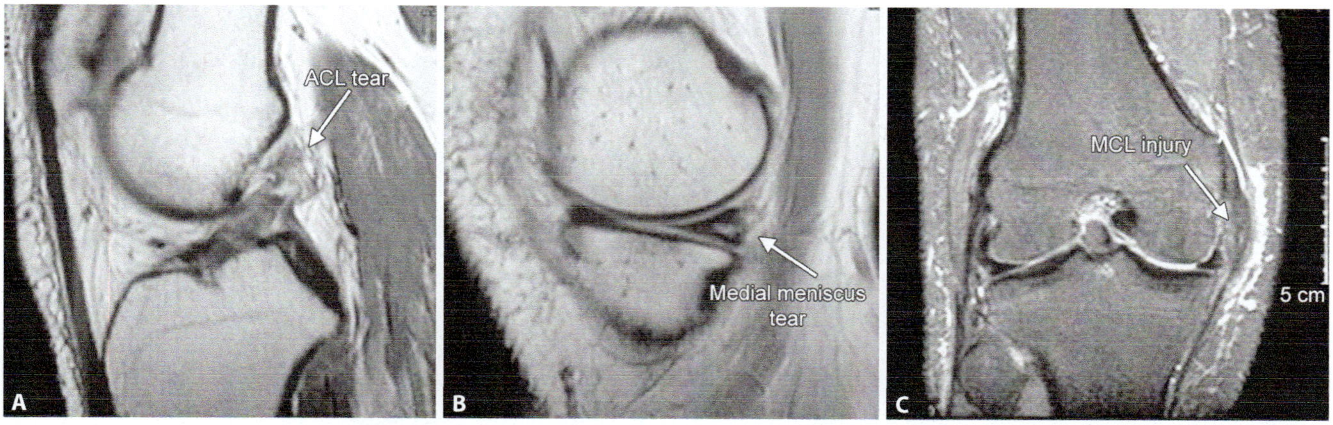

Figs. 22A to C: (A and B) T2W sagittal; and (C) STIR coronal MR images showing anterior cruciate ligament tear, medial meniscus tear, and injury of the medial collateral ligament—O'Donoghue triad.

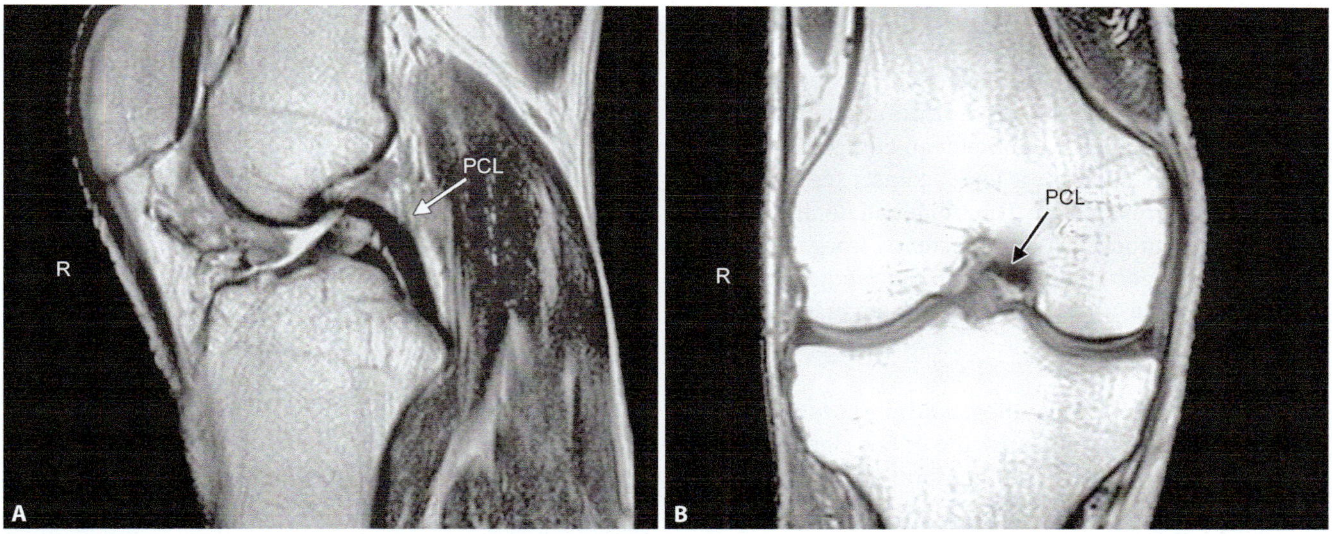

Figs. 23A and B: (A) T2W sagittal MR image of knee showing normal posterior cruciate ligament (PCL) as a band-like structure of low-signal intensity having an arcuate shape; (B) T1W coronal MR image showing the normal PCL as a triangular structure within the intercondylar notch.

provides central support to the knee joint and protects against excessive posterior translation of tibia, stabilizes the joint against excessive varus and valgus stress, and restricts external rotation of tibia.

MR Appearance

On MRI, the PCL is normally depicted as a band-like structure of low signal intensity. In sagittal images, it has an arcuate shape with the knee in neutral position **(Figs. 23A and B)**.

PCL Injury

MR findings of PCL injury are anatomic disruption, increased signal intensity in the ligament, and redundancy of an avulsed ligament.[44]

Injuries to the PCL are classified as **(Figs. 24A to C)**:

- *Grade I* is consistent with intraligamentous edema and hemorrhage and appears as foci of increased signal in a ligament with otherwise intact borders.
- *Grade II* injuries represent partial tears.
- *Grade III* abnormalities represent complete tears.

Aggressive surgical treatment of PCL tears is recently becoming more common since chronic knee instability with early degenerative arthritis has become better appreciated with chronic injuries of the PCL.

MEDIAL STRUCTURES OF THE KNEE

Anatomy

Medially, the supporting structures of the knee are arranged in three layers. The invested deep fascia of the sartorius muscle, which overlies the gastrocnemius muscle, forms the most superficial layer.[45] The tibial

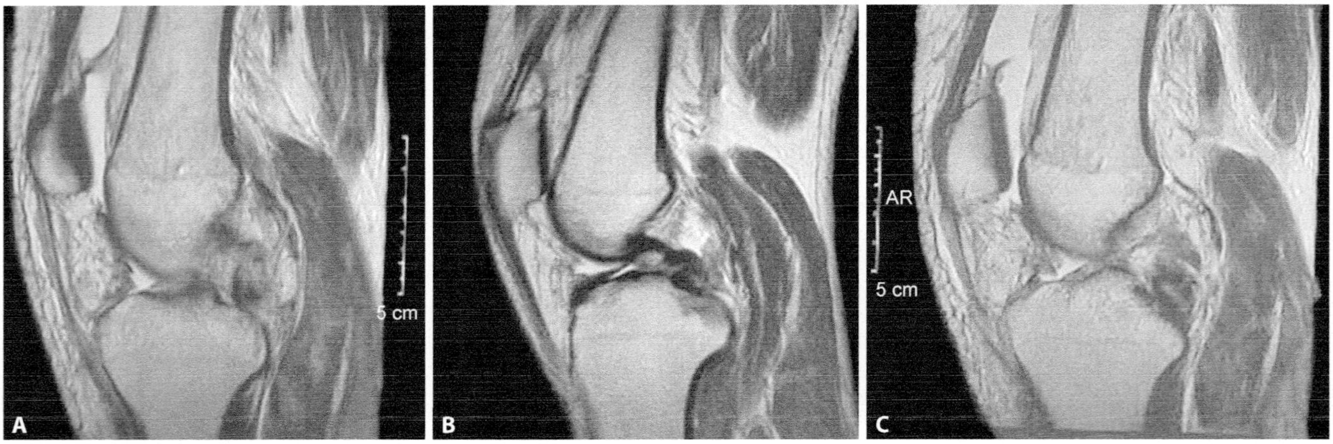

Figs. 24A to C: T2W sagittal MR images showing (A) grade I tear of the posterior cruciate ligament seen as intraligamentous edema and hemorrhage; (B) Grade II tear seen as partial tear of the tibial attachment; and (C) Grade III tear seen as a complete disruption of the ligament.

collateral ligament and the superficial component of the MCL forms the middle layer. The deepest layer is comprised of the meniscofemoral and meniscotibial ligaments, which constitute the deep components of the MCL. The MCL stabilizes the knee against excessive valgus force and hyperextension. The tibial collateral ligament, the primary support structure, extends from the medial epicondylar region of the femur to the medial surface of the proximal tibia and spans about 8–9 cm in length.[46]

Magnetic Resonance Imaging

On MRI, the MCL is best displayed on coronal images and appears as a smooth structure of low signal intensity that extends from the medial femoral epicondyle to the proximal tibial metaphysis **(Fig. 25)**. At the level of the joint line, the superficial and deep portions of the ligament are separated by a bursa and surrounding fat which should not be mistaken for a localized meniscocapsular separation.

MCL Injury

Twisting injuries cause a large number of MCL injuries.

- In grade I injury, a slight contour irregularity or thickening of the ligament may be seen but there is no discontinuity of its fibers. Edema and hemorrhage are identified in the soft tissue and subcutaneous fat paralleling the MCL **(Figs. 26A and B)**.
- In grade II, discontinuity of some fibers may be evident.
- In grade III, frank discontinuity of all its fibers is seen **(Figs. 27A and B)**. Two findings that may be encountered on conventional radiography are predictive of underlying MCL injury. Pellegrini-Stieda disease or calcification around the medial femoral condyle represents chronic partial or complete tears of the MCL.[47] The reverse Segond fracture is an avulsion fracture of medial tibial plateau at the attachment of the deep fibers of the MCL. This finding is associated with PCL disruption and peripheral medial meniscal tear.

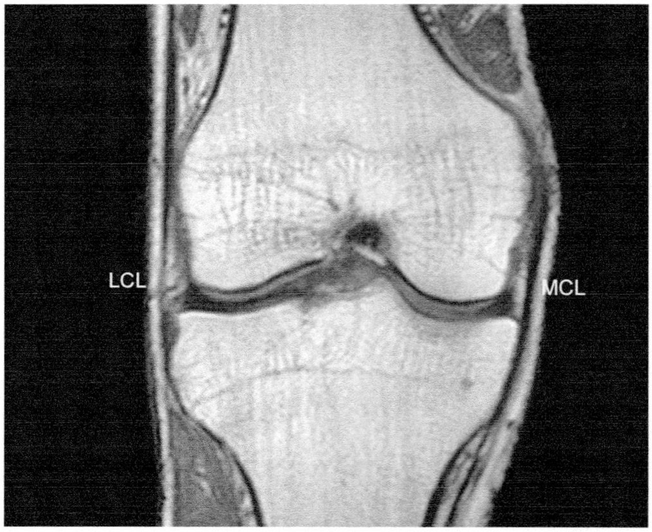

Fig. 25: T1W coronal MR image of the knee showing the normal medial collateral ligament (MCL) as a low-signal intensity structure that extends from the medial femoral epicondyle to the proximal tibial metaphysis.

CORNER-BASED ANATOMY OF THE KNEE

The secondary stabilizers of the knee can be thought of in terms of "corner"-based anatomy. The corners of the knee include PLC, PMC, ALC, and AMC or the extensor mechanism of the knee.

Posterolateral Corner of the Knee

Of all the corners about the knee, the PLC has received the greatest attention. Once regarded as the "dark side of the knee", the fine anatomic details of the region have now been elucidated owing to the advances in imaging.[48] Timely diagnosis and interventions of the PLC injuries are imperative to prevent chronic knee instability, cartilage damage, and failed ligament reconstruction.

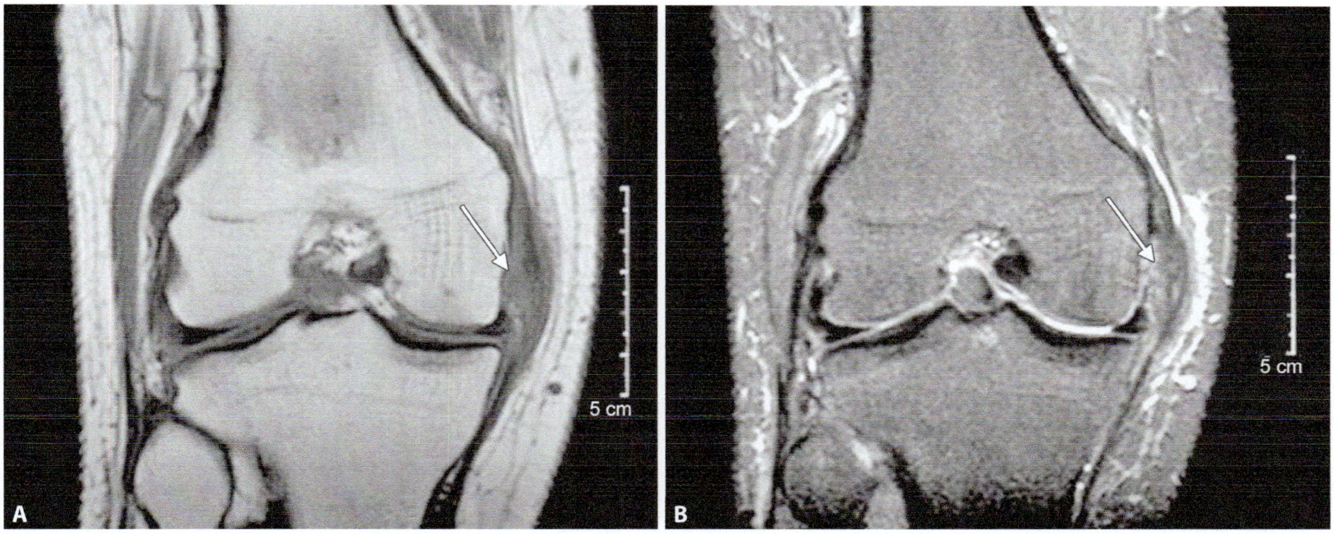

Figs. 26A and B: (A) T1W coronal MR; and (B) STIR coronal images showing grade I medial collateral ligament (MCL) injury as edema and hemorrhage in the soft tissue and subcutaneous fat paralleling the MCL with slight contour irregularity of the ligament.

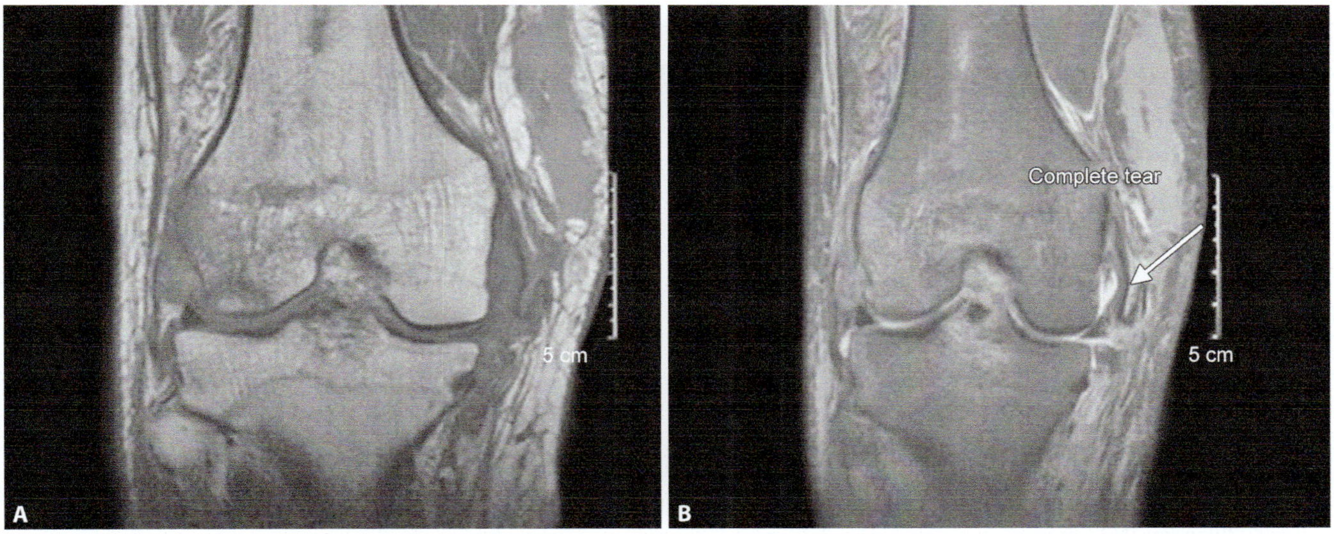

Figs. 27A and B: (A) TIW; and (B) STIR coronal MR images showing a complete disruption of the medial collateral ligament (MCL) with extensive edema and hemorrhage in the adjacent soft tissues and subcutaneous fat. Extensive bone marrow contusions are also noted—complete MCL tear.

Anatomy

The PLC of the knee is composed of ligaments, muscles, and tendons that are static and dynamic restraints to posterior translation, varus angulations, and external rotation of the knee. Also called the arcuate ligament complex, they include the fibular ligament or lateral collateral ligament (LCL), popliteus muscle and tendon, popliteofibular ligament, biceps femoris tendon, fabellofibular ligament, and the arcuate ligament. The components are summarized in **Box 1**.

The fibular collateral ligament or LCL is 5-7 cm long, arising from a tubercle on the lateral femoral condyle directly above the groove of the popliteus tendon origin. It inserts on the lateral surface of the head of the fibula, joining the biceps femoris tendon to form the conjoined tendon **(Figs. 28A and B)**. The main function of the LCL is to stabilize the knee against varus forces.[50]

Box 1: Components of the posterolateral corner.[48,49]

- Fibular collateral ligament
- Popliteus tendon and muscle complex
- Arcuate ligament
- Fabellofibular ligament
- Posterolateral joint capsule
- Popliteofibular ligament

The fabellofibular ligament courses from the fibular styloid process to the fabella, a normal sesamoid bone within the lateral gastrocnemius tendon. The arcuate

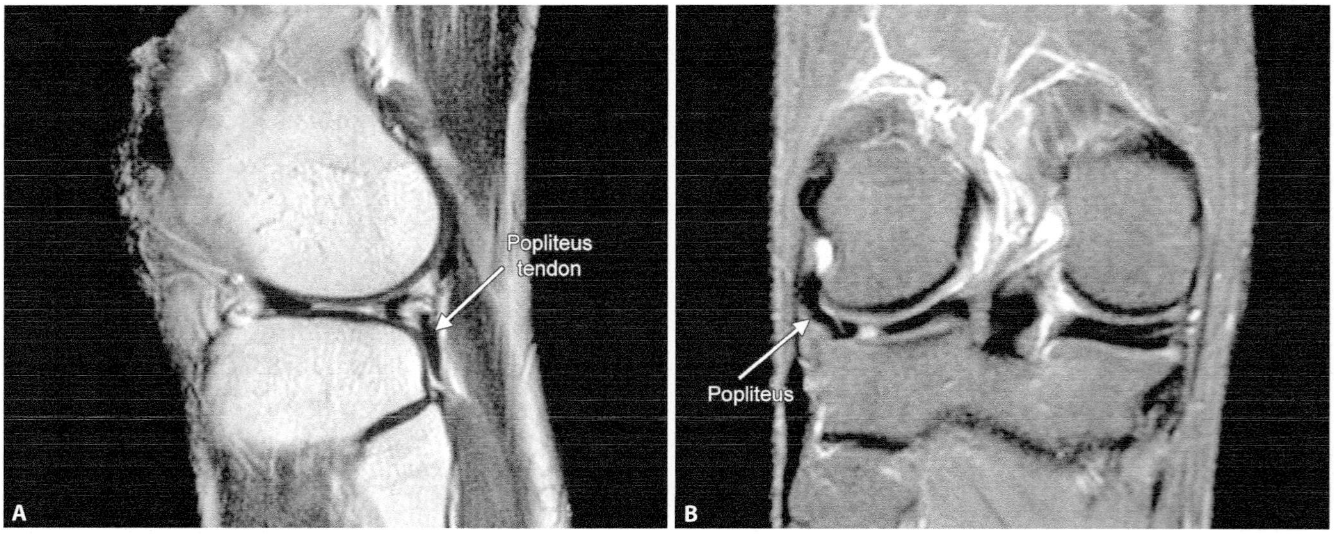

Figs. 28A and B: (A) Proton density sagittal; and (B) STIR coronal MR images of the knee showing the popliteal muscle that arises as a tendon from the lateral femoral condyle just anterior and inferior to the lateral collateral ligament, courses in a posteromedial direction to insert at the medial aspect of tibia, attaches to the lateral meniscus forming the popliteomeniscal ligament, and has a third attachment site on the styloid process of the fibula.

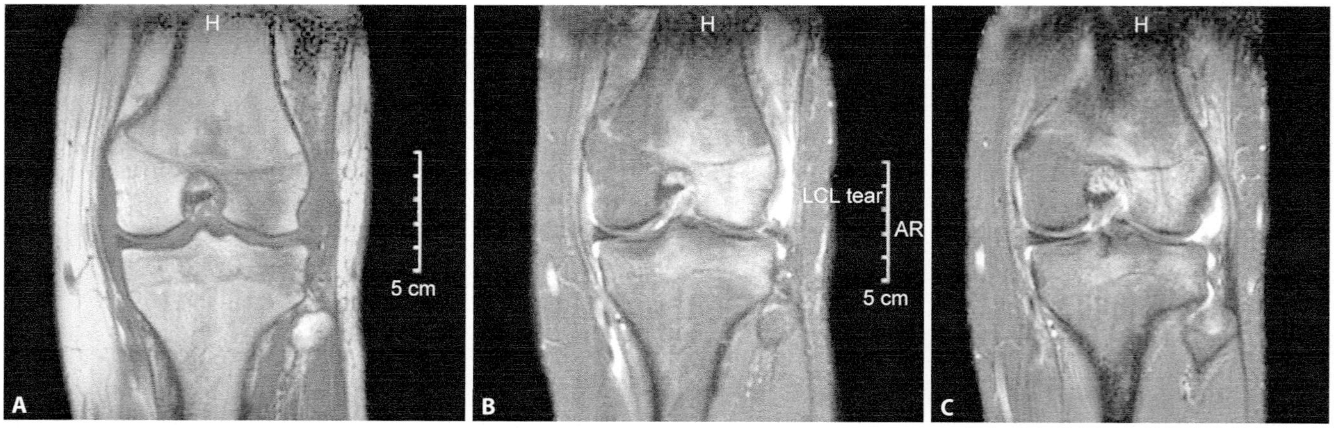

Figs. 29A to C: (A) T1W; and (B and C) STIR coronal MR images showing complete discontinuity and retraction of the fibers of the lateral collateral ligament (LCL) producing a ribbon-like deformity. Extensive contusions are seen in the lateral femoral condyle and lateral aspect of the tibial plateau—complete LCL tear.

ligament is a Y-shaped structure that represents thickening of the posterolateral joint capsule.[49]

Magnetic Resonance Imaging

The LCL is most vulnerable when a varus force is applied to the knee when it is in flexion or internal rotation. The LCL is best visualized in entirety in the coronal plane. It is seen as low-signal intensity structures on all pulse sequences and nearly uniform in thickness. Soft tissue edema characterizes the MRI findings associated with acute LCL injuries. Contour changes, such as thickening and irregularity, are more typical of subacute or old injuries. Complete tears with discontinuity and retraction of the fibers may produce a ribbon-like deformity of the LCL **(Figs. 29A to C)**. Most complete ruptures involve the conjoined tendon and may produce a small avulsion of the styloid process of the fibular head. When this occurs, marrow edema in the proximal fibula is usually evident on T2W and STIR images.

Most injuries involving the posterolateral structures are optimally depicted using a coronal oblique plane that is oriented parallel to the popliteus tendon.[51] Acute injuries of the popliteus muscle most commonly involve the myotendinous junction, whereas avulsion injuries of fibular insertion are less common. When the popliteal tendon tears, hemorrhage and edema in the muscle and tendon produce focal and high signal on T2W sequences. Edema of the adjacent soft tissue structures can also be observed. Complete tears of the popliteal tendon cause enlargement of the muscle belly and the retracted tendon terminates abruptly. Isolated popliteal injuries are rare because most are associated with concomitant injuries

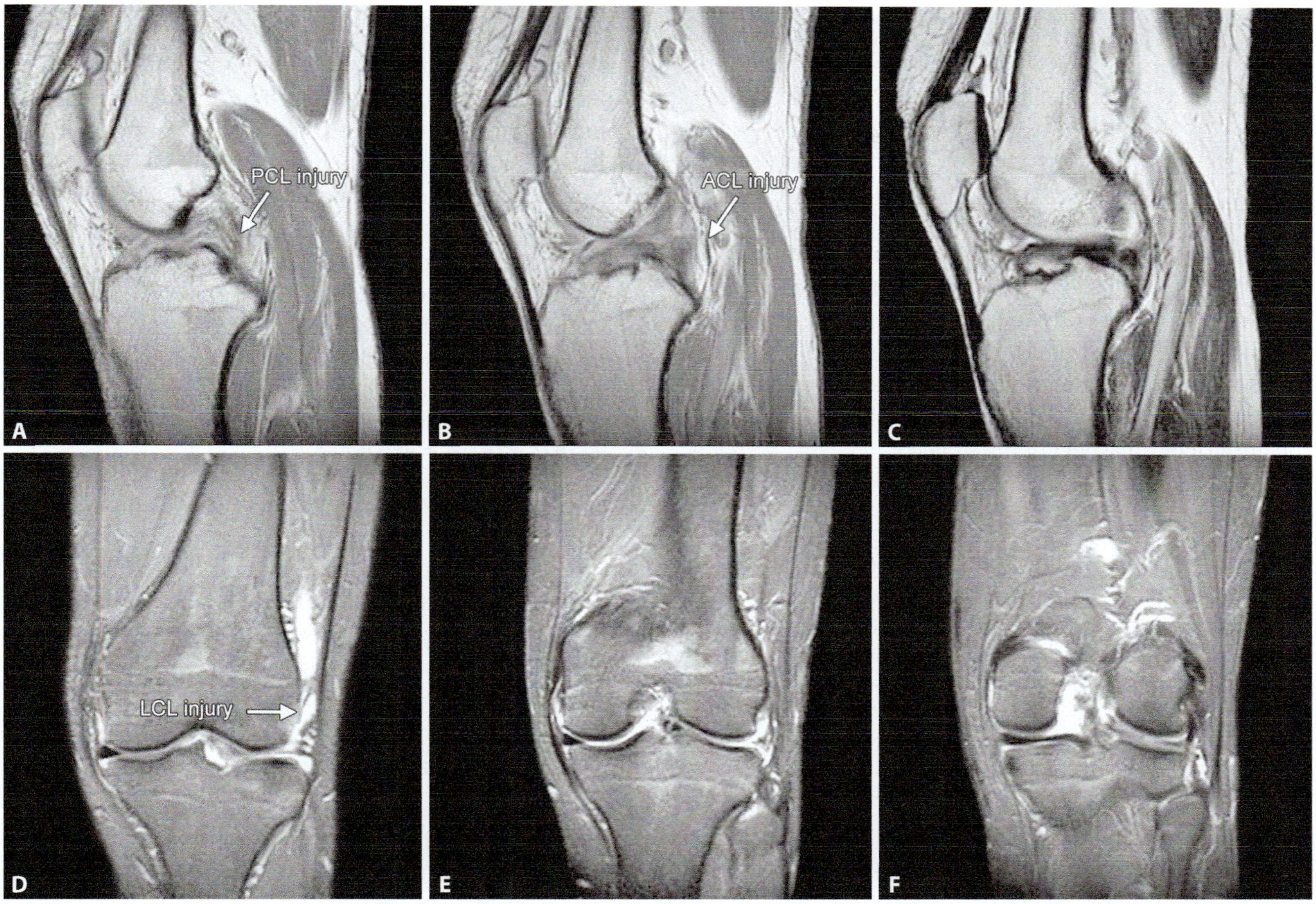

Figs. 30A to F: (A to C) T2W sagittal; and (D to F) STIR coronal MR images showing a tear of the posterior cruciate ligament (PCL), anterior cruciate ligament (ACL), and lateral collateral ligament (LCL)—multiligament injury of the knee.

of the arcuate ligament complex. PLC injuries are very often associated with cruciate ligament injuries, more commonly with the PCL **(Figs. 30A to F)**.

Posteromedial Corner of the Knee

Anatomy

The tendon of the semimembranosus muscle and the posterior oblique ligament are the main support structures in the posteromedial aspect of the knee.[52] The posterior oblique ligament is formed by the union of the posterior fibers of the MCL and the medial capsular ligament. The semimembranosus muscle originates from the posterolateral portion of the ischial tuberosity, and inserts on the posteromedial surface of the medial tibial condyle. The components of PMC are enumerated in **Box 2**.

Box 2: Components of the posteromedial corner.[53]

- Semimembranosus tendon and aponeurotic expansions
- Posterior oblique ligament
- Posteromedial capsule
- Oblique popliteal ligament
- Posterior horn medial meniscus
- Deep components of medial collateral ligament complex (meniscofemoral and meniscotibial)

Magnetic Resonance Imaging

Posteromedial corner injuries usually result from a valgus stress combined with rotational forces. The semimembranosus tendon is the largest tendon in the popliteal fossa. It has a fusiform configuration and appears uniformly hypointense on all imaging sequences. A strain of the semimembranosus tendon is manifested by loss of continuity at the insertion and high signal on T2W and STIR sequences owing to edema and hemorrhage. Accompanying fluid within the tendon sheath is a common finding. A focus of marrow edema may be present when the posterior oblique ligament avulses.

Anterolateral Corner of the Knee

Normal Anatomy

Anterolateral corner of the knee includes the anterolateral ligament (ALL), the iliotibial band (ITB), the anterior oblique band (AOB) of the LCL, and the capsular ligament **(Box 3)**.

Box 3: Components of the anterolateral corner.

- Anterolateral ligament
- Iliotibial band
- Anterior oblique band
- Capsular ligament

Together, these structures contribute to anterior and posterolateral stability. The ALL arises from the femur and courses anteroinferiorly to attach at anterolateral aspect of proximal tibia. The ITB is an extension of the tensor fasciae latae with distal attachments to the lateral femoral condyle, the lateral patella, and the tubercle of Gerdy at the anterolateral aspect of the tibia.

Iliotibial Band Injury

Iliotibial band injury is the most common injury to the ALC. Tearing most often involves the posterior fibers that interdigitate with the AOB. These are usually well demonstrated on coronal MR images.

Segond Fracture

The Segond fracture, or avulsion of the anterolateral aspect of the lateral tibial plateau, is a radiographic entity that signifies underlying trauma to the ALC structures of the knee. These lesions such as all anterolateral corner injuries, are highly suggestive of the presence of an underlying ACL tear (75–100%), meniscal tear (66–75%) or PLC injury.

Iliotibial Band Friction Syndrome

Iliotibial band friction syndrome (ITBFS) refers to lateral knee pain arising from the friction that occurs as the ITB passes over the lateral femoral epicondyle during repetitive flexion and extension of the knee. This injury is seen most often in individuals who participate in long-distance running and cycling. On MR images, ill-defined signal abnormality signifying soft tissue edema is present within the fat deep to the ITB.

POSTERIOR STRUCTURES OF THE KNEE

Anatomy

The gastrocnemius, soleus, and plantaris muscles form the superficial muscles of the calf. The gastrocnemius muscle arises as two heads from the posterior surface of the medial and lateral femoral condyles. The tendons of the gastrocnemius muscles along with the soleus tendon form the Achilles tendon, which inserts on the posterior tubercle of the calcaneus. The primary action of the gastrocnemius muscle is plantar flexion of the foot but also serves as a passive supportive structure of the posterior joint capsule.

Magnetic Resonance Imaging

Gastrocnemius injuries are most commonly caused by hyperextension of the knee or when the tibia posteriorly dislocates during knee flexion.[54] Acute injuries of the proximal gastrocnemius include interstitial edema of the myotendinous junction and surrounding soft tissues.[55] Occasionally, an intramuscular hematoma forms a space-occupying mass in the muscle. MRI can assess the chronicity of the hematoma by the general appearance of the products of hemoglobin degradation. A complete rupture of the gastrocnemius head is associated with retraction of the muscle belly.

KNEE DISLOCATIONS

A dislocation of the knee is a severe injury that is caused by high-energy trauma, such as motor vehicle and motorcycle accidents, falls, and industrial accidents. Knee dislocations are important because they produce extensive disruption of the ligaments that stabilize the knee and the surrounding soft tissue structures, including the popliteal artery.[56]

Magnetic Resonance Imaging

A knee dislocation is classified according to the position of the tibia relative to the femur. There are five different types of dislocations—(1) anterior, (2) posterior, (3) lateral, (4) medial, and (5) posterolateral. Posterior and posterolateral dislocations have a high association with complete tears of the popliteus and conjoined tendons, manifested by retraction, hemorrhage, and muscle edema. In general, both cruciate ligaments are likely to be torn. Complete disruption of one or both of the collateral ligaments is expected with this severe injury. Concomitant meniscal injury is also common. Frequently, the pattern of bone contusions allows definition of the type of knee dislocation. This is an important observation because posterior and posterolateral dislocations have a high association with peroneal nerve injury.[56] Neurovascular injury is the most dreaded complication of knee dislocation. It can result in irreversible neurologic deficits with consequent limb loss. Being relatively fixed in the popliteal fossa, the popliteal artery is at an increased risk in up to 40% of dislocations. Amputation rate is as high as 85% if revascularization is not done within 8 hours.

ANTERIOR STRUCTURES OF THE KNEE OR THE EXTENSOR MECHANISM OF THE KNEE

Anatomy

The main soft tissue structures in the anterior aspect of the knee are the components of the extensor mechanism and include the quadriceps tendon, patellar tendon, and the medial and lateral patellar retinacula.[57] The four muscle

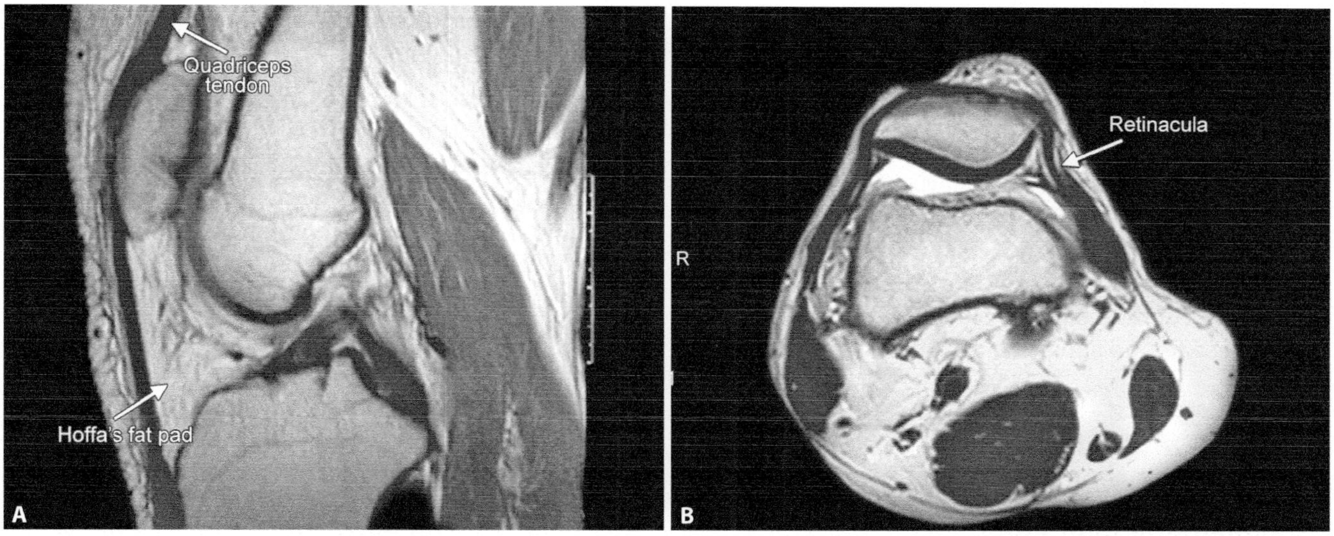

Figs. 31A and B: (A) T2W sagittal MR image showing the normal quadriceps tendon inserting on the superior pole of the patella, the patellar tendon, and the infrapatellar Hoffa's fat pad; (B) T2W axial MR image showing the medial and lateral patellar retinacula.

groups that form the quadriceps tendon include the rectus femoris, vastus lateralis, vastus medialis, and the vastus intermedius. The quadriceps tendon inserts on the superior pole of the patella and causes extension of the knee joint **(Fig. 31A)**. The medial and lateral patellar retinacula are extensions of the vastus medialis and lateralis, respectively and contribute to passive stabilization of the patella **(Fig. 31B)**.

The layers of the quadriceps tendon can be visualized best in sagittal plane on MRI as uniform low-signal intensity bands with intervening higher signal intensity fat separating each layer. The layered configuration of the quadriceps tendon enables discrimination between partial and full tears. Discontinuity of any of the tendinous layers is consistent with partial tears often involving the rectus femoris component. Transection of all the layers is diagnostic of a complete rupture and may be associated with a mass of edematous tissue and hemorrhage seen as high signal on T2W images.[58] A patella baja (low-riding patella) and undulating appearance of the patellar tendon is associated.

The patellar tendon also has homogeneous low-signal intensity appearance except for small occasional triangular areas of intermediate signal intensity directly below the patella and adjacent to the tibial tuberosity. The normal thickness of the tendon does not exceed 7 mm in its proximal part. A large collection of adipose tissue, the infrapatellar fat pad of Hoffa, rests just posterior to the patellar tendon. The patellar tendon ruptures less frequently than the quadriceps tendon.

Patellar Tendonitis (Jumper's Knee)

Most patellar ligament injuries are the result of repetitive forced extension of the knee as seen in the context of basketball, volleyball, soccer, tennis, and track events—hence the name jumper's knee. This form of injury manifests as thickening and partial tearing of the proximal patellar tendon and is well seen on sagittal MR images as increased tendon thickness greater than 7 mm or as intrasubstance high-signal intensity. Similar changes can be seen in both symptomatic and asymptomatic individuals. In symptomatic patients, the findings may be accompanied by patellar tracking disorders in as many as 45% of patients.

Acute Patellar Tendon Disruption

A minority of patellar ligament injuries are complete tendon disruption resulting from acute macrotrauma in the setting of sports-related activity. This most commonly occurs near the patellar attachment and is best seen on sagittal MR images as discontinuity of the patellar ligament with buckling of the tendon, retraction of the patella, and fluid signal in the intervening gap.

Patellar Tendon-lateral Femoral Condyle Friction Syndrome

Patellar tendon-lateral femoral condyle friction syndrome refers to the constellation of MRI findings that correspond to the clinical entity known as fat pad impingement syndrome. Affected patients are both athletes and nonathletes who experience chronic anterior knee pain that localizes to the inferior patellar pole on physical examination. The etiology is unknown, but it is likely related to friction onto the fat interposed between the patellar ligament and the lateral femoral condyle due to abnormal patellar tracking or alignment. MRI findings include abnormal obliteration of the fat planes, abnormal signal, and enhancement within the lateral soft tissues of the inferior patellofemoral joint. Most patients demonstrate patellar alignment abnormality, such as patella alta or lateral subluxation. Patients typically respond well to conservative treatment, which usually entails taping the superior pole of the patella.

Retinacular tears are characterized by areas of high signal on T2W and STIR sequences secondary to edema and hemorrhage.[59] The medial retinaculum is thinner than the lateral and frequently tears. The avulsed free end of the retinaculum is often frayed and thickened and fluid may dissect around a muscular slip of the vastus medialis muscle.

PATELLOFEMORAL JOINT AND KINEMATIC MRI

Patellofemoral Joint Anatomy

The shape of the patella and femoral trochlear groove is important for the function of the patellofemoral joint.

Patellar shape: Wiberg has proposed a three-part classification to encompass the majority of patellar facet configurations. In type I configuration, both facets are gently concave, symmetrical, and nearly equal in size. In type II, which is the most common, the medial facet is smaller than the lateral. In type III configuration, the medial facet is distinctly markedly smaller with marked lateral predominance.[60] Dysplastic patellar shapes have a variety of unusual configurations and are commonly observed with chondromalacia, recurrent dislocation, and patellofemoral instability.

The medial stabilizers prevent lateral subluxation of patella and include the medial patellar retinaculum and the medial patellofemoral ligament. The lateral stabilizers include the lateral patellar retinaculum and the lateral patellofemoral ligament.

MRI of Patellar Instability

The predisposing factors for patellar instability include trochlear dysplasia, excessive lateral distance between the tibial tubercle and the trochlear groove (lateralization of tibial tuberosity), and patella alta. For a safe tracking of the patella throughout the range of patellofemoral flexion, the femoral sulcus must be deep enough and the lateral trochlea high enough. Patellar dislocation is characterized by a complete loss of contact between the patellofemoral joint surfaces with the patella dislocating laterally in almost all cases.

Trochlear Dysplasia

This refers to a flattening of the joint surface. It can be evaluated on MR imaging by measuring the lateral trochlear inclination, trochlear facet asymmetry or trochlear depth.[61]

Lateral Trochlear Inclination

The most superior section showing trochlear cartilage is selected from axial section. A line is drawn along the subchondral bone of the lateral trochlear facet and another along the posterior aspect of the femoral condyles. The angle between the two lines is then measured. An inclination angle of less than 11° suggests trochlear dysplasia **(Figs. 32A and B)**.[61]

Trochlear Facet Asymmetry

This is calculated as the ratio of the length of the medial trochlear facet to the length of lateral trochlear facet. A trochlear facet ratio of less than 40% indicates trochlear dysplasia **(Figs. 33A and B)**.

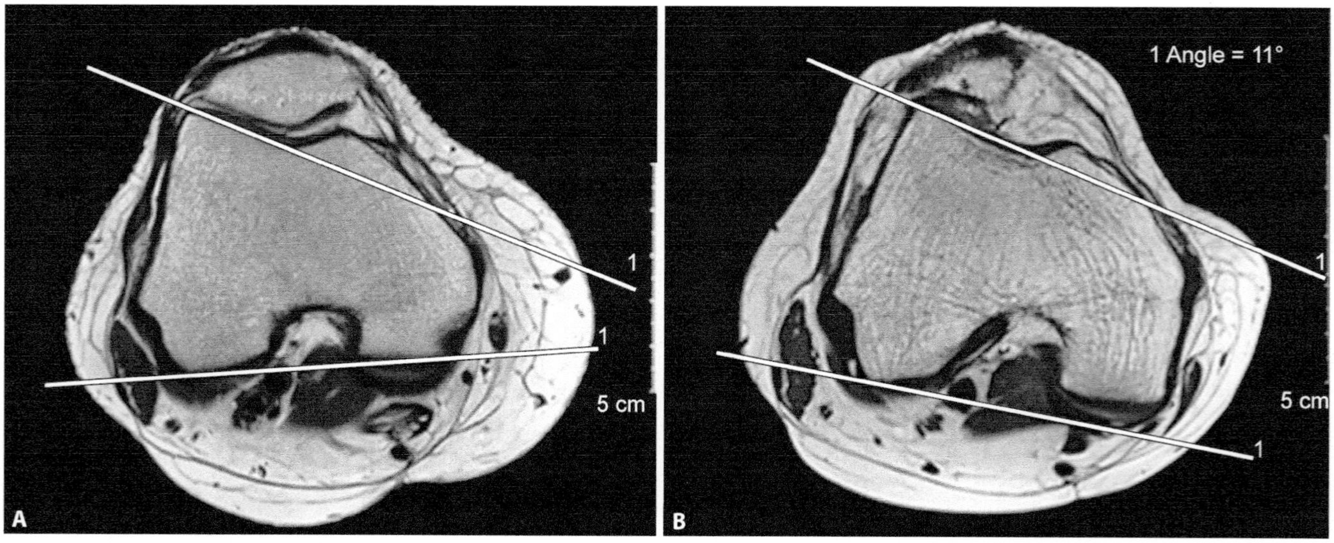

Figs. 32A and B: MR images showing the normal trochlear inclination (A) and abnormal (<11°) in a case (B).

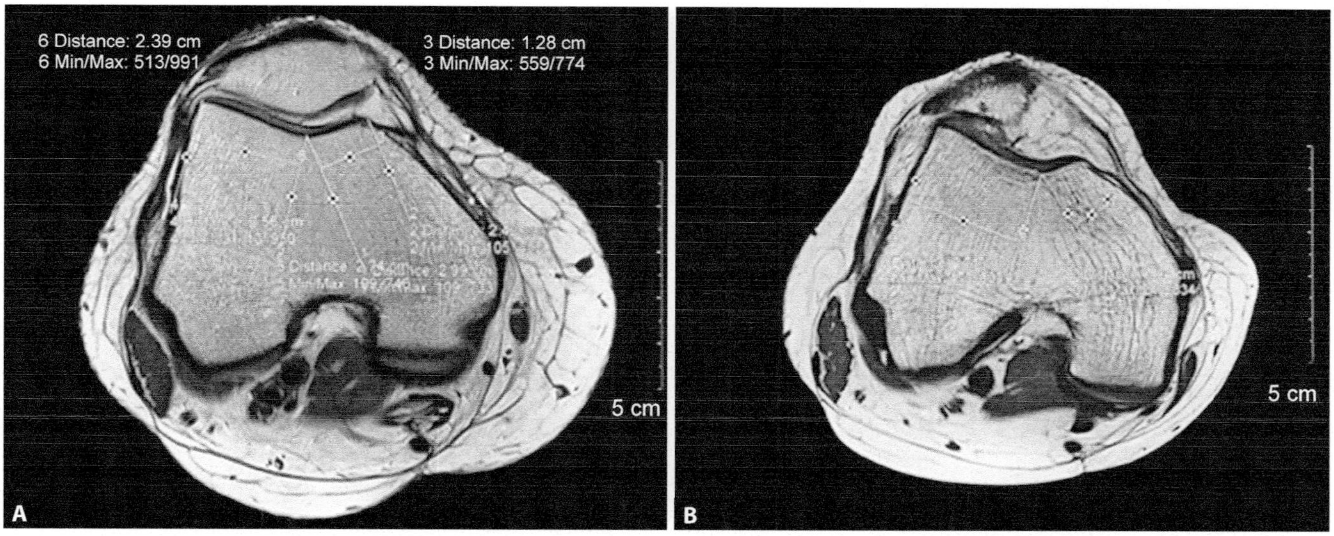

Figs. 33A and B: MR images showing the normal trochlear facet ratio (>40%) in a case (A); (B) Abnormal facet ratio (<40%) seen in another.

Trochlear Depth

If the depth of the trochlear groove is less than 3 mm, it is indicative of trochlear dysplasia.[61]

Sulcus Angle

The femoral trochlear groove provides a mechanical restraint that helps stabilize and serve as a guide for the patella as it articulates with the groove during joint function. In the axial plane, the posterior apex of a normal patella is centered directly above the intercondylar femoral sulcus. The sulcus angle is formed by the highest points of the medial and lateral femoral condyles and the lowest point of the intercondylar sulcus and measures 138° ± 6° **(Figs. 34A and B)**. Shallow sulcus angles (larger sulcus angle measurements) predispose to patellar instability.

Distance from Tibial Tubercle to Trochlear Groove[61]

A distance between tibial tubercle and trochlear groove less than 15 mm is normal, distances between 15 and 20 mm are borderline and distances of more than 20 mm are indicative of lateralization of tibial tuberosity **(Figs. 35A and B)**. This causes the patella to be pushed laterally during flexion predisposing to lateral dislocation.

Patella Alta and Patella Baja

In the sagittal plane, the patella is in normal position when in semiflexion of the knee the greatest diagonal length of the patella approximately equals the distance between the inferior pole of the patella and the tibial tuberosity (patellar tendon length). A truly high-riding patella (patella alta) most commonly results from a patellar tendon tear but is also associated with lateral patellar subluxations, recurrent dislocations, and spastic neuromuscular disorders[61] **(Figs. 36A to C)**. A low-riding patella (patella baja or profunda) occurs in quadriceps tendon rupture but is also found with paralytic neuromuscular disorders, achondroplasia, and juvenile rheumatoid arthritis (JRA).

Kinematic MRI

Kinematics is a term to describe movement of a body without reference to force or mass. Although conventional computed tomography (CT) and cine CT have also been used to perform kinematic studies of the patellofemoral joint, kinematic MRI has the advantage of showing the various soft tissue components (i.e., medial and lateral retinacula, patellar tendon, quadriceps muscles) that are involved in the stability and function of the joint.

Techniques

Incremental, passive positioning technique: The technique involves obtaining multiple axial images at different section locations and both the patellofemoral joints are passively flexed into incremental positions using a nonferromagnetic positioning device. The use of a special positioning device is crucial because direct anterior or lateral pressure may occur with the patient placed in prone position that is sufficient to displace the patella and give an erroneous appearance of patellar subluxation.

The MR images are obtained using a T1W spin echo, or spoiled gradient echo pulse sequences at several different slice locations while the joint is progressively flexed at 5° increments from 5° to 30°. This procedure should be repeated at three different section locations so that the entire excursion of the patella can be evaluated as it articulates with the femoral trochlear groove.[60]

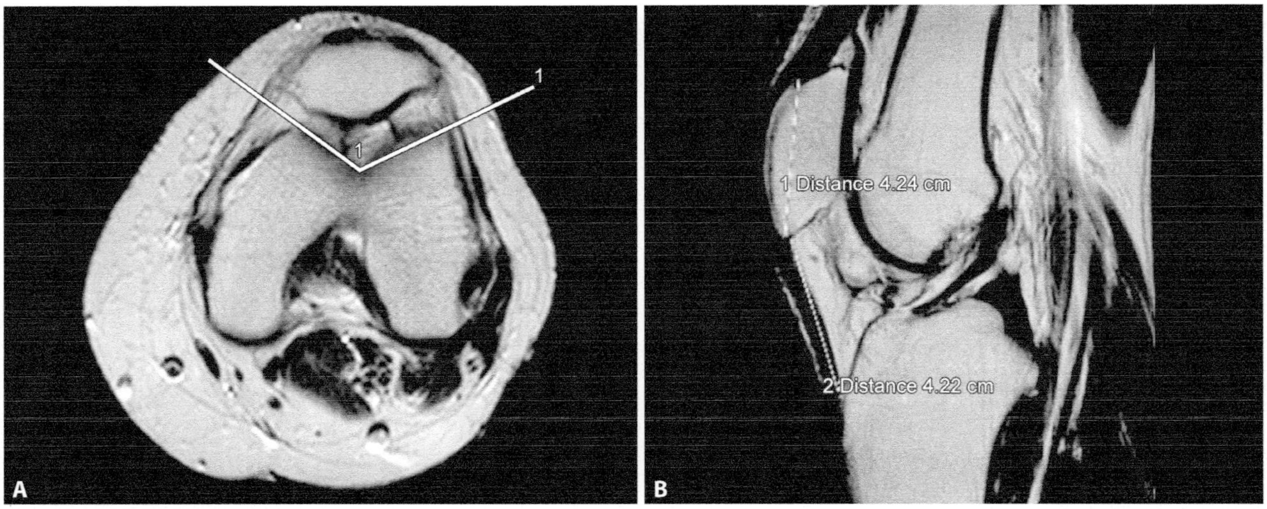

Figs. 34A and B: (A) T1W axial image showing the normal sulcus angle formed by the highest points of the medial and lateral femoral condyles and the lowest point of the intercondylar sulcus; (B) T2W sagittal MR image showing the normal position of the patella (the greatest diagonal length of the patella equals the patellar tendon length).

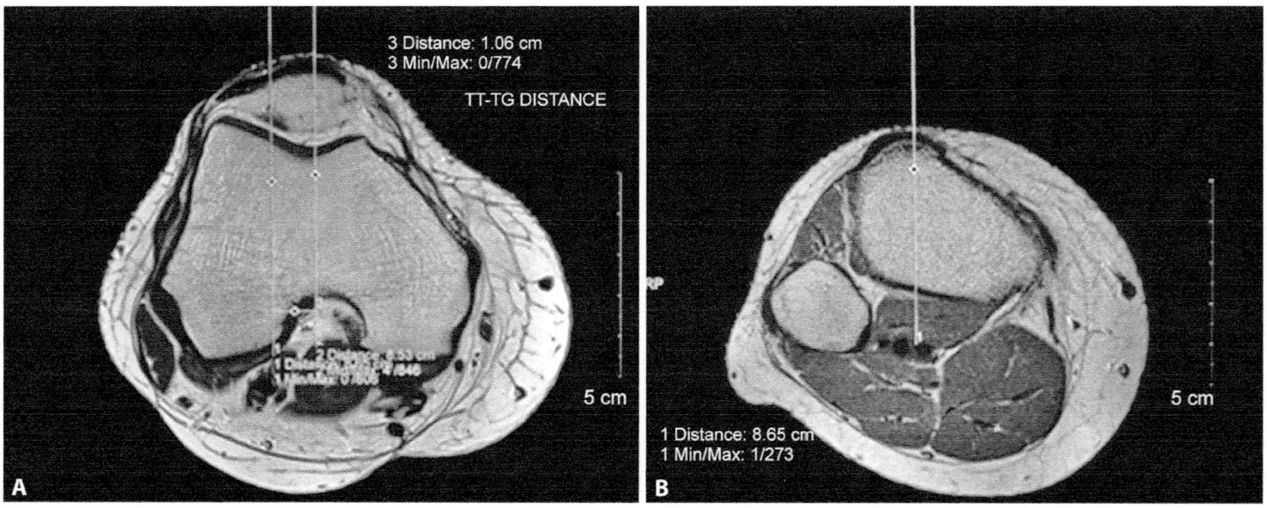

Figs. 35A and B: MR images showing the normal tibial tubercle to trochlear groove distance <15 mm.

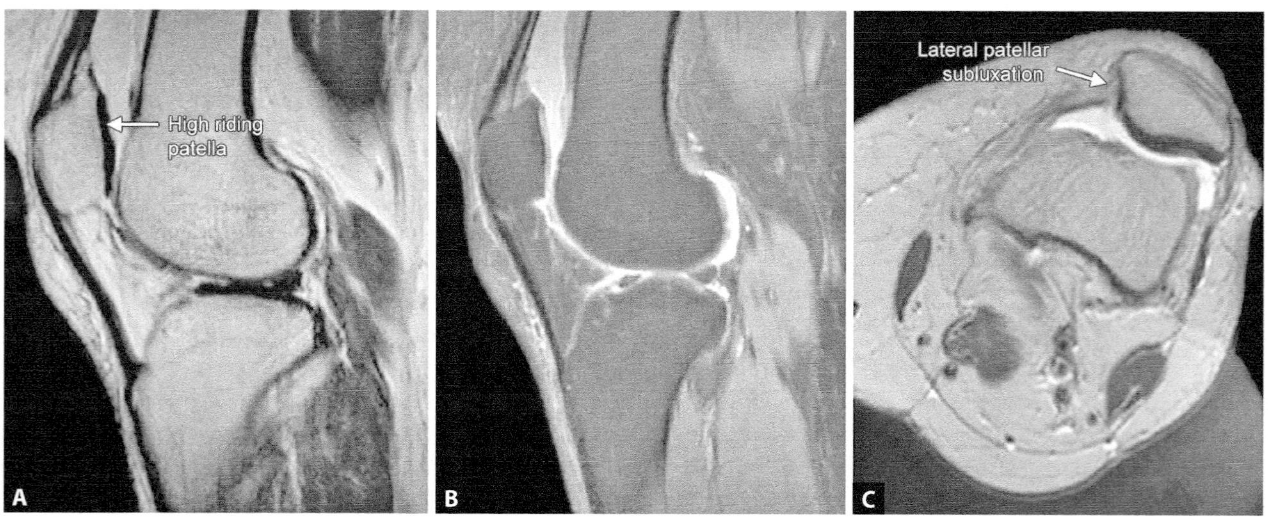

Figs. 36A to C: (A) Proton density; and (B) T2W fat suppressed sagittal MR images showing a high-riding patella with (C) Axial T2W MR image revealing a lateral patellar subluxation—patella alta.

Active movement or dynamic technique: Faster MRI techniques, e.g., ultrafast spoiled gradient recalled acquisition in the steady state (GRASS), turbo fast low-angle shot (FLASH) have been developed recently that provide significant improvements in temporal resolution and allow images to be obtained during active or dynamic movement of the patellofemoral joint. MR images typically are obtained at a temporal resolution of one image per second or faster using these fast scan techniques. The primary advantage of using active movement kinematic MRI technique is that the patellofemoral joint may be examined in terms of influence of the activated muscles and other related soft tissue structures on patellar alignment and tracking. Compared with the incremental, passive positioning technique, a more physiological examination is obtained and in certain instances, abnormal patellar tracking is more apparent during active movement. Dynamic MRI has the potential to characterize and quantify mechanics of internal structures in vivo.

Motion triggered cine technique: In this technique, a special nonferromagnetic device incorporates a trigger system that senses the motion of the patella. The patient is placed supine on the positioning device and a single patellofemoral joint is flexed and extended repeatedly while gradient echo images are obtained using a circular surface coil.

Active movement, loaded technique: In this, active movement against an externally applied load or resistance is applied.[62] With the patient in prone position, the movement against this resistance primarily requires activation of the extensor mechanism of the knee. This method enables identification of abnormalities that may not be observed during unloaded examination.

Abnormalities that may be seen on kinematic MR include lateral or medial subluxation of patella and lateral patellar tilt or excessive lateral pressure syndrome.

Kinematic MR study can be combined with routine MR study of the knee since both the procedures can be completed within an acceptable time and can provide a more thorough examination of the knee especially in cases of suspected patellofemoral incongruency.

Weight-bearing MRI of the Knee

Imaging in nonrecumbent position under physiological stress allows detection of load-induced physiological and pathological variations. WB-MRI is dedicated open MR unit in which the patient is positioned standing upright or sitting.[63] Such systems allow flexion and extension views to be obtained (multipositional MRI). This instrument enables detection of unstable meniscal lesions as there occurs a modification of the meniscal morphology resulting in a posterior subluxation of the posterior horn of the medial meniscus in unstable lesions during passage from supine to upright position. Upright MRI also allows one to understand patellofemoral kinematics. This helps in understanding the etiology of patellofemoral pain, differentiates non-maltrackers from maltrackers, and helps improve treatment for patellofemoral instability by pinpointing the exact cause.[63]

MRI OF THE ARTICULAR CARTILAGE

The articular surfaces of the knee are covered by hyaline cartilage. By deforming under pressure, the articular cartilage greatly increases the effective contact area between femoral condyles and tibial plateaus, significantly decreasing the pressure transmitted across these joints. The menisci are also helpful in distributing forces across the knee joint. The cartilaginous matrix of articular cartilage allows the knee to withstand large local pressures up to 5 times the normal pressures.

Initial evaluation of the articular cartilage used primarily T1W images. Because of its hydropic composition, normal hyaline cartilage demonstrates intermediate signal intensity on T1W images compared with the low signal intensity of the cortex and fibrocartilaginous menisci. On conventional T2W images also, hyaline cartilage displays an intermediate signal intensity. In the presence of joint effusion, T2W images create an arthrogram like effect with hyperintense synovial fluid improving the delineation of thinner cartilage surfaces (e.g., medial and lateral compartments). There is poor contrast, however, between articular cartilage and subchondral bone on conventional T2W images and in the absence of joint effusion, surface or contour irregularities may not be resolved.

STIR and gradient echo images can also depict morphological changes of the articular cartilage. With STIR image contrast, it is possible to differentiate the brighter signal intensity of fluid from intermediate-to-high signal intensity of articular cartilage. This sequence is also useful in demonstrating early changes of subchondral bone in areas of overlying articular cartilage damage. Areas of fluid within articular cartilage fissures and fragmentation can also be visualized on STIR images. Gradient echo imaging is useful with respect to imaging geometry, speed, and contrast. 3D imaging significantly improves SNR at high spatial resolution. With gradient echo techniques, articular cartilage demonstrates high signal intensity. However, articular cartilage and articular fluid show similar high-signal intensity, and significant cartilaginous injuries may be missed using gradient echo techniques if joint fluid and articular cartilage are isointense.

The demand for improved preoperative detection and characterization of articular cartilage damage has resulted in recent improvements in the accuracy of MRI of articular cartilage with use of sequences optimized for articular cartilage evaluation. Fat suppressed T2W

FSE techniques are useful in separating the cartilage-fluid interface and identifying early changes of articular cartilage degeneration **(Fig. 37A)**.[64] A fat suppressed three-dimensional spoiled gradient echo technique (3D SPGR) is also used.[65-67] The sequence, dual echo steady state (DESS), combines the principles of heavily T2W steady state sequence and gradient echo imaging **(Fig. 37B)**. 3D MR pulse sequences commonly used for articular cartilage have different vendor specific abbreviations as given in the **Table 1**.[68]

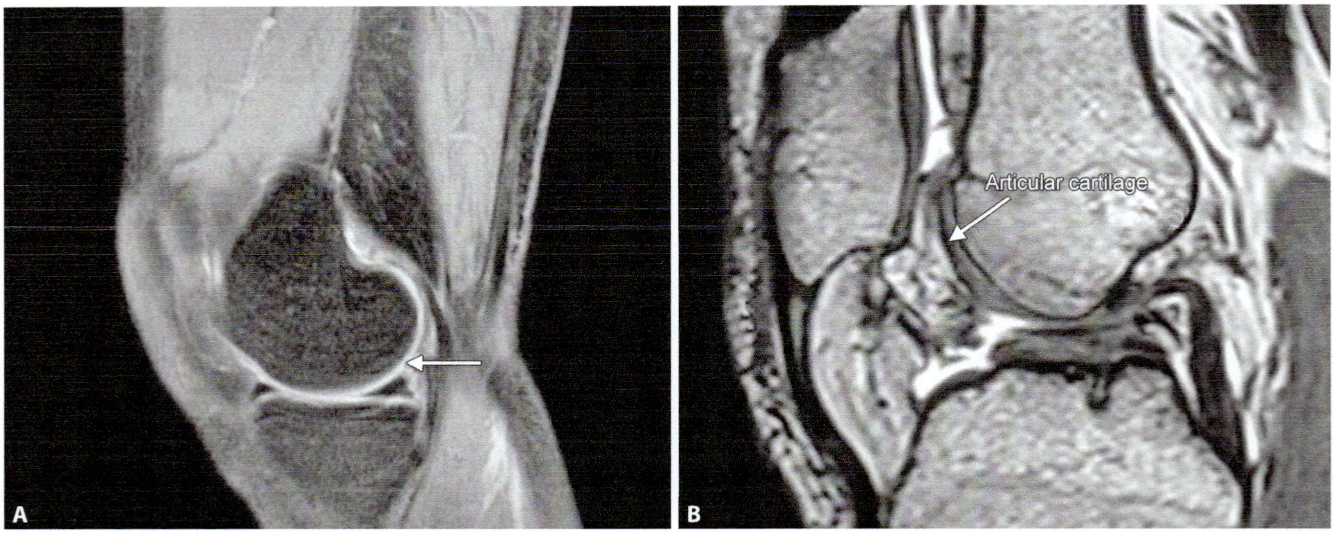

Figs. 37A and B: (A) Sagittal fat suppressed T2W MR image showing the articular cartilage as high-signal intensity; (B) DESS sequence for articular cartilage showing the intermediate gray signal articular cartilage. The thickness of the cartilage varies with the thickest cartilage seen at the patella and thinnest seen at the tibial plateau.

Table 1: Three-dimensional MRI pulse sequences commonly used in musculoskeletal imaging.

Sequences	*Fluid signal intensity*	*Vendor abbreviation*		
		GE	*Siemens*	*Philips*
GRE-based sequences				
Spoiled GRE	Dark	SPGR (Spoiled gradient-recalled echo)	FLASH (Fast low-angle shot)	T1 FFE (Fast field echo)
Steady-state sequences				
Postexcitation refocused (Coherent gradient echo)	Bright	GRASS (Gradient-recalled acquisition in steady state), Fast MPGR (Multiplanar gradient-recalled)	FISP (True fast imaging with steady-state free precession)	FFE (Fast field echo)
Fully refocused (bSSFP)	Bright	FIESTA (Fast imaging using steady-state free acquisition)	True FISP (true fast imaging with steady-state free precession)	Balance FFE (Fast field echo)
Pre-excitation refocused (Steady-state free precession)	Bright	SSFP (Steady-state free precession)	PSIF (reversed FISP) (reverse fast imaging with steady-state free precession)	T2 FFE (Fast field echo)
Derivative bSSFP	Bright	VIPR-SSFP (Vastly undersampled isotropic projection steady-state free precession)		
Dual/multiecho steady-state balanced imaging	Bright	MENSA (Multiecho in steady-state acquisition)	DESS (Dual-echo in steady state)	
Spin-echo-based sequences				
Fast spin-echo	Variable	CUBE, XETA (Extended echo train acquisition)	SPACE (Sampling perfection with application optimized contrast with different flip-angle evolutions)	VISTA (Volume isotropic turbo spin-echo acquisition)

Source: Adapted from Naraghi A, White LM. Three-dimensional MRI of the musculoskeletal system. Am J Roentgenol. 2012;199(3):W283-93.68

The new 3D FSE sequences such as SPACE from Siemens, VISTA from Philips, and 3D MVOX (multivoxel) from Hitachi provide contrast that equals the 2D FSE sequences in contrast, offer submillimeter isotropic resolution, can be reconstructed in any imaging plane, and have a scan time which is shorter than the scan time needed to acquire three 2D sequences.[68]

All three imaging planes are useful, however, the sagittal plane is the best single plane for evaluation of articular cartilage because it provides near orthogonal images of most of the articular cartilage surfaces in the knee. Intra-articular contrast or MR arthrography is useful for detection of loose bodies or for evaluation of osteochondral defects for assessment of integrity of overlying articular cartilage.

MRI Assessment of Articular Cartilage Injury

Arthroscopic grading system for correlation with MR findings is:

- Minimal articular cartilage change with localized softening and minimal or no break in the articular surface.
- Areas of fibrillation or fissuring with an irregular roughened surface.
- Definite fibrillation with fissuring extending to the subchondral region and a classic "crab meat" appearance.
- Absence of articular cartilage with possibly eburnated subchondral bone.

MR can thus be used for grading and determining the extent of cartilage damage.[69,70] MR also has a role in the follow-up of cartilaginous injuries. Arthroscopy is too invasive for follow-up of these lesions.[60]

Chondromalacia Patellae

The term chondromalacia patellae meaning softening of the patellar cartilage is widely used to designate a clinical syndrome of retropatellar pain, patellofemoral crepitus, and quadriceps wasting which is associated with softening or fibrillation of the articular cartilage of patella.[71] The clinical observations that symptoms are self-limiting, may settle spontaneously, and that chondromalacia patellae does not progress to fully-developed OA in later life, suggest that the two diseases are different entities. Patients with chondromalacia patellae have cartilaginous thinning, focal signal or focal contour defects in the patellar cartilage on T2W MR images.

Osteoarthritis

Osteoarthritis affects the knee more frequently than any other joint. The MR findings in degenerative arthrosis/osteoarthritis vary from osteophytic spurring to compartment collapse, denuded articular cartilage, torn and degenerative meniscal fibrocartilage, and diminished marrow signal intensity in areas of subchondral sclerosis **(Figs. 38A to C)**. The various alterations in the subchondral bone microstructure associated with the different stages of OA include:[72]

- *Bone marrow edema-like lesions*: Bone marrow edema-like lesions (BMELs) are defined on MRI as monocystic subchondral areas of ill-defined hyperintensity on STIR and T2W sequences and areas of hypointensity on T1W sequences. BMELs may increase or decrease over time and larger BMELs are seen more frequently in subjects who have pain.[73]
- *Subchondral cyst-like lesions*: These lesions have a characteristic appearance on MRI and are seen as well-defined round areas of fluid like signal intensity on nonenhanced imaging. They are a consequence of traumatic bone necrosis following impact of two opposing articular surfaces.
- *Synovitis*: Synovitis occurs not only as a secondary phenomenon related to cartilage degeneration but also plays a role in the progression of cartilage loss. Synovial inflammation is believed to contribute to pain in patients who have knee OA.

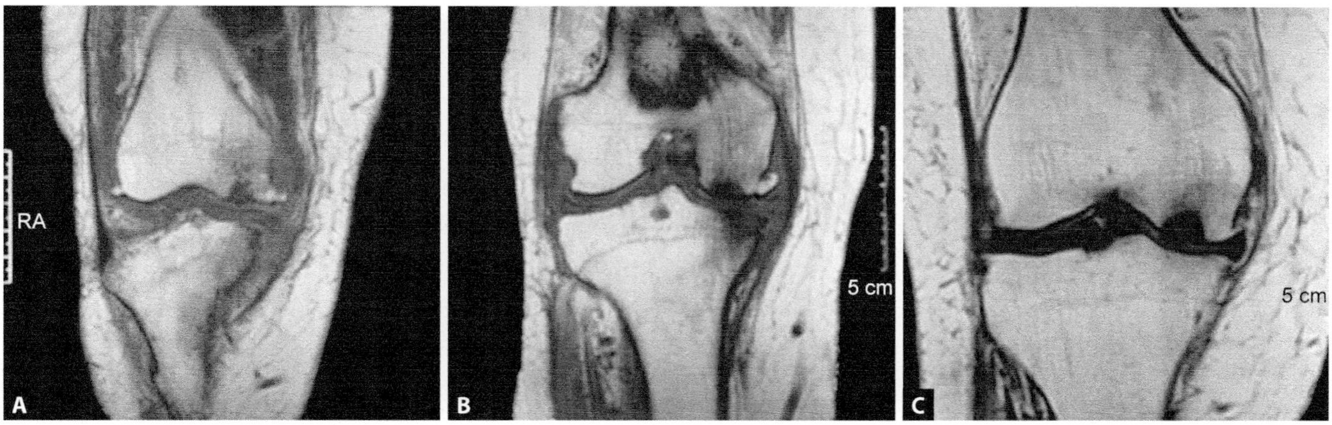

Figs. 38A to C: T1W coronal MR images of the knee showing osteophytic spurring, denuded articular cartilage, mild medial compartment collapse, and subchondral sclerosis—osteoarthritis.

- *Joint effusion*: Joint effusion is commonly detected in patients who have moderate-to-advanced OA and reflects synovial activation secondary to ligament injury, loose bodies, hyaline cartilage deterioration, and meniscal damage. Only contrast-enhanced images can differentiate between synovium and joint effusion.
- *Subchondral bone attrition*: Subchondral bone attrition is defined as a depression or flattening of the subchondral bony surface unrelated to gross fracture. It is considered to be a predictor of knee pain in cases of OA.
- *Periarticular cysts*: A wide spectrum of periarticular cystic lesions may be encountered in knee OA like parameniscal cysts and ganglion cysts may be seen. Ganglion cysts are viscous synovium filled masses with mucopolysaccharide rich contents. Septations are common within ganglia. There is usually a connection or stalk traceable to the joint.
- *Loose bodies*: Chondral fragments (intermediate-signal intensity) and loose bodies (high-signal intensity of marrow fat) may be associated with more advanced degenerative disease. A T1W image in at least one plane should be included in the study to improve the identification of loose bodies that contain marrow fat. The exclusive use of fat suppressed sequences may lead to the loose bodies being missed. In addition to the patellofemoral, medial, and lateral compartments of the knee, changes in the tibiofibular joint which may also be affected by degenerative arthrosis are well seen by MRI **(Figs. 39A to D)**.

The ability of MRI to accurately assess hyaline cartilage surfaces may give MR an advantage over plain film radiography in preoperative planning for joint replacement procedures, especially in unicondylar arthroplasties for OA.[74] Therapeutic techniques such as chondrocyte transplantation requires high resolution and volumetric MRI studies for accurate identification of focal articular cartilage defects and generalized cartilage loss. Creation of cartilage models by 3D MR image rendering may be helpful for preoperative planning of orthopedic surgical procedures in advanced cases of OA. Also, tailored MRI producing high spatial and contrast resolution images is proving to be an important tool in the early detection and surveillance of progression of OA.[75]

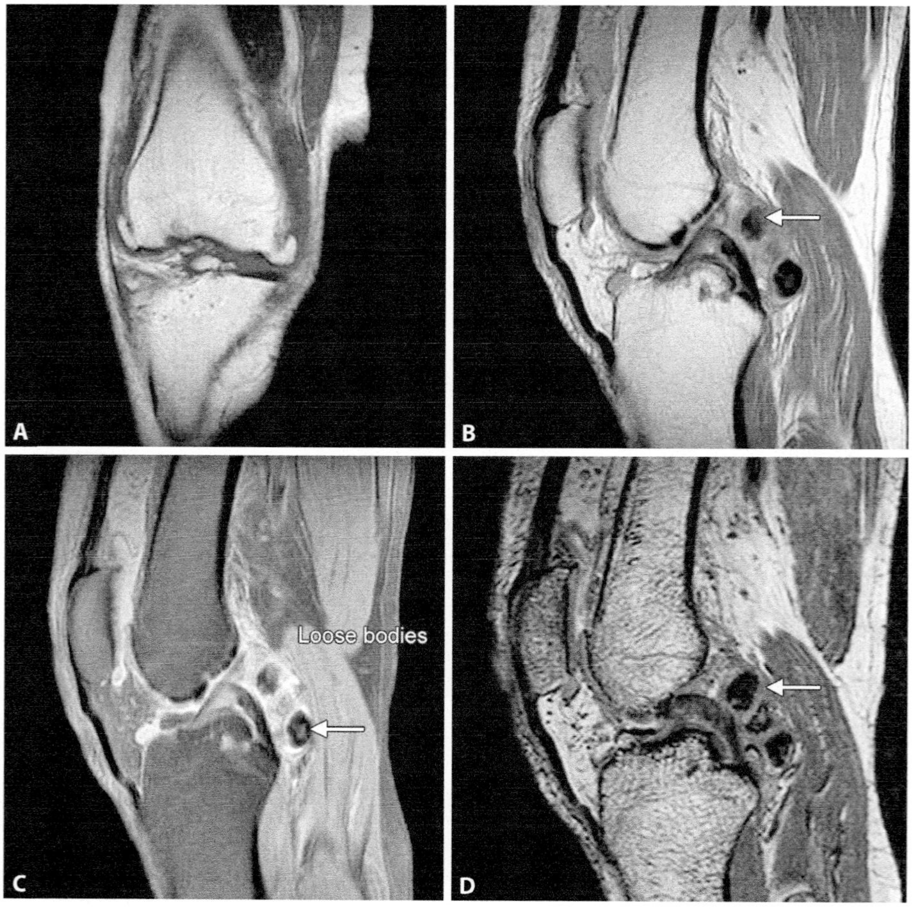

Figs. 39A to D: (A) T1W coronal; (B) T2W sagittal; (C) Fat suppressed T2W sagittal; and (D) Double echo steady state sequence showing osteophytic spurring at femur, patella, and multiple loose bodies. The loose bodies show high-signal marrow fat on T1W image (A) with signal suppression on fat suppressed image (B).

NOVEL SEQUENCES AND TECHNIQUES FOR DETECTION OF EARLY OSTEOARTHRITIS

Biochemical MR Imaging of Knee Articular Cartilage/Compositional MRI[76]

The various routine MRI sequences allow for an evaluation of the morphology of articular cartilage but do not provide much information about its biochemical properties **(Figs. 40A and B)**. The main constituents of the articular cartilage are an extracellular matrix composed of 80% water, proteoglycan molecules, and type II collagen fibers. The biochemical changes of early OA include a decrease in the proteoglycan content, an increase in the free water content, and a disorganization of the collagen fibers.[76] The MR techniques which allow a study of these early biochemical changes include T1 rho and T2 mapping **(Figs. 40C to E)**.

T1 Rho

In T1 rho mapping, a low power RF pulse follows the critical RF pulse for a user defined time period called the spin lock time (TSL). As a result, the protons relax with a

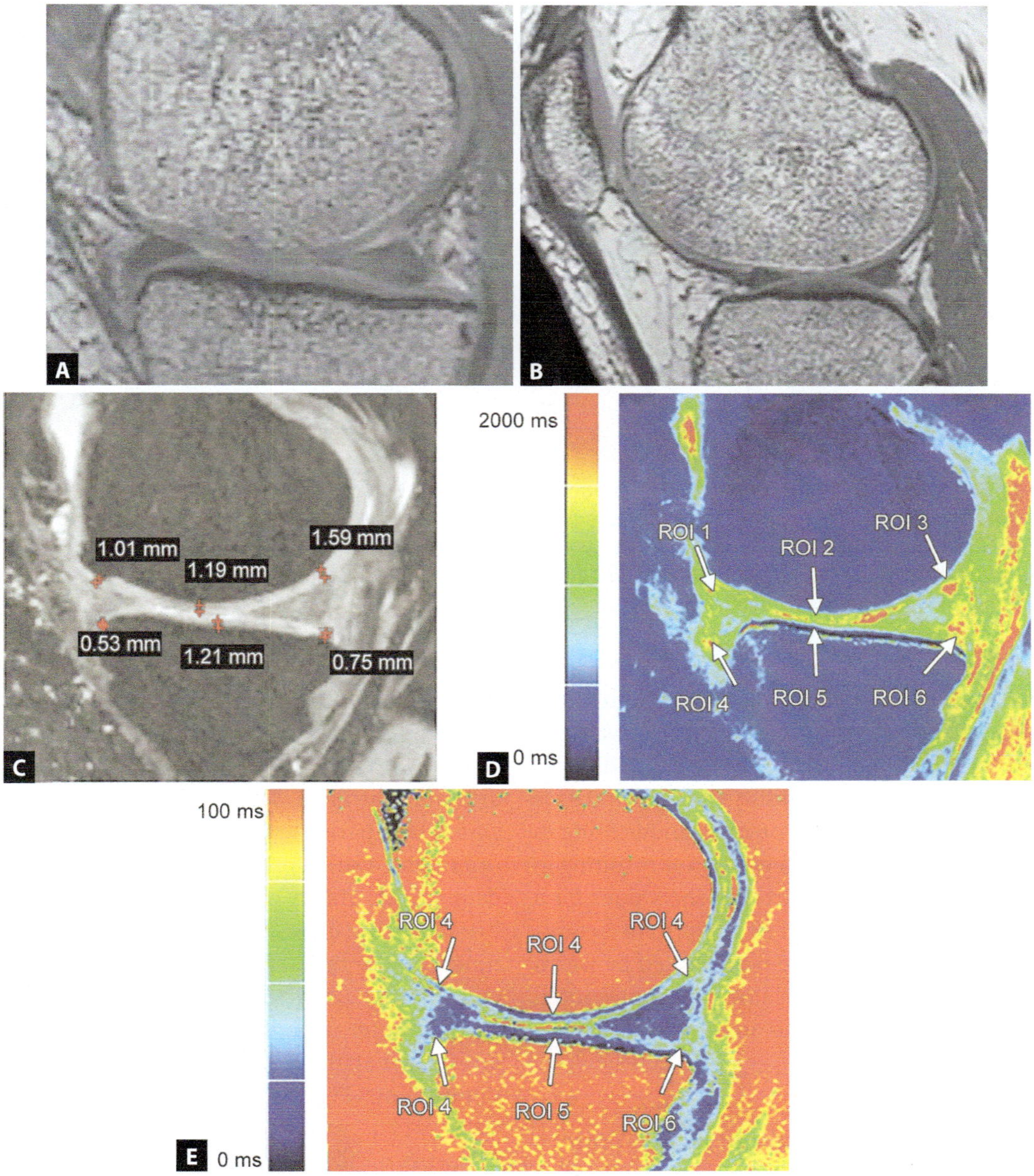

Figs. 40A to E: (A) T1W sagittal SPGR image shows thinning of medial femoral and tibial articular cartilage; (B) T1W sagittal SPGR image shows thinning of lateral femoral and tibial articular cartilage; (C) T2W sagittal double echo steady state image showing medial femorotibial compartment (average thickness of articular cartilage in MFC ~1.28 mm and MTC ~0.83 mm); (D) Corresponding color coded sagittal T1 map of medial femor-tibial compartment [average T1 relaxation time of articular cartilage (in ROI 1, 2, and 3) for MFC ~1068.54 ms and (in ROI 4, 5, and 6) MTC ~957.8 ms]; (E) Color-coded sagittal T2 map of medial femorotibial compartment [average T2 relaxation time of articular cartilage (in ROI 1, 2, and 3) for MFC ~63.25 ms and (in ROI 4, 5, and 6) for MTC ~59.14 ms].

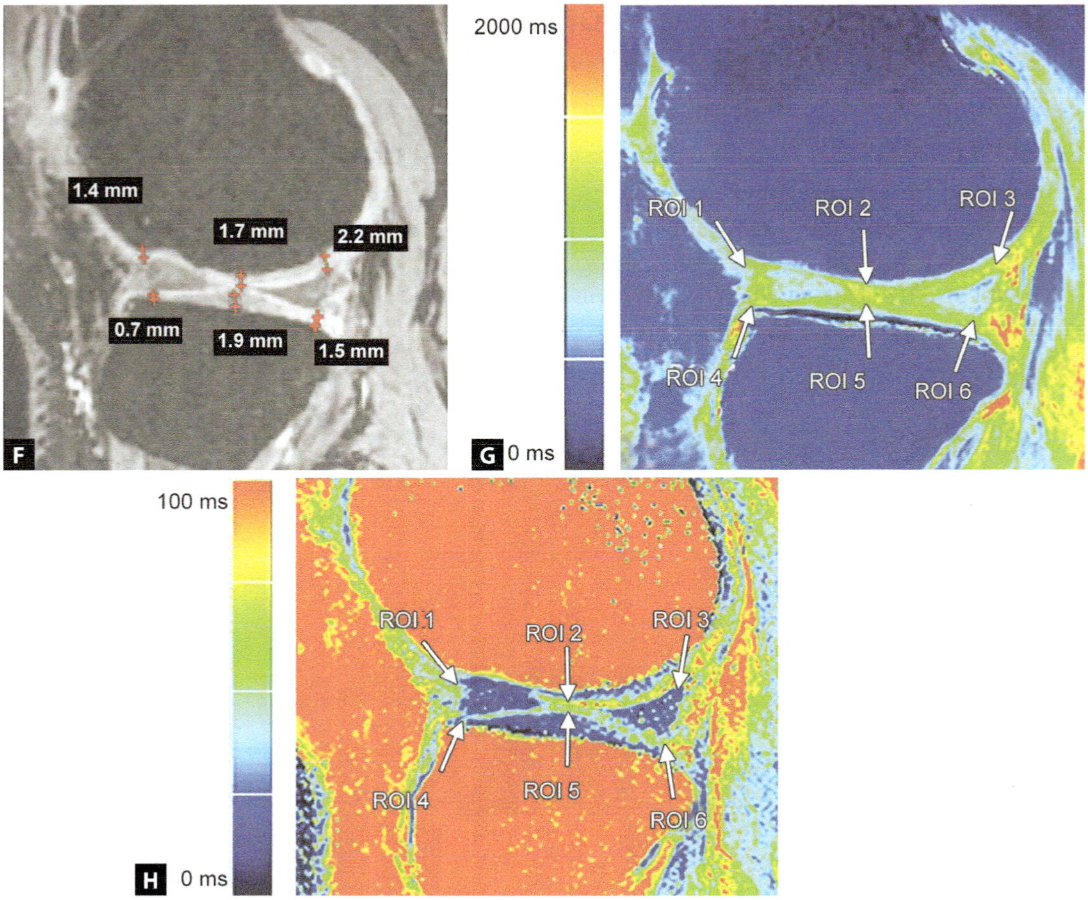

Figs. 40F to H: (F) T2W sagittal double echo steady state image showing lateral femorotibial compartment (average thickness of articular cartilage in LFC ~1.76 mm and LTC ~1.36 mm); (G) Corresponding color-coded sagittal T1 map of lateral femorotibial compartment [average T1 relaxation time of articular cartilage (in ROI 1, 2, and 3) for LFC ~1098.39 ms and (in ROI 4, 5, and 6) for LTC ~1098.89 ms]; (H) Color-coded sagittal T2 map of lateral femorotibial compartment [average T2 relaxation time of articular cartilage (in ROI 1, 2, and 3) for LTC ~60.6 ms and (in ROI 4, 5 and 6) for LTC ~65.54 ms].

different time constant called T1 rho rather than the time constant T2 of conventional MR imaging.[77] T1 rho value of a given tissue is always higher than the corresponding T2 value of the tissue for a given RF pulse strength. In cases of early OA, there is depletion of proteoglycan resulting in fewer water molecules bound to proteoglycans resulting in increased T1 rho values. The acquired T1 rho values for a region of cartilage can be displayed in the form of a color-coded map. High T1 rho values are represented by warm colors (red tones) and low T1 rho values are represented by cool colors (blue tones) **(Figs. 40F to H)**.

T2 Mapping

In normal healthy articular cartilage, water protons are bound by well-organized collagen fibers allowing for a rapid dephasing and hence low T2 values. T2 values are reflective of the collagen disorganization and increased water content that begins with OA in addition to the proteoglycan depletion.[77] T2 mapping can also be represented in the form of a color coded map, similar to the T1 rho maps with the red tones standing for high T2 values and blue tones standing for low T2 values. T2 mapping also permits differentiation among the three zones of articular cartilage. The superficial zone shows a higher signal compared to the deep layers owing to the more organized radial orientation of collagen fibers in the deep layers. This zonal differentiation is important as the osteoarthritic changes affect the more superficial layers much before the deeper layers. T1 rho and T2 mapping can also be used to study the degeneration of fibrocartilaginous structures like menisci in addition to the articular cartilage and both provide complementary information **(Figs. 40I to N)**.

Cartigram

T2 maps can be automatically generated by MR scanner when a special sequence is applied, e.g., Cartigram on General Electric MR scanners. T1 rho and T2 maps can also be generated using postprocessing methods like voxel-based relaxometry.

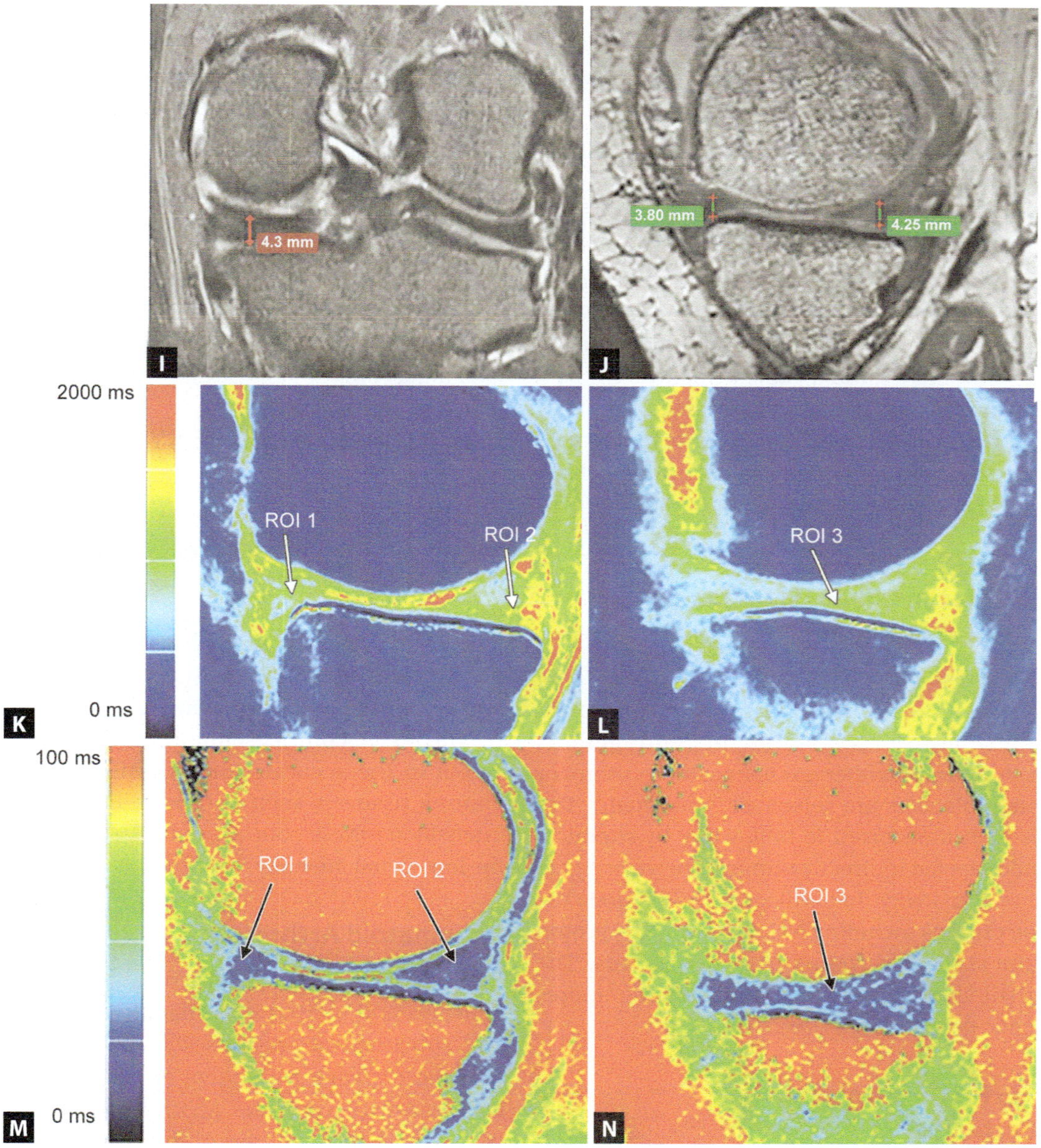

Figs. 40I to N: (I) T1W coronal STIR image shows average thickness of body of medial meniscus; (J) T1W sagittal SPGR image shows average thickness of anterior and posterior horn of medial meniscus; (K and L) Color-coded sagittal T1 maps show average T1 relaxation time (in ROI 1, 2, and 3) of medial meniscus ~924.79 ms; (M and N) Color-coded sagittal T2 maps show average T2 relaxation time (in ROI 1, 2, and 3) of medial meniscus ~25.54 ms.

Quantitative Cartilage Imaging—Delayed Gadolinium-enhanced MRI of Cartilage

The normal cartilage is rich in glycosaminoglycans (GAG) which have negatively charged carboxyl and sulfate groups. Negatively charged contrast agents such as Gd-DTPA are injected intravenously or (intra-articularly) and these get distributed in the cartilage by diffusion. Because both GAG and gadolinium are negatively charged, gadolinium diffuses to articular cartilage in inverse proportion to local GAG concentration. Gd-based contrast agents thus show only a minimal enhancement in the normal healthy cartilage, owing to the high GAG concentration and accumulate in areas of cartilage loss with low GAG content.[78] The protocol consists of intravenous administration of Gd-DTPA (0.2 mmol/kg), 10 minutes of cycling or exercise to enhance its distribution and image acquisition 90 minutes (1–2 hours) using a 3D inversion recovery spoiled gradient echo sequence. Since there is a delay between contrast administration and image acquisition, the technique is called delayed gadolinium-enhanced MRI of cartilage (dGEMRIC). The concentration of Gd-DTPA in cartilage can be quantified and these quantitative findings have a particularly important role in evaluating early OA where changes are still reversible. dGEMRIC uses a T1 mapping technique after intravenous application of Gd-DTPA. dGEMRIC has been found helpful in monitoring therapy and interventions such as cartilage repair and oral medications.[79]

Sodium Imaging

Owing to the GAG content of the cartilage being negatively charged, cations such as Na^+ are attracted in the cartilaginous interstitial matrix. Thus the GAG content can be estimated using the sodium content. This, however, requires a dedicated sodium MRI which suffers from low SNR because of very low sodium concentration (~260–400 times lower than proton concentration in healthy cartilage). Sodium MRI, thus, has a limited clinical applicability as it requires dedicated coils, has low SNR, limited resolution, and long acquisition time (15–30 minutes). Further improvements in hardware and software combined with high field imaging at 7 T are required to make sodium MRI clinically feasible.[79,80]

Glycosaminoglycan Chemical Exchange Saturation Transfer Imaging

This is the newest compositional cartilage imaging technique. In chemical exchange saturation transfer (CEST) experiments, exogenous or endogenous compounds containing either exchangeable protons or exchangeable molecules are selectively saturated.[80] The saturation is then transferred to bulk water by chemical exchange and detected indirectly through the water signal with enhanced sensitivity. In cartilage, CEST exploits the exchangeable protons including NH, OH, and NH_2 proton groups on the GAG side chains of proteoglycans. The technique is still in the experimental stages and requires higher magnetic field strengths like 7 T.

Ultrashort Echo Time Imaging of Articular Cartilage

Tissues with a very short transverse relaxation time (T2) include bone, ligaments, tendons, menisci, and calcified cartilage. When conventional MR sequences are used, the signal from the tissues with a short T2 decays very rapidly. The result of the rapid decay is that signal from these tissues is zero or close to zero by the time the receive mode of a clinical MR system is enabled. The tissues thus appear hypointense in conventional MRI. Ultrashort echo time (UTE) sequences use TEs of <100 ms. These pulse sequences enable materials with short T2 to be assessed. UTE imaging in the knee enables detection of subtle matrix alterations and holds promise in the diagnosis of early degenerative changes.

In Vivo Diffusion MRI

Water mobility is restricted in the intact collagen network. In early degenerative disease of articular cartilage, an increased mobility of water is found leading to increased apparent diffusion coefficient values. Diffusion tensor imaging can measure the diffusion anisotropy of cartilage and provide information on the mechanical function of articular cartilage. It is a promising technique but requires sophisticated and high field imaging making it less suitable for routine clinical application.

Hybrid MRI

A combination of PET and MRI (PET/MRI) allows a combination of structural and molecular (metabolic) imaging techniques for the detection of early OA.[79]

EVALUATION OF THE SYNOVIUM

Synovial reaction and proliferation are characterized on MR images by changes in the contour of synovial reflections. Although the synovium cannot be imaged directly, a corrugated surface along Hoffa's infrapatellar fat pad is evident in the early stages of synovial irritation. This irregular infrapatellar fat pad sign is seen in patients with RA, pigmented villonodular synovitis (PVNS), hemophilia, and hemorrhagic effusions with reactive synovium.

Gd-DTPA contrast-enhanced T1W MR images are useful in the accurate identification of pannus tissue. Pannus tissue is seen as an area of increased signal intensity on these contrast-enhanced images adjacent to the low-signal intensity joint fluid.[81]

Rheumatoid Arthritis

Rheumatoid arthritis (RA) typically presents with joint effusions and bony and cartilaginous erosions. Marginal and subchondral erosions with diffuse loss of hyaline articular cartilage are evident on both medial and lateral femoral articular surfaces. An irregular fat pad may be seen in the more active stages of the disease. Hypertrophied synovial masses remain relatively low in signal intensity on T1W and T2W images. The Gd-DTPA contrast-enhanced images are useful in identifying the pannus or granulation tissue that grows on the surfaces of articular cartilage in RA **(Figs. 41A to D)**.[81]

The ability to map out pannus is useful in examining patients with inflammatory arthritis when synovectomy is considered. MRI determined synovial membrane and effusion volumes are sensitive markers and predictors of disease activity and treatment outcome in RA. Osteonecrosis and infarcts in rheumatoid arthritis can also be identified on MR scans before radiographic changes are evident.

Tuberculosis of the Knee

Magnetic resonance imaging is excellent for detecting early changes of tuberculosis. Synovial proliferation

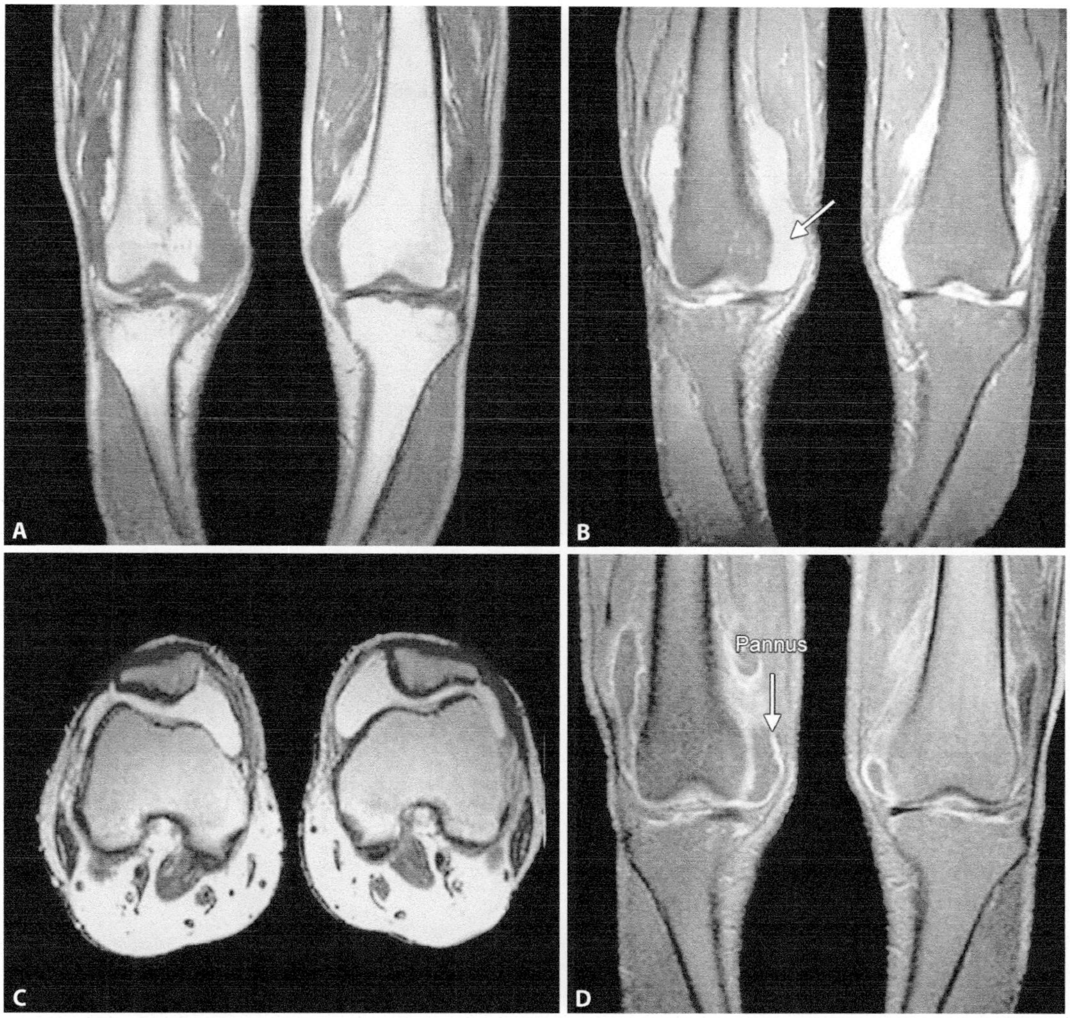

Figs. 41A to D: (A) T1W coronal; (B) STIR coronal; (C) Axial T2W; and (D) Postcontrast T1W coronal images showing joint effusion with enhancing pannus growing on the surface of the articular cartilage in both the knees—rheumatoid arthritis.

seen in TB is typically hypointense on T2W images. On administration of IV contrast, the hypertrophied synovium is intensely enhancing. Marrow edema, osteomyelitis, cortical erosions, myositis, cellulitis, abscesses, and skin ulceration/sinus formation can be seen in the bone and adjacent soft tissues **(Figs. 42A to C)**.

Juvenile Rheumatoid Arthritis

In JRA or Still's disease, MRI studies demonstrate synovitis with irregularity of Hoffa's infrapatellar fat pad in the early stage. Articular cartilage erosions and synovial hypertrophy can also be identified. Hypoplastic menisci, with small anterior and posterior horns and body, have also been described in patients with JRA on MR studies. An enlarged epiphysis, widening of the intercondylar notch, and squaring of the inferior margin of the patella are radiographic findings also detected on MR. MR evaluation of signs of disease progression such as pannus tissue changes may be a cost-effective way of monitoring the effectiveness of therapy. MR studies may also be used for serial follow-up of functional status in patients with JRA.

Pigmented Villonodular Synovitis

Pigmented villonodular synovitis may also affect the knee. PVNS may present as a focal mass but more frequently is monoarticular. Histologically, the lesions present with fibrous synovial proliferation, infiltration by histiocytes, multinucleated giant cells and hemosiderin laden macrophages, and hemosiderin staining of the synovium presumably from recurrent hemorrhage. These lesions present on MRI as characteristic proliferative synovial focal masses containing hypointense signal on all pulse sequences **(Figs. 43A to D)**. The signal loss results from proton dephasing from local magnetic field inhomogeneity caused by magnetic susceptibility effects of the iron containing byproducts of hemoglobin. Bony erosions are better visualized on MR than on plain films.[5,60]

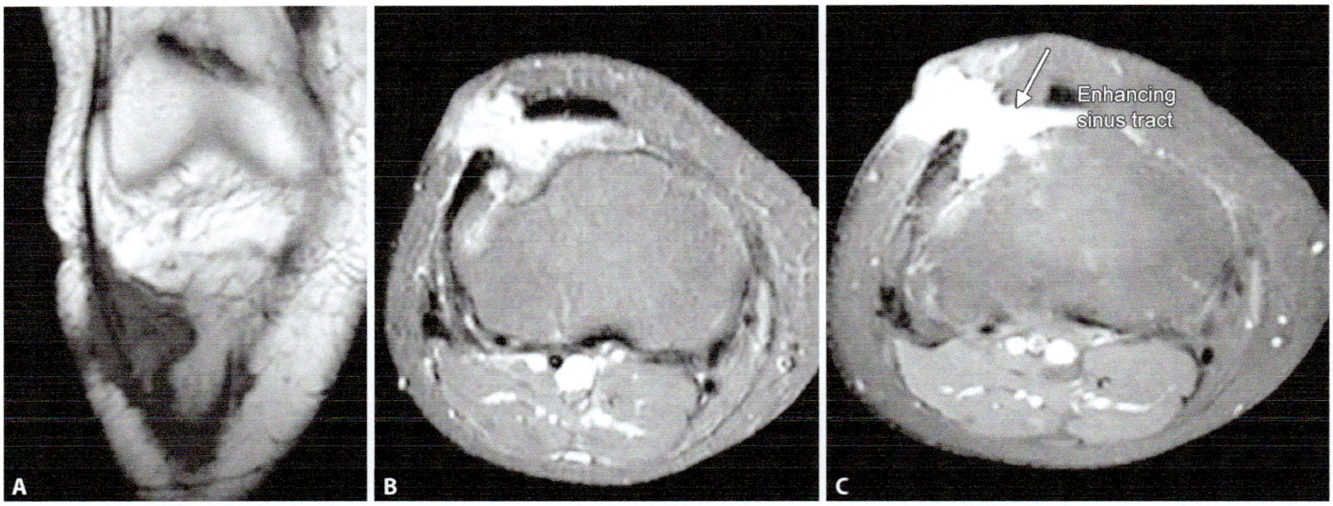

Figs. 42A to C: T1W coronal (A) and postcontrast T1W axial (B and C) MR images showing irregularity of the lateral tibial plateau with enhancing synovium and an enhancing sinus tract from the bone to the skin surface—tuberculosis.

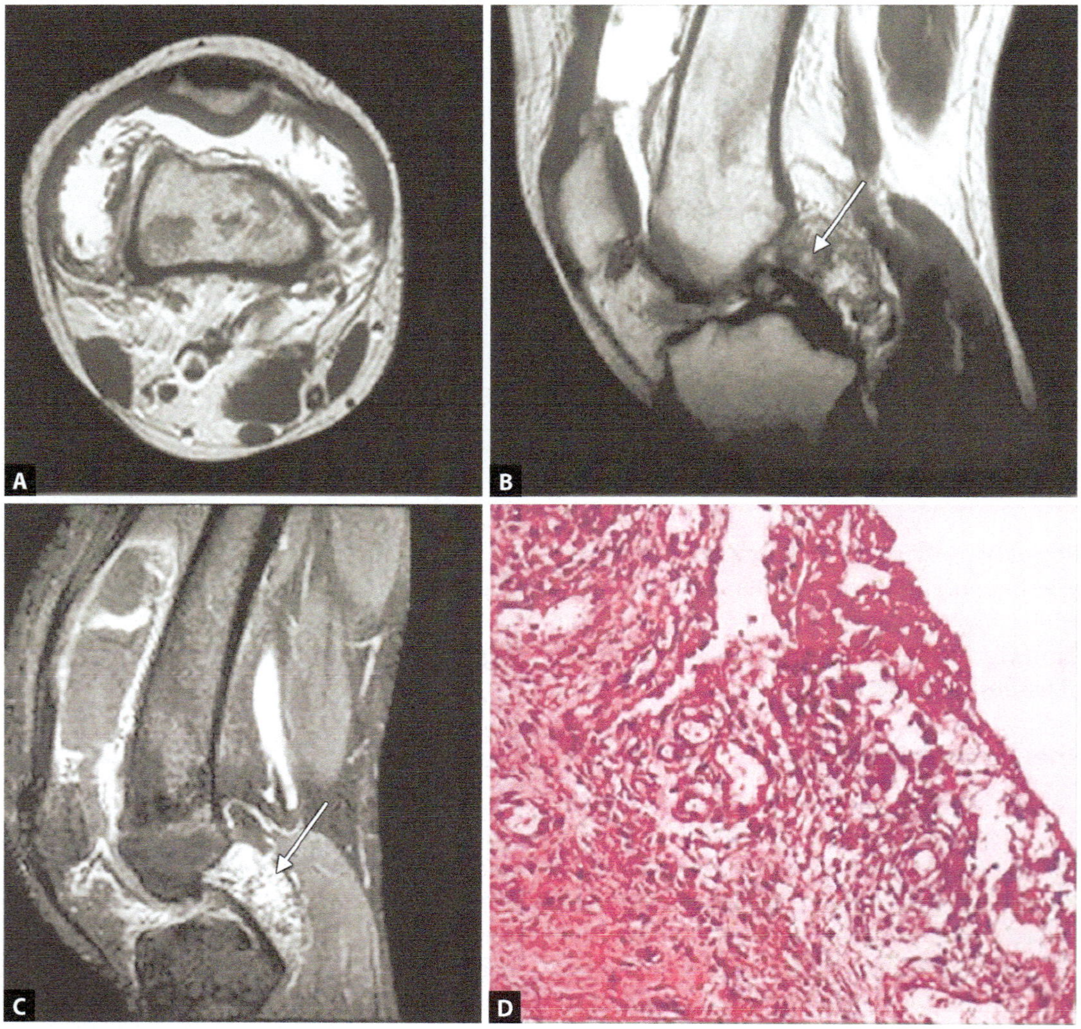

Figs. 43A to D: (A) Axial T2W; and (B) Sagittal images showing synovial thickening and associated effusion with scattered low signal areas of hemosiderin within. Low signal mass seen posterior to posterior cruciate ligament (PCL); (C) Postcontrast image showing enhancement of the thickened synovium and the focal mass posterior to PCL; (D) Biopsy showing histiocytes with hemosiderin pigment—pigmented villonodular synovitis.

Hemophilia

Subchondral and intraosseous cysts or hemorrhage can be identified on coronal and sagittal MR images. Hemosiderin and fibrous tissue formed from repeated episodes of joint hemorrhage demonstrate low-signal intensity on T1W and T2W images **(Figs. 44A to C)**. Signal loss in these conditions is usually more uniform in its involvement of the joint synovium and focal masses characteristic of PVNS are not usually seen in chronic hemorrhagic conditions.

Synovial Chondromatosis of the Knee

It is a process associated with metaplastic changes within the synovium that produce multiple cartilaginous islands in the synovium. These cartilaginous islands may become dislodged producing both calcified and noncalcified loose bodies. Lesions contain enough calcium to be detected on plain films. They are low in signal intensity on all MR pulse sequences.

Deferiprone-induced Arthropathy

Deferiprone (DFP) is widely used as an iron chelator in thalassemia patients. The arthropathy consists of musculoskeletal stiffness, joint pain, and joint effusion. Arthroscopy reveals excess iron in the synovium and cartilage. MRI in these cases reveals irregular thickening of the cartilage with subchondral erosions and cartilage intrusions in the subchondral defects. Synovial thickening and enhancement, synovial bands, and effusions have been described. The symptoms decrease with dose reduction or temporary discontinuation of drug **(Figs. 45A to C)**.

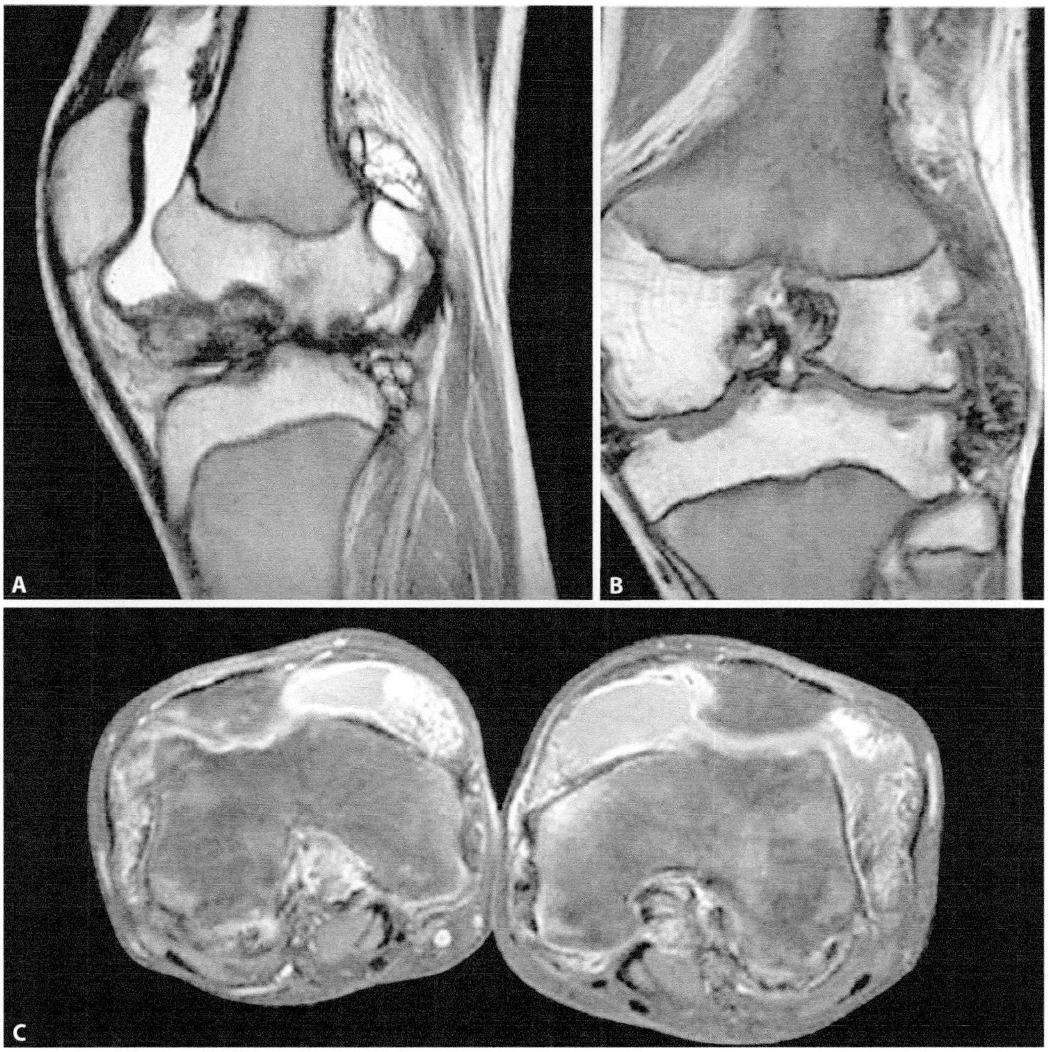

Figs. 44A to C: (A) Sagittal T2W; (B) Coronal T1W; and (C) Postcontrast T1W axial MR images showing thickening of the joint synovium with low signal areas within due to hemosiderin and fibrous tissue. There is fuzziness and irregularity of the articular margins. Changes are seen in both the knees—hemophilic arthropathy.

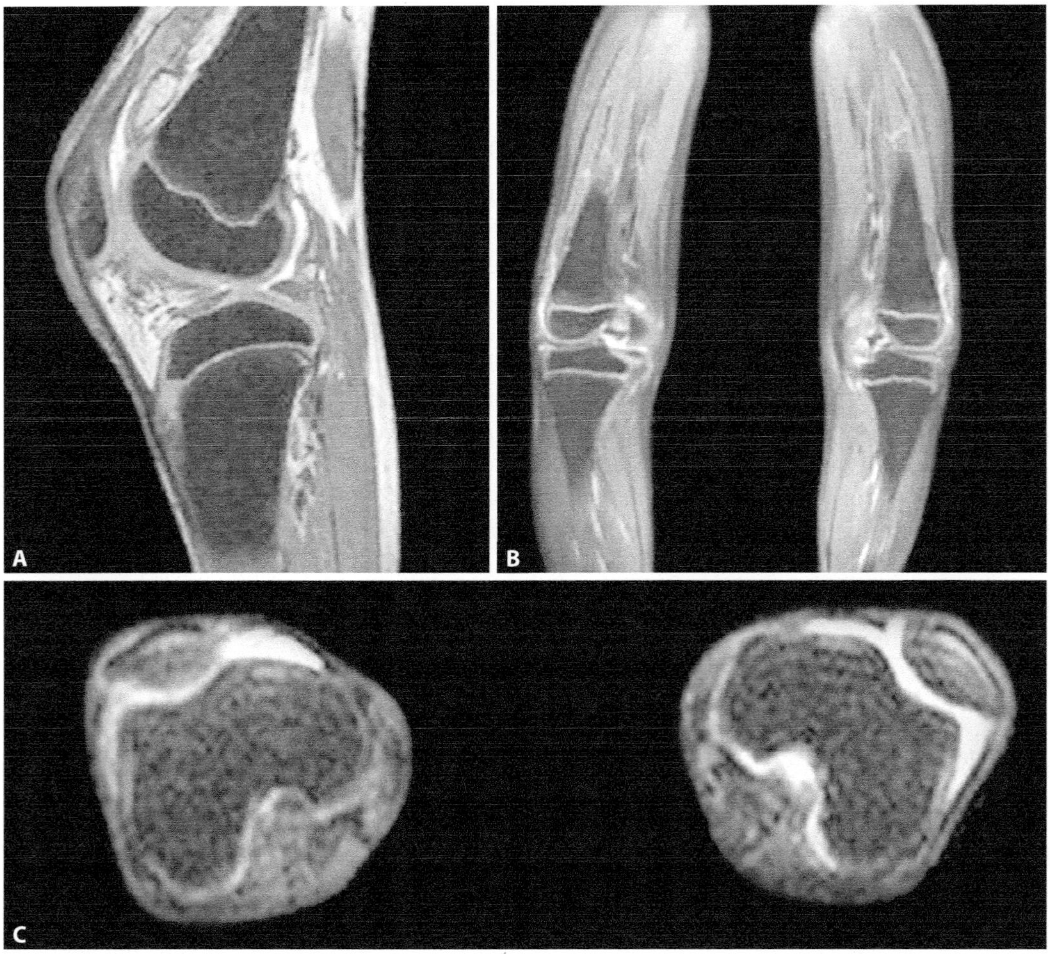

Figs. 45A to C: Sagittal (A) and coronal (B) GE images showing black out in the metaphyseal marrow, irregular thickening of the articular cartilage of femoral condyles, and patella with synovial thickening; (C) Postcontrast image showing synovial thickening and enhancement—deferiprone-induced arthropathy.

TRAUMATIC BONE MARROW ABNORMALITIES OF THE KNEE

The ability of MRI to detect clinically significant bony injuries that are undetected on radiographic studies has probably been MRI's most important attribute in clinical practice. MRI may be very helpful in evaluating patients with acute knee pain. Occult bony injuries are an important component of the cause of symptoms. Lynch has classified bony injuries as:[60]

Lynch type I: An acute impaction force on a bone results in marrow hemorrhage and edema, disruption of trabeculae, and interstitial fluid leakage within the marrow space. On MRI, these type I bony injuries known as bone bruises/contusions are identified by the vague, geographic, edema-like pattern hypointense on T1 and hyperintense on T2 and STIR images **(Fig. 46)**. Majority of the bone bruises show signal resolution at 3 months. A minority <5% fail to resolve by 3 months probably secondary to repetitively applied trauma. A method of grading severity of marrow

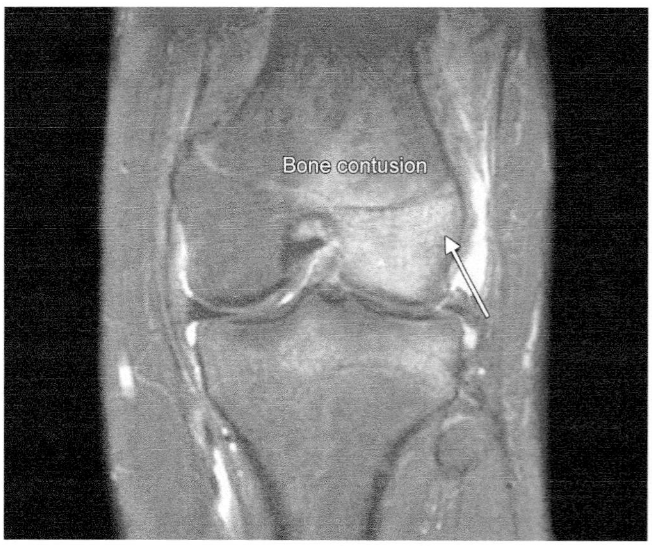

Fig. 46: STIR coronal MR image in a case of trauma showing areas of geographic bone marrow edema seen as hyperintense signal in the lateral femoral condyle and the posterolateral tibial plateau—type I bony injury.

edema, particularly trauma-induced marrow edema, is based on diffusion imaging. Diffusion imaging represents a precise method of evaluating water movement. Trabecular disruption leads to increased multidirectional movement of water, hence a recorded change in marrow diffusion is an objective marker of the severity of marrow injury. A high recorded diffusion coefficient can be used as an early indicator of severe marrow injury and can be optimally managed by a nonweight bearing regimen.[82] Five classic contusion patterns have been described in the knee include:

1. The *pivot shift injury* occurs in skiers and American football players as a result of rapid deceleration with simultaneous change in direction. The tibia undergoes external rotation with the knee in flexion. On MRI, bone bruises are seen in the posterolateral tibial plateau and midportion of the lateral femoral condyle. This pattern is highly suggestive of an ACL injury.[83]
2. The *dashboard injury* occurs in passengers in automobiles who undergo traumatic impact of the anterior proximal tibia with the dashboard while their knee is in flexion. An identical injury pattern can result from a fall onto bent knee. This injury will manifest on MRI as a bone contusion at the site of impact. A significant association has been demonstrated with injury to the PCL.
3. *Hyperextension injury* of the knee occurs with a direct blow to the anterior tibia on to the planted foot, results in "kissing contusions" of the anterior aspect of the proximal tibia and the distal femur. This finding on MRI is suggestive of additional trauma to the PCL, ACL, or menisci.
4. The *clip injury* results from pure valgus stress onto the partially flexed knee joint. Classically, this injury is seen in American football players who experience a blow to the lateral knee with the foot planted. It may also occur in a pedestrian struck by a car. The direct impact to the lateral knee will result in bone contusion at the lateral femoral condyle and lateral tibial plateau. The distractive forces at the medial joint compartment may result in coexisting MCL and medial meniscal tears (O'Donoghue triad). A smaller contusion in the medial femoral condyle at the MCL attachment may also be present as a result of the avulsive stress. Small contusion at the posterior lip of the medial tibial plateau has been described and attributed to contrecoup impaction as the knee relocates following the ACL tear.
5. *Lateral patellar dislocation* occurs in the setting of internal rotation of the femur with the knee in flexion. The resultant contraction of the quadriceps tendon in this configuration causes the patella to dislocate laterally. Bone contusions occur at the inferomedial patella and the anterior aspect of the lateral femoral condyle from the contact that occurs on relocation.

Lynch type II: These lesions reveal an interruption in the cortical bone on T1W scans **(Fig. 47A)**. These are seen as regions of increased signal intensity on T2W images and those lesions usually represent acute traumatic injuries with medullary hemorrhage and edema.

Lynch type III: Lesions present as regions of profound signal loss immediately adjacent to the cortical bone on both T1W and T2W scan. Type III lesions most likely represent degenerative type subchondral sclerosis.[74]

Acute and Chronic Avulsive Injuries

Distraction injuries result in a small avulsion fracture related to a tendinous, ligamentous or capsular attachment on the bone. The associated marrow edema is much less extensive than the marrow edema seen with an impaction injury because cortical rather than medullary bone is involved.[84] The avulsed fragment is difficult to detect on MRI as the disproportionate edema and hemorrhage in the adjacent soft tissues masks the small osseous fragment. An example is Segond fracture. A Segond fracture represents an avulsion of the lateral tibial rim at the attachment site of the lateral capsular ligament **(Fig. 47B)**. Although the fracture fragment is typically small, cortical and obscured by soft tissue edema, this injury is important to identify because it indicates substantial meniscoligamentous injury and anterolateral instability of the knee which may cause long-term disability if not recognized.

Thigh and shin splints cause traction periostitis.[85] In addition to the expected periosteal edema or fluid, MRI reveals marrow edema and even cortical signal abnormalities that indicate osseous stress injuries of varying degrees.

Fatigue and Insufficiency Fractures

Fatigue fractures occur when abnormal stress is applied to normally mineralized bone whereas insufficiency fractures result from normal activities applied to the weakened bone. MRI reveals a spectrum of findings from periosteal edema alone to progressively severe marrow edema **(Figs. 48A and B)** to a hypointense fracture line in cancellous or cortical bone. MR has been advocated as a problem-solving modality in suspected stress fracture in a patient[86] with negative plain radiographs and equivocal bone scan. MR may secure the diagnosis if the fracture line is identified.

Stress Fractures

Stress fractures can result from either normal stress placed on deficient bone, as would occur in the osteoporotic elderly individual or, excessive stress placed on normal bone, as would occur in the running, jumping, or hurdling athlete.

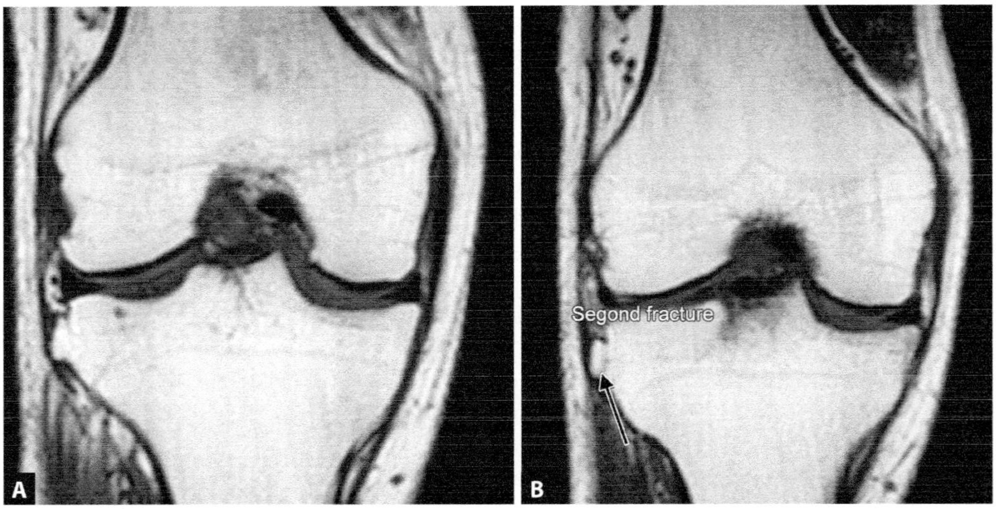

Figs. 47A and B: T1W coronal images showing an interruption in the cortical bone seen as linear low signal in the tibial spine—Grade II bony injury. Also seen is avulsion of the lateral tibial rim slightly below the level of the joint—Segond fracture.

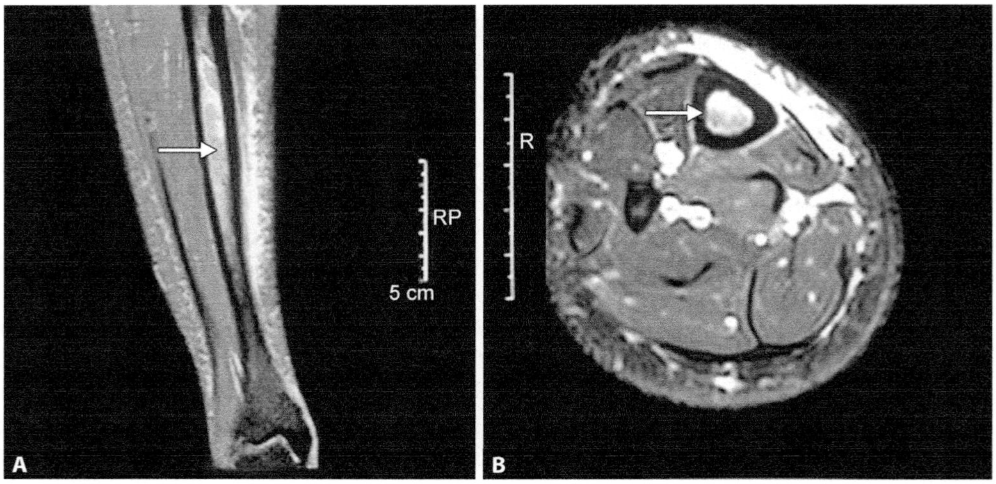

Figs. 48A and B: (A) STIR coronal; and (B) STIR axial images showing edema in the subcutaneous tissues, extensive bone marrow edema seen as hyperintense signal with no evidence of cortical irregularity or periosteal reaction—stress fracture in tibia.

Radiography is unreliable for detecting these lesions, particularly in the early stages. MRI, with a reported sensitivity and specificity as high as 88% and 100%, respectively, is the modality of choice. On MRI, stress fractures appear as as linear low-signal intensity bands, away from the joint on T1W and T2W images. Increased signal intensity may be seen around the impacted fracture site on T2W images, reflecting the associated edema.

OSTEOCHONDRAL LESIONS OF THE KNEE

The term "osteochondral lesion" refers to a localized abnormality of the articular cartilage and subchondral bone. This may be seen as a scalloped defect along the articular surface of the bone.

Spontaneous Osteonecrosis

As the name implies, spontaneous osteonecrosis of the knee (SPONK/SONK) is a condition that affects the knee and results in an area of subchondral necrosis. Although long thought to represent a form of primary osteonecrosis, recent studies have concluded that this lesion is actually a subchondral insufficiency fracture (SIF) that results in a devitalized segment of bone between the fracture line and overlying articular cartilage.[87] The primary event is thus a SIF followed by secondary necrosis limited to the area between the fracture line and the subchondral bone. SONK is basically a SIF that progresses into collapse. Hence, the term spontaneous osteonecrosis is a misnomer and is a condition completely different from primary osteonecrosis of the knee.

Spontaneous osteonecrosis is a distinct clinicopathological entity characterized by an older age of onset (most commonly an elderly woman), an abrupt onset of symptoms, acute onset of pain, a predilection for the weight bearing surface of medial femoral condyle, and a unique MRI appearance. The patients who develop osteonecrosis are elderly and osteoporotic. The osteoporotic bone is susceptible to microfracture leading to accumulation of fluid within the subchondral bone seen as extensive edema on the MR images. Initial radiographs are often normal in spontaneous osteonecrosis even though the pain is severe, and the patient is unable to ambulate. On MRI, extensive edema-like signal is seen in the medial femoral condyle along with a linear subchondral focus of low-signal intensity that represents the insufficiency fracture[88] **(Figs. 49A and B)**. A length of 14 mm and a thickness of 4 mm for these subchondral low-signal intensity areas are indicative of evolution to collapsed osteonecrosis. Deeply located low signal lines with respect to subchondral bone also indicate irreversible osteonecrosis. Medial meniscal tears have also been reported in association with spontaneous osteonecrosis.

This entity needs to be differentiated from osteochondritis dissecans (OCD) and from transient bone marrow edema syndrome. The lesion in OCD is typically in a different location on the lateral aspect of medial femoral condyle.[89] Histologically, the osteochondritic lesion is composed of hyaline articular cartilage covering a metabolically active ossific nucleus. The lesion in osteonecrosis consists of dead bone. Loose bodies are a frequent result of osteochondritis—in fact they may be the presenting symptom in OCD but they are unusual in osteonecrosis.[90]

Juvenile and Adult Osteochondritis Dissecans[91]

Osteochondritis dissecans is an idiopathic focal alteration of subchondral bone that carries the risk for instability and disruption of adjacent articular cartilage. OCD may result in premature OA. While acute traumatic osteochondral lesions first affect the articular cartilage and the bone later ("outside in" mechanism), OCD lesions involve the cartilage later (inside out mechanism). The condition manifests itself either in childhood (juvenile OCD) or middle age (adult OCD), but the most frequent age of onset is preadolescence. Several theories have been postulated for its etiology. It has been suggested by some to result from repetitive trauma that causes shear forces across the cartilage. The alternative theory, more popular recently, is that OCD is an avascular lesion attributed to an insufficient end arterial blood supply to the subarticular trabeculae and poor anastomoses with the neighboring systems resulting in the infarctions of small wedge-shaped pieces of bone immediately beneath the articular cartilage. Whatever be the etiology, the insult causes a disturbance of a small area of epiphyseal growth plate which results in localized delay or cessation of normal ossification. The affected epiphyseal segment remains cartilaginous while the rest of the epiphysis continues to ossify and expand in a centrifugal fashion. This creates an appearance of a radiolucent crater which basically represents hindered cartilage ossification and is called a "progeny" segment. The progeny segment may later develop laminar calcifications in the deep areas or may ossify partially or completely.[91] When the OCD lesion cannot withstand forces applied to the joint, it separates from the "parent" bone. The sequence of events is as follows 5 cleft/rim at the interface between the fragment and adjacent bone -> fragment instability -> disruption of the bone and overlying articular cartilage -> fragment separation. The fragment may separate completely to form a loose body or it may remain in its crater in the femoral condyle.

The typical location of an OCD lesion is the lateral aspect of the medial femoral condyle. Radiographic findings include a geographic subchondral lucency along the nonweight bearing surface of the medial femoral condyle.

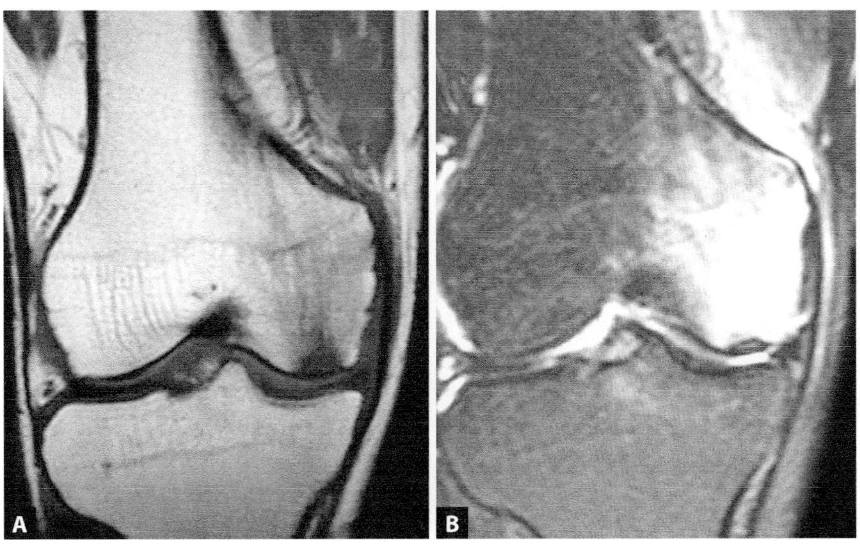

Figs. 49A and B: (A) T1W coronal; and (B) STIR coronal MR images showing extensive marrow edema in the medial femoral condyle along with a crescentic subchondral focus of low-signal intensity—spontaneous osteonecrosis of the knee.

MRI plays an important role in detecting the lesion if plain films are normal. It usually shows a crescentic or ovoid focus of subchondral signal abnormality. MRI can also allow characterization of various tissue components of the progeny fragment. Gradient recalled echo sequences show nonmineralized portions of the fragment. The primary concern when evaluating a focus of OCD is whether the fragment of subchondral bone is unstable or stable. The four signs of instability described on MRI include **(Figs. 50A to C)**:

1. T2W MR images reveal a high-signal intensity rim at the interface between the fragment and adjacent bone.
2. Fluid-filled cysts beneath the lesion.
3. A high-signal intensity line extending through the articular cartilage overlying the lesion.
4. A focal osteochondral defect filled with joint fluid.

All four criteria when present indicate a 100% sensitivity and 100% specificity for instability in adult OCD. However, these criteria are not specific for juvenile OCD. These criteria have been revised for juvenile OCD with the addition of three secondary signs:[91]

1. A high-signal intensity rim surrounding a juvenile OCD lesion indicates instability only if it has the same signal intensity as that of joint fluid.
2. A second outer rim of T2W low-signal intensity.
3. Multiple breaks in the subchondral bone plate on the T2W MR images.

The rim of fluid-filled signal intensity surrounding an OCD lesion represents a cleft filled with fluid between the parent bone and progeny. The outer rim of low-signal intensity represents fibrous tissue and subchondral cysts should be multiple and larger than 5 mm for the lesion to be unstable.

MRI of the knee is an excellent diagnostic tool that provides information about the composition, integrity, and stability of the OCD segment.

These osteochondral lesions may predispose to OA. An assessment of the overlying articular cartilage is important to guide appropriate treatment. Once OA occurs, it may be impossible to determine the original cause and treatment options may be limited to joint replacement.

Transient Bone Marrow Edema Syndrome (Transient Osteoporosis)

Transient bone marrow edema syndrome (also known as transient osteoporosis) was first described in the hip. In the knee, the lateral femoral condyle is usually involved, although involvement of the medial femoral condyle and tibial plateau has also been described. Affected patients present with an acute onset of pain usually not associated with trauma. Resolution of pain and edema usually takes place within 6 to 12 months. Long-term sequelae do not occur. MRI findings include diffuse edema (low signal on T1W images and high signal on T2W or STIR sequences) without a focal area of signal abnormality typical of osteonecrosis.[92]

There is a considerable difference in clinical prognosis and treatment of transient osteoporosis as compared to spontaneous osteonecrosis. Hence, it is important to differentiate between these two entities. The differentiating features include:

- Absence of low-signal intensity in subchondral areas on T2W MR images is indicative of complete reversibility.
- Absence of focal deformity of the epiphyseal contour is indicative of complete reversibility.
- Spontaneous osteonecrosis of the knee typically involves medial femoral condyle while transient osteoporosis is more commonly seen in the lateral femoral condyle.

MISCELLANEOUS LESIONS

Bursae[1]

Several bursae may be seen around the knee joint. At times, these can mimic intra-articular pathology and need to be differentiated.

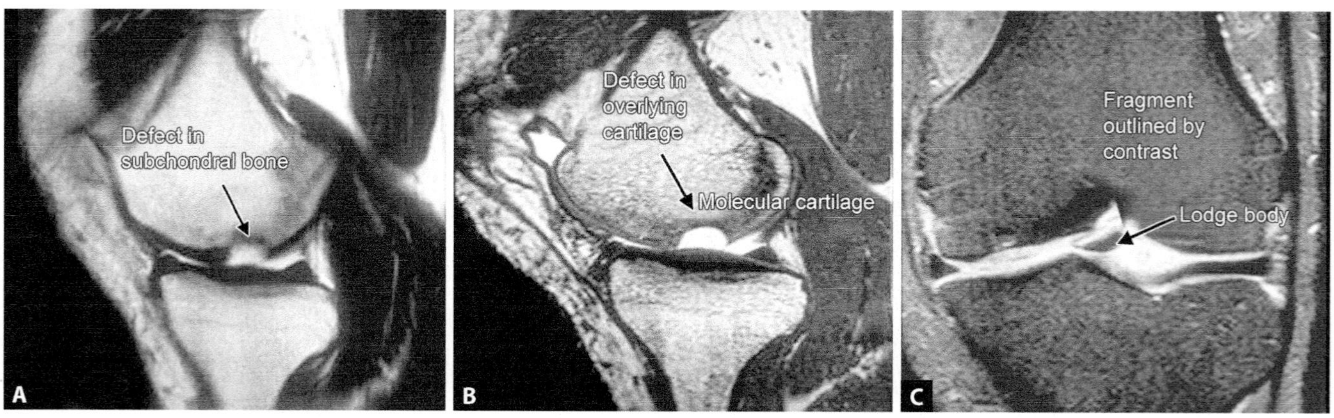

Figs. 50A to C: (A) Sagittal T2W; (B) DESS sagittal plane images showing a defect in the subchondral bone and overlying cartilage; and (C) Indirect MR arthrography showing the displaced fragment outlined by contrast—osteochondritis dessicans.

Popliteal (Baker's Cysts)[4]

Popliteal (Baker's cysts) of the gastrocnemius semimembranosus bursae arise between medial head of the gastrocnemius muscle and the more medial semimembranosus tendon. A narrow neck connecting the cyst to the joint may be seen on axial images **(Figs. 51A and B)**. Popliteal cysts may arise from any condition that causes an increase in synovial fluid within the joint and are frequently seen in association with tears of the posterior horn of the medial meniscus.[60] Popliteal cysts at times can become very large and cause compartment syndrome. The rupture in the adjacent musculature can cause intense inflammation, mimic deep vein thrombosis, and be very symptomatic.

Prepatellar Bursa

Also called the housemaid's knee, prepatellar bursitis is a common cause of anterior knee pain. It is seen as a fluid collection anterior to the patella.

Pes Anserinus Bursa

Also called the "goose's foot" (webbed foot appearance), it refers to the configuration of the insertion of the pes tendons on to the tibia. Gracilis, sartorius, and semitendinosus constitute the pes anserinus tendons. The bursa lies beneath the tendons and on being inflamed may be seen to extend proximally toward the joint. Pes Anserinus bursitis is seen just below the joint line on the anteromedial tibia.[4]

Semimembranosus-tibial Collateral Ligament Bursa

This bursa occurs on the joint line and drapes like a horseshoe over the semimembranosus tendon. It may mimic a meniscal cyst but no connection to a meniscus is, however found.

Tibial Collateral Ligament Bursa

This lies deep to the MCL and extends vertically above and below the joint line. The finding of the fluid being well contained and cyst like rather than being diffusely distributed separates it from meniscocapsular separation.

Medullary Infarction

Several factors, e.g., steroids, trauma, vasculitis are known to predispose to the development of focal areas of medullary infarction. Medullary infarcts result in geographic areas of ischemic and devitalized marrow that produce a characteristic MRI appearance; a geographic focus of typically heterogeneous signal within the marrow that is surrounded by characteristic low-signal intensity, serpentine border on T1W images. This border often demonstrates a classic double-line sign on T2W images. This is one of the few medullary lesions that usually contain some central fat. The presence of central fat is characteristic of this lesion.

Reflex Sympathetic Dystrophy

The exact cause of reflex sympathetic dystrophy (RSD) is unclear but it is believed to represent sequelae from hyperactivity of the sympathetic nervous system. In many cases, it occurs after a recent episode of trauma. It results in circulatory changes and may progress to muscle atrophy, contractures, pale skin, and loss of hair on the extremity. MRI reveals diffuse, patchy bone marrow edema, which does not progress to the subchondral collapse seen in osteonecrosis. MRI findings which suggest the diagnosis

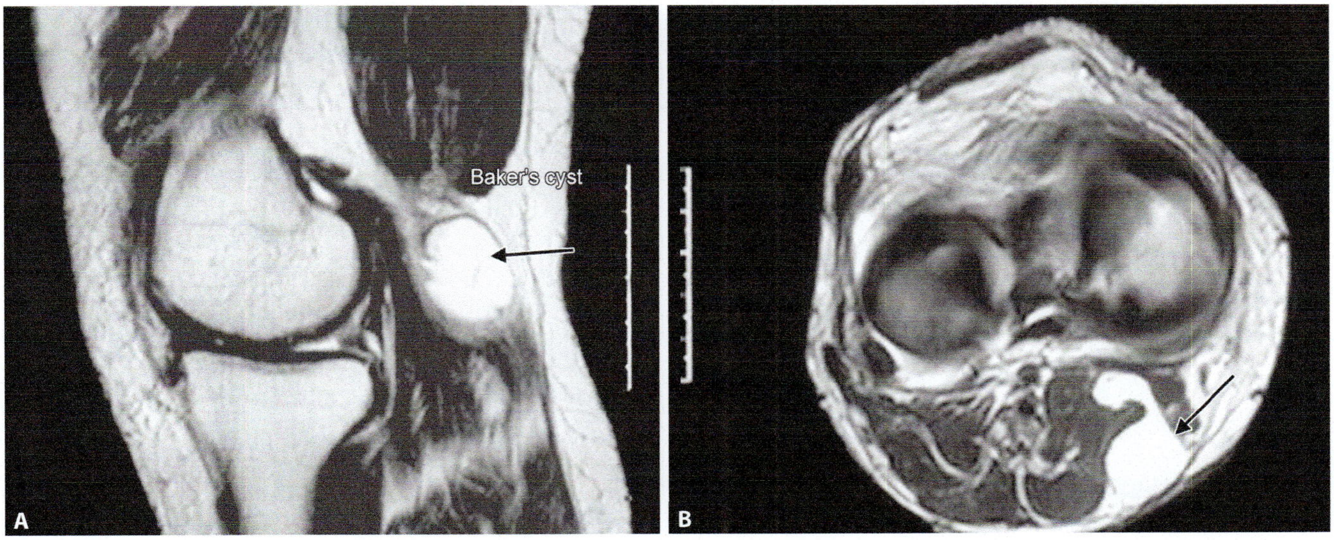

Figs. 51A and B: (A) T2W sagittal; and (B) T2W axial MR images of the knee showing fluid intensity cystic structure between the medial head of gastrocnemius and the more medial semimembranosus tendon—popliteal/Baker's cyst.

of RSD include skin thickening, contrast enhancement, muscular atrophy, soft tissue edema, and joint effusions.[93]

BONE INFECTIONS

Capsular distension and joint effusions can be seen in MR scans of infected joints but are nonspecific findings.[94] A septic joint may be further characterized by intra-articular debris and synovitis from hematogenous seeding. In cases of osteomyelitis, the metaphysis, an active site of bone formation in children may show signal abnormalities (low signal on T1, bright signal on T2 or STIR images) restricted to this region. Marrow infiltration and soft tissue extension of osteomyelitis can be demonstrated using STIR and fat suppressed T2W image **(Figs. 52A to D)**. Supportive findings include overlying cortical destruction and an abscess or fistula extending to bone. A low-signal intensity rim sign has been described in chronic infection resulting from trauma. This rim of fibrous tissue or reactive bone displays low signal on all pulse sequences and surrounds the area of active bone disease.

Magnetic resonance is also used to evaluate subacute osteomyelitis including Brodie's abscess. In Brodie's abscess, the focus of involvement of osteomyelitis is hyperintense on STIR and fat suppressed T2W images. The sclerotic margin displays low signal on all pulse sequences and there may be fluid in communication with the central infected focus.[5]

BONE NEOPLASMS

Magnetic resonance imaging has become an important component in the evaluation of primary bone neoplasms because of its ability to detect and accurately determine the local extent of disease. MRI and MR spectroscopy may also be helpful in following a patient's response to therapy. Osteogenic sarcoma is one of the most common primary bone tumors emanating from the distal femur. The extent of intramedullary disease is best defined with T1W spin echo or STIR images while T2W images may provide information about full extent disease and edema into the soft tissues. Encasement of major

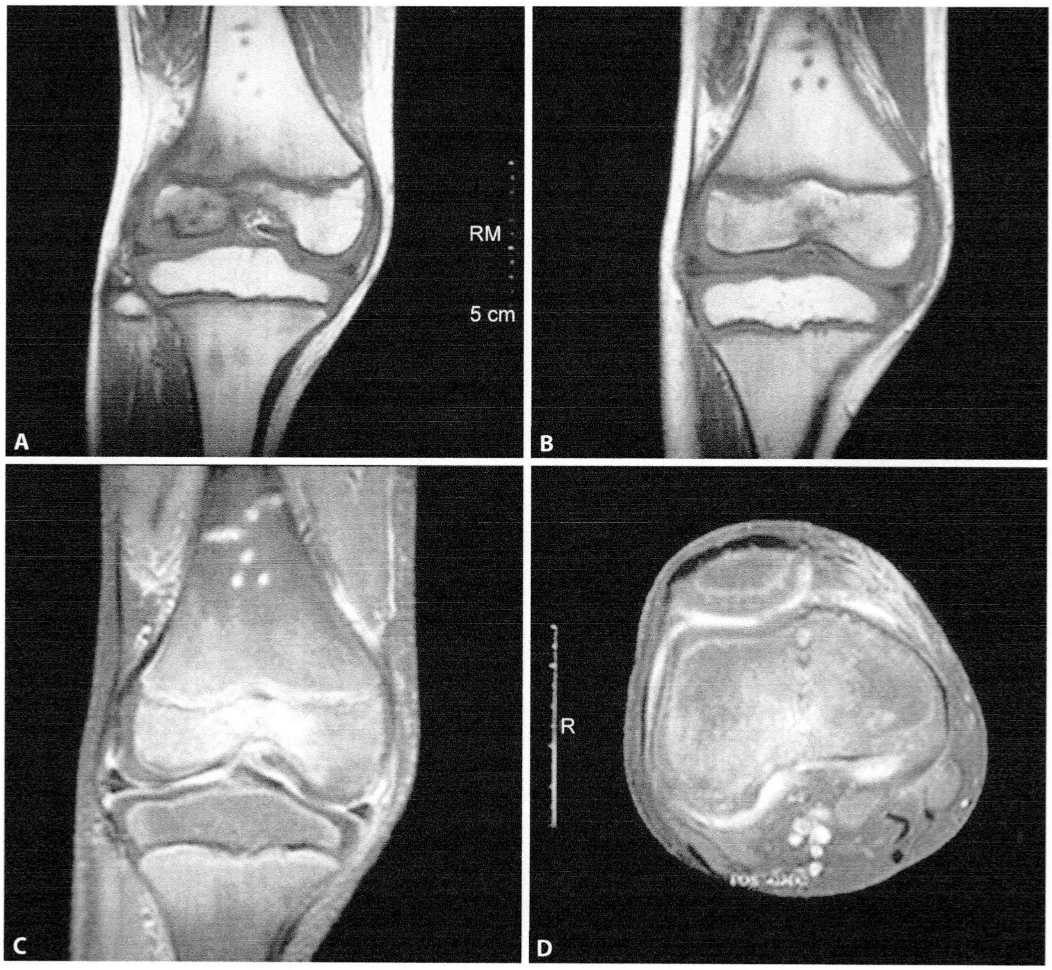

Figs. 52A to D: T1 coronal (A) and (B) postgadolinium coronal (C) postgadolinium T1 axial (D) images showing erosion of the articular margin of femur, fuzziness of the articular margins, marrow signal alteration, joint effusion, and thick enhancing synovium—septic arthritis.

vessels and nerves as well as involvement of multiple muscular compartment may all be evaluated by MR and may decrease the efficacy of limb salvage surgery **(Figs. 53A to D)**.[95]

Infiltrative neoplasms such as leukemia and lymphoma may present with knee pain indistinguishable from that caused by internal derangements of knee. These lesions need to be distinguished from signal inhomogeneity of normal marrow bone in metaphyses caused by variations in extent of hematopoietic marrow. Most types of marrow pathology result in signal intensity that is lower than that of skeletal muscle or intervertebral disc on T1W images whereas hematopoietic marrow demonstrates signal intensity that is slightly higher than that of skeletal muscle or disc on T1W images (owing to the relatively high amount of fat present even in red marrow). Other features of red marrow include signal intensity that parallels the signal intensity of other areas of known hematopoietic marrow, bilateral symmetry, scattered foci of fatty signal within the region of concern, and an abrupt margination at the level of a closed physis. Also, in contrast to the normal hematopoietic marrow, infiltrative disorders usually present a homogeneous low signal intensity mass on T1W images and show well-defined margin.

Magnetic resonance imaging is also helpful in evaluating benign bony neoplasms. MRI characterizes the components of an osteochondroma better than other imaging techniques such as CT. The cartilaginous cap is well-visualized by MRI and should be less than 1 cm in the non-neoplastic disease.[51]

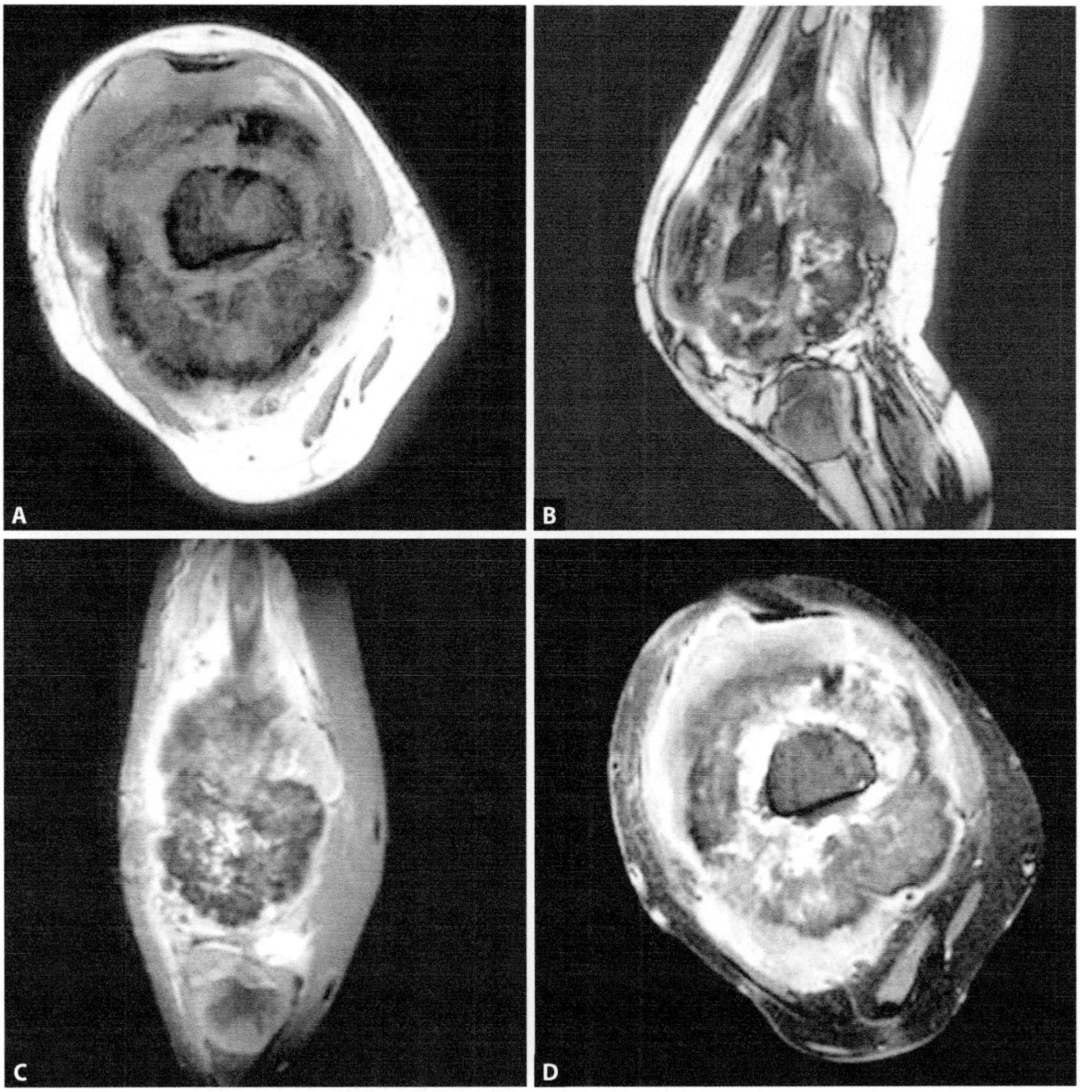

Figs. 53A to D: (A) T1 axial; (B) T2 sagittal; (C) T1 postcontrast coronal; and (D) Axial MR images showing an irregular circumferential heterogeneous mass arising from the lower metadiaphyseal region of femur with cortical destruction, spiculated periosteal reaction, new bone formation, infiltration of medulla and multicompartment muscle involvement. Skip/metastatic focus also seen in upper tibia—osteogenic sarcoma lower end femur.

MR ARTHROGRAPHY

Intra-articular contrast material enhances the diagnostic capabilities of MRI especially in the depiction of small structure and subtle disease.

Technique

The direct MR arthrographic technique does not differ from conventional arthrography. The knee is placed in a slightly bent, recumbent position for the usually used anterolateral access. The patella is pulled laterally and the puncture is made mid-patella or above with the needle entering the joint beneath the surface of the patella. To be able to fill the knee joint with a small volume of dissolved contrast medium, compression is applied to the soft tissues 15–20 cm above the joint cavity with an elastic bandage to prevent entry of the contrast medium into the suprapatellar recess. The injection is carried out under sterile conditions. The total amount of the dilute contrast mixture (Gd-DTPA) injected should be 30–40 mL. After the injection, active and passive movements of the knee joint are carried out several times to achieve uniform distribution in the joint. An arthrographic effect or indirect MR arthrography can also be achieved with joint fluid enhancement following intravenous injection of Gd-DTPA. This method is referred to as indirect MR arthrography since no articular injection is required. The role of MR arthrography is in the following lesions:

- *Meniscal lesions*: MR arthrography has been shown to have a greater accuracy than conventional MRI for the detection of meniscal retears.[96] Because gadolinium-based contrast material has a lower viscosity than synovial fluid, it is more likely to be imbibed into a small cleft and thereby highlight the presence of a tear.
- *Cartilage lesions*: Administration of intra-articular contrast agent allows excellent delineation of the cartilage surface and provides good discrimination of cartilaginous lesions which have been graded from I to IV.[97] MR arthrography allows detection of grade II to IV lesions, however, grade I lesions still remain difficult to detect by arthrography since grade I lesions have no surface abnormality that is detected by intra-articular Gd-DTPA solution. On delayed sequences, however, an enhancement effect in cartilaginous areas with altered intrachondral structures can be observed. This is caused by diffusion of contrast material into the hyaline cartilage, although the thickness and surface of the cartilage may still appear normal in grade I lesions.
- *Osteochondritis dissecans*: OCD is a lesion that characteristically affects the articular cartilage and subchondral bone with the potential of fragmentation and separation. Early detection of osteochondral lesion is desirable because the onset of degenerative arthritis in patients with OCD is estimated to occur 10 years earlier than in normal individuals. Management and prognosis of these osteochondral lesions depend on the stability of the fragment within its bony crater and the status of the overlying articular cartilage. MR arthrography is more accurate than MR in staging these osteochondral lesions of the knee.[98]
- *Intra-articular bodies*: The knee is affected most commonly by intra-articular bodies. These may consist of bone, cartilage or both bone and cartilage. Imaging is necessary to confirm the clinical diagnosis and to localize these bodies before surgery, because intra-articular bodies may be missed during arthroscopy. Radiography and conventional tomography are useful only when radiopaque intra-articular bodies are present. MR arthrography has the greatest sensitivity (86%) which is significantly more sensitive than conventional MRI.[99]
- *Plica synovialis*: The three plicae of the knee (suprapatellar plica, medial patellar plica, and infrapatellar plica) are remnants of the embryologic synovium that separate the joint into different compartments during gestation. Partial plical remnants are often identified at arthroscopy but are incidental findings without clinical significance. Some plicae may persist into adult life and cause anterior knee pain, clicking, catching or locking of the knee when these plicae become inflamed and thickened by trauma or overuse.

The mediopatellar plica which extends from underneath the quadriceps and slides over the medial femoral condyle with knee movement is of great pathologic importance. The plica is usually attached closely to the femoral condyle and is not visualized when there is insufficient synovial fluid to outline. Differentiation between knee injuries and mediopatellar plica is important to avoid unnecessary arthroscopy. MR arthrography enables assessment of thickened plicae and should be considered as an alternative to diagnostic arthroscopy in patients with mediopatellar plica.[100]

POSTOPERATIVE EVALUATION OF THE KNEE

New developments and improvements in the ligamentous and meniscal surgery and cartilage repair procedures have led to an increased incidence of these procedures being performed. Subsequently there is an increase in the postoperative imaging studies and it is imperative for the radiologist to know the normal imaging appearance and complication of these procedures.

Imaging of the ACL Graft

The most commonly injured ligament in the knee is the ACL. ACL-deficient knees can result in changes in mechanics causing secondary meniscal and cartilage injury. Hence, reconstruction of ACLs is being undertaken more commonly. FSE is preferred over conventional spin echo because of the decreased metallic artifact seen with FSE.[101] An addition, an oblique sagittal scan, is often performed in the plane of the graft to allow better visualization of the ACL graft on one slice. Use of thinner 3 mm sections reduces volume averaging artifacts and provides better delineation of the neoalignment. An ACL neoalignment is considered intact if a smooth well-defined low-signal intensity band is seen along its entire course on both T1W and T2W images. The MR criteria used to assess disruption are contour irregularity, increased signal intensity within the ligament on T2W images, and discontinuity of the ligament.

Graft Rupture

Spontaneous graft rupture is rare and is frequently secondary to trauma. The same criteria used to diagnose a torn native ACL are used to diagnose a ruptured ACL graft and include discontinuity of normal fibers **(Figs. 54A and B)** and abnormal signal intensity within the substance of the graft which is usually fluid signal intensity interrupting the graft.

Graft Impingement

Graft impingement occurs when the graft abnormally contacts either the wall or the roof of the intercondylar notch. Impingement can lead to stretching, erosion, remodeling, and tearing of the graft.

In impingement, MRI shows the tibial tunnel to project anterior to a line drawn along the intercondylar roof and extended to the tibial plateau (Blumensaat's line). The distal two-thirds of the graft show increased signal intensity on T2W images,[102] however, this is never fluid signal intensity unlike in graft rupture.

Arthrofibrosis

Following ACL reconstruction loss of terminal extension (extension lag) is one of the major causes of morbidity. One of the major etiologies causing extension lag is localized anterior arthrofibrosis. In this condition, a focal fibrous nodule develops anterior to the distal portion of the ACL within the intercondylar notch. The nodule physically impairs terminal extension of the knee. The bluish discoloration of this rounded lesion resembles an eyeball on arthroscopy and has been named the cyclops lesion.[103] Cyclops lesion can be identified on MRI. On T1W and PD-weighted images, nodular intermediate-signal intensity mass is seen at the anterior distal aspect of the graft in the intercondylar notch. On T2W images, the nodule has a heterogeneous but predominantly low-signal intensity.

Postoperative Meniscus

The criteria for diagnosing meniscal tears in the virgin meniscus do not apply to the post-meniscectomy knee because there can be residual abnormal signal intensity and morphology. This is especially important when greater than 25% of the meniscus is removed in which the remaining meniscus can appear foreshortened with an irregular margin. In addition, abnormal signal can also be seen in stable meniscal remnants. The specificity of these findings for meniscal retear is lower than that for tears in nonoperative menisci. Several studies have reported an accuracy of 66–80% in the postoperative meniscus.[96]

Signal changes within the meniscus at a site distant from the original tear, *fluid signal intensity* in the meniscus remnant and a displaced fragment are specific signs of a meniscal retear but are not very sensitive. Direct MR arthrography increases the accuracy of diagnosing retears of the postoperative meniscus.

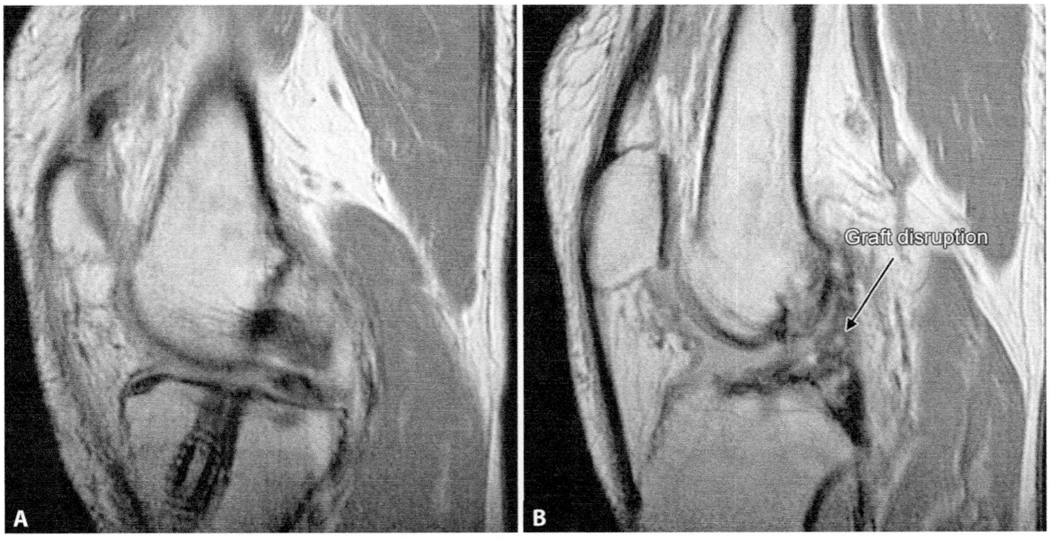

Figs. 54A and B: T2W sagittal MR images in a postoperative knee with anterior cruciate ligament graft showing discontinuity of the graft fibers with high-signal intensity within—graft disruption.

Postoperative Articular Cartilage

The development of new cartilage repair procedures that transplant or potentially reform hyaline-like articular cartilage has led to an accurate noninvasive evaluation of the cartilage lesions following repair procedures.

Magnetic resonance imaging has been used to assess incorporation of grafts, assess vascularity of grafts, evaluate the congruency between the graft and the native cartilage and bone, and assess the donor site. One complication associated with this procedure is incongruence of the graft. Other complications include loose bodies, avascular necrosis of the donor site, and condylar fracture which are all detected by MRI.

Autologous chondrocyte implantation involves harvesting chondrocytes from the relative nonweight bearing surfaces such as intercondylar notch. The chondrocytes are grown *ex vivo* and replaced into the periosteal covered site of the cartilage defect. Chondrocytes progress through several stages. Initially in the proliferative stage there is formation of a jelly-like substance. The second stage (7–12 weeks), known as the transition stage, involves formation of a type II collagen framework. From 13 weeks to 3 years, the maturation stage involves remodeling of the collagen framework resulting in firm hyaline tissue. MRI can assess the rate of and characteristics of growth cartilage and its incorporation within the native cartilage. The state of the underlying subchondral bone can also be assessed by MRI.

Magnetic resonance imaging and arthroscopy are complementary examinations for follow-up of autologous chondrocyte implants in knee. Arthroscopy is better used for assessing the cartilage surface and MR is better used for assessing lesions deep within the cartilage and underlying bone.[104,105]

ARTIFICIAL INTELLIGENCE IN THE EVALUATION OF KNEE PATHOLOGY[106]

The integration of artificial intelligence (AI) algorithms into the workflow of MSK radiology has the potential to improve diagnostic accuracy, reduce reader fatigue, expedite cases with urgent findings, and provide decision support. The CNNs or convolutional neural networks can detect pathology (tear of ligaments/meniscus, cartilage lesion), help in classification (grading OA on knee radiographs, meniscal tears), and provide cartilage and meniscus segmentation. AI thus holds the potential for lesion detection, characterization, and disease monitoring but a lot of work is needed to achieve this.[106]

CONCLUSION

Magnetic resonance imaging is clearly the imaging modality of choice for detecting and exploring joint, osseous, and soft tissue injuries in the knee. MRI plays a pivotal role in making a precise diagnosis and then guiding treatment decisions. It is also extremely helpful in imaging the postoperative knee and in determining the response to therapy. It should be the goal of any radiologist who interprets MRI examinations of the knee to be able to recognize not only the normal anatomy and accurately diagnose pathology but also to develop a better grasp of the surgical implications of the imaging findings. By thinking like an arthroscopist, one can provide a more clinically relevant report and by doing so, add value to the workup of a patient with any knee pathology.

REFERENCES

1. Reicher MA, Bassett LW, Gold RH. High resolution MRI of the knee joint. Pathologic correlations. AJR. 1985;145(5):903-9.
2. Reicher MA, Hartzman S, Duckwiler GR, Bassett LW, Anderson LJ, Gold RH. Meniscal injuries. Detection using MR imaging. Radiology. 1986;159(3):753-7.
3. Hartzman S, Reicher MA, Bassett LW, Duckwiler GR, Mandelbaum B, Gold RH. MR imaging of the knee. Chronic disorder. Radiology. 1987;162:553-7.
4. Kaplan PA. Knee. In: Kaplan PA, Helms CA, Dussault R, Anderson MW, Major NM (Eds). Musculoskeletal MRI, 1st edition. US: WB Saunders; 2001.
5. Stoller DW, Cannon WD, Anderson LJ. The knee. In: Stoller DW (Ed). Magnetic Resonance Imaging in Orthopaedics and Sports Medicine, 2nd edition. Philadelphia: Lippincott Raven; 1997.
6. Ariyachaipanich A, Bae WC, Statum S, Chung CB. Update on MRI pulse sequences for the knee: Imaging of cartilage, meniscus, tendon and hardware. Semin Musculoskeletal Radiol. 2017;21(2):45-62.
7. Bassett GC. The meniscus. Orthopaedics. 1992;15:35-42.
8. Koski JA, Ibarra C, Rodeo SA, Warren RF. Meniscal injury and repair. Clinical status. Orthop Clin North Am. 2000;31:419-35.
9. Escobedo EM, Hunter JC, Zink-Brody GC, Wilson AJ, Harrison SD, Fisher DJ. Usefulness of turbo spin-echo MR imaging in the evaluation of meniscal tears. Comparison with a conventional spin echo sequence. Am J Roentgenol. 1996;167(5):1223-7.
10. Kowalchuk RM, Kneeland JB, Dalinka MK, Siegelman ES, Dockery WD. MRI of the knee. Value of short echo time fast spin echo using high performance gradients versus conventional spin echo imaging for the detection of meniscal tears. Skeletal Radiol. 2000;29(9):520-4.
11. Helms CA, Laorr A, Cannon WD. The absent bow-tie sign in Bucket handle tears of the menisci in knee. Am J Roentgenol. 1998;170(1):57-61.
12. Ryu KN, Kim IS, Kim EJ, Ahn JW, Bae DK, Sartoris DJ, et al. MR imaging of tears of discoid lateral menisci. Am J Roentgenol. 1998;171(4):963-7.
13. Yu JS, Cosgarea AJ, Kaeding CC, Wilson D. Meniscal flounce MR imaging. Radiology. 1997;203(2):513-5.
14. Schnarkowski P, Tirman PF, Fuchigami KD, Crues JV, Butler MG, Genant HK. Meniscal ossicle: radiographic and MR imaging findings. Radiology. 1995;196(1):47-50.

15. Hajek PC, Gylys Morin VM, Baker LL, Sartoris DJ, Haghighi P, Resnick D. The high signal intensity meniscus of the knee magnetic resonance evaluation and *in vivo* correlation. Invest Radiol. 1987;22(11):883-90.
16. Kaplan PA, Nelson NL, Garvin KL, Brown DE. MR of the knee. The significance of high signal in the meniscus that does not clearly extend to the surface. Am J Roentgenol. 1991;156(2):333-6.
17. Davis SJ, Teresi LM. The "Notch" sign: meniscal contour deformities as indicators of tear in MR imaging of the knee. J Comput Assist Tomography. 1990;14:975-80.
18. Seung JY, Seunghun L, Song Y. Two slice touch rule in meniscal tear. Radiology. 2016;280(2):649-50.
19. Campbell SE, Sanders TG, Morrison WB. MR imaging of meniscal cysts: incidence, location and clinical significance. Am J Roentgenol. 2001;177(2):409-13.
20. Harper KW, Helms CA, Lambert HS III, Higgins LD. Radial Meniscal tears: significance incidence and MR appearance. AM J Roentgenol. 2005;185(6):1429-34.
21. Tuckman GA, Miller WJ, Remo JW, Fritts HM, Rozansky MI. Radial tears of the menisci: MR findings. Am J Roentgenol. 1994;163(2):395-400.
22. Ozkor G, Circi E Gone U, Irgit K, Pourbagher A, Tandogan RN. Radial tears in the root of the posterior horn of the medial meniscus. Knee Surg Sports Traumatol Arthrosc. 2008;16(9):849-54.
23. Wright DH, De Smet AA, Norris M. Bucket handle tears of the medial and lateral menisci of the knee: value of MR imaging in detecting displaced fragments. Am J Roentgenol. 1995;165(3):621-5.
24. Singson R, Feldman F, Staron R, Kiernan H. MR imaging of displaced meniscal bucket handle tear of the medial meniscus. Am J Roentgenol. 1991;156(1):121-4.
25. Rao N, Patel Y, Opsha O, Chen Q, Owen J, Eisemon E, et al. Use of the V-sign in the diagnosis of bucket handle meniscal tear of the knee. Skeletal Radiol. 2012;41(3):293-7.
26. Belzer JP, Cannon WD. Meniscus tears: treatment in the stable and unstable knee. J Am Acad Orthop Surg. 1993;1(1):41-7.
27. Nguyen JC, Smet A, Graf BK, Rosas HG. MR imaging based diagnosis and classification of meniscal tears. Radiographics. 2014;34(4):981-99.
28. Bergin D, Hochberg H, Zoga AC, Qazi N, Parker L, Morrison WB. Indirect soft tissue and osseous signs on knee MRI of surgically proven meniscal tears. Am J Roentgenol. 2008;191(1):86-92.
29. Vahey TN, Bennett HT, Arrington LE, Shelbourne KD, Ng J. MR imaging of the knee: pseudotear of the lateral meniscus caused by the meniscofemoral ligament. Am J Roentgenol. 1990;154(6):1237-9.
30. Watanabe AT, Carter BC, Teitelbaum GP, Seeger LL, Bradley WG Jr. Normal variations in MR imaging of the knee: appearance and frequency. Am J Roentgenol. 1989;153(2):341-4.
31. Peterfy CG, Janzen DL, Tirman PF, van Dijke CF, Pollack M, Genant HK. Magic-angle phenomenon: a cause of increased signal in the normal lateral meniscus on short TE MR images of the knee. Am J Roentgenol. 1994;163(1):149-54.
32. Henning CE, Lynch MA. Current concepts of meniscal function and pathology. Clin Sports Med. 1985;4(2):259-64.
33. Matava MJ, Eck K, Totty W, Wright RW, Shively RA. Magnetic resonance imaging as a tool to predict meniscal reparability. Am J Sports Med. 1999;27(4):436-43.
34. Reicher MA, Hartzman S, Bassett LW, Mandelbaum B, Duckwiler G, Gold RH. MR imaging of the knee traumatic disorders. Radiology. 1987;162(2):547-51.
35. Crues JV, Mink J, Levy TL, Lotysch M, Stoller DW. Meniscal tears of the knee: accuracy of MR imaging. Radiology. 1987;164(2):445-8.
36. Bencardino JT, Rosenber ZS, Brown RR, Hassankhani A, Lustrin ES, Beltran J. Traumatic musculotendinous injuries of the knee: diagnosis with MR imaging. Radiographics. 2000;20:103-20.
37. Lee JK, Yao L, Phelps CT, Wirth CR, Czajka J, Lozman J. Anterior cruciate ligament tears. MR imaging compared with arthroscopy and clinical tests. Radiology. 1988;166(3):861-4.
38. Chan WP, Peterfy C, Fritz RC, Genant HK. MR diagnosis of complete tears of the anterior cruciate ligament of the knee: importance of anterior subluxation of tibia. Am J Roentgenol. 1994;162(2):355-60.
39. Kaplan PA, Gehl RH, Dussault RG, Anderson MW, Diduch DR. Bone contusions of the posterior lip of the medial tibial plateau (countercoup injury) and associated internal derangements of the knee at MR imaging. Radiology. 1999;211(3):747-53.
40. Graf BK, Cook DA, De Smat AA, Keene JS. Bone bruises on magnetic resonance imaging evaluation of anterior cruciate ligament injuries. Am J Sports Med. 1993;21(2):220-3.
41. Tung GA, Davis LM, Wiggins ME, Fadale PD. Tears of the anterior cruciate ligament: primary and secondary signs at MR imaging. Radiology. 1993;188(3):661-7.
42. Vanhoenacker F, Vos ND, Dyck PV. Common mistakes and pitfalls in magnetic resonance imaging of the knee. Journal of the Belgian Society of Radiology. 2016;100(1):1-17.
43. Covey DC, Sapega AA. Anatomy and function of the posterior cruciate ligament. Clin Sports Med. 1994;13(3):509-18.
44. Hansford BG, Yablon CM. Multiligamentous injury of the knee: MRI diagnosis and injury pattern. Semin Musculoskeletal Radiol. 2017;21(2):63-74.
45. D Maesaneer M, Von Roy F, Lenchik L, Barbaix E, De Ridder F, Osteaux M. Three layers of the medial capsular and supporting structures of the knee: MR imaging-anatomic correlation. Radiographics. 2000;20:83-9.
46. Schweitzer MS, Tran D, Deely DM, Hume EL. Medial collateral ligament injuries: evaluation of multiple signs, prevalence and location of associated bone bruises and assessment with MR imaging. Radiology. 1995;194(3):825-9.
47. Mendes LF, Preeterklieber ML, Cho JH, Garcia GM, Resnick DL, Chung CB. Pellegrini Stieda disease: A heterogeneous disorder not synonymous with ossification/calcification of the tibial collateral ligament—anatomic and imaging investigation. Skeletal Radiol. 2006;35(12):916-22.
48. Rosas HG. Unraveling the posterolateral corner of the knee. Radiographics. 2016;36(6):1776-91.
49. Jadhav S, Mone S, Riascos R, Lemos DF, Swischuk LE. Comprehensive review of the anatomy, function and

imaging of the popliteus and associated pathologic conditions. Radiographics. 2014;34(2):496-513.
50. Recondo JA, Salvador E, Villanua JA, Barrera MC, Gervás C, Alústiza JM. Lateral stabilising structures of the knee: functional anatomy and injuries assessed with MR imaging. Radiographics. 2000;20:91-102.
51. Yu JS, Salonen DC, Hodler J, Haghighi P, Trudell D, Resnick D. Posterolateral aspect of the knee: improved MR imaging with a coronal oblique technique. Radiology. 1996;198(1):199-204.
52. Loredo R, Hodler J, Pedowitz R, Yeh LR, Trudell D, Resnick D. Posteromedial corner of the knee: MR imaging with gross anatomic correlation. Skeletal Radiol. 1999;28(6):305-11.
53. Lundqnist RB, Matcuk GR, Schein AJ, Skalski MR, White EA, Forrester DM, et al. Posteromedial corner of the knee: the neglected corner. Radiographics 2015,35(4):1123-37.
54. Hayes CW, Brigido MK, Jamadar DA, Propeck T. Mechanism based pattern approach to classification of complex injuries of the knee depicted at MR imaging. Radiographics. 2000;20:121-34.
55. Menz MJ, Lucas GL. Magnetic resonance imaging of a rupture of the medial head of the gastrocnemius muscle. J Bone Joint Surg Am. 1991;73(8):1260-1.
56. Yu JS, Goodiwn D, Salonen D, Pathria MN, Resnick D, Dardani M, et al. Complete dislocation of the knee: Spectrum of associated soft tissue injuries depicted by MR imaging. Am J Roentgenol. 1995;164(1):135-9.
57. Yu JS, Petersilge C, Sartoris DJ, Pathria MN, Resnick D. MR imaging of injuries of the extensor mechanism of the knee. Radiographics. 1994;14(3):541-51.
58. Nance EP, Kaye JJ. Injuries of the quadriceps mechanism. Radiology. 1982;142(2):301-7.
59. Quinn SF, Brown TR, Demlow TA. MR imaging of patellar retinacular ligament injuries. J Magn Reson Imaging. 1993;3(6):843-7.
60. Crues JV, Manji SA, Shellock FG. Knee. In: Stark D, Bradley WG (Eds): Magnetic Resonance Imaging, 3rd edition. US: Mosby; 1999.
61. Diederichs G, Issever AS, Scheffler S. MR Imaging of patellar instability. Radiographics. 2010;30(4):961-81.
62. Shellock FG, Mink JH, Deutsch AL, Foo TK, Sullenberger P. Patellofemoral joint: identification of abnormalities with active movement 'unloaded' versus 'loaded' kinematic MR imaging techniques. Radiology. 1993;188(2):575-8.
63. Bruno F, Barile A, Arrigoni F, Laporta A, Russo A, Carotti M, et al. Weight bearing MRI of the knee: a review of advantages and limits. Acta Biomed. 2018;89:78-88.
64. Bradella MA, Tirman PFJ, Peterfy CG, Zarlingo M, Feller JF, Bost FW, et al. Accuracy of T2 weighted fast spin-echo MR imaging with fat saturation in detecting cartilage defects in the knee: comparison with arthroscopy in 130 patients. AJR. 1999;172(4):1073-80.
65. Hardy PA, Recht MP, Piraino DW. Fat suppressed MRI of articular cartilage with spatial-spectral excitation pulse. J Magn Reson Imaging. 1998;8(6):1279-87.
66. Disler DG, McCauley TR, Kelman CG, Fuchs MD, Ratner LM, Wirth CR, et al. Fat suppressed three-dimensional spoiled gradient-echo MR imaging of hyaline cartilage defects in the knee: comparison with standard MR imaging and arthroscopy. Am J Roentgenol. 1996;167(1):127-32.
67. Erickson SJ, Waldochmidt JG, Czervionke LF, Prost RW. Hyaline cartilage truncation artifact as a cause of trilaminar appearance with fat suppressed three dimensional spoiled gradient recalled sequences. Radiology. 1996;201(1):260-4.
68. Naraghi A, White LM. Three-dimensional MRI of the musculoskeletal system. Am J Roentgenol. 2012; 199(3):W283-93.
69. Kijowski R, Blankenpaker DG, Davis KW, Shinki K, Kaplan LD, De Smet AA. Comparison of 1.5 and 3.0 T MR imaging for evaluating the articular cartilage of the knee joint. Radiology. 2009;250(3):839-48.
70. Wong S, Steinbach L, Zhao J, Stehling C, Ma CB, Link TM. Comparative study of imaging at 3.0 T versus 1.5 T of the knee. Skeletal Radiol. 2009;38(8):761-9.
71. McCauley TR, Kier R, Lynch KJ, Jokl P. Chondromalacia patellae: diagnosis with MR imaging. Am J Roentgenol. 1992;158(1):101-5.
72. Crema MD, Roemer FW, Marra MD, Guermazi A. MR Imaging of intra and periarticular soft tissues and subchondral bone in knee osteoarthritis. Radiol Cl N Am. 2009;47(4):687-701.
73. Kijowski R, Stanton P, Fine J, Smet AD. Subchondral bone marrow edema in patients with degeneration of the articular cartilage of the knee joint. Radiology. 2006;238(3):943-9.
74. Waldochmidt JG, Braunstein EM, Buckwalter KA. Magnetic resonance imaging of osteoarthritis. Rheum Dis Clin North Am. 1999;25:451-65.
75. Buckwalter JA, Mankin HJ. Articular cartilage repair and transplantation. Arthritis Rheum. 1998;41:1331-42.
76. Le J, Peng Q, Sperling K. Biochemical magnetic resonance imaging of knee articular cartilage: T1 rho and T2 mapping as cartilage degeneration biomarkers. Ann NY Acad Sci. 2016;1383(1):34-42.
77. Sophia Fox, Bedi AJA, Rodeo SA. The basic science of articular cartilage: structure, composition and function. Sports Health. 2009;1(6):461-8.
78. Link TM, Stahl R, Woertler K. Cartilage imaging, motivation, techniques, current and future significance. Eur Radiol. 2007;17(5):1135-46.
79. Hayashi D, Roemer FW, Guermazi A. Recent advances in research imaging of osteoarthritis with focus on MRI, ultrasound and hybrid imaging. Clin Exp Rheumatol. 2018;36:S43-52.
80. Schmitt B, Zbyn S, Stelzeneder D, Jellus V, Paul D, Lauer L, et al. Cartilage quality assessment by using glycosaminoglycan chemical exchange saturation transfer and 23Na MR Imaging at 7 T. Radiology. 2011;260(1):257-64.
81. McGonagle D, Gibbon W, O'Connor P, Green M, Pease C, Emery P. Characteristics magnetic resonance imaging entheseal changes of knee synovitis in spondyloarthropathy. Arthritis Rheum. 1998;41(4):694-700.
82. Sanders TG, Medynski MA, Feller JF, Lawhorn KW. Bone contusion patterns of the knee at MR imaging: footprint of the mechanism of injury. Radiographics. 2000;20:135-51.
83. Baltazar R, Ma C, Shankman S, Beltran J. Knee. In: Haaga JR, Dogra VS, Forsting M, Gilkeson RC, Kwon HA H,

Sundaram M (Eds). CT and MRI of the Whole Body, 5th edition. US: Mosby; 2009.

84. Palmer WE, Levine SM, Dupuy DE. Knee and shoulder fractures: Association of fracture detection and marrow oedema on MR images with mechanism of injury. Radiology. 1997;204(2):395-401.
85. Anderson MW, Ugalde U, Batt M, Gacayan J. Shin splints: MR appearance in a preliminary study. Radiology. 1997;204(1):177-80.
86. Anderson MW, Greenspan A. Stress fractures. Radiology. 1996;199(1):1-12.
87. Yamamoto T, Bullough PG. Subchondral insufficiency fracture of the femoral head and medial femoral condyle. Skeletal Radiol. 2000;29(1):40-4.
88. Frosberg PK, Braunstein EM, Buckwalter KA. Osteonecrosis, transient osteoporosis and transient bone marrow edema. Radiol Clin North Am. 1996;34(2):273-91.
89. Hughston JC, Hergenroeder PT, Courtenay BG. Osteochondritis dissecans of the femoral condyles. J Bone Joint Surg. 1984;66(9):1340-8.
90. DeSmet A, Fisher DR, Graf BK, Lange. Osteochondritis dissecans of the knee: value of MR imaging in determining lesion stability and the presence of articular cartilage defects. Am J Roentgenol. 1990;155(3):549-53.
91. Gorbachova T, Melenevsky Y, Cohen M, Cerniglia BW. Osteochondral lesions of the knee: differentiating the most common entities at MRI. Radiographics. 2018;38(5):1478-95.
92. Wambeek N, Munk PL, Lee MJ, Meek RN. Intra-articular regional migratory osteoporosis of the knee. Skeletal Radiol. 2000;29(2):97-100.
93. Schweitzer ME, Mandel S, Schwartzman RJ, Knobler RL, Tahmoush AJ. Reflex sympathetic dystrophy revisted: MR imaging findings before and after infusion of contrast material. Radiology. 1995;195(1):211-4.
94. Graif M, Schweitzer ME, Deely D, Matteucci T. The septic versus nonspecific inflamed joint: MRI characteristics. Skeletal Radiol. 1999;28(11):616-20.
95. Sundaram M, McGuire MH, Herbold DR. Magnetic resonance imaging in planning limb salvage surgery for primary malignant tumours of bone. J Bone Joint Surg. 1986;68:809-19.
96. Applegate GR, Flannigan BD, Tolin BS, Fox JM, Del Pizzo W. MR diagnosis of recurrent tears in the knee: Value of intra-articular contrast material. Am J Roentgenol. 1993;161(4):821-5.
97. Kramer J, Recht MP, Imhof H, Stiglbaüer R, Engel A. Postcontrast MR arthrography in assessment of cartilage lesions. J Comput Assist Tomography. 1994;18(2):218-24.
98. Kramer J, Stiglbauer R, Engel A, Prayer L, Imhof H. MR contrast arthrography in osteochondrosis dissecans. J Comput Assist Tomography. 1992;16(2):254-60.
99. Brossmann J, Priedler KW, Daenen B, Pedowitz RA, Andresen R, Clopton P, et al. Imaging of osseous and cartilaginous intra-articular bodies in the knee: Comparison of MR imaging and MR arthrography with CT and CT arthrography in cadavers. Radiology. 1996;200(2):509-17.
100. Kobayashi Y, Murkami R, Tajima H, Yamamoto K, Ichikawa T, Mase Y, et al. Direct MR arthrography of plica synovialis mediopatellaris. Acta Radiol. 2001;42(3):286-90.
101. Schatz JA, Potter HG, Rodeo SA. MR imaging of anterior cruciate ligament reconstruction. Am J Roentgenol. 1997;169:223-8.
102. Howell SM, Berns GS, Farley TE. Unimpinged and impinged anterior cruciate ligament grafts: MR signal intensity measurements. Radiology. 1991;179(3):639-43.
103. Recht MP, Piraino DW, Cohen MA, Parker RD, Bergfeld JA. Localised anterior arthrofibrosis (cyclopos lesion) after reconstruction of the anterior cruciate ligament: MR imaging findings. Am J Roentgenol. 1995;165(2):383-5.
104. Ho YY, Stanley AJ, Hui JH, Wang SC.. Postoperative evaluation of the knee after autologous chondrocyte implantation: what Radiologists Need to Know. Radiographics. 2007;27(1):207-20.
105. Gnannt R, Chhabra A, Theodoropoubs JS, Hodler J, Andreisek G. MR imaging of postoperative knee. Journal of Magnetic Resonance Imaging. 2011;34(5):1007-21.
106. Garwood ER, Tai R, Joshi G, Watts V GJ. The use of Artificial Intelligence in the evaluation of knee pathology. Semin Musculoskeletal Radiol. 2020;24(1):21-9.

CHAPTER

20

Magnetic Resonance Imaging of Ankle

Anindita Sinha, Mahesh Prakash

INTRODUCTION

Ankle joint is formed by the lower end of tibia, fibula, and talus and is a hinge joint allowing plantar flexion and dorsiflexion. The ankle mortise is formed by the medial and lateral malleoli and tibial plafond articulating with the talar dome or trochlea of talus, which is broader anteriorly, making the foot more stable in dorsiflexion. The lower ankle joint is formed by the talus articulating with the calcaneus forming the subtalar joint and the navicular **(Fig. 1)**. The subtalar joint allows inversion and eversion of the foot **(Figs. 2A and B)**. The ankle joint is stabilized by ligaments on the lateral [anterior and posterior talofibular and calcaneofibular ligaments (CFL)], medial (deltoid), and plantar aspects. Ankle injuries are the most common indication for imaging the ankle joint, and inversion injuries are most common with tear of the lateral ligaments; most commonly anterior talofibular ligament. Chronic pain as a result of previous injury leading to instability and impingement and congenital or acquired causes of flat foot are among the other common indications. Differentiating between infection and neuropathic joint in diabetic foot is also a major diagnostic concern. Detailed knowledge of osseous, ligamentous and tendon, and neurovascular anatomy in the various compartments (anterior, medial, lateral, and posterior) is a prerequisite for proper diagnosis.

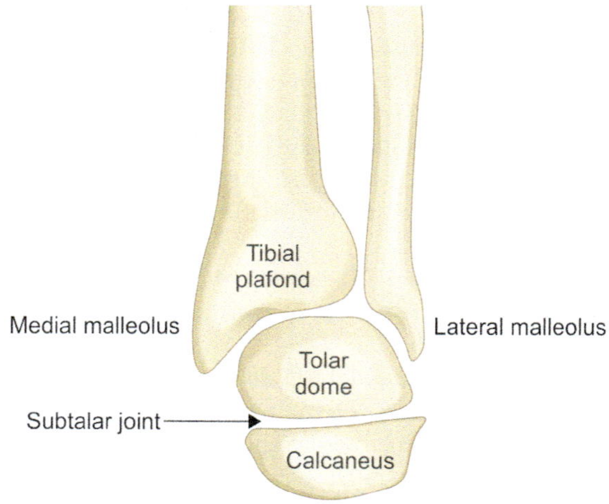

Fig. 1: Ankle joint.

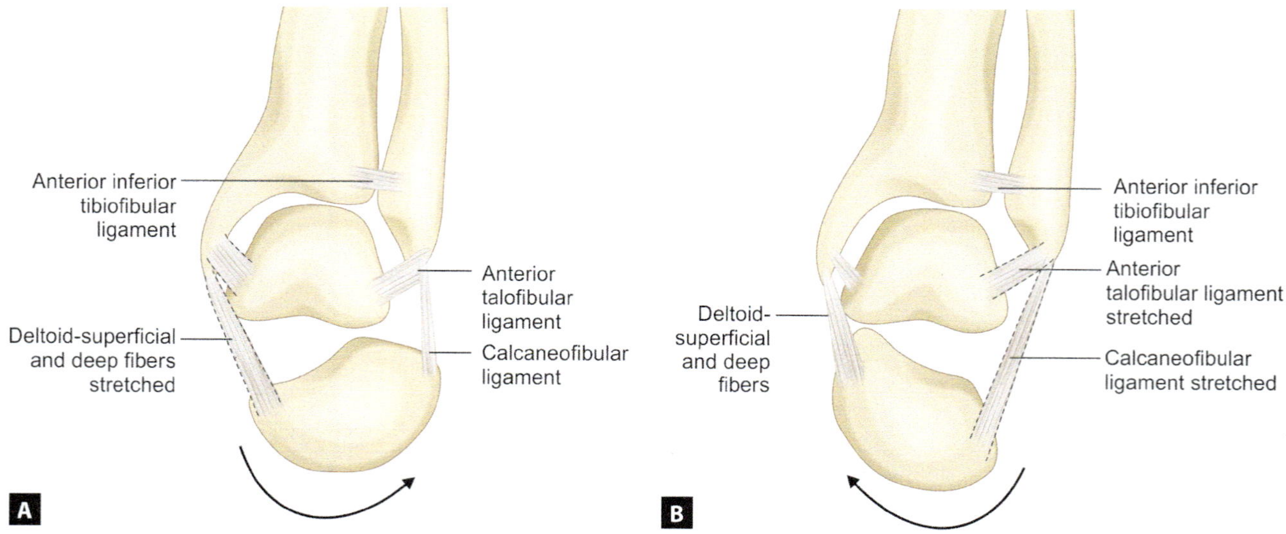

Figs. 2A and B: Eversion (A) and inversion (B) injuries of the foot. Inversion injuries (B) are much more common than eversion injuries.

IMAGING PROTOCOLS/TECHNICAL FACTORS

An ideal magnetic resonance (MR) technique should yield images with good contrast and spatial resolution of the osseous and soft tissue structures of the ankle.

Patient Positioning and Coils

1.5 or 3.0 T scanners are the most common MR units for musculoskeletal (MSK) imaging. Conventional closed bore, open bore, and extremity units are used for ankle imaging. Closed-coupled coil should be used to achieve optimal signal-to-noise ratios and spatial resolution. Standard extremity coil is routinely used.

The patient is placed supine with foot in the neutral position. The foot should be at right angle to the lower leg or 20° plantar flexion. The foot should be supported and immobilized with padding or straps to maintain the alignment and prevent movement.

With surface coils, it is recommended to use FOV (field of view) of 8–16 cm and 256 × 256 or 256 × 192 matrix. Foot and ankle are not scanned simultaneously and hence an ankle MRI should not include the toes, and a forefoot examination should not include the ankle.

Slice Thickness

A 2–4 mm slice thickness with 0.2–0.5 mm interslice gaps is best for defining complex foot and ankle anatomy.

Imaging Planes and Pulse Sequences

Coronal, axial, and sagittal image planes are commonly used for foot and ankle examination.

An ankle protocol includes T1-weighted axial and sagittal images, proton density (PD) and T2-weighted images in the sagittal plane, STIR sequence in the axial and sagittal plane.

The scan planning is initially done on axial or sagittal localizer with sagittal plane preferred.[1]

Axial images are first obtained (most valuable), parallel to the axis of the calcaneus, covering from distal tibial metadiaphyseal junction to the distal most part. Base of the metatarsals should be included in the axial images.

Coronal images are acquired next perpendicular to the axials. The coronal images should cover the base of the metatarsals. Next on the axial scout images, sagittal images are planned covering from lateral to medial malleolus.[1]

Sagittal images are best used to evaluate Achilles tendon, sinus tarsi, and plantar fascia. Axials of ankle are best for evaluation of tibiofibular ligaments, anterior and posterior talofibular ligaments (PTFLs), spring ligament complex, and the osseous structures.

Coronal images of ankle are best for detailed review of the deltoid ligaments, deep and superficial CFL, and the tarsal tunnel.

MAGNETIC RESONANCE ANATOMY

- *Anterior*: From medial to lateral the structures are **(Figs. 3A and B)**—
  - Tendons of tibialis anterior (TA), extensor hallucis longus (EHL), extensor digitorum longus (EDL)
  - Anterior tibial artery located between EHL and EDL
  - Deep peroneal nerve crosses the artery from medial to lateral.
- *Lateral* **(Figs. 3 to 6)**:
  - Ligaments:
    - Anterior talofibular ligament—attaches on anterior margin of fibular malleolus and on the talus it attaches just anterior to lateral articular surface—anterior talofibular ligament (ATFL) is the weakest and most frequently torn ligament in ankle sprains.
    - Posterior talofibular ligament—thick and striated and infrequently torn.
    - Calcaneofibular ligament—descends vertically deep to the peroneal tendons to attach to the trochlear tubercle on the lateral surface of calcaneum.
  - Tendons—peroneus longus and peroneus brevis:
    - Peroneus longus—attaches to plantar surface of the base of medial cuneiform and first metatarsal and is located behind the peroneus

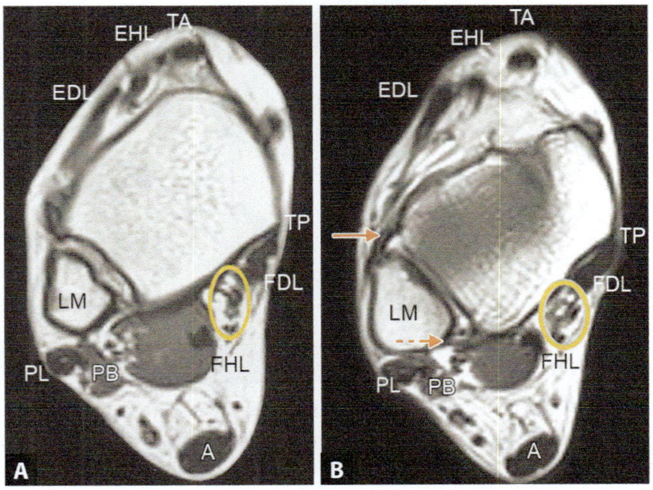

Figs. 3A and B: Anterior tendons from medial to lateral-tibialis anterior (TA), extensor hallucis longus (EHL), and extensor digitorum longus (EDL). Peroneus longus (PL) and peroneus brevis (PB) seen posterior to lateral malleolus (LM); peroneus brevis tendon is smaller and flat. Medial group of tendons are tibialis posterior (TP), flexor digitorum longus (FDL), and flexor hallucis longus (FHL) most posteromedially. Lower section of inferior tibiofibular joint shows the anterior inferior tibio-fibular ligament (AITFL) (arrow) and posterior inferior tibio-fibular ligament (PITFL) (dashed arrow). The neurovascular bundle is between FDL and FHL (oval). Achilles tendon (A) shows mild focal anterior convexity which may be a normal finding.

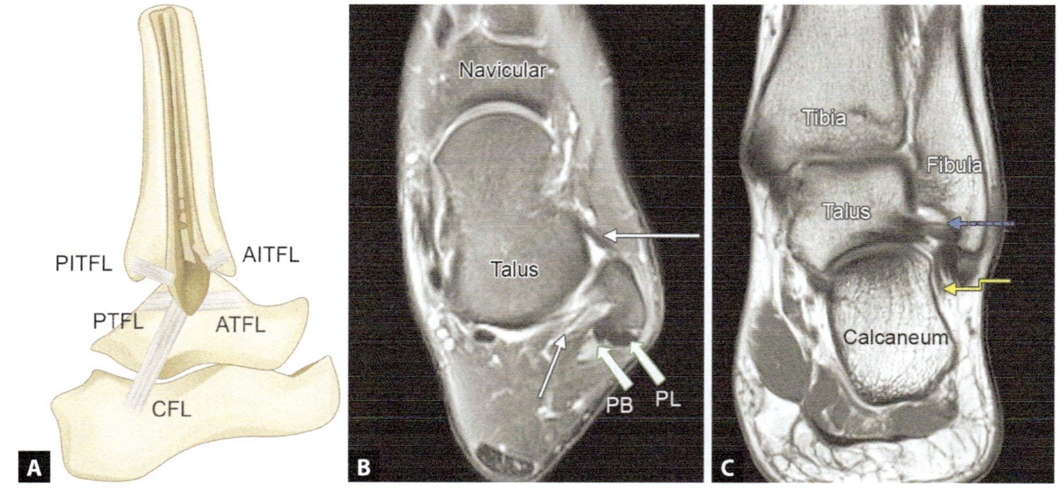

Figs. 4A to C: (A) Ligaments on the lateral aspect of the ankle. Anterior and posterior inferior tibiofibular ligaments (AITFL and PITFL) or syndesmotic ligaments, anterior and posterior talofibular ligaments (ATFL and PTFL), and calcaneofibular ligament (CFL); (B) Axial PD-weighted fat-saturated image shows the thin hypointense ATFL (arrow), and the striated appearance of PTFL (small arrow); (C) Coronal PD-weighted image shows the PTFL (dashed arrow) and the CFL (step arrow) abutting the lateral margin of the calcaneus deep to the peroneal tendons. The peroneal tendons are seen behind the fibular retromalleolar groove, which here is flat and not concave. The peroneus brevis (PB) is anteromedial and peroneus longus (PL) is larger.

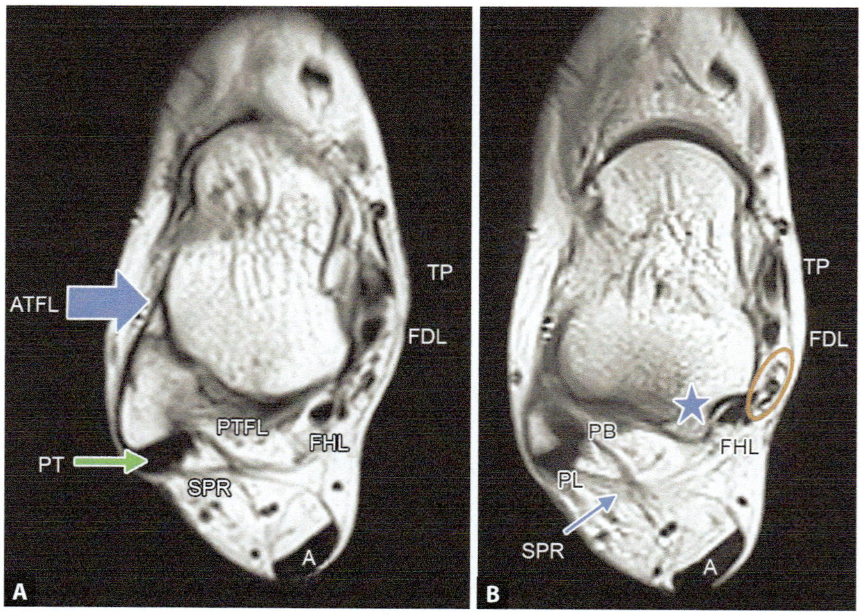

Figs. 5A and B: Axial proton density-weighted images at the level of lateral malleolar fossa demonstrates the uniform thickness hypointense band of anterior talofibular ligament (ATFL-arrow) from the anterior ridge of lateral malleolus to the lateral surface of talus. Note that tibia is not seen at the level of ATFL. The striated and thicker posterior tibiofibular ligament (PTFL) is seen posteriorly. PTFL is rarely torn in isolation. The peroneal tendons are seen behind the lateral malleolus which has a flat retromalleolar groove in this case. The peroneal tendons (PT in A) are enclosed within a thin triangular hypointense fascial layer known as superior peroneal retinaculum (SPR-arrow in B). Posteriorly the hypointense Achilles tendon with a concave anterior margin is seen. Medially from anterior to posterior the tibialis posterior tendon (TP), flexor digitorum longus (FDL) is visualized. The posterior tendon of flexor hallucis longus (FHL) lies behind the neurovascular bundles of posterior tibial artery and nerve (oval) and lodges between posterior tubercles of talus (*).

brevis tendon and on axial sections is rounded in shape.

- Peroneus brevis—attaches to base of the fifth metatarsal. Located just posterior to fibular retromalleolar groove, and is adjacent to bone. Peroneus brevis tendon is smaller and flatter on axial views.
- Both tendons are enclosed in a thin sheath known as superior peroneal retinaculum (SPR) superiorly at malleolar level, which extends

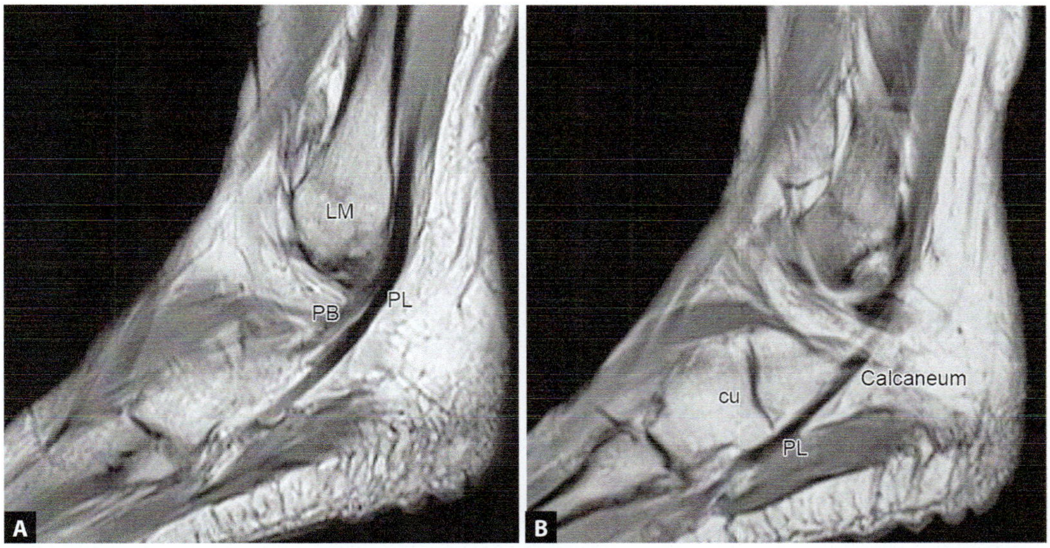

Figs. 6A and B: Sagittal proton density-weighted images show peroneus longus tendon (PL) coursing behind lateral malleolus (LM). Peroneus brevis is seen anteriorly (PB). A more medial sagittal section shows the peroneus longus curving around groove in cuboid (cu); the tendon in this area is intermediate in signal intensity due to magic angle artefact.

from the posterior fibular ridge laterally to the calcaneus or Achilles tendon posteriorly.
- Due to their curved course, both tendons can show magic angle effect with artefactual high signal mimicking a tear or tendinopathy on short TE images.

- *Superior peroneal retinaculum:* It encases and stabilizes the peroneal tendons at the level of the retromalleolar groove. SPR is visible on MRI as a thin hypointense band extending from the lateral malleolus to the lateral calcaneus.

- *Medial* **(Figs. 3A and B)**:
  - Tendons of **T**ibialis posterior, flexor **D**igitorum longus, flexor **H**allucis longus (FHL)
  - Posterior tibial **A**rtery
  - Tibial **N**erve
  - Arrangement is **T**om **D**ick **A**nd **H**arry from anterior to posterior
  - Deltoid ligament—a triangular/fan-shaped ligament from medial malleolus—is divided into **(Figs. 7 and 8)**:
    - *Superficial layer*:
      - Extends from medial malleolus to navicular, spring ligament, calcaneus
      - Tibiocalcaneal, tibiospring, tibionavicular
    - *Deep layer*:
      - Extends from medial malleolus to talus
      - Anterior tibiotalar and posterior tibiotalar (thickest)
      - Stronger than superficial layer
  - Spring ligament **(Figs. 9A to D)**:
    - One of the important stabilizers of medial longitudinal arch of foot and stabilizes talar head

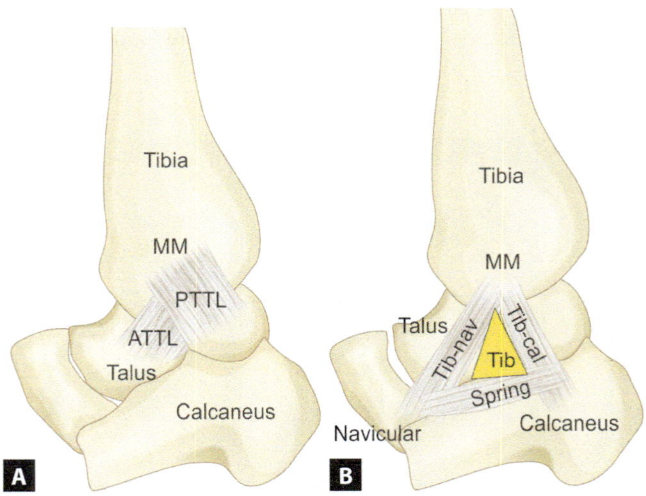

Figs. 7A and B: Diagrammatic representation of the deltoid ligament: (A) The deep deltoid ligament attaching the tibia to the talus—the anterior (ATTL) and posterior tibiotalar ligament (PTTL); (B) Components of the deep deltoid ligaments—from anterior to posterior-tibionavicular (Tib-nav), tibiospring (Tib), and tibiocalcaneal ligaments (Tib-cal). (MM: medial malleolus).

    - Has three components:
      - Superomedial calcaneonavicular—from sustentaculum tali to medial portion of navicular bone—most important ligament
      - Two other components are the inferoplantar longitudinal calcaneonavicular ligament and medioplantar oblique calcaneonavicular ligament

- *Posterior* **(Figs. 3 and 10)**:
  - *Achilles tendon* is formed by soleus, medial, and lateral head of gastrocnemius.
  - It inserts into calcaneal tuberosity.

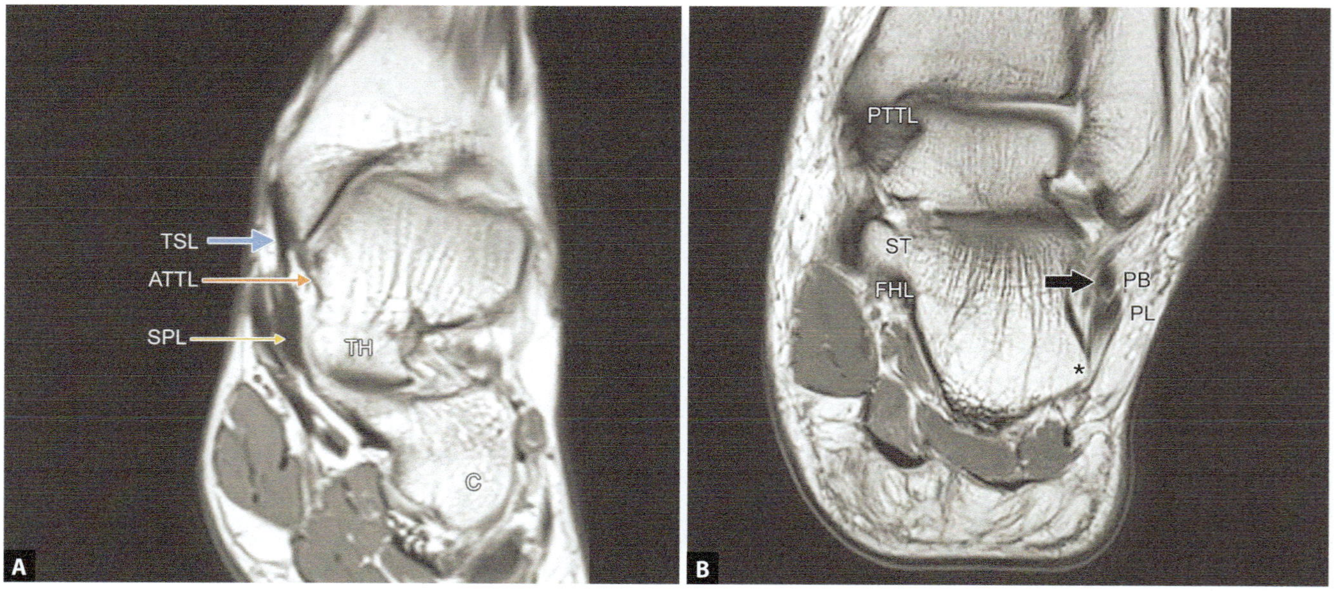

Figs. 8A and B: Coronal T1-weighted image (A) shows thin strand of anterior tibiotalar ligament (ATTL)—a deep portion of the deltoid ligament, which is very thin and variably seen. The tibiospring ligament (TSL), part of the superficial deltoid, attaches to the spring ligament (SPL) near the talar head (TH); (B) On a more posterior section, the striated posterior tibiotalar ligament (PTTL) is seen. On the lateral aspect, the calcaneofibular ligament (CFL) (arrow) can be seen in its entirety attaching to the calcaneal tuberosity (*) deep to the peroneal tendons [peroneus brevis and peroneus longus (PB and PL)].

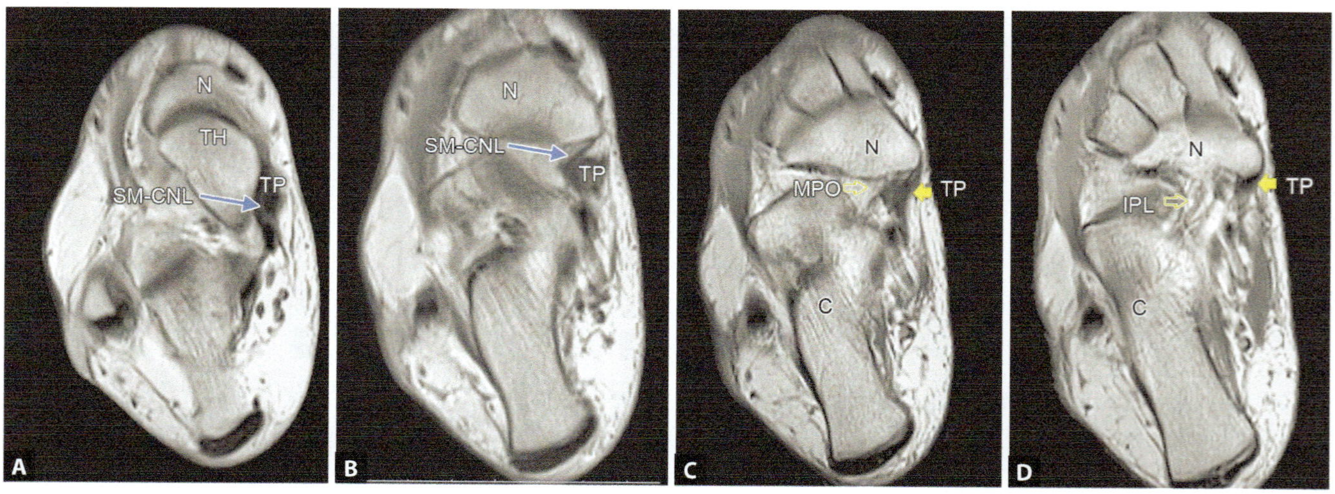

Figs. 9A to D: Spring ligament: (A and B) Axial proton density-weighted consecutive images show the hypointense band of superomedial calcaneonavicular ligament (SM-CNL) deep to the tibialis posterior (TP) tendon, adjoining the medial aspect of the talonavicular joint. Talar head (TH) and navicular bone is marked N; (C and D) Hypointense band of medioplantar oblique calcaneonavicular (MPO) and inferoplantar longitudinal (IPL) calcaneonavicular portions of the spring ligament. Navicular bone is marked by (N) and calcaneum by (C). The tibialis posterior has attached to the tuberosity of navicular (TP). Posteriorly the Achilles tendon attachment is seen at the calcaneal tuberosity.

- The tendon does not have a lining synovial sheath, but is surrounded by fibrous connective tissue known as paratendon.
- The myotendinous junction is formed in mid-calf and tendon length is around 15 cm.
- MRI appearance is hypointense on all sequences.
- Best seen in axial and sagittal views
- Axial—anterior margin is concave. Sagittal—tendon margins are parallel.
- Bursa around Achilles tendon:
  - Retro-Achilles bursa—behind Achilles tendon
  - Retrocalcaneal bursa—in front of the anterior margin of distal Achilles tendon between tendon and posterior calcaneus.

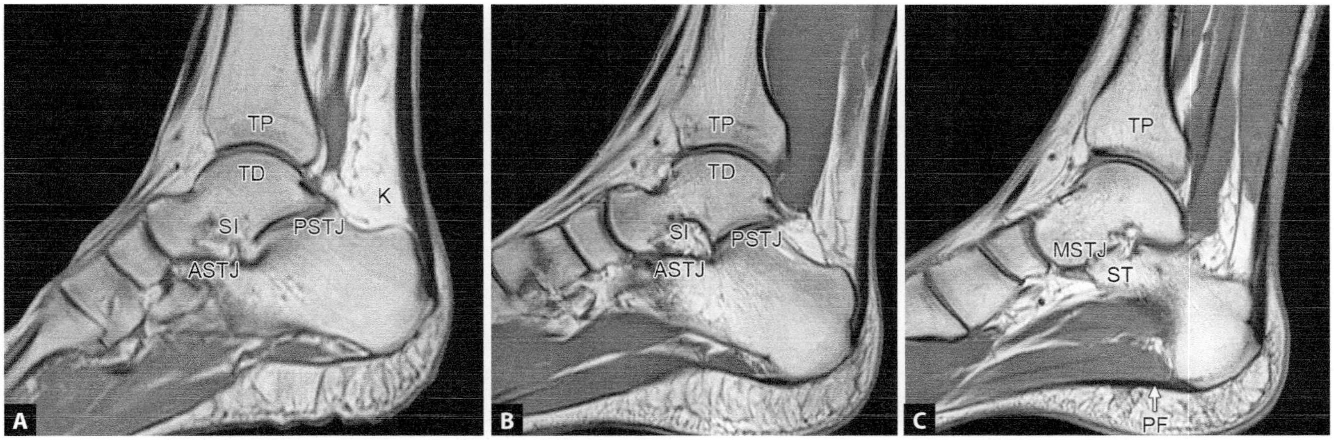

Figs. 10A to C: Sagittal proton density-weighted images show Achilles tendon-straight and hypointense and attaching to calcaneal tuberosity. The Kager's fat pad (K) is seen anterior to Achilles tendon. The anterior, middle, and posterior subtalar joints (talocalcaneal joints) are marked ASTJ, MSTJ, and PSTJ. The middle subtalar joint is formed by the articular facet of sustentaculum tali (ST). In these medial sections the hypointense plantar fascia (PF) is seen at calcaneal attachment. The fat and interosseous ligaments of a portion of the sinus tarsi (SI) are also seen. The tibial plafond (TP) and talar dome (TD) form the tibiotalar joint.

- Plantaris tendon—may be present medial to Achilles tendon and inserts within or anteromedial to Achilles tendon insertion on calcaneus. An intact plantaris can simulate a partial tear of a completely torn Achilles tendon.
- Kager's fat pad is a triangular area seen anterior to Achilles tendon.

Joints (Figs. 1 and 10)

The ankle joint is formed by three joints:

1. Tibiotalar joint (talocrural or ankle joint mortise)—formed by tibial plafond, dome of talus, and medial and lateral malleolus
2. Subtalar joint formed between the talus and calcaneum (there are three articulations—anterior, middle, and posterior)
3. Inferior tibiofibular joint (joined by syndesmotic ligaments—anterior and posterior inferior tibiofibular ligament) **(Fig. 1B)**.

Achilles Tendon Pathologies

Achilles tendon is the strongest and largest tendon in the body. Achilles tendon injuries are common and can be due to acute trauma or due to chronic overuse in athletes.

Acute Injuries

Acute tendon injuries are most commonly seen due to sudden forced ankle movement in elderly otherwise fit individuals. Spontaneous acute rupture is seen in individuals with connective tissue disorders or diabetes.

Chronic Injuries

Tennis leg rupture of the myotendinous junction of the medial head of gastrocnemius or a myofascial injury is more common than a plantaris rupture. Fluid signal is seen between medial head of gastrocnemius and soleus.

Tendinopathy/Tendinosis

- Achilles tendinopathy can appear as focal or diffuse thickening with loss of normal anterior concavity in axial plane. Signal may remain hypointense or become hyperintense in mucoid degeneration.[2,3]
- Achilles paratendinopathy—diffuse thin fluid is seen around the Achilles tendon, since the tendon itself does not have a true synovium-lined tendon sheath but is surrounded by fibrous connective tissue to allow for its gliding action **(Figs. 11A and B)**.

Tendon Ruptures

- Partial or complete ruptures of the Achilles tendon are caused by acute sudden dorsiflexion.
- Site prone to tear is a relatively avascular zone 2–6 cm proximal to insertion.
- Patients with pre-existing connective tissue disorders or diabetes are prone to tendon rupture following minor trauma.
- MRI appearance—a fluid-filled gap is seen between the torn ends. Hemorrhage with heterogeneous signal may be present. Tendon itself may be thickened in cases of pre-existing tendon degeneration **(Figs. 12A to C)**.
- Partial tears can be longitudinal split tears.
- Chronic tears with intervening fibrotic tissue may make diagnosis difficult.[2,4,5]

Haglund's Syndrome (Fig. 13)

- Haglund's syndrome causes posterior ankle pain and is caused by ill-fitting shoes pressing the retro-Achilles bursa against the posterior calcaneal tuberosity.

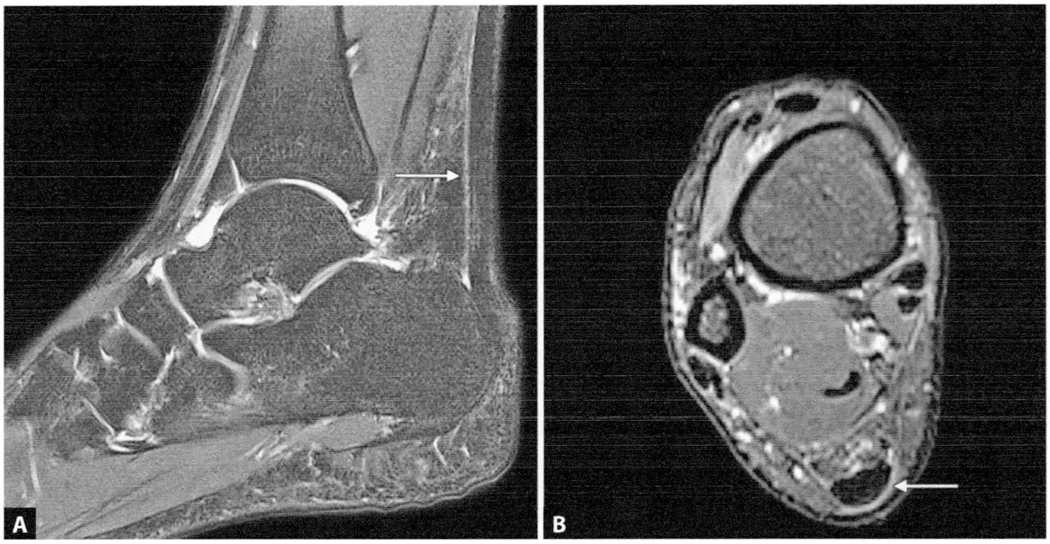

Figs. 11A and B: Achilles paratendinosis: Sagittal and axial T2-weighted images show a thin sliver of fluid (arrow) surrounding the Achilles tendon, which remains hypointense and maintains its anterior concave margin on axial sections.

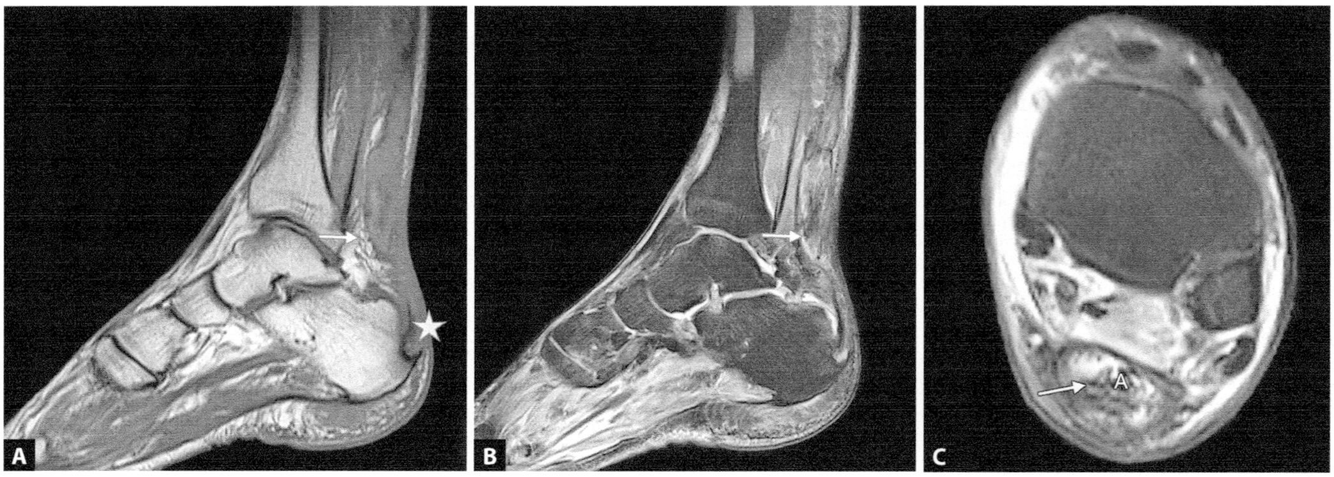

Figs. 12A to C: Complete tear of Achilles tendon (A) with hemorrhage-sagittal T1-weighted and T2-weighted images shows heterogeneous T1 hyperintense area (arrow) 4 cm from insertion of the Achilles tendon (*). This is heterogeneously hypointense on T2-weighted image (arrow in B), due to hemorrhage. The tendon insertion is also hypointense and shows erosion and sclerosis of the calcaneal tuberosity, suggesting a pre-existing tendinopathy with enthesitis. A gap is seen between the proximal and distal ends of the torn tendon (arrow in B). Intratendinous thickening and heterogeneity is seen on axial images (C).

- Chronic irritation causes edema or enlargement of the calcaneal tuberosity (Haglund's deformity).
- Fluid-filled retrocalcaneal and retro-Achilles bursa can be seen.
- Achilles tendinosis can be associated with Haglund's syndrome.

Achilles Tendon Xanthomas

- Achilles tendon xanthomas present as painless soft tissue masses, may often be present bilaterally.
- Histopathologically, they are lipid-laden macrophages due to cholesterol deposits in tissues—may be associated with familial hypercholesterolemia and cerebrotendinous xanthomatosis.[6]
- MRI appearance:
  - Diffuse or focal tendon enlargement with speckled appearance is seen on MRI.
  - The lesions are hyperintense on T1- and T2-weighted images.[6]
- Differential diagnosis includes tendinopathy and gout.

Peroneal Tendon Pathologies

- Peroneal tears or tendinopathies are seen in athletic young individuals as well as in elderly and are often associated with other injuries.
- Common presentations are lateral hind foot pain, popping or snapping in patients with peroneal subluxations or dislocations.

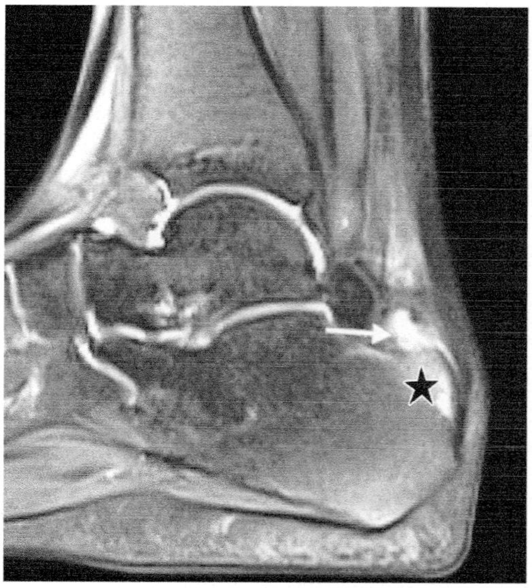

Fig. 13: Haglund's syndrome. Edema and prominence of the calcaneal tuberosity (*) with retrocalcaneal bursitis (arrow).

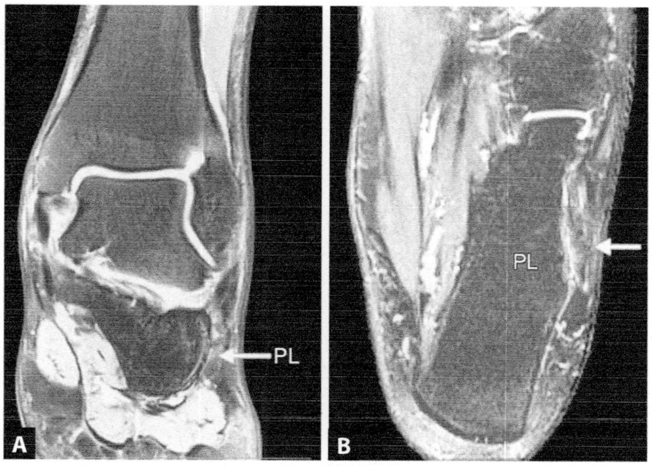

Figs. 14A and B: Peroneal tendinopathy. Coronal (A) and axial (B) T2-weighted fat-saturated images show tendinopathy of peroneus longus (PL) just beyond the peroneal tubercle. The tendon appears intermediate in signal intensity (arrow) and has a thin sliver of fluid surrounding it.

- Peroneus brevis tendon tears/tendinopathies.
- Overuse and friction against an abnormally-shaped retromalleolar groove is a common cause.
- *Shape of retromalleolar groove:* Retromalleolar groove is generally concave. Flat or convexity or irregular protuberance posteriorly causes chronic injury especially in the peroneus brevis located adjacent to fibular malleolus.[7]

Tendinopathy (Figs. 14A and B)

- Common sites of friction are:
  - Peroneal tubercle of the calcaneus—a bony prominence on the lateral surface of the calcaneum that separates the peroneus brevis from the peroneus longus—enlargement >5 mm is associated with chronic tears or tendinopathies.
  - Cuboid notch—where the peroneus longus turns toward the plantar aspect of the foot toward its ultimate insertion to the plantar aspect of base of medial cuneiform and first metatarsal.
- Patients with rheumatoid arthritis, psoriatic arthritis, and diabetes are prone to tendinopathies.
- *MR appearance:* Tendon is thickened with increased intrasubstance signal abnormality.[8]

Tenosynovitis

- Peroneal tenosynovitis can be postinfective or post-traumatic (acute trauma associated with CFL injury causes false-positive appearance of tenosynovitis due to accumulation of joint fluid within the tendon sheath)
- Chronic inflammatory arthritis is a risk factor for tenosynovitis.
- Patients present with pain, tenderness, and swelling along the lateral ankle
- *MRI appearance:* Fluid distension of the tendon sheath (a sliver of fluid is normal; >3 mm thickness of fluid is a sign of tenosynovitis)
- The fluid signal may be heterogeneous; low-signal intensity bands may be seen in stenosing tenosynovitis
- Peroneal tendons may be thickened
- Synovial enhancement is commonly seen on postcontrast images.[8]

Peroneal Tendon Injuries

- Tendon injuries are often associated with ankle sprains and can be easily overlooked
- Preexisting tendinopathy and microtrauma are other predisposing factors for tendon tears
- Partial tears can be associated with tendon thinning or thickening—a thickened tendon makes it difficult to differentiate between a thickened partially torn tendon and a tendinopathy
- Complete tears show discontinuity.

Peroneus Brevis Tears (Figs. 15A to D)

- Peroneus brevis is prone to tears due to friction between retromalleolar groove and anteriorly peroneus longus posteriorly.
- This anterior position against the retromalleolar groove makes the peroneus brevis more prone to tendinopathies and tears than the peroneus longus.[7]
- Predisposing factors include associated tears of ATFL, flat, convex or irregular retromalleolar groove, accessory muscle, low lying muscle belly of peroneus brevis and injuries and tears of superior peroneal retinaculum.

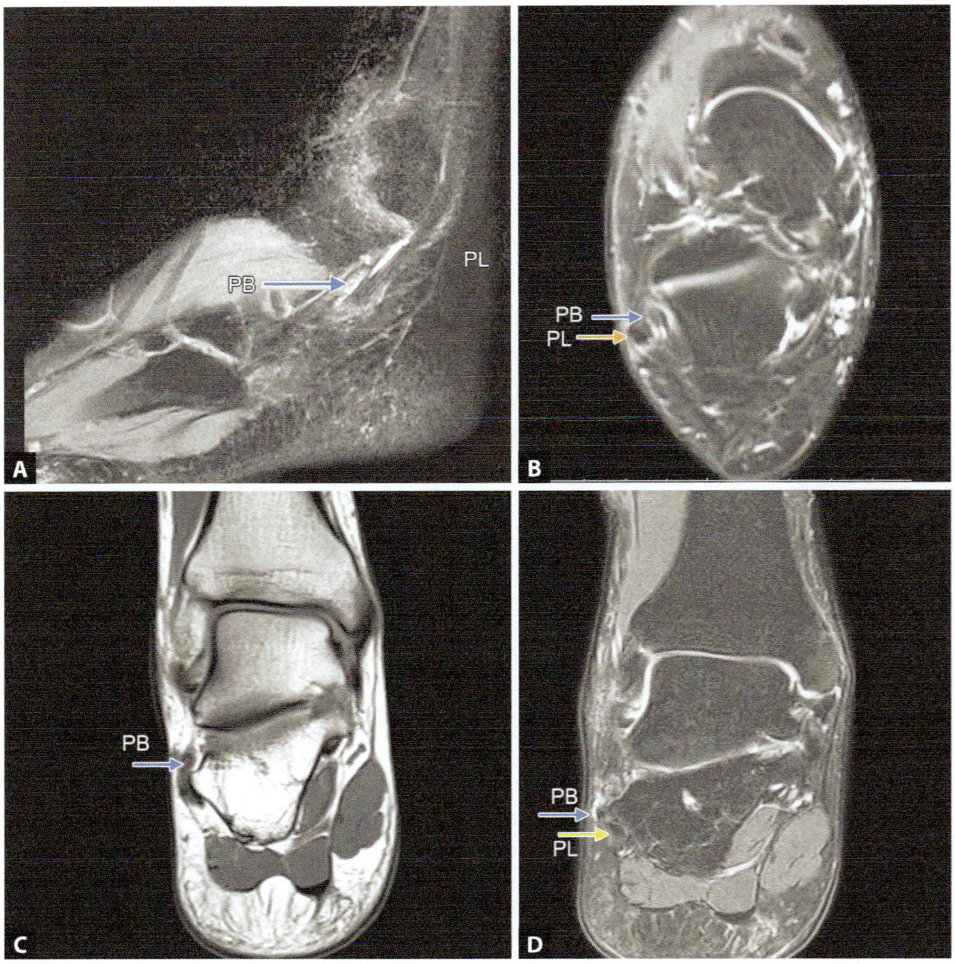

Figs. 15A to D: Partial tear of peroneus brevis (PB) tendon. On sagittal T2-weighted fat-saturated images there is partial fluid-filled discontinuity within the peroneus brevis, which may appear sometimes due to volume averaging on the sagittal images (A). However, tendon is thinned and shows a linear intermediate signal due to partial tear on axial T2-weighted fat-saturated image (B) and also on coronal proton density-weighted and T2-weighted fat-saturated images (C and D). (PL: peroneus longus)

- *MRI appearance*:
  - *Boomerang or "C" shape:* A boomerang or "C" shaped peroneus brevis tendon engulfs the peroneus longus.
  - *Split tear:* Tears may progress to a longitudinal split with two separate tendon components of peroneus brevis and tendon of peroneus longus subluxating anteriorly between the torn tendon components (intrasheath subluxation).[8,9]

Peroneus Longus Tears

- Peroneus longus tears can also be partial or complete split tears at ankle or mid foot.
- Peroneus longus tears are less common than peroneus brevis tears and are often associated with peroneus brevis tears.
- Partial tears are more common in retromalleolar region and complete tear in midfoot at the point of the tendon curving around the cuboid on toward its plantar course.[8]
- Osseous abnormalities accompanying peroneus longus tears on MRI are:[7-9]
  - Hypertrophied peroneal tubercle
  - Edema of cuboid
  - Avulsion fracture of os peroneum (with separation of the avulsed fragments by >2 mm)
  - The entire os peroneum may be edematous and dislocated posteriorly from its normal position near the lateral calcaneocuboid joint.

Subluxation/Dislocation/SPR Injuries (Figs. 16A and B)

- Peroneal tendon subluxation and dislocations result from injury to the superior peroneal retinaculum.
- SPR injuries result from acute trauma in athletic individuals and mimic ankle sprain.
- SPR injuries can occur at the fibular attachment, with a complete tear or stripping off of the periosteum. A bony avulsion from lateral malleolus can also be present. Anterolateral subluxation or dislocation of the

peroneal tendons may occur into the pouch formed by the stripped off periosteum.

- Transient peroneal subluxations can be difficult to identify on MRI, and dynamic ultrasound is essential to demonstrate the subluxation.
- Secondary evidence with hyperintensity along the retinaculum and nonvisualized or partially visualized retinaculum, edema along the adjacent lateral malleolus suggest retinacular injuries.[9]

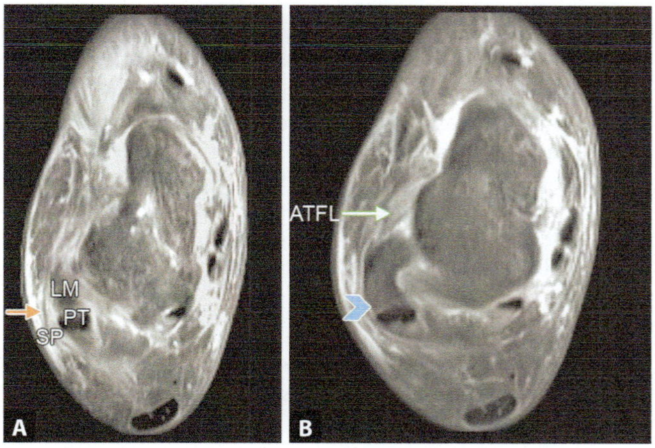

Figs. 16A and B: Acute SPR injury and ATFL injury. (A) The superior peroneal retinaculum is hyperintense and stripped off from the lateral malleolus (LM) (small arrow); peroneal tendons (PT) are not subluxated and remain behind lateral malleolus. A superior axial proton-density-weighted image (B) reveals a thickened, hyperintense, and torn anterior talofibular ligament at fibular attachment. The retromalleolar fossa is flat (arrowhead in B). Extensive edema seen along medial aspect of joint. (ATFL: anterior talofibular ligament; SPR: superior peroneal retinaculum)

Medial Compartment Tendon Abnormalities (Figs. 17A to C)

- *Tibialis posterior:* Tibialis posterior tenosynovitis, tendinopathies, and tears cause adult-acquired flat foot (planovalgus).
- Tendon dysfunction is common in elderly females. Patients present with chronic pain in the medial side of the arch of foot.
- Tibialis posterior tendon sheath normally contains a sliver of fluid, however, circumferential fluid >2 mm in thickness suggests tenosynovitis.
- Tenosynovitis progresses to tendinopathy and tears.
- Tendinopathy is characterized by fusiform enlargement of tendons and mild-to-moderate increased signal on T2-weighted images.[10,11]
- Complete tears of tibialis posterior are uncommon; partial or interstitial tears are more common and present as thinning and intrasubstance hyperintensity.
- Normal tibialis posterior is double the size of FHL and thinner than TA or combined diameters of peroneal tendons.
- Healed partial tears can present with hypertrophic thickening due to fibrotic scarring.
- A mixed hypertrophic-atrophic pattern of chronic tears can also be seen with hypertrophic proximal tendon.[11,12]

Ligament Injuries—Lateral

- *Mechanism of injury*: Plantar flexion with inversion causes the typical "ankle sprain."
- *Indications for imaging*: Most acute ankle sprains are not imaged. Indications for imaging are in professional

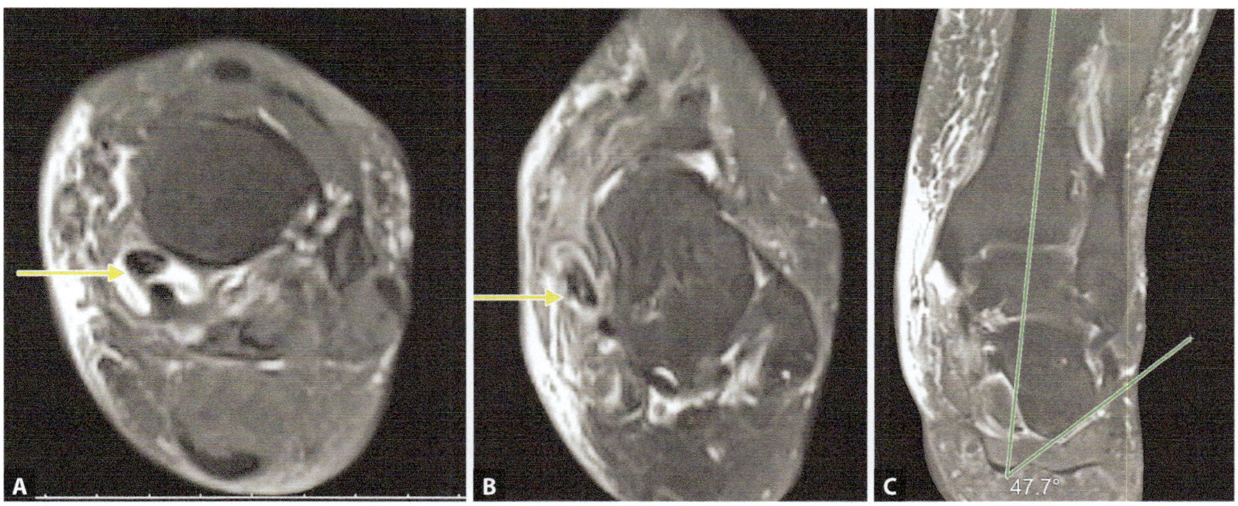

Figs. 17A to C: Tibialis posterior tenosynovitis with partial split tear and valgus deformity. Fluid seen surrounding the proximal tibialis posterior (arrow in A) in the axial T2-weighted fat-saturated image. Distal axial section shows intratendinous increased signal due to an interstitial tear (arrow in B). The patient presented with progressive flat foot due to posterior tibial dysfunction and had calcaneal valgus (C).

athletes and to rule out syndesmotic injury, prolonged pain or ankle instability.

- *Ligaments most commonly torn*—ATFL and CFL. PTFL is the strongest and is rarely torn except in severe trauma associated with dislocations.

Anterior Talofibular Ligament and Posterior Talofibular Ligament

- ATFL is the weakest and the commonly injured ligament.
- *MRI appearance*: Normal ATFL has a hypointense band-like appearance on all pulse sequences and attaches to anterolateral aspect of lateral malleolar tip and lateral surface of talar neck. A striated appearance due to interposed fat may be seen.
- Normal PTFL is the thickest and has a striated appearance.
- PTFL attaches to malleolar fossa of fibula and posterolateral tubercle on posterior surface of talus.
- Low-grade ATFL injuries result in interstitial tear with intermediate intraligamentous signal intensity and intra- and periligamentous edema on proton density and fat saturated T2-weighted images.
- Injured ligament is seen as thickened, irregular, lax and wavy, or discontinuous ligament with intraligamentous or periligamentous edema.[13]
- Partial tear is seen as a focal discontinuity within the ligament.
- Full thickness tears can cause thinned out appearance or complete discontinuity at attachment or midsubstance of the ligament **(Figs. 17 and 18)**.
- Bright rim sign of tiny hyperintense foci at the torn site of attachment of ATFL has been reported by Lee et al.[14]
- Healing of ATFL tear takes 6–12 months and imaging appearances vary from ill-defined intermediate edematous signal with thickening of the ligament in initial stages to a more hypointense well-defined ligament with decrease in thickening as the scar tissue matures.[13]
- MRI has a 76–84% accuracy and 83–92% sensitivity in the diagnosis of chronic ATFL tears. Redundant or discontinuous ligament is more likely to be associated with instability.[13]
- *PTFL injuries*: PTFL is normally striated and hyperintense. This normal appearance should not be mistaken for a tear.

Calcaneofibular Ligament

- CFL is the second common ligament to be torn in inversion injuries after ATFL.
- CFL connects the lower tip of the lateral malleolus with the trochlear eminence on the lateral calcaneal surface.
- It has a vertical oblique course, best seen deep to the peroneal tendons.

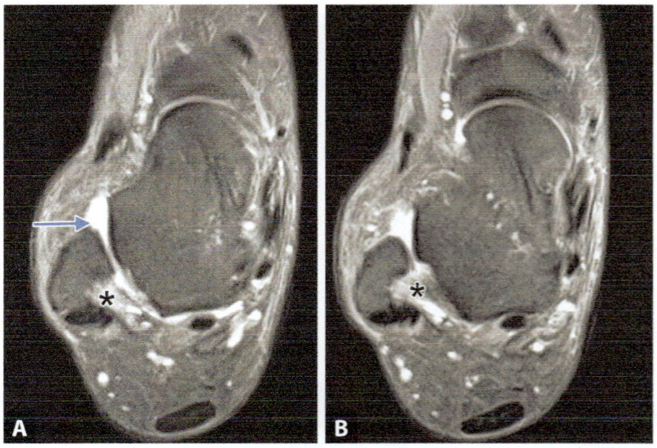

Figs. 18A and B: ATFL complete tear-nonvisualized ATFL (arrow in A) in a case of chronic tear. PTFL (*) is normal and striated in appearance (B). Another patient with thickened and heterogeneous wavy PTFL with loss of striation due to acute partial tear. No discontinuity seen either at attachment sites or within the ligament. Complete ATFL tear was also seen in this patient. (ATFL: anterior talofibular ligament; PTFL: posterior talofibular ligament)

- *MRI appearance*: It is best seen as a 6–8 mm hypointense structure deep to peroneal tendons and parallel to and adjacent to calcaneal lateral wall on axial and coronal images.
- Tears can cause thickening and intermediate- or high-signal intensity with indistinct ligament, irregular wavy margins medial to peroneal tendons as well as fluid within the peroneal tendons **(Figs. 19A and B)**.
- In complete tears, the peroneal tendons about the lateral surface of the lateral malleolus.
- *Anatomical classification of ankle sprains*:[15]
  - First degree sprain—a partial or complete tear of the ATFL
  - Second degree sprain—partial or complete tearing of the both the ATFL and CFL
  - Third degree sprain—injury to all of the lateral ligaments, including the PTFL.

Syndesmotic Ligaments[16]

- *Injury of distal tibiofibular syndesmotic ligaments:* Anterior inferior tibiofibular ligament, posterior inferior tibiofibular ligament, and interosseous ligament injury result in high ankle sprain.
  - *Anterior-inferior tibiofibular ligament (AITFL)* inserts between anterior aspect of lateral malleolus and fibular tubercle on the anterolateral aspect of inferior tibia **(Fig. 3B)**
  - Posterior-inferior tibiofibular ligament (PITFL) attaches at the posterior tubercle of tibia and posterior lateral malleolus **(Fig. 3B)**.
  - *Interosseous ligament* is the thickened inferior portion of the interosseous membrane.[16]

- *Mechanism of injury* is hyperdorsiflexion and external rotation, commonly seen in footballers.
- *Radiography* is essential and may show avulsion fractures of lateral process or posterolateral talar process, talar dome, base of 5th metatarsal, and ankle fractures. Fibular fractures are commonly associated with syndesmotic injury so radiographs of both ankle and proximal tibiofibular joint are needed to detect Maisonneuve fractures.[13]
- AITFL is the most frequently injured syndesmotic ligament. Normal ligament is band like.
- *MRI appearance*:[16,17] Normal AITFL is hypointense on all pulse sequences.

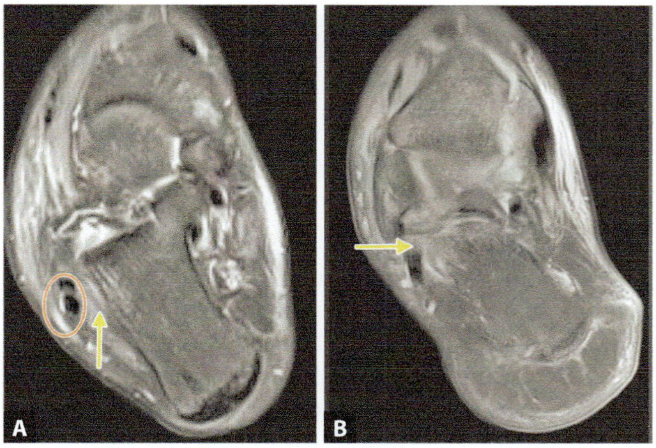

Figs. 19A and B: Calcaneofibular ligament tear. Axial and coronal proton density-weighted fat-saturated images show intermediate signal of the CFL medial to the peroneal tendons with periligamentous edema. The acutely kinked course on coronal images suggests a mid-substance tear. Adjacent osseous edema at the calcaneal attachment is seen. Peroneal tendons (oval) are intact. (CFL: calcaneofibular ligament)

- Adjacent osseous edema or osteochondral injury may be present.
- Fluid tracking up the tibiofibular recess above the level of the talar dome for a height of >1 cm is also indicative of syndesmotic ligament injury.
- Ankle arthrography may help in demonstrating intra-articular gadolinium extending high up into the recess.

Ligament Injuries—Medial (Figs. 20A to C)

- Deltoid ligament injuries comprise 15% of ligament injuries of ankle.[18]
- Common mode of injury is eversion.
- Lateral malleolar fracture and lateral talar dislocation are commonly associated.
- Avulsion fractures of medial malleolus at the site of superficial ligamentous attachment may be found.
- Lateral ligament complex injuries and syndesmotic injuries are also frequently found along with deltoid ligament injury.

Anatomy

- *Deep component:*
    - *Anterior tibiotalar ligament*—the thinnest and variably present in 50% of the population.
    - It attaches to the anterior tip of the anterior colliculus of medial malleolus and to fovea of the talus just distal to anterior part of medial articular surface.
    - *Posterior tibiotalar ligament*:[18] This is the thickest medial ligament; it originates from posterior surface of anterior colliculus of medial malleolus, intercollicular groove and posterior colliculus. It inserts into medial surface of talus under the medial articular facet, posteriorly extending up to the posteromedial tubercle of talus.

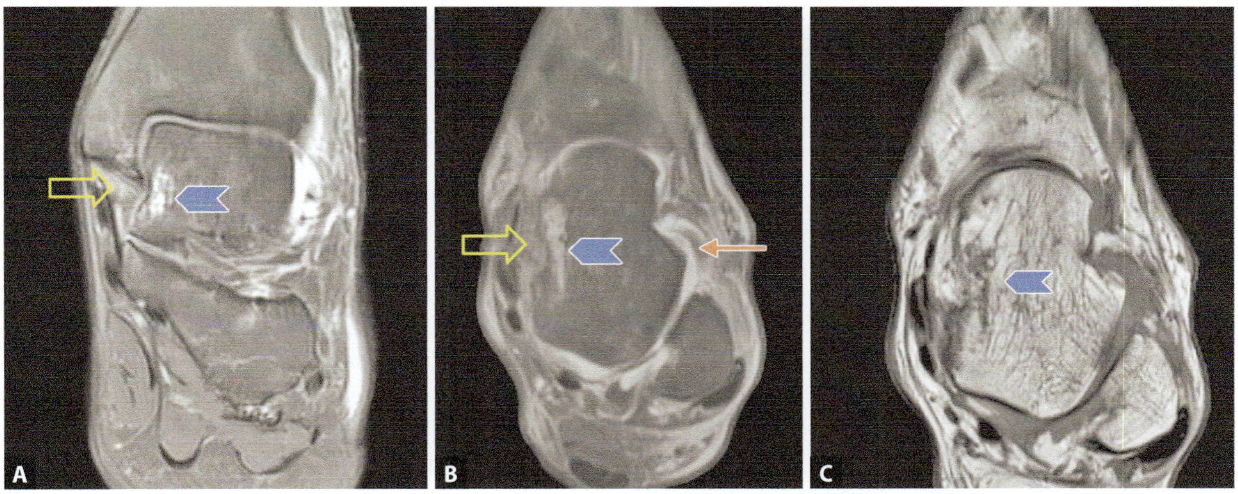

Figs. 20A to C: Deep deltoid injury with complete ATFL tear. Coronal and axial proton-density weighted fat saturated image (A) shows hyperintensity within the posterior tibiotalar ligament (arrow) with bone bruise (arrowhead) along medial margin of talus. The linear hypointense microtrabecular fractures are better appreciated on T1-weighted images (arrowhead in C). A completely torn ATFL is seen (small arrow). (ATFL: anterior talofibular ligament)

- *MRI of tear*:[18] Focal tears are more common than full thickness tears.
- Hematoma, complete absence of ligament, and soft tissue edema are seen in full thickness tears.
- The most common site of tear of the superficial component is at medial malleolus and that of the deep posterior tibiotalar component is at the talar attachment.[19]

Deltoid ligament injuries are also found in chronic lateral ankle instability, which causes recurrent ankle sprain after a single episode of lateral sprain.[20]

Ankle Impingement

- Ankle impingements can occur due to post-traumatic synovitis, malunion, recurrent sprain, scarring, and osseous abnormalities.[21]
- *Anatomical locations of impingement:* Impingements can be anterior, anteromedial, anterolateral, posterior, and posteromedial.
- Clinically patients present with painful and restricted range of motion.

Anterior Impingement

- Patients present with restricted dorsiflexion.
- Anterior impingement occurs at the anterior recess between talar dome and anterior tibial plafond **(Fig. 21)**.
- Commonly seen in football players due to repeated dorsiflexion.
- Radiographs show osteophytes from anterior inferior margin of tibial plafond and from talar neck (forming a talar beak); however, these traction spurs may also be asymptomatic.[22]
- MRI is useful for diagnosing soft tissue abnormalities like anterior capsular and synovial thickening and fibrous bands in addition to anterior osteophytes.[23,24]

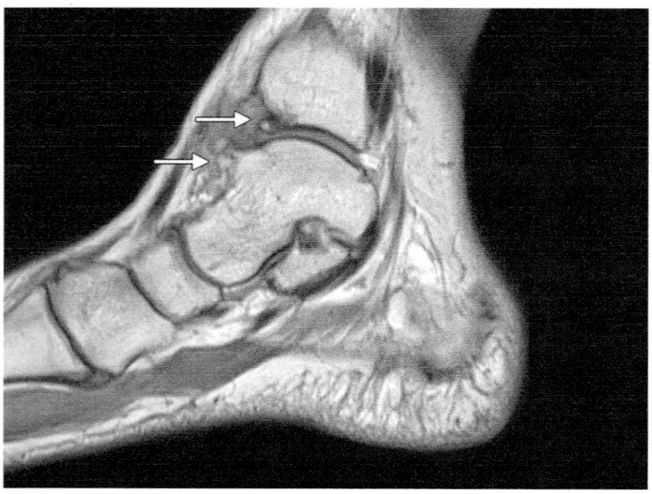

Fig. 21: Anterior impingement. Sagittal T1-weighted image shows osteophytes from anterior tibial plafond and from adjacent dome of talus.

Anterolateral Impingement

- Uncommon and is a diagnosis of exclusion in patients presenting with chronic anterolateral ankle pain exacerbated on dorsiflexion accompanied by swelling
- Usually caused by prior inversion injuries of the ankle
- Pain is caused by pathology in anterolateral recess
- Anatomical boundaries of anterolateral recess—anteriorly—ATFL
- Superiorly—anterior inferior tibiofibular ligament, medially-tibia, laterally fibula
- Normal content is minimal fluid
- Impingement can occur due to chronic synovial proliferation or torn or thickened ATFL or fibrotic tissue
- The fibrotic tissue can appear like triangular meniscus—known as meniscoid lesion
- Osteophytes in anterolateral tibial plafond can also cause impingement.[24]

Differential diagnosis of lateral ankle pain—peroneal tendon pathologies (tendinopathy, tears or subluxations), sinus tarsi syndrome, osteoarthritis, and ganglia.[21]

Anteromedial Impingement

- Uncommon cause of anteromedial ankle pain
- Caused by injury to anterior tibiotalar ligament (component of deep deltoid ligament), leading to thickening, soft tissue (meniscoid lesion), osteophytes or spurs along talar dome or anteromedial tibial plafond or medial malleolus

Posterior Impingement (Figs. 22A and B)

- Posterior impingement is clinically characterized by posterior ankle pain on plantar flexion.
- Commonly seen due to chronic repetitive injury in football players due to repeated plantar flexion causing impingement soft tissues between posterior calcaneal process and posterior tibia.
- Osseous abnormalities associated with posterior impingement include elongated lateral posterior process of talus (Stieda process) or os trigonum (formed by failure of fusion of the secondary ossification center of the lateral process).
- Edema of the posterior process or os trigonum can be seen.
- Soft tissue abnormalities include posterior capsular thickening, injuries of posterior talofibular, and tibiofibular ligament.[25]

Tarsal Coalitions (Figs. 23A to C)

- Patients with tarsal coalitions may be asymptomatic or present with hind-foot pain or flat foot.
- Calcaneonavicular and talo-calcaneal coalitions are most common; calcaneocuboid or talonavicular coalitions or multiple tarsal coalitions are rare.

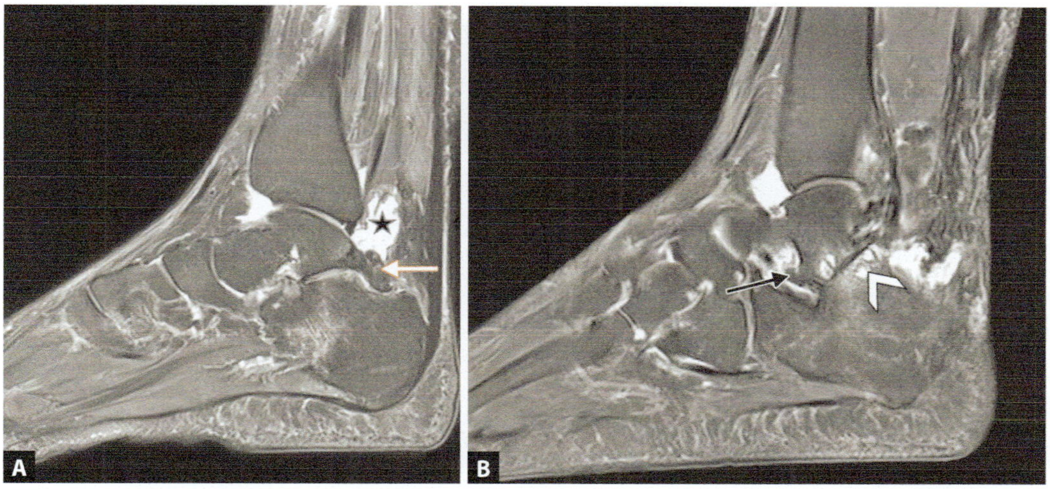

Figs. 22A and B: Posterior impingement due to elongated Stieda process (arrow in A) with osteophytes with subtalar arthritis (arrowhead). Complete replacement of sinus tarsi fat is also seen with edema and osteophytes (black arrow in B). Adventitious bursitis is seen superior and posterior to the Stieda process (* in A).

- X-ray—45° internal oblique view can easily diagnose calcaneonavicular coalitions, with typical elongation of anterior process of calcaneus forming the "ant-eater sign." Reverse ant-eater sign is used to describe a hyperplastic navicular and a "drunken waiter" sign or C sign to describe a dysplastic sustentaculum tali.[26]
- Coalitions can be fibrous (hypointense on T2-weighted images), cartilaginous [hyperintense on T2-weighted images or osseous (bone marrow signal)]. Joint space is reduced or irregular and hypointense in fibrous coalitions, and obliterated in cases of osseous coalitions.[27]
- Bone marrow edema adjacent to the involved joint may be found and may lead to diagnosis of unsuspected coalition.[27]
- Sagittal MR images best depict the calcaneonavicular coalition.
- Coronal sections are best to visualize talocalcaneal coalitions, which generally involves the middle facet of talocalcaneal joint.
- CT and X-ray may be normal in patients with fibrous or cartilaginous coalitions, whereas MRI can directly show the area of abnormality.[27,28]

Adult-acquired Flat Foot[10]

- Acquired flat foot deformity in adults occurs due to lesions in the stabilizers of the medial side of the ankle-deltoid ligament complex, spring ligament or posterior tibial tendon.[10]
- Spring ligament consists of superomedial calcaneonavicular ligament, medioplantar oblique calcaneonavicular ligament, and inferoplantar longitudinal calcaneonavicular ligament.
- Superomedial calcaneonavicular ligament is the most frequently injured important component.
- MRI shows thickening and heterogeneity of the ligament (>6 mm) or thinned out or discontinuity within the ligament.[10]
- Adult-acquired flat foot is often associated with posterior tibial tendinopathy or tears.

Bones

Avascular Necrosis of Talus (Figs. 24A to C)

- *Anatomical considerations* predisposing to avascular necrosis (AVN)—talus is predominantly covered by cartilage (60%) with a tenuous arterial supply through the bare areas of the bone, predisposing it to ischemia in cases of traumatic disruption of blood supply.[29]
- *Atraumatic AVN*—predisposing factors include corticosteroid intake, alcoholism, SLE, renal transplant, and hyperlipidemia.
- *Traumatic AVN*—occurs most commonly as a sequelae of displaced talar neck fracture with subtalar dislocation. Associated ankle joint dislocation or talonavicular dislocation increases risk of AVN to 100%. Talar body fractures also have a high risk of AVN and a worse prognosis.[29]
- *"Hawkins sign"*—a linear radiolucent area parallel to talar dome is a well-described sign on radiographs; post-traumatic "Hawkins sign" implies an area of revascularization with reduced chances of AVN.
- However, radiographs are insensitive in early AVN, where ischemic or necrotic bone and healthy bone cannot be differentiated.
- *MRI* is sensitive in detecting bone marrow edema in early AVN.[29]
- T1-weighted images show the typical serpiginous low-signal intensity line in the talar dome.
- On T2-weighted images, a hyperintense line demarcating avascular bone is seen.

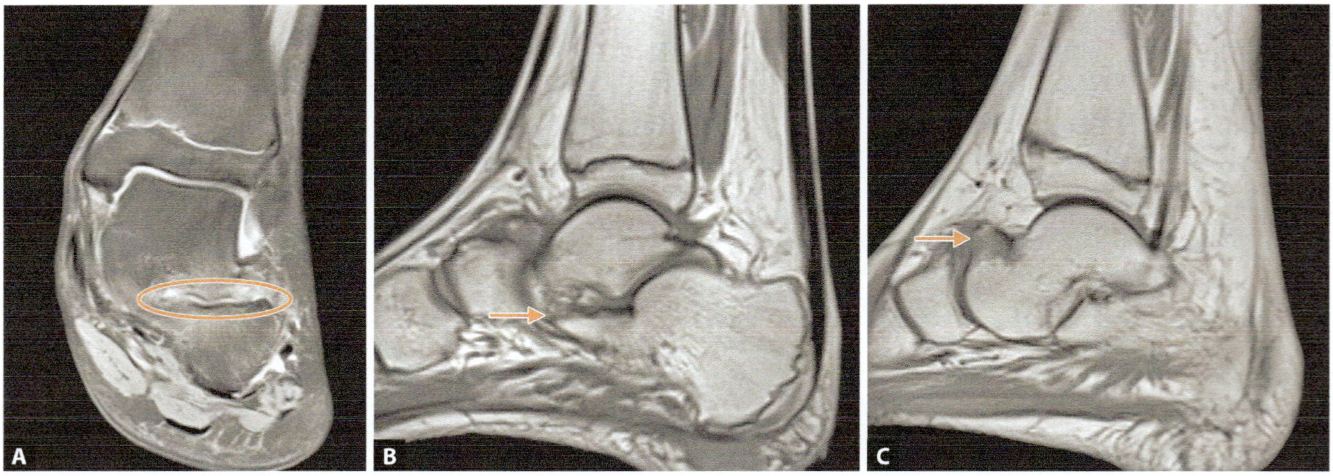

Figs. 23A to C: Coalition of anterior facet of talocalcaneal joint (oval in A) with absence of normal cartilage signal and irregular decreased joint space. (B) An elongated anterior process of calcaneus is seen (arrow). A talar beak is also seen (arrow in C).

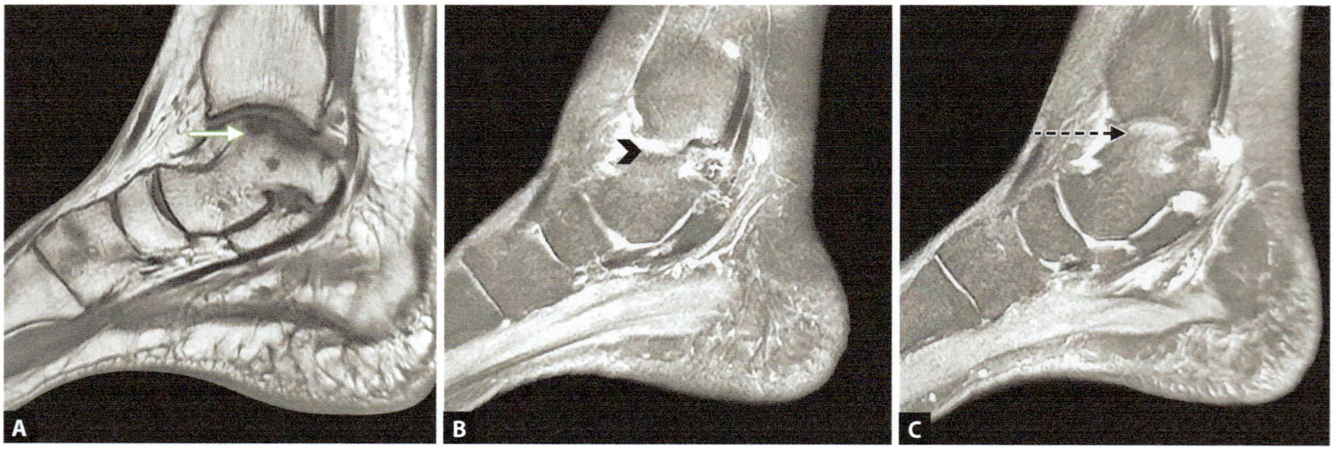

Figs. 24A to C: AVN of talus. (A) Sagittal T1-weighted image shows a subchondral area of hypointensity in the talar dome (arrow). On PD-weighted fat-saturated images (B and C), subchondral hyperintensity is seen in the talar dome (dashed arrow) along with subchondral collapse (arrowheads) and articular cartilage loss. (AVN: avascular necrosis)

- Advanced AVN presents with articular cartilage damage and subchondral collapse **(Figs. 24A to C)**.[29]
- Other bones of foot prone to AVN are navicular and heads of metatarsals (Freiberg disease).

Osteochondral Lesions of Talus

- Osteochondral lesions of the talus have a predilection for the medial talar dome, (due to greater frequency of inversion injuries) and are areas of articular cartilage and subchondral bone changes.
- Osteochondral lesions denote a wide spectrum of changes including bone marrow edema to osteochondral fragment to osteoarthritic changes.[30]
- Clinical symptoms vary and patient can remain asymptomatic and this lesion can be incidentally detected.
- Patients can also present with persistent pain and instability.
- Lesions can be associated with acute as well as chronic injuries.[31]
- Routine radiographs may miss subtle lesions and weight bearing views and mortise views are recommended
- MRI demonstrates both articular cartilage changes as well as the condition of the subchondral bone.
- Articular cartilage in ankle is thinner and more difficult to assess but has the same trilaminar appearance with intermediate signal (higher on fat-saturated sequences).
- The innermost of basal layer of cartilage is relatively hypointense and adjacent subchondral bone is linear and hypointense.[31]
- Chondral damage can be limited to fissuring (which is difficult to detect without high resolution imaging) and fragmentation.
- Frank delamination of the basal layer of chondral cartilage leads to a flap which can remain in situ without any displacement.[31]

- Hyperintense fluid signal cleft may be found with minimal displacement. Since the fluid which insinuates may be minimal and intermediate in signal, these changes are difficult to appreciate.
- Underlying bone may be normal or show edema or an osteochondral fracture in acute injury.
- Chronic changes may be in the form of subchondral bone cysts or subchondral sclerosis **(Fig. 25)**.[31]

Degenerative

- Osteoarthritis (OA) of ankle joint is rare as compared to osteoarthritis of knee and most cases are idiopathic and occur in younger individuals.
- Post-traumatic osteoarthritis can also occur, after osteochondral injury with cartilage damage and ligamentous injuries **(Figs. 26A to C)**.

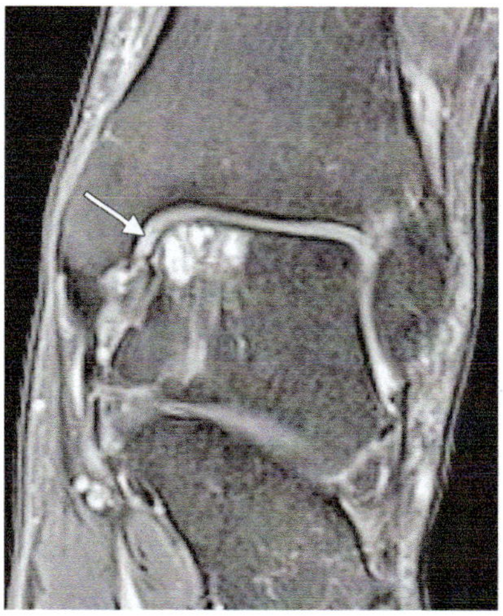

Fig. 25: Osteochondral lesion talus: Subchondral bone cysts in the medial talar dome with overlying cartilage showing loss of the trilaminar appearance and an area of hyperintensity (arrow). No definite osteochondral flap is seen.

- *MRI findings* include bone marrow edema around tibiotalar and talofibular joint. Subtalar joint arthritis may cause periarticular bone marrow edema around talus and calcaneum.
- Bone marrow changes may be absent in early osteoarthritis even with radiographic evidence of OA.[32]

Nerve Entrapment-Tarsal Tunnel Syndrome

- *Anatomical boundaries*—tarsal tunnel is a fibro-osseous tunnel located on medial side of ankle.[1]
- It is bounded laterally by talus and sustentaculum tali of calcaneus, medially by flexor retinaculum and abductor hallucis muscle.
- *Contents*—tibialis posterior, FHL, flexor digitorum longus, posterior tibial artery, and tibial nerve
- *Clinical presentation* of tarsal tunnel syndrome—burning and pain in sole and toes.
- *Common causes* are compression of posterior tibial nerve by ganglion cyst, tenosynovitis, neurogenic tumors, pannus, fibrosis, and varicosities **(Fig. 27)**. Post-traumatic scarring and hind foot valgus can also cause tarsal tunnel syndrome. Many cases are idiopathic.[33]
- *MRI findings* depend on the cause. Ganglion cysts are common.

Sinus Tarsi Syndrome

- *Anatomical boundaries*—sinus tarsi is a cone-shaped space located between talus and calcaneus, open laterally.
- *Contents*—fat, neurovascular structures, cervical ligament, interosseous ligament, and joint capsule insinuation from posterior subtalar joint.
- *Clinical presentation*—sinus tarsi syndrome is characterized by lateral ankle pain and instability.

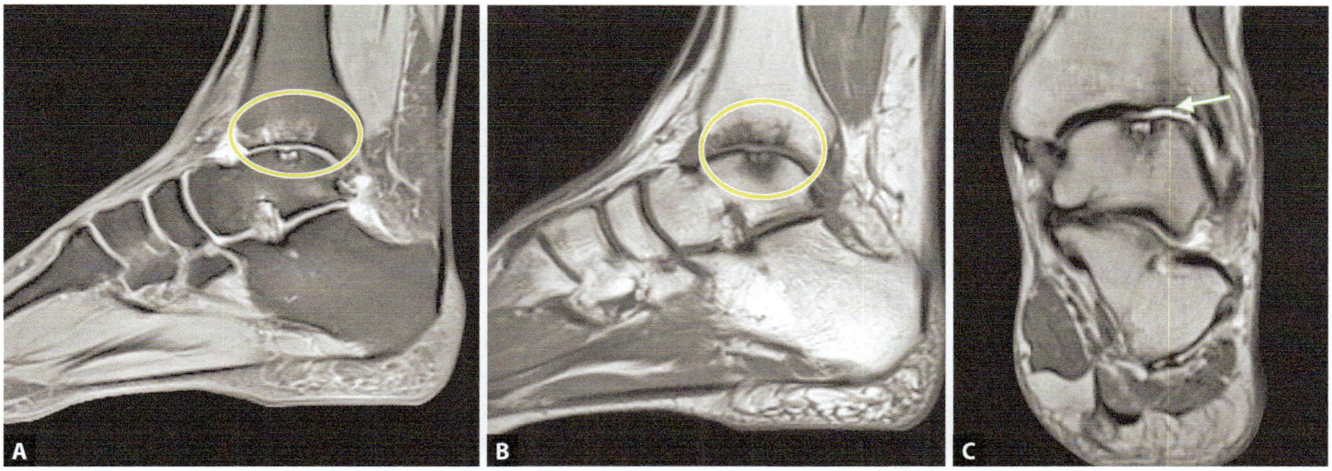

Figs. 26A to C: Degenerative arthritis with osteochondral lesion of talus. Subchondral cysts and edema seen in tibial plafond and talar dome (oval in A) with subchondral sclerosis (oval in B). There is an osteochondral lesion in mid-talar dome with subchondral cyst and mild flattening of talar dome. Cartilage denudation seen on coronal T2-weighted image (arrow in C).

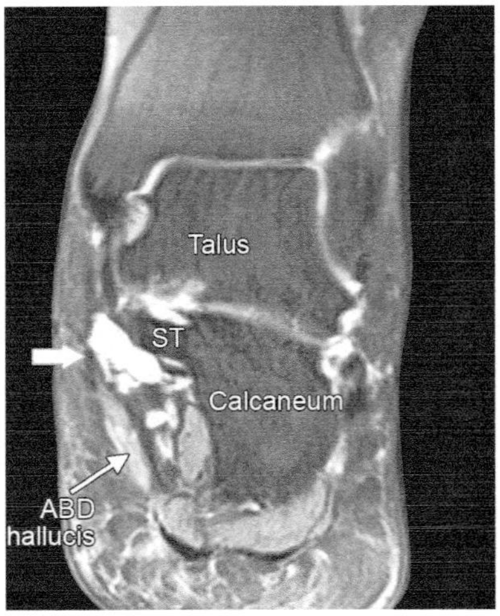

Fig. 27: Tarsal tunnel syndrome. Lobulated ganglion cyst (large arrow) causing mass effect on the tarsal tunnel. (ABD hallucis: abductor hallucis; ST: sustentaculum tali).

- *Cause*—chronic inversion injuries with disruption of the cervical and interosseous ligaments along with injuries to lateral ligaments; inflammatory arthritis.
- *MRI findings*—complete obliteration of fat in the sinus tarsi replaced by high-signal intensity due to fluid or low signal in fibrosis (partial obliteration of fat is nonspecific)
- In the setting of acute ankle sprain, fluid or hemorrhage may accumulate in sinus tarsi, and should not be diagnosed as sinus tarsi syndrome.[1]

Infections

Untreated infectious arthritis causes rapid destruction of articular cartilage.[34] MRI is sensitive in detecting osteomyelitis as early as 1–2 days after infection. Osteitis with hypointense signal on T1-weighted images is the earliest finding.

In patients with diabetic neuropathy, a common indication for imaging is differentiating between neuropathic joint (Charcot's neuropathic osteoarthropathy) and osteomyelitis or osteomyelitis complicating neuropathic joint. MRI is sensitive and more specific than bone scintigraphy. Negative MRI rules out Charcot's neuroarthropathy.[35]

Early stages can present with subchondral bone marrow edema with or without microfractures on MRI, and early diagnosis is important for early offloading of the ankle joint to prevent chronic damage. The pattern of involvement can be tarsometatarsal, tarsal or subtalar, and ankle joints. Early stages progress to marked muscle and soft tissue edema **(Figs. 28A and B)**.[36] Untreated patients progress to chronic stage with subluxation, dislocation, and fractures with joint distension with debris and fluid. In later stages, MRI can be useful for diagnosing complications like infections with intraosseous or soft tissue abscesses, sinus tracts or causes of internal derangement due to ligament or tendon tears or tendinopathy due to impingements caused by subluxations or dislocations.[36]

Atypical infections like actinomycosis (actinomyces is a filamentous bacteria) or eumycetomas (true fungi) are chronic granulomatous suppurative infections of the foot with typical clinical presentation of blackish or yellowish granular discharge through draining sinuses depending upon the causative agent. A dot-in-circle sign has been described in mycetomas, which are a hypointense speck within a hyperintense lesion.[37]

Inflammatory Arthritis

The ankle is affected by rheumatoid arthritis, seronegative arthropathies, reactive arthritis as well as gout. Erosions and synovitis and bone marrow edema along with effusions are seen earlier with MRI than on radiographs. Seronegative arthropathy and reactive arthritis presents with enthesitis with edema at insertion of Achilles tendon with or without tendinopathy along with plantar fasciitis **(Figs. 29A and B)**. MRI appearance of gouty arthritis with gouty tophi is nonspecific with hypointensity or intermediate signal on T1-weighted sequences and heterogeneous signal on T2-weighted images.[38] Erosions and synovitis are also seen.

Plantar Fasciitis (Figs. 30A and B)

- The plantar fascia originates from the plantar aspect of calcaneal tuberosity.
- It has three components—a central portion which originates from medial aspect of calcaneal tuberosity and medial and lateral expansions.[1]
- Normal thickness should not exceed 4 mm near the calcaneal attachment.[1]
- Clinical symptoms—pain or tenderness on the plantar aspect of ankle near plantar fascia attachment. Middle-aged women and patients with seronegative arthropathy are prone to develop this condition.[1]
- MRI appearance of plantar fasciitis—thickening of the plantar fascia near calcaneal attachment with high signal on T2-weighted sequences.
- Adjacent calcaneum may show edema or erosions.

Tumors

Tumors of the ankle and foot are rare.

Osseous tumors: Tumors of distal tibia and fibula most commonly seen are nonossifying fibromas, giant cell tumors **(Figs. 31A and B)**, aneurysmal bone cysts, enchondromas, and osteochondromas.[39]

Intraosseous lipoma and simple bone cyst are typically found anteriorly in midportion of calcaneus, whereas giant cell tumors and aneurysmal bone cysts are

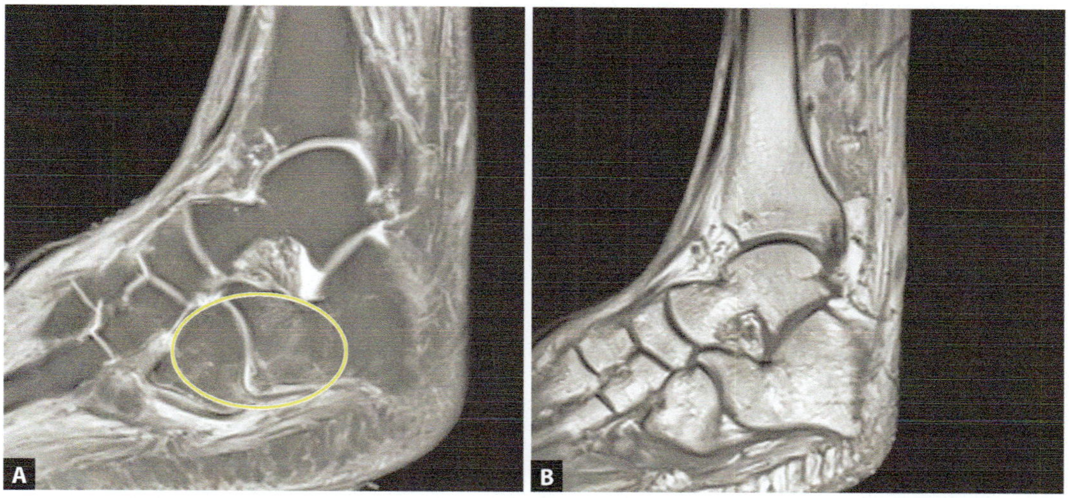

Figs. 28A and B: Early Charcot's neuroarthropathy with subarticular bone marrow edema at calcaneocuboid joint (oval in A) which is showing patchy hyperintensity in sagittal PD-weighted fat-saturated sequence (A). No hypointensity seen on sagittal T1-weighted image (B) suggesting absence of infection. Extensive muscle and soft tissue edema is seen.

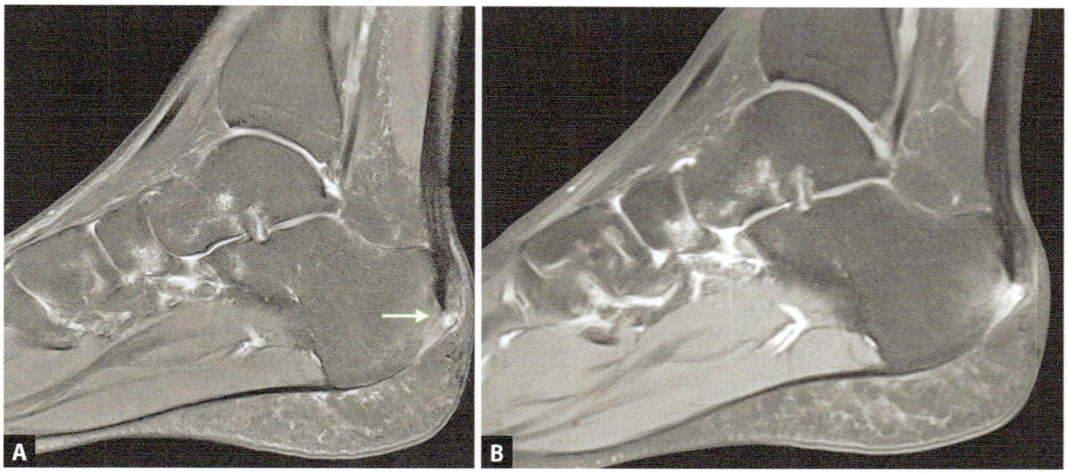

Figs. 29A and B: Seronegative arthropathy with enthesitis at Achilles tendon insertion (arrow in A) on sagittal PD-weighted fat-saturated image, with subarticular bone marrow edema in subtalar joint and navicular, which shows enhancement on postcontrast T1-weighted fat-saturated images (B).

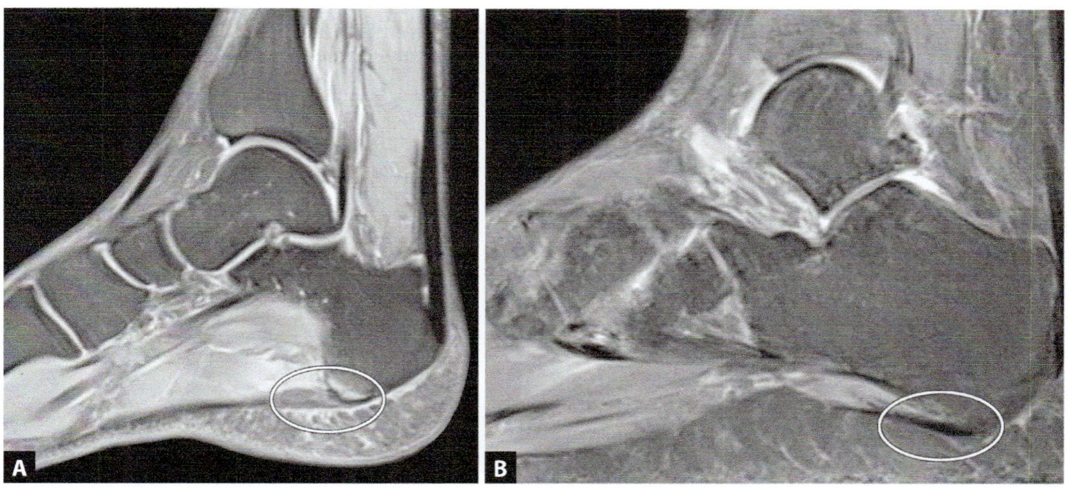

Figs. 30A and B: (A) Plantar fasciitis. The plantar fascia (oval) is thickened and hyperintense on the PD fat-saturated sagittal sequence. Adjacent bone marrow edema is seen in the calcaneum; (B) Normal hypointense thin plantar fascia.

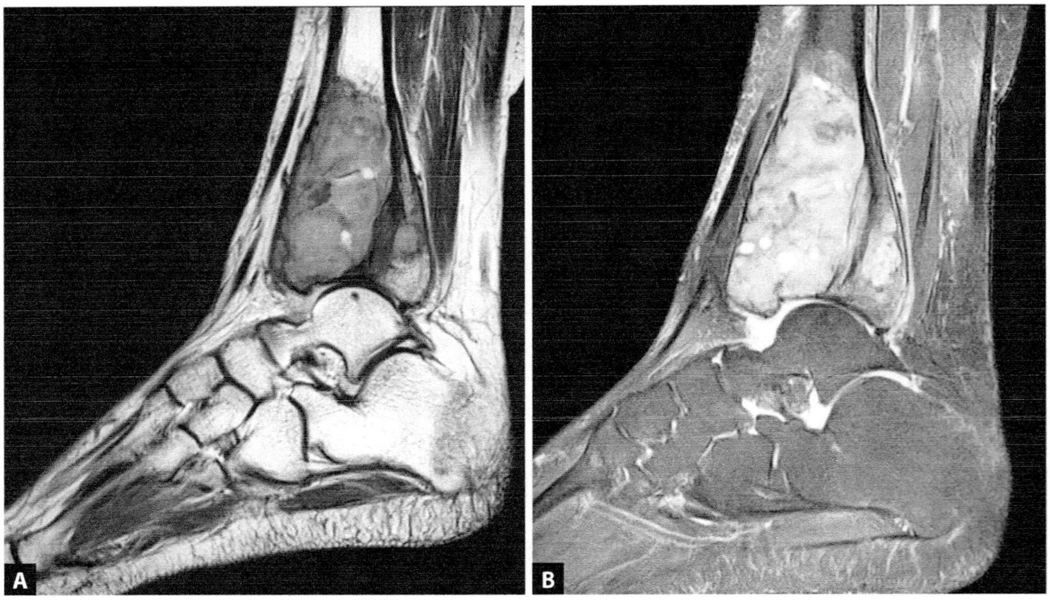

Figs. 31A and B: Giant cell tumor of the lower end of tibia: (A) A subarticular mildly expansile lesion with hypointense margins and predominantly hypointense internal contents with few hyperintense areas on sagittal T1-weighted image; (B) The lesion is hyperintense on sagittal T2-weighted fat-saturated image. No cortical breech or soft tissue is noted.

located posteriorly. Ewing's sarcoma and osteosarcoma rarely can involve the ankle and foot.[1] In the older adult, chondrosarcoma is common.[40]

Soft Tissue Tumors

Benign—plantar fibromatosis, vascular malformations, ganglion cysts, giant cell tumors of the tendon sheath, pigmented villonodular synovitis, and neurogenic tumors are common benign soft tissue tumors of the ankle and foot.

Malignant tumors—synovial sarcomas, epithelioid sarcomas, and pleomorphic sarcomas the common soft tissue are common soft tissue sarcomas in the ankle and foot.[40]

REFERENCES

1. Helms C, Major N, Anderson M, Kaplan PE, Dussault R, (Eds). Musculoskeletal MRI, 2nd edition. USA: Saunders; 2009. p. 435.
2. Schweitzer ME, Karasick D. MR imaging of disorders of the Achilles tendon. Am J Roentgenol. 2000;175(3):613-25.
3. Tam KF, Lui TH. MR imaging of the Achilles tendon after surgical repair. Open Orthop J. 2017;31(11):697-703.
4. Pierre-Jerome C, Moncayo V, Terk MR. MRI of the Achilles tendon: A comprehensive review of the anatomy, biomechanics, and imaging of overuse tendinopathies. Acta Radiol. 2010;51(4):438-54.
5. Lawrence DA, Rolen MF, Abi Morshed K, Moukaddam H, Moukaddam H. MRI of heel pain. Am J Roentgenol. 2013;200(4):845-55.
6. Griffith JF, Hu M, Yeung DKW, Guo P, Lam SL, Xiao F, et al. Achilles tendon xanthomas: Fat-water separation at baseline and after treatment. Radiology. 2017;285(3):876-84.
7. Schubert R. MRI of peroneal tendinopathies resulting from trauma or overuse. Br J Radiol. 2013;86(1021):20110750.
8. Taljanovic MS, Alcala JN, Gimber LH, Rieke JD, Chilvers MM, Latt DL. High-resolution US and MR imaging of peroneal tendon injuries. Radiographics. 2015;35 (1):179-99.
9. Wang XT, Rosenberg ZS, Mechlin MB, Schweitzer ME. Normal variants and diseases of the peroneal tendons and superior peroneal retinaculum: MR imaging features. Radiographics. 2005;25(3):587-602.
10. Mengiardi B, Pinto C, Zanetti M. Spring ligament complex and posterior tibial tendon: MR anatomy and findings in acquired adult flatfoot deformity. Semin Musculoskelet Radiol. 2016;20(1):104-15.
11. Schweitzer ME, Karasick D. MR imaging of disorders of the posterior tibialis tendon. Am J Roentgenol. 2000;175(3):627-35.
12. Schweitzer ME. Magnetic resonance imaging of the foot and ankle. Magn Reson Q. 1993;9(4):214-34.
13. Linklater JM, Hayter CL, Vu D. Imaging of acute capsuloligamentous sports injuries in the ankle and foot: Sports imaging series. Radiology. 2017;283(3):642-65.
14. Lee MH, Cha JG, Lee YK, Choi GC, Paik SH, Lee HK, et al. The bright rim sign on MRI for anterior talofibular ligament injury with arthroscopic correlation. Am J Roentgenol. 2012;198(4):885-90.
15. Rosenberg ZS, Beltran J, Bencardino JT. From the RSNA refresher courses. Radiological Society of North America. MR imaging of the ankle and foot. Radiographics. 2000;20:S153-79.
16. Evans JM, Schucany G. Radiological evaluation of a high ankle sprain. Proc (Bayl Univ Med Cent). 2006;19:402-5.
17. Brown KW, Morrison WB, Schweitzer ME, Parellada JA, Nothnagel H. MRI findings associated with distal tibiofibular syndesmosis injury. Am J Roentgenol. 2004;182(1):131-6.
18. Mengiardi B, Pinto C, Zanetti M. Medial collateral ligament complex of the ankle: MR imaging anatomy and findings

in medial instability. Semin Musculoskeletal Radiol. 2016;20(1):91-103.
19. Jeong MS, Choi YS, Kim YJ, Kim JS, Young KW, Jung YY. Deltoid ligament in acute ankle injury: MR imaging analysis. Skeletal Radiol. 2014;43(5):655-63.
20. Chun KY, Choi YS, Lee SH, Kim JS, Young KW, Jeong MS, et al. Deltoid ligament and tibiofibular syndesmosis injury in chronic lateral ankle instability: Magnetic resonance imaging evaluation at 3T and comparison with arthroscopy. Korean J Radiol. 2015;16(5):1096-103.
21. Berman Z, Tafur M, Ahmed SS, Huang BK, Chang EY. Ankle impingement syndromes: An imaging review. Br J Radiol. 2017;90(1070):20160735.
22. Stoller SM, Hekmat F, Kleiger B. A comparative study of the frequency of anterior impingement exostoses of the ankle in dancers and nondancers. Foot Ankle. 1984;4(4):201-3.
23. Haller J, Bernt R, Seeger T, Weissenback A, Tuchler H, Resnick D. MR-imaging of anterior tibiotalar impingement syndrome: agreement, sensitivity and specificity of MR imaging and indirect MR-arthrography. Eur J Radiol. 2006;58(3):450-60.
24. Cerezal L, Abascal F, Canga A, Pereda T, García-Valtuille R, Pérez-Carro L, et al. MR imaging of ankle impingement syndromes. Am J Roentgenol. 2003;181(2):551-9.
25. Robinson P, White LM. Soft-tissue and osseous impingement syndromes of the ankle: Role of imaging in diagnosis and management. Radiographics. 2002;22(6):1457-71.
26. Nalaboff KM, Schweitzer ME. MRI of tarsal coalition: Frequency, distribution, and innovative signs. Bull NYU Hosp Jt Dis. 2008;66(1):14-21.
27. Guignand D, Journeau P, Mainard-Simard L, Popkov D, Haumont T, Lascombes P. Child calcaneonavicular coalitions: MRI diagnostic value in a 19-case series. Orthop Traumatol Surg Res. 2011;97(1):67-72.
28. Newman JS, Newberg AH. Congenital tarsal coalition: Multimodality evaluation with emphasis on CT and MR imaging. Radiographics. 2000;20(2):321-32.
29. Pearce DH, Mongiardi CN, Fornasier VL, Daniels TR. Avascular necrosis of the talus: A pictorial essay. Radiographics. 2005;25(2):399-410.
30. Posadzy M, Desimpel J, Vanhoenacker FM. Staging of osteochondral lesions of the talus: MRI and cone beam CT. J Belg Soc Radiol. 2017;101(S2):1.
31. Linklater JM. Imaging of talar dome chondral and osteochondral lesions. Top Magn Reson Imaging. 2010;21(1):3-13.
32. Nakamura Y, Uchiyama S, Kamimura M, Komatsu M, Ikegami S, Kato H. Bone alterations are associated with ankle osteoarthritis joint pain. Sci Rep. 2016;6:18717.
33. Erickson SJ, Quinn SF, Kneeland JB, Smith JW, Johnson JE, Carrera GF, et al. MR imaging of the tarsal tunnel and related spaces: normal and abnormal findings with anatomic correlation. Am J Roentgenol. 1990;155(2): 323-8.
34. Pioro MH, Mandell BF. Septic arthritis. Rheum Dis Clin North Am. 1997;23(2):239-58.
35. Rogers LC, Frykberg RG, Armstrong DG, Boulton AJ, Edmonds M, Van GH, et al. The Charcot foot in diabetes. J Am Podiatr Med Assoc. 2011;101(5):437-46.
36. Mautone M, Naidoo P. What the radiologist needs to know about Charcot foot. J Med Imaging Radiat Oncol. 2015;59(4):395-402.
37. Sarris I, Berendt AR, Athanasous N, Ostlere SJ. MRI of mycetoma of the foot: Two cases demonstrating the dot-in-circle sign. Skeletal Radiol. 2003;32(3):179-83.
38. Gandikota G, Glazebrook KN, Jacobson JA. Advanced imaging in gout. Am J Roentgenol. 2013;201(3):515-25.
39. Toepfer A, Harrasser N, Recker M, Lenze U, Pohlig F, Gerdesmeyer L, et al. Distribution patterns of foot and ankle tumors: A university tumor institute experience. BMC Cancer. 2018;18:735.
40. Mascard E, Gaspar N, Brugières L, Glorion C, Pannier S, Gomez-Brouchet A. Malignant tumours of the foot and ankle. EFORT Open Rev. 2017;2(5):261-71.

SECTION

6

Miscellaneous MSK-trauma/Soft Tissue/Nerve/Prosthetics Imaging

CHAPTER

21

Radiological Evaluation of Appendicular Trauma

Atin Kumar, Devasenathipathy Kandasamy, Arun Kumar Gupta

INTRODUCTION

Skeletal trauma is one of the most common forms of injuries suffered by people in everyday life. The extremities are the most often affected. The emergency radiologist plays a key role in the workup of such patients as the initial evaluation requires radiographic examination. The radiograph has to be well-performed and accurately interpreted. It provides diagnostic evidence of the presence of fracture or dislocation along with the severity and extent of the trauma. The radiographs are also essential to check for accuracy of fracture reduction and to monitor bone healing.

CLINICAL EVALUATION

The features pointing toward underlying fracture include deformity, swelling, ecchymosis, marked local tenderness, abnormal mobility and crepitus on palpation, and impairment of function. It is important to assess the state of the circulation and neural integrity in the limb distal to the fracture, both at the time of initial presentation and after any intervention.

The radiologist should also be aware of the mechanism of the injury as well as the time interval from the injury to the radiographic examination. This helps the radiologist to know what and where to look for in the radiograph. The radiologist can also look for specific injuries that are known to be associated with the mechanism of the injury.

RADIOLOGICAL EVALUATION

Definitions and Classification

A *fracture* is a disruption in the continuity of the bone. A *dislocation* is a complete disruption of a joint with loss of congruity between the articular surfaces. *Subluxation* is a minor disruption of the joint where some part of the articular surfaces remain in contact.

The fractures are clinically classified into open or closed fractures. The open fractures are those which penetrate the overlying skin and the fracture site is exposed to the external environment whereas closed fractures are those with intact overlying skin and hence no exposure to the environment. This makes the open fractures amenable to the risk of infection because of contamination by microorganisms.

The radiographic evaluation of fracture should work on the basic principle of obtaining at least two views of the involved bone, ideally perpendicular to each other, with each view including two joints adjacent to the involved bone. This helps the radiologist eliminate the risk of missing an associated dislocation or subluxation at a site remote from the apparent primary injury. Additional views should be obtained if there is any doubt or in specific situations like an oblique view for scaphoid fracture. It is estimated that about 5% of fractures are seen only on one view and about 5% of fractures require additional views to be detected **(Figs. 1A and B)**. In children, especially if there is involvement of the ossification centers which are not fused, it may be necessary to obtain a radiograph of the normal, unaffected side for comparison.

The complete radiographic evaluation of a trauma patient should consist of:

- Osseous evaluation
- Soft tissue evaluation

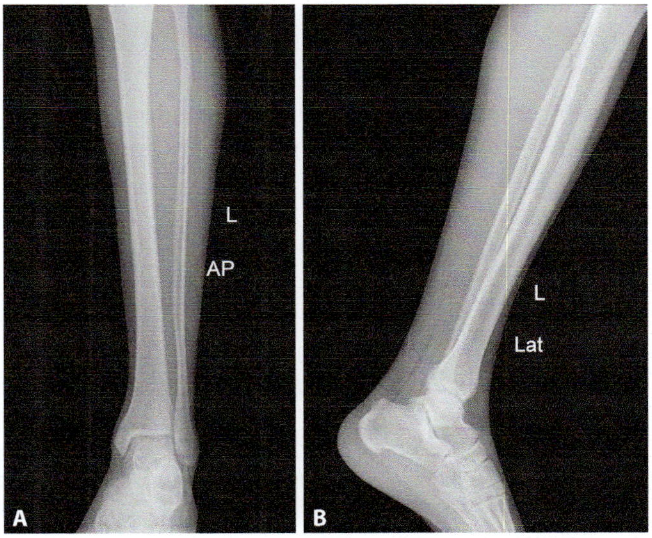

Figs. 1A and B: Anteroposterior (AP) and lateral (Lat) radiographs of the leg show a fracture of the upper shaft of fibula which is visualized only on the lateral view and is almost not seen on the AP view.

Osseous Evaluation

Presence or Absence of Bony Injury

A careful examination of all the bones included in the radiograph must be done for detection or ruling out a fracture. A fracture can appear as any of the following—an obvious disruption in continuity of bone, abnormal line of radiolucency, cortical irregularity or increase in bone density (due to impacted or compression fractures). Sometimes the fracture may be "occult" which are clinically suspected but are not visualized on the initial radiograph. They may be detected subsequently on a follow-up radiography or scintigraphy. Scaphoid fractures are an example.

Anatomic Location and Extent of the Fracture

When describing a fracture it is important to specify the location within the long bone. In case of a fracture involving shaft of a long bone it should be described whether it is located in proximal, middle or distal thirds of bone, or at junction of any two parts. It can also be described in terms of involvement of anatomic point of reference, e.g., supracondylar fracture of humerus. For fractures located near bone ends, mention should be made of any intra-articular extension as this will alter the subsequent management of the patient.

Types of Fracture

Complete or incomplete: The fracture is classified as complete if it involves the entire width of the bone to involve both the cortices and incomplete if only some of the bony trabeculae are completely severed while others are bent or remain intact.[1] Incomplete fractures are more likely to be seen in children. Angular deformities are common without any displacement in incomplete fractures **(Table 1)**.

The complete fractures are further classified as:

- *Simple*: One fracture line separating the bone into two fragments.
- *Comminuted*: Two or more fracture lines with three or more fragments. A "butterfly" fragment can be seen if a small triangular fragment gets isolated on the concave side of the injury.

Table 1: Fracture types.

Complete fracture	*Incomplete fracture*
• Simple—one fracture line, two bony fragments • Comminuted—two or more fracture lines with three or more fragments	• Greenstick—cortical break in convex side, intact concave side • Torus—compression fracture in concave side • Plastic bowing—no fracture, just bowing seen

The incomplete fractures can be of following types:

- *Greenstick (Hickory stick) fractures* ***(Figs. 2A and B)***: Fractures occurring due to angulation forces primarily in infants and young children below 10 years of age because of the relatively greater component of pliable woven bone. The fracture affects the tension or the convex side of the bone. The bone bends with the convex side showing a horizontal break in the continuity of the cortex whereas the other concave side remains intact.[1] The greenstick fractures heal without any complications in most instances.
- *Torus (buckling) fractures*: Fractures occurring due to longitudinal compressive forces over a soft bone of young child. The fracture affects the compressive (concave) side of the bone. The cortex bulges outward due to compressive forces at the site of injury. They occur mostly in the metaphysis and are very painful.[1]
- *Plastic bowing fractures* ***(Figs. 3A and B)***: No true fracture is seen. It occurs when the force on the bone is not sufficient enough to cause a cortical disruption but instead leads to bowing of the bone.

Direction of the Fracture Line

This is described with respect to the longitudinal axis of the bone.[2] Based on this, the fractures can be classified into:

- *Transverse fracture* ***(Figs. 4A and B)***: The fracture line is perpendicular to the long axis of the bone. In long bones it occurs as a result of angulation force. This type of fracture is usually stable and unlikely to be displaced after reduction.
- *Oblique fracture*: The fracture line runs oblique to the long axis of the bone and the angle is <90°.
- *Spiral fracture* ***(Fig. 5)***: The fracture line turns and twists around the shaft and encircles it at least once. It occurs as a result of twisting force to the limb. This type of fracture is prone to be displaced after reduction.[2]

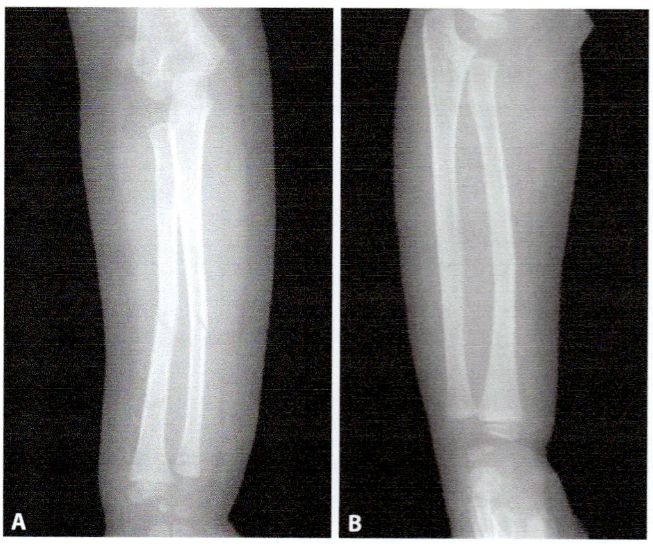

Figs. 2A and B: Anteroposterior and lateral radiographs of the forearm show greenstick fractures of the shaft of radius and ulna.

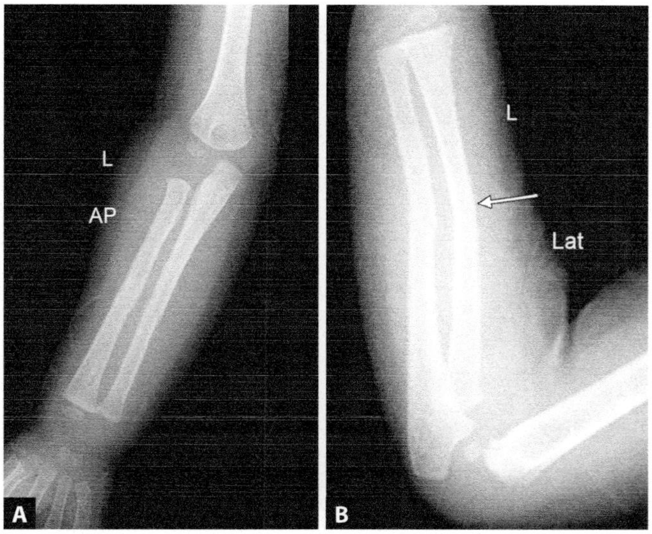

Figs. 3A and B: Anteroposterior and lateral radiographs of the forearm show plastic bowing fracture without an obvious cortical break in the midshaft of radius (arrow). A complete fracture of the adjacent ulna is associated.

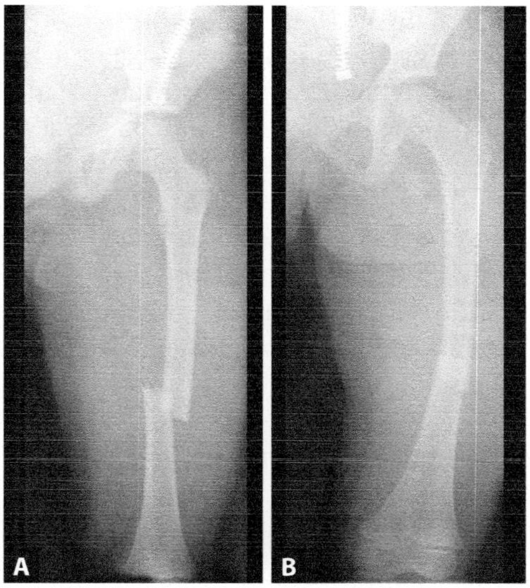

Figs. 4A and B: Anteroposterior and oblique radiographs of the left thigh show a transverse fracture of the shaft of ulna with overriding of the bone fragments.

Spatial Relationship of the Fragments

This is described in terms of apposition/displacement, alignment/angulation, rotation and distraction/overriding.

- *Apposition*: It refers to the state of bony contact at the fracture site and the resultant shift of the fragments relative to each other. This classifies fractures into undisplaced and displaced. The displacement is described with reference to the direction of shift of the distal fragment. An undisplaced fracture with a fine fracture line is termed as "hairline" fracture.
- *Alignment*: It refers to the position of the distal fragment with respect to the proximal fragment. It can be lateral/medial displacement or tilt/angulation. The angulation of the distal fragment medially is termed "varus" and laterally is termed "valgus"
- *Rotation*: It refers to the rotation of the distal fragment over the longitudinal axis. It can be internal or external rotation. To comment on rotation, the proximal and distal joints must be included in the radiograph.
- *Overriding/distraction*: A longitudinal separation of the bony fragments in the long axis of the bone with resultant increased distance between the two fragments is termed distraction. If the bony fragments overlap on each other, it is termed overriding and leads to foreshortening of the limb **(Figs. 4A and B)**.

Presence of Special Features

The special features that need to be commented upon in a radiograph include:

- *Impaction*: When the two fragments are driven into each other. This occurs due to compressive forces.

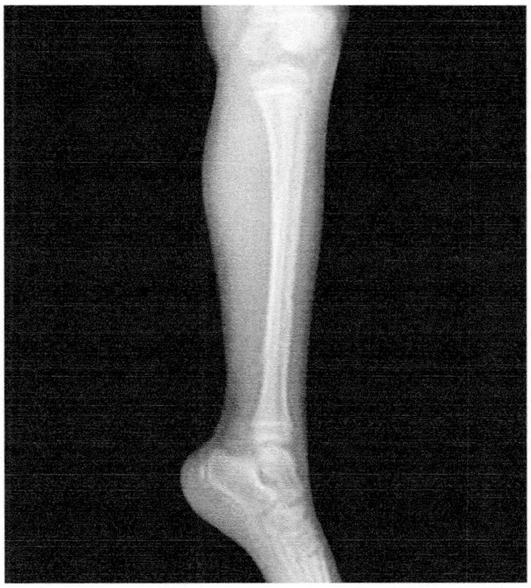

Fig. 5: Lateral radiograph of the leg showing a spiral fracture through the lower shaft of tibia.

The classical radiolucent fracture line is not seen but instead a subtle radiopaque line is seen at the site which may be the only marker of the fracture. It is important to obtain additional views in this situation in case of a doubt.

- *Depression*: It represents an inward bulging of the outer bony surface. It is a type of impaction fracture. This gives rise to a "double cortical line". It is seen most commonly at tibial plateau and radial head in extremities and in frontal bone in the skull.
- *Compression*: It represents an impaction fracture involving the spinal vertebral body due to hyperflexion forces.

- *Avulsion*: It involves tearing away of a portion of the bone usually at insertion of a muscle or ligament due to forceful pulling. The frequent sites are tuberosities of tubular bones, elbow, lateral metatarsal and lower cervical spinous processes. A small cortical avulsion is termed a "flake" fracture. "Chip" or "corner" fracture represents avulsion of a small fragment of bone from the corner of a phalanx or other short or long tubular bone. Corner chip fractures at metaphyseal ends in children should raise the suspicion of battered baby syndrome.

Presence of Associated Abnormalities of the Adjacent Joints

It may be commonly associated with certain types of mechanisms of injuries and some specific fractures. Examples include a femoral shaft fracture associated with hip joint dislocation, a lower end tibial fracture associated with upper end fibula fracture, etc. The joints may be dislocated or subluxated. When dislocation is associated with a fracture, it is termed as fracture dislocation. A fracture through a joint surface may involve the cartilage only (chondral fracture) or cartilage and underlying bone (osteochondral fracture).

Presence of Special Types of the Fractures

The fractures may be due to excessive stress or due to underlying bone weakening disorder. A normal classical fracture occurs due to excessive trauma to a normal bone without underlying abnormality. The ends of the fracture are sharply marginated and the adjacent bone appears healthy in acute settings. However, if the underlying bone is weakened by a localized (tumor) or systemic disease process (osteopenia due to any cause, metastases, multiple myeloma), then even a normal trauma (which is otherwise insufficient to cause fracture) can lead to a fracture. Such fractures are termed "pathological fractures." These fractures are usually transverse with smooth margins. A "stress (fatigue)" fracture is caused by repetitive stress on normal bone. The stress itself is insufficient to cause fracture but over a period of time it leads to the development of fracture. These are commonly seen in runners, dancers, and gymnasts. The metatarsals, tibia, and fibula are commonly affected bones. These fractures become radiologically evident about 2–4 weeks after trauma as a faint transverse radiolucent line often surrounded by a callus **(Figs. 6A and B)**. "Insufficiency fractures" are special type of fractures which occur as a result of chronic repetitive normal stress on a pathological (often osteoporotic) bone. They can occur even with normal walking in a person with underlying osteopenia. They occur commonly in patients of osteomalacia, Paget's disease, and rickets. Radiographically they are seen as linear lucencies on the convex surface of the bone that are oriented perpendicular to the long axis of the bone. They are often multiple and bilateral.

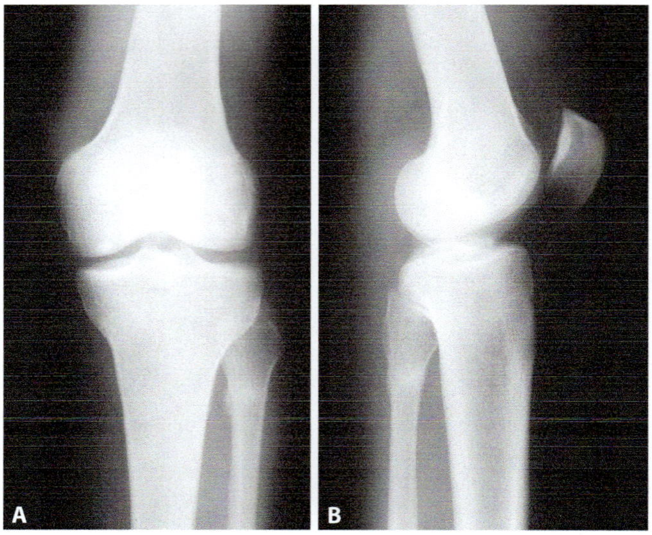

Figs. 6A and B: Anteroposterior and lateral radiographs of the knee joint show a stress fracture of the proximal shaft of fibula.

Table 2: Salter-Harris classification of physeal injuries.

Types	*Imaging features*
Type 1	Fracture through the growth plate. The radiograph appears normal
Type 2	Fracture through the displaced growth plate with involvement of the metaphysis. The metaphyseal fragment is known as the "Thurston Holland" sign. This type is the most common seen in about 75% of cases
Type 3	Fracture through the growth plate with involvement of the epiphysis. The resultant intra-articular fracture often requires open reduction treatment
Type 4	Obliquely oriented vertical fracture passing though the metaphysis, growth plate, and epiphysis
Type 5	Crush fracture leading to compressive deformity of the growth plate. The initial radiographs are normal. Subsequently due to growth arrest there occurs progressive angulation deformity. Hence, it is advisable to follow-up these children for at least 2 years following injury

Involvement of Growth Plate/Physis: Seen in Children

These fractures result in growth arrest and deformity. The *Salter-Harris* classification is used most commonly for such fractures.[3] This classifies the physeal injuries into the five types **(Table 2)**.

Radiographs may not detect the epiphyseal injuries or their displacement especially if only one side alone is radiographed. Hence, it is important to radiograph the opposite limb for comparative evaluation.

Soft-tissue Evaluation

- *Soft-tissue swelling*: Almost always present adjacent to the site of acute fracture.
- *Obliteration or displacement of fat stripes*: Also gives a clue to underlying soft tissue swelling associated with a fracture. Commonly seen in fractures around the wrist joint.
- *Joint capsular swelling*: May be seen due to joint effusion/hemarthrosis secondary to an intra-articular fracture. The capsular distension is also evident by bulging of fat planes around it. It is a good sign to detect fractures near elbow joint. If there is leak of bone marrow fat from within the medullary cavity into the joint along with blood (lipohemarthrosis), then a fat-fluid level may be visualized. It is better evident on computed tomography (CT) or magnetic resonance imaging (MRI).

FRACTURE HEALING

The pathological process of healing of fractures occurs in following phases which last for about 10 days each.[4]

- Circulatory or inflammatory phase—it comprises:
  - Stage of hematoma
  - Stage of subperiosteal and endosteal cellular proliferation
  - Stage of callus formation
- Consolidation or reparative phase
- Remodeling or mechanical phase.

Radiologically, the fracture line shows increase in its width in the first few days due to resorption of its margins. In the next 2–4 weeks the healing occurs by formation of callus. In cases of simple undisplaced fractures the healing occurs by primary union wherein the predominant callus formation is endosteal (internal) which obliterates the fracture line. In cases of complex displaced fractures the healing occurs by secondary union wherein the predominant callus formation is periosteal (external). The callus is initially radiolucent when it contains fibrous tissue and cartilage. At this stage the fracture may be clinically united. Gradually the callus gets remodeled and also gets ossified to give the radiodense white line appearance consistent with radiographic union. In a young adult the total process takes around 4–6 weeks while it may take up to 12 weeks in elderly.[5]

COMPLICATIONS OF FRACTURE

The various complications occur at multiple time intervals postinjury. They are divided into immediate, intermediate, and delayed complications **(Table 3)**.

Table 3: Complications of fractures.

Immediate complications	*Intermediate complications*	*Delayed complications*
• Vascular injury • Nerve and soft tissue injury • Compartment syndrome • Fat embolism • Gas gangrene	• Infection • Post-traumatic ossification • Sudeck's post-traumatic osteodystrophy • Post-traumatic osteolysis • Synostosis	• Abnormal healing process • Avascular necrosis • Disuse osteoporosis • Post-traumatic arthritis

Immediate Complications

- *Vascular injury*: Most commonly with penetrating trauma, sharp bony fragments in open or comminuted fractures or even due to operative manipulation. The popliteal artery, distal superficial femoral artery, and the brachial artery are involved most frequently.
- *Nerve and soft tissue injury*: The adjacent nerves, muscles, ligaments, and tendons may show varying severity of injury.
- *Compartment syndrome*: Results from increased pressure within a muscular compartment secondary to hemorrhage and edema. It leads to muscle necrosis and may be limb or life threatening. Anterior compartment of leg and anterior compartment of forearm are common sites.
- *Fat embolism*: Associated with fracture of a major bone most commonly femur. Usually, it is not of any clinical significance as it occurs in minor degree. It leads to emboli of fat globules from the bone marrow into the vessels and get lodged in small vessels of lung and brain. There is a classical symptom free period of about 2 days between the injury and symptoms of fat embolism. It is clinically evident by cerebral disturbance, drowsiness, coma, tachypnea, dyspnea, and petechial rash over the body.[6,7] Chest radiograph may reveal bilateral diffuse air space consolidation in peripheral distribution with normal sized heart. Brain changes are best evident on MRI in the form of bilateral small T2-hyperintense lesions in deep white matter and corpus callosum which may show restricted diffusion.[8]
- *Gas gangrene*: Occurs in open wounds which get infected by *Clostridium perfringens*.

Intermediate Complications

- *Infection*: It occurs in the form of osteomyelitis and is seen in open fractures and those which have undergone operative intervention. Most commonly by *Staphylococcus aureus*. Tibia and femur are the frequently involved bones.
- *Post-traumatic ossification* ***(Fig. 7)***: It is also known as myositis ossificans which is a misnomer as there is no infective lesion of the muscle. It is heterotopic bone formation occurring deep to the muscles. The common sites are elbow and thigh. The new bone formation

occurs in the hematoma beneath the stripped periosteum and the joint capsule. The children are more prone as the periosteum is loosely attached and gets stripped following trauma. On radiograph the classical hallmark is the clearly recognizable pattern of its evolution over a period of 2 months. At the end of 2 months when the lesion is fully formed, the characteristic zonal appearance may be seen. The central part is radiolucent representing immature bone formation. It is surrounded by a dense peripheral zone of ossification. The outermost part of this ossification zone shows definite well-organized cortical bone. A thin lucent zone may separate this cortical layer from the ossific mass. If the ossification reaches up to the bone surface it mimics parosteal osteosarcoma. CT and MRI may help to confirm the diagnosis. Biopsy is conformatory.[9]

- *Sudeck's post-traumatic osteodystrophy*: Also known as reflex sympathetic dystrophy syndrome or post-traumatic painful osteoporosis. The hands or feet are commonly involved. The patient presents about 2 months after injury with extremely painful and tender swollen extremity which hyperemic and glossy with marked stiffness of the small joints. Colles' fracture is the most common cause in upper limb. The radiograph shows diffuse soft-tissue swelling with gradually progressive patchy osteoporosis which is more than that expected by disuse osteoporosis. The bone scan may show diffuse area of increased uptake.
- *Post-traumatic osteolysis*: It refers to dissolution of bone following trauma. Most commonly involves distal end of clavicle and pubic bones.
- *Synostosis*: It may occur between bones which are closely opposed such as radius-ulna and tibia-fibula.

Delayed Complications

- *Abnormal healing process*: These occur secondary to multiple factors including inadequate blood supply, distraction, inadequate immobilization, interposition of soft tissues, infection, and pathological weakness of bone. The term delayed union is used to describe a fracture which does not unite within a reasonable period of time (16–18 weeks) depending on patient's age and the fracture site. Nonunion is diagnosed if the fracture fails to unite. The most common sites are midclavicle, ulna, and tibia. The radiograph shows characteristic features after few months which include rounding of fracture edges, smoothening of margins with sclerosis, gap between the two fragments, demonstration of mobility (on serial stress radiographs or on fluoroscopy), lack of callus formation, and pseudoarthrosis **(Figs. 8A and B)**. Pseudoarthrosis refers to formation of false joint-like cavity with synovial-like capsule between the ends of the two fragments. If formed, a pseudoarthrosis requires refracture and removal for the process of healing. Malunion refers to a union of fracture fragments in an imperfect anatomical position which results in unacceptable deformity. It usually requires surgical correction.
- *Avascular necrosis* ***(Fig. 9)***: It is also known as osteonecrosis. It occurs due to loss of blood supply secondary to fracture. The process may take months to years. The most commonly affected bones are femoral head, scaphoid, humeral head and talus. On radiograph it appears as a sharply defined dense bone in contrast to the surrounding disuse osteoporosis. This progresses to loss of height of the involved part with shrunken, crumpled appearance. Bone scan with ^{99m}Technetium may be helpful. MRI shows the features earliest.

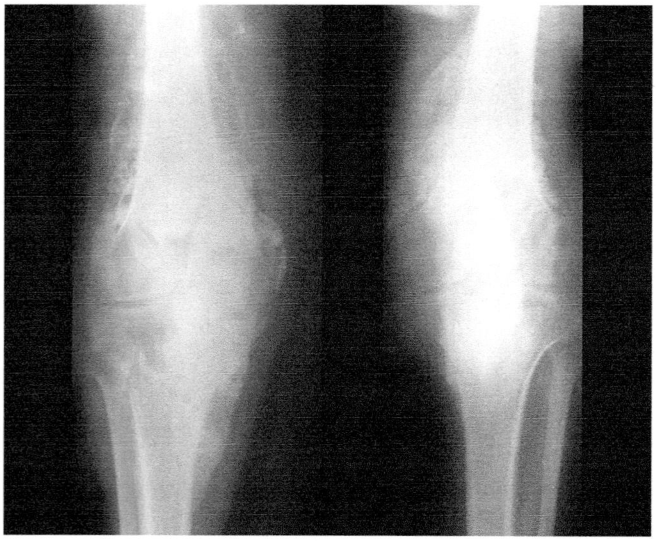

Fig. 7: Anteroposterior radiograph of the bilateral knee joints shows extensive soft tissue ossification around bilateral knee joints suggestive of myositis ossificans.

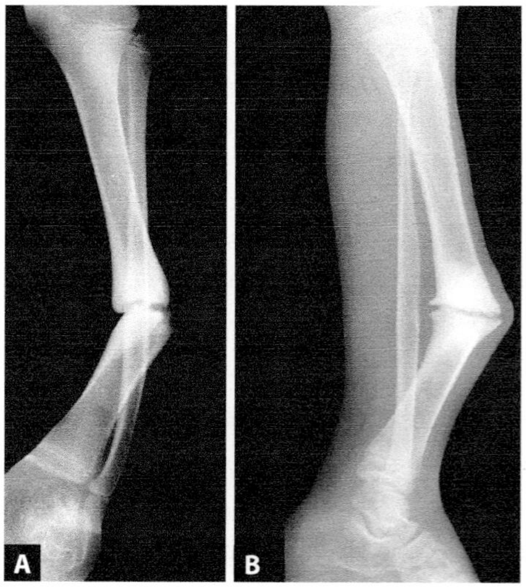

Figs. 8A and B: Anteroposterior and lateral radiographs of the leg. 6 months after trauma shows an old nonunited fracture of the shaft of tibia with rounding of fracture edges, marginal sclerosis, gap between the fracture ends and formation of pseudoarthrosis.

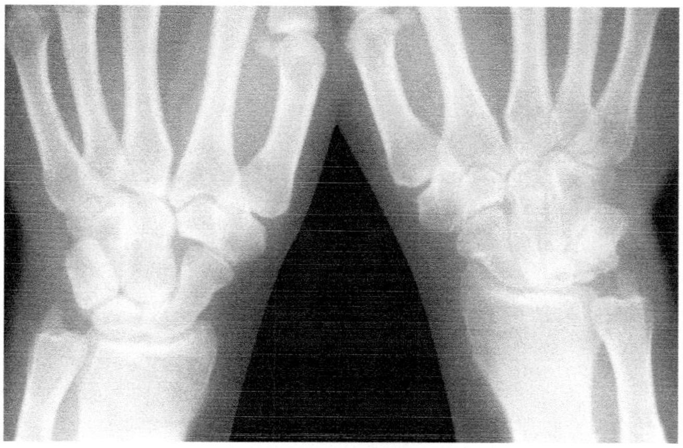

Fig. 9: Posteroanterior radiograph of the bilateral wrist joints. The left lunate is showing an old fracture with marked sclerosis of the bone consistent with avascular necrosis (Kienböck's disease).

- *Disuse osteoporosis*: Mild-to-moderate degree osteoporosis secondary to pain and immobilization.
- *Post-traumatic arthritis*: Degenerative changes in the joint. The predisposing factors include intra-articular fracture, malaligned fracture and avascular necrosis. Seen most commonly in weight bearing joints such as knee, hip and ankle.

IMAGING MODALITIES

Plain radiograph: It is the first-line investigation for any skeletal trauma of the extremities. A minimum of two radiographic projections ideally perpendicular to each other should be acquired to conclusively rule out fracture. Additional views are taken if necessary. The detailed radiographic evaluation has been discussed earlier.

Ultrasonography: It has been shown to have an increasing role in the detection of fractures in the acute setting of trauma as well as monitoring of fracture healing. It is also helpful in joint pathologies for detection of effusion (hemarthrosis), ligaments, and tendinous injuries.

Radioisotope scanning: With ^{99m}Technetium diphosphonate is useful in detection of occult fractures. The scan may take become positive after 24 hours in acute setting. It is also helpful in detection of stress fractures.

Computed tomography: It is markedly superior to radiograph for detection of bony injuries. It is reserved for areas of complex bony anatomy or where the radiographs are equivocal. Multiplanar reformats in all three planes gives a complete overview of the presence and extent of the bony injury along with its relation to surrounding structures. In addition, the soft tissues can also be well evaluated which gives it an added advantage over radiographs. It is commonly used to assess fractures of tibial plateau, ankle, and epiphyseal injuries. In addition it can assess complications such as vascular injury by CT angiography.

Magnetic resonance imaging: It has become the investigation of choice for detailed evaluation of injuries of joints and soft tissues. It has advantages of excellent depiction of soft tissue injuries including those of ligaments, tendons, menisci, and cartilage besides detection of bony injuries by marrow edema. It can detect subtle bone injuries such as occult fractures and bone contusions which may sometimes not be evident on both radiographs and CT. It is also the best modality to detect complications such as avascular necrosis. Use of contrast MR arthrography also enables better depiction of articular and periarticular injuries such as those related to labrum, cartilage, and menisci.

UPPER LIMB TRAUMA

Dislocation of the Shoulder

Glenohumeral joint is the most common joint of the body to dislocate. It is seen usually in adults and elderly. It is classified into subtypes depending upon the direction of displacement of the humeral head into anterior, posterior, superior and inferior direction.

Anterior dislocation: It is the most frequent (95% cases). The humeral head can dislocate anteriorly to lie in subglenoid, subcoracoid, or subclavicular position. The subglenoid dislocation is accompanied by fracture of greater tuberosity whereas subcoracoid dislocation can occur without bony injury and is prone to recurrence **(Fig. 10)**. The Hill-Sachs defect (impaction of the humeral head) and avulsion of the inferior glenoid rim (Bankart's lesion) are often seen especially with recurrent dislocations. Magnetic resonance imaging with MR arthrography is more sensitive in detecting these lesions.[10]

Posterior dislocation: It occurs as a result of violent muscle contraction as in epileptic convulsion or following electric shock.

Inferior dislocation: It is also known as *luxatio erecta*. It occurs secondary to severe hyperabduction trauma with humeral head locked in abduction under the subglenoid position.

Superior dislocation: It is rare. It occurs secondary to considerable force and most commonly occurs secondary to rotator cuff tear.

The radiological evaluation of shoulder dislocation should consist of a true anteroposterior and a transscapular view since it may be missed in the anteroposterior views with internal and external rotation which are routinely done for any shoulder pathology.[11] The AP view can diagnose a shoulder dislocation but the anterior and posterior varieties cannot be differentiated on it.

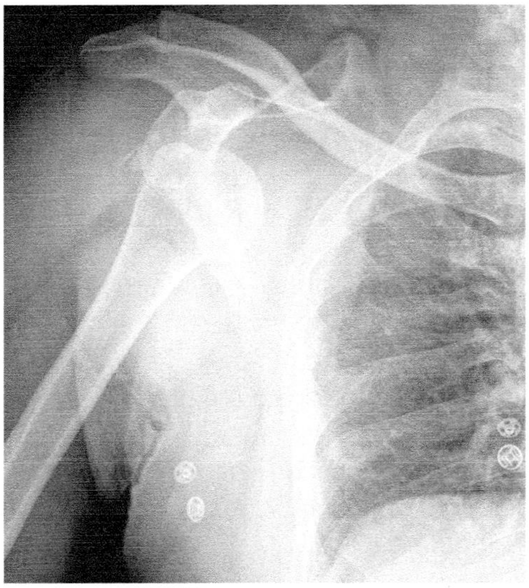

Fig. 10: Anteroposterior radiograph of the right shoulder shows anteroinferior dislocation of the right humerus.

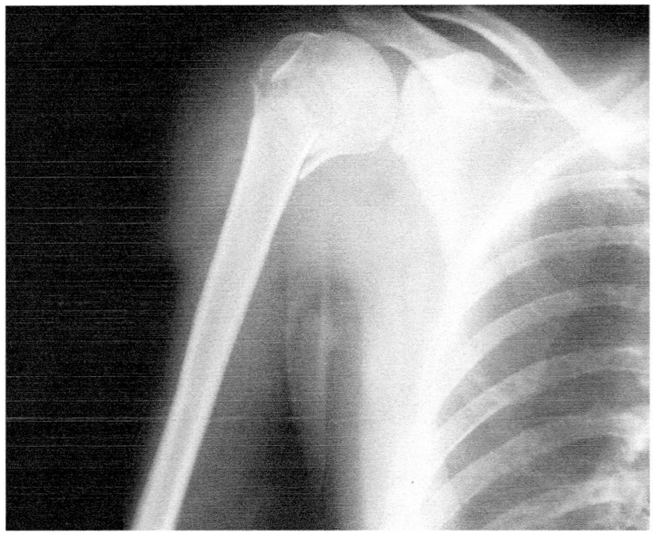

Fig. 11: Anteroposterior radiograph of the right arm shows fracture at the surgical neck of the humerus.

Fracture of the glenoid rim or the greater tuberosity may be seen in this view. Recurrent anterior dislocations would show the Hill-Sachs deformity. In posterior dislocations, on AP radiograph the normal parallelism between the humeral head and the anterior rim of glenoid is absent. The "light bulb" or the "tennis racquet" appearance on the AP view along with widening of the joint space more than 6 mm are clue to diagnosis of posterior dislocation of shoulder. Since the head is fixed in internal rotation, there occurs no change in the appearance of the head on external rotation view.[12]

Fracture of the Neck of Humerus

The frontal AP views of the shoulder with humerus in internal and external rotation are usually sufficient to detect majority of humeral fractures. The fractures of the neck are described by Neer classification[13] which includes four different areas of involvement—the anatomic neck, surgical neck, greater tuberosity, and lesser tuberosity. The total number of fractures and their angulations are taken into account to classify the fractures into four parts—1, 2, 3, and 4. The fragments are considered displaced if there is at least 1 cm of separation or 45° angulation. Most common (80%) are one part fractures. The surgical neck which lies immediately distal to the tuberosities is the most commonly fractured region **(Fig. 11)**. The axillary nerve may be involved by these fractures. It is important to note that an impacted fracture can be easily overlooked in this region. Undisplaced fractures in this region may be managed conservatively. However, significant displacement of the greater or lesser tuberosity is an indication for surgical repair.

Fracture of the Shaft of Humerus

These can involve the proximal, middle, or distal shaft of the humerus. The fracture orientation can be transverse, oblique, or spiral. There can be marked angulation, overlap, or displacement of the fragments. Transverse fracture of the middle shaft is the most common fracture in this region. A fracture in the proximal shaft should be carefully evaluated to look for underlying pathology as metastatic deposits are common in this part of the bone.

Fracture of the Distal Humerus

The fractures of this region are classified according to their relationship with humeral condyles and the shape of the fracture line.

- *Supracondylar fractures*: The fracture line runs superior to the level of condyles. This is seen most commonly in children after fall on outstretched hand. The distal fragment is displaced and angulated posteriorly. The lateral view shows the displacement and the fracture best. Elevation of anterior and posterior fat pads is also indirect signs of underlying fracture. The fracture may be associated with development of Volkmann's ischemic contracture. The brachial artery may also be injured.
- *Intercondylar fractures*: The fracture line runs between the medial and lateral condyles and extends into the supracondylar region to form a "T" or "Y" configuration. This is more commonly seen in adults. If the fracture involves both condyles it is termed transcondylar fracture.
- *Condylar fractures*: Fracture running through either of the lateral or medial humeral condyle. Fracture of the lateral condyle is the second most common

fracture of this region in children and can often result in nonunion. The ulnar nerve may be injured in lateral condyle fractures. If a small fragment gets detached it can lead to loose body within the joint.

- *Epicondylar fractures*: They are avulsion injuries of the epicondyles due to strong pull of the flexor or extensor tendons. The medial epicondyle fractures are seen in sportspersons with throwing action. In children, due to the apophysis being unossified, the fracture may not be radiologically evident.

Dislocation of the Elbow

It is the most common joint to be dislocated in children and third most common in adults (after shoulder and interphalangeal joints).[14] The most common type is posterior or posterolateral dislocation which describes the position of the radius and ulna relative to the humerus **(Figs. 12A and B)**. It is often associated with fractures of the radial head, coronoid process, capitulum, or the medial epicondyle. Post-traumatic ossification can also be seen following posterior dislocations.

The other form of dislocation of the elbow is "pulled elbow." It occurs in young children less than 5 years of age due to traction to the elbow as in lifting the child from the floor by holding the hand. It leads to slippage of the humeral head out of the annular ligament. It leads to immediate crying of the child with forearm held in midpronation. It is not evident radiographically. The treatment involves just simple supination of the forearm.

Fracture of the Head and Neck of Radius

It is the most common injury of the elbow region in young adults and occurs due to fall on outstretched hand. It usually is a hairline fracture oriented vertically involving the articular surface. Since the fracture is often nondisplaced, it is sometimes difficult to visualize on routine AP and lateral views of the elbow. Displacement of anterior and posterior fat pads on the lateral view may aid in the diagnosis. The presence of posterior fat pad is a more reliable and consistent indicator of underlying fracture of the radial head. The radial neck fracture is usually an impacted fracture at its junction with the head. Comminuted fractures of the radial head are often dealt with complete excision of the radial head surgically.

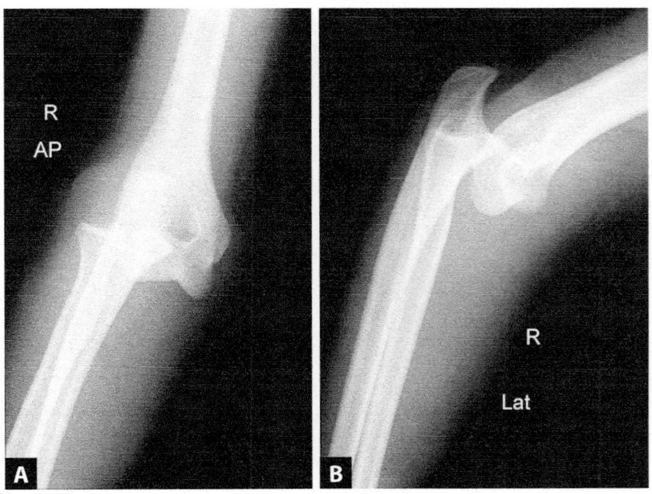

Figs. 12A and B: Anteroposterior and lateral radiographs of the elbow show posterolateral dislocation of the elbow.

Fracture of the Upper End of Ulna

Olecranon fractures are the second most common fractures of this region in adults. They occur after fall on the point of elbow. The fracture line is best visualized on lateral view. The coronoid process may rarely be fractured in association with posterior dislocation of the elbow or by avulsion by brachialis muscle.

Fractures of the Shaft of Radius and Ulna

The radius and ulna can be fractured in isolation but are both fractured in association in a large number of patients when it is called both bones ("B-B") fracture. The fractures of this region are prone to displacement with angulation and rotation and hence often require surgical correction. There are increased chances of compartment syndrome after fractures of this region.

A fracture of the proximal ulnar shaft with dislocation of the radial head is known as *Monteggia fracture-dislocation* **(Figs. 13A and B)**.

An isolated fracture of distal ulnar shaft is termed as *Nightstick* or *Parry fracture*.

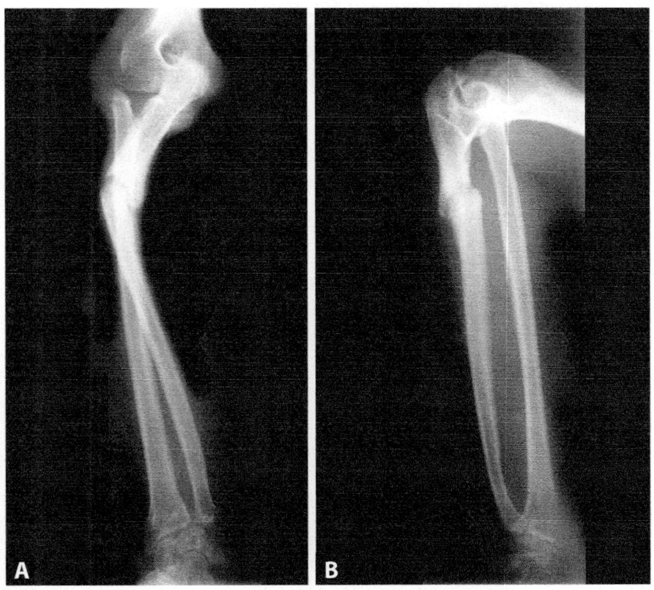

Figs. 13A and B: Anteroposterior and lateral radiographs of the forearm show an old nonunited fracture of the upper shaft of ulna with dislocation of the radial head consistent with *Monteggia fracture-dislocation*.

A fracture of the distal shaft of radius at the junction of middle and distal third with dislocation of the distal radio-ulnar joint is termed as *Galeazzi* or *"reversed" Monteggia fracture*.

Fractures of the Distal End of Radius

Fractures of the distal part of radius are common injuries of adulthood especially in females.[15]

A fracture of the distal end of radius with posterior angulation of the distal fragment is termed as *Colles' fracture* **(Figs. 14A and B)**. The fracture line is seen around 2–3 cm proximal to the articular surface of the radius. The distal fragment is tilted dorsally so that on lateral view it gives rise to classical "dinner-fork" deformity. A fracture of ulnar styloid process is associated in 60% of cases. Complications include malunion and Sudeck's post-traumatic osteodystrophy.

A fracture of the distal radius with anterior angulation of the distal fragment is termed as *Smith's fracture* or *Reversed Colles' fracture.*

A fracture of the posterior rim of the distal radial articular surface with associated proximal dislocation of the carpus is termed *Barton's fracture.* The involvement of volar radial rim is termed *Reverse Barton's fracture.*

Fracture of the radial styloid process is termed *Chauffeur's fracture.*

A fracture through the distal radial epiphysis is common in children. The epiphysis gets slipped posteriorly and is usually associated with a small metaphyseal fracture making it a Type 2 Salter Harris injury. This is equivalent to a *Colles' fracture* of adult.

Fractures of the Carpal Bones

Scaphoid is the most common carpal bone to be fractured. It is usually seen in adults with fall on outstretched hand. Clinically, there is tenderness in the anatomical snuffbox. The standard views to detect a scaphoid fracture include PA, lateral, external oblique, and a PA view with ulnar deviation.[16] About 70% of fractures involve the waist of scaphoid followed by proximal and distal poles **(Figs. 15A and B)**. Nondisplaced fractures are difficult to identify. If there is high clinical suspicion but no fracture line is visible on initial radiograph, then precautionary immobilization is done and the radiograph is repeated after 2 weeks. The fracture line may be better evident by this time. A bone scan may detect the fracture earlier. Fractures through the waist or proximal to it make the proximal part of scaphoid prone to avascular necrosis as the nutrient artery enters the bone through the distal part of the waist. The chances of avascular necrosis increase with more proximal fracture line. The avascular part is seen as more dense compared to the rest of the bone and the other surrounding bones. The scaphoid fractures are also more prone to nonunion.

Triquetrum is the second most common carpal bone to be fractured. An avulsion fracture at the site of attachment of the radiocarpal ligament is termed *Fischer's fracture.* It is identified on lateral radiograph of the wrist.

Lunate fractures are uncommon. *Kienböck's disease* is avascular necrosis of the lunate which may be secondary to a fracture **(Fig. 9)**.

Dislocation of the Wrist

Dislocations affecting the wrist are mainly of two types:

1. Single carpal dislocations
2. Multiple carpal dislocations.[17]

Single Carpal Dislocations

Lunate dislocation is the most common of all carpal bones. The lunate displaces anteriorly with forward tilt so that the concave lower articular surface faces anteriorly. This is best seen on the lateral view.

The scaphoid is the second most common bone to subluxate. It usually undergoes rotatory subluxation so

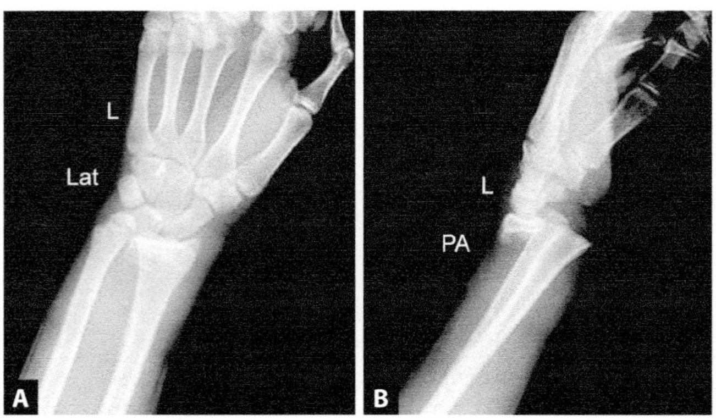

Figs. 14A and B: Posteroanterior and lateral radiographs of the hand show Colles' fracture of the radius.

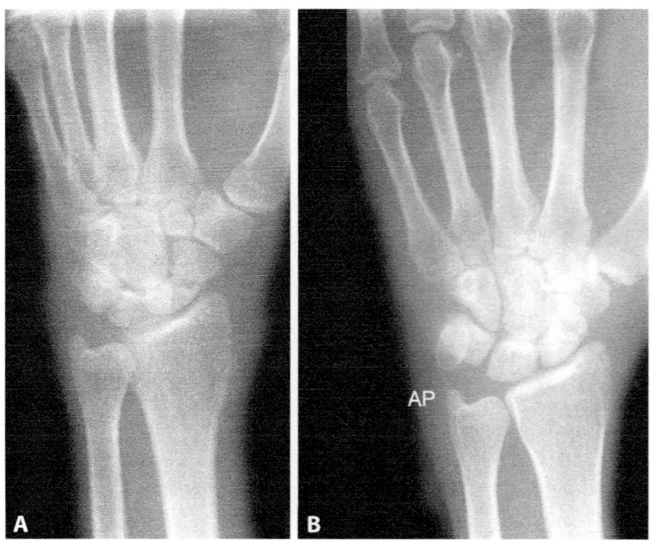

Figs. 15A and B: Posteroanterior and oblique radiographs of the wrist joint show a fracture through the waist of scaphoid bone.

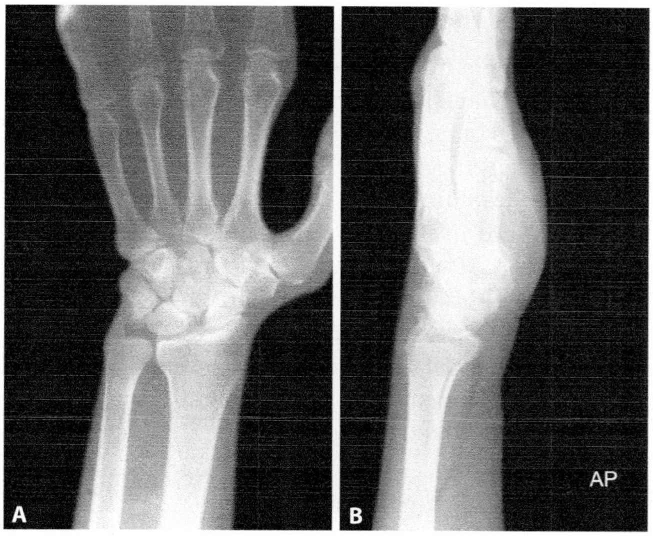

Figs. 16A and B: Posteroanterior and lateral radiographs of the wrist show scapholunate dislocation with increased distance between the scaphoid and lunate (*Terry Thomas sign*) and signet ring appearance of the scaphoid.

that it rotates anteriorly and moves laterally to cause scapholunate dissociation. The distance between the scaphoid and lunate on AP view is increased to more than 4 mm (known as *Terry Thomas sign*). In addition the scaphoid appears small and circular in shape (*signet ring sign*) **(Figs. 16A and B)**.

Multiple Carpal Dislocations

The most common in perilunate dislocation where the lunate bone maintains its spatial relationship with the radius but rest of all the carpal bones get dislocated dorsally. It is best visualized on lateral view. This type of dislocation may be associated with fracture of the scaphoid.

Fractures and Dislocations of the Hand

Posteroanterior, lateral, and oblique projections are the most commonly used views to image injuries of this region. Collimated views may be required if a single digit is to be evaluated.

Among the metacarpals, the first metacarpal base is most commonly injured. An oblique intra-articular fracture through the base of first metacarpal with dorsal and radial displacement of the shaft is known as *Bennet's fracture.* A comminuted Bennet's fracture is termed *Ronaldo's fracture.* A transverse fracture of the neck of the fifth metacarpal with volar angulation of the distal fragment is termed *Boxer's fracture.*

Fractures of the phalanges are more common than metacarpal fractures. An avulsion chip fracture at the base of distal phalanx at the insertion of extensor tendon leads to *Mallet finger* with the finger fixed in moderate flexion and cannot be extended.

LOWER LIMB TRAUMA

Dislocations of the Hip

The dislocations of the hip are classified as posterior and anteriors dislocations.[18]

Posterior Dislocation

It is the most common type accounting for approximately 80% of hip dislocations. It occurs when there is a blow to the knee with hip in flexed position. The femoral head displaces posteriorly to lie outside the acetabulum on its lateral and superior aspect. This often produces a fracture of the posterior acetabular rim with rarely a small fracture of the anterior femoral head. These fractures are best seen on CT scan. The sciatic nerve may also be injured. Clinically, there is medial rotation of the leg with limb shortening.

Anterior Dislocation

It accounts for about 15% of hip dislocations and is caused by forced abduction and extension of the femur. Clinically the limb is seen to lie in abduction. The head may be dislocated anteriorly and superiorly (subspinous or iliac type) with the femur extended and abducted or the head may get dislocated anteriorly and inferiorly (obturator type) with the femur abducted and externally rotated. The acetabulum usually does not show any fracture.[19]

Fractures of the Proximal Femur

Fracture of the neck of femur is a common injury seen in elderly especially in females with underlying osteoporosis.[20] Complications include avascular necrosis, osteoarthritis, and nonunion. AP view of pelvis, coned AP view of ipsilateral hip, and horizontal beam lateral view are the usual radiographs for detection. The fractures of this region are classified into intracapsular and extracapsular types depending upon the relationship of the fracture line to the joint capsule.

Intracapsular Fractures

The intracapsular fractures include all fractures above the level of trochanters. They account for about 60% of all proximal femoral fractures. The intracapsular fractures are more prone to undergo nonunion and avascular necrosis.

Subcapital fracture occurs at the junction of head with neck and is the most common type of intracapsular fracture. These fractures may be impacted without displacement or may show variable degrees of displacement.

Midcervical fracture at the middle part of the neck and basicervical fractures just above the level of trochanters are the other types of intracapsular fractures. These regions may be more commonly fractured with underlying pathological lesion.

Extracapsular Fractures

These include all fractures at or below the level of the trochanters.

The intertrochanteric fractures constitute of a fracture line running obliquely to involve both the trochanters **(Fig. 17)**. These fractures are generally comminuted. These fractures unite easily without significant complications.

The trochanteric fractures involve avulsion injuries of the greater or the lesser trochanter.

Subtrochanteric fractures occur below the level of the trochanters or may be seen as an extension of intertrochanteric fractures. It is usually seen in younger patients with significant trauma or superimposed over pathological bone in elderly.

Fractures of the Shaft of Femur

These occur at all ages and are a result of severe violence. The fracture orientation may be spiral, oblique, or transverse. The fractures may be associated with significant soft tissue hemorrhage. The femoral artery may commonly get injured most commonly at the level of the adductor canal. Radiograph should always include both the proximal hip and the distal knee joint because of high incidence of ipsilateral associated injuries.

The supracondylar fracture of the femur produces posterior angulation and displacement of the distal fragment due to the pull of the gastrocnemius muscle.

The condylar fractures often involve the articular surface and need to be corrected to prevent delayed osteoarthritis. The condyles may be injured in isolation or there may be extension of a supracondylar fracture into the intercondylar area with a "T" or "Y" configuration. Injury of the popliteal artery must be looked for with these fractures.

Fractures of the Patella

The patella gets fractured either by direct trauma or by indirect mechanism of strong quadriceps contraction. Direct trauma often leads to a comminuted fracture while the quadriceps mechanism usually results in a transverse or oblique fracture **(Figs. 18A and B)**. The transverse fracture line is at the mid part. These fractures at best visualized on AP and lateral view except a rare vertical fracture which may be seen only on the sunrise or the skyline view. A superolateral accessory ossification center in a bipartite patella may simulate an acute fracture but can be differentiated by its typical location, well-defined sclerotic margins, and being bilateral.

Dislocation of the Patella

The patella most commonly dislocates laterally. It may occur secondary to a sudden change in direction while dancing or running or may occur following direct trauma. The dislocation is usually transient and gets reduced easily. The patella may rarely get dislocated in vertical direction with locking in the intercondylar notch or in horizontal direction with inversion and locking of superior pole of patella in the knee joint.

The dislocations may be associated with an osteochondral fragment on the medial facet of the patella or the lateral femoral condyle. CT scan may be required for the diagnosis as the fragment needs to be removed to prevent future occurrence of osteoarthritis.

Fractures of the Proximal Tibia

Fracture of the lateral tibial plateau is much more common than that of the medial tibial plateau **(Figs. 19A and B)**. It is also known as bumper fracture as is commonly seen in

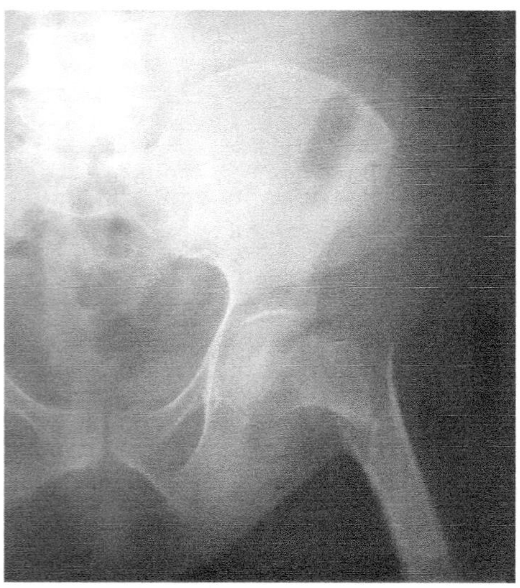

Fig. 17: Anteroposterior radiograph of the left hip joint shows an intertrochanteric fracture of the left femur.

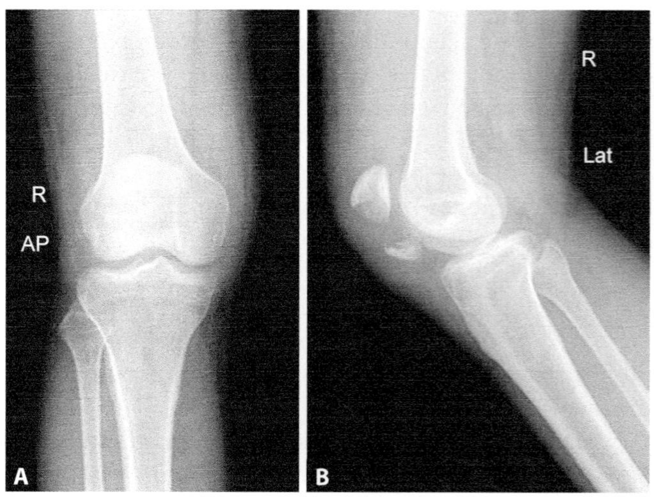

Figs. 18A and B: Anteroposterior and lateral radiographs of the knee joint show a fracture through the mid part of patella with separation of the fracture fragments due to associated muscle pull.

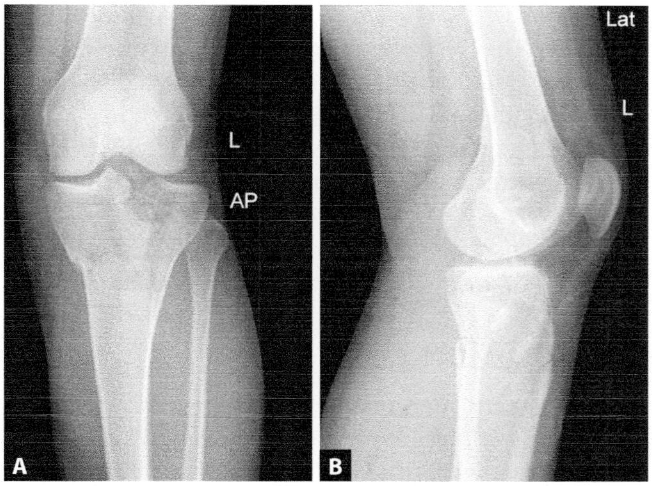

Figs. 19A and B: Anteroposterior and lateral radiographs of the knee joint show fracture of the lateral tibial plateau extending into the proximal metaphysis.

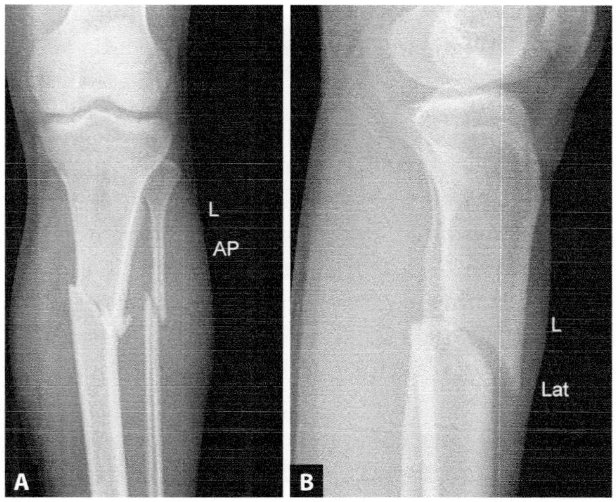

Figs. 20A and B: Anteroposterior and lateral radiographs of the proximal leg show fractures of upper shafts of both tibia and fibula.

car accidents but this mechanism constitutes only 25% of etiology.[21] It may be more commonly seen in various other injury mechanisms including vertical compression and twisting. The common classification followed is the Hohl classification:[22] Type 1 is a vertical split of the joint margin, Type 2 is a compression of lateral plateau by impaction of lateral femoral condyle, Type 3 is a split peripheral vertical fracture with compression of the medial articular surface of the lateral tibial plateau, Type 4 is fracture of medial tibial plateau, and Type 5 is bicondylar fracture with "Y" or "T" configuration.

These fractures may be associated with ligament injuries. Hence, on radiograph it is important to look for avulsion fractures at the site of ligamentous attachments. Lipohemarthrosis may be seen in tibial plateau fractures and is identified on horizontal beam lateral radiograph. CT scan and MRI are often indicated to look for the exact extent of the fracture and the associated ligamentous injuries.

An avulsion fracture of the lateral tibial plateau at the site of attachment of the iliotibial tract is termed as *Segond fracture*. It is commonly associated with injuries of the anterior cruciate ligament and meniscal injuries.

Fractures of the anterior and posterior tibial spine (intercondylar eminence) usually result from avulsion injuries at the origin of anterior and posterior cruciate ligaments.

Fractures of the Shaft of Tibia and Fibula

Fractures of shaft of the tibia are often associated with fractures of fibula **(Figs. 20A and B)**. The fibular fracture is commonly at upper- and middle-third region whereas the tibial fractures are usually at middle and lower-third region. Hence, it is important to image the complete length of both bones in the radiograph so as to avoid missing associated fracture. The fractures of this region are prone to development of compartment syndrome.

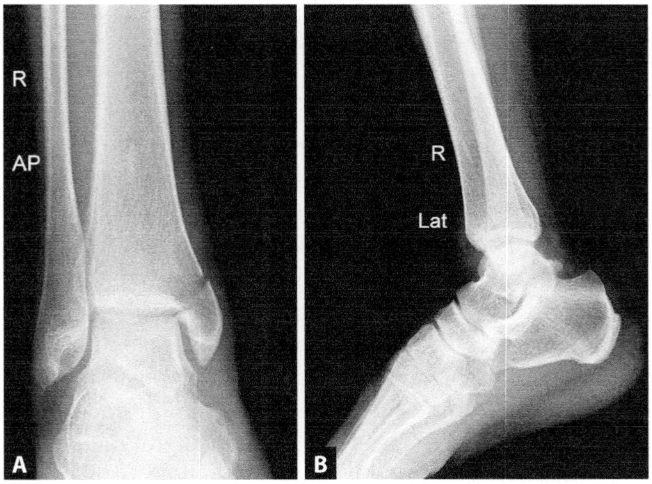

Figs. 21A and B: Anteroposterior and lateral radiographs of the ankle joint show a transverse fracture of the medial malleolus.

An undisplaced spiral fracture in a child around 2 years of age is called as toddler's fracture.

Midshaft of the tibia along with proximal tibial metaphysis, fibular shaft, and femoral neck are the common sites for stress fractures. They are seen in athletic individuals or those involved in strenuous running. Clinically, it presents with pain during activity with relief on rest.

Fractures of the Distal Tibia and Fibula

Fractures of the medial and lateral malleoli occur due to adduction and abduction injuries. The medial malleolus fractures are generally transverse or oblique whereas those of the lateral malleolus are usually spiral **(Figs. 21A and B)**. There may also be avulsion injuries at the malleoli.

The distal tibiofibular joint may also show diastasis associated with the malleolar fractures.

Fractures of the Talus

Fractures of the talus are second only to the calcaneus as a site of injury in the ankle region. Most common injuries are the avulsion fractures. It occurs at the anterosuperior part of the talar neck at the site of attachment of the joint capsule. The other common type of fracture is the vertical fracture of the talar neck occurring in an automobile accident. Such fractures are often complicated by avascular necrosis of the proximal part of talus. The likelihood of developing avascular necrosis increases with more anterior neck fracture. The talar dome is also a common site for development of osteochondral fractures.[23] These occur in typical location of middle third of lateral margin or posterior third of the medial margin of talar dome. If there is doubt in detection of osteochondral fractures on plain radiograph, CT scan can be done which clearly shows the fracture line.

Fractures of the Calcaneum

The calcaneus is the most frequent tarsal bone to get injured. About 75% of the fractures are intra-articular with involvement of the subtalar joint and the rest 25% are extra-articular.[24,25] The intra-articular fractures are most commonly caused by fall from height and are compression fractures. They are often bilateral (10%) and/or associated with fractures of the thoracolumbar spine. These fractures usually have associated depression of the posterior facet of the subtalar joint. The subtle compression fractures of the calcaneum can be best detected on lateral radiograph of ankle by measuring the Böhler's angle. It is the angle between a line joining the superior most part of anterior process of calcaneum to the superior point of posterior facet and a line joining the superior point of posterior facet to posterosuperior margin of calcaneum tuberosity. Normally the angle between these two lines ranges from 28° to 40°. A Böhler's angle of less than 28° represents a depression of the calcaneus and hence a fracture. The extra-articular fractures are mainly avulsion injuries and may involve the anterior process (most common), superior aspect of tuberosity, plantar aspect of tuberosity, or the sustentaculum tali. The extra-articular fractures are usually managed conservatively whereas significant involvement of articular surface of subtalar joint is an indication for operative repair.[26,27]

Dislocations of the Foot

The talus is the most common foot bone to dislocate. The dislocation may involve the talotibial, talocalcaneal (subtalar), and the talonavicular joints.

Lisfranc's dislocation is a dislocation at tarsometatarsal junction. The second, third, and fourth metatarsals dislocate laterally, with or without associated fractures. Fracture of the base of second metatarsal is characteristic. The first metatarsal may dislocate laterally with other metatarsals (homolateral type) or may deviate medially (divergent type).

Chopart's dislocation is medial dislocation of the talonavicular and calcaneocuboid joints of the foot.

CONCLUSION

For an accurate interpretation of a radiograph of skeletal trauma, it is important for the radiologist to be aware of the clinical details including the time interval from injury and mechanism of injury. The traumatized region should always be imaged in at least two different planes with inclusion of both the proximal and distal joints to the injured bone. A knowledge of the common injuries, their radiographic manifestations, the special radiographic views for that region if any, the pitfalls in diagnosis and the associated injuries is paramount for the radiologist. It is important not to miss an injury not only because of the treatment implications but also because many of these are medicolegal cases in which the radiograph forms part of concrete irrefutable radiological evidence. Comparative evaluation with the contralateral normal limb may be required especially in children. The use of other imaging modalities including ultrasound, CT, MRI, and scintigraphy may be indicated in specific situations as and when indicated. The radiologist also has a role in the detection of post-traumatic early and delayed complications during the follow-up of the patient.

REFERENCES

1. Felson B. Roentgenology of Fractures and Dislocations. New York: Grune and Stratton; 1978.
2. Rogers LF. Radiology of Skeletal Trauma, Vols 1 and 2, 3rd edition. Philadelphia PA: Churchill Livingstone; 2002.
3. Dalinka MK. Imaging of skeletal trauma. In: Hodler J, Zollikofer CL, Von Schulthess GK (Eds). Musculoskeletal Diseases 2009–2012. Milano: Springer; 2009.
4. Salter RB, Harris WR. Injuries involving the epiphyseal plate. J Bone Joint Surg. 1963;45:587.
5. Cruess RL, Dumont J. Current concepts, fracture healing. Can J Surg. 1975;18:403.
6. Hulth A. Current concepts in fracture healing. Clin Orthopaed. 1989;249:265.
7. Bulger EM, Smith DG, Maier RV, Jurkovich GJ. Fat embolism syndrome: a 10-year review. Arch Surg. 1997;132:435-9.
8. Shaikh N, Parchani A, Bhat V, Kattren MA. Fat embolism syndrome: clinical and imaging considerations: Case report and review of literature. Indian J Crit Care Med. 2008;12:32-6.

9. Gupta B, Kaur M, D'souza N, Dey CK, Shende S, Kumar A, et al. Cerebral fat embolism: a diagnostic challenge. Saudi J Anaesth. 2011;5(3):348-52.
10. Bashir WA, Aziz A, Jidaal I. Imaging of skeletal extremity trauma: a review. Trauma. 2014;16(4):300-17.
11. Nuovo MA, Norman A, Chumas J, Ackerman LV. Myositis ossificans with atypical clinical, radiographic, or pathologic findings: a review of 23 cases. Skeletal Radiol. 1992;21:87-101.
12. Workman TL, Burkhard TK, Resnick D, Goff WB 2nd, Balsara ZN, Davis DJ, et al. Hill Sach lesion: comparison of detection with MR imaging, radiography and arthroscopy. Radiology. 1992;185:847.
13. Pavlov H, Freiberger RH. Fractures and dislocations about the shoulder. Semin Roentgenol. 1978;13:85-91.
14. Kerr R. Diagnostic imaging of upper extremity trauma. Radiol Clin North Am. 1989;27(5):891-908.
15. Neer CS II. Displaced proximal humeral fractures. Part 1-classification and evaluation. J Bone Joint Surg (Am). 1970;52:1077.
16. Linscheid RL, Wheeler DK. Elbow dislocations. JAMA. 1965;194:1171.
17. Goldfarb CA, Yin Y, Gilula LA, Fisher AJ, Boyer MI. Wrist fractures: What the clinician wants to know. Radiology. 2001;219:11-28.
18. Munk PL, Lee MJ, Logan PM, Connell DG, Janzen DL, Poon PY, et al. Scaphoid bone waist fractures, acute and chronic: Imaging with different techniques. Am J Roentgenol. 1997;168:779-86.
19. Fisher MR, Rogers LF, Hendrix RW. A systematic approach to the diagnosis of carpometacarpal dislocations. Radiographics. 1982;2:612-27.
20. Newberg AH, Greenstein R. Radiographic evaluation of tibial plateau fracture. Radiology. 1978;126:319.
21. Epstein HC. Traumatic dislocations of the hip. Clin Orthop. 1973;92:116.
22. Erb RE, Steele JR, Nance EP Jr, Edwards JR. Traumatic anterior dislocation of the hip: spectrum of plain film and CT findings. Am J Roentgenol. 1995;165:1215-9.
23. Hohl M. Tibial condylar fractures. J Bone Joint Surg (Am). 1967;49:1455.
24. David S. Textbook of Radiology and Imaging, 7th edition. London: Churchill Livingstone; 2003. pp. 1371-416.
25. Canale ST, Belding RH. Osteochondral lesions of the talus. J Bone Joint Surg (Am). 1980;62A:97-102.
26. Greenspan A. Imaging of the foot and ankle. Curr Opin Orthop. 1996;7:61-8.
27. Karasick D. Fractures and dislocations of the foot. Semin Roentgen. 1994;24:152.

CHAPTER 22

Imaging of Soft Tissue Tumors

Ashu Seith Bhalla, Ankur Goyal, Priyanka Naranje

INTRODUCTION

Soft tissue tumors (STTs) encompass a wide spectrum of entities. Patients often present with nonspecific clinical findings, such as an ill-defined soft tissue swelling or a discrete palpable mass, with or without accompanying tenderness or pain. With equivocal clinical findings, imaging can confirm the presence of a soft tissue mass or identify a suspected "mass" as normal tissue. The objectives of initial imaging evaluation are detecting the suspected lesion, establishing a diagnosis or formulating a differential diagnosis and radiological staging (if the lesion is neoplastic). The evaluation of STTs has undergone dramatic evolution with advances in magnetic resonance imaging (MRI). Soft tissue sarcoma (STS) is a broad term used for tumors of mesenchymal origin and encompasses the various subtypes described in the classification below. While these constitute <1% of malignancies encountered in the adults, the incidence is more in children which is approximately 12%.[1]

CLASSIFICATION

The classification currently followed for STTs is the 4th edition of the WHO classification (2013).[2] This system is based not only on the histopathological features but also clinical behavior and molecular and genetic features.[3] The broad categories of STT according to WHO classification are illustrated in **Flowcharts 1 and 2**. Further two of these groups also include tumors of uncertain differentiation and undifferentiated sarcomas (or unclassified).

The WHO classification is based on the tissue that the tumor morphology is similar to (e.g., smooth muscle/skeletal muscle) and not necessarily the one that it arises from. Apart from histopathology, immune histochemistry (IHC) and molecular techniques (for genetics) govern the diagnosis.

Immune Histochemistry

Some important IHC markers are summarized in **Table 1**.

Molecular Studies

Common methods employed for detecting genetic mutations include FISH (fluorescence in situ hybridization) and RT-PCR (reverse transcriptase polymerase chain reaction). Affected chromosomes include EWSR1 with various translocations of the gene described in Ewing's sarcoma, clear cell sarcoma, among others.[4]

Each of the groups of classification includes numerous entities. This chapter focuses on common lesions and/or those with characteristic imaging appearances.

Flowchart 1: Groups of soft tissue tumors (STTs) according to the WHO classification.

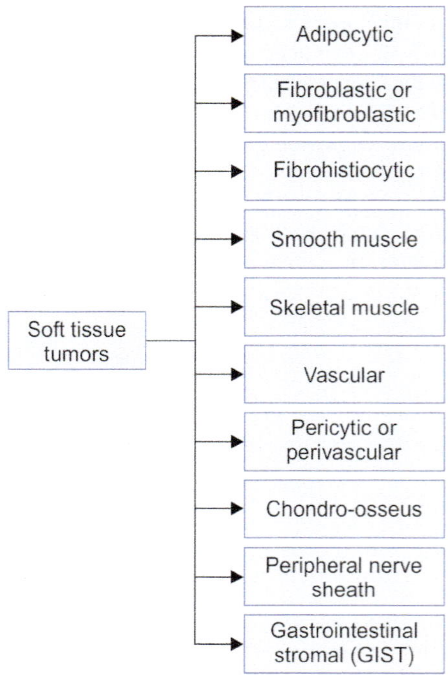

Flowchart 2: The WHO classification based on biological behavior (applies to each category).

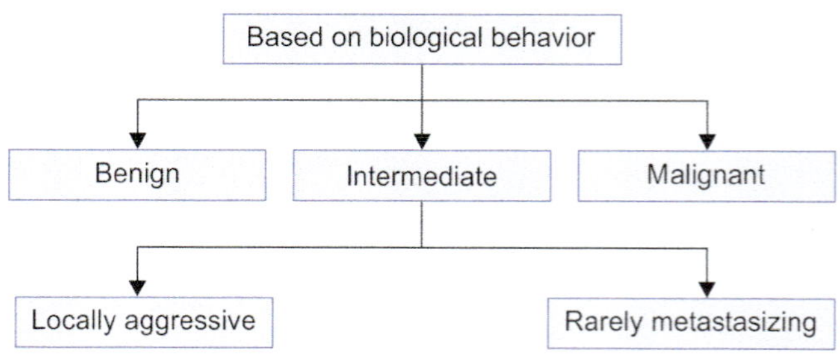

Table 1: Important immune histochemistry markers.

Desmin	*S-100*	*Cytokeratin*
Myogenic differentiation • Rhabdomyosarcoma • Leiomyosarcoma	• Nerve sheath tumors • Ossifying fibromyxoid tumor	*Rare* • Synovial sarcoma • Epitheloid sarcoma • Absent in fibrosarcoma

ADIPOCYTIC TUMORS

This group forms the most frequently encountered STTs. Classification of these tumors is shown in **Table 2**.

Lipoma

Majority of adipocytic tumors are benign and lipoma is the most common.[5] Numerous chromosomal aberrations have been reported in these tumors with HMGA2 protein truncation being one of the effects.[6] Typical patient profile is that of an overweight, middle aged person; though these are encountered at any age including children. Most of these tumors do not cause pain unless they compress nerves. The classical lipoma on imaging displays an appearance of homogeneous fatty lesion similar to subcutaneous fat **(Figs. 1A to F)**. Fine septae may be present. Many categories of lipomas are often discussed.[7]

Based on location: Superficial or deep, with the division based on the fascia covering the muscles. In the deep lipomas, parosteal or intramuscular forms are known. Lipoma arborescens occurs in relation to synovial lining of a joint.

Based on capsule: Lipomas may have a capsule (encapsulated). Those without capsule can appear infiltrative with infiltrative intramuscular lipoma being one form. These can be challenging to differentiate from liposarcomas (LPSs).

Based on content: Lipomas may have a mixed histology with other components such as bone or cartilage.

Lipoblastoma

Lipoblastoma is a rare tumor encountered typically in infants or early childhood (less than 3 years). It is mostly painless; however, nerve compression can result in pain or even Horner's syndrome (in cervicothoracic tumors) or even thoracic cage compression in case of large tumors. Appendicular location is commoner than trunk or head and neck.

Unlike lipoma, the tumor is composed of immature fatty tissue, which on MRI shows less hyperintensity (on T1WI) compared to mature fat. Also, there may be components of myxoid or fibrous tissues found within, further giving it a heterogeneous appearance. The tumor is known to regress spontaneously or mature into a lipoma, as the child grows. Hence, this should be kept in mind when a decision regarding surgery or conservative approach is taken. On imaging and even histology, the lesion resembles an LPS **(Figs. 2A to C)**; however, the typical age of presentation aids in the distinction. A diffuse, infiltrative form of the neoplasm is referred to as "lipoblastomastosis."[8]

Other Benign Tumors

Other benign adipocytic tumors mostly include entities, which have elements of other tissues and include:

- *Angiolipoma*: Mature fatty tissue with small vessels. Small subcutaneous lesions, often multiple **(Figs. 1A to F)**.
- *Myolipoma*: Mature fat plus mature smooth muscles. Deep location is more frequent.
- *Chondroid lipoma*: Chondroid or myxoid matrix with mature fat.
- *Spindle cell lipoma (SCL)*: Synonym pleomorphic lipoma, more frequent in men.
- *Lipomatosis of nerve (LN)*: Synonym fibrolipomatous hamartoma. The most common location of this lesion is the wrist, occurring in relation to median nerve/ branches.
- *Lipomatosis*: These lesions involve proliferation of mature adipose tissue in various locations (often deep) in an infiltrative manner **(Figs. 3A to D)**. These can be part of spectrum of "overgrowth syndromes" when involving an extremity.
- *Hibernoma*: Neoplasm of brown fat which is seen in neck or back and can resemble LPS on imaging.

Liposarcoma

The classification of LPS group of tumors is shown in **Flowchart 3**.

Intermediate well-differentiated liposarcoma/atypical lipomatous tumor: The tumors of this grade can be locally aggressive, have a higher recurrence rate but do not metastasize, unless they evolve into a high-grade sarcoma which is seen up to 17% of those in the retroperitoneum (RP).[9]

On imaging, while the predominant component of the mass remains fatty (as in lipomas), there is presence of thick septations (>2 mm) which may be nodular, with or without nonfatty components appearing as soft tissue attenuation (<2 cm) **(Figs. 4 and 5)**. Calcifications can be

Table 2: Classification of adipocytic tumors.

Benign	*Intermediate (locally aggressive)*	*Malignant*
• Lipoma • Lipomatosis • Lipoblastoma • Angiolipoma	• Atypical lipomatous tumor • Well-differentiated liposarcoma	Liposarcoma • Dedifferentiated • Myxoid • Pleomorphic • NOS

(NOS: not otherwise specified).

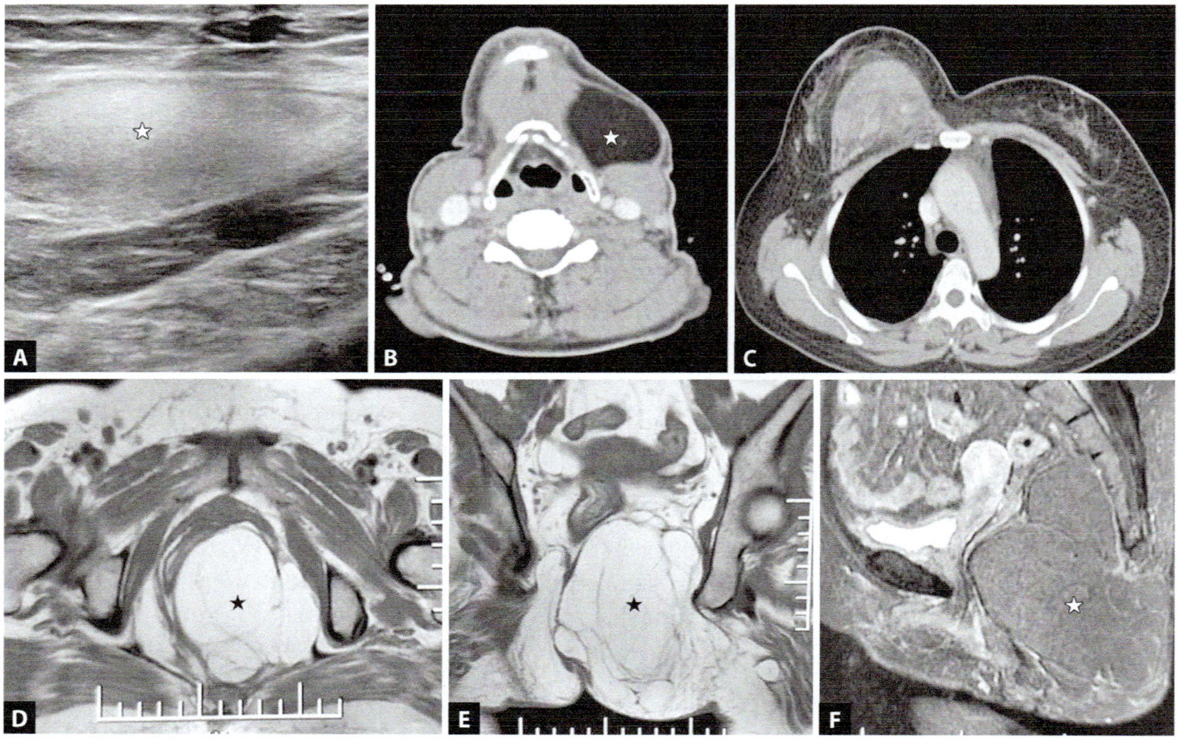

Figs. 1A to F: Lipomas. (A) Ultrasound image shows homogeneously echogenic lesion (asterisk) in the gluteal subcutaneous location, suggestive of lipoma; (B) Axial computed tomography (CT) image shows homogeneous fat-attenuation lesion (asterisk) anterior to left sternocleidomastoid; (C) Axial CT image shows heterogeneous lesion in RT chest wall (retromammary location) with mixed soft tissue and fat attenuation with prominent vessels. Histology revealed angiolipoma; (D) Axial; and (E) Coronal T1-weighted (T1W) magnetic resonance (MR) images show fat signal intensity hyperintense lesion (asterisks) in left ischiorectal fossa with thin septations, suggestive of lipoma; (F) There is complete suppression of lesion signal on fat-suppressed image.

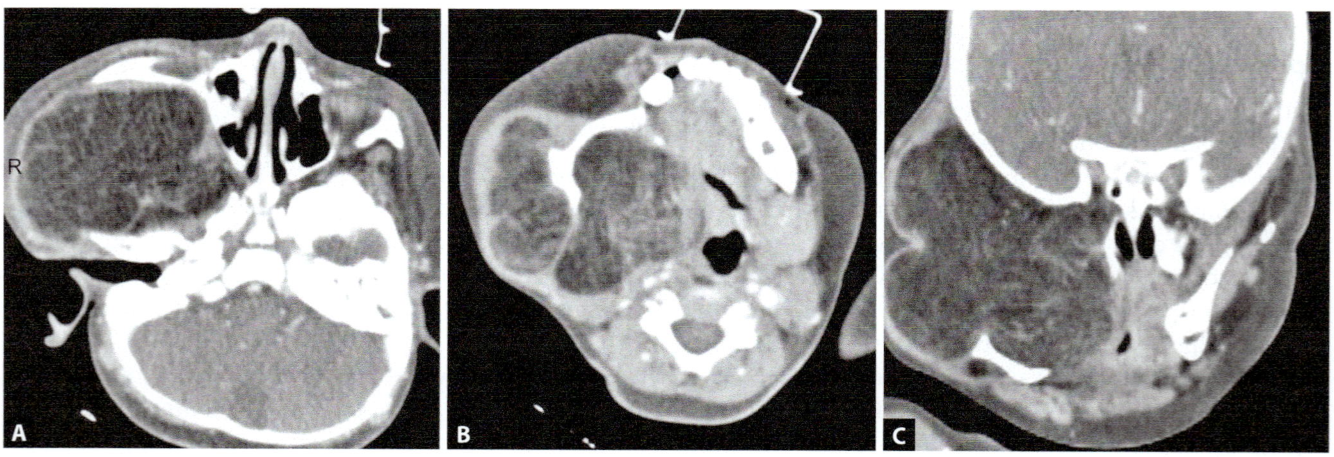

Figs. 2A to C: Lipoblastoma. (A and B) Axial; and (C) Coronal contrast-enhanced computed tomography (CECT) images in an infant show fat attenuation infiltrative lesion in RT face and infratemporal fossa with septations within, suggesting the diagnosis of lipoblastoma.

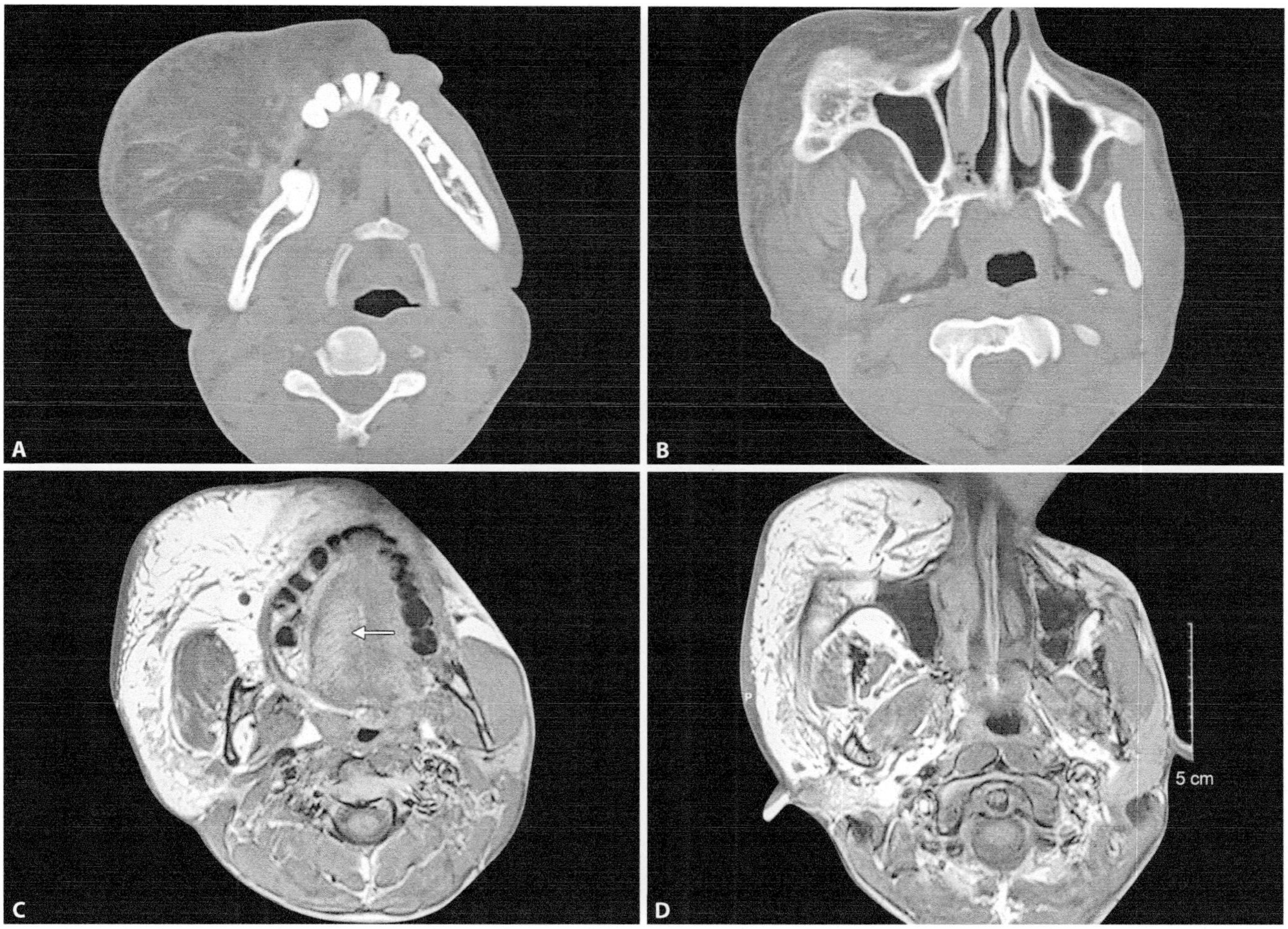

Figs. 3A to D: Lipomatosis. (A and B) Axial computed tomography (CT) images show diffuse fatty hypertrophy involving the right side of face, predominantly in subcutaneous region but also involving mastication muscles and parotid. There is bony overgrowth of the maxilla as well; (C and D) T1-weighted (T1W) magnetic resonance (MR) images better show hyperintense fat signal intensity. The right part of tongue also shows lipomatosis (arrow).

Flowchart 3: Classification of liposarcoma.

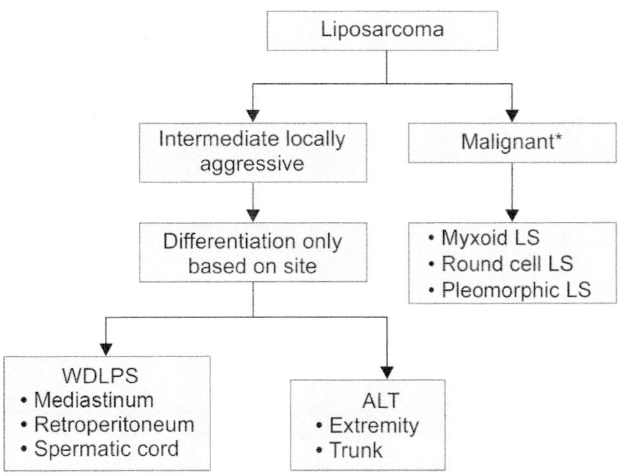

(WDLPS: well-differentiated liposarcomas; ALT: atypical lipomatous tumor; LS: liposarcoma)

*Among these, pure myxoid LPSs are low-grade sarcomas, others are high grade.

seen in up to one-third of the masses on CT. Further most fatty lesions in RP or mediastinum are well-differentiated liposarcoma (WDLPS) rather than a benign lipoma. Management is surgical, i.e., wide local excision (WLE).

Well-differentiated liposarcoma and atypical lipomatous tumor (ALT) are similar on histology and molecular markers (positive for MDM 2, HMGA2, CDK4); the only differentiation being based on site. ALT refers to tumors in extremity and trunk which are easier to resect **(Figs. 4A to D)**; WDPLS are lesions in mediastinum/ RP wherein complete resection is challenging due to involvement of vital structures, and hence has higher recurrence rate and poor prognosis.

Malignant liposarcoma

Dedifferentiated liposarcoma: The most common site of dedifferentiated liposarcoma (DDLPS) is RP, occurring in elderly patients. The tumor can arise de novo or result from dedifferentiation of WDPLS. Essentially the nonfatty

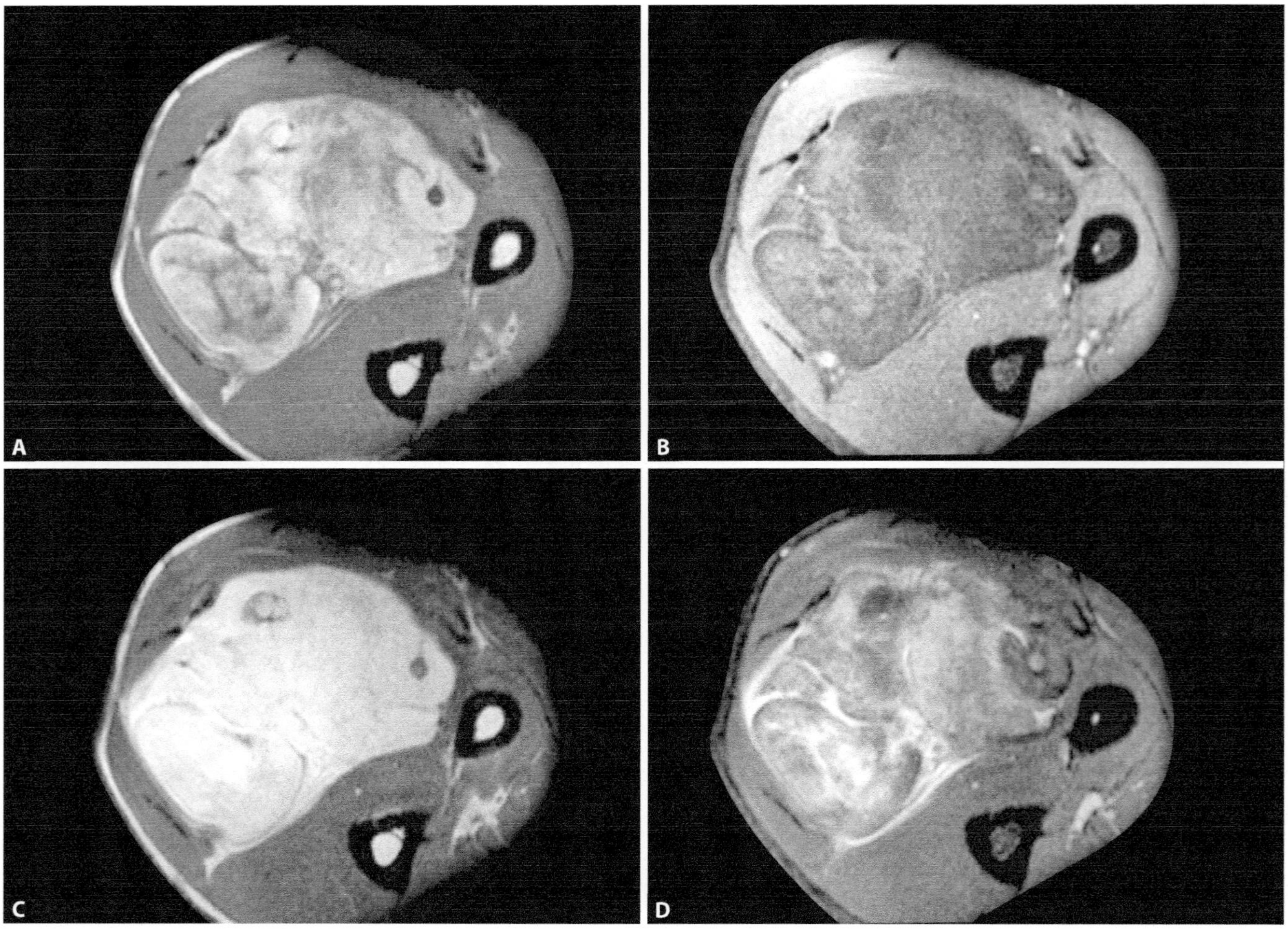

Figs. 4A to D: Atypical lipomatous tumor. (A) Axial T1-weighted (T1W); (B) T1W fat-suppressed; (C) T2-weighted (T2W); and (D) T2W fat-suppressed images depict large intramuscular heterogeneous lesion showing fat signal intensity areas which are suppressed on fat-saturated (FS) images. There are intermingled areas of soft-tissue signal intensity as well which appear hyperintense on T2W FS image (D). Histology revealed atypical lipomatous tumor.

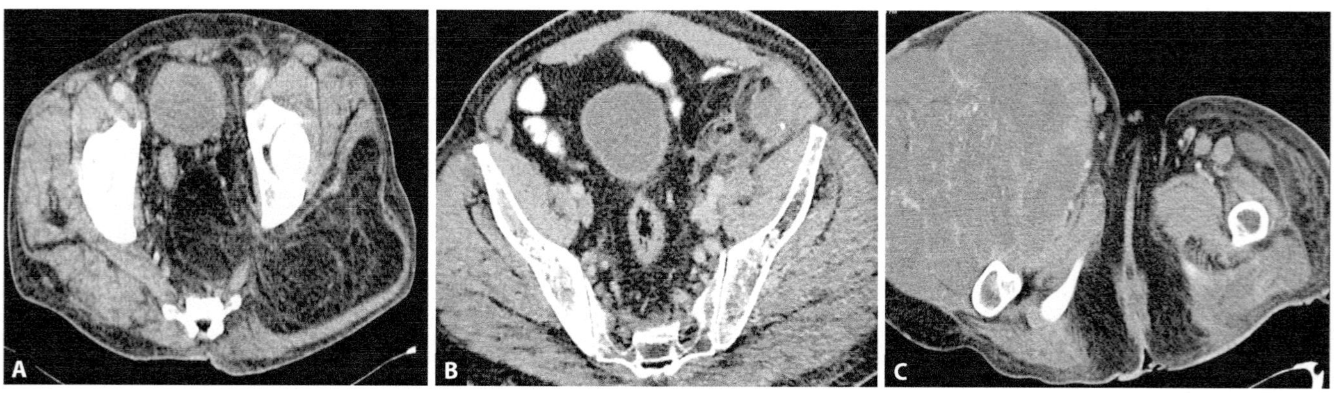

Figs. 5A to C: Liposarcomas. (A) Axial contrast-enhanced computed tomography (CECT) image shows fat-attenuation lesion in the left hemipelvis herniating into gluteal region with thin soft-tissue strands within in a case of well-differentiated liposarcoma; (B) Ill-defined lesion in left side of pelvis with relatively demarcated areas of fat and soft-tissue attenuation, (latter >2 cm and nodular) along with a speck of calcification. Histology revealed dedifferentiated liposarcoma; (C) Myxoid liposarcoma shows a large hypodense enhancing mass in the right thigh without any evident fat on imaging.

component is malignant and of variable histology, e.g., rhabdomyosarcoma (RMS) or osteosarcoma. Four morphological types of appearance are described.[10]

- *Category I*: Mainly fatty, nonfatty part is small.
- *Category II*: Mainly nonfatty, fatty part is small.
- *Category III*: Both the components are well delineated, lying adjacent to each other **(Figs. 5A to C)**.
- *Category IV*: Similar to III but both components are mainly nonfatty.

Treatment of choice is WLE; however, likelihood of incomplete resection is high.

Myxoid liposarcoma/round cell liposarcoma: Pure myxoid LPS is a low-grade sarcoma that typically occurs in the extremities, in the deep location (typically thigh), and in younger patients. It has a characteristic MR appearance with T1 hypointensity and striking high T2 signal, resembling a myoma or even a cyst. The lesion however shows contrast enhancement **(Figs. 5A to C)**. These lesions can have a round cell component, with myxoid and round cell LPS being considered two ends of same spectrum. Those tumors with more than 5% component being round cell are considered as high grade.[8] Such tumors have a more heterogeneous MR signal and poor prognosis. Myxoid LS shows a high propensity for extrapulmonary metastasis (bone/soft tissues).

Pleomorphic liposarcoma: This variant of LPS is a high-grade sarcoma encountered in extremities off middle aged patients and less commonly in the RP/mediastinum.[11] Among the three variants of malignant LPS, this form has the lowest incidence. On imaging, it is mostly a soft tissue nonfatty mass measuring more than 10 cm, with areas of necrosis and hemorrhages. Fatty component is the small, and differentiation from other STS is often not possible. It is an aggressive lesion with high incidence of pulmonary metastases.

The imaging differences between lipoma, WDLPS, and malignant LPS are summarized in **Table 3**.

FIBROBLASTIC OR MYOFIBROBLASTIC TUMORS

This group of tumors is more common in children than adults.[12] **Table 4** enumerates the entities constituting fibroblastic or myofibroblastic tumors. The more common entities are discussed in **Figures 6 to 8**.

Myositis Ossificans

This is the most commonly encountered lesion in this group, and is reparative process in majority of the patients. The frequent sites being skeletal muscles, tendons, and fat, wherein there is formation of metaplastic bone. There are three subtypes of myositis ossificans (MO).

1. Post-traumatic (most common, three-fourths of the patients)[13]
2. Nontraumatic
3. Myositis ossificans progressive.

Post-traumatic Myositis Ossificans

The stages observed on imaging reflect the progressive ossification on histology. The time period stated is in the relationship to the time of trauma **(Table 5; Figs. 7 and 8)**.

Table 3: Differentiating imaging features of lipoma, well-differentiated liposarcoma (WDLPS), and malignant liposarcoma (LPS).

	Lipoma	*WDLPS*	*Malignant LPS*
Attenuation	• Homogeneous • Fat • Thin septae • <2 mm	• Soft tissue, nonfatty components (<2 cm) • Thick septae (nodular/interrupted) • >2 mm	• Soft tissue component • >2 cm • Large size • Myxoid LPS: Typical T2 hyperintensity • *High-grade sarcomas*: Large size (>10 cm) • Necrosis, hemorrhage, size of fatty component small
Location	Rare in mediastinum/RP	Mediastinum/RP	*DDLPS*: RP/mediastinum *Myxoid/Pleomorphic*: Extremities

Table 4: Classification of fibroblastic or myofibroblastic tumors.

Benign	*Intermediate (locally aggressive)*	*Intermediate (rarely metastasizing)*	*Malignant*
• Fasciitis – Nodular – Proliferative • Myositis ossificans • Fibrous hamartoma of infancy • Calcifying fibrous tumor	• Fibromatosis – Palmar/plantar – Desmoid type – Lipofibromatosis	• Dermatofibrosarcoma • Protuberans – Solitary fibrous tumor – Inflammatory myofibroblastic tumor – Infantile fibrosarcoma	• Adult fibrosarcoma • Myxoid fibrosarcoma

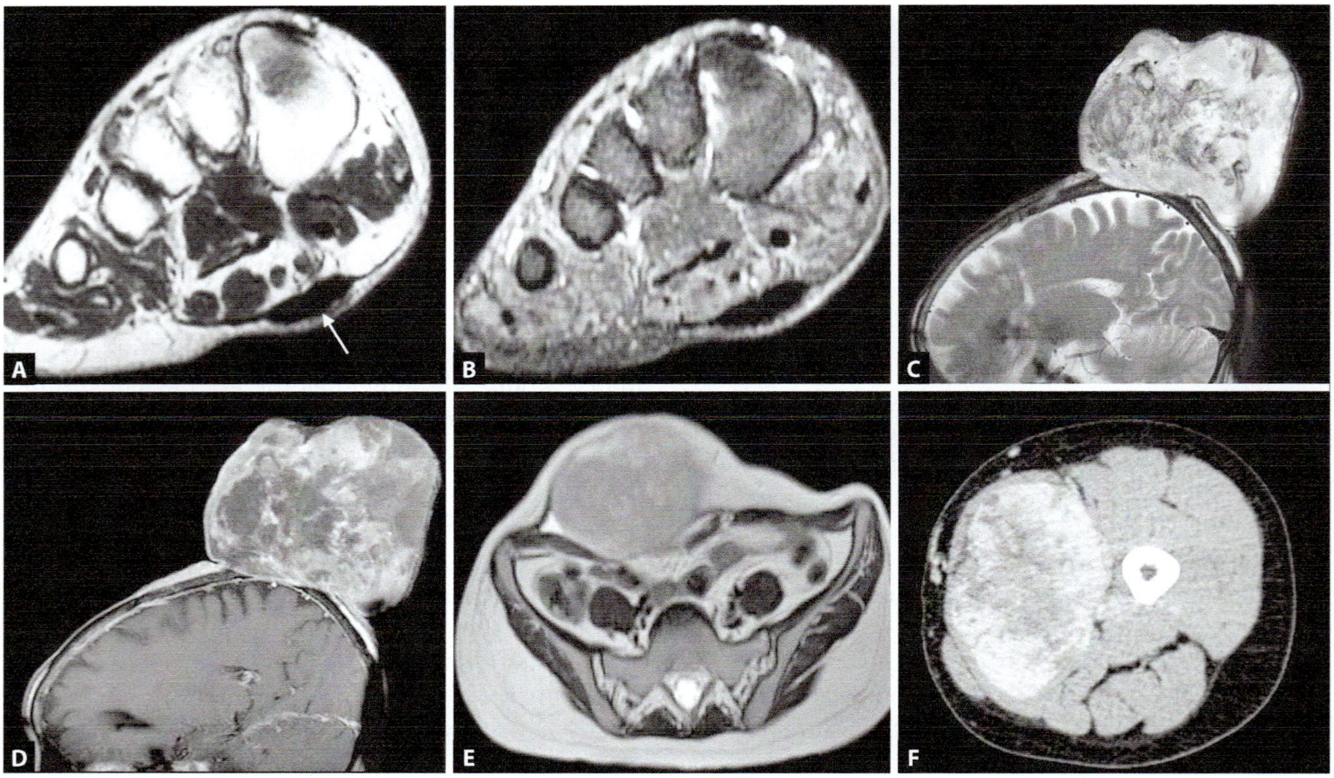

Figs. 6A to F: Myofibroblastic tumors. (A) T2-weighted (T2W); and (B) T2W fat-saturated (FS) images show hypointense nodular thickening of plantar fascia (arrows) in a case of plantar fasciitis; (C) Sagittal T2W; and (D) Postcontrast images show heterogeneous appearing large tumor in case of dermatofibrosarcoma protuberans; (E) Axial T2W image shows intermediate signal intensity mass arising from abdominal wall in case of fibromatosis; (F) Axial contrast-enhanced computed tomography (CECT) image in a case of solitary fibrous tumor shows intensely enhancing thigh mass.

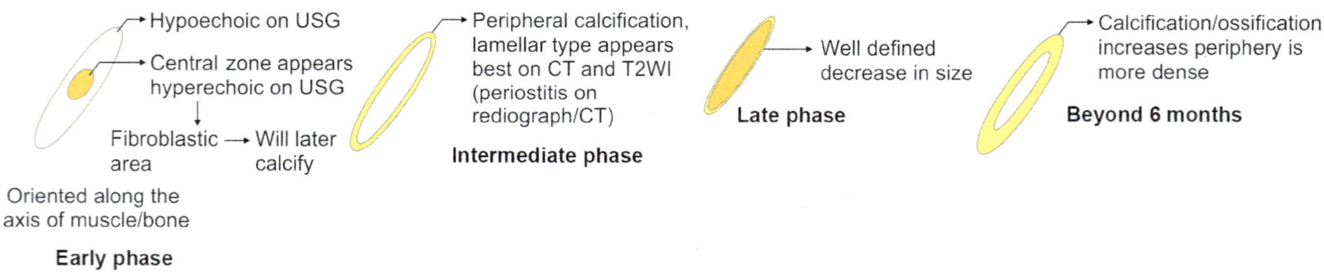

Fig. 7: Schematic diagram showing phases of post-traumatic myositis ossificans. (CT: computed tomography; T2WI: T2-weighted image; USG: ultrasonography)

In the early phase, clinically and radiologically, it is difficult to differentiate the lesions from other tumors including sarcomas. Patients present with swelling, pain, erythema, and even fever.

Features that aid in distinction from STSs on MRI in early phase include:

- Surrounding edema
- Long axis of lesion
- Periostitis
- Peripheral rim enhancement, however can be diffuse
- Intact bone cortex.

As the lesion matures, the peripheral calcification and subsequent increasing ossification is best seen on T2-weighted images. Also edema and periostitis resolve with time and the size of lesion decreases.

Nontraumatic Myositis Ossificans

Synonym: Pseudomalignant myositis ossificans

This form of MO occurs in patients with burns or long-standing paralysis (beyond 2 months). It is more frequent in adults and typically occurs below the level of paralysis, also connective tissues are involved more than skeletal muscle.

Myositis Ossificans Progressiva

Synonym: Fibrodysplasia ossificans progressiva

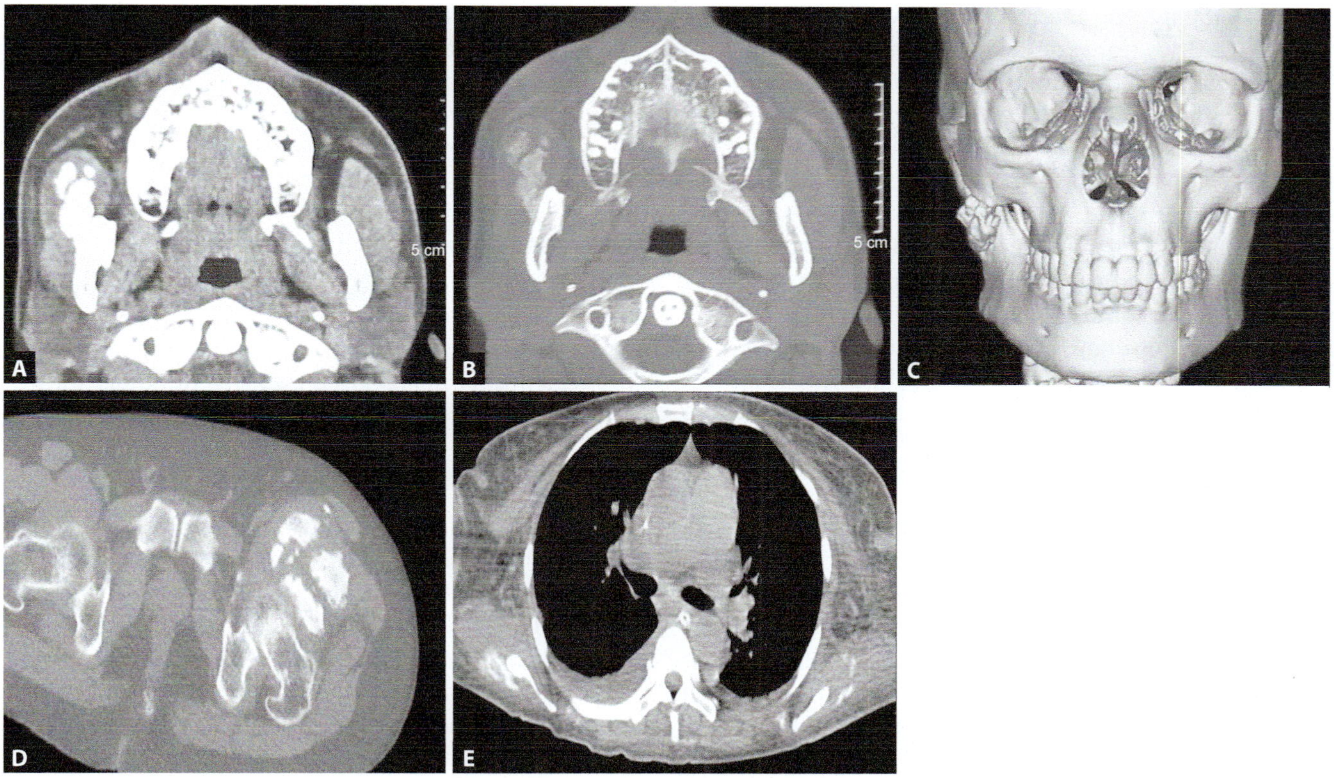

Figs. 8A to E: Myositis ossificans. (A) Axial soft tissue; and (B) Bone window computed tomography (CT) images show chunky calcification in the right masseter in a case of myositis ossificans. Periphery is denser than the center; (C) Volume-rendered image depicts the calcified lesion; (D) Myositis ossificans in muscles of the anterior thigh, separate from the underlying bone; (E) Another case of myositis ossificans with calcified lesions in both shoulder girdles.

Table 5: Imaging appearance of myositis ossificans according to various phases.

Phases	*Time frame*	*Imaging appearance*
Early proliferative phase	Less than 3 weeks	• Nonspecific soft tissue • Along the long axis of muscle/bone
Intermediate phase (calcification plus ossification)	3–7 weeks	Peripheral calcification
Mature ossification phase	More than 7 weeks	• Progressive fall in calcification, increase in ossification • Clear margins • Size reduction (beyond 6 months)

This is an autosomal dominant inherited disorder of the connective tissues resulting from mutation of *ACVR1* gene.[14] In early childhood, patients present with recurrent episodes of soft tissue swellings. These are associated with pain and followed by a trivia trauma. These eventually develop heterotropic ossification. Some characteristic features are:

- Multiple compartment involvement.
- Skeletal muscles, fascia, and ligaments/tendons can be involved.
- *Progression*: Axial to appendicular; cranial to caudal.

The condition is not treatable and patients have severe limitation of mobility, and eventually difficulty in breathing, resulting in mortality. The disease begins in early childhood, and worsens significantly by second or third decade of life.

Desmoid Fibromatosis

Desmoid fibromatosis (DF) is a locally aggressive tumor encountered in children and young adults (it has a bimodal peak—one in first decade and then in third decade). It is common in extremities, truncal region, and less frequent in head and neck. If the lesion develops in a preexisting fibroma, it has a more aggressive behavior. Association with familial adenomatous polyposis/Gardner syndrome is described.[15] Also, intra-abdominal lesions are more aggressive.

On imaging, the masses can be well-delineated or infiltrative. The stroma of the tumors may predominantly have a stroma that is composed of collagen, or one that is predominantly mucous. The imaging appearance will vary accordingly. Collagen-rich tumors are hypoechoic on USG and show posterior acoustic shadowing, have similar attenuation to muscles on CT, T1 hypointense with variable T2 signal (collagen rich—hypointense, cellular—hyperintense). Mucus-rich tumors are also T1 hyperintense. Tumor may cause scalloping/pressure erosion of adjoining bone. Another sign described on imaging is the "fascial tail sign"—these results from extension of the neoplasm along the fascia.[12] Significant, heterogeneous contrast enhancement is seen on MR.

Management strategy:

- *Conservative*: Clinicoradiological follow-up
- *Chemotherapy*: Rapidly growing tumor or those in critical location
- *Surgical resection*: Only if surgery is possible without undue morbidity
- Recurrence rates are high and particularly higher in those with neurovascular bundle involvement.

Inflammatory Myofibroblastic Tumor

Inflammatory myofibroblastic tumor (IMT), earlier called inflammatory pseudotumor, is an intermediate grade tumor (rarely metastasizing type). Up to one-fourth of the tumors recur post resection, but metastases is rare.[13] It is encountered most commonly in 1st to 3rd decades of life with common sites being chest, head and neck, and abdomen. The tumor secretes interleukins which are inflammatory mediators and can hence be associated with systemic symptoms.

The tumor is composed of fibroblasts and myofibroblasts in combination with lymphocytes, plasma cells as well as eosinophils. It is this variable combination of fibrotic and cellular elements which will govern the imaging appearance, particularly the T2 signal. These tumors can be large and are characterized by moderate enhancement, which is characteristically persistent. Calcification is frequent **(Figs. 9A to D)**.[16]

In the chest, peripheral tumors are more common than central ones, though IMT may occur in both locations **(Figs. 9A to D)**. In the abdomen, infiltration of soft tissues around the porta (in case of liver IMT) and bowel involvement (in mesenteric/omental location) is described.[17] Surgery is the treatment of choice, though recurrence is frequent. Chemotherapy is only employed in case of unresectable neoplasms.

FIBROHISTIOCYTIC TUMORS

The term used for these tumors by WHO classification is "so-called fibrohistiocytic tumors." The term "so-called" has been attached to the tumors, as HPE IHC and genetic analysis show that these tumors do not arise from histiocytes but only resemble them.[18] The term MFH or malignant fibrous histiocytoma is now eliminated from this category, and only four neoplasms are included. Entities under this group are enumerated in **Table 6.**

Tenosynovial Giant Cell Tumor

Tenosynovial giant cell tumor (TSGCT) basically arise from the synovium lining joints, tendon sheaths, or even bursae, hence, can be extra-articular or intra-articular. These are further divided into localized or diffuse forms[19] **(Table 7 and Fig. 9)**.

SMOOTH MUSCLE TUMORS

This group includes two entities: (1) leiomyoma (benign) and (2) leiomyosarcoma (malignant). Leiomyomas are most frequent in the uterus and the GI tract, with other sites including soft tissues being rare. These have a nonspecific MR appearance, and calcification may be seen in leiomyomas but is rare in the leiomyosarcomas. Leiomyosarcomas are larger and more heterogeneous with necrosis. Both the tumors tend to remodel bone (rather than cause permeative destruction).

PERICYTIC (PERIVASCULAR) TUMORS

These tumors resemble pericytes, which are contractile smooth muscle cells located around vessels and include glomus tumors, myopericytoma, and angioleiomyoma. Glomus tumors in this category are not the same as paragangliomas (also called "glomus"). Glomus tumors of this form occur in the extremities, with less frequent site being paranasal sinuses. These tumors are rare and occur in middle age/elderly, are intensely enhancing, unencapsulated, and locally aggressive lesions **(Figs. 9A to D)**. The tumors are iso/hypointense on T2WI.[20]

Angioleiomyoma is typically encountered in middle-aged females and displays flow voids and avid enhancement due to its mixed composition.

SKELETAL MUSCLE TUMORS

The benign tumor in this group is rhabdomyoma and the malignant neoplasm is RMS.

Rhabdomyosarcoma

Rhabdomyosarcoma is frequent in the pediatric age group, particularly in children less than 10 years of age, among whom it constitutes about half of the STSs.[21] It is a high-grade, small round cell neoplasm, with the more differentiated components resembling skeletal muscle. On IHC, tumors are positive for desmin and myogenin. The types of RMS are illustrated in **Flowchart 4**. The main differences between the major types are enlisted here.[22]

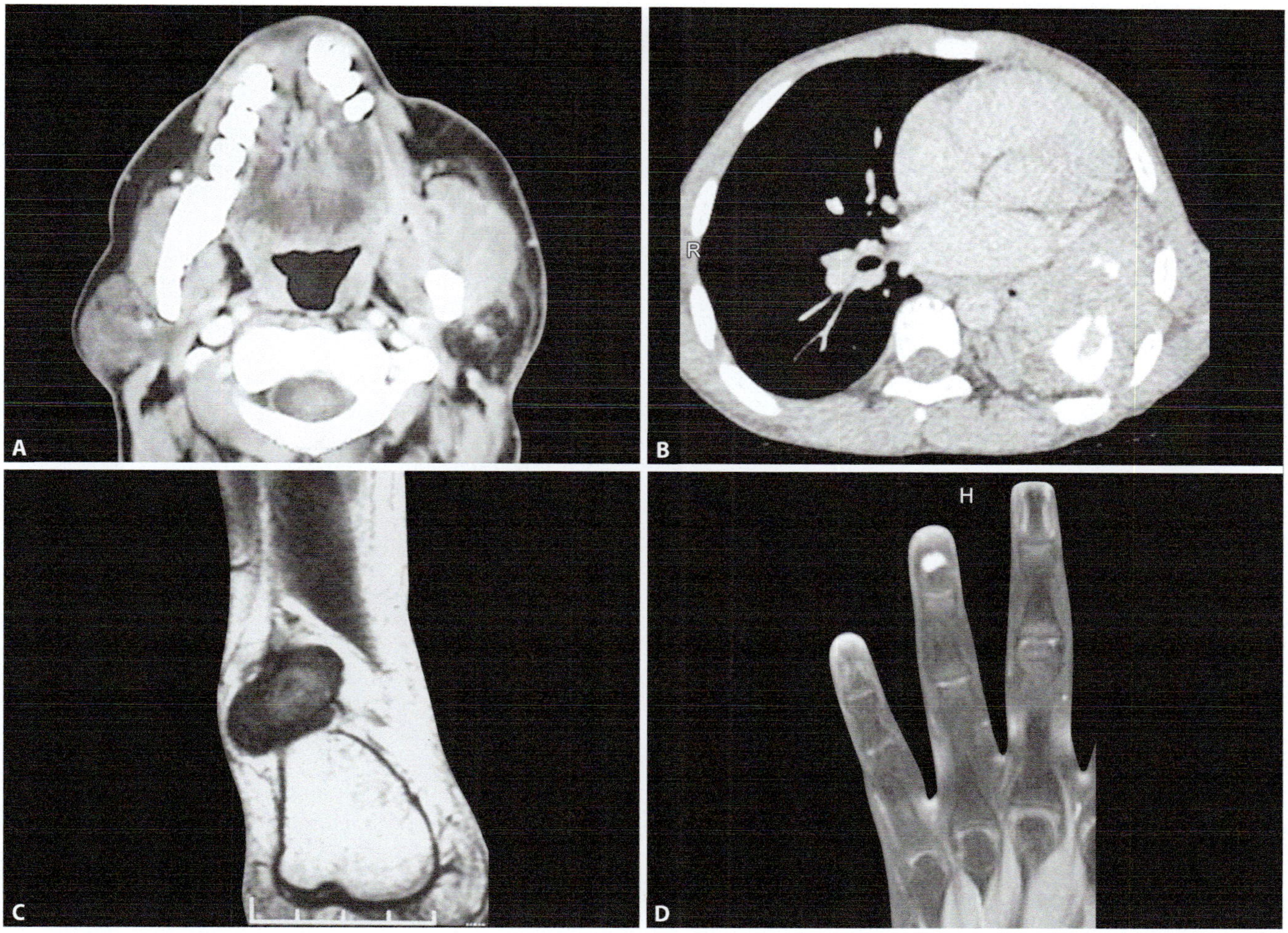

Figs. 9A to D: Inflammatory pseudotumor, giant cell tumor, and glomus tumor. (A) Axial contrast-enhanced computed tomography (CECT) image shows bulky left masseter with fatty replacement of ipsilateral parotid. Biopsy revealed inflammatory myofibroblastic tumor (IMFT); (B) Another patient with chest IMFT shows large mass filling in the left thoracic cavity with chunky calcification; (C) Coronal T2-weighted (T2W) image shows round hypointense lesion posterior to the ankle joint, suggestive of localized giant cell tumor; (D) Postcontrast coronal image shows intensely enhancing subcentimetric lesion in soft tissues of the finger tip, suggesting glomus tumor.

Table 6: So-called fibrohistiocytic tumors.

Benign	*Intermediate (rarely metastasizing)*	*Malignant*
Tenosynovial giant cell tumor	Plexiform fibrohistiocytic tumor	No entity
Deep benign fibrous histiocytoma	Giant cell tumor of soft tissue	

Embryonal RMS

- More common (more than two-thirds)
- Younger age group
- Better prognosis.

Alveolar RMS

- Less than one-third cases
- Older group
- Worse prognosis.

Head and neck is the most common site (over one-third cases), followed by genitourinary or extremities **(Figs. 10A to D)**. In the head and neck, masses may be orbital, parameningeal (involving skull base), or nonparameningeal. Common genitourinary sites include bladder, prostate, or vagina. Other sites include biliary, trunk, thorax, or extremities. RMS is an aggressive neoplasm and is frequently metastatic with common sites being pulmonary, osseous, or lymph nodal. These can be associated with Li-Fraumeni syndrome or DICER1 syndrome among other predisposing factors.

The imaging appearance of RMS is nonspecific. It is the presence of a soft tissue mass in described locations that is aggressive with no fatty component in a young patient that raises the suspicion. Embryonal forms can cause bowing of adjoining bones, while bone destruction is seen in up to one-fifth of the patients. Calcification is uncommon. Necrosis is seen in alveolar and pleomorphic forms, while the embryonal type is mostly homogeneous.

Table 7: Clinical and imaging features of localized and diffuse forms of tenosynovial giant cell tumor (TSGCT).

	Localized TSGCT	*Diffuse TSGCT*
Synonym	• GCT of tendon sheath • Nodular tenosynovitis	• Diffuse type GCT • Pigmented villo-nodular synovitis/tenosynovitis
Behavior	Benign	Locally aggressive (nonmetastasizing)
Age	• 30–50 years • F>M	<40 years
Location	Hand	• Large joints • Knee, hip, elbow, shoulder
Presentation	• Slow growth • Painless	Painful, tender
Radiograph/CT	• Soft tissue mass, well defined • Pressure erosion of adjoining bone	• Ill-defined soft tissue mass • No calcification • Bone erosion • Joint effusion • Joint space preserved • Bone density normal
USG	• Solid • Well defined • Hypoechoic • Homogeneous/heterogeneous • Adjoining a tendon/joint • Internal vascularity+	• Ill defined • Joint effusion+
MRI (modality of choice)	• *T1WI*: Low intermediate • *T2WI*: Variable • Hypointense foci (hemosiderin deposits) • *Gradient echo*: Blooming • *CEMR*: Diffuse enhancement	• Similar features • *Synovial thickening:* Diffuse or plaque like or nodular • Subchondral cysts/erosions • Effusion with septae
Recurrence rates	Less	More
Treatment of choice	Excision	Wide excision

Flowchart 4: Histological subtypes of rhabdomyosarcoma (RMS).

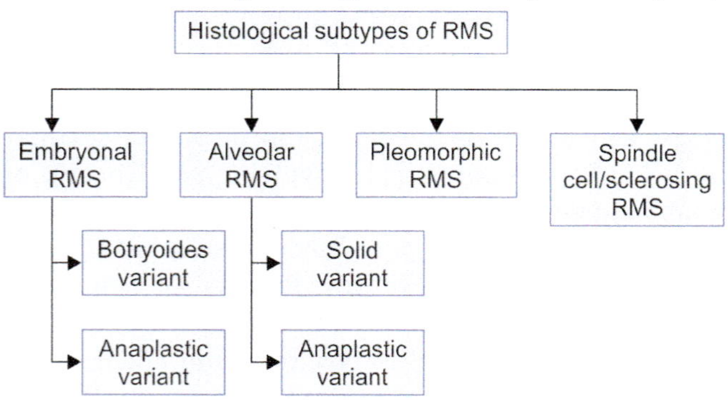

MR signal is also nonspecific. The lesion may show flow voids. Contrast enhancement is moderate **(Figs. 10A to D)** and the pleomorphic form may show "ring like" enhancement. Staging is similar to other STS, as is addressed later in the chapter.

VASCULAR TUMORS

The discussion on this group of tumors encompasses concepts both from the WHO classification as well as the ISSVA (International Society for Study of Vascular Anomalies) classification, primarily the ISSVA concepts[23] **(Table 8).**

Infantile Hemangioma

Superficial infantile hemangioma is associated with skin discoloration (strawberry mark) while in deep lesions overlying skin/mucosa maybe normal. It is encountered during infancy or neonatal period, increases during the next few months, and then regresses. It is characterized by the following phases **(Table 9)**. Beta-blockers have shown to be effective in proliferating phase.[24] These tumors are often GLUT-1 positive.[25]

Congenital Hemangioma

It includes two forms: (1) rapidly involuting congenital hemangioma (RICH) and (2) noninvoluting CH (NICH). The main difference between IH, RICH, or NICH is the age of presentation/regression. CH tumors peak at birth or in some instances have already begun to involute by that

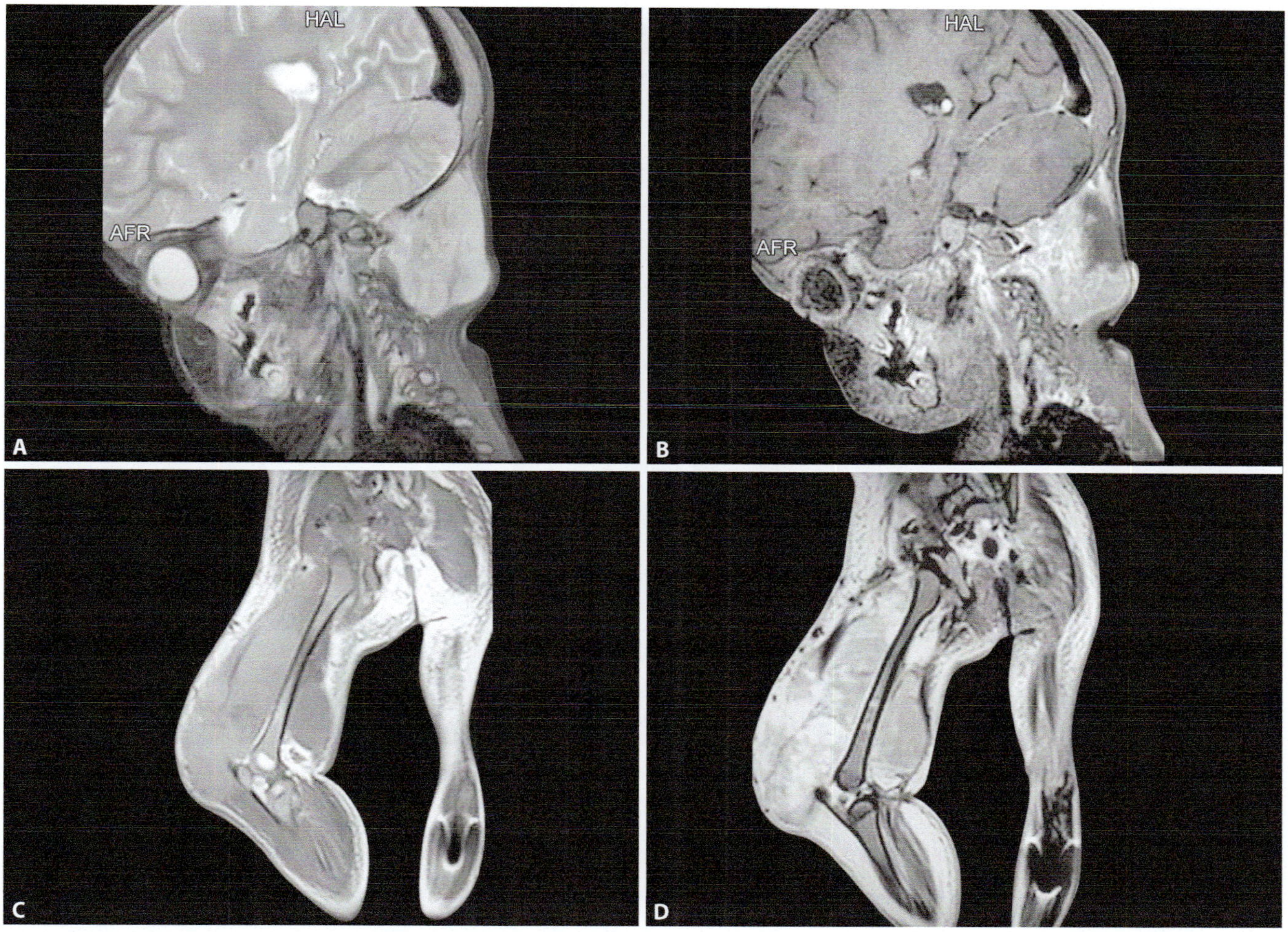

Figs. 10A to D: Rhabdomyosarcoma. (A) Sagittal T2-weighted (T2W); and (B) Postcontrast magnetic resonance (MR) images show mildly hyperintense mass in the soft tissues of the neck, showing heterogenous contrast enhancement; (C) Sagittal T1-weighted (T1W); and (D) T2W MR images in another child show large heterogeneous thigh mass in a case of alveolar rhabdomyosarcoma.

Table 8: Vascular tumors.

Benign	*Intermediate (locally aggressive)*	*Intermediate (rarely metastasizing)*	*Malignant*
Hemangioma	Kaposiform hemangioendothelioma	Hemangioendothelioma • Retiform • Composite • Pseudomyxogenic	Epitheloid hemangioendothelioma Angiosarcoma

Table 9: Imaging appearance of infantile hemangioma according to phases.

Phases	*Period*	*USG*	*MRI*
Proliferative phase	• Neonatal/early infancy • Up to about one and a half years of age	• Well defined mass with variable echogenicity (low or high) • Lobulated • Doppler–arterial flow	• Well defined • Lobulated – *T1WI*: hypo/isointense – *T2WI*: Hyperintense • Flow voids • Early, persistent enhancement
Involuting phase	• After 1 year • Continues for years • Slow regression	Decrease in size and vascularity	• Decrease in size • T2 hyperintensity and enhancement reduce • Fatty replacement

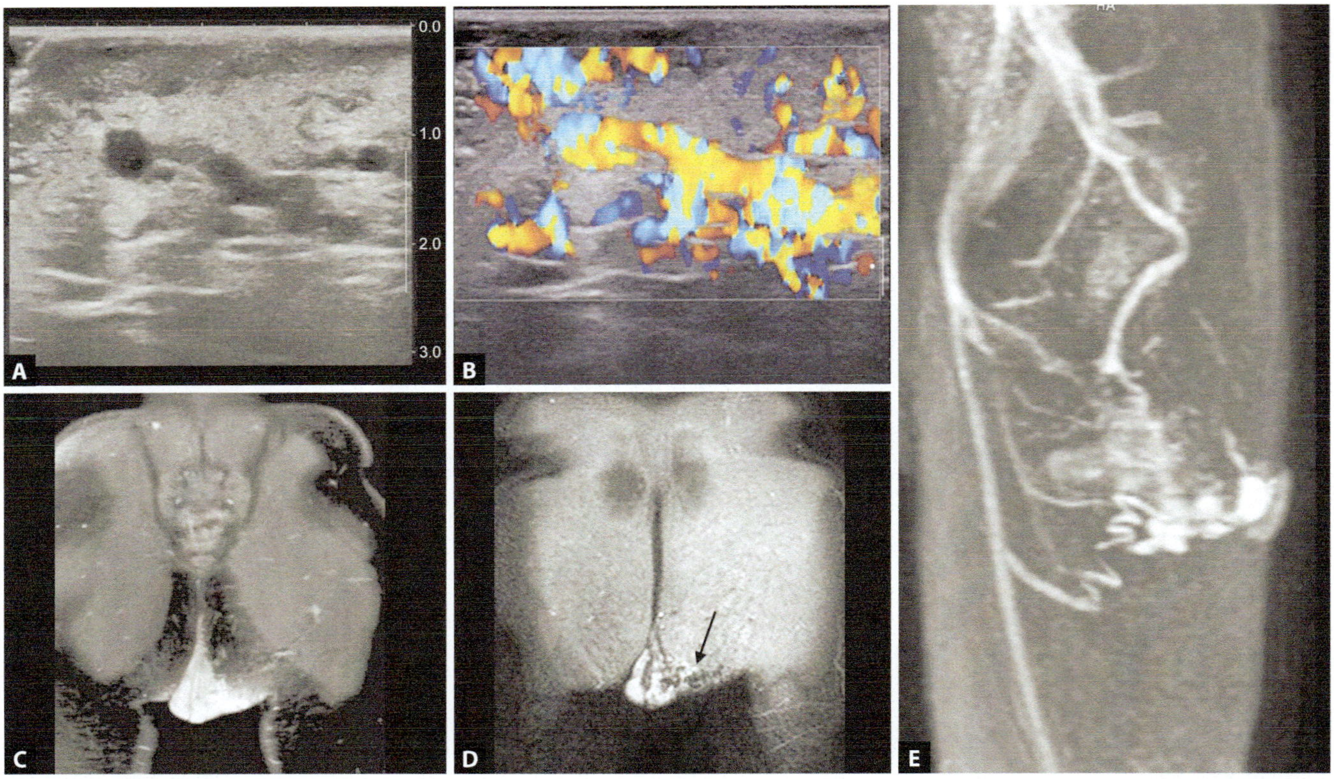

Figs. 11A to E: Lobular capillary hemangioma in a young female patient. (A) Gray-scale ultrasound image shows echogenic mass with anechoic vascular channels, showing intense color flow on Doppler image (B); (C and D) Coronal short tau inversion recovery (STIR) images show hyperintense mass involving skin, subcutaneous tissues in perineal region with flow voids (arrow); (E) Time-resolved magnetic resonance (MR) angiography depicts early intense enhancement with arteriovenous shunting.

time. The rapidly involuting form completely regresses by about 1 year of age. NICH on the other hand does not regress.[26] CH tumors are usually GLUT-1 negative.

While imaging features of CH and IH are broadly similar, CH displays some differences:

- More heterogeneity
- Ill-defined margins
- Aggressive features on angiography-aneurysms or arteriovenous shunts **(Figs. 11A to E)**
- Calcification may be present.

Kaposiform Hemangioendothelioma

Kaposiform hemangioendothelioma (KHE) is so-called due to its resemblance to Kaposi's sarcoma on pathology. It is a locally aggressive neoplasm which occurs in infants or children. KHE has an association with Kasabach-Merritt syndrome (a consumption coagulopathy with thrombocytopenia). On imaging, the tumors are similar to hemangiomas but has ill-defined infiltrative margins and may show osseous invasion.[27] The tumor does not metastasize.

Angiosarcoma

Angiosarcoma is a locally aggressive tumor, which occurs most frequently in skin, followed by soft tissues or bone. It is more common in the elderly. Tumor has both vascular/lymphatic components. The tumor displays early and widespread metastases, with lung being the most common site. On imaging, it shows similar features as the other vascular tumors. However, it displays a restriction on diffusion due to high cellularity.[28] A variant described is the "Stewart-Treves syndrome," wherein the neoplasm arises in post-treatment breast carcinoma patients with lymphedema of long duration.

Table 10: Chondro-osseous tumors.

Benign	*Malignant*
Soft tissue chondroma	• Mesenchymal chondrosarcoma • Extraskeletal osteosarcoma

CHONDRO-OSSEOUS TUMORS

The presence of characteristic chondroid/osteoid matrix in extra-osseous masses alerts to the possibility of these tumors. Soft tissue chondro-osseous neoplasms are uncommon/rare tumors encountered in the extremities or head and neck **(Table 10)**.

GASTROINTESTINAL STROMAL TUMORS

The discussion of this tumor is beyond the scope of this chapter.

PERIPHERAL NERVE SHEATH TUMORS

The subtypes of peripheral nerve sheath tumors (PNSTs) are given in **Table 11**.

Benign Peripheral Nerve Sheath Tumors

Of the PNSTs, benign tumors constitutes almost a tenth of all STT. Both schwannomas and neurofibromas share a similar imaging appearance; however, many differential features are also described. Both the tumors are well circumscribed, longitudinally oriented in the direction of nerve and may be homogeneous/heterogeneous **(Figs. 12 and 13)**. The key differences among them are:

- Nerve is eccentric in schwannomas, hence separable; but located within the tumor in neurofibromas.
- Heterogeneity, necrosis, and cystic degeneration are more frequent in schwannomas **(Figs. 13A to D)**.
- Schwannomas are encapsulated tumors, neurofibromas are not. Pseudocapsule can be present.
- "Split-fat sign" can be seen in both, much more often in schwannoma. It refers to the presence of fat around the tumor.[29]
- On MRI, both are iso/hypointense (to muscle) on T1-weighted images, and mildly hyperintense on T2-weighted images with moderate enhancement.

Table 11: Benign and malignant peripheral nerve sheath tumors (PNSTs).

Benign	*Malignant*
• Schwannoma • Neurofibroma – Plexiform neurofibroma • Granular cell tumor	• Malignant PNST • Malignant triton tumor

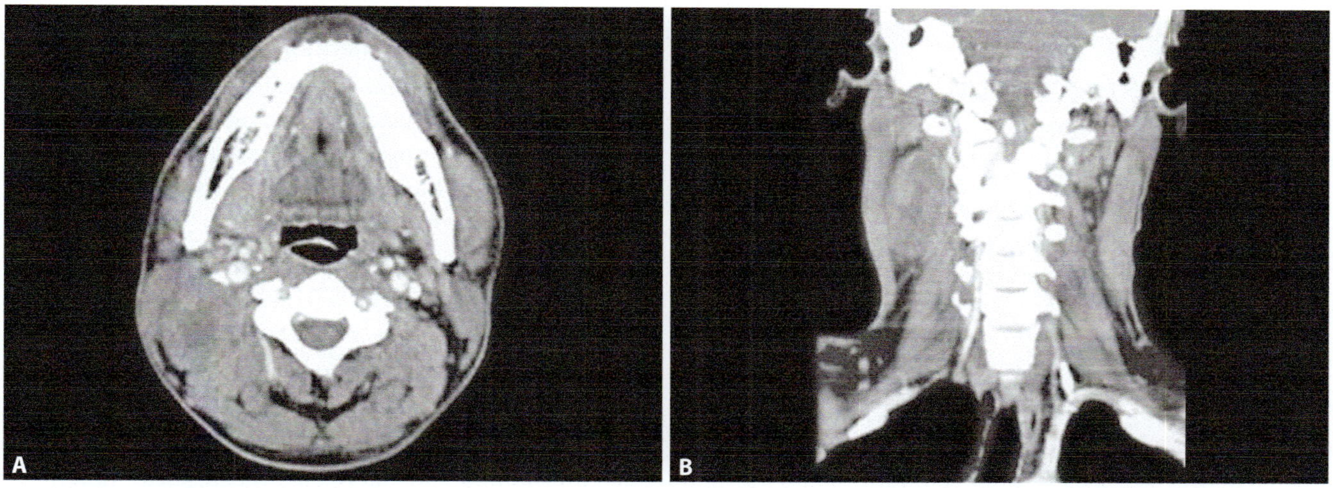

Figs. 12A and B: Neurogenic tumor. Contrast-enhanced computed tomography (CECT) images show a longitudinally ovoid, heterogeneous right carotid space mass lesion displacing the vessels anteriorly, suggestive of vagal neurogenic tumor.

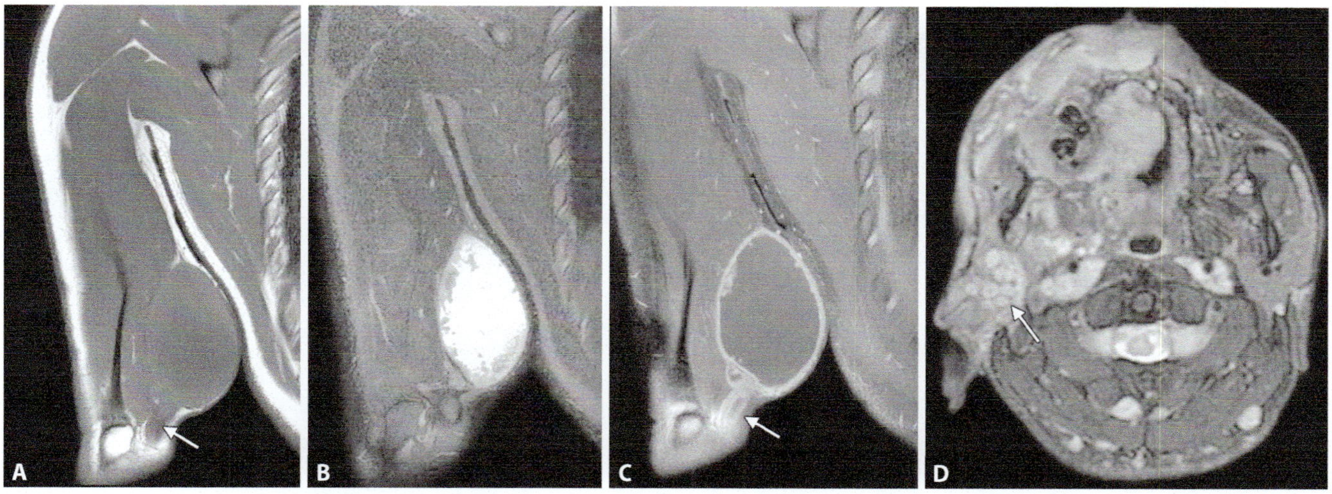

Figs. 13A to D: Schwannoma and plexiform neurofibroma. (A) Coronal T1-weighted (T1W); (B) T2-weighted (T2W); and (C) Postcontrast images show longitudinal ovoid lesion, in continuity with the ulnar nerve (arrow), brightly hyperintense on T2W image and showing peripheral contrast enhancement in case of ulnar nerve schwannoma; (D) Another patient with plexiform neurofibroma of the right side of face shows central hypointensity of target sign (arrow).

- "Target sign" on MR may be seen in neurofibromas, which refers to low-signal intensity in the center (fibrocollagenous tissue), with hyperintense periphery (myxoid areas) on T2-weighted image **(Figs. 13A to D)**.

Malignant Peripheral Nerve Sheath Tumors

Malignant PNSTs (MPNSTs) can be challenging to differentiate from benign PNSTs on imaging. The features that suggest malignancy are:

- Large size
- Loss of definition of margins (even if partial or focal) should is the suspicion of MPNST
- Rapidly increasing size
- Heterogeneity and necrosis.

Malignant PNSTs are more frequent in patients with neurofibromatosis (NF-1) and can often developed in preexisting benign PNST. Multiple PNSTs are encountered in NF-1 both in soft tissues and deeper locations (chest and abdomen).

TUMORS OF UNCERTAIN DIFFERENTIATION

These include uncommon/rare entities such as acral fibromyxoma, hemosiderotic fibrolipomatous tumors, and synovial sarcoma. Among these, the malignant counterpart synovial sarcoma is the most frequently encountered.

Synovial Sarcoma

Synovial sarcoma (SS) is an intermediate to high-grade, slow-growing STT, which occurs most frequently in young adults, particularly seen around the joints, especially in popliteal fossa. It does not arise in intra-articular location or synovial structures, but tends to occur near the joints. Pathologically, the cells resemble the normal synovium but stain for epithelial markers and have monophasic, biphasic, or poorly differentiated subtypes. Over 90% of cases demonstrate t(X;18) translocation which is highly specific for SS.[30]

Imaging features are nonspecific, but a juxta-articular soft tissue mass with calcification (which is seen in 30% of cases) in a young patient is very suggestive of SS. On CT or MRI, the tumor shows lobulated margins and heterogeneity with presence of hemorrhage, septations, calcification, or fluid levels **(Figs. 14A to C)**. Such marked heterogeneity gives rise to the "triple sign" which represents the cystic degeneration; and high-signal on T2WI along with presence of hypointense internal fibrotic bands and calcifications. "Bowl of grapes" sign arise due to presence of multiple fluid–fluid levels secondary to recurrent bleeds. Bone involvement can occur in the form of extrinsic erosion or periosteal reaction.

The tumor has high metastatic potential and cannon ball pulmonary metastasis is well known.[31] SS most commonly affects the lower extremities, and is less commonly seen in head and neck region, and is rare in chest wall and viscera. Management constitutes surgery along with pre- and postoperative radiotherapy/chemotherapy. SS has a tendency to locally recur (30–50% local recurrence rates).[30]

UNDIFFERENTIATED/UNCLASSIFIED SARCOMAS

This category contains only malignant lesions not included in the other categories. The types of undifferentiated sarcomas include spindle cell, pleomorphic, round cell, epitheloid, and NOS (not otherwise specified). Prior to 2013, these were labeled as "malignant fibrous histiocytoma."

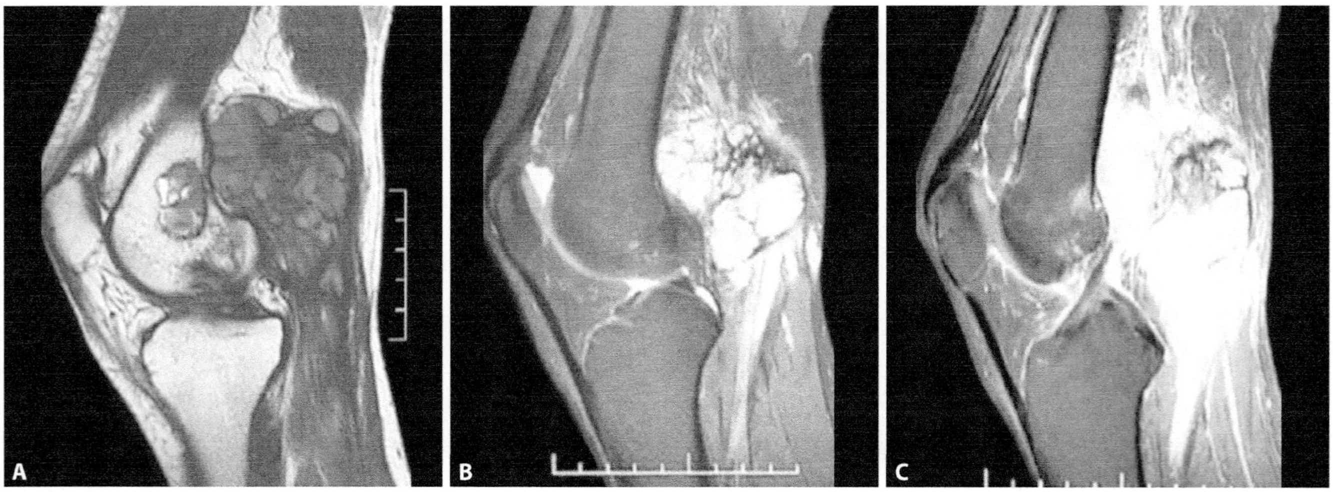

Figs. 14A to C: Synovial sarcoma. (A) Sagittal T1-weighted (T1W); (B) T2-weighted (T2W); and (C) Postcontrast magnetic resonance (MR) images of a young male show a heterogeneous, solid, lobulated extra-articular mass located just behind the knee joint. The lesion is brightly hyperintense on T2W image and shows intense enhancement. Intraosseous extension is seen into the adjoining femur.

Staging of Soft Tissue Sarcomas

American Joint Committee on Cancer (AJCC), 8th edition, staging system is recommended for staging of STS.[32] Similar to bone tumors, STS staging also accounts grade based on histopathology (G); in addition to primary tumor (T), lymph nodes (N), and metastases (M). STS are considered under four categories, based on location:

1. Trunk and extremity
2. Head and neck
3. Retroperitoneum
4. Visceral.

Tumor Grades

The AJCC staging system includes three tumor grades, based on the French Federation of Cancer Centers Sarcoma Group (FNCLCC) system: high grade (poorly differentiated) is the highest grade 3, followed by intermediate grade (moderate differentiated 2), and low- or well-differentiated which is labeled as grade 1.

Steps of Staging (Flowchart 5)

T Stage

T stage definition differs according to the site of the tumor. Tx category is common to all sites, i.e., that the tumor is not assessable. **Table 12** shows the T descriptors according to site.

Size refers to largest tumor dimension.

The staging of STS is applicable to most histological subtypes; however, some unusual tumors/sites have been excluded from the common staging system. The discussion of these entities and of gastrointestinal stromal tumor is beyond the scope of this chapter.

The stage groupings are essentially dependent on the stage and histological grade (G), as presence of positive nodes or metastases places the tumor in stage III or IV depending on site **(Table 13)**. There are some differences in the staging systems advocated by AJCC and UICC (Union for International Cancer Control). In this chapter, the AJCC system is followed for discussion. The 8th edition introduced two new sites: (1) "Head and neck" and (2) "Abdomen and thoracic visceral organs." While separate T descriptors for these sites have been detailed **(Table 12)**, separate stage groupings have not been given. The only difference in stage groupings of trunk, extremity vs. RP is that in the latter N1 is placed in III B group.

In the head and neck region, T4 category has been further divided based on which surrounding organs are infiltrated.

Flowchart 5: Steps of staging.

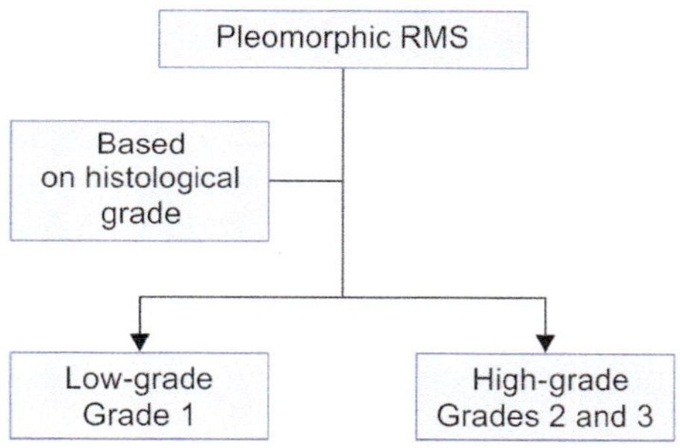

Table 12: T descriptor according to various sites.

T descriptor	*Trunk/Extremity/RP*	*Head and neck*	*Abdominal and thoracic visceral organs*
T0	No primary tumor	No primary tumor	No primary tumor
T1	Size ≤ 5 cm	Size ≤ 2 cm	Limited to the organ
T2	Size > 5 cm, ≤10 cm	Size > 2 cm, ≤4 cm	Spread beyond the organ
T3	Size >10 cm, ≤15 cm	Size > 4 cm	Infiltration of a different organ
T4	Size >15 cm	When there is surrounding infiltration/invasion	Multifocal

Table 13: Staging groups.

Applicable to trunk and extremities					
Stage I		*Stage II*	*Stage III*		*Stage IV*
A	B		A	B	
T1	T2–T4	T1	T2	T3	N1 or M1 with any T
Gx or G1	Gx or G1	G2 or G3	G2 or G3	G2 or G3	
Applicable to retroperitoneum					
Similar	Similar	Similar	Similar + any T, any G N1 included		M1 (any T any G)

- *T4a*: Orbit, skull base or dura, viscera, facial bones, pterygoid muscles.
- *T4b*: Invasion of cerebral parenchyma, carotid artery, prevertebral muscle, perineural spread (to CNS).

On the other hand, the subdivision of T4 category in abdomen and thoracic is based on number sites involved: 2 sites being T4a, 3–5 sites being T4b, and more than 5 sites being T4c.

IMAGING MODALITIES AND APPROACH

Ultrasonography

Ultrasonography (USG), due to its obvious advantages, is advocated as the first level screening modality for evaluation of soft tissue masses **(Box 1)**.[33] Although, it suffers from limitations, particularly in evaluation of deep seated lesions, it can categorize several lesions definitely avoiding biopsy or further evaluation **(Table 14)**. Addition of tissue harmonic imaging, compound imaging, and Doppler is advocated depending on nature of lesion. USG is also useful for image-guided interventions. Elastography is an adjunct tool to high-resolution USG in the evaluation of soft tissue lesions. Assessment of stiffness of masses using elastography helps in their characterization.[34] Contrast-enhanced US (CEUS) has been shown to have some role in characterization of STTs into benign and malignant forms. One of the studies have shown an inhomogeneous pattern of contrast uptake, and arterial phase enhancement is associated with high risk of malignancy.[35]

Algorithmic approach to choice of imaging modalities for evaluation of suspected STT is outlined in **Flowchart 6.**[36]

MRI

Magnetic resonance imaging is the work-horse of imaging of STTs. It may be performed upfront if clinical suspicion of malignancy is high (primary MRI), or subsequent to another imaging modality.[37] MRI aids in both characterization and tumor mapping **(Table 14).**

Some lesions which can be clearly diagnosed on MRI. These include the list given under USG. Additional lesions which can be diagnosed on MR include:

- Hamartoma
- Myositis ossificans
- PVNS
- Muscle tears.

Further, the MR signal also guides further diagnosis **(Flowchart 7)**.

Box 1: Lesions that can be labeled as clearly benign on USG.

- Cystic lesions
  - Simple cyst
  - Ganglion cyst
  - Bursae
- *Lipoma*: If superficial, well defined, stable in size
- Vascular malformations
- Superficial fibromatosis
- Superficial nerve sheath tumors in known patients of neurofibromatosis
- Motor neuroma
- Aneurysms

CT Scan

Computed tomography has been largely replaced in the evaluation of soft tissue masses, except when MRI is contraindicated or unavailable. It can be performed upfront (primary CT) for abdominal/pelvic/retroperitoneal or thoracic masses; or subsequent to USG. In intrathoracic lesions it is often the preferred primary modality. It may be required even subsequent to MRI even, for better assessment of calcification/ossification/bone involvement in abdominal or chest masses.

Radiographs

Plain radiography may be performed initially if the distinction from an osseous origin mass is unclear clinically. It is mostly used as a "complimentary modality" to USG/MRI to better visualize calcification/ossification in the soft tissue mass; or underlying osseous involvement. It is mostly used for appendicular lesions for this purpose; with CT being the preferred modality for truncal lesions.

Table 14: Magnetic resonance (MR) acquisition protocol.

System	*1.5 T or 3 T (minimum 1 T)*
FOV (field of view)	Not only include complete lesion but also adjoining edema plus normal surrounding tissues Skin markers can be used
Matrix	≥256
Slice thickness	3 mm or 4 mm depending on tumor size
Sequences	
Precontrast T1W	Axial
Fat-sat fluid sensitive sequences (e.g., STIR)	Parallel to tumor long axis
T2W: Fat saturated (FS) or PD-FS	Axial
Intravenous gadolinium-based contrast	Preferable to use unless contraindicated *Dose*: 0.1 mm/kg
Postcontrast T1W FS	In long axis and in one additional plane Subtraction images should be generated
Dynamic contrast enhanced MR	Optional
Diffusion weighted imaging	b-values 400–1000

Flowchart 6: Choice of imaging modalities for evaluation of suspected soft tissue tumors (STT).

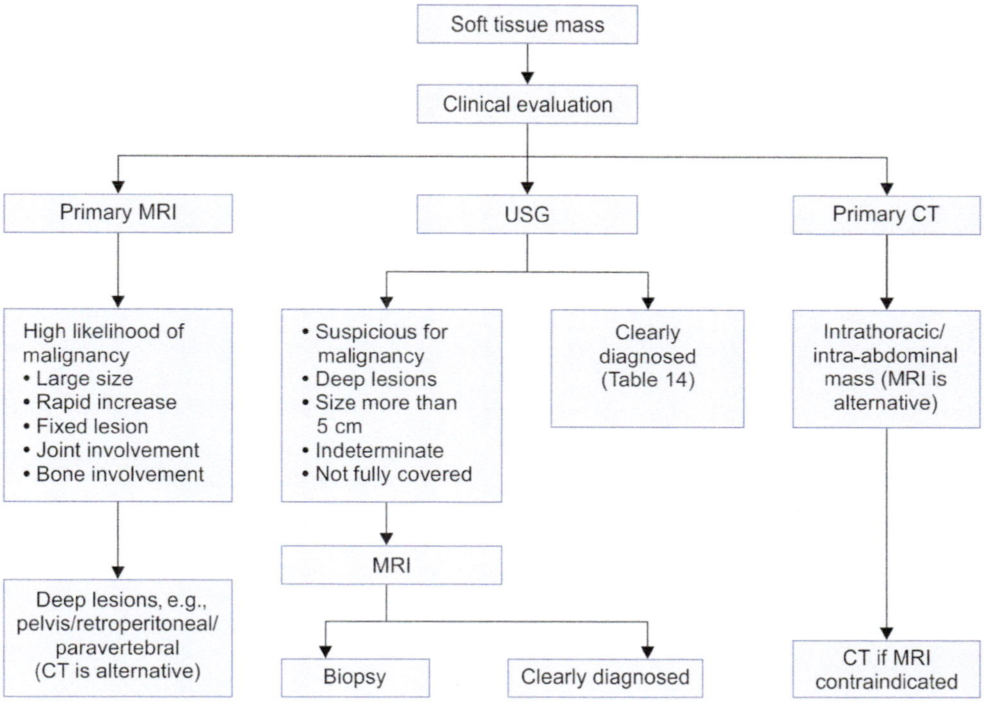

Flowchart 7: Approach based on magnetic resonance (MR) signal.

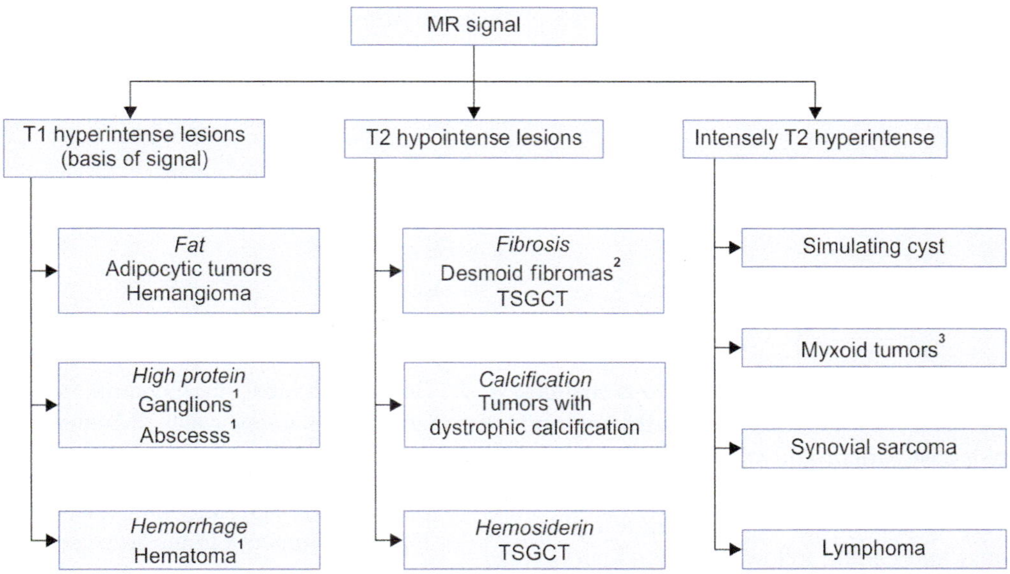

[1]Not neoplasms.
[2]*Fibromas*: Plantar fibroma, elastofibroma, fibrosarcoma.
[3]*Myxoid tumors*: Myxoid LPS, intramuscular myxoma.

Biopsy

Biopsy is indicated in all masses suspicious for malignancy and in indeterminate masses. In suspected malignant masses recommended gauge of the biopsy needle is a minimum of 14 G. Also, at least 3–4 cores should be obtained. FNAC is not adequate for diagnosis. Also, biopsy should be performed where facility for appropriate molecular/genetic evaluation is available besides histopathology. If not, patient may require a rebiopsy at a specialist center. Currently, image-guided biopsies are preferred over excision biopsy, unless the lesion is small (<2 cm).

STRUCTURED REPORTING FORMAT

Ultrasound and MRI would suffice for evaluation of most soft tissue lesions, while plain radiographs and CT are

Table 15: Systematic reporting of USG and MRI of soft tissue masses.

USG	
Morphology: Echogenicity of lesion	• Cystic • Solid • Mixed solid cystic
Margins	Well-defined/ill-defined/infiltrative
For solid masses	• Homogeneous • Heterogeneous with necrosis
For cystic lesion	• Internal echoes • Septae • Walls
Vascularity	
Calcification	Posterior acoustic shadowing (Present/absent)
Size	In all three dimensions
Location or relationship to/ infiltration of adjoining structures	• Fascia (superficial and deep) • Compartment • Adjoining bone/joints • Vessels and nerves
Elastography strain ratio	
MRI	
T1WI signal	Hypointense, intermediate, hyperintense
T2WI signal	Hypointense, intermediate, hyperintense
DWI	Restricted/Facilitated (ADC value)
Postgadolinium enhancement pattern	Homogeneous/heterogeneous/rim
Capsule/pseudocapsule	±
Peritumoral edema/surrounding infiltration	±
Satellite lesion/multiple lesions	±
Nodes	± with size and location
Any specific sign if present	e.g., split-fat sign, target sign
T stage	In case of STS
N stage	In case of STS

useful adjuncts to demonstrate associated osseous changes or matrix mineralization/ossification. MRI is the method of choice for their assessment and staging but MRI does not provide histologic diagnosis. Soft tissue involvement is often underestimated by CT. Indeterminate lesions will require biopsy and careful follow-up. Once histology has confirmed that a lesion is malignant, CT scanning of thorax is required to determine the presence or absence of intrapulmonary metastases. Use of a structured reporting format enhances the quality of the report. The structured reporting format of USG/MRI of soft tissue lesions is shown in **Table 15.**

In addition, morphological features as detailed under USG should also be mentioned in the MRI report.

REFERENCES

1. Siegel RL, Miller KD, Jemal A. Cancer statistics, 2020. CA Cancer J Clin. 2020;70(1):7-30.
2. Fletcher C, Bridge J, Hogendoorn P, Mertens F. World Health Organization Classification of Tumours of Soft Tissue and Bone, 4th edition. Lyon: IARC Press; 2013.
3. Vilanova JC. WHO classification of soft tissue tumors. In Vanhoenacker FM, Parizel PM, Gielen JL (Eds). Imaging of Soft Tissue Tumors. Chcam: Springer; 2017. pp.187-96.
4. Wei S, Henderson-Jackson E, Qian X, Bui MM. Soft tissue tumor immunohistochemistry update: Illustrative examples of diagnostic pearls to avoid pitfalls. Arch Pathol Lab Med. 2017;141(8):1072-91.
5. Bancroft LW, Kransdorf MJ, Peterson JJ, O'Connor MI. Benign fatty tumors: Classification, clinical course, imaging appearance, and treatment. Skeletal Radiol. 2006;35(10):719-33.
6. Dreux N, Marty M, Chibon F, Vélasco V, Hostein I, Ranchère-Vince D, et al. Value and limitation of immunohistochemical expression of HMGA2 in mesenchymal tumors: About a series of 1052 cases. Mod Pathol. 2010;23(12):1657-66.
7. Burt AM, Huang BK. Imaging review of lipomatous musculoskeletal lesions. SICOT J. 2017;3:34.

8. Gupta P, Potti TA, Wuertzer SD, Lenchik L, Pacholke DA. Spectrum of fat-containing soft-tissue masses at MR imaging: The common, the uncommon, the characteristic, and the sometimes confusing. Radiographics. 2016;36(3): 753-66.
9. Weiss SW, Rao VK. Well-differentiated liposarcoma (atypical lipoma) of deep soft tissue of the extremities, retroperitoneum, and miscellaneous sites. A follow-up study of 92 cases with analysis of the incidence of "dedifferentiation". Am J Surg Pathol. 1992;16(11):1051-8.
10. Hong SH, Kim KA, Woo OH, Park CM, Kim CH, Kim MJ, et al. Dedifferentiated liposarcoma of retroperitoneum: Spectrum of imaging findings in 15 patients. Clin Imaging. 2010;34(3):203-10.
11. El Ouni F, Jemni H, Trabelsi A, Ben Maitig M, Arifa N, Ben Rhouma K, et al. Liposarcoma of the extremities: MR imaging features and their correlation with pathologic data. Orthop Traumatol Surg Res. 2010;96(8):876-83.
12. Sargar KM, Sheybani EF, Shenoy A, Aranake-Chrisinger J, Khanna G. Pediatric fibroblastic and myofibroblastic tumors: a pictorial review. Radiographics. 2016;36(4):1195-214.
13. Coffin CM, Alaggio R. Fibroblastic and myofibroblastic tumors in children and adolescents. Pediatr Dev Pathol. 2012;15(1 Suppl):127-80.
14. Giacopelli F, Cappato S, Tonachini L, Mura M, Di Lascio S, Fornasari D, et al. Identification and characterization of regulatory elements in the promoter of ACVR1, the gene mutated in Fibrodysplasia Ossificans Progressiva. Orphanet J Rare Dis. 2013;8:145.
15. Ferrari A, Alaggio R, Meazza C, Chiaravalli S, Vajna de Pava M, Casanova M, et al. Fibroblastic tumors of intermediate malignancy in childhood. Expert Rev Anticancer Ther. 2013;13(2):225-36.
16. Patnana M, Sevrukov AB, Elsayes KM, Viswanathan C, Lubner M, Menias CO. Inflammatory pseudotumor: The great mimicker. AJR Am J Roentgenol. 2012;198(3): W217-27.
17. Kim SJ, Kim WS, Cheon JE, Shin SM, Youn BJ, Kim IO, et al. Inflammatory myofibroblastic tumors of the abdomen as mimickers of malignancy: Imaging features in nine children. AJR Am J Roentgenol. 2009;193(5):1419-24.
18. Kang HS. So-Called Fibrohistiocytic Tumors, 1st edition. Singapore: Springer; 2017.
19. Gouin F, Noailles T. Localized and diffuse forms of tenosynovial giant cell tumor (formerly giant cell tumor of the tendon sheath and pigmented villonodular synovitis). Orthop Traumatol Surg Res. 2017;103(1S):S91-S7.
20. Razek AA, Huang BY. Soft tissue tumors of the head and neck: imaging-based review of the WHO classification. Radiographics. 2011;31(7):1923-54.
21. Jawad N, McHugh K. The clinical and radiologic features of paediatric rhabdomyosarcoma. Pediatr Radiol. 2019;49(11):1516-23.
22. Leiner J, Le Loarer F. The current landscape of rhabdomyosarcomas: An update. Virchows Arch. 2020;476(1): 97-108.
23. Nozaki T, Matsusako M, Mimura H, Osuga K, Matsui M, Eto H, et al. Imaging of vascular tumors with an emphasis on ISSVA classification. Jpn J Radiol. 2013;31(12):775-85.
24. Léauté-Labrèze C, Dumas de la Roque E, Hubiche T, Boralevi F, Thambo JB, Taïeb A. Propranolol for severe hemangiomas of infancy. N Engl J Med. 2008;358(24): 2649-51.
25. Restrepo R, Palani R, Cervantes LF, Duarte AM, Amjad I, Altman NR. Hemangiomas revisited: The useful, the unusual and the new. Part 1: overview and clinical and imaging characteristics. Pediatr Radiol. 2011;41(7):895-904.
26. Restrepo R, Palani R, Cervantes LF, Duarte AM, Amjad I, Altman NR. Hemangiomas revisited: The useful, the unusual and the new. Part 2: endangering hemangiomas and treatment. Pediatr Radiol. 2011;41(7):905-15.
27. Gruman A, Liang MG, Mulliken JB, Fishman SJ, Burrows PE, Kozakewich HP, et al. Kaposiform hemangioendothelioma without Kasabach-Merritt phenomenon. J Am Acad Dermatol. 2005;52(4):616-22.
28. Walker EA, Salesky JS, Fenton ME, Murphey MD. Magnetic resonance imaging of malignant soft tissue neoplasms in the adult. Radiol Clin North Am. 2011;49(6):1219-34, vi.
29. Kakkar C, Shetty CM, Koteshwara P, Bajpai S. Telltale signs of peripheral neurogenic tumors on magnetic resonance imaging. Indian J Radiol Imaging. 2015;25(4):453-8.
30. Murphey MD, Gibson MS, Jennings BT, Crespo-Rodríguez AM, Fanburg-Smith J, Gajewski DA. From the archives of the AFIP: Imaging of synovial sarcoma with radiologic-pathologic correlation. Radiographics. 2006;26(5):1543-65.
31. Bakri A, Shinagare AB, Krajewski KM, Howard SA, Jagannathan JP, Hornick JL, et al. Synovial sarcoma: Imaging features of common and uncommon primary sites, metastatic patterns, and treatment response. AJR Am J Roentgenol. 2012;199(2):W208-15.
32. Tanaka K, Ozaki T. New TNM classification (AJCC eighth edition) of bone and soft tissue sarcomas: JCOG Bone and Soft Tissue Tumor Study Group. Jpn J Clin Oncol. 2019;49(2):103-7.
33. Catalano O, Varelli C, Sbordone C, Corvino A, De Rosa D, Vallone G, et al. A bump: What to do next? Ultrasound imaging of superficial soft-tissue palpable lesions. J Ultrasound; 2019.
34. Li S, Liu L, Lv G. Diagnostic value of strain elastography for differentiating benign and malignant soft tissue masses. Oncol Lett. 2017;14(2):2041-4.
35. De Marchi A, Prever EBD, Cavallo F, Pozza S, Linari A, Lombardo P, et al. Perfusion pattern and time of vascularisation with CEUS increase accuracy in differentiating between benign and malignant tumours in 216 musculoskeletal soft tissue masses. Eur J Radiol. 2015;84(1):142-50.
36. Wu JS, Hochman MG. Soft-tissue tumors and tumorlike lesions: A systematic imaging approach. Radiology. 2009;253(2):297-316.
37. Manaster BJ. Soft-tissue masses: Optimal imaging protocol and reporting. Am J Roentgenol. 2013;201(3):505-14.

CHAPTER 23

Imaging of Peripheral Nerves

Mahesh Prakash, Harish Bhujade, Anindita Sinha

INTRODUCTION

The peripheral nervous system (PNS) consists of nerves, ganglions, receptors which carry signal from central nervous system to the peripheral organs and vice-versa. There are many acquired, traumatic, or rarely congenital conditions which are seen in PNS. Traditionally, clinical examination and electrophysiological studies are the mainstay to make diagnosis of disorders of PNS. However, due to the patchy distribution of conduction block and slow conduction, accurate diagnosis is challenging in certain cases on electrophysiological studies.[1] The accuracy of electrophysiological studies may be affected by a many other factors such as age, gender, built, temperature, and body mass index.[2] Accurate diagnosis of peripheral nerve disorders is very important to guide correct patient management.[3] Many neuropathies are often remain undiagnosed on clinical examination or nerve conduction studies. Imaging of PNS is not only useful in direct demonstration of nerves but also helpful in assessing surrounding tissue.[3] Recent advances in high resolution ultrasound (US) and magnetic resonance imaging (MRI) permit precise evaluation and diagnosis of various diseases of peripheral nerves.[4] Improvements in technology (developments in transducer materials, enhanced software, higher fields MR scanner and availability of MR selective sequences) permit accurate diagnosis of various disorders of PNS. Especially the MR neurography, which is a noninvasive technique, allows assessment of the underlying cause of injury and differentiate between surgically curable and noncurable etiologies.[5]

ANATOMY OF PERIPHERAL NERVOUS SYSTEM

The nerve consists of multiple axons, which is covered by a tissue layer known as endoneurium. Many axons are grouped together to form the fascicles. Every fascicle is surrounded by tissue layer known as perineurium. These bundles of fascicles are covered by a tissue layer known as epineurium which is outermost layer of nerve **(Fig. 1)**. The PNS consists of spinal nerves and cranial

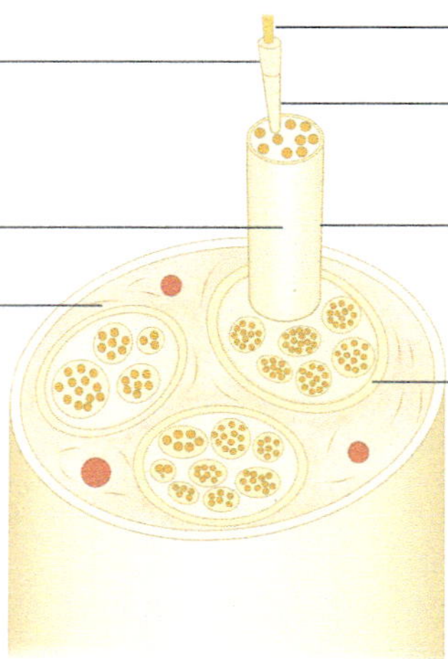

Fig. 1: Anatomy of nerve.

nerves. The dorsal and ventral roots of spinal nerves composed of sensory and motor axons, respectively. The spinal nerves divided into anterior (ventral) and posterior (dorsal) rami innervating muscles and the skin. These rami are hybrids containing sensory and motor fibers.

CURRENT IMAGING IN PERIPHERAL NERVOUS SYSTEM

Radiological imaging of PNS is very good in assessing the size, appearance, course, and continuity of nerves and also in evaluating surrounding soft tissue and bones. The indications of imaging of PNS include localization of the pathology, visualization of anatomical definition of a nerve, traumatic grading of the nerve injury, response to therapy, evaluation of radiation injury to a nerve or plexus, and evaluation of cases of chronic pain. Preprocedural imaging is also helpful for planning of image-guided intervention. Evaluation of PNS mainly depends on US and MRI.

Conventional Radiography

Conventional radiography has very limited role, may be useful to look for bony abnormalities.[6] It is initial screening technique to rule out any osseous or joint pathology.

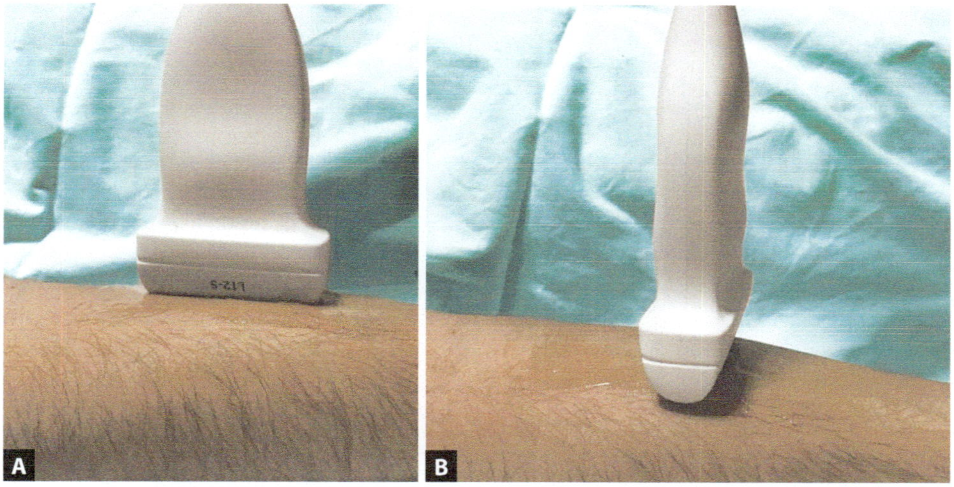

Figs. 2A and B: Ultrasound (US) technique is showing position of transducer in long (A) and short axis (B).

Computed Tomography

The role of computed tomography (CT) in imaging of PNS is often limited to assessment of bony structures. It is useful in diagnosis of nerve compression by osseous pathology[6] CT angiography can be sometimes useful in cases of nerve compression by vascular causes or aberrant vessel. The peripheral nerve tumors can be visible on CT imaging, however, it is inferior to MRI in characterization and origin of peripheral nerve masses.[7] The larger peripheral nerve such as sciatic nerve may be seen on CT, however, morphology of nerve and various pathologies cannot be assessed due to poor contrast resolution.[8]

Ultrasound

A recent advancement in high-resolution US has made increase use of US for initial assessment of peripheral nerve. Newer high end on US machine and higher frequency linear transducer enables better visualization of peripheral nerves.[9] The special resolution of US is comparable to MRI and scores over MRI due to ability of US to perform dynamic study, cost effective, and easy availability and less time consuming. However, there is long learning curve in accurate assessment of PNS to make accurate diagnosis.

Technique

High frequency linear transducer with 12–18 MHz is generally used to assess the peripheral nerves. The nerves are assessed by placing the transducer on skin surface in transverse and longitudinal sections **(Figs. 2A and B)**. Proper depth and focus are of utmost importance for optimal visualization of nerves. An extended field of view and panoramic view **(Fig. 3)** are helpful for entire nerve length visualization. Color Doppler study is useful for assessing the vascularity of nerve pathology. Normal nerve shows no or minimal vascularity on Doppler. Dynamic scanning is the most useful to identify the neuropathy due to instability. The advantages and limitation of US are mentioned in **Table 1**.

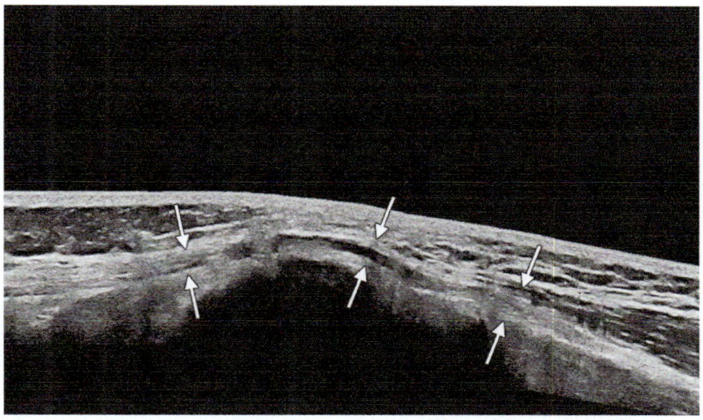

Fig. 3: Ultrasound (US) panoramic view shows extended length of ulnar nerve (arrows) in arm and forearm.

US Appearance

In transverse plane, nerve appears as round to oval with hypoechoic areas corresponding to fascicles separated by hyperechoic interfascicular perineum (honey-combing appearance). In longitudinal plane, it appears as bundles of hypoechoic linear areas with hyperechoic lines in between, corresponding to perineurium giving fibrillary appearance.[10] The epineurium is seen as thin hyperechoic layer surrounding in nerve **(Figs. 4A and B)**. On US, nerves show minimal anisotropy compared to tendons. US assessment of peripheral nerve includes size of nerve, echotexture, fascicular morphology, course and continuity of nerve, vascularity of nerve, and status of adjacent structures. Abnormal nerve may show diffuse or focal nerve enlargement, enlarged fascicles, loss of fascicular pattern, or increased vascularity on Doppler study **(Figs. 5A and B)**. Perineural soft tissue changes can also be assessed on US. In addition, US can identify changes in muscle such as muscle atrophy in denervation when compared to contralateral side.[11]

Table 1: Advantages and limitations of ultrasound (US) and magnetic resonance imaging (MRI).

Imaging	*Advantages*	*Limitations*
US	• Very good spatial resolution • Dynamic assessment • Low cost • Easily available • Nonionizing • US-guided procedures or biopsy • Quick	• Operator dependent • Long learning curve • Deeper structures cannot be evaluated • Poor resolution in obese patients • Bony lesion may not be seen
MRI	• Excellent contrast and spatial resolution • Three dimensional • Deeper structures can be evaluated • Less operator dependent • Evaluation of muscles • Bony lesions/marrow edema can be seen • Research potential	• Higher cost • Contraindications to MR (Pace maker, claustrophobia, MR incompatible implants) • Long duration time • Static examination

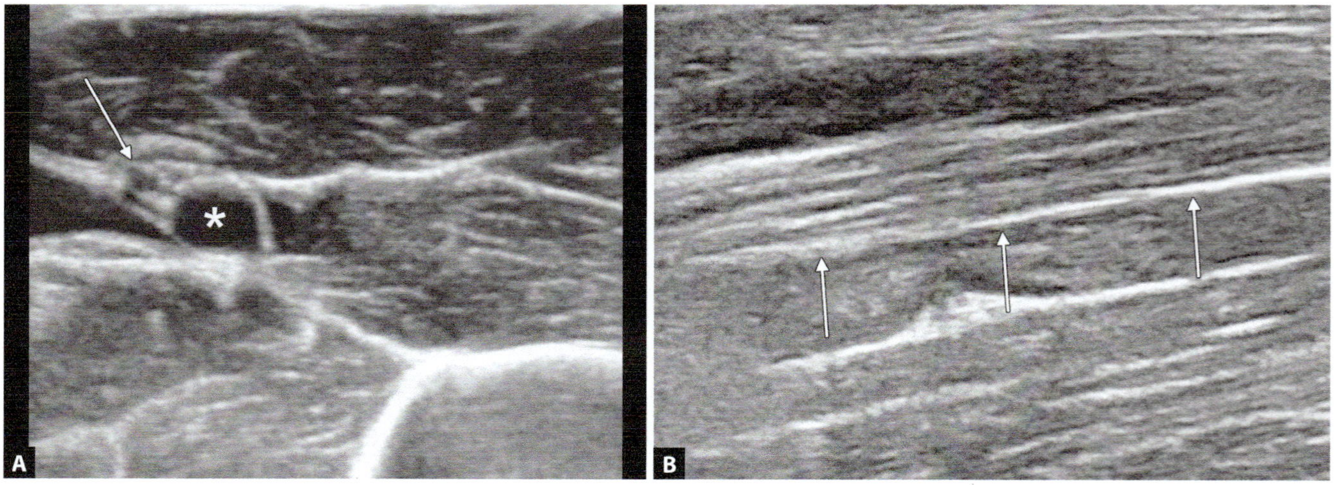

Figs. 4A and B: Ultrasound (US) appearance of normal nerve. (A) Short axis image showing honeycomb appearance of median nerve (arrow); (B) Long-axis image showing fascicular pattern of median nerve (arrows). Star (*) depicts brachial artery.

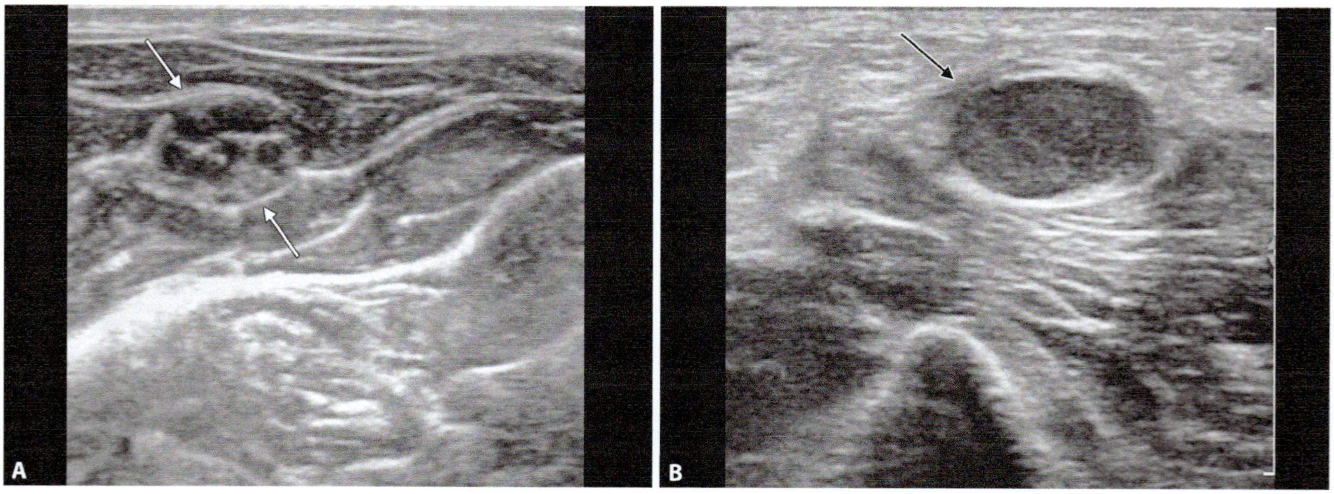

Figs. 5A and B: Abnormal US appearance of nerve. (A and B) The images show thickening with fascicular enlargement (white arrows) (A) and loss of fascicular pattern (black arrow) (B).

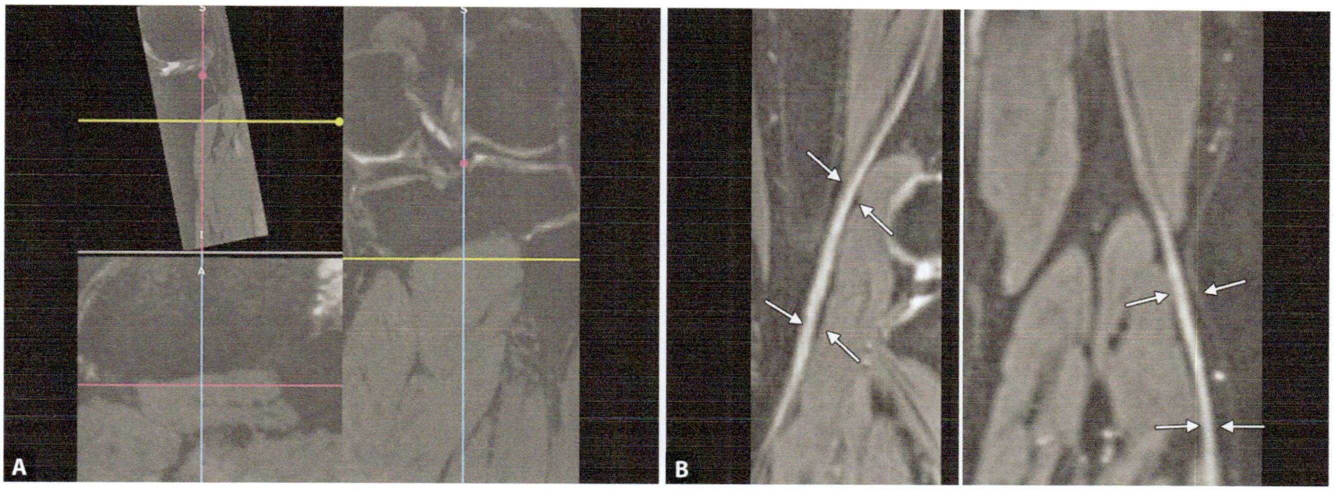

Figs. 6A and B: (A) Multiplanar reconstruction (MPR) technique; (B) Curved MPR images show better visualization of course of nerve (arrows).

Magnetic Resonance Imaging

Magnetic resonance imaging is a noninvasive, radiation-free technique and useful in direct visualization of peripheral nerve trunk. Due to high special resolution of MRI, the fascicular patter can be identified. Perineural soft tissue and deeper structures can be easily evaluated on MRI. It is less operator dependent as compared to US. The advantages and limitation of MRI are mentioned in **Table 1**. The MR protocols for nerve imaging may be different at various institutes or organizations. The routine sequences for MR neurography at our institute are given here.

- T1W nonfat suppressed axial
- T2W fat-suppressed axial
- T2 W fat-suppressed coronal or sagittal (optional)
- T2 space (sampling perfection with application optimized contrast)
- 3D PSIF (reversed FISP, fast imaging with steady-state free precession)
- Diffusion-weighted imaging (DWI)/diffusion tensor imaging (DTI)
- Postcontrast T1W fat-saturated axial and coronal (on case basis in infection/inflammatory conditions or tumors).

The MR neurography is often done by using heavily T2-weighted acquisition with long echo times (>90 ms) and saturation bands to decrease signal from surrounding vascular structure.[12] The 3D diffusion-weighted PSIF (reversed FISP) sequence is also obtained using heavily T2-weighted MR technique with suppression of adjacent the vessel signal. Additionally, 3D sequences enable formation of multiplanar reconstruction (MPR) and maximum intensity projection (MIP) images **(Figs. 6A and B)**.

"Magic angle phenomenon," similar to tendons, can be seen in nerves, when their orientation is at around 55° angle to magnetic field in T2-weighted sequences with long TE.[13] The magic angle signal changes should be considered while reading MR images, especially when only abnormal nerve signal present and there are no associated changes.

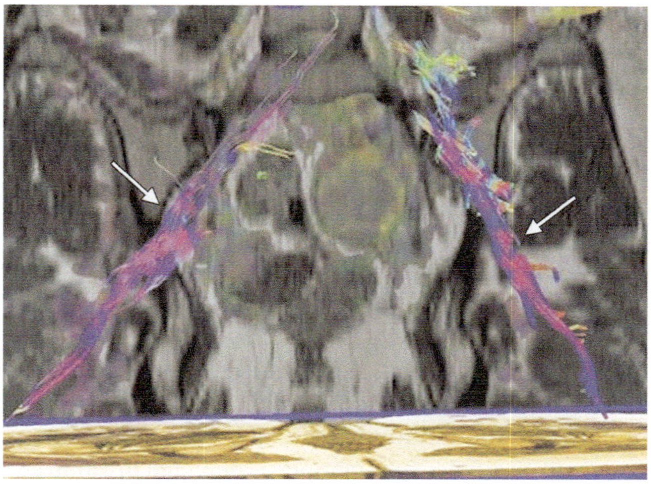

Fig. 7: Diffusion tensor imaging with tractography of bilateral sciatic nerves (arrows).

Intravenous gadolinium can be useful to see enhancement when there is breach in blood brain barrier. It is especially helpful in infectious or inflammatory and neoplastic conditions of nerve. Normally, the nerve shows little or no contrast enhancement.[14]

Diffusion tensor imaging uses tissue anisotropy to produce images. The measurements caused by water molecules motion in anisotropic media is used to give information about architecture and orientation of tissues. The DWI can be useful in the evaluation of larger peripheral nerves compared to smaller nerves.[15,16] Tractography is the mathematical rendered technique derived from DTI used to obtain 3D images of fiber tracts and evaluation of the course and direction of nerve fibers **(Fig. 7)**.[17,18] It consists

Table 2: Normal and abnormal appearance of nerve on magnetic resonance neurography.[22]

Features	*Normal nerve*	*Abnormal nerve*
Size of nerve	Similar to adjacent arteries, gradually decreases distally	Focal or diffuse enlargement, larger than adjacent arteries
Signal intensity	Isointense to skeletal muscle on T1- and T2-weighted imaging; isointense to minimally hyperintense on STIR and fat-suppressed T2-weighted imaging	Hyperintense on T2-weighted imaging similar to adjacent veins
Fascicular morphology	Seen on T1- and T2-weighted imaging	Enlargement or disruption of single or multiple fascicles
Course	Smooth without focal deviations, outlined by perineural fat	Focal or diffuse deviations, discontinuity
Continuity	Maintained	Discontinuous or complete transaction
Postcontrast	Absent except in areas of deficient blood-nerve barrier, such as dorsal nerve root ganglion	Present in tumors and infections because of disruption of blood-nerve barrier
Perineural fat	Preserved best seen on T1 non-FS	Effaced

(FS: fat saturated)

of mean apparent diffusion coefficient (ADC) and mean fractional anisotropy (FA). Fiber tracking acquisition uses a spin-echo single-shot diffusion-weighted EPI sequence with fat suppression. Color coding is given to the direction of anisotropic structures. Any disease or injury to the nerve fibers will change nerve architecture which can be depicted by this technique.[19,20] The tractography is currently useful for evaluation of large nerve bundles.

The MR evaluation of peripheral nerves includes assessment of signal intensity of nerves, size of nerve, morphology or fascicular pattern, course and continuity of nerves, perineural fat and surrounding soft tissue, status of muscles, and tendons.[21] The appearance of nerve on magnetic resonance neurography is depicted in **Table 2.**[22]

Signal Intensity

On T1WI, normally nerves have intermediate signal intensity compared to muscles **(Fig. 8A)**. Nonfat-saturated T1 images are best to evaluate the nerve anatomy and course. On T2WI normal nerves show isointense signal intensity to that of muscle.[11] On fluid sensitive fat-suppressed sequences such as SPAIR, T2WIFS or STIR sequences peripheral nerves show as isointense or minimally hyperintense to that of muscle **(Fig. 8B)**. PSIF sequence suppressed the signal from adjacent vascular structures and nerve appears minimally hyperintense with clear demarcation **(Fig. 8C)**. Increased signal intensity on fluid-sensitive sequences which is similar to adjacent vessels suggests nerve pathology. Most of the nerve tumors appears hyperintense on fluid-sensitive sequences and hypo- to isointense T1 images.

Size and Fascicular Pattern of Peripheral Nerve

The neural injury/neuropathy is suggested by presence of enlargement or thinning of nerve, enlarged single or multiple fascicles, loss of the normal fascicular appearance, or ill-defined perifascicular fat. The anatomic changes can be easily picked up on MR in large nerve such as sciatic, median, or ulnar nerve. Fascicular pattern of larger nerve are often visible on axial nonfat-saturated T1- and T2-weighted images.

Course and Continuity

Normal peripheral nerves have regular course without any lump or bumps. Branches of peripheral nerve normally directed to supplying muscles. The peripheral nerves have well-defined margins surrounding by perineural fat which can easily identified on nonfat saturated T1- and T2-weighted images. Normal variant in course of peripheral nerve sometime can be seen in form of bifid nerve.[23] The abnormal nerve may have deviated course or discontinuous which can be seen on MR neurography. However, one should be careful for interpreting MR artifacts such as metallic artifacts as nerve pathology.

Perineural Fat

There is layer of fat surrounding the nerve trunk, which can be easily seen in T1- or T2-weighted images. At times it may be difficult to recognize perineural fat in poorly build individuals. Increased signal intensity of perineural fat is often seen on fluid-sensitive sequences like STIR images in cases of inflammatory pathologies.

Muscles

In acute setting, muscle denervation is best depicted by the STIR or T2 fat-suppressed sequences which occur due to muscle edema.[24] There are minimal changes in T1-weighted images in acute setting. The early stages there is increase in extracellular fluid within the muscles which show increase signal intensity. However, muscle bulk is not

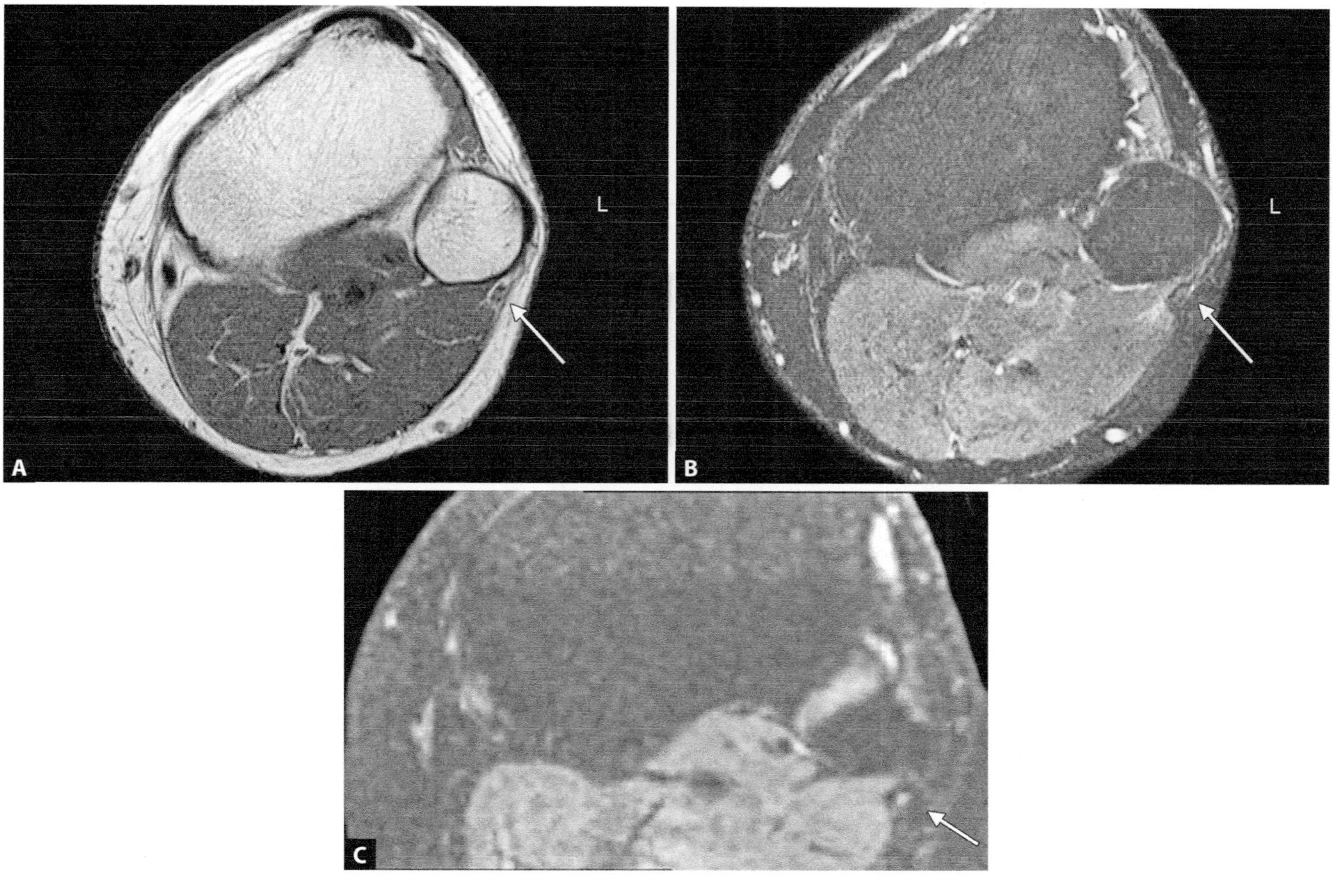

Figs. 8A to C: Normal MR appearance of nerve. (A and B) Nonfat-suppressed T1 weighted image and fat-suppressed T2-weighted image showing common peroneal nerve (arrows) at the level of fibular neck. Note the hyperintense perineural fat on T1WI; (C) PSIF sequence shows minimally hyperintense normal nerve with clear demarcation (arrow).

affected in early stages. Nerve injury leads to denervation of the muscles supplied by the nerve. Identification of denervated muscles helps to recognize the peripheral nerve involved and also helps to differentiate between other muscle pathologies such as myositis, muscle infections, or infarcts.

In chronic denervation, there is muscle atrophy and fatty replacement of muscles. This leads to increased T1-signal intensity on nonfat-saturated images. There is also increased signal intensity on T2-weighted images and STIR images. Reduced muscle bulk can be identified easily if comparison is made to contralateral side.

Specific Peripheral Nerve Pathologies

Nerve Injury

Peripheral nerve injury occurs due to trauma, various mechanisms of traction, shear stress and ischemia, in isolation or combination.[19] The various imaging features depend on congestion of nerve, edema, fibrosis, and axonal damage.

Wallerian degeneration is response to nerve injury distal to site of nerve injury by the axon, Schwann cell, and macrophages. It starts immediately within few minutes after the nerve injury. Initially there is degeneration of axon with increase in immune and inflammatory response distal to site of injury followed by the regrowth of axon stump toward distal stump. If regeneration of nerve may take months to years, if regeneration does not happen, the injury segment is replaced by fibrous tissue. There is focal swelling of axon stump known as neuroma.[25] The classification of nerve injury was given by Seddon, who categorized nerve injuries into three grades, from least to most severe, as neurapraxia, axonotmesis, and neurotmesis **(Fig. 9, Table 3)**.[19,26,27] The neuropraxia refers to the transient nerve conduction block causing transient sensory and motor loss followed by full rapid and complete recovery. Axonotmesis referred to damage to axon but intact epineurium. In neurotmesis there is complete transaction or discontinuity of nerve. The Sunderland classification **(Table 3)** is currently used by most of the surgeons. It has five grades and these grades are similar to Seddon classification of increasing severity of nerve injury. Dellon and MacKinnon described the sixth grade that includes incomplete or mixed nerve damages.[28] In incomplete damage, a part of the nerve

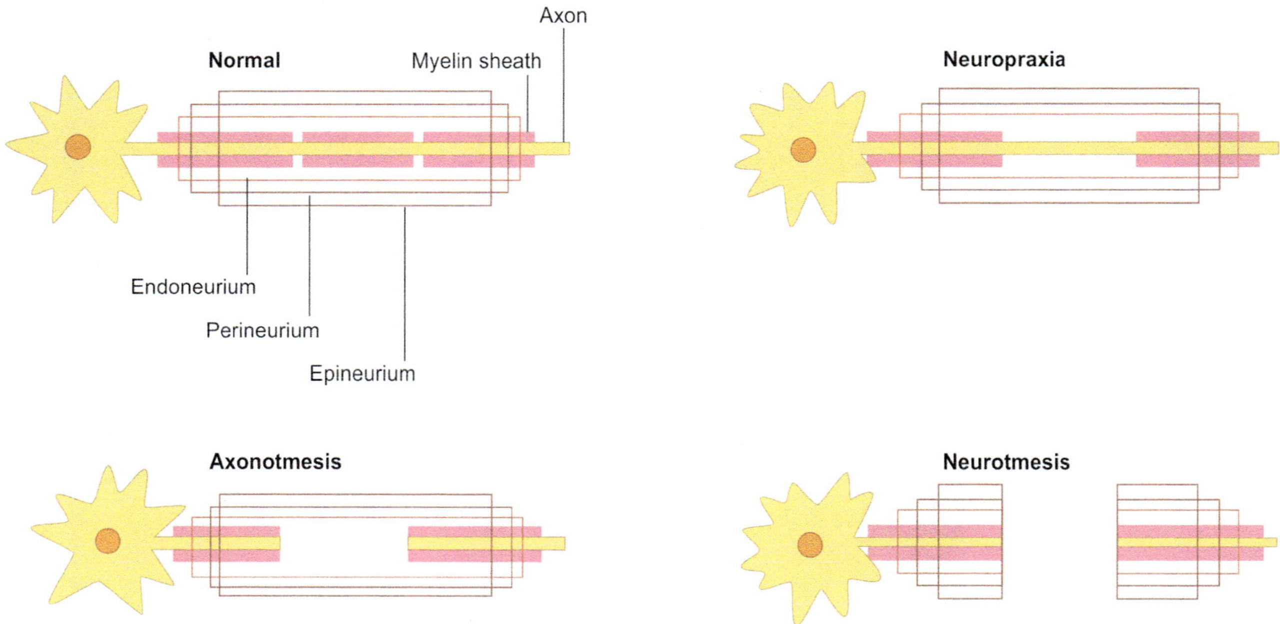

Fig. 9: Grading of nerve injury.

Table 3: Seddon and Sunderland classifications of peripheral nerve injury with the magnetic resonance (MR) and ultrasound (US) features.[26,27]

Sunderland (Grade)	*Seddon*	*Nerve injury*	*MR features*	*US features*
I	Neuropraxia	Focal demyelination	Nerve: Hyperintense ± increased caliber	Nerve: Hypoechoic ± increased caliber
II	Axonotmesis	Axon	Nerve: Hyperintense ± increased caliber. Expanded fascicles Denervation changes in muscles	Nerve: Hypoechoic ± increased caliber Expanded fascicles
III	Axonotmesis	Axon endoneurium	Nerve: Hyperintense ± increased caliber. Expanded fascicles (More marked than grade II) Denervation changes in muscles	Nerve: Focal hypoechogenicity with increase in caliber with muscle: Altered echogenicity of the denervated muscles
IV	Axonotmesis	Axon endoneurium perineurium	Nerve: Neuroma at ends with discontinuous fascicles Denervation changes in muscles	Nerve: Hypoechoic neuroma in continuity with the nerve with loss of fascicular pattern Muscle: Altered echogenicity of the denervated muscles
V	Neurotmesis	Complete nerve transection	Nerve: End bulb neuroma with separation Denervation changes in muscles	Nerve : Hypoechoic neuroma at end with surrounding heterogenicity Muscle: Altered echogenicity of the denervated muscles
VI	Neurotmesis	Mixed level of injury	Combination of above findings Fibrosis with sudden signal changes of the nerves.	Nerve: Hypoechoic enlarged with mixed findings of fibrosis, discontinuity or neuroma formation

fibers (circumference) is damaged while the rest of the fibers are intact. In mixed nerve damages, all tissues of the nerve are involved. The recovery of nerve injury depends on type of damage and severity of every nerve fiber.

In neurapraxic injury, the nerve may appear as swollen with hypoechoic appearance on US **(Fig. 10)** and hyperintense on T2 fat-suppressed and PSIF sequences **(Figs. 11A and B)**. In axotomies, the nerve appears

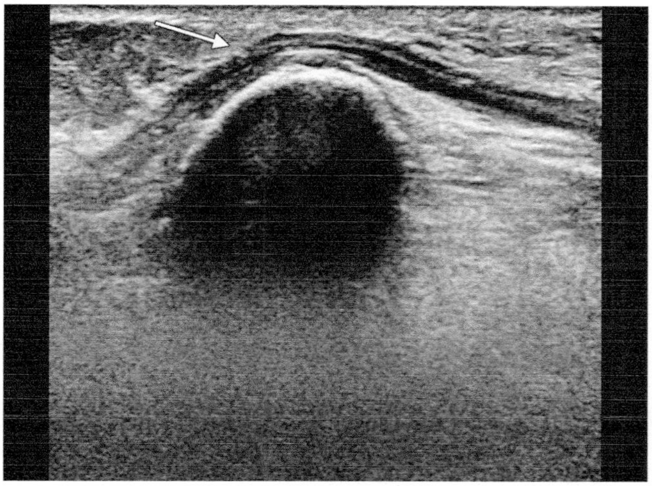

Fig. 10: High-resolution ultrasound (US) of ulnar nerve shows hypoechoic appearance of nerve (arrow) in stretch injury (neuropraxia).

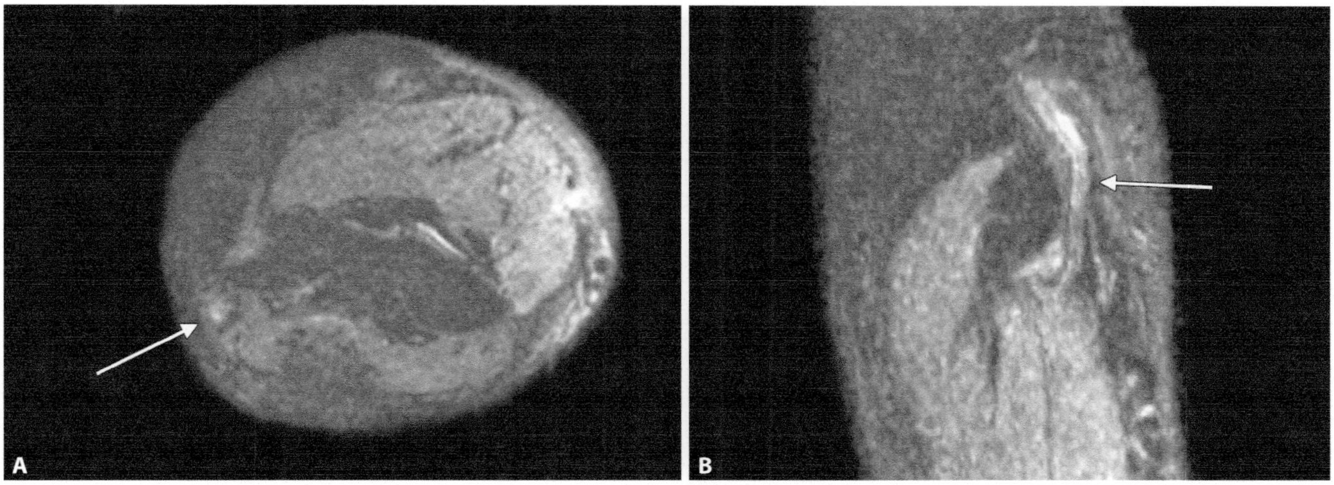

Figs. 11A and B: Neuropraxia of ulnar nerve. 3D PSIF axial (A) and sagittal (B) reconstruction shows patchy hyperintensities in ulnar nerve without disruption (arrows).

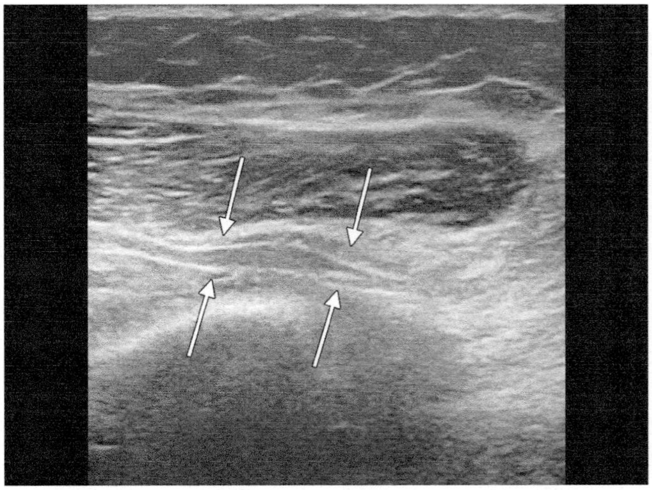

Fig. 12: High-resolution ultrasound (US) in post-traumatic case shows ulnar nerve injury with neuroma in continuity of nerve (arrows).

swollen and hypoechoic with enlarged fascicles on US and MR with more marked findings than neuropraxic injury. Neuroma-in-continuity is seen as fusiform hypoechoic thickened nerve with decreased nerve echotexture on US **(Fig. 12)** and fusiform thickened hyperintense nerve on MRI **(Figs. 13A and B)**.[26] The complete disruption of nerve fibers can be identified on US in cases of transaction injury due to glass and sharp objects, etc. A neuroma formation can be seen at both ends of transacted nerve which appear as hypoechoic thickening or a bulbous mass at nerve ends **(Figs. 14 and 15)**. High resolution US or MR neurography, both can depict the nerve injury. The various features of imaging are given in **Table 3**.

Nerve Compression

Nerve compression can occur due to kinetic and static causes. Kinetic compression often arises during motion

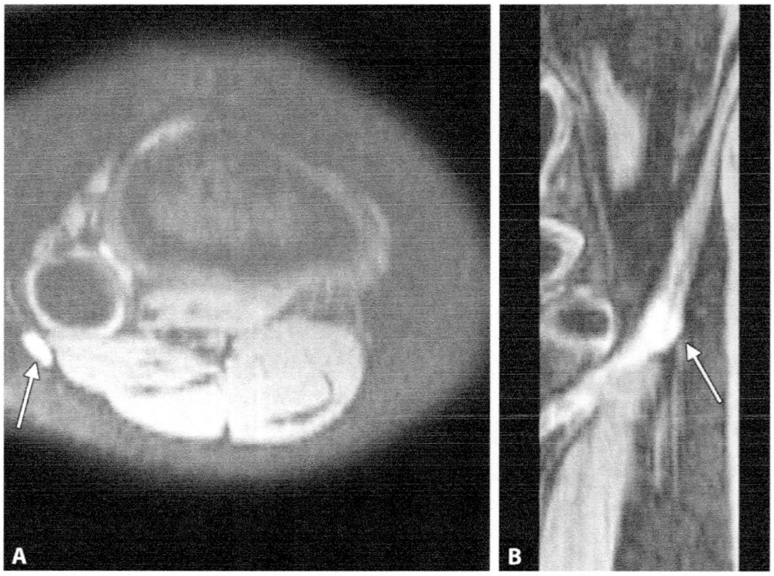

Figs. 13A and B: Neuroma in continuity. 3D PISF axial (A) and coronal reformatted (B) MR neurography images show focal fusiform thickening (arrows) of common peroneal nerve near fibular head with continuation of nerve fibers.

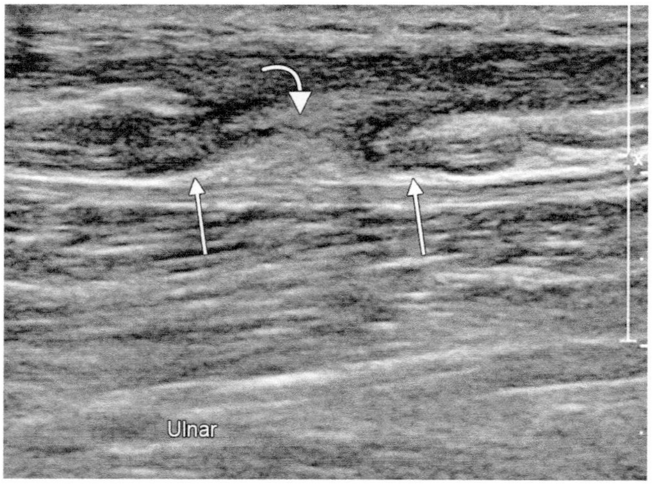

Fig. 14: High-resolution ultrasound (US) in post-traumatic case show complete transaction of ulnar nerve (curved arrow) in forearm with end nerve neuroma formation at both ends (white straight arrows).

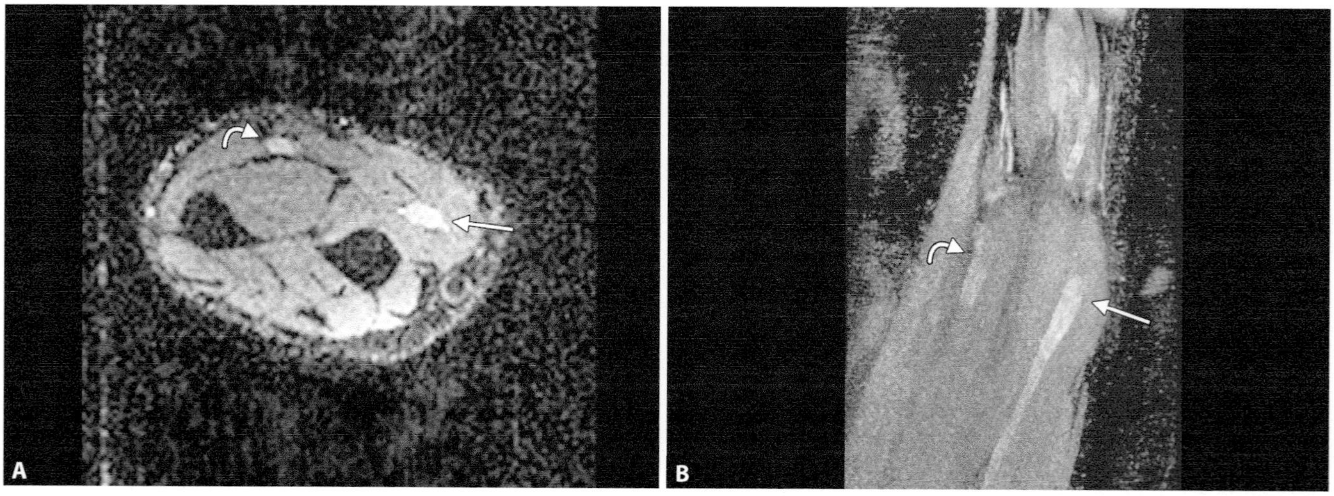

Figs. 15A and B: Cut injury at the level of forearm. 3D PSIF axial (A) and coronal reconstructed neurography images (B) show complete transaction of median (straight arrows) and ulnar nerve (curved arrows) with end neuroma formation.

or mobility of joints. Static causes include compression of nerve by adjacent tissue, which may be pathological such as infections, tumor, bony fragment, or aberrant/ anomalous in nature.[4] Commonly, the compression occur at specific locations where the nerves passes through the anatomic space or tunnels such as cubital and carpal tunnels **(Figs. 16 to 18)**, or in an unspecified location where a space occupying lesion can cause compression of the nerve **(Figs. 19 and 20)**. Mostly, the sensory component is arranged in periphery compared to the motor component in the mixed nerves. Therefore, nerve compression is more likely to have early sensory signs. Presently, the peripheral nerve compression is commonly graded based on symptoms, clinical examination results,

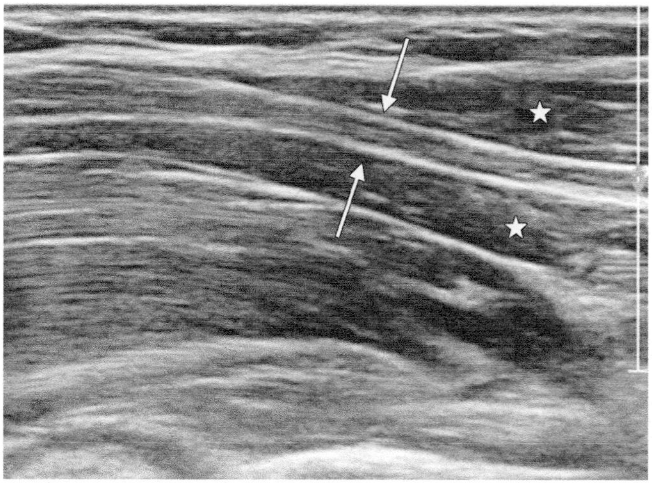

Fig. 16: High-resolution ultrasound (US) (long axis) showing compression of median nerve (white arrows) between two heads of pronator teres (stars).

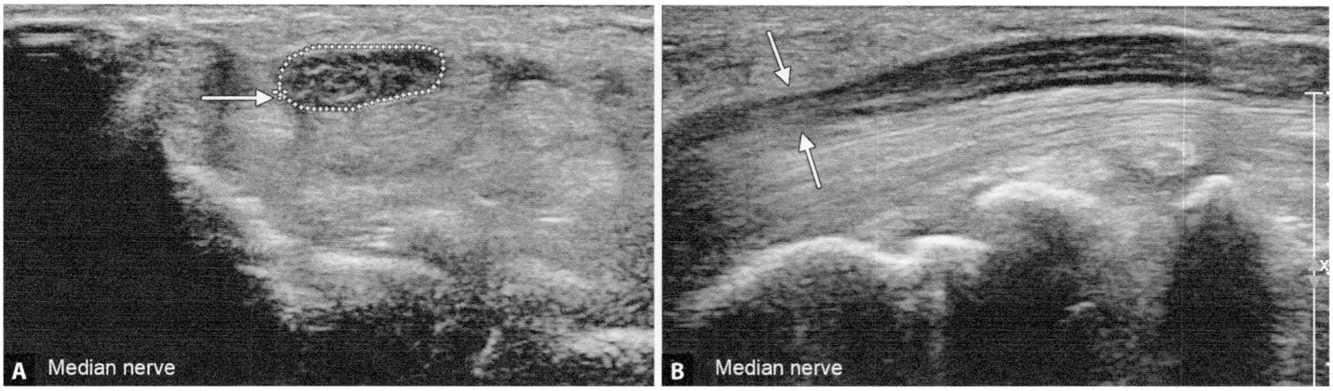

Figs. 17A and B: Carpal tunnel syndrome. High-resolution ultrasound (US), short axis (A) and long axis (B) shows increased cross sectional area of median nerve (arrow in A) with typical compression at flexor retinaculum (arrows in B).

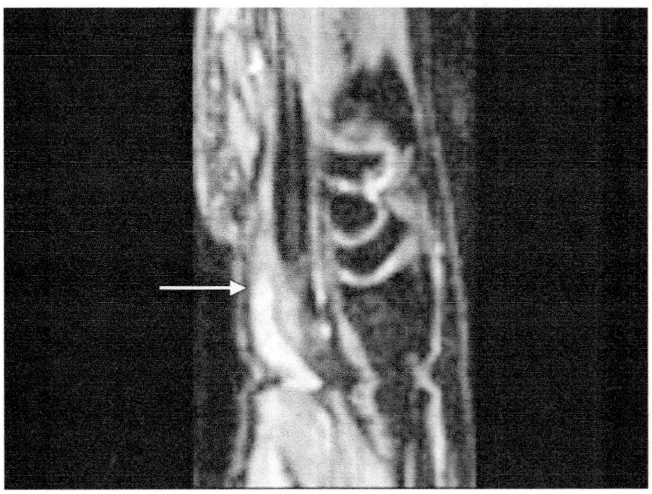

Fig. 18: Sagittal reformatted 3D PSIF images of wrist show focal enlargement and hyperintensity of median nerve (arrow) in carpal tunnel syndrome.

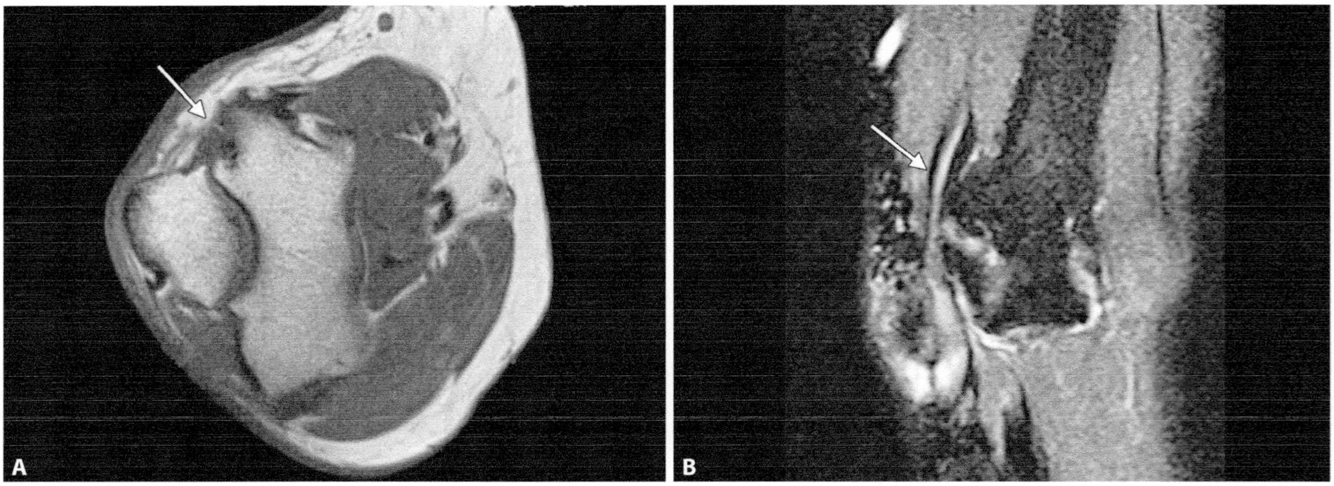

Figs. 19A and B: Compression of ulnar nerve at cubital fossa. Axial nonfat-suppressed T1-weighted image (A) and oblique fat-suppressed T2-weighted image (B) showing compression of ulnar nerve (arrows) by osteophytes and fibrotic tissue due to old injury of elbow.

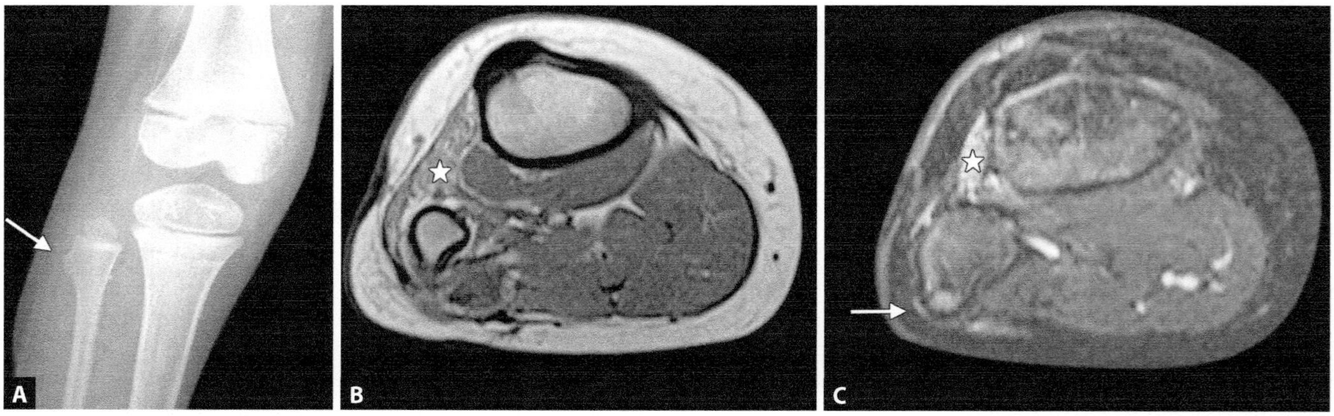

Figs. 20A to C: Nerve compression due to osteochondroma. AP radiograph of knee (A), axial T1 nonfat-suppressed image (B) and axial T2 fat-suppressed image (C) showing compression of common peroneal nerve (white arrow) by fibular osteochondroma (black arrow) with denervation changes (atrophy, increased T1 signal and fatty infiltration) in extensors muscles (stars).

and electrodiagnostic findings. The various tunnels and known entrapment sites along the course of the commonly imaged peripheral nerves are described in **Table 4**.[29]

The compression of nerve can be detected on careful examination with high resolution US. Various US features of compression include thinning of nerve or reduction in diameter or cross sectional area, enlargement of nerve proximal or distal to compression site.[9] The nerve cross-sectional area can be calculated on US. In larger-sized nerves such as sciatic, median, ulnar nerves or common peroneal nerve, loss of fascicular morphology can be seen. For smaller nerve, careful examinations with higher frequency transducer (17–24 MHz) are very useful in assessment of morphology of nerve.

Nerve Infections

Mycobacterium leprae is the causative organism of a chronic disease "leprosy," which is common cause of curable peripheral neuropathy. The ulnar nerve is often involved in leprosy. Other nerves such as median, posterior auricular, fibular, and posterior tibial nerves are also involved. The disease process causes enlargement of nerve which can be detected on imaging US or MRI.[30] Subacute phase may show calcifications of nerve in leprosy. On US, the abnormal nerve appears as hypoechoic enlarged nerve with enlarged fascicles **(Figs. 21A and B)**, loss of fascicular pattern, or asymmetry of fascicles **(Figs. 22 and 23)**.[31,32] Color Doppler can be helpful which may show increased vascularity in lepromatous nerve **(Figs. 22A and B)**. Sometimes, infection of nerve results in abscess formation which appears as homogeneous fusiform collection hyperintense T2 and hypointense on T1 images. DWIs may show central diffusion restriction **(Figs. 24A to C)**. US shows hypoechoic collection along the course of nerve in cases of nerve abscess. Pyogenic infections of nerve are often direct extension of infection from adjacent tissue **(Fig. 25)**.

Table 4: Various sites of compression of peripheral nerves.[29]

Nerve	*Sites*	*Remarks*
Ulnar nerve	• The arcade of Struthers • Medial epicondyle at the entry the cubital fossa • Within the cubital fossa • Proximal forearm at pronator teres • Guyon canal	The arcade of Struthers, a fibrous space posteriorly made up of intermuscular septum, the internal brachial ligament, deep fascia
Median nerve	• Distal arm by Struthers ligament • At elbow by biceps aponeurosis • At Elbow between two heads of the pronator teres. • Proximal forearm by flexor digitorum superficialis muscle • Carpal tunnel by retinaculum	Struthers ligament is a fibrous residue, between anteromedial distal humerus to medial epicondyle in 2.7 % individuals The most common nerve entrapment is carpal tunnel syndrome
Radial nerve	• At radial head between the brachioradialis and joint capsule • At radial neck by the leash of Henry, branches of the radial recurrent artery • Margin of the extensor carpi radialis brevis muscle • The arcade of Frohse • At wrist (Wartenberg syndrome)	The arcade of Frohse is a thick tendinous proximal margin of the superficial head of the supinator Wartenberg syndrome or cheiralgia paresthetica, is entrapment of the superficial branch of the radial nerve in the distal forearm or wrist
Femoral nerve	At the level of the inguinal ligament • The iliacus compartment • At Groin in hernia repair, femoral puncture, gynecological and hip surgeries	Iliacus compartment, a space between the ilio-psoas and iliacus fascia
Sciatic nerve	• Greater sciatic notch (piriformis muscle syndrome) • At the level of the ischial tuberosity by the biceps femoris	The sciatic nerve at greater sciatic notch may compressed by the pyriformis muscle or its pathology, known as piriformis syndrome
Common peroneal nerve	• Fibular neck. • Proximal attachment of peroneus longus	Extrinsic compression, stretching or trauma can cause nerve injury at these sites
Posterior tibial nerve	Tarsal tunnel (Tarsal tunnel syndrome)	Tarsal tunnel syndrome caused by trauma (fracture, surgery, and scarring), adjacent tissue pathologies (tumor, ganglia, varicosities), anomalous muscles and foot deformities
Interdigital nerve	Intermetatarsal space (Morton neuroma)	The entrapment of the nerve against the transverse metatarsal ligament or nerve ischemia causes formation of neuroma

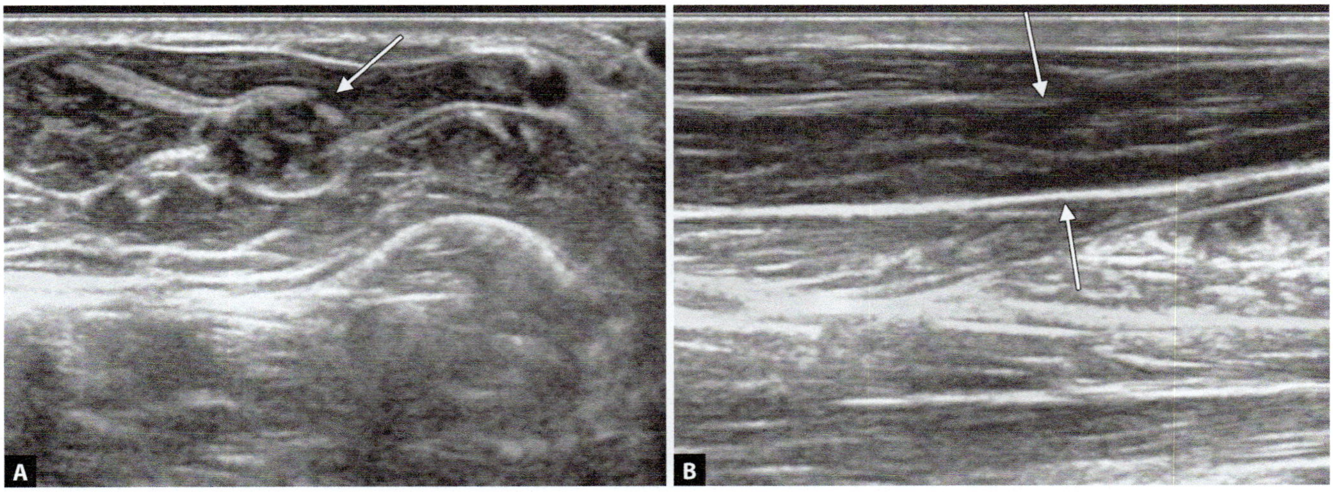

Figs. 21A and B: Leprotic neuropathy of ulnar nerve. High-resolution ultrasound (US) short axis (A) and long axis (B) shows diffuse enlarged ulnar nerve with symmetric enlargement of fascicles (white arrows).

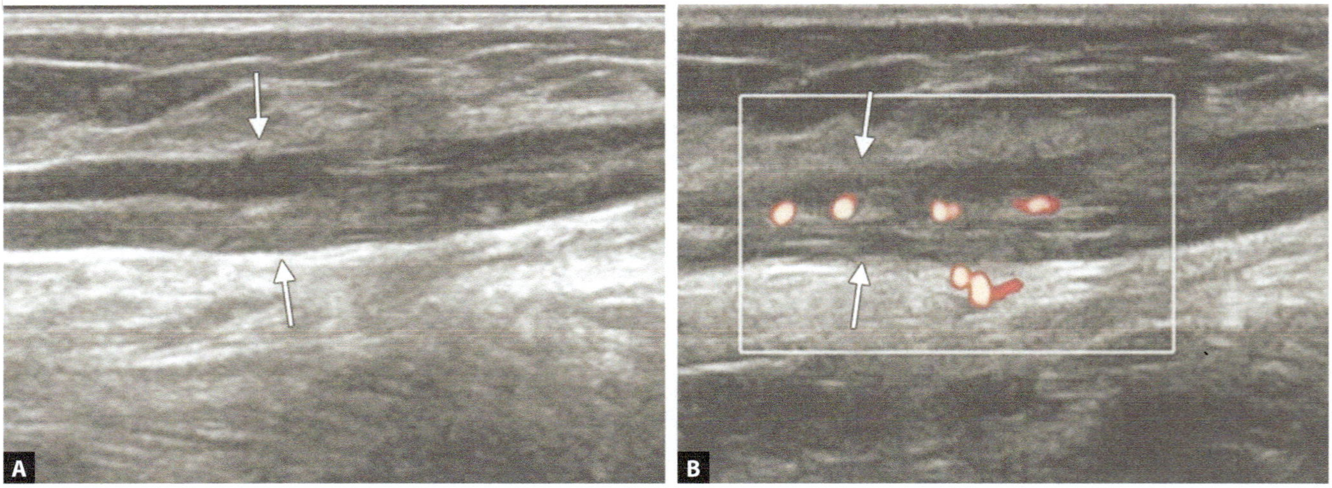

Figs. 22A and B: Asymmetric fascicular pattern. High-resolution ultrasound (US) long axis, gray scale (A) and color Doppler (B) images showing enlarged thickened ulnar nerve with asymmetric fascicles (arrows in A) with increased color flow (arrows in B) in leprotic neuropathy.

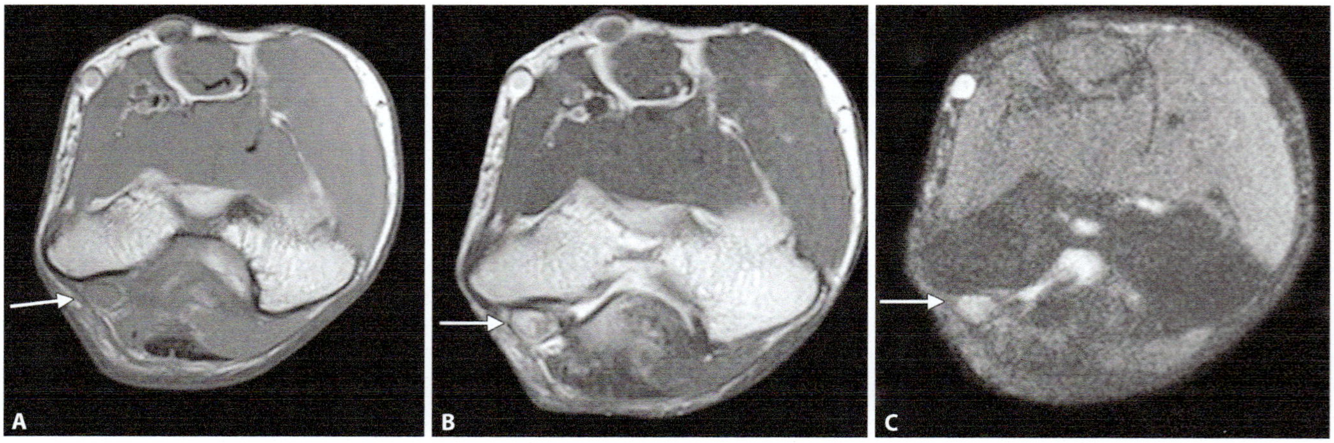

Figs. 23A to C: MRI of leprotic nerve. Axial T1 nonfat suppressed (A), T2 nonfat-suppressed (B) and T2 fat-suppressed (C) images showing enlarged and thickened ulnar nerve with asymmetric fascicles (arrows) in leprotic neuropathy.

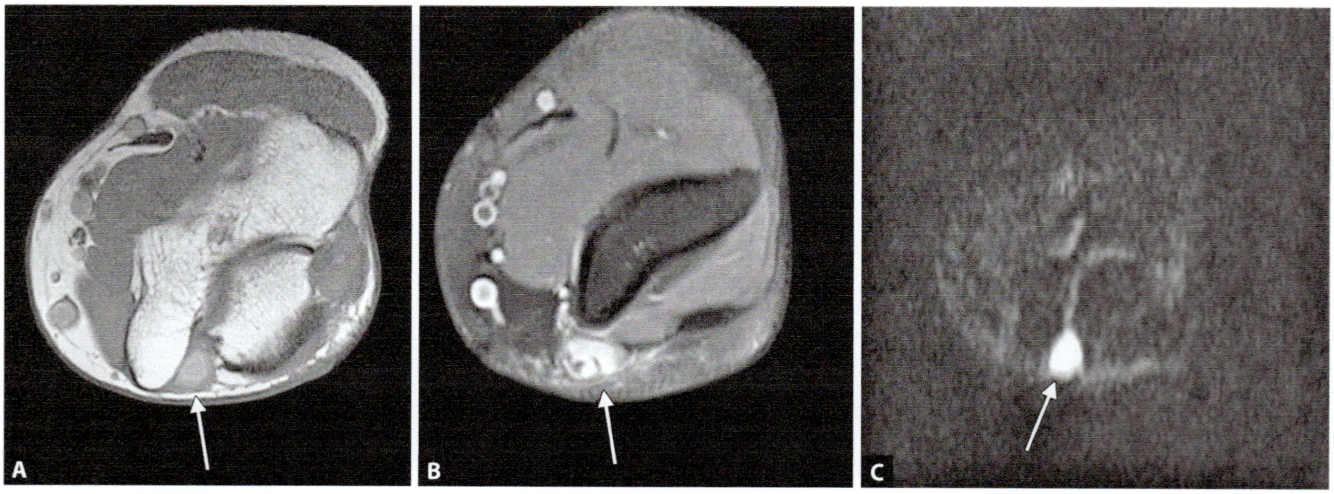

Figs. 24A to C: MRI of leprotic nerve abscess. (A and B) Axial T1 nonfat-suppressed and PD fat-suppressed images at elbow level showing T1 hypointense and PD hyperintense lesion in ulnar nerve (arrows); (C) DWI shows diffusion restriction within the abscess (arrow).

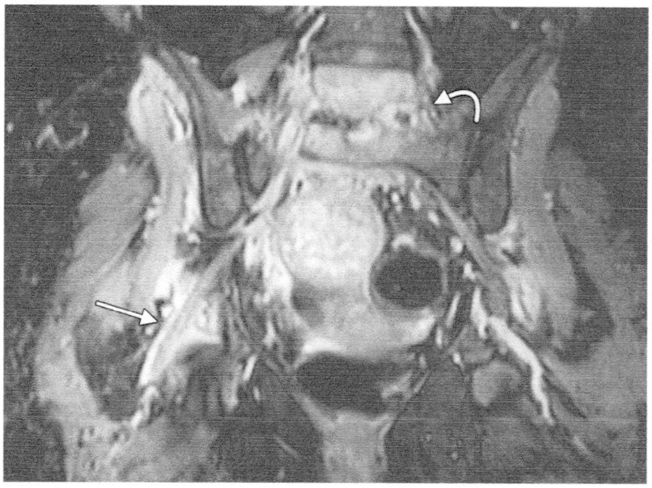

Fig. 25: Pyogenic infective neuritis: T2 fat-suppressed coronal MR image shows hyperintensity of sciatic nerve (straight arrow) with surrounding inflammation in case of pyogenic discitis (curved arrow) and pyogenic collections. Sciatic nerve was secondarily involved.

Nerve Tumors and Tumor-like Conditions

Peripheral nerve sheath tumor (PNST) is the most commonly seen tumor of peripheral nerve. If regional muscle denervation changes are seen in the adjacent or distal to the tumor, one should look for the PNST. Also the large mass tends to impinge the nerve may lead to muscle denervation changes. The nerve tumor is suggested by the "tail sign" (where the mass tapers at one end) or "fusiform-shaped" tumor (where the mass tapers at both ends), "fascicular sign" (enlarged nerve fibers seen in cross-section as multiple small ring-like shapes), target sign (central low signal due to collagenous tissue with peripheral myxoid change on a fluid-sensitive sequence), and "split-fat sign" (fat separating the tumor from adjacent muscles, best seen at tapering margins of the tumor showing its slow growth consequently leading to displacement of the perineural fat planes) **(Figs. 26A to C)**.[25] These lesions show diffuse homogeneous enhancement.[33] Different features of common PNSTs are depicted in **Table 5**.[34]

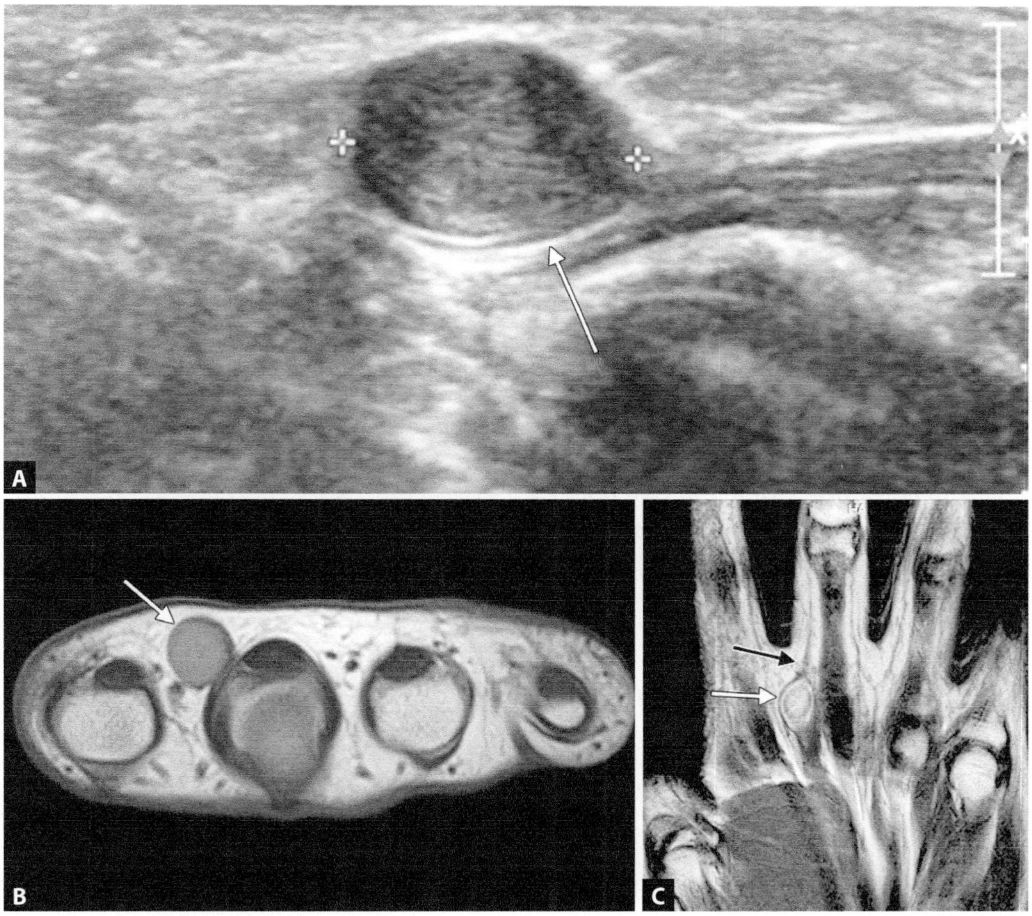

Figs. 26A to C: Schwannoma of digital nerve. High-resolution US in long axis (A) show well-defined fusiform hypoechoic lesion along the course of digital nerve. MRI of same patient: Axial T1 nonfat-suppressed (B) and coronal T2 nonfat-saturated section (C) showing well-defined T1 hypointense and T2 hyperintense "fusiform" lesion with "target sign" (white arrow) and "tail sign" (black arrow) along the course of digital nerve of hand.

Table 5: Imaging characteristics of common nerve tumors.[34]

Imaging features	*Neurofibroma*	*Schwannoma*	*MPNST*
Location	Central	Eccentric	Central
Target sign	+++	+	-
Fascicular sign	+++	+++	+/-
Split fat sign	+++	+++	-
T2 hyperintense thin rim	+	++	-
Cystic degeneration	+/-	++	+/-
Surrounding fat strandings	-	-/+	++
Hemorrhage	-	++	+++
Enhancement	Central and homogeneous	Peripheral, may be heterogeneous	Heterogeneous, with areas of necrosis
Adjacent tissue invasion	-	-	++

(MPNST: malignant peripheral nerve sheath tumor)

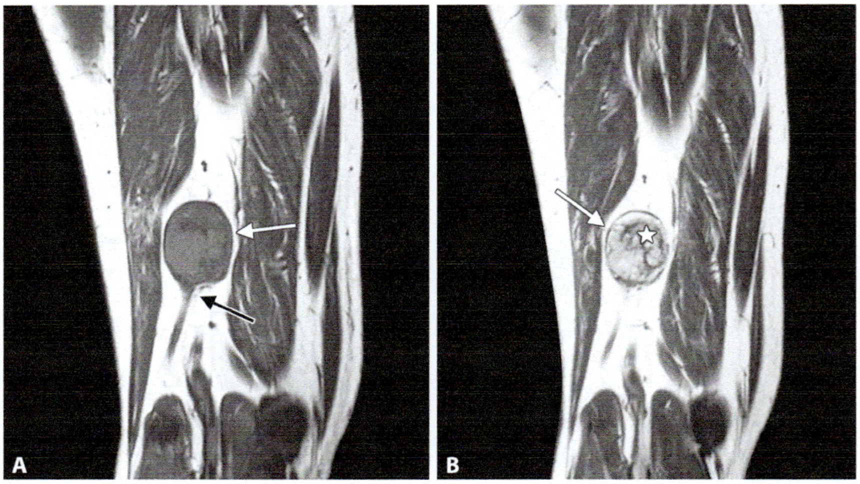

Figs. 27A and B: Coronal nonfat-suppressed T1 (A) and T2 (B) images of thigh showing eccentric well-defined T1-hypointense and T2-hyperintense lesion (white arrows) suggestive of Schwannoma. Note is made of tail sign (black arrow) and few hemorrhagic areas are also seen within the lesion (star).

The ultrasound appearance of peripheral nerve masses are seen as hypoechoic fusiform soft tissue lesion along the course of nerve. The entry or exit of nerve may be seen on careful US examination. The most of the tumors of PNS are generally benign. Heterogeneous appearance of tumor on US may be due to internal hemorrhages or cystic changes.

Schwannoma is more prevalent than neurofibroma, and often shows cystic changes, calcification, and internal hemorrhage **(Figs. 27 and 28)**. Slow growth, stability on follow-up, or underlying history and genetics are useful indicators of benign diagnosis.

Plexiform neurofibroma shows diffuse infiltrative mass lesion and/or associated skin thickening. Plexiform neurofibroma or schwannoma may additionally show "bag of worms" appearance.[35] Schwannomatosis is characterized by numerous schwannomas without bilateral acoustic neuromas. It is a distinct entity from

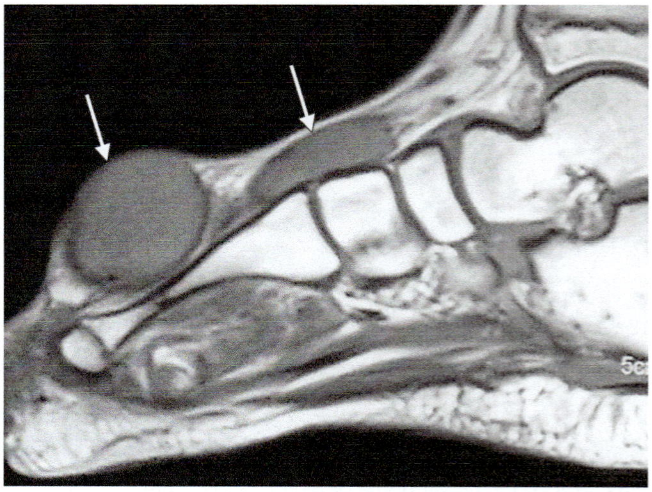

Fig. 28: Neurofibromas. Sagittal T1 nonfat-suppressed section of foot in known case of neurofibromatosis showing T1 hypointense well-defined variable sized and shaped lesions on dorsum of foot.

NF type II which shows acoustic neuromas and exhibits different genetic aberrations.

Malignant PNST can occur in a sporadic fashion (older age and less aggressive) or as part of NF type I (earlier age, increased incidence, and more aggressive). The imaging features which suggest malignant lesion includes large size (>5 cm), heterogeneous appearance, internal hemorrhage and/or necrosis, local tissue invasion or extracompartmental extension, surrounding edema, heterogeneous enhancement **(Fig. 29)**, and low ADC values on DTI (<1.1 mm^2/s) with disrupted and disorganized tracts on tractography.[36]

In lymphoma, there is diffuse infiltration of nerve with nodularity **(Fig. 30)**. The postcontrast MR shows homogeneous contrast enhancement. Diagnosis is often made on nerve biopsy.

Fibrolipomatous hamartomas of nerves is a rare tumor-like condition, characterized by fatty deposition within nerve sheaths. The median nerve is the most commonly affected. Macrodactyly is seen into 30–35% of the cases with involvement of median nerve. On MR neurography, there is prominent serpentiform fascicles bounded by fibrous and fatty tissue within the expanded nerve sheath **(Figs. 31A and B)**.[37,38]

Interdigital neuroma or Morton's neuroma may present with chronic foot pain due to vascular compromised or entrapment of the digital nerve in web spaces of foot against the transverse intermetatarsal ligament (commonly 3rd web space).[39] On US, it appears as hypoechoic ill-defined soft tissue lesion in web space. It may show internal vascularity on Doppler. On MR neurography, it shows hypointense to intermediate signal

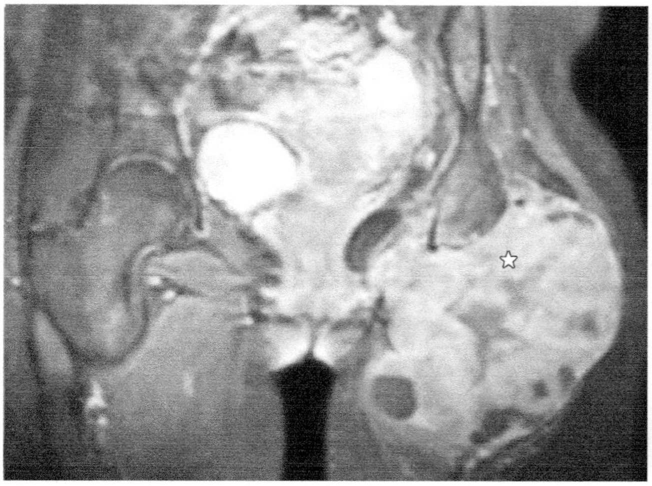

Fig. 29: Malignant peripheral nerve sheath tumor. Postcontrast T1FS coronal section showing heterogeneously enhancing lobulated mass lesion (star) in hip region extending along sciatic notch with local infiltrations of adjacent muscles and bones.

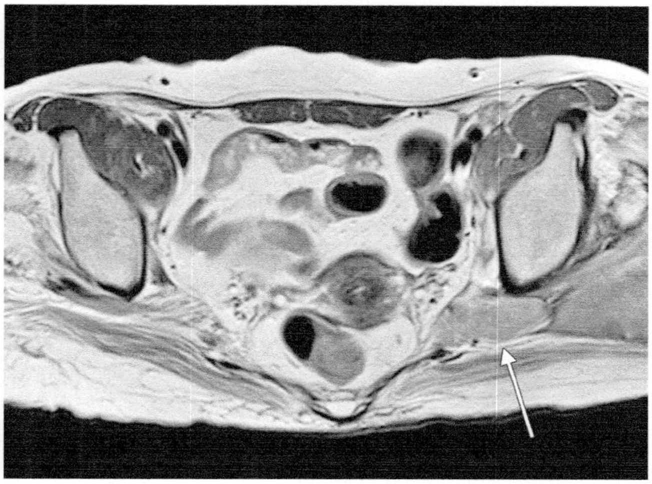

Fig. 30: Lymphomatous involvement of nerve. Axial T2 nonfat-suppressed image showing minimally hyperintense signal intensity with diffuse nodular enlargement of sciatic nerve in known case of lymphoma.

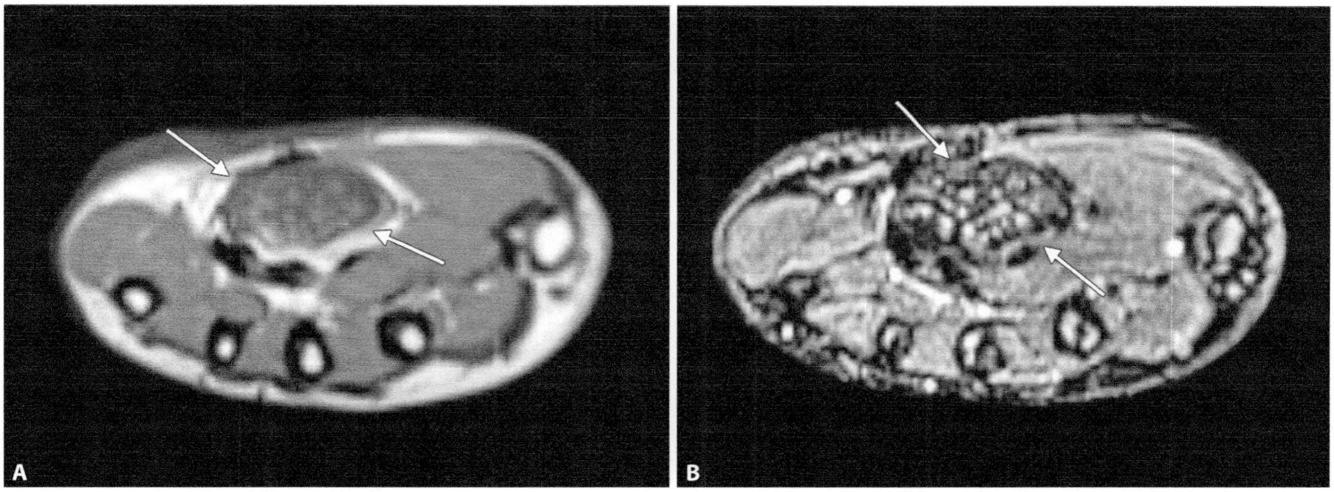

Figs. 31A and B: Fibrolipomatous hamartoma of median nerve. Axial T1 nonfat-suppressed (A) and T2 fat-suppressed (B) images of hand showing grossly enlarged median nerve (arrows) with fatty deposition giving cable-like appearance.

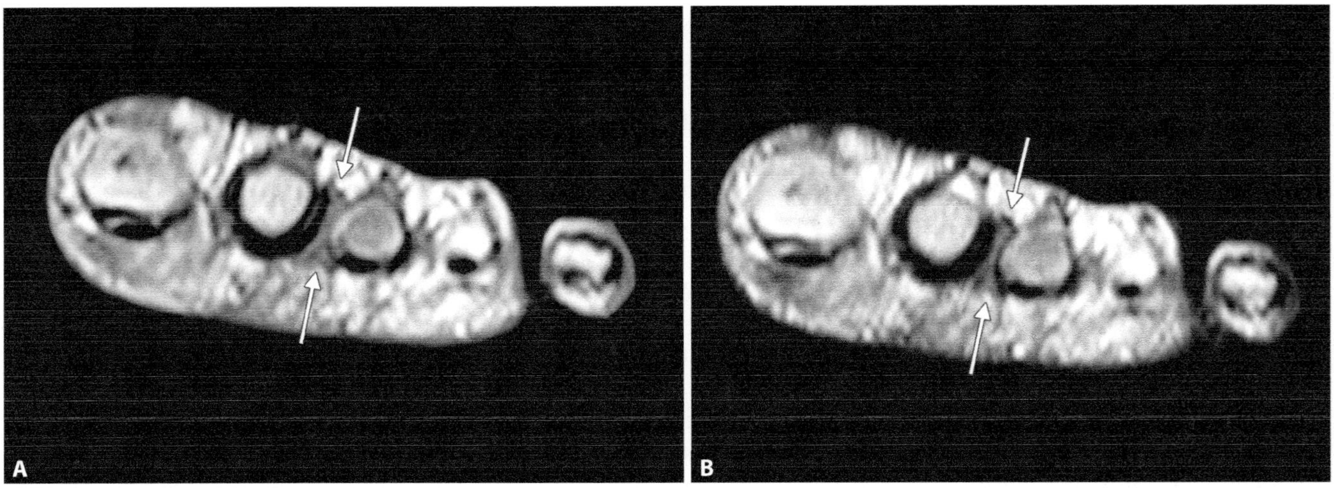

Figs. 32A and B: Morton's neuroma: Coronal nonfat-suppressed T1 (A) and T2 (B) images of forefoot showing hypointense lesion in 2nd intermetatarsal web space (arrows).

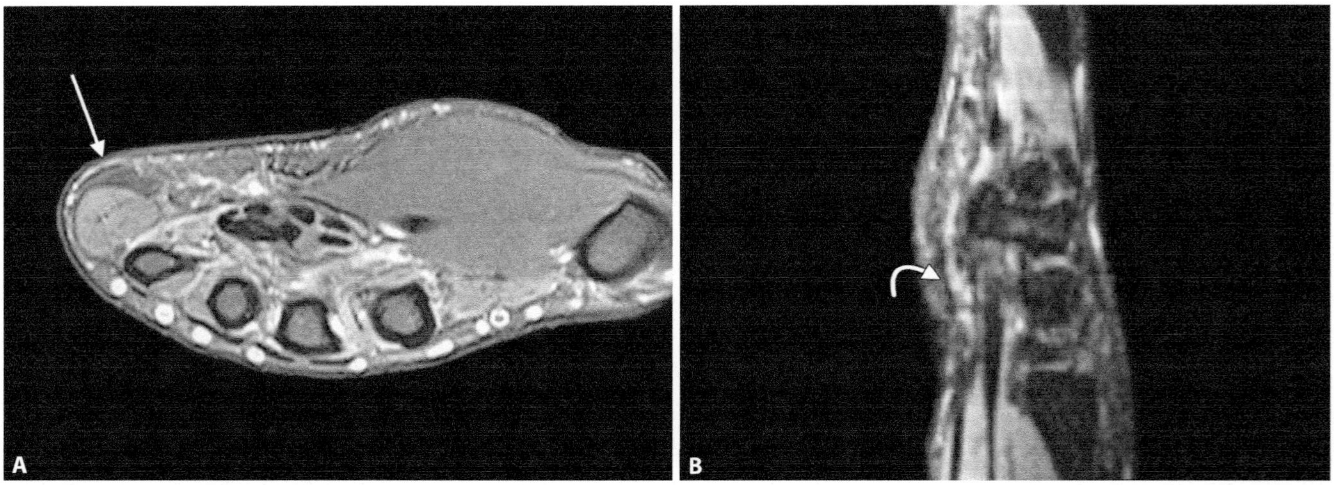

Figs. 33A and B: Chronic inflammatory demyelinating neuropathy (CIDP) involving ulnar nerve. Axial T2 fat-suppressed (A) and 3D PSIF sagittal reformatted (B) images showing atrophy and denervation edema of hypothenar muscles (straight arrow) and nodular hyperintense ulnar nerve (curved arrow).

on T1-weighted images and hypointense on T2-weighted images **(Figs. 32A and B)**. T2 hypointensity can be used to differentiate Morton's neuroma from other lesions of web spaces like bursitis or Schwannoma. On postcontrast MR images, it often shows variable contrast enhancement.[40]

Systemic Etiologies of Neuropathy

Multiple systemic disease can cause neuropathy such as Guillain-Barré syndrome (GBS), chronic inflammatory demyelinating neuropathy (CIDP), multifocal motor neuropathy (MMN), Hirayama disease, drug-induced neuropathy, metal toxicity, hereditary neuropathy (Charcot-Marie-Tooth disease), vasculitis, diabetes mellitus, thyroid disease, deposition disease (amyloidosis), neurocutaneous syndromes, hyperlipidemia, etc. Clinical examinations with electrophysiologic studies are helpful for the diagnosis of these disorders.[41] Imaging is useful for exclusion or confirmation of neuropathy. Imaging plays important role to detect superimposed complications, such as secondary lymphoma (nodular lesions in the nerve). Multiple nerve abnormalities or multifocal nerve disease, diffuse disease, abnormality at unexpected sites of nerve, nodularity or focal/multifocal nerve thickening points to the diagnosis of lymphoma, amyloid deposition, or neurocutaneous syndrome.[41]

There are useful clinical and biochemical tests in the diagnosis of systemic etiologies. These includes history, nature and course of weakness, blood work up, autoimmune work up, cerebrospinal fluid (CSF) analysis, and history of drug intake, etc.

In GBS, apart from specific clinical features, MR shows diffuse nerve thickening and increased signal intensity of affected nerves on T2/STIR sequences, such as in cauda equina nerve roots.[42] In CIDP, on imaging there is diffuse or patchy nerve thickening **(Figs. 33A and B)**.[43]

In CMT type 1A, pseudo masses may be seen mimicking neurofibromatosis.[44] Vasculitis or chemotherapy-induced neuropathy causes bilateral patchy nerve involvement, often seen in sciatic nerve. In diabetes mellitus, there is diffuse nerve thickening, increase signal intensity, and intraepineurial fat deposition. Amyloidosis is usually presenting with bilateral sciatic nerve thickening with or without nodularity and patchy enhancement. Neurocutaneous syndromes show diffuse nerve thickening and multifocal nodularity.[41]

Radiation Neuropathy

Postradiation neuritis or neuropathy may be seen in patient who underwent radiation therapy for other diseases. Radiation neuropathy may be seen after some period (weeks to years) postradiation therapy. It is generally diagnosis of exclusion. The severity of radiation neuropathy depends on dose of radiation exposure.[45] The affected nerve shows nonspecific features on imaging such as enlargement of nerve **(Figs. 34A to C)**.

RECENT ADVANCES IN PERIPHERAL NERVE IMAGING

Microneurography

In microneurography, very high magnetic fields (>9 T) with powerful gradients (400 mT/m) and coils are used which provides very high special resolution. This is similar to use of higher frequency US, which increases the spatial resolution.[46]

Dedicated Contrast Media

The contrast agents can be helpful in MR assessment of peripheral nerve:

- Superparamagnetic MR contrast agents (SPIO: Endorem or Resovist) and ultrasmall superparamagnetic contrast agents (USPIO: Sinerem), having iron oxide particles and have their affinity for the macrophage which gives hypointense signal on gradient-echo sequences through a paramagnetic effect.[25,47]
- Gadofluorine have affinity to demyelinating area of injured nerve, which gives low T1 signal until remyelination is over. It has high sensitivity and specificity in detecting focal demyelinating areas. This can be useful in post-therapy follow-up of demyelinating diseases.[25,48]

Contrast-enhanced Ultrasound

The contrast-enhanced US may be useful in peripheral nerve imaging, providing quantitative measures of PNS perfusion. The applications have been suggested, particularly in trauma cases to monitor grafted nerve injuries[49]

Elastography

Ultrasound elastography is a measure of the elasticity of tissues. It is a noninvasive technique in which both qualitative and quantitative evaluation of nerve tissue constitution can be done.[50] Many studies found that in peripheral neuropathy, the nerve rigidity increases due to loss of less rigid myelin and restoration with connective tissue. The qualitative evaluation is represented by the color coded mapping. The quantitative shear modulus maps can be measured by shear-wave velocities in meters per second or tissue elasticity in kilopascals **(Fig. 35)**.

Spinal Ganglion Morphometry

In a study by West et al., they showed quantification of spinal ganglion volume corresponded to with histological quantification, which corresponded to the number of nerve cell bodies.[51] The loss of neurons corresponds to decrease in spinal ganglion volume which may be useful in objective and early method of measuring sensory neuronal injury.

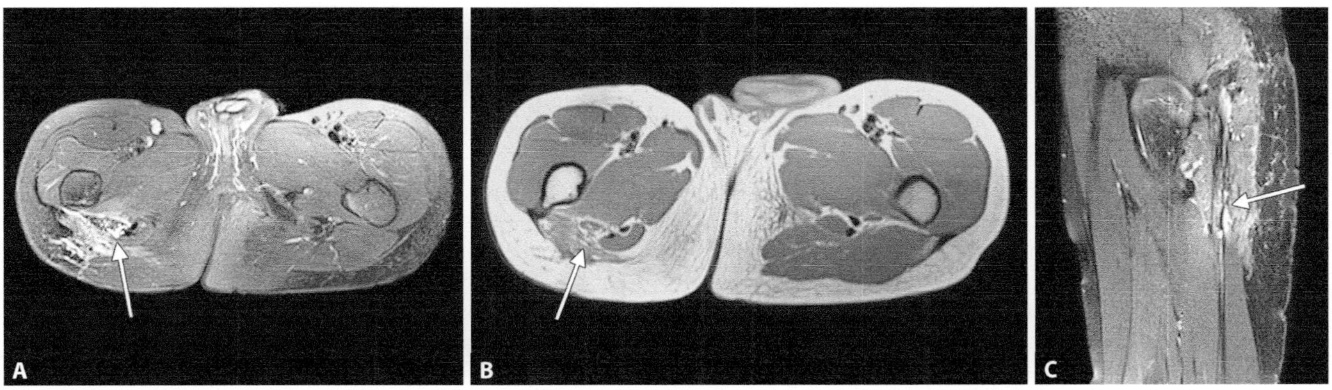

Figs. 34A to C: Radiation neuropathy of right sciatic nerve. Axial T2 fat-suppressed (A) and axial T1 nonfat-suppressed (B) and sagittal T2 fat-suppressed (C) images shows mildly thickened right sciatic nerve with heterogeneous signal. This patient received radiotherapy for malignant tumor thigh and hip region.

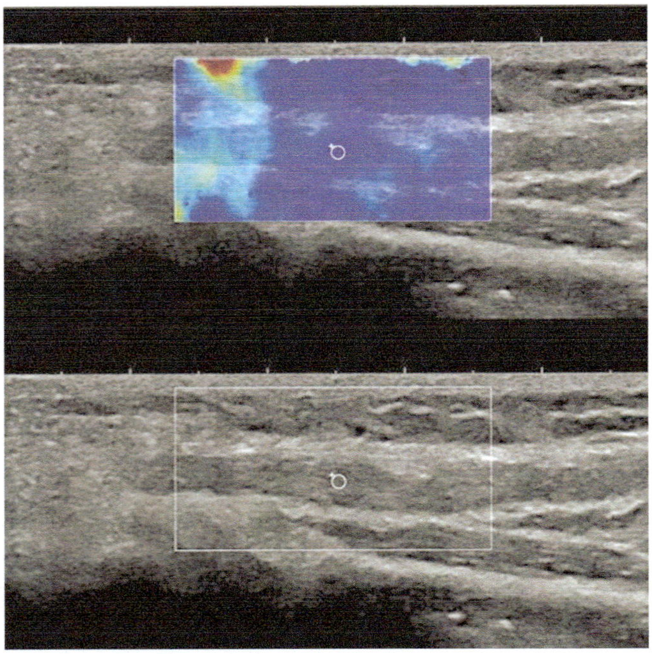

Fig. 35: Elastography of ulnar nerve. Shear-wave elastographic images with color mapping in case of leprotic neuropathy.

In chronic inflammatory demyelinating polyneuropathy, inherited neuropathies or lymphomatous infiltration of nerve, there is increase in volume of spinal ganglion.[25]

MR Spectroscopy

The contrast resolution (~7–10 mm) of MRS is not promising in imaging of PNS at present. The muscle metabolism was studied by Baldassarri[52] in nerve regeneration using 31P MRS to specify high-energy metabolites and calculate muscle pH. The study showed that muscle tissue pH was alkaline in the denervation phase and returned to normal after reinnervation.

REFERENCES

1. Franssen H, Wieneke GH, Wokke JH. The influence of temperature on conduction block. Muscle Nerve. 1999;22:166-73.
2. Grant GA, Goodkin R, Maravilla KR, Kliot M. MR neurography: diagnostic utility in the surgical treatment of peripheral nerve disorders. Neuroimaging Clin N Am. 2004;14(1):115-33.
3. Goedee HS, van der Pol WL, Hendrikse J, van den Berg LH.. Nerve ultrasound and magnetic resonance imaging in the diagnosis of neuropathy. Curr Opin Neurol. 2018;31:526-33.
4. Möller I, Miguel M, Bong DA, Zaottini F, Martinoli C. The peripheral nerves: Update on ultrasound and magnetic resonance imaging. Clin Exp Rheumatol. 2018;114(5):145-58.
5. Petchprapa CN, Rosenberg ZS, Sconfienza LM, Cavalcanti CF, Vieira RL, Zember JS. MR imaging of entrapment neuropathies of the lower extremity part 1. The pelvis and hip. Radiographics. 2010;30:983-1000.
6. Hochman MG, Zilberfarb JL. Nerves in a pinch: Imaging of nerve compression syndromes. Radiol Clin North Am. 2004;42(1):221-45.
7. Pilavaki M, Chourmouzi D, Kiziridou A, Skordalaki A, Zaram-poukas T, Drevelengas A. Imaging of peripheral nerve sheath tumors with pathologic correlation: Pictorial review. Eur J Radiol. 2004;52(3):229-39.
8. Floch H, Naux E, Pham Dang C, Dupas B, Pinaud M. Computed tomography scanning of the sciatic nerve posterior to the femur: Practical implications for the lateral mid-femoral block. Reg Anesth Pain Med. 2003;28(5):445-9.
9. Ellis JRC, McNally EG, Scott PM. Ultrasound of peripheral nerves. Imaging. 2002;14(3):217-22.
10. Martinoli C, Bianchi S, Derchi LE. Ultrasonography of peripheral nerves. Semin Ultrasound CT MR. 2000;21:205-13.
11. Kim S, Choi JY, Huh YM, Song HT, Lee SA, Kim SM, et al. Role of magnetic resonance imaging in entrapment and compressive neuropathy-what, where, and how to see the peripheral nerves on the musculoskeletal magnetic resonance image: Part 2. Upper extremity. Eur Radiol. 2007;17(2):509-22.
12. Maravilla KR, Bowen BC. Imaging of the peripheral nervous system: Evaluation of peripheral neuropathy and plexopathy. Am J Neuroradiol. 1998;19(6):1011-23.
13. Chappell KE, Robson MD, Stonebridge-Foster A, Glover A, Allsop JM, Williams AD, et al. Magic angle effects in MR neurography. Am J Neuroradiol. 2004;25:431-40.
14. Martinoli C, Derchi LE, Bertolotto M, Gandolfo N, Bianchi S, Fiallo P, et al. US and MR imaging of peripheral nerves in leprosy. Skeletal Radiol. 2000;29:142-50.
15. Takahara T, Hendrikse J, Yamashita T, Mali WP, Kwee TC, Imai Y, et al. Diffusion-weighted MR neurography of the brachial plexus: Feasibility study. Radiology. 2008;249(2):653-60.
16. Zhang ZW, Song LJ, Meng QF, Li ZP, Luo BN, Yang YH, et al. High-resolution diffusion-weighted MR imaging of the human lumbosacral plexus and its branches based on a steady-state free precession imaging technique at 3T. Am J Neuroradiol. 2008;29(6):1092-4.
17. Hiltunen J, Suortti T, Arvela S, Seppä M, Joensuu R, Hari R. Diffusion tensor imaging and tractography of distal peripheral nerves at 3T. Clin Neurophysiol. 2005;116:2315-23.
18. Skorpil M, Karlsson M, Nordell A, Peripheral nerve diffusion tensor imaging. Magn Reson Imaging. 2004;22:743-5.
19. Chhabra A, Madhuranthakam AJ, Andreisek G. Magnetic resonance neurography: Current perspectives and literature review. Eur Radiol. 2018;28:698-707.
20. Kabakci N, Gürses B, Firat Z, Bayram A, Uluğ AM, Kovanlikaya A, et al. Diffusion tensor imaging and tractography of median nerve: Normative diffusion values. Am J Roentgenol. 2007;189:923-27.
21. Hormann M, Traxler H, Ba-Ssalamah A, Mlynarik V, Shodaj-Baghini M, Kubiena H, et al. Correlative high-resolution MR-anatomic study of sciatic, ulnar, and proper palmar digital nerve. Magn Reson Imaging. 2003;21(8):879-85.
22. Chhabra A, Andreisek G, Soldatos T, Wang KC, Flammang AJ, Belzberg AJ, et al. MR neurography: Past, present, and future. Am J Roentgenol. 2011;197:583-91.

23. Kraus E, Tenforde AS, Beaulieu CF, Ratliff J, Fredericson M. Piriformis syndrome with variant sciatic nerve anatomy: A case report. PMR. 2016;8(2):176-9.
24. Kamath S, Venkatanarasimha N, Walsh MA, Hughes PM. MRI appearance of muscle denervation. Skeletal Radiol. 2008;37:397-404.
25. Ohana M, Moser T, Moussaoui A, Kremer S, Carlier RY, Liverneaux P, et al. Current and future imaging of the peripheral nervous system. Diagnos Intervent Imag. 2014;95:17-26
26. Chhabra A, Ahlawat S, Belzberg A, Andreseik G. Peripheral nerve injury grading simplified on MR neurography: as referenced to Seddon and Sunderland classifications. Indian J Radiol Imaging [Serial Online]. 2014;24:217-24.
27. Agarwal A, Chandra A, Jaipal U, Bagarhatta M, Mendiratta K, Goyal A, et al. Can imaging be the new yardstick for diagnosing peripheral neuropathy?—a comparison between high resolution ultrasound and MR neurography with an approach to diagnosis. Insights Imaging. 2019; 10:104.
28. Mackinnon S, Dellon AL. Diagnosis of nerve injury. Surgery of the peripheral nerve. New York: Thieme Publications; 1988. pp. 74-8.
29. Miller TT, Reinus WR. Nerve entrapment syndromes of the elbow, forearm, and wrist. Am J Roentgenol. 2010;195: 585-94.
30. Benedetti PF, Anderson MW, Maselli R, Rogero GW. Hypertrophic peripheral neuropathy due to leprosy: MR features. J Comput Assist Tomogr 1994;18:995-6.
31. Zaidman CM, Al-Lozi M, Pestronk A. Peripheral nerve size in normals and patients with polyneuropathy: An ultrasound study. Muscle Nerve. 2009;40(6):960-6.
32. Martinoli C, Schenone A, Bianchi S, Mandich P, Caponetto C, Abbruzzese M, et al. Sonography of the median nerve in Charcot-Marie-Tooth disease. Am J Roentgenol. 2002;178(6):1553-6.
33. Bhargava R, Parham DM, Lasater OE, Chari RS, Chen G, Fletcher BD. MR imaging differentiation of benign and malignant peripheral nerve sheath tumors: Use of the target sign. Pediatr Radiol. 1997;27:124-9.
34. Kakkar C, Shetty CM, Koteshwara P, Bajpai S. Telltale signs of peripheral neurogenic tumors on magnetic resonance imaging. Indian J Radiol Imaging. 2015;25:453-8.
35. Wilkinson LM, Manson D, Smith CR. Best cases from the AFIP: Plexiform neurofibroma of the bladder. Radiographics 2004; 24:S237-S242.
36. Li CS, Huang GS, Wu HD, Chen WT, Shih LS, Lii JM, et al. Differentiation of soft tissue benign and malignant peripheral nerve sheath tumors with magnetic resonance imaging. Clin Imaging. 2008;32:121-7.
37. Walker CW, Adams, BD, Barnes CL, Roloson GJ, Fitzrandolph RL. Case report 667. Fibrolipomatous hamartoma of the median nerve. Skeletal Radiol. 1991;20:237-9.
38. Choi W, Jung JY, Song IS, Lee JS, Lee TJ, Jung YY, et al. Fibrolipomatous hamartoma of digital branch of the median nerve without macrodystrophy: Two case reports with magnetic resonance imaging findings. J Korean Soc Radiol. 2012;67(6):483-7
39. Bencardino J, Rosenberg ZS, Beltran J, Liu X, Marty-Delfaut E. Morton's neuroma: Is it always symptomatic? AJR Am J Roentgenol. 2000;175 (3): 649-53.
40. Espinoza N, Schmitt JW, Saupe N, Maquieira GJ, Bode B, Vienne P, et al. Morton neuroma: MR imaging after resection-postoperative MRI and histologic findings in asymptomatic and symptomatic metatarsal spaces. Radiology. 2010;255:850-6.
41. Chhabra A. Peripheral MR neurography. Neuroimaging Clin North Am. 2014;24(1):79-89.
42. Sureka J, Cherian RA, Alexander M, Thomas BP. MRI of brachial plexopathies. Clin Radiol. 2009;64:208-18.
43. Bradley LJ, Wilhelm T, King RH, Ginsberg L, Orrell RW. Brachial plexus hypertrophy in chronic inflammatory demyelinating polyradiculoneuropathy. Neuromuscul Disord. 2006;16:126-31.
44. Cartwright MS, Brown ME, Eulitt P, Walker FO, Lawson VH, Caress JB. Diagnostic nerve ultrasound in Charcot-Marie Tooth disease type 1B. Muscle Nerve. 2009;40(1):98-102.
45. Mondrup K, Olsen NK, Pfeiffer P, Rose C. Clinical and electrodiagnostic findings in breast cancer patients with radiation-induced brachial plexus neuropathy. Acta Neurol Scand. 1990;81:153-8.
46. Bilgen M, Heddings A, Al-Hafez B, Hasan W, McIff T, Toby B, et al. Microneurography of human median nerve. J Magn Reson Imaging. 2005;21(6):826-30.
47. Bendszus M, Stoll G. Caught in the act: In vivo mapping of macrophage infiltration in nerve injury by magnetic resonance imaging. J Neurosci. 2003;23(34):10892-6.
48. Wessig C, Jestaedt L, Sereda MW, Bendszus M, Stoll G. Gadofluorine M-enhanced magnetic resonance nerve imaging: Comparison between acute inflammatory and chronic degenerative demyelination in rats. Exp Neurol. 2008;210(1):137-43.
49. Wang Y, Tang P, Zhang L, Guo Y, Wan W. Quantitative evaluation of the peripheral nerve blood perfusion with high frequency contrast-enhanced ultrasound. Acad Radiol. 2010;17(12):1492-7.
50. Zakrzewski J, Zakrzewska K, Pluta K, Nowak O, Miłoszewska-Paluch A. Ultrasound elastography in the evaluation of peripheral neuropathies: A systematic review of the literature. Pol J Radiol. 2019;84:e581-e591
51. West CA, Davies KA, Hart AM, Wiberg M, Williams SR, Terenghi G. Volumetric magnetic resonance imaging of dorsal root ganglia for the objective quantitative assessment of neuron death after peripheral nerve injury. Exp Neurol. 2007;203(1):22-33.
52. Baldassarri AM, Zetti G, Masson S, Gatti S, Albani AP, Ferla G, et al. Magnetic resonance (MR) imaging and MR spectroscopy of nerve regeneration and target muscle energy metabolism in a model of prosthesis-guided reinnervation in rats. Acad Radiol. 1995;2(2):128-34.

CHAPTER

24

Imaging in Prosthetic Joints

Ankur Goyal, Shivanand Gamanagatti

INTRODUCTION

Most commonly performed orthopedic procedures include fracture fixations and joint arthroplasties.[1] Thus, there is a need for the radiologist to know about the imaging interpretation of commonly performed arthroplasties. The common indications of arthroplasty include severe pain due to advanced osteoarthritis, postinflammatory or infective arthritis, complex fractures, and avascular necrosis.[1] Neuropathic joint, morbid obesity, and active infection are the usual contraindications.

This chapter focuses on basic concepts of arthroplasty and imaging evaluation of three most commonly performed prosthetic joints, namely hip, knee, and the shoulder. First and foremost, we should be able to recognize the proper positioning of the implant and secondly any associated complications.

BASIC CONCEPTS

The purpose of arthroplasty is to alleviate the joint pain while preserving function, stability, and mobility.

Primary fixation of an implant is based on tight press-fit with the stem being inserted more than the bony crevice. This compression generates hoop stress, providing stability. *Secondary or definitive fixation* is due to bony ingrowth, providing anchorage for longevity of the implant.

Osseointegration refers to formation of lamellar bone around the implant, which enables tight fit. If the degree of motion at the implant-bone interface is <20 mm, then there is predominantly bone formation at the interface, stabilizing the implant. Motion >150 mm leads to formation of fibrous tissue and 40–150 mm leads to both bone and fibrous tissue formation. The center of the prosthesis needs to be placed in anatomical position without any offset. Any deviation leads to increased wear and loosening of the implant.

Wearing in refers to loss of material of the articulating prosthesis surfaces when they slide against each other under load. This is the most common cause of implant failure. Wear in produces particulate debris, inciting foreign body reaction, osteolysis, and asymmetric joint space narrowing.

Prosthesis leads to diminution of normal stress from the periprosthetic bone leading to osteopenia (Wolff's law) and is known as *stress shielding*. This bone loss leads to failure of osseointegration and it is the most common cause of implant loosening. It is more pronounced with large or long implants or those with extensive porous-coated stems.

Resistance of the implant to a particular degree of motion is referred to as *constraint*. Accordingly, implants may be fully constrained (restricted motion in a particular axis), semiconstrained or nonconstrained (allow full movement in a particular axis). For example, in knee, nonconstrained prostheses retain the cruciate ligaments; semiconstrained ones include large anterior tibial spine and corresponding rectangular space to prevent posterior tibial subluxation; and constrained prostheses are hinged ones used in tumors and revision arthroplasties.

Conformity refers to the degree of the geometric articulation fit between the prosthetic components. Greater conformity means more contact area, resulting in reduced stress and wear but more deformation of polyethylene and early loosening.

Modularity refers to the option of adding stems, augmentations, and wedges to the implant components so as to customize the prosthesis intraoperatively.

Custom prosthesis refers to preoperatively designed implant which is different from the standard one to cater to the specific needs of the patient. One example is long-stem implant in limb salvage procedures in case of tumors **(Fig. 1A)**.

Fixation of the prosthesis to the underlying bone may be done with bone cement [polymethylmethacrylate (PMMA)] or without (cementless/uncemented implants; **Fig. 1B**). In latter, implants are specially textured and porous coated (hydroxyapatite or titanium) to promote bony fixation. Cemented implants are used when the bone is fragile (osteopenia/postinflammatory arthritis) and enable early weight-bearing. However, they are prone to loosening.

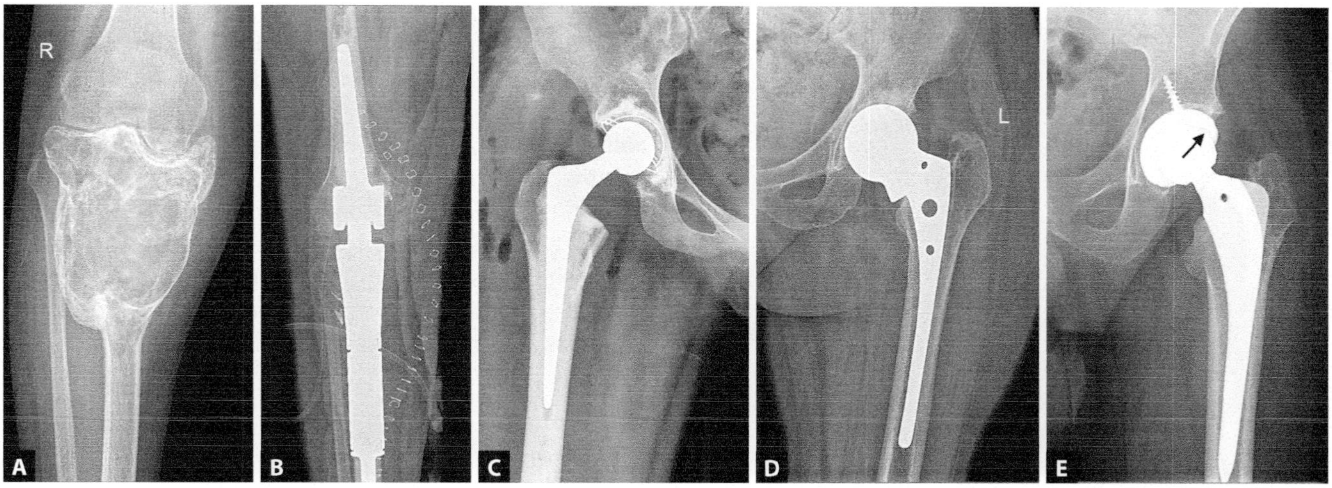

Figs. 1A to E: (A) Radiograph depicts expansile lytic soap-bubble lesion in proximal tibia in a case of giant cell tumor; (B) Radiograph shows custom hinged prosthesis with long-stem implant; (C) Radiograph following total hip arthroplasty shows cemented fixation of both femoral (metal) and acetabular components (polyethylene) in total hip replacement (THR); (D) Radiograph shows noncemented fixation of femoral stem which articulates with native acetabulum in unipolar hemiarthroplasty; (E) Radiograph depicts bipolar hemiarthroplasty, where acetabular component is fixed using a screw. Arrow denotes radiolucent polyethylene cup at the articulation of the prosthetic femoral head and the acetabulum.

PROSTHETIC MATERIALS

Commonly used prosthetic materials include metal, ceramics, polyethylene, and bone cement. Metals used in making the implants include stainless steel, titanium, and alloys based on titanium and cobalt. Smaller crystal size provides better strength and resistance. However, there may be long-term harmful effects of metal ions and loosening due to allergic response.

Ultra-high-molecular-weight polyethylene (UHMWPE) plastic has high strength, chemically inert, biocompatible with good fatigue resistance.

Ceramics (aluminum or zirconium oxide) are harder than metals and resistant to oxidative wear, but more susceptible to breakage. Ceramics have the lowest wear rate.[2]

Bearing (contact) surfaces can be made of polyethylene, metal or ceramic and accordingly the implant combinations (nomenclature) can be of the following types:

- Hard-on-soft (metal on polyethylene or ceramic on polyethylene)
- Hard-on-hard (metal-on-metal, ceramic-on-ceramic and metal-on-ceramic).

Most commonly used combination is metal-on-polyethylene **(Fig. 1C)**. For example, in hip prosthesis, femoral stem is metallic, head can be metallic or ceramic, cup is metallic or of polyethylene, and cup liner is usually ceramic or polyethylene.

The particulate polyethylene debris due to wear-in can however result in aseptic loosening of the implant. To decrease the particulate debris from abrasive wear, hard-on-hard combinations were developed to improve the life of implant.

Fixation materials include PMMA cement, calcium phosphate ceramic-coating or porous metal surfaces and promote osseointegration **(Figs. 1D and E)**. Bone cement is used less as an adhesive and more to fill the space between the implant and the bone.[2] Porous metal surface, fiber mesh, and sintered microsphere beads allow bony ingrowth whereas textured surface allows bony ongrowth. Surfaces can be textured by grit blasting with aluminum oxide or plasma spraying.[2] Bioactive coatings (hydroxyapatite) also promote bone growth.

IMAGING MODALITIES

Radiographs

Radiographs are very useful for initial assessment as well as postoperatively to look for type of prosthesis, alignment of components and to look for complications such as osteolysis, loosening, and implant failure and fractures **(Figs. 2A and B)**. Serial radiographs are very useful to identify stress shielding, implant wear in and loosening. Various measurements can be done on radiographs for early detection of implant offset.

Computed Tomography

Computed tomography (CT) provides comprehensive multiplanar evaluation with high spatial resolution. This is helpful for assessment of acetabular and femoral neck version, measuring rotational alignment of knee prosthesis **(Fig. 3A)**, assessing periprosthetic bone **(Fig. 3A)**, evaluation of collections and masses, and taking treatment decisions for revision surgery.

However, the beam hardening artifacts are a major problem and hamper with the image interpretation

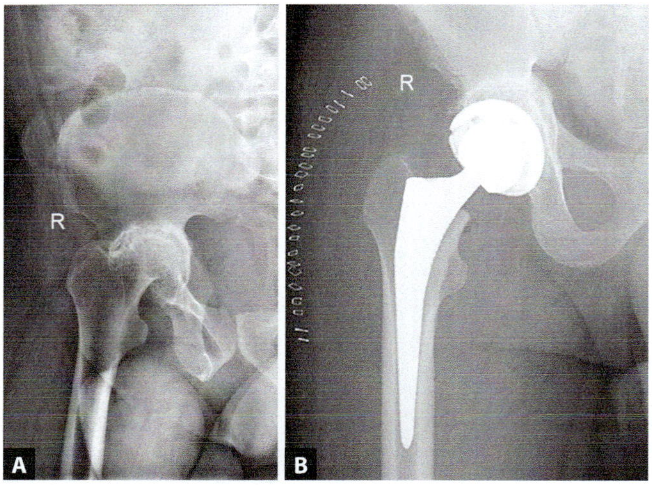

Figs. 2A and B: (A) Frontal radiograph shows severe osteoarthritis on right hip; (B) Immediate postoperative radiograph after bipolar hemiarthroplasty (metal-on-polyethylene bearing surfaces).

(Fig. 3B). **Table 1** depicts the factors affecting metal-related artifacts. Thus, the methods to reduce them include: Increasing tube voltage (kVp) and tube current and exposure time product (mAs), using narrow detector collimation and low pitch, using lower frequency or iterative deblurring reconstruction algorithms, increasing section thickness while scrolling and using extended CT scale technique for multiplanar reformation (MPR) and wide window settings to accentuate border of osseous structures.[3] It may be kept in mind that most of these remedies also increase the radiation dose to the patient.

Ultrasound

Sonography is an excellent modality for evaluation of periprosthetic soft tissues. Any adjacent collections or effusions can be assessed and aspirated **(Figs. 4A and B)**. Ultrasound is also useful in distinguishing aseptic

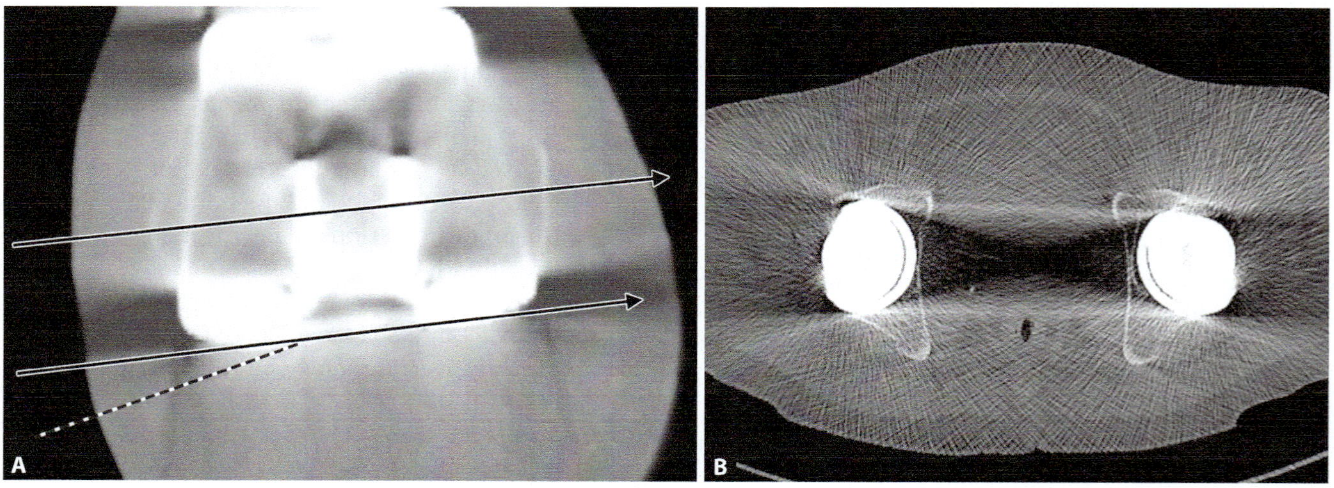

Figs. 3A and B: (A) Axial thick multiplanar reconstruction (MPR) image shows the transepicondylar line and femoral component posterior condylar line drawn to measure femoral component rotation post-knee arthroplasty; (B) Axial computed tomography (CT) image postbilateral total hip replacement (THR) shows beam hardening artifacts.

Table 1: Factors which affect metal-related artifacts on computed tomography (CT).

Factor	*Effect*
Metal composition	Titanium < Stainless steel < Cobalt-chrome (more dense metal produces more artifacts)
Prosthesis shape	More artifacts with complex shape
Orientation	More artifact along the long axis in axial plane
Collimation	Less artifact with narrow collimation
Pitch	Less artifact with low pitch (most important parameter affecting image quality in prosthesis cases)
Tube voltage (kVp)	Less artifact with high kVp
Tube current and exposure time product (mAs)	Less artifact with high mAs
Reconstruction algorithm	Less artifact with lower spatial frequency algorithm ("smooth" images)
Reconstruction section thickness	Less artifacts with thicker sections

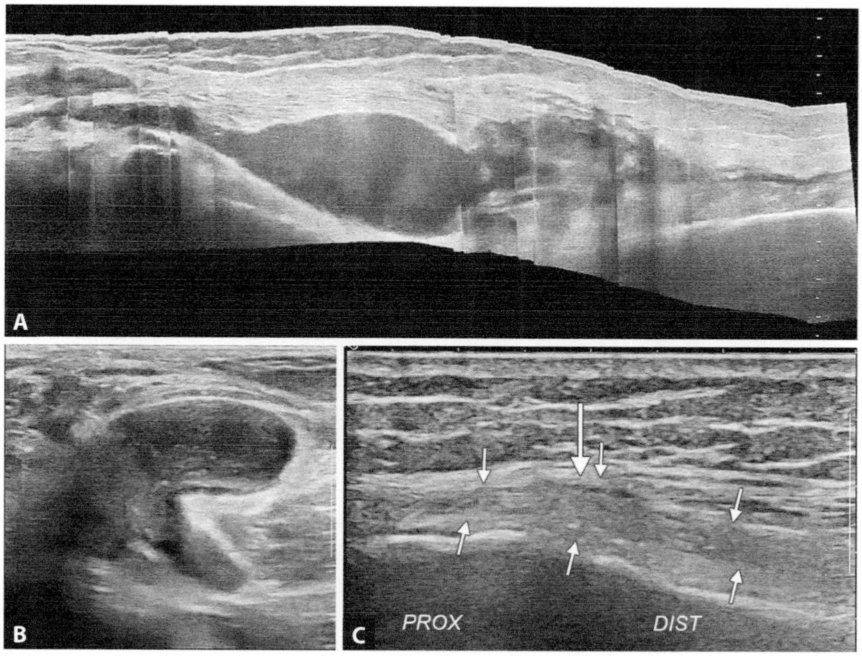

Figs. 4A to C: (A) Extended field-of-view panoramic ultrasound image shows large fluid collection in a patient who underwent total hip replacement (THR) 1 month ago. Aspiration revealed purulent material; (B) Another patient with Baker's cyst post-THR showing echogenic debris within; (C) Ultrasound of common peroneal nerve in another patient who developed foot drop post-THR. There is focal bulkiness of the nerve (long arrow) with preserved fibrillar architecture and continuity suggesting neuropraxia.

loosening from infection. It is also useful in evaluation of any nerve compression or hematoma in the immediate postoperative period **(Fig. 4C)**.

Magnetic Resonance Imaging

The indications of magnetic resonance imaging (MRI) in prosthetic joint imaging include:

- Evaluation of adjacent soft tissues
- Metallosis or particle disease **(Fig. 5)**
- Infection
- To assess tendon or muscle injuries
- Characterize collections and masses.

Most of the metallic implants used nowadays are MR compatible. However, metallic components cause artifacts by inducing magnetic field heterogeneity **(Fig. 5)**. This leads to in-plane distortion (pileup artifacts and signal loss, latter due to T2* dephasing), poor fat suppression, geometric distortion through section distortion. These artifacts are more on 3T compared with 1.5T and also depend on the type of prosthesis (size, shape, and configuration) and metal (titanium < cobalt-chromium < stainless steel).

Methods to Reduce Metal Artifacts in MRI

- Long axis of the prosthesis to be positioned parallel to the magnetic field and frequency encoding direction along the long axis of the implant.
- Fast spin echo with long echo-train length and short echo time (TE).
- Increasing the receiver bandwidth (reduces geometric distortion) and image matrix size.
- Reducing the field-of-view (FOV).
- Reducing slice thickness (reduces through section distortions).
- Fast spin-echo sequences with long echo-train length are least susceptible to metal artifacts and should be preferred over gradient-echo sequences.
- Short-tau inversion recovery (STIR) and Dixon-based fat suppression produce lesser artifacts than spectral fat suppression.

Based on these methods, the first integrated approach to reduce in-plane MR artifacts was described by Olsen et al. and termed metal artifact reduction sequences (MARS).[4] The typical MARS protocol includes STIR coronal, T1 and T2 spin-echo axial and proton-density coronal images. WARP includes multidirectional view-angle tilting (VAT) to further optimize MARS, however it results in image blurring.

Artifacts due to metal in the adjacent plane (through-plane artifacts) can be reduced by using special multispectral sequences such as multiacquisition variable-resonance image combination (MAVRIC) or slice-encoding for metal artifact correction (SEMAC). The former uses multiple overlapping acquisitions at different frequencies while the latter uses an additional slice-encoding gradient to fast spin echo. MAVRIC uses multiple frequency-selective excitations, multidirectional VAT, computational postprocessing, and reduces in-plane

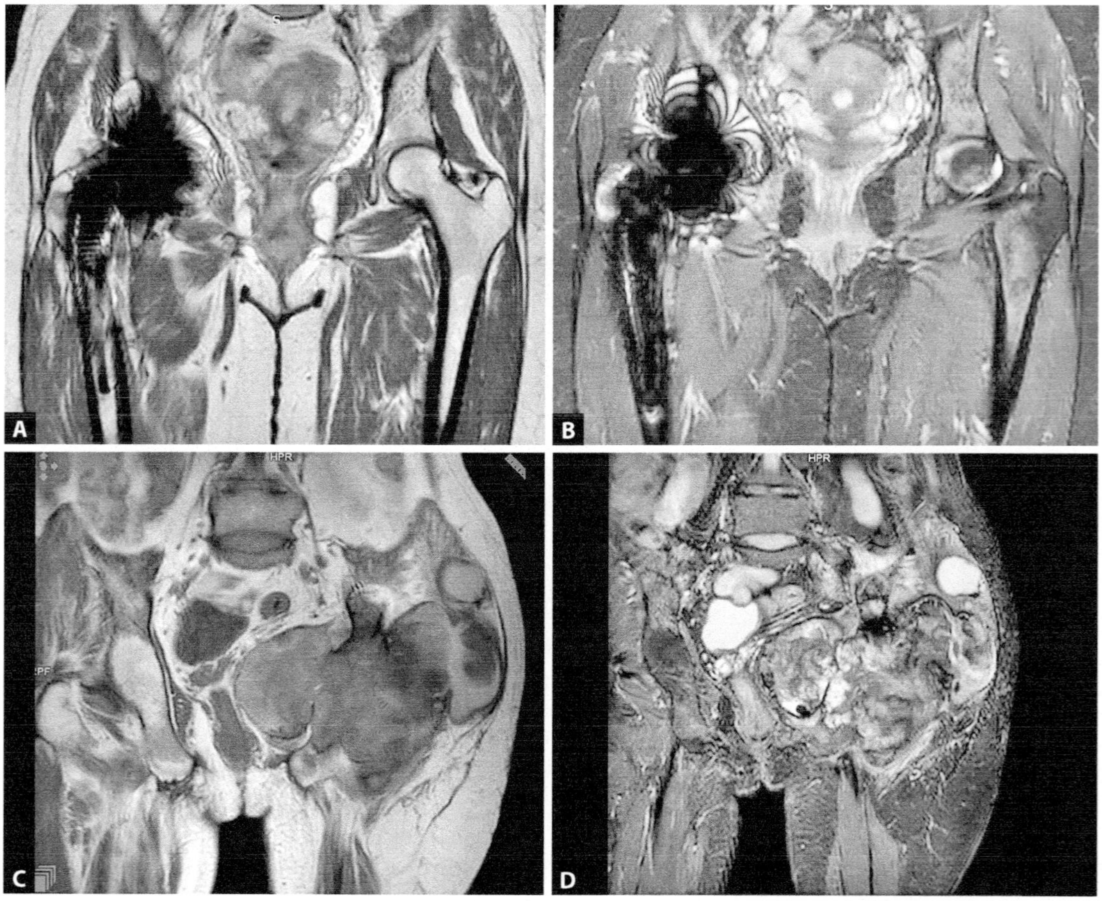

Figs. 5A to D: (A) Coronal T2-weighted (T2W) and (B) Fat-suppressed T2W images show susceptibility artifacts due to metal component, exaggerated in (B); (C and D) Coronal T1W and short-tau inversion recovery (STIR) images show large hypointense mass around the hip prosthesis due to metallosis.

artifacts as well. SEMAC is a two-dimensional (2D) fast spin-echo sequence where there is phase encoding in the third dimension (Z-axis) for each slice so that exact delineation of the distortion due to magnetic susceptibility is there.[4]

Nuclear Medicine Scans

Various scintigraphy techniques are available for evaluation of postimplant complications. A standard three-phase bone scan is sensitive to detect failed joint replacement. Combining gallium scintigraphy enables differentiation between infection and aseptic loosening of the implant with moderate accuracy **(Figs. 6 and 7)**. Radiolabeled leukocyte scintigraphy is however the investigation of choice to identify neutrophil-mediated processes **(Figs. 6 and 7)**. Combined in vitro labeled leukocyte or bone marrow scintigraphy is the gold standard imaging modality to diagnose infection with higher accuracy than even ^{18}F-fluorodeoxyglucose-positron-emission tomography (FDG-PET) and single photon emission computed tomography (SPECT).

COMMON ARTHROPLASTIES: INDICATIONS, TERMINOLOGY, AND MEASUREMENT

The common indications of any arthroplasty include severe pain due to osteoarthritis, ankylosis secondary to prior infection/inflammatory arthritis/trauma, complex fractures, avascular necrosis, and tumors around the joint.

Hip Arthroplasty

Hip arthroplasty is of two types. *Total hip replacement or arthroplasty (THR/THA)* means replacing both the femoral and acetabular articulating surfaces and is usually done when both native surfaces are abnormal and is the most common type of hip arthroplasty. There are two components in THR implants: an acetabular part and a stemmed femoral part with head **(Fig. 8)**. Former is fixed after removing the acetabular articular cartilage and the underlying sclerotic bone. Latter is fixed after removing the femoral head and neck and reaming the intramedullary cavity.[2] Hybrid THR comprises cemented femoral part and uncemented acetabular part whereas reverse hybrid THR employs reverse fixation.[2]

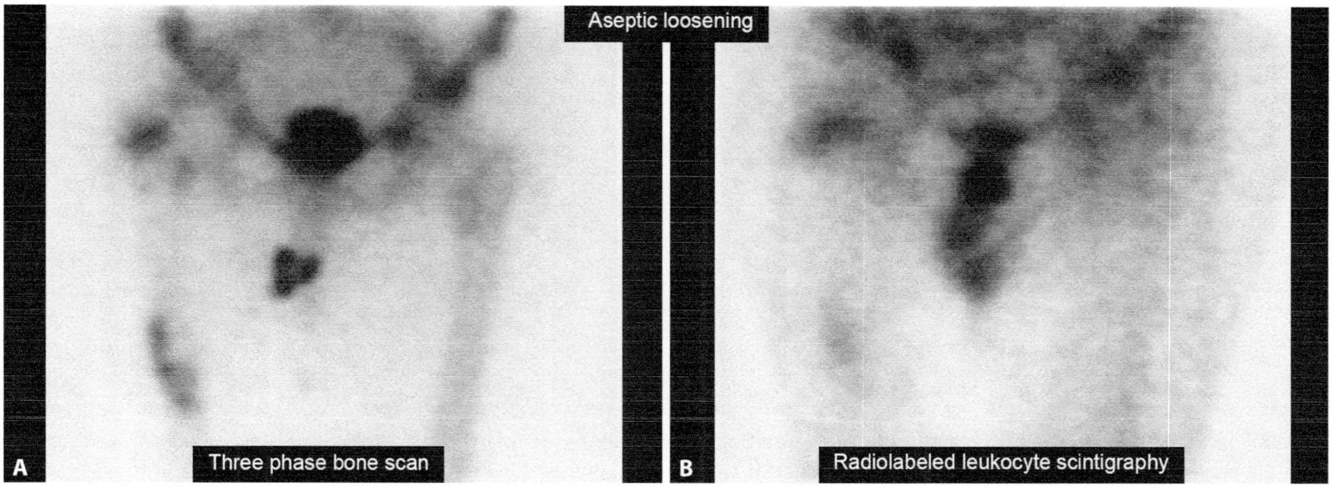

Figs. 6A and B: (A) Bone scan shows increased periprosthetic uptake on right side but no significant uptake is seen on leukocyte scintigraphy (B). This was a case of aseptic loosening of total hip replacement (THR).

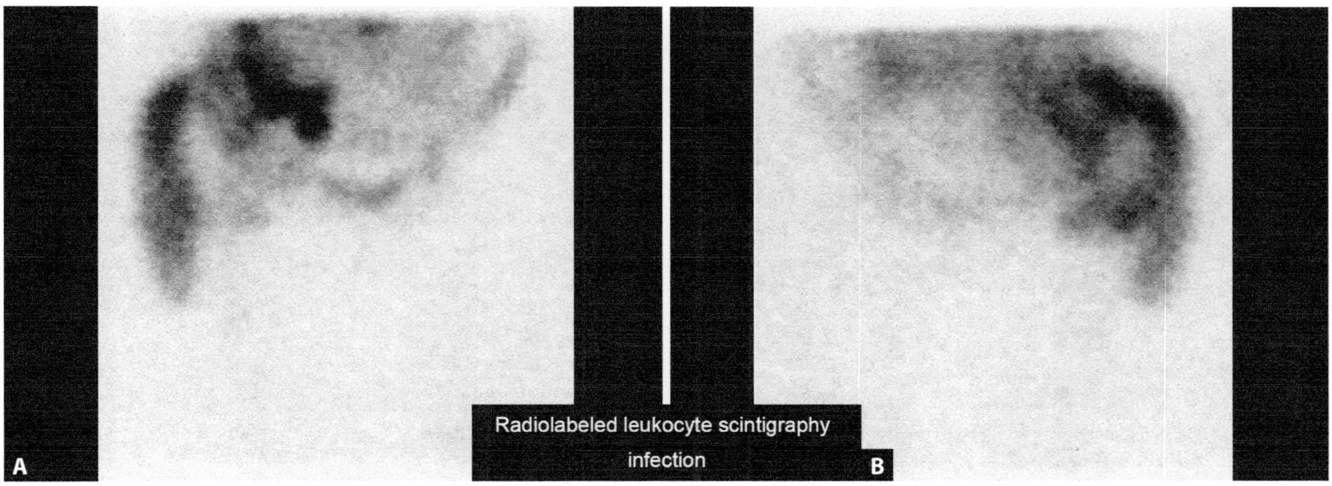

Figs. 7A and B: Leukocyte scintigraphy in periprosthetic infection shows increased uptake on right side (A is anterior projection and B is posterior projection).

Hemiarthroplasty or partial hip replacement refers to replacing the femoral head which articulates with native acetabular cartilage (done in case of severe subcapital femoral neck fractures). Hemiarthroplasty may employ unipolar prosthesis (no movement within the implant) or bipolar prosthesis (movement occurs between the implant components; **Figs. 8A and B**). Bipolar hip implant has two parts: a femoral stem with head and a polyethylene-lined acetabular cap **(Fig. 8B)**. Thus, motion can occur between the head and acetabular cap as well as between the cap and the native acetabulum. Bipolar implants have better longevity (due to less wear of the acetabular articular cartilage), less prone to dislocation and can be more easily converted to THR later in life. Thus, unipolar hemiarthroplasty of hip is commonly done only in elderly patients (with limited life expectancy) for intracapsular hip fractures.[1]

In *resurfacing arthroplasty*, only the articular surface is replaced and the underlying bone is retained to reduce complications but the pain relief is suboptimal. Resurfacing arthroplasty can be done for both the articular surfaces (resurfacing THA) or only the femoral head (resurfacing hemiarthroplasty) and is usually employed in young active patients **(Figs. 8D and E)**.

In the initial postoperative evaluation of hip arthroplasty patient, following measurements are commonly done: Femoral stem alignment, acetabular version, and femoral anteversion.

Femoral Stem Alignment

On anteroposterior (AP) radiograph, femoral stem should be along the axis of femoral shaft (neutral alignment) with tip in center of the femoral shaft **(Fig. 9A)**. Varus malpositioning leads to implant failure. In resurfacing

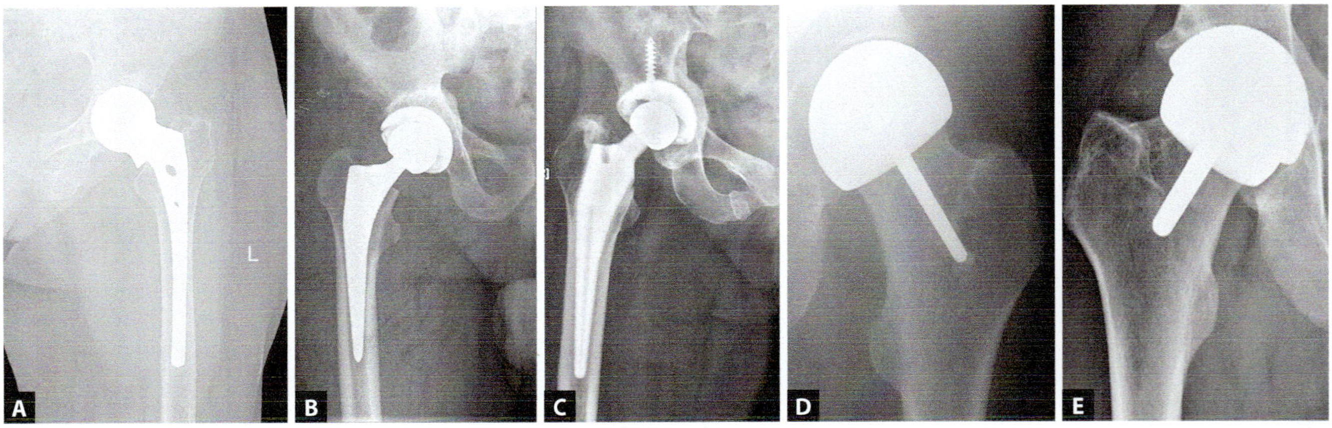

Figs. 8A to E: Different types of hip arthroplasty: (A) Unipolar noncemented hemiarthroplasty; (B) Bipolar hemiarthroplasty. Native sclerotic acetabulum is preserved with acetabular articular cartilage evident as thin lucency between acetabulum and the acetabular cup; (C) Total hip replacement (THR; acetabular component is attached to reamed acetabulum); (D) Resurfacing hemiarthroplasty; (E) Resurfacing total hip arthroplasty.

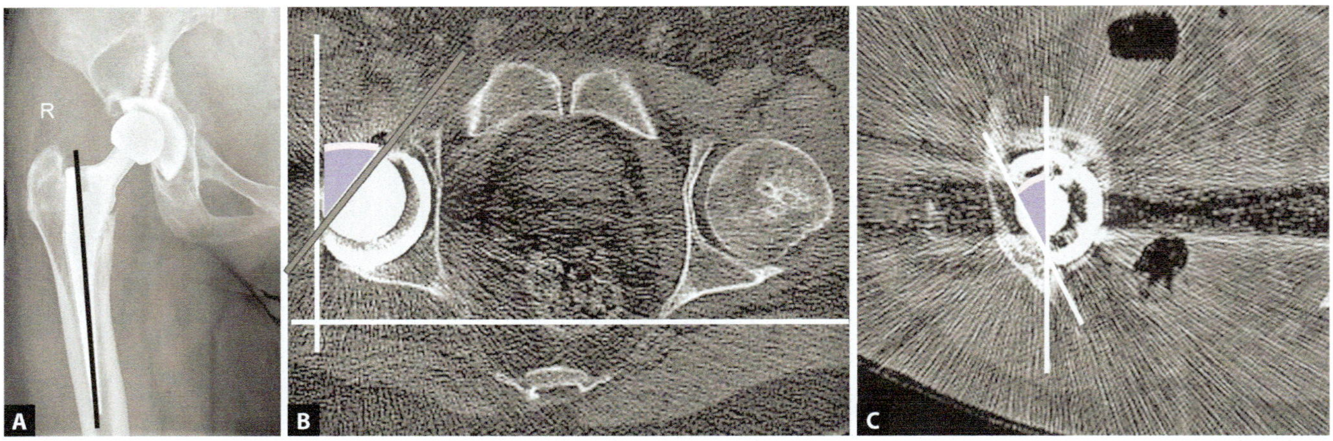

Figs. 9A to C: Measurements in hip arthroplasty: (A) Anteroposterior (AP) radiograph shows normal alignment of femoral stem along the shaft; (B) Acetabular anteversion angle measurement on CT; (C) Acetabular retroversion.

arthroplasty, femoral implant is placed in mild valgus position (5–10°) relative to femoral neck.[5]

Acetabular Version

The angulation of the acetabular axis from the coronal plane on a lateral radiograph is termed acetabular anteversion. Normal values are 5–25° to allow adequate flexion. Excessive anteversion predisposes to anterior dislocation while retroversion makes the prosthesis prone to posterior dislocation. On CT, one line is drawn between the lateral anterior and posterior margins of the acetabular component and another line (sagittal plane) is drawn perpendicular to the line connecting two identical points on either side of pelvis (interischial line) and the corresponding angle is measured **(Figs. 9B and C)**.[6] Normal range is same as in radiographs.

Femoral Version

Femoral component version is calculated on CT as the angle between femoral head-neck line (between center of head and neck of femoral prosthesis) and posterior intercondylar line (between posterior aspect of medial and lateral femoral condyles; **Fig. 10**). Normal range of femoral neck anteversion is 10–20°. It is also termed femoral antetorsion or femoral neck version.

Knee Arthroplasty

Knee arthroplasty is resurfacing arthroplasty in which articular surfaces are resurfaced using metal and polyethylene. Unlike hip, knee arthroplasty always involves replacement of both the opposing joint surfaces. There are three compartments in the knee joint: medial, lateral, and patellofemoral. *Unicompartmental arthroplasty (partial knee replacement or hemiarthroplasty)* is mostly done for isolated medial compartment arthritis (medial compartment arthroplasty; **Fig. 11**).[1] Patellofemoral arthroplasty is reserved for trochlear dysplasia or malalignment of the patellofemoral joint; however, has not shown encouraging results.[1]

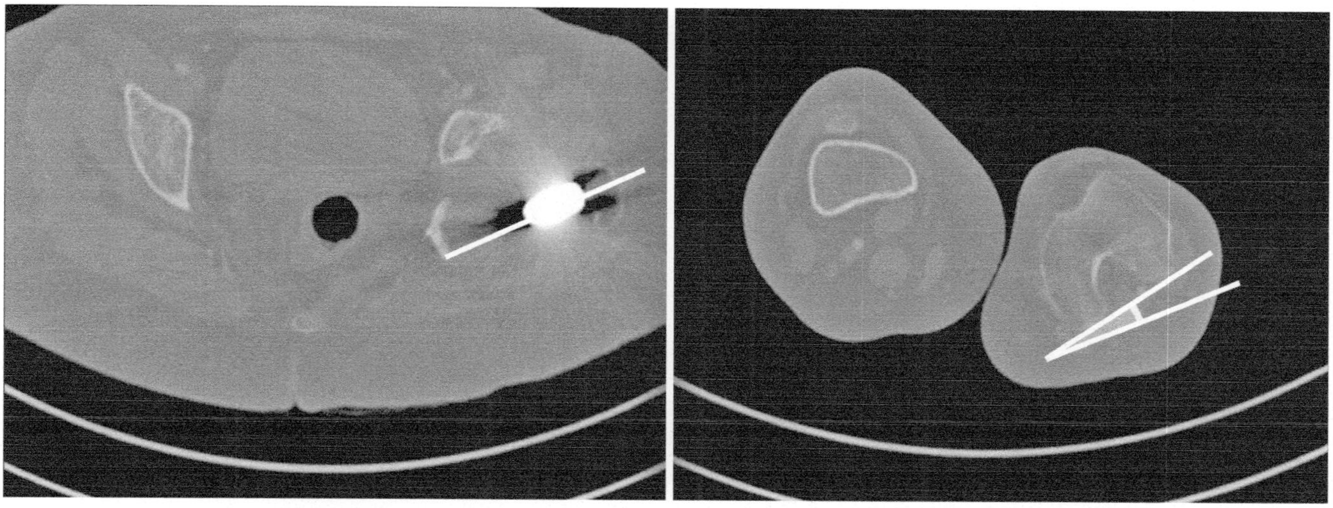

Fig. 10: Measurement of femoral anteversion (angle between the femoral neck line and posterior condylar line).

Total knee replacement (TKR) includes replacing femoral, tibial, and patellar articular surfaces (tricompartmental replacement; **Fig. 11**). Multiradius metal component replaces the surface of both the femoral condyles as well as the trochlear notch, tibial component is high-density polyethylene commonly with metal backing and patellar surface is replaced by polyethylene (with or without metal backing).

Multiple designs of TKR implants are available. *Cruciate-retaining implants* are most commonly used; they preserve the posterior cruciate ligament (PCL), are nonconstrained and done in patients with healthy surrounding muscles and ligaments.

Cruciate-substituting arthroplasty employs semi-constrained implants and done when there is ligament injury or deformed knee joint. PCL is resected and posterior stability is provided by including a post or spine in the tibial polyethylene which articulates with a box-like defect in the center of femoral component. Mobile-bearing designs allow additional motion between the tibial polyethylene and tibial metal component in the region of tibial spacer.

Constrained (hinged) prostheses are used in case of tumors and revision surgeries **(Figs. 1A and B)**. The stem of these implants can be cemented, noncemented or anchored with screws.

Computed tomography enables accurate measurement of rotational alignment of tibial and femoral components. *Rotational alignment of femoral component* is determined by measuring angle between transepicondylar line (connecting lateral epicondyle with base of medial sulcus adjacent to medial epicondyle) and femoral prosthesis posterior condylar line **(Fig. 3A)**. Normal is mild internal rotation. Abnormal femoral rotation leads to increased tibiofemoral wear and dislocations.

Tibial component rotation refers to angle subtended between the tibial component line and tibial tubercle line, measured at the geometric center of proximal tibia.[7] A perpendicular line is drawn to the posterior surface of tibial component and is termed tibial component line. In the next caudal section, the geometric center of proximal tibia is established. The next caudal section through tibial tubercle is superimposed on the geometric center image and then a line is drawn from the apex of tibial tubercle to the geometric center. Following this, the tibial component image is also superimposed and angle between the tibial tubercle line and tibial component line is measured to assess the rotational position of tibial component.

Shoulder Arthroplasty

Similar to hip, hemiarthroplasty consists of only humeral component (metallic stem with modular head) articulating with native glenoid and in total arthroplasty it articulates with glenoid component **(Figs. 12A and B)**.[1] Former is done in case of proximal humeral fractures or severe rotator cuff tears where glenoid is normal. Resurfacing humeral head implants are also available. Glenoid component is of two types: polyethylene with wire loop (keeled) or metal (pegged). Former is cemented while latter is secured by screws. The functionality of shoulder implant depends on the competency of the rotator cuff and these prostheses are less constrained than those of the hip. Another type is reverse total shoulder arthroplasty, in which metal sphere is fixed on glenoid and plastic socket forms humeral cap, done in patients who requires shoulder arthroplasty but their rotator cuff muscles are either atrophic or damaged **(Fig. 12C)**.

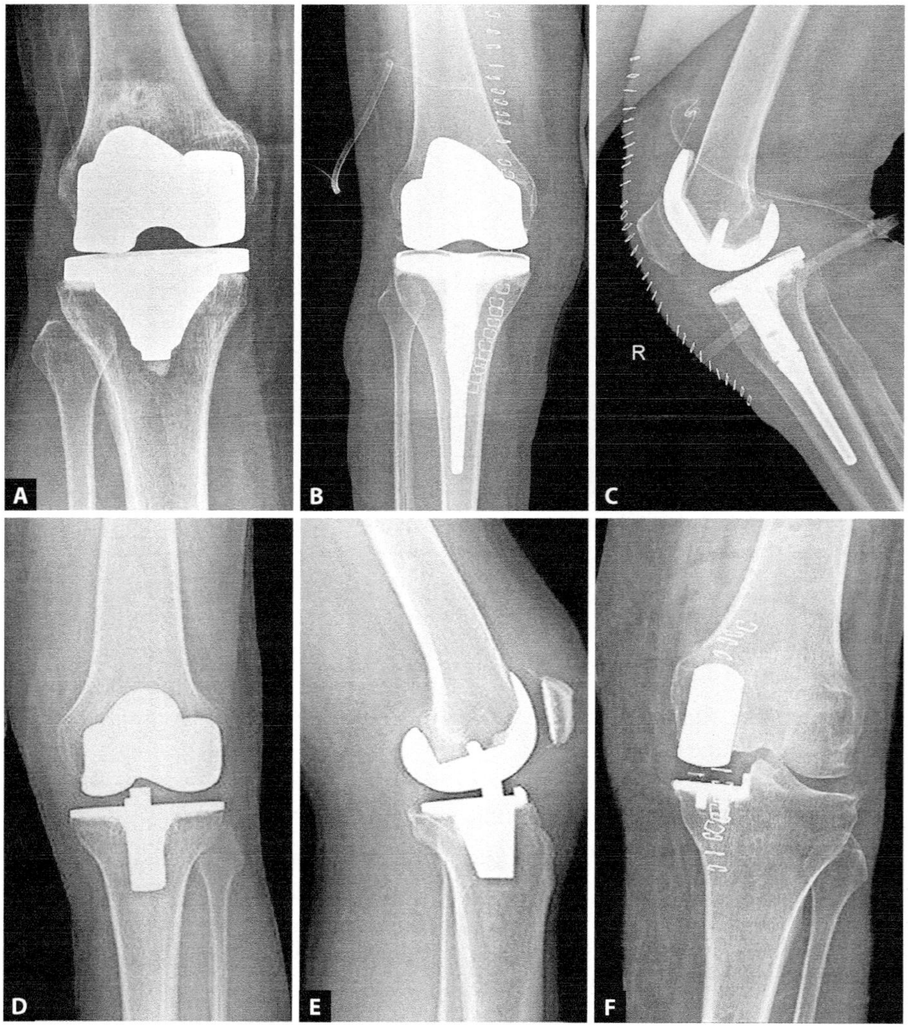

Figs. 11A to F: Different types of knee arthroplasty: (A) Cemented total knee replacement (TKR) with cruciate retaining arthroplasty; (B and C) Cemented long-stem tibial implant in TKR (cruciate retaining arthroplasty); (D and E) Cruciate substituting arthroplasty; (F) Medial joint hemiarthroplasty.

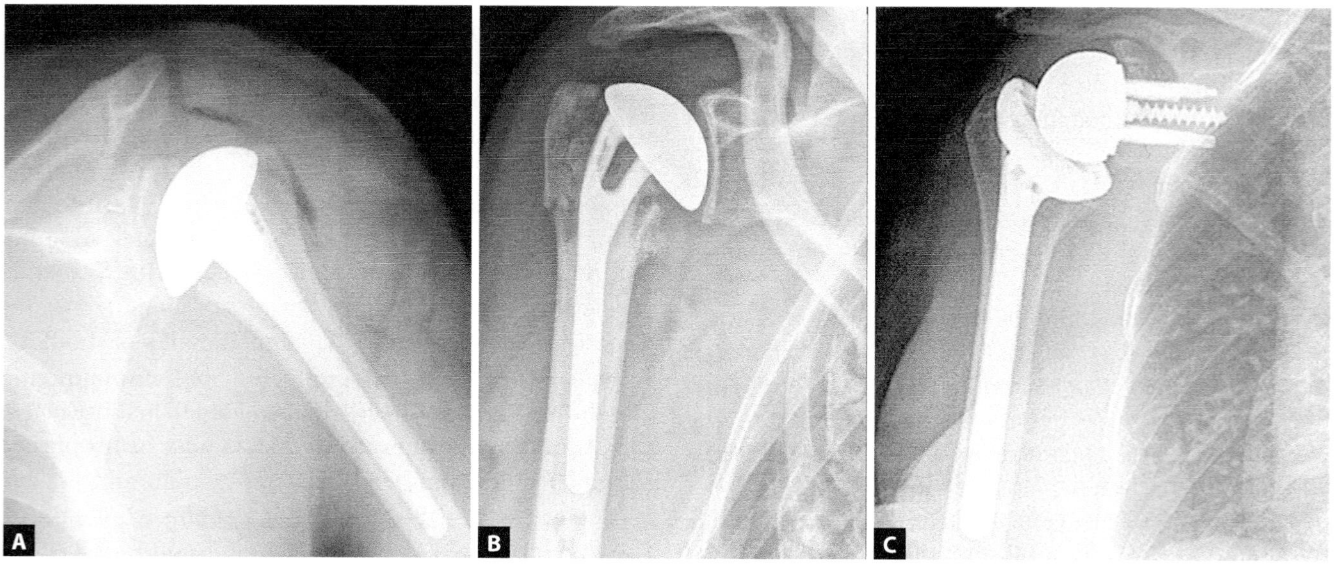

Figs. 12A to C: Types of shoulder arthroplasty: (A) Total shoulder arthroplasty; (B) Hemiarthroplasty for proximal humeral fractures; (C) Reverse shoulder arthroplasty.

COMPLICATIONS

Complications occur due to failure of fixation, failure of implant material or wear and tear **(Figs. 13A to D)**.

Polyethylene Wear

Abnormal loading stress on the implant leads to wear of the polyethylene on the superolateral aspect of the hip. This is the most common cause of arthroplasty failure. The normally expected molding is in superomedial aspect and leads to slight polyethylene thinning in the area of weight-bearing (known as creep). While creep is normal postoperative phenomenon, wear is pathological. Wear results in loss of particulate debris from the prosthetic surface due to abrasion, adhesion, or fatigue. Scratching over of one surface by another is termed abrasion. Transient bonding of the bearing surfaces due to poor lubrication is known as adhesion. Fatigue refers to excessive stress on the implant material, more than the mechanical limits. Loss of the particle debris leads to asymmetric joint space narrowing and eventual metal-on-metal contact. Also, the debris incites foreign body granulomatous reaction, manifested in the form of synovitis and osteolysis **(Flowchart 1)**.

Classification of wear is as follows:

- *Type 1*: Normal.
- *Type 2*: One articulating surface is worn (thinning of polyethylene liner so that metal backing is exposed and articulates with prosthetic head).
- *Type 3*: Third-body (fragment) interposition and abrasion between normal articulating surfaces.
- *Type 4*: Articulation or motion between two nonbearing surfaces.

Particle disease on MRI manifests as intermediate high-signal intensity collections on T2-weighted (T2W) images with synovial thickening (represented by peripheral T2-hypointense foci; **Fig. 13**) and areas of bone lysis (cortical thinning or disruption).

Osteolysis

It refers to bony resorption around the prosthesis and is an important cause of aseptic loosening, eventually requiring revision surgery. Osteolysis results because of poor initial fixation, mechanical stress leading to poor fixation or due to granulomatous reaction to particulate debris from the prosthesis and is common in THR than TKR due to larger particles in former. In the knee, tibial component failure is more common.

Loosening can occur at the implant-bone interface, implant-cement or cement-bone interface. Patients present with chronic persistent pain and there may be mild increase in serum inflammatory markers.

Imaging shows periprosthetic lucency >2 mm or progressive increase in lucency on serial radiographs, especially at the margins of the implant **(Figs. 13 and 14)**. There may be fracture of the cement mantle, bead shedding (punctate metal pieces around the bony

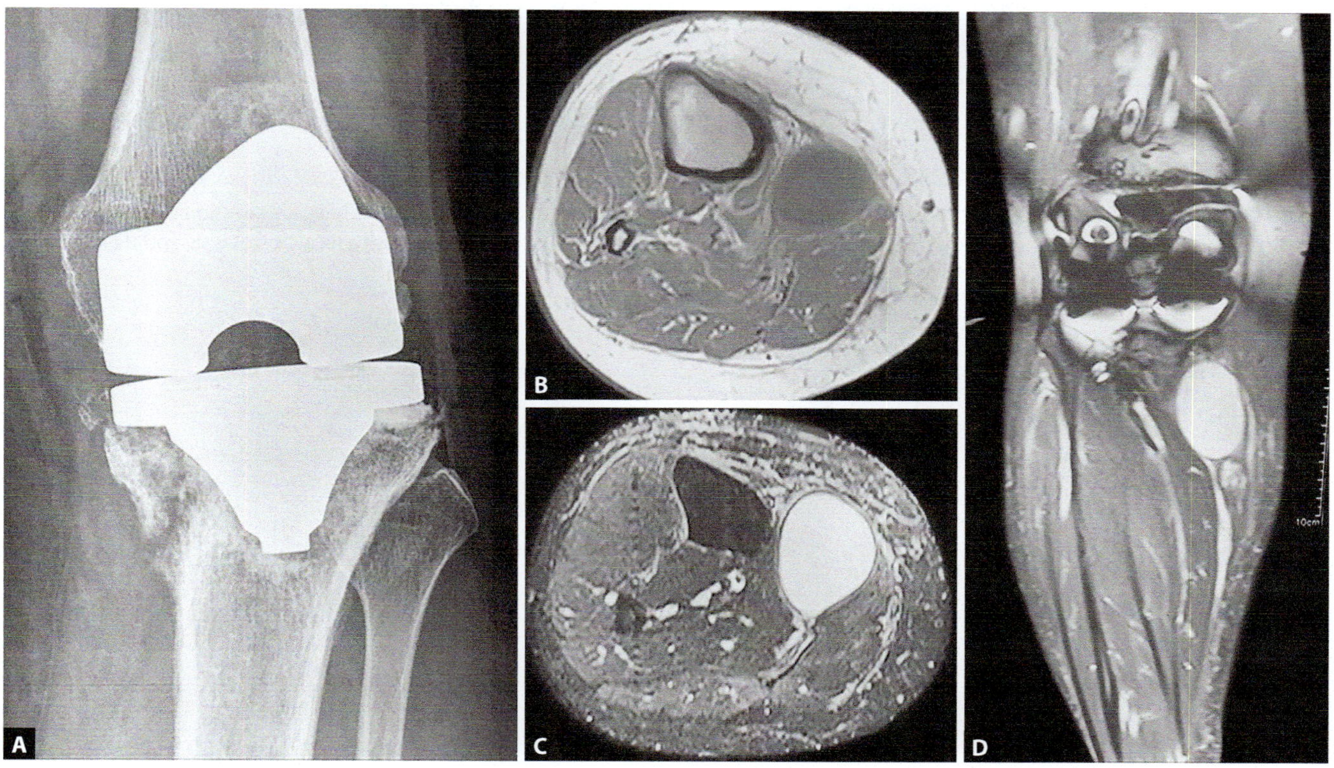

Figs. 13A to D: Complications of joint prosthesis: (A) Aseptic loosening of tibial component with periprosthetic fracture and implant malalignment; (B) Axial T1-weighted (T1W); (C) T2W; and (D) Short-tau inversion recovery (STIR) coronal images showing periprosthetic fluid collection.

ingrowth) and pedestal formation (sclerosis in medullary cavity distal to the tip of implant) as well. Progressive increase in periprosthetic radiolucency and component motion, fracture, change in position or migration is highly suggestive of aseptic loosening. However, this entity has to be differentiated from infection. Prior researchers have suggested standard zones to describe the location of periprosthetic lucencies on radiographs (three zones from lateral to medial for acetabular component on AP view, 7 zones each on AP and lateral views for the femoral component, 7 zones for tibial component; **Figs. 15A to C**).[8,9]

Flowchart 1: An algorithmic approach to show how polyethylene wear leads to failure of implant.

Polyethylene wear
↓
Foreign body reaction: Particle disease
↓
Aseptic loosening
↓
Implant failure
↓
Revision surgery

Infection

Infection is a mimicker of aseptic loosening and may be difficult to differentiate. Infection also leads to osteolysis and loosening of the implant with resultant change in position or migration. Diagnosis may be aided by increased erythrocyte sedimentation rate (ESR), C-reactive protein (CRP), leukocyte counts or joint aspiration may be needed. Demonstration of sinus tract on CT or MRI communicating with the implant clinches the diagnosis **(Figs. 16A to D)**. Presence of bone erosions, periosteal reaction, or collection in the soft tissues is suggestive of infection

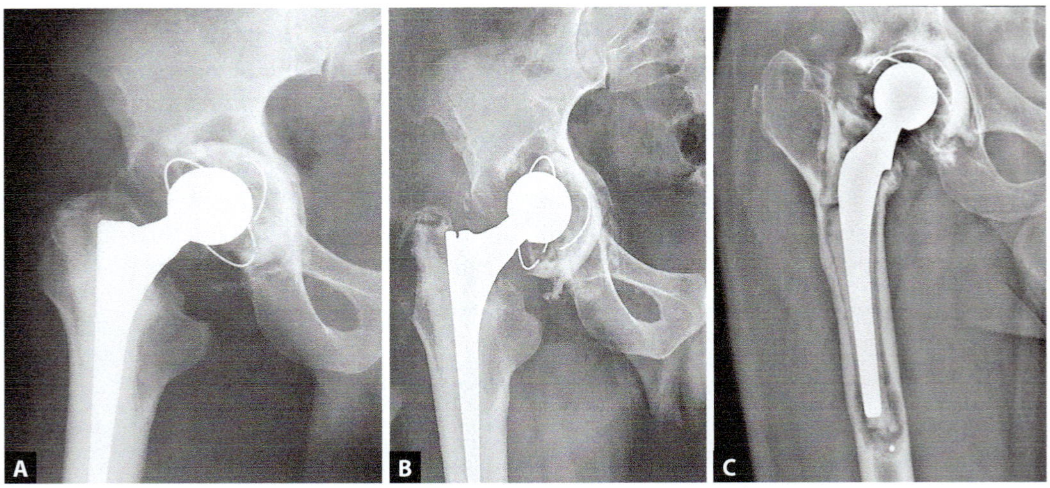

Figs. 14A to C: Complications of joint prosthesis: (A and B) Serial radiographs show development of lucency around acetabular implant (due to particle disease) causing osteolysis, protrusio, and implant failure; (C) Another patient with aseptic osteolysis and development of periprosthetic radiolucency.

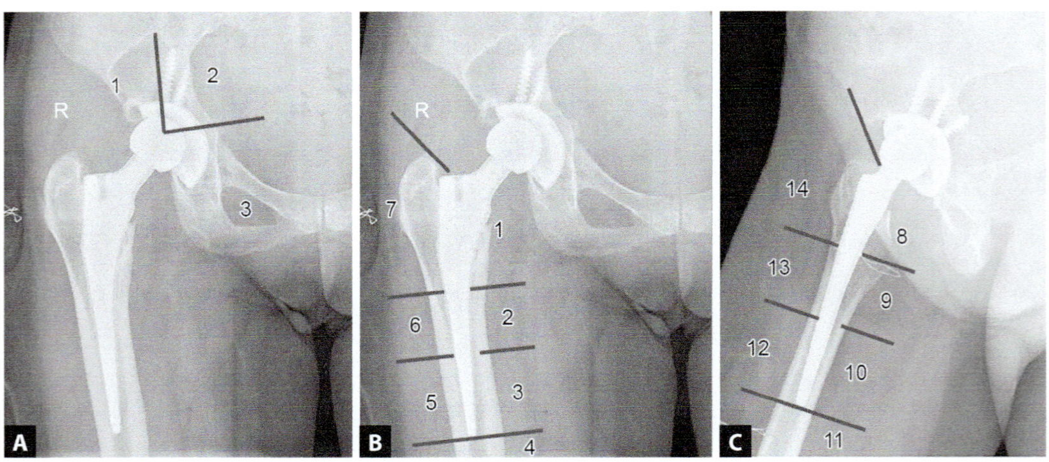

Figs. 15A to C: (A and B) Anterioposterior (AP); and (C) Lateral radiographs showing three zones to describe acetabular lucency, seven zones for femoral lucency on frontal and seven zones on lateral projection.

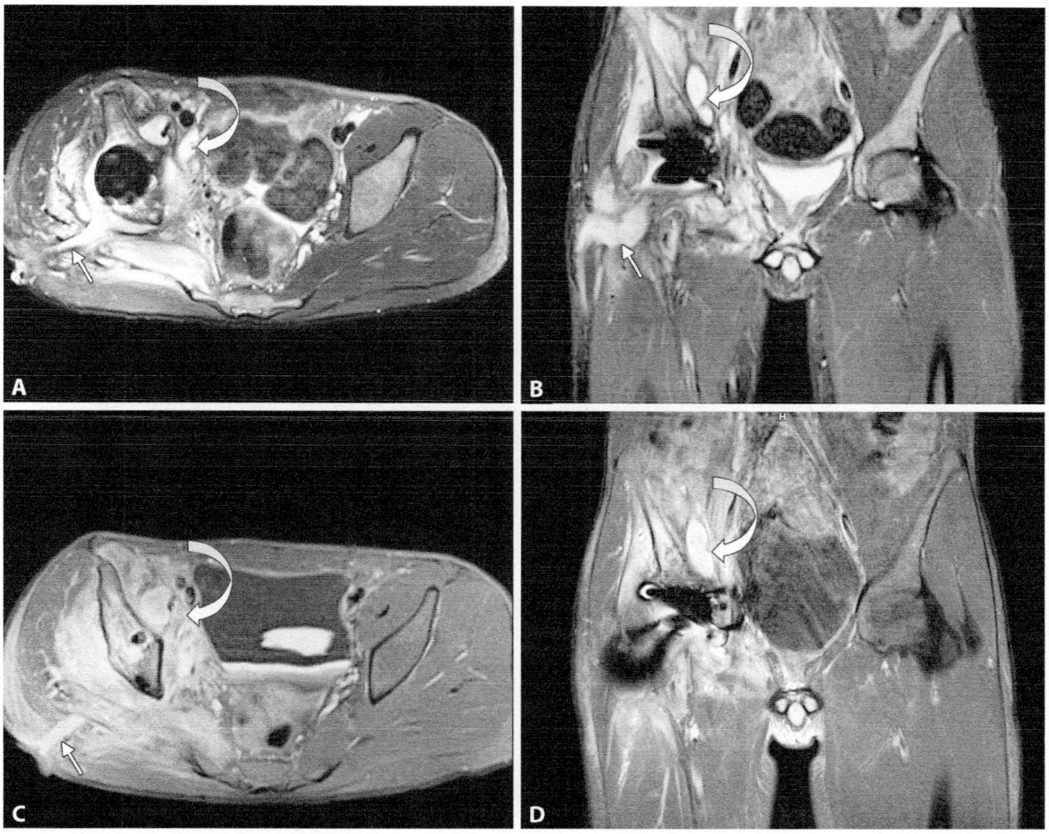

Figs. 16A to D: (A) Axial short-tau inversion recovery (STIR); (B) Coronal STIR; (C) Axial; and (D) Coronal postcontrast magnetic resonance (MR) images show presence of right hip synovitis and soft tissue edema. Note made of multiple fluid collections and lymphadenopathy (curved arrows) in addition to sinus tract reaching the skin (arrow), suggesting active infection.

but not commonly seen. Ultrasound or MRI may show collections and joint effusions which may be aspirated under ultrasound guidance. Associated marrow and soft tissue edema is often present and serves to differentiate from sterile collections.[4] Radionuclide imaging is helpful and leukocyte bone marrow scintigraphy is the imaging gold standard to diagnose infection.

Instability

The causes of prosthetic instability include implant failure either due to aseptic loosening or infection, pre-existing deformity, component malalignment or tears of the ligaments and tendons.[10] In knee, mediolateral instability is the most common. Plain radiographs play important role in identifying instability. Ultrasound helps to identify ligament and tendon injuries especially quadriceps and patellar tendon ruptures.

Fracture/Dislocation

Fractures can occur intraoperatively or after surgery secondary to trauma. In the hip, femoral component is more prone to fracture while in TKR, patella has the maximum propensity to fracture followed by femur and tibia. The propensity of implant fractures has reduced because of the use of high strength metal alloys. Fracture of the femur may occur in THR during the placement of the stem of the femoral implant. Causes of fracture include osteolysis, osteoporosis, falls in elderly patients or prosthetic malalignment **(Figs. 17A and B)**. Dislocation is rare after primary arthroplasty; however, is common in revision THR.[11]

Metallosis/Pseudotumors

Toxicity of metal ions can incite lymphocyte predominant immunological response (similar to type 4 hypersensitivity reaction). This is known as adverse reaction to metal debris or metallosis and histologically it is known as aseptic lymphocyte-dominated vasculitis-associated lesion (ALVAL).[4] These present as mass-forming collections, known as pseudotumors, which are neither neoplastic nor infective. Metal-on-metal THRs are the usual culprits with elevated serum chromium and cobalt levels (>17 μg/L and >19 μg/L respectively) in corresponding prosthesis associated with metallosis. Radiographs may show soft tissue density mass around the implant, which can cause erosions or bony destruction, and may mimic

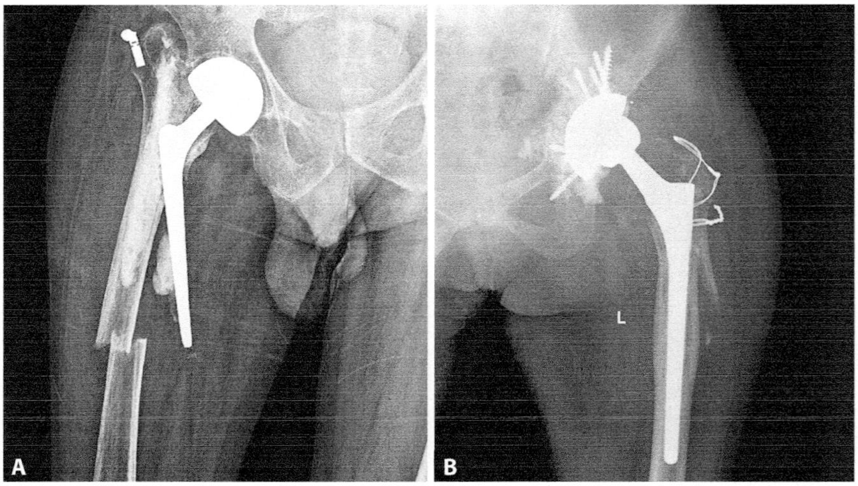

Figs. 17A and B: Postimplant periprosthetic fractures: (A) Radiograph shows fracture femoral shaft; (B) Osteolysis in femoral neck with fracture proximal shaft.

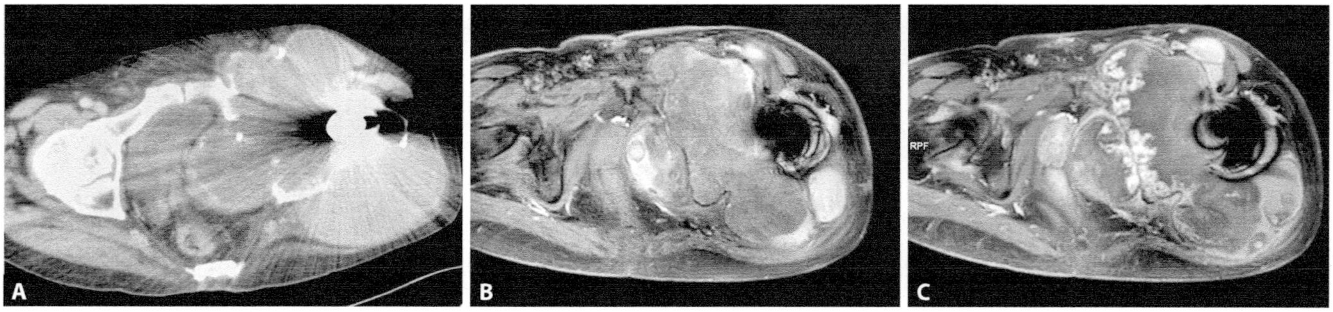

Figs. 18A to C: (A) Axial computed tomography (CT) image shows large destructive mass post left total hip replacement (THR) causing expansion and bone lysis; (B) Axial T1-wighted fat-suppressed image shows heterogeneous signal mass with peripheral hyperintensity; (C) Axial postcontrast image shows heterogeneous enhancement of soft tissue mass. Aspiration revealed sterile viscous dark colored fluid, consistent with the diagnosis of pseudotumor.

like aggressive bone tumor **(Figs. 18A to C)**. Ultrasound demonstrates these lesions as collections which may be anechoic or filled with echogenic debris and associated synovial thickening. On MRI, these lesions usually have a well-defined T2-hypointense wall. The contents are usually hypointense on T2W and hyperintense on T1W images **(Figs. 5 and 18)**.

Heterotopic Ossification

Another complication of joint prosthesis (especially hip) is heterotopic ossification and risk factors include elderly (>65 years) age, male gender, seronegative spondyloarthropathy, and diffuse idiopathic skeletal hyperostosis. It is graded as per Brooker classification, which depends of the extent of involvement of the space between the femur and pelvis.

Soft Tissue Injury

There may be injury to the tendon and muscles leading on to tears and tendinosis, especially at the myotendinous junctions. Predisposed structures include abductor tendons of the hip, the iliopsoas, quadriceps, and patellar tendon and the rotator cuff tendons of the shoulder.[4]

CONCLUSION

With increasing number of joint replacements performed these days, it is imperative for the radiologists to be aware of the normal expected postoperative findings and interpret any abnormality diligently for early detection of complications. Radiographs are the most commonly used imaging modality and serial follow-up is important. Ultrasound, CT, and metal-suppression MRI are used for further evaluation and leukocyte scintigraphy is helpful to diagnose infection.

REFERENCES

1. Taljanovic MS, Jones MD, Hunter TB, Benjamin JB, Ruth JT, Brown AW, et al. Joint arthroplasties and prostheses. Radiographics. 2003;23(5):1295-314.
2. Mulcahy H, Chew FS. Current concepts of hip arthroplasty for radiologists: part 1, features and radiographic assessment. AJR Am J Roentgenol. 2012;199(3):559-69.

3. Roth TD, Maertz NA, Parr JA, Buckwalter KA, Choplin RH. CT of the hip prosthesis: appearance of components, fixation, and complications. Radiographics. 2012;32(4):1089-107.
4. Talbot BS, Weinberg EP. MR imaging with metal-suppression sequences for evaluation of total joint arthroplasty. Radiographics. 2015;36(1):209-25.
5. Vanrusselt J, Vansevenant M, Vanderschueren G, Vanhoenacker F. Postoperative radiograph of the hip arthroplasty: what the radiologist should know. Insights Imaging. 2015;6(6):591-600.
6. Fujishiro T, Hayashi S, Kanzaki N, Hashimoto S, Kurosaka M, Kanno T, et al. Computed tomographic measurement of acetabular and femoral component version in total hip arthroplasty. Int Orthop. 2014;38(5):941-6.
7. De Valk EJ, Noorduyn JCA, Mutsaerts EL. How to assess femoral and tibial component rotation after total knee arthroplasty with computed tomography: a systematic review. Knee Surg Sports Traumatol Arthrosc. 2016;24(11):3517-28.
8. DeLee JG, Charnley J. Radiological demarcation of cemented sockets in total hip replacement. Clin Orthop Relat Res. 1976;121:20-32.
9. Johnston RC, Fitzgerald RH, Harris WH, Poss R, Müller ME, Sledge CB. Clinical and radiographic evaluation of total hip replacement. A standard system of terminology for reporting results. J Bone Joint Surg Am. 1990;72(2):161-8.
10. Fritz J, Lurie B, Potter HG. MR imaging of knee arthroplasty implants. Radiographics. 2015;35(5):1483-501.
11. Manaster BJ. From the RSNA refresher courses. Total hip arthroplasty: radiographic evaluation. Radiographics. 1996;16(3):645-60.

SECTION

7

Breast Imaging and Interventions

CHAPTER

25

A Systematic Approach to Imaging of Breast Lesions

Smita Manchanda, Smriti Hari, Manisha Jana, Arun Kumar Gupta

INTRODUCTION

Imaging plays a crucial role in the early detection and accurate diagnosis of breast cancer, the first-line investigations being mammography and ultrasound (US). Magnetic resonance imaging (MRI) has a high sensitivity for breast pathology and is a valuable second-line investigation. Mammographic early detection of breast cancer has proven reduction in mortality.[1] In the screening setup, the sensitivity of mammography in detection of breast malignancy is in the range of 83–95%.[2] But in radiographically dense breasts, this sensitivity decreases to as low as 30–48%.[3]

IMAGING TECHNIQUES

MAMMOGRAPHY

Mammography is technically challenging as it requires excellent soft tissue contrast, high spatial resolution, and wide image latitude especially in denser breasts combined with a low radiation dose. The mammography equipment and technique has to account for the wide variation in breast size and also the relative amounts of fat, glandular and stromal tissue. Also, there is a low inherent contrast between normal and abnormal breast tissue.

Mammography Equipment

Dedicated mammography X-ray equipment **(Fig. 1)** with following features is necessary for producing high-quality images:

- *Tube current:* As high as possible to keep exposure time short.
- *Target-filter combination:* Molybdenum target with 0.03 mm molybdenum filter.
  - *Special X-ray tubes with molybdenum or rhodium anodes:* Low energy X-rays required necessary to achieve high tissue contrast.
  - *Adding filters at the source of the X-ray beam:* This removes the very low energy photons which are likely to be absorbed in the breast (do not contribute in the image formation).
- *Peak kilovoltage (kVp):* Range 26–30 kV.

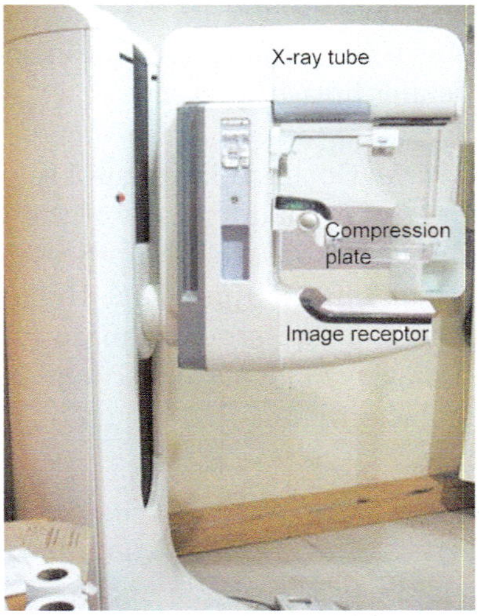

Fig. 1: Mammography equipment. Modern mammography machines automatically select target/filter combination, peak kilovoltage (kVp) and tube current according to breast density and the thickness of the compressed breast.

- High spatial resolution is essential to identify microcalcifications measuring in the order of 100 μm.
  - Small focal spot of the X-ray tube (0.3 mm for routine mammography and 0.1 mm for magnification mammography).
  - High-resolution film-screen combinations.
- Grids are used to reduce scattered radiation and to increase contrast, especially in the dense or thick breast.
- *Automated exposure control:* Modern equipment automatically selects target/filter combination, kVp and tube current according to breast density and the thickness of the compressed breast, e.g., higher energy X-ray spectrum for large breasts for sufficient penetration. These devices also control the exposure duration so that the optimum optical density of the mammograms is maintained over a wide range of breast densities and sizes. The automatic exposure control device (phototimer or ionization chamber) is normally positioned 3 cm posterior to the nipple, where the most dense glandular tissue is likely to be seen.

- *Single side emulsion film with a single intensifying screen:* For optimum resolution. Specially designed cassettes ensure good film-screen contact.
- *Breast compression:* Good breast compression with radiolucent compression paddle is essential for mammography. This results in uniform thickness and hence uniform exposure and density in most parts of the breast. Separation of the overlapping tissues improves their visualization. Firm compression of the breast closer to film/image receptor also helps to reduce the geometric blur and magnification. As the breast is stabilized, the movement blur is also reduced. Mammography cannot be performed if breast compression is not possible (example in uncooperative women, tender breasts, presence of wound or recent surgery).
- *Quality control:* Good quality control is essential and includes periodic maintenance of the equipment, positioning and exposure, film processing, viewing conditions and the interpretation. The requirements of mammography are probably more stringent than any other imaging modality for accurate detection and disease characterization.

Mammography Projections

The standard mammographic evaluation consists of two orthogonal images for basic imaging evaluation of each breast: (1) mediolateral oblique (MLO) view and (2) craniocaudal (CC) view. The entire breast cannot be included in any single mammographic view. More breast tissue is shown on the MLO projection than on any other view.

Mediolateral Oblique View

It is obtained with the tube angled at 45° to the horizontal, with compression applied obliquely across the chest wall, perpendicular to the long axis of the pectoralis major muscle **(Fig. 2A)**.

Craniocaudal View of Breast

It is obtained with a vertical X-ray beam. The breast is pulled up and forward, away from the chest wall and compression is applied from above **(Fig. 2B)**. It demonstrates the subareolar, medial and lateral portions of the breast; however, tissue in the posterolateral aspect of the breast may not be documented completely. The criteria for well-positioned MLO and CC views are given in **Box 1**.

Supplementary Views

These can be taken to solve specific diagnostic problems.

Rolled view: These separate normal fibroglandular elements into their individual components. The breast tissue is "rolled" and compressed in the same projection in which the finding was first noted. On the rolled view, true masses will retain their shape and persist; whereas if it is separated into its normal fibroglandular components, it represents a summation shadow.

Magnification view ***(Figs. 4A and B):*** Magnification is required for analysis of microcalcifications and the margins of small mass lesions. This can be done by increasing the film-object distance, producing an "air gap", and using a fine focal spot to increase resolution.

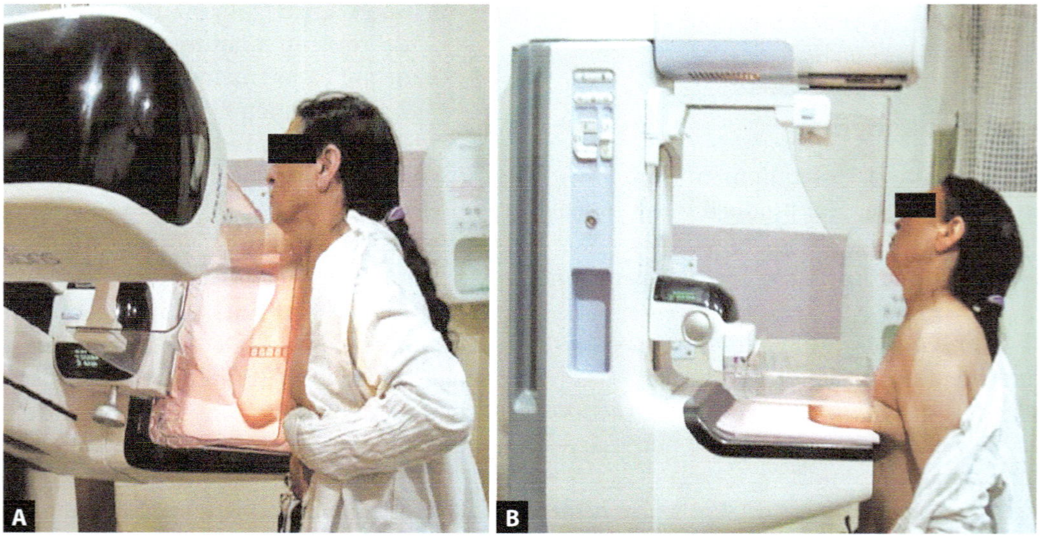

Figs. 2A and B: Positioning for mediolateral oblique (MLO) and craniocaudal (CC) views. (A) MLO view. The MLO view is obtained with the tube angled at 45° to the horizontal, with compression applied obliquely across the chest wall, perpendicular to the long axis of the pectoralis major muscle; (B) CC view. Positioning is achieved by pulling the breast up and forward, away from the chest wall, with compression applied from above.

Box 1: Criteria for well-positioned mediolateral oblique (MLO) and craniocaudal (CC) views.

Criteria for a well-positioned MLO view ***(Fig. 3A)***:
- Nipple to be seen in profile
- Pectoralis muscle should extend inferior to the posterior nipple line (PNL)
(PNL is an imaginary line drawn from the nipple to the pectoralis muscle or film edge and is perpendicular to pectoralis muscle)
- Visible open inframammary fold
- No superimposition of skin folds on the breast

Criteria for a well-positioned CC view ***(Fig. 3B)***:
- Nipple to be demonstrated in profile
- The PNL on the CC view is drawn from the nipple to the pectoralis muscle or film edge. Length of PNL on the CC view should be within 1 cm of its length on the MLO view

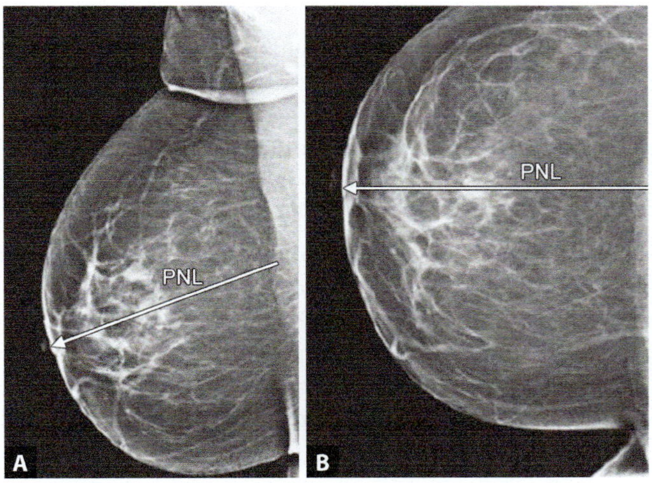

Figs. 3A and B: Well-positioned mediolateral oblique (MLO) and craniocaudal (CC) views. (A) A well-positioned MLO view should include breast tissue from high in the axilla to just below the inframammary fold. The pectoralis muscle should extend inferior to the posterior nipple line (PNL) an imaginary line drawn from the nipple to the pectoralis muscle or film edge and perpendicular to the pectoralis muscle; (B) An adequately positioned CC view should demonstrate the subareolar, medial and lateral portions of the breast. The PNL on the CC view is drawn from the nipple to the pectoralis muscle or film edge. The length of the PNL on the CC view should be within 1 cm of its length on the MLO projection.

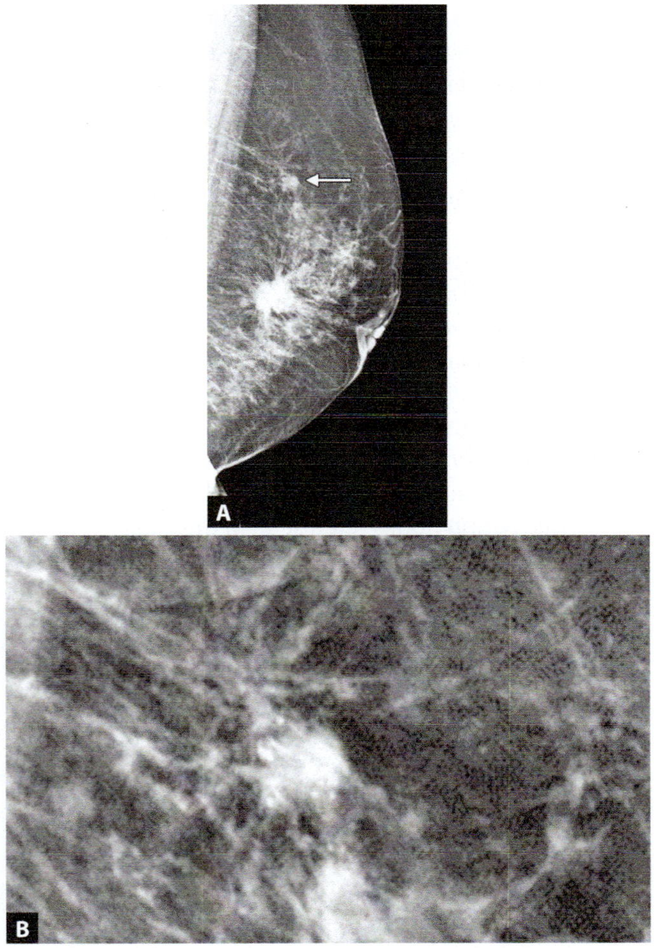

Figs. 4A and B: Left mediolateral oblique (MLO) (A) and magnification mammography (B). Margins of the mass in upper outer quadrant of left breast (arrow in A) are better seen on magnification mammography.

Spot compression view: This is obtained by using a small compression paddle with or without magnification. Compression displaces the breast tissue overlying a small lesion and there is better delineation of morphologic features. Spot compression view also helps to differentiate the cause of asymmetrical soft tissue shadows as normal glandular tissue or underlying mass lesion.

Extended craniocaudal view: This view is performed by rotating the patient's body to display the lateral or medial breast tissue better than possible with a standard CC view. When the patient is rotated medially, the lateral part of the breast and axillary tail is brought over the film and the medial portion of the breast is excluded. This well demonstrates the tissue in most posterolateral part of the breast. For medial breast lesions, the patient is rotated laterally to bring the medial part of the breast over the film and the outer breast tissue is excluded.

Indications for Mammography

Mammography is not usually done in pregnant or lactating women and is generally avoided in women below 30 years of age. The major indications for mammography are listed in **Box 2**.

Normal Mammographic Anatomy

There are 15–20 lobes in the breast. A single lactiferous duct drains each lobe and repeatedly branches within breast. Terminal ducts are the distal most branches and they have extralobular and intralobular portions **(Fig. 5)**. Lobule is formed by the intralobular portion and the acini.

The lobule and extralobular duct form the terminal ductal lobular unit (TDLU). This TDLU is the site of beginning of most malignant and benign disease of the breast.

Mammographic Appearance

It depends on the relative amounts of fat and glandular tissue.

- *Young woman's breast:* Large amount of glandular tissue (soft tissue density)
- *Older women:* Involution of glandular tissue has occurred and mostly fatty density.

Normal lymph node: An oval or lobulated dense mass with a radiolucent fatty hilum.

- *Intramammary lymph nodes:* Within the breast in the upper outer quadrant
- Normal lymph nodes often seen in the axilla.

Box 2: Indications for mammography.

- Screening asymptomatic women age ≥ 50 years
- Screening asymptomatic women aged ≥ 35 years with high risk of developing breast malignancy
  - Women with have one or more first-degree relatives diagnosed with premenopausal breast malignancy
  - Women with histologic risk factors at previous surgery, e.g., atypical ductal hyperplasia
- Symptomatic women aged 35 years with breast lump or any other clinical evidence of breast tumor
- For occult primary tumor, search in patients presenting with metastases
- Postoperative surveillance of breast following local excision of breast cancer
- Breast lump in a male

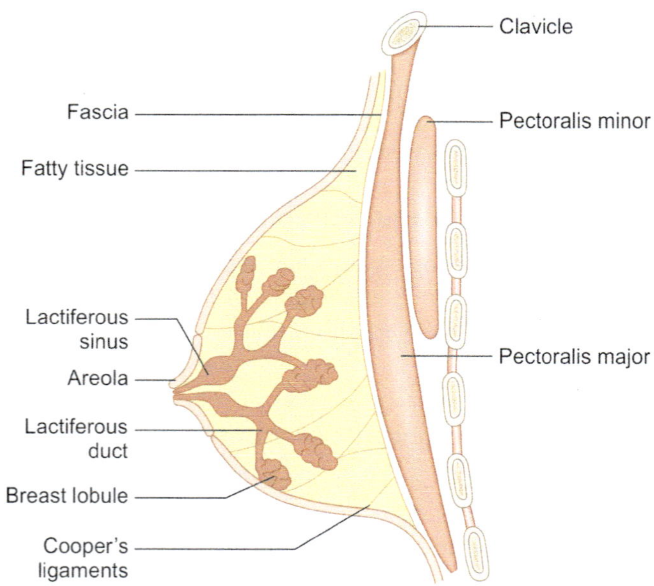

Fig. 5: Schematic representation of the breast anatomy.

Nipple:

- Usually everted
- Should be seen in profile on at least one mammographic view (retroareolar region can be visualized without superimposition of nipple)
- It can be inverted since birth as a normal variant
- Recent nipple inversion is of concern for a retroareolar mass.

Interpretation and Reporting of Mammograms

Viewing:

- Ideally on console [two-dimensional (2D) and tomosynthesis images]

Films:

- In optimum lighting conditions and exclude light from around the films and inessential light in the viewing room
- Check for correct labeling and for radiographic quality
- Standard MLO and CC views studied with right and left breast films "back to back"
- Essential to examine the symmetry of breast tissue.

Breast Imaging—Reporting and Data System

The American College of Radiology (ACR) has devised the Breast Imaging-Reporting and Data System (BI-RADS) for mammogram, US, and MRI. This is a standardized method to describe the morphology of breast lesions and categorize these findings in a definite report. For this lesion description and assessment, there is a lexicon of descriptive terms and the main intention is to provide a common language and ensure consistency in reports. Currently the 5th edition, which was released in 2013, is in use.[4]

Breast Density

The breast density/composition is an evaluation of the relative amounts of fat and fibroglandular tissue in the breast and should be evaluated first while interpreting a mammogram. It is important to remember that the diagnostic accuracy of mammogram falls with increased density of breast. In the 4th edition of ACR lexicon, percentage values of fibroglandular tissue were assessed and reported in increments of 25%. The current ACR BI-RADS divides breast composition into four major categories (from least dense to most dense) based on visual assessment of the mammographic density **(Box 3)**.

Box 3: ACR BI-RADS categories of breast density **(Figs. 6A to D)**.

- Breast tissue almost entirely fatty
- Scattered fibroglandular tissue
- Heterogeneously dense breasts
- Extremely dense breast (lowers the sensitivity of mammograhy)

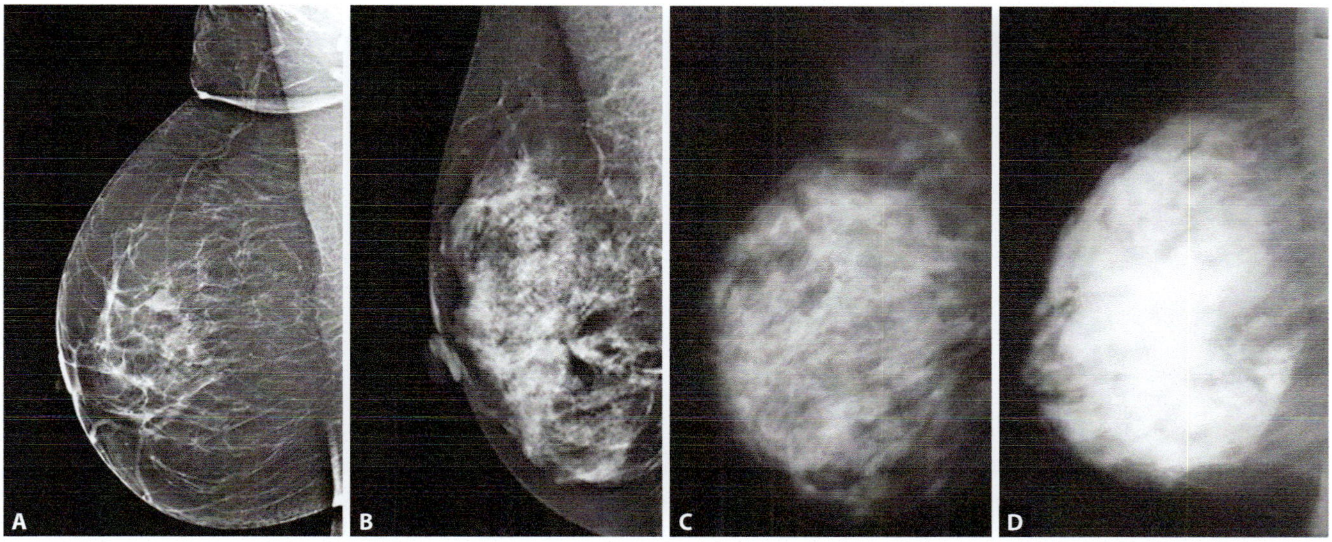

Figs. 6A to D: The American College of Radiology (ACR) categories of breast parenchymal density. (A) Category A: breast tissue almost entirely fatty; (B) Category B: scattered fibroglandular tissue; (C) Category C: heterogeneously dense breasts; (D) Category D: extremely dense breast.

Table 1: ACR BI-RADS mass descriptors in mammography.

Characteristic	*Term*	*Description*
Shape	Round	Spherical
	Oval	Elliptical
	Irregular	Neither round nor oval
Margin	Circumscribed	Margins form a sharp, abrupt transition with the surrounding tissue
	Obscured	Normal surrounding tissue hides the true edge of the lesion
	Microlobulated	Short undulations at the surface of the lesion
	Indistinct	Demarcation between the mass and surrounding tissue is not clearly defined
	Spiculated	Sharp lines radiating from the margins of the mass
Density	High	High density relative to glandular parenchyma
	Equal	Similar density relative to glandular parenchyma
	Low	Less dense relative to glandular parenchyma
	Fat containing	Internal lucent area suggestive of fat

The abnormal mammographic finding is then categorized as a mass, calcification, architectural distortion or asymmetry. Other findings include intramammary lymph node, skin lesion, and solitary dilated duct.

Mass

A breast mass is defined as a three-dimensional (3D) space-occupying lesion, seen in two mammographic views (ACR BI-RADS lexicon). Mass evaluation is optimally done in a spot compression magnification view in which the mass is superimposed over the surrounding fat.

Mass should be described under the following headings:

- Size, morphology (shape, margin), density, associated calcifications, associated features, and location **(Table 1)**.

Size and Location: This should be clearly mentioned in the report in terms of quadrant and approximate clock of position.

Morphology:

Shape: The shape of a mass may be round, oval or irregular **(Figs. 7A to C)** and as the shape becomes more irregular, the probability of malignancy increases. It is important to note that lobular shape descriptor is no longer used according to the ACR 5th edition.[5,6] Hence, a mass with two or three lobulations will be oval and further morphological description would be in terms of margins.

Margins: The margins can be circumscribed (sharply defined), obscured, microlobulated, indistinct or spiculated **(Figs. 8A to E)**. In general, this margin categorization is from least suspicious to most suspicious

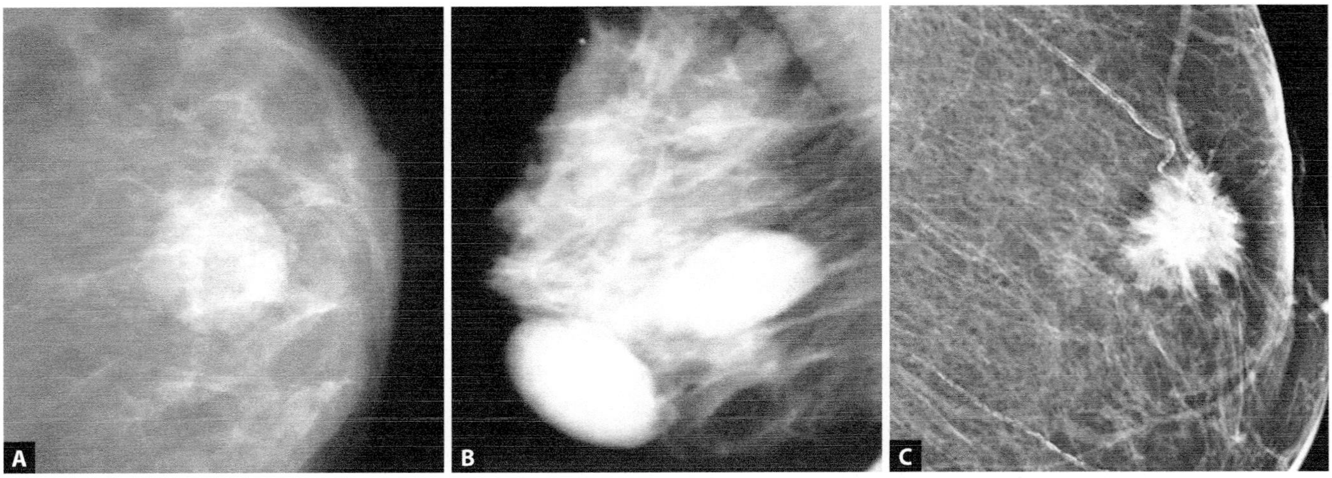

Figs. 7A to C: The American College of Radiology Breast Imaging-Reporting and Data System (ACR BI-RADS) descriptors for mass shape on mammography. (A) Round; (B) Oval; (C) Irregular.

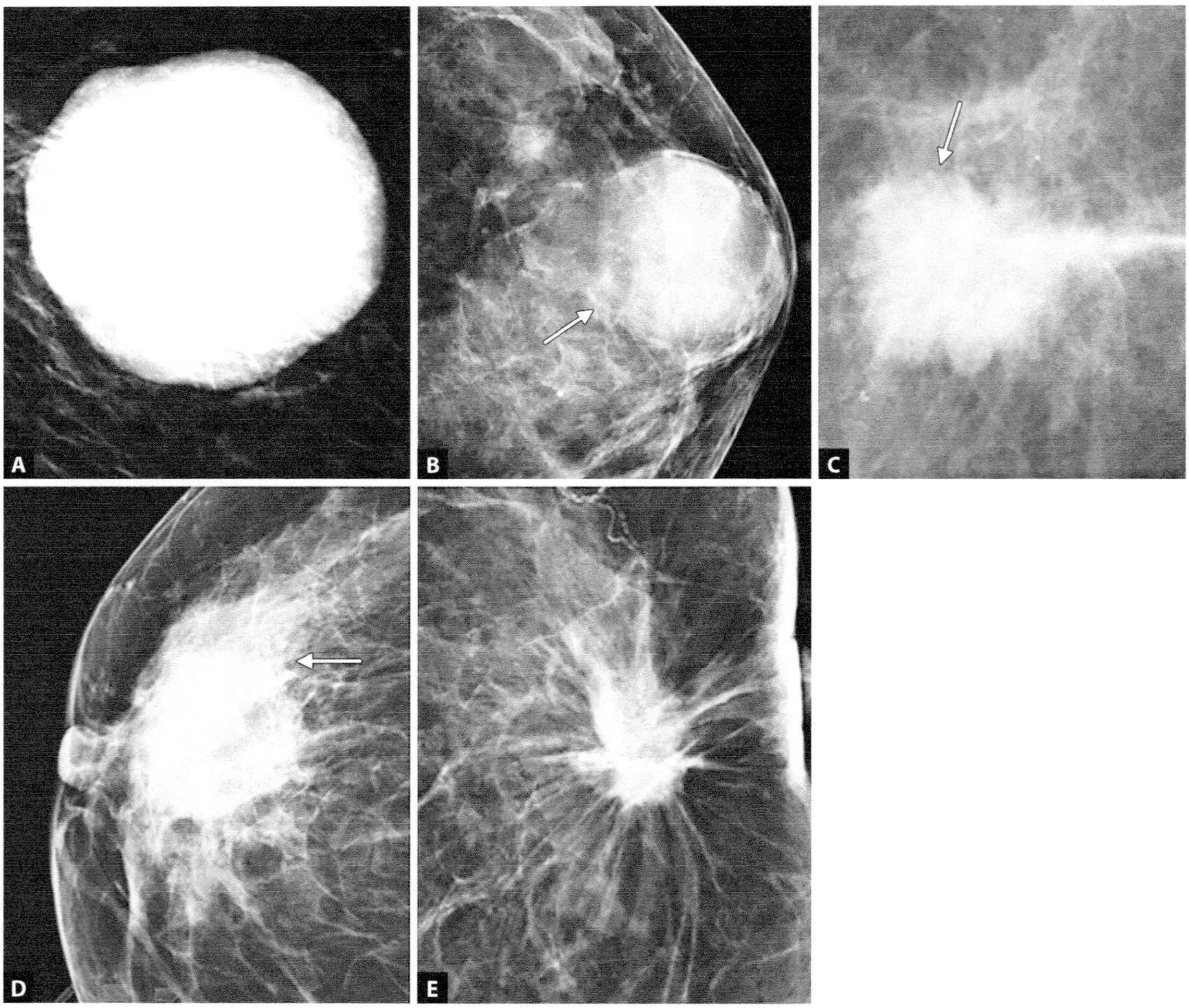

Figs. 8A to E: ACR BI-RADS descriptors for mass margins on mammography. (A) Circumscribed (sharply defined); (B) Obscured (arrow); (C) Microlobulated (arrow); (D) Indistinct (arrow); (E) Spiculated.

for malignancy. Benign masses have *well-circumscribed* borders as these do not invade tissue margins. Term *obscured margin* is used when all or part of the margin abuts glandular parenchyma and cannot be evaluated precisely. *Microlobulations* are small undulations and are suspicious for malignancy.

Breast cancers invade basement membrane and extend into surrounding glandular tissue resulting in irregularly shaped masses with indistinct or spiculated margins. *Spiculated margin* is highly suspicious for malignancy and is characterized by thin lines radiating from the central portion of the mass. Intense fibrotic reaction to tumor or growth of the cancer into surrounding glandular tissue can result in spiculations.

Density: Density is termed as high, equal or low relative to glandular breast parenchyma **(Figs. 9A to C)**. Density of the mass is not effective in characterization of the masses. Exception is fat-containing masses which are always benign and are described as such. The term "radiolucent" has been omitted in the current lexicon.

Calcification

Calcifications are commonly encountered on mammograms but majority of these are the result of benign processes. For description of calcifications, the following descriptors are used: morphology, distribution, associated features, and location.[6,7]

Morphology: Calcifications are broadly classified into typically benign calcifications and those of suspicious morphology **(Table 2)**.

Benign calcifications ***(Figs. 10A to F)****:* Most benign calcifications are >0.5 mm. Typically benign calcifications include lucent-centered calcifications (skin calcifications or fat necrosis), vascular calcifications, popcorn calcifications of involuted fibroadenoma, eggshell or rim calcifications, long rod-like ductal calcifications and coarse dystrophic calcifications. The new lexicon includes eggshell and lucent-centered calcifications under the term "rim". The term "round" includes round and punctate calcifications.

Suspicious morphology category ***(Figs. 11A to D)****:* Amorphous: Tiny, roundish "flake-like" particles too small and vague to characterize further, 27% probability of malignancy. Edges not as sharply defined as in the pleomorphic category. These are often difficult to detect as their density is only slightly higher than surrounding glandular tissue.[5]

Coarse heterogeneous: Irregular, conspicuous and > 0.5 mm, 13% probability of malignancy.

Fine pleomorphic: Varying in shape and density, irregular, < 0.5 mm (microcalcifications), 50% probability of malignancy.

Fine linear or fine-linear branching (casting) calcifications: These form an irregular cast of the duct and appear as little broken needles with sharp ends or "dot-dash" appearance with both linear and round shapes, 78% probability of malignancy. Ductal carcinoma in situ (DCIS) develops in breast duct epithelium, remains within the duct basement membrane, and grows along the duct. Individual calcifications form within the DCIS tumor because of cell death and necrosis in the comedo form of DCIS.

Distribution: The distribution of calcifications **(Table 2 and Figs. 12A to D)** within the breast often may allow benign and malignant categorization. The TDLU is the anatomic site of origin of most intraductal carcinomas. Thus, calcifications oriented in a "linear" or multiple linear ("segmental") orientation are more suspicious. For example, linear or segmental arrangements of coarse heterogeneous calcifications are more worrisome than a regional distribution of the same calcifications.[5,7]

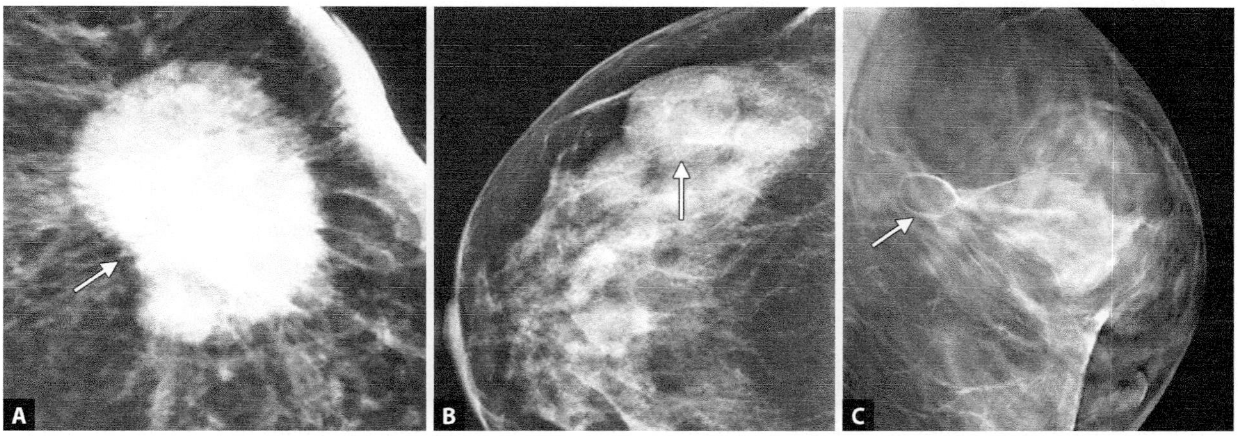

Figs. 9A to C: ACR BI-RADS descriptors for mass density (as compared to the fibroglandular parenchyma) on mammography. (A) High-density mass (arrow); (B) Isodense mass (arrow); (C) Fat attenuation (arrow).

Table 2: Specific ACR BI-RADS terms for description of calcifications.

Characteristic	*Term*	*Description*
Distribution	Segmental	Five or more calcifications in a cubic centimeter of tissue constitutes a cluster
	Linear	Fine-linear branching pattern produced by calcification of necrotic cancer cells within a duct
	Grouped	Calcifications within a single duct network of a lobe
	Regional	Randomly distributed calcifications not conforming to a duct and usually occupying a quadrant or more
	Diffuse	Randomly distributed calcifications throughout the entire breast
Morphology (typically benign)	Skin	Sharply defined with lucent center
	Vascular	Parallel tram-track calcification
	Coarse or "popcorn-like"	Characteristic of involuting fibroadenoma
	Large rod-like	Secretory calcifications—calcified debris in the duct lumen (solid rods), calcified inflammatory reaction around a duct (lucent-centered rods)
	Round	Concretions formed in the acini of microcystically dilated lobules
	Rim	Very thin, benign calcifications that appear as calcium deposited on the surface of a sphere
	Dystrophic	Large (>0.5 mm), irregular (post-trauma or radiotherapy)
	Milk of calcium	
	Suture	Typically linear or tubular in appearance, and knots are frequently visible
Suspicious morphology	Amorphous	Round or flake-shaped deposits those are too small or hazy to characterize
	Coarse heterogeneous	Irregular, dense calcifications >0.5 mm in size
	Fine pleomorphic	Irregular, vary in size and shape, and are <0.5 mm
	Fine linear or fine-linear branching	Thin, discontinuous, irregular particles that form in a linear pattern and are < 1 mm in width (calcifications of necrotic tumor in the lumen of a duct that is irregularly involved by breast cancer)

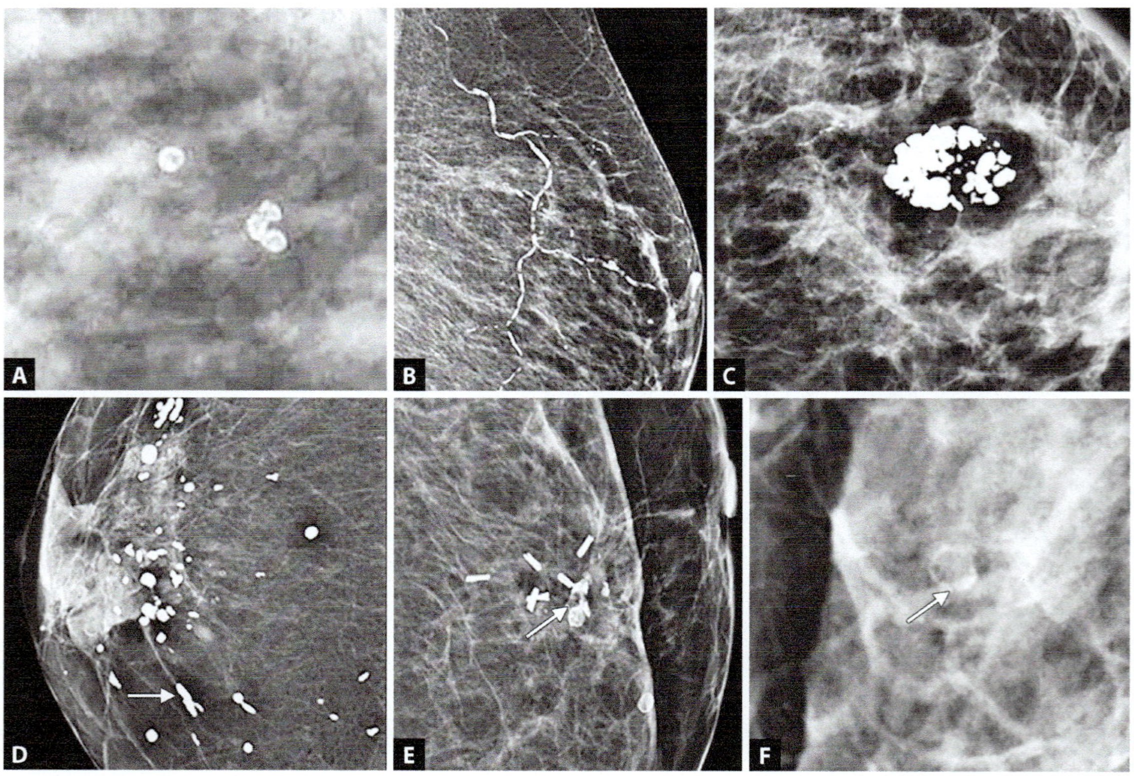

Figs. 10A to F: Typically benign calcifications. (A) Lucent-centered calcifications consistent with skin calcifications; (B) Vascular calcification; (C) Popcorn calcifications within involuted fibroadenoma; (D) Large rod-like (arrow) and round calcifications; (E) Coarse dystrophic calcifications (arrow) and sutures seen in a postoperative breast; (F) Milk of calcium (secretory) (arrow).

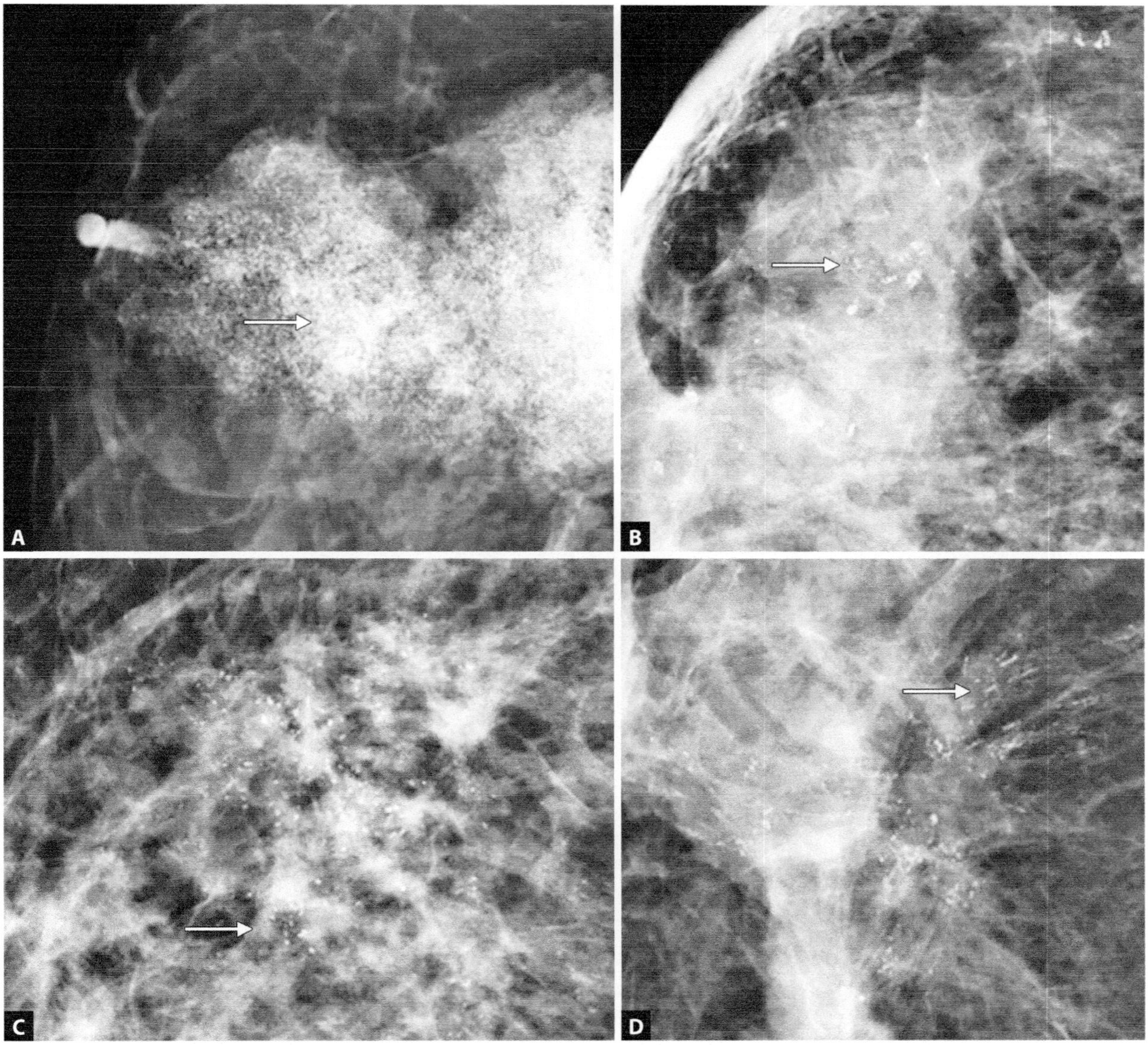

Figs. 11A to D: Calcifications of suspicious morphology. (A) Amorphous (arrow); (B) Coarse heterogeneous (arrow); (C) Fine pleomorphic (arrow); (D) Fine linear or fine-linear branching (arrow).

Grouped microcalcifications occupy <1 cm^3 of tissue and are composed of at least five elements. The new lexicon also includes "a larger number of calcifications within 2 cm of each other" under this category of grouped calcifications.

Architectural Distortion

Architectural distortion implies focal distortion/tethering of trabeculae, focal spiculations and retraction of parenchyma.

Imaging: Architectural distortion is characterized by multiple thin, straight lines or spiculations radiating from an area with no obvious features of an underlying mass or focal asymmetry **(Fig. 13)**. It is important to remember that these radiating spicules can also be seen from the edge of a mass or focal asymmetry where it is a margin descriptor. At times, it is difficult to differentiate spiculated mass from architectural distortion; however, the presence of these radially oriented lines is highly suspicious for malignancy.

Differential diagnosis:[5,6] This includes radial scar/complex sclerosing lesion, malignancy and postoperative scarring. In absence of surgical history, this finding requires a histological diagnosis.

Asymmetries

It is important to differentiate an asymmetry versus a focal asymmetry versus a mass.[6]

Asymmetry: Soft tissue finding identified only on one view, without matching tissue in a similar location in the contralateral breast.

Focal asymmetry and mass: These are seen on two views at a comparable depth with similar density and shape.

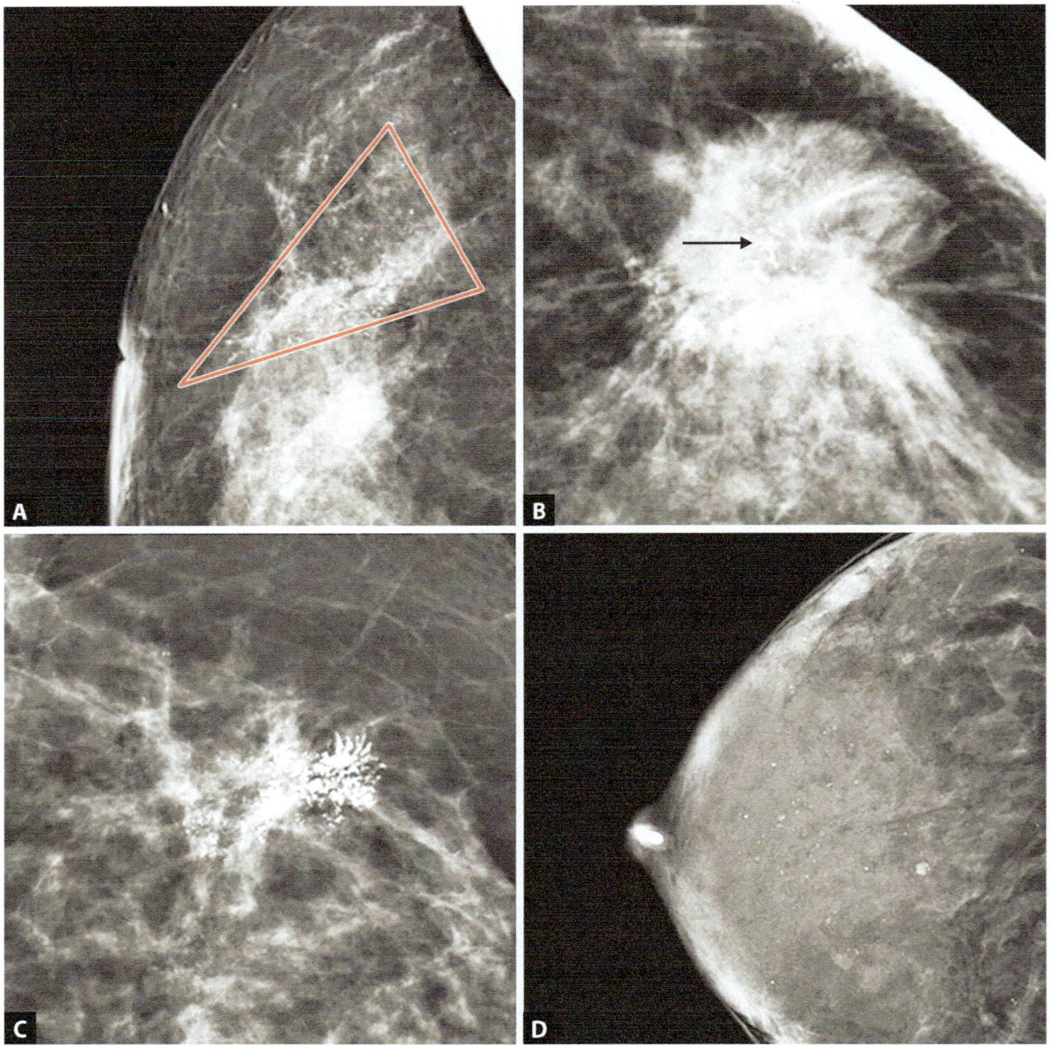

Figs. 12A to D: ACR BI-RADS descriptors for distribution of calcifications. (A) Segmental; (B) Linear (arrow); (C) Grouped; (D) Diffuse.

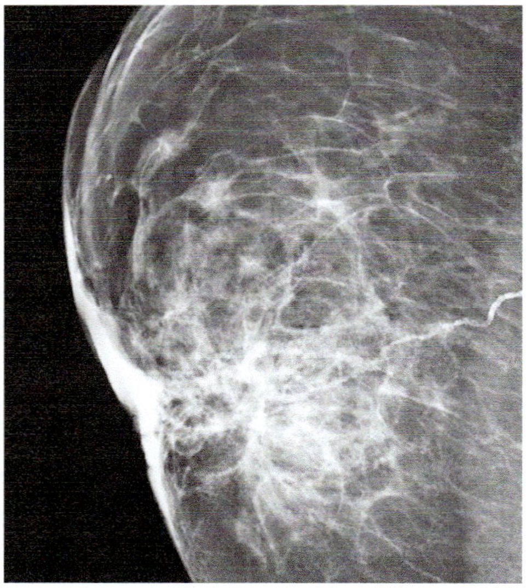

Fig. 13: Architectural distortion (postoperative breast). Mammogram showing multiple thin, straight lines radiating from a central area that does not have features of a mass. There is associated focal skin thickening and retraction.

Mass: Consistent convex margins

Focal asymmetry: It lacks convex outward borders on both views **(Figs. 14A and B)** and usually confined to a small area of the breast.[6]

Global asymmetry: In a larger portion of the breast (>1 quadrant). It can be a normal variation or secondary to the effects of hormone replacement therapy (HRT).

Developing asymmetry: This is a new term introduced in the ACR 5th edition and is defined as "a focal asymmetry which is new or becomes more conspicuous over time". Developing asymmetry is of concern because if seen at screening mammography, there is 12.8% risk for malignancy and persistence at diagnostic mammography carries a 26.7% risk for malignancy.[8]

Associated Features

Certain associated features have been described in the 5th edition for further characterization of mass, calcification

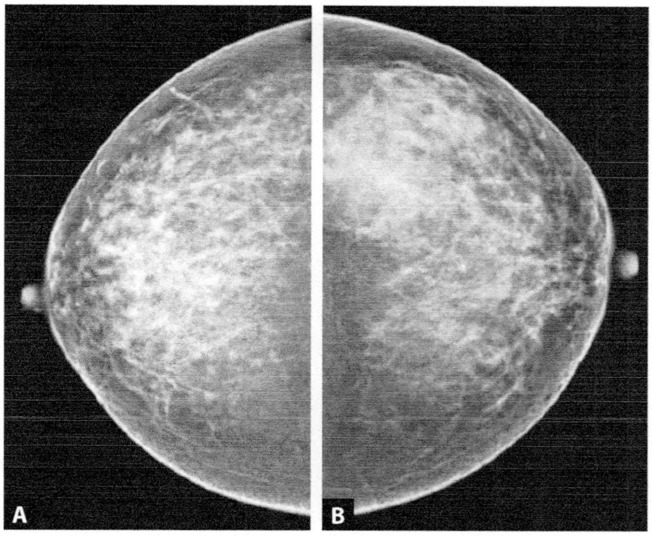

Figs. 14A and B: (A and B) Focal asymmetry. Bilateral craniocaudal (CC) views showing focal asymmetry in the left breast outer quadrant which was also seen on the mediolateral oblique (MLO) view. Ultrasound showed a suspicious mass. Invasive ductal carcinoma on histopathology.

and asymmetry. These include nipple retraction, skin retraction, trabecular thickening, skin thickening, axillary lymphadenopathy, architectural distortion, and calcifications.

Location of Lesion

This should include laterality, the depth of lesion, distance from nipple and quadrant and clock face.[4]

Special Cases

The terms intramammary lymph node, solitary dilated duct and skin lesion are the same as in BI-RADS fourth edition. Asymmetric tubular structure is no longer used now.[5,6] Breast edema and axillary lymph nodes are detailed here.

Breast edema: Breast edema is recognized on mammograms as diffusely increased density and coarse trabecular pattern in an enlarged breast with thickened skin. The causes of an edematous breast are:

- Primary breast cancer. Lymphatic spread from an advanced primary tumor or inflammatory carcinoma can lead to breast edema.
- Axillary lymph node metastasis.
- Breast abscess.
- Radiotherapy (RT). Postradiotherapy treatment there is gradual progression of breast edema which reaches a maximum at 6 months. There is resolution approximately 18 months after RT treatment.
- Cardiac or renal failure: unilateral or bilateral breast edema.

Abnormal axillary lymph nodes:

Normal lymph nodes:

- Commonly seen on mammograms
- Typically, well-defined with central lucency (fatty hilum) and peripheral soft tissue attenuation
- Intramammary lymph nodes: Commonly in the upper outer quadrant with similar features.

Pathological lymph nodes:

- Enlarged and show loss of central fatty lucency
- Benign conditions like infection, sarcoidosis
- Malignant conditions like lymphoma, leukemia or metastasis.

Calcification in lymph nodes:

- Metastatic lymph nodes from breast cancer: Microcalcification
- Tubercular nodes: Coarse calcification.

ACR BI-RADS Assessment Categories

The mammographic findings are categorized from BI-RADS 0 to BI-RADS 6, which are primarily aimed for communication of significance of the mammographic findings to the referring physician and to recommend the most appropriate management[4-6] **(Table 3)**.

Mammographic Assessment is Incomplete

Category 0—Incomplete evaluation: This category needs additional evaluation by imaging and/or comparison with previous mammograms.

Mammographic Assessment is Complete—Final Categories

Category 1—Negative: In this category, there is nothing specific to mention. Both the breasts are symmetric and there is no evidence of any mass, suspicious calcification or architectural distortion.

Category 2—Benign finding: This category is also a normal assessment; however, lesions with characteristically benign findings are described here. This includes multiple secretory calcifications and involuting or calcified fibroadenomas. The fat-containing lesions (oil cysts, galactoceles, lipomas, hamartomas) also have characteristic appearances.

Other findings like intramammary lymph nodes, implants, vascular calcifications, or postoperative changes (architectural distortion/sutures) can also be mentioned in this category clearly stating that there is no mammographic evidence of malignancy.

Category 3—Probably benign finding: A finding in this category would have >0% chance of malignancy but <2%. This includes a nonpalpable well-circumscribed mass on mammogram, or cluster of punctate calcifications or a

Table 3: ACR BI-RADS mammographic assessment categories.

Category	*Description*	*Likelihood of malignancy*	*Examples*	*Next step in evaluation*
0	Incomplete; need additional imaging evaluation, or comparison with previous examinations	Unknown	Asymmetry, mass, calcifications on screening mammography	Special mammographic views, US, MRI; obtain previous examinations
1	Negative	No mammographic evidence of malignancy	Normal mammography	Routine screening
2	Benign finding	No mammographic evidence of malignancy	Intramammary lymph node, oil cyst, vascular calcifications, calcifying fibroadenoma	Routine screening
3	Probably benign finding	<2%	Benign-appearing solid mass or clustered calcifications	Follow-up imaging (mammography or US) at 6 and 12 months
4	Suspicious abnormality	5–95%	Complex or solid mass, indeterminate clustered calcifications	Biopsy
5	Highly suggestive of malignancy	>95%	Spiculated mass	Biopsy
6	Known malignancy	100%	Biopsy-proven	Definitive treatment

focal asymmetry. It is essential to document lesion stability on an initial short-term interval follow-up at 6 months; followed by additional examinations till long-term 2- or 3-year stability is documented.[7]

Category 4—Suspicious abnormality: In this category, the probability of malignancy is large from 5 to 95% and it is further subdivided into 4A, 4B, and 4C.

BI-RADS 4A category: Lesions with a very low probability for malignancy. They are sampled but a malignant histopathology report is not expected. In these cases, a 6-month follow-up after a benign biopsy is suitable. Examples: palpable, partially circumscribed solid mass with sonography features suggestive of a fibroadenoma, a breast abscess or a palpable complicated cyst.

BI-RADS 4B category: Lesions with an intermediate probability of malignancy. Biopsy is recommended and close radiopathological correlation is warranted. If there is a benign biopsy report, follow-up depends on the concordance between imaging and pathological features.

For example, a partially circumscribed mass with ill-defined margins with a fibroadenoma result is satisfactory, but in case of a diagnosis of papillary lesion, surgery should be advised.

BI-RADS 4C category: These findings are of moderate concern, but not classical for malignancy and a malignant biopsy result is expected in this category. In case of a benign result, 6-month follow-up is essential to rule out a false-negative report.

Examples of findings placed in this category are recent cluster of fine pleomorphic calcifications solid, irregular masses with ill-defined margins.

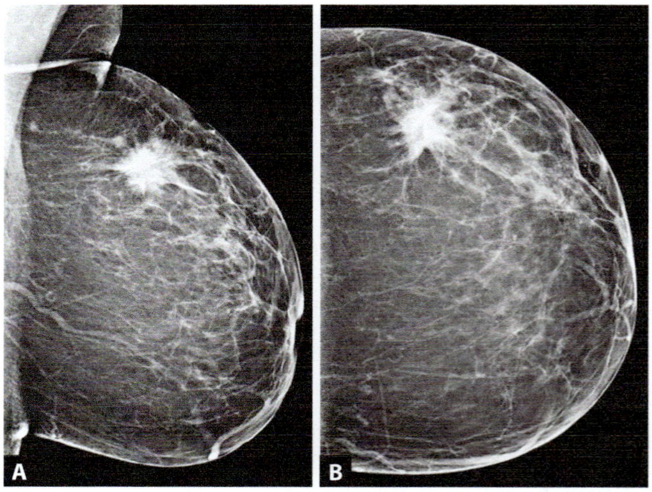

Figs. 15A and B: Illustrative example for ACR BI-RADS mammographic assessment categories. (A) Craniocaudal (CC) view; (B) Mediolateral oblique (MLO) view. High density, irregular shaped mass with spiculated margins in upper outer quadrant of left breast. Highly suggestive of malignancy lesion—BI-RADS 5.

Category 5—Highly suggestive of malignancy: Findings typical for classic breast cancers, with a >95% likelihood of malignancy.

Examples of findings suggestive of this category are: segmental or linear arrangement of fine-linear calcifications; spiculated, irregular high-density mass or irregular spiculated mass **(Figs. 15A and B)** with associated pleomorphic calcifications.

Category 6—Known biopsy-proven malignancy: In this category, lesions are identified on the imaging study of patients with biopsy diagnosis of malignancy.

Digital Mammography

Full-field digital mammography (FFDM) is now gradually replacing screen-film (conventional) mammography. The diagnostic yield is increased by newer applications of digital mammography like digital breast tomosynthesis (DBT) and contrast-enhanced mammography.

Full-field Digital Imaging

Digital systems may be direct radiography (DR) units, which have a built-in digital detector, thus completely replacing screen-film mammography (SFM) or computed radiography (CR) units, which consist of add-on digital conversion detectors that only replace the screen-film cassette system in a screen-film unit.

Computed Radiography Systems

These use photostimulable phosphor imaging plates that can be loaded into a conventional bucky assembly. Image acquisition in CR is a two-stage process and requires transfer of the CR plate to the readout device. The CR mammography screen and cassettes are different from CR radiography and have higher detective quantum efficiency (DQE) and reduced noise. The CR image can be displayed on a high-resolution monitor or printed on film.

Digital Radiography Systems

The digital detector converts the X-rays into digital signals and replaces the film and are of two types.

1. *Indirect digital detectors*: These convert X-rays into light and then into a digital signal. These detectors use photostimulable phosphors, amorphous silicon or charge-coupled devices (CCDs).
2. *Direct digital detectors*: Also known as flat panel detectors, they use a photoconductive material that is able to directly convert X-ray photons into a digital image. Examples include amorphous selenium detectors and crystal silicon detectors.[9]

The overall design of the mammography unit (including X-ray tube, gantry, compression paddles), technique of doing the mammography and amount of radiation involved remains similar to those of the film-screen mammography.

Radiation Dose

The mean glandular dose in FFDM is comparable to or less than SFM. The average single view mean glandular dose for FFDM is 1.86 mGy, which is 22% lower than the average film-screen mammography mean glandular dose of 2.37 mGy.[10]

Advantages and Applications of the Digital Mammography

Digital mammography images are available for immediate viewing and dark room, which is frequently a major source of image degradation and artifacts, is eliminated. The advantages of digital mammography over SFM are:

- Better contrast characteristics and dynamic range. There is no loss of contrast in over or underexposed portions of the digital image and similar contrast is seen over the entire dynamic range of the detector.
- Postprocessing such as manipulations of the brightness, contrast, zoom-pan and edge enhancement and adjustment of image display.
- Better archival, storage and communication, i.e. picture archiving and communication system (PACS) and telemammography.

When compared with the SFM, major limitations of digital mammography are the cost and lower spatial resolution. FFDM systems have spatial resolutions from 5 to 10 lp/mm, whereas the SFM combinations have a linepair resolution of 18–20 lp/mm. This lower spatial resolution of FFDM is compensated by an increase in contrast resolution. The digital system has wider dynamic range and hence it can record and differentiate minor variations in contrast better than SFM.

Newer applications of the digital mammography are exciting. These include computer-aided detection (CAD) and diagnosis, DBT and dual-energy contrast-enhanced mammography.

Computer-aided Detection

Computer-aided detection is a computer software system that is designed to aid the film reader by highlighting the areas of concern (calcifications and masses). The software highlights the suspicious areas for careful evaluation by the radiologist. The CAD thus decreases the chances of overlooking these abnormalities. It may help inexperienced radiologists, and also acts as a second opinion to the experienced radiologists. Use of CAD in screening setups increases the cancer detection rates.[11] There is lower specificity with high false-positive rates.

Digital Breast Tomosynthesis

The dense glandular tissue may hide an underlying mass, or it may simulate a mass when none exists. DBT is a digital imaging technique, which helps to distinguish glandular breast tissue from true lesions, especially in dense breasts. It is more helpful in characterization of asymmetries, architectural distortion and masses than in the assessment of calcifications.[12]

Multiple projections are acquired at different depths by a digital detector from a mammographic X-ray source that

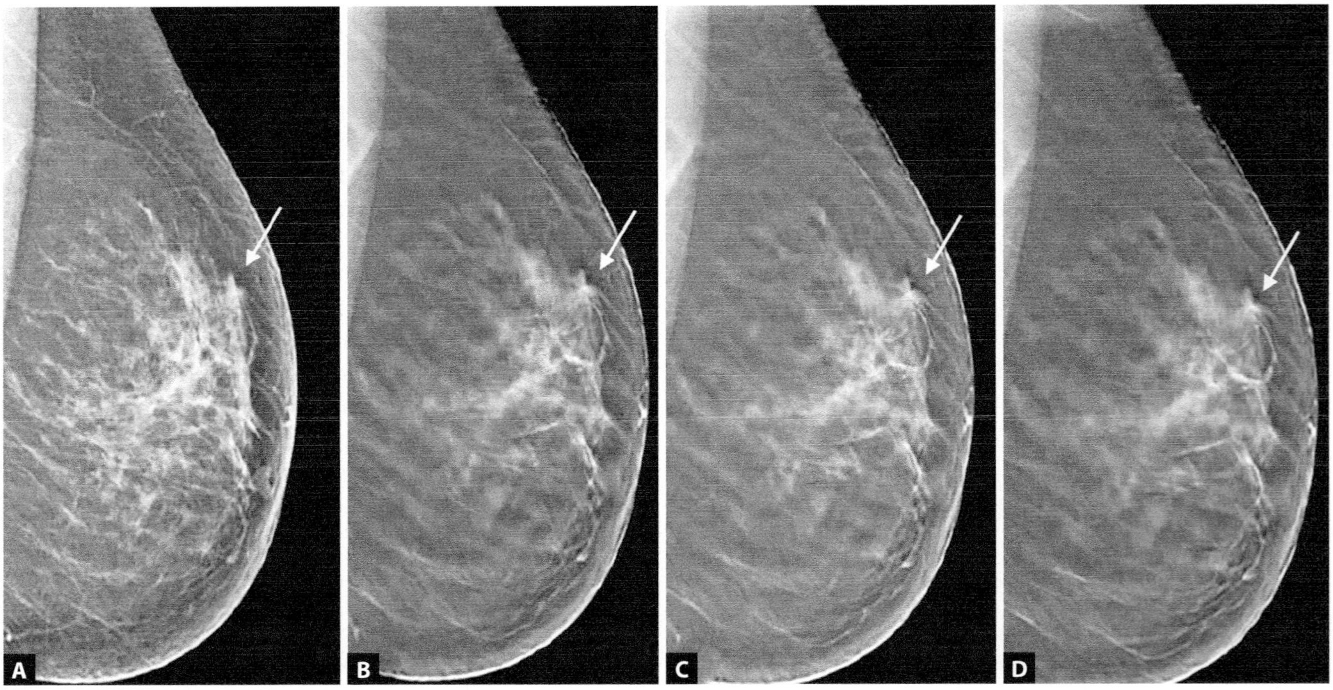

Figs. 16A to D: Digital breast tomosynthesis. (A) Conventional mediolateral oblique (MLO) view shows a subtle area of architectural distortion (arrow) in the upper part of right breast; (B to D) 1-mm thin contiguous tomographic slices convincingly show the irregular spiculations radiating from this area (arrows), thus increasing the diagnostic confidence.

moves gradually in a small arc over the compressed breast. These projection image datasets are reconstructed using specific algorithms in the form of sections similar to the CT. Each individual slice presents a planar mammogram in either the CC or MLO view. As each reconstructed slice may be as thin as 0.5 mm, masses and mass margins that may otherwise be superimposed with out-of-plane structures are more visible in the reconstructed slice **(Figs. 16A to D)**.

As the technique involves number of exposures compared to single exposure per view for nontomosynthesis FFDM, the radiation dose is slightly increased. However, all FFDM systems produce DBT images with dose below the Food and Drug Administration (FDA) limit of 300 millirad (mrad) per exposure.

The potential benefits of DBT include an increase in screening sensitivity, improvement in lesion size at detection, better characterization, and decrease in recall rates.[13] It is useful in both screening and diagnostic evaluation of the breast. The primary benefit of DBT is for evaluation of noncalcified mammographic findings such as masses, distortion and asymmetries.

BREAST ULTRASOUND

Ultrasound is the most valuable adjunct to mammography for the diagnosis of breast diseases. The additional advantages include lack of ionizing radiation, easy availability and low cost. US can be used as a primary imaging modality; and a secondary adjunct modality for targeted evaluation of any lesion detected on mammography/MRI.

Technique

Breast US should be performed with linear high-frequency transducers. The center frequency should be 10 MHz, with frequency ranging as high as 17 MHz in the near field and as low as 5 MHz deeper in the image field, thus enabling greater penetration of the posterior breast tissue and pectoralis muscle. The patient is examined in the supine oblique position. The side being examined is raised and the arm is placed above the head to ensure that the breast is evenly distributed over the chest wall. If the US is being done as a targeted examination, proper area to scan must be determined from the mammogram or clinical examination. The direction of scanning is in the transverse and longitudinal directions. A systematic approach should be followed (e.g., center to periphery). Scanning in the radial (parallel to the ducts) and antiradial (perpendicular to ducts) planes is of value in demonstrating ductal abnormalities. If lesion is identified, its presence should be confirmed with 90° rotation of the transducer. The morphology of the lesion should be carefully assessed. For the purpose of accurate follow-up, it is crucial to consistently and completely document the lesion size and location. The specific location, including laterality (right or left breast), the clock-face location, and the distance from the nipple, should be accurately annotated on the images and documented in the reports. The length of

Table 4: Indications for breast ultrasound (US).[14]

Definite	*Possible*	*Inappropriate*
• Screening in high-risk population (where MRI could not be performed) • First investigation in any young patient (<40 years) with clinical breast abnormality • Pregnancy and lactation with clinical breast abnormality • Suspicious abnormality in MRI or mammography • Locoregional staging in diagnosed breast cancer (when MRI is not done) • Breast cancer patients receiving neoadjuvant treatment, for monitoring (when MRI could not be done) • Surgical scar abnormality after mastectomy or conservation surgery • Symptomatic patients with breast implants • Patients with suspicious nipple discharge, recent onset nipple inversion/skin thickening/inflammatory changes • Percutaneous breast intervention guidance	• 40–74 years age group women with dense breast; as an adjunct to mammography • Patients who previously have had a mammographically occult tumor • Normal clinical examination; in the setting of complaint of lump palpable by the patient • New onset noncyclical breast pain • Intraoperative ultrasonography (USG)	• Screening average risk young patients (<40 years) • As a sole investigation for screening in average risk patients >40 years; replacing mammography • As a sole investigation in follow-up in previous breast cancer patients, without mammography • Asymptomatic breast implants • Diffuse premenstrual breast pain

the transducer face (footprint), usually between 3.5 and 5 cm, can be used to estimate the distance from the nipple. Extended field of view (FOV) imaging is a helpful tool to image large lesions that extend beyond the width of the transducer footprint or to better depict relationships among multiple lesions. Evaluation of the nipple and retroareolar region requires should be done carefully. It is often helpful to place the transducer slightly off center to the nipple and then use angulation to image the retroareolar tissues. "Rolled nipple" technique is another maneuver of visualization of retroareolar area. Whenever in doubt; a comparison with the contralateral side should be done to exclude any artifacts or normal variation.

Investigations into the use of Doppler US of breast lesions have produced mixed results. Because Doppler technique relies on increased vascularity (which can be seen in both benign and malignant lesions), significant overlap of positive findings is not unexpected. As color Doppler equipment has become more and more sensitive, vascular signals can been found in normal, benign, and malignant tissue. Penetrating vessels are more likely to be present in malignant tumors.[14] There are several potential causes of false-positive Doppler results (inflammatory lesions, recent fine-needle aspiration, and some vascular fibroadenomas) and false-negative results (poorly vascularized tumors, insensitive Doppler parameters, and incidental cancers) on color Doppler US.

Indications for Breast Ultrasound

In current clinical practice, the indications for breast US can be in two broad categories: (1) screening and (2) diagnostic. The European Society of breast imaging has divided the indication into three categories: (1) definite, (2) possible, and (3) inappropriate[14] **(Table 4)**. US is indicated in young (30–35 years) high-risk women who cannot undergo MRI screening for various reasons. In older high-risk women, US can be used as an adjunct to mammographic screening.[15] BRCA mutation carriers are more prone to develop radiation-induced cancers; hence, US is a suitable modality in screening them, especially at a young age.[16]

In the absence of a suspicious clinical lesion, a negative US and mammography has a very high negative predictive value for malignant disease. Main disadvantage of US is that its performance is operator-dependent and can be time consuming. Whereas mammogram is superior to US in lesion detection in older women with fatty breast composition; US is superior in lesion detection in dense breasts. It should be kept in mind that US is not always an alternative to mammography; rather they play a complementary role.

Normal Anatomy

The skin, which is normally 1–3 mm thick, appears as two parallel echogenic lines. The subcutaneous fat layer is demonstrated superficially as hypoechoic tissue compared to the glandular tissue from which it is separated by a well-defined scalloped margin. Normal ducts are often visible in the subareolar region, as anechoic tubular structures. The US appearance of the glandular tissue depends on how much involution of the glandular tissue has taken place. The young glandular breast contains a well-defined layer of glandular tissue, within which round or oval well-defined, hypoechoic fat lobules may be present. As involution takes place, more of the breast is composed of fat. In the completely involuted breast, US shows hypoechoic fat lobules separated by fine curvilinear septa of increased echogenicity. Fat lobules can be distinguished by their unique spindle shape, which merges with the rest of the parenchyma at different angles and planes of imaging. By contrast, masses remain discrete with distinctive borders in all planes of imaging. Deep to the glandular tissue, a retromammary fat layer is seen and behind this pectoral muscle can be seen sharply demarcated by its echogenic fascia. Costochondral cartilages appear as hypoechoic oval masses deep to the muscle and calcified ribs show prominent shadowing. Beneath the thoracic wall, a linear echogenic interface can be seen that includes chest wall, pleura, and lung border. Anatomic structures that can be seen in axilla include blood vessels, lymph nodes, and the proximal portions of the pectoral muscles.

ACR BI-RADS Ultrasound Lexicon Descriptors

The 5th edition of ACR BI-RADS lexicon has been in use since its release in 2014[4] **(Table 5)**. US BI-RADS category was first introduced in the 4th edition of BI-RADS lexicon in 2003.

On US, a mass is evaluated by its shape, orientation, margin, echo pattern and posterior features. A mass can be oval, round or irregular **(Figs. 17A to C)**. By definition, orientation refers to the relationship the mass has to the skin **(Figs. 18A and B)**. In general, benign solid masses are parallel to the skin. When a mass is taller than it is wide, it is a suspicious sonographic finding. When describing mass margins, the most important distinction is between circumscribed and noncircumscribed margins **(Figs. 19A to E)**. Circumscribed margins are well defined or sharp, with an abrupt transition between the lesion and the surrounding tissue. Noncircumscribed margins encompass the remaining margin descriptors, including microlobulated, indistinct, angular, and spiculated. Microlobulated margins demonstrate a scalloped appearance. Indistinct margins are not clearly demarcated from the surrounding tissue. Angular margins demonstrate sharp corners, often with acute angles, in distinction from spiculated margins, which appear more as lines projecting from a mass. The BI-RADS US descriptors shown to have a high predictive value for benignity include a circumscribed margin (90%), parallel orientation (78%), and an oval shape (78%).[17] The features most predictive of malignancy are an irregular shape (62%), spiculated margins (86%), and nonparallel orientation (69%). The internal echogenicity of the mass may be anechoic, hyperechoic, complex cystic and solid, hypoechoic, isoechoic or heterogeneous **(Figs. 20A to D)**. The patient's fat should serve as the internal control to which the echogenicity of all lesions should be compared. Generally, lesions that are hyperechoic to the subcutaneous fat are benign. Because a majority of both malignant and benign solid breast masses are hypoechoic, other features, such as margin characteristics, establish the level of suspicion.

Posterior features **(Figs. 21A and B)** may or may not be seen when imaging solid masses. Posterior acoustic shadowing is a suspicious finding and may be seen in cases of invasive carcinoma, postoperative scar, complex sclerosing lesion, or macrocalcifications. Posterior enhancement is an indeterminate US finding that can be associated with a variety of entities, including simple cysts, complicated cysts, fibroadenoma, papilloma, complex cystic mass, invasive ductal carcinoma, and lymphoma.

In the 5th edition of ACR BI-RADS Atlas, there are a few changes which are highlighted in **Table 6**.[5,6]

After complete US evaluation, the appropriate ACR BI-RADS category should be assigned to guide further management **(Table 7)**.

Challenges in Assigning Final Assessment Categories and the Influence of Clinical Factors

For a lesion with benign characteristics, although data support follow-up of probably benign lesions, an important clinical factor that influences BI-RADS final assessment categorization is the age of the patient. For an older patient, the threshold for biopsy should be lowered, and biopsy may be warranted even in the setting of probably benign imaging features.

Despite benign imaging features at US or mammography, palpable solid lesions are frequently subjected to biopsy, which leads to a large number of benign results of biopsies and incurs both financial and psychologic costs. Recent data support the fact that a solid mass need not be subjected to biopsy simply because it is palpable.[18] For palpable masses with benign imaging characteristics, the range of reported negative predictive values is 97–100%.[19] Therefore, such lesions should be managed with short-interval follow-up rather than with biopsy.

There are situations in which clinical factors are more important than the imaging appearance of a lesion. An abscess often demonstrates a complex internal echo pattern and can be indistinguishable from an invasive carcinoma. However, in the correct clinical setting (a young lactating patient with clinical signs of infection and a mass that is tender to palpation), the likelihood of malignancy is low and it should be categorized as a BI-RADS 3 lesion with recommendation of follow-up.

Contrast-enhanced Ultrasound

During the last few years, US contrast agents have been developed that increase blood echogenicity and improve US image quality by detection of slow and low-volume blood flow in small tumor vessels (<5 mm) within the focal

Table 5: ACR BI-RADS ultrasound lexicon descriptors for breast lesions.

Characteristic	*Term*	*Description*
Shape	Oval	Elliptical (may include 2–3 undulations)
	Round	Spherical
	Irregular	Neither round nor oval in shape
Orientation	Parallel	Wider than tall
	Not parallel	Taller than wide
Margin	Circumscribed	Well-defined or sharp margin with an abrupt transition between the lesion and the surrounding tissue
	Angular	Some or all of the margin has sharp corners, often forming acute angles
	Indistinct	No clear demarcation between a mass and its surrounding tissue
	Microlobulated	Short cycle undulations impart a scalloped appearance to the margin of the mass
	Spiculated	Margin characterized by sharp lines projecting from the mass
Echo pattern	Anechoic	Without internal echoes
	Hyperechoic	Increased echogenicity relative to fat
	Complex cystic and solid	Mass contains both anechoic and echogenic components
	Isoechoic	Same echogenicity as fat
	Hypoechoic	Decreased echogenicity relative to fat
	Heterogeneous	Heterogeneous hypo- and hyperechoic appearance
Posterior features	No posterior acoustic features	No posterior shadowing or enhancement
	Enhancement	Increased posterior echoes
	Shadowing	Decreased posterior echoes; edge shadows are excluded
	Combined pattern	
Associated features	Duct changes	Abnormal caliber
	Edema	Increased echogenicity of surrounding tissue
	Architectural distortion	Disruption of normal anatomic planes
	Skin thickening/retraction	Normal skin is 2 mm or less in thickness except in the periareolar area and lower breast
	Vascularity (absent/internal vascularity/ vessels in rim)	Doppler US signal in a mass
	Elasticity assessment (soft/ intermediate/hard)	Elasticity value measurement of the mass in comparison with the adjacent breast tissue
Calcifications	Calcification within a mass	Echogenic foci within a mass
	Calcifications outside a mass	Echogenic calcific foci outside the mass
	Intraductal calcifications	Echogenic foci within the ducts
Special cases	Clustered microcysts	A cluster of tiny anechoic foci 2–3 mm in diameter with thin intervening septations and no discrete solid components
	Simple cyst	Completely anechoic cyst
	Complicated cysts	Cysts having homogeneous, low-level echoes. May also have fluid-fluid, or fluid debris levels
	Mass in or on skin	These masses are clinically apparent and may include sebaceous or epidermal inclusion cysts, keloids, moles and neurofibromas
	Lymph nodes	Bean-shaped, well-defined with an echogenic hilum
	Foreign body including implants	
	Vascular abnormalities	Arteriovenous malformations or Mondor's disease
	Postsurgical fluid collection	Anechoic fluid collection (seroma) or collection with variable degree of internal echoes (hematoma)
	Fat necrosis	Well-circumscribed echogenic lesion/anechoic cystic lesion (oil cyst) with rim calcification

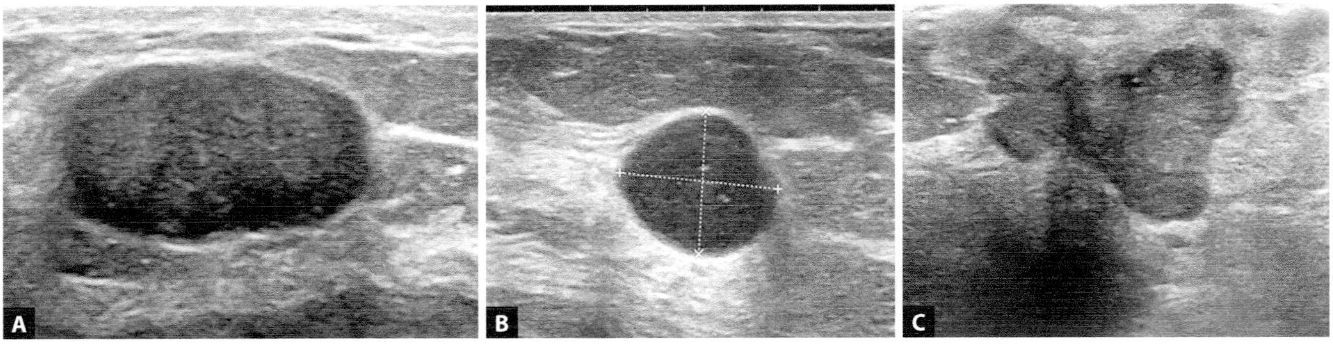

Figs. 17A to C: ACR BI-RADS descriptors for mass shape on ultrasound. (A) Oval; (B) Round; (C) Irregular.

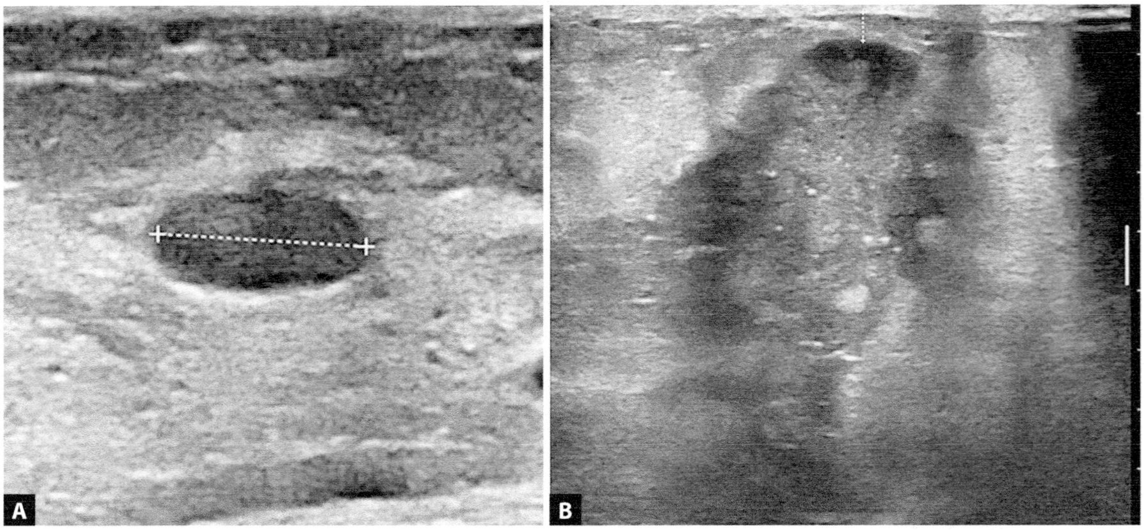

Figs. 18A and B: Orientation of a mass to skin on ultrasound. (A) Parallel orientation (wider than taller); (B) Antiparallel orientation (taller than wider).

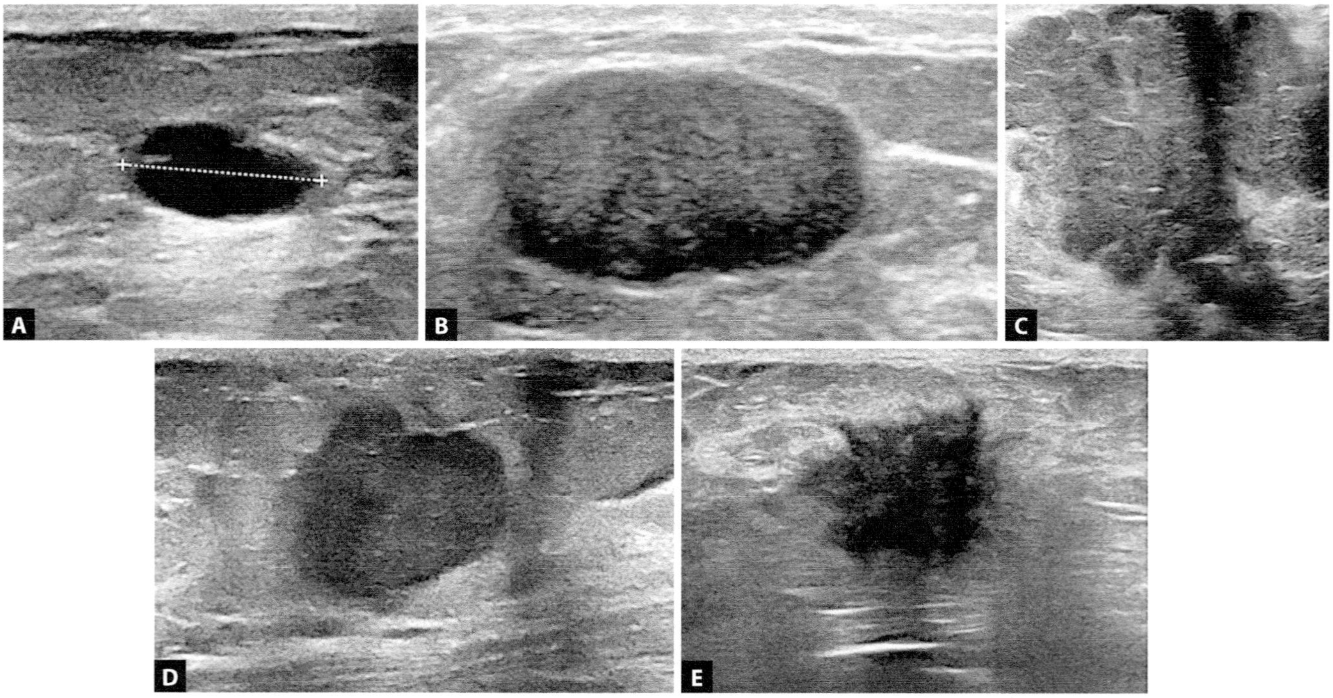

Figs. 19A to E: ACR BI-RADS descriptors for mass margins on ultrasound. (A) Circumscribed; (B) Microlobulated; (C) Indistinct; (D) Angular; (E) Spiculated.

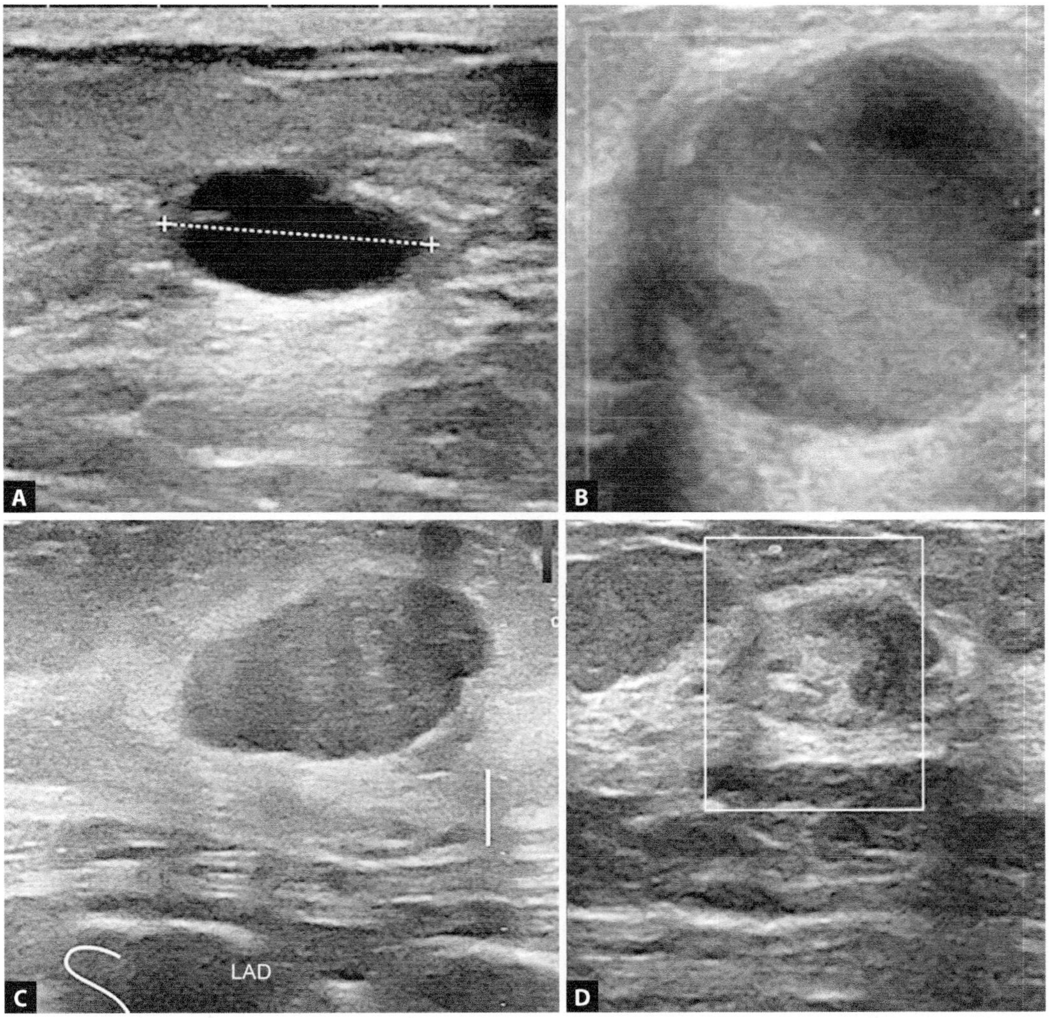

Figs. 20A to D: ACR BI-RADS descriptors of mass echogenicity. (A) Anechoic; (B) Complex solid cystic; (C) Hypoechoic; (D) Hyperechoic. (LAD: left anterior descending)

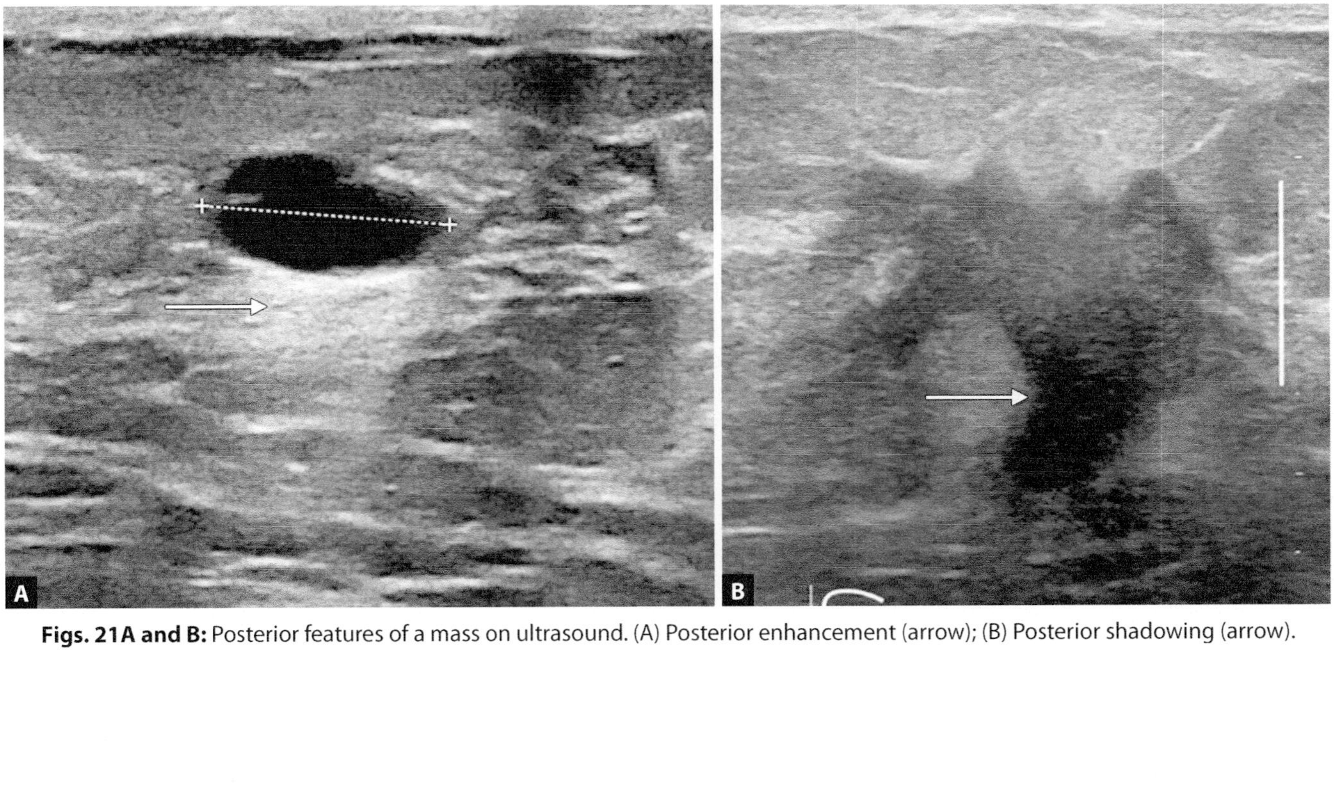

Figs. 21A and B: Posterior features of a mass on ultrasound. (A) Posterior enhancement (arrow); (B) Posterior shadowing (arrow).

Table 6: Modifications in ACR BI-RADS 5th edition ultrasound lexicon.

Section	4th edition	5th edition	Change
Background echotexture	Background echotexture • Homogeneous background echotexture-fat • Homogeneous background echotexture-fibroglandular • Heterogeneous	Tissue composition • Homogeneous background echotexture-fat • Homogeneous background echotexture-fibroglandular • Heterogeneous	Renamed as "tissue composition"
Masses	Lesion boundary		Omitted
	Echo pattern • Anechoic • Hyperechoic • Complex • Hypoechoic • Isoechoic	Echo pattern • Anechoic • Hyperechoic • Complex cystic and solid • Hypoechoic • Isoechoic • Heterogeneous	"Complex" renamed as "complex cystic and solid" Addition: "Heterogeneous"
	Surrounding tissues • Ducts • Changes in Cooper's ligaments • Edema • Architectural distortion • Skin thickening • Skin retraction/irregularity	Associated features • Architectural distortion • Duct changes • Skin changes • Edema • Vascularity • Elasticity assessment	Moved to another category "Associated features" after a few changes
Calcifications	• Macrocalcifications • Microcalcifications – In a mass – Outside a mass	• Calcification in a mass • Calcification outside a mass • Intraductal calcification	Micro/macrocalcification differentiation omitted "Intraductal" category added
Special cases	• Clustered microcysts • Complicated cyst • Mass in or on skin • Foreign body • Lymph nodes	• Simple cyst • Clustered microcysts • Complicated cyst • Mass in or on skin • Foreign body • Lymph nodes • Vascular abnormality • Postsurgical fluid collection • Fat necrosis	New conditions added

lesions in the breast. Commonly used US contrast agents include Sonovue (sulfur hexafluoride microbubbles coated with phospholipids) and Levovist (galactose microparticles coated with palmitic acid). Various studies involving contrast-enhanced US (CEUS) in breast masses have shown differences in the vascularity pattern in benign and malignant lesions. Malignant lesions tend to have greater number of vessels, irregular vessels running to the center of the mass and greater enhancement **(Figs. 22A and B)**. In spite of being in clinical use for quite a long duration,[20,21] it is still listed as "upcoming applications"; and not recommended in the current EFSUMB guidelines.[22]

Ultrasound Elastography

Elasticity assessment has been introduced in the present ACR BI-RADS lexicon 5th edition.

Ultrasound elastography explores the simple principle of tissue response to a given amount of external pressure; a harder tissue (breast malignancies tend to be scirrhous and therefore harder) resists deformation by external pressure and hence retains its original shape while benign lesions are softer and get easily deformed by external pressure.

Elastography can be broadly divided into two categories: (1) static US elastography and (2) shear wave elastography (SWE). Static US elastography requires external application of pressure by the operator and provides a color-coded map of elasticity that is superimposed on the real-time grayscale image. SWE is a new quantitative technique of obtaining elastography images where an acoustic radiation force impulse (ARFI) is induced in the tissues by a focused US beam and an ultrafast imaging sequence captures in real-time the propagation of the resulting shear waves. The production

Table 7: ACR BI-RADS ultrasound assessment categories.

Category	*Description*	*Likelihood of malignancy*	*Examples*	*Next step in evaluation*
0	Incomplete; need additional imaging evaluation, or comparison with previous examinations	Unknown	Postoperative scar/recurrence	MRI; obtain previous examinations
1	Negative	No ultrasound evidence of malignancy	Normal ultrasound	Negative findings at US do not exclude breast cancer in the setting of a suspicious mammographic finding. If the patient is being evaluated for a palpable abnormality and the findings with both US and mammography are negative, the report should stress the importance of clinical assessment and further management should be based on the clinical level of concern
2	Benign finding	No ultrasound evidence of malignancy	Simple cysts, breast implants, stable postsurgical changes, and probable fibroadenomas noted to be unchanged at successive US studies	Routine screening
3	Probably benign finding	<2%	A solid mass with circumscribed margins, an oval shape, and parallel orientation	Follow-up imaging (mammography or ultrasound) at 6 and 12 months
4	Suspicious abnormality	3–95%	Solid masses with benign features (e.g., fibroadenomas) if the lesion is clinically palpable. Complicated cysts and some complex cystic and solid masses (e.g., clinically apparent abscesses)	Fine-needle aspiration, percutaneous or surgical biopsy
5	Highly suggestive of malignancy	>95%	Spiculated mass	Percutaneous or surgical biopsy
6	Known malignancy	100%	Biopsy-proven	Definitive treatment

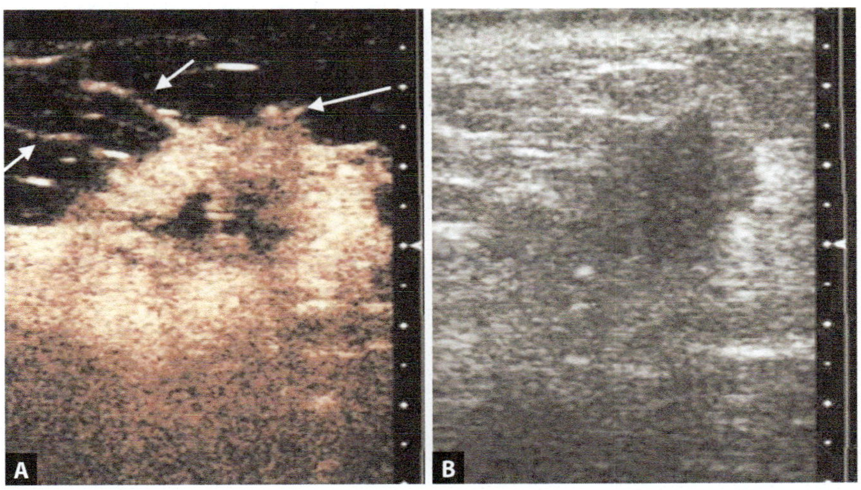

Figs. 22A and B: Contrast-enhanced ultrasound in a 43-year-old lady with invasive ductal carcinoma. Ultrasound image obtained 30 seconds after contrast injection shows intense early enhancement of the irregular mass lesion with ductal extension (arrows).

of ARFI impulse by the probe rather than the operator (as in static US elastography) means SWE is more reproducible than static elastography.

The parameters measured in a quantitative SWE **(Fig. 23)** are listed in **Table 8**. The region of interest (ROI) placement in 2D SWE should be done with caution, as it affects the measurement parameters. Invasive breast cancers have been shown to be stiffer than benign or normal tissues. Various studies[23-25] have provided wide cutoff elasticity values for differentiation of benign from malignant masses [33.3–80 kPa (median, 59.35 kPa) for E_{mean}; 46.7–93.8 kPa (median, 79.25 kPa) for E_{max}]. Addition of SWE to grayscale US can improve the sensitivity and specificity in reclassifying BI-RADS category 3 and 4a lesions.[26]

Three-dimensional SWE is a new technique in which volumetric color-coded tissue stiffness maps are generated upon a single acquisition. Studies have demonstrated that

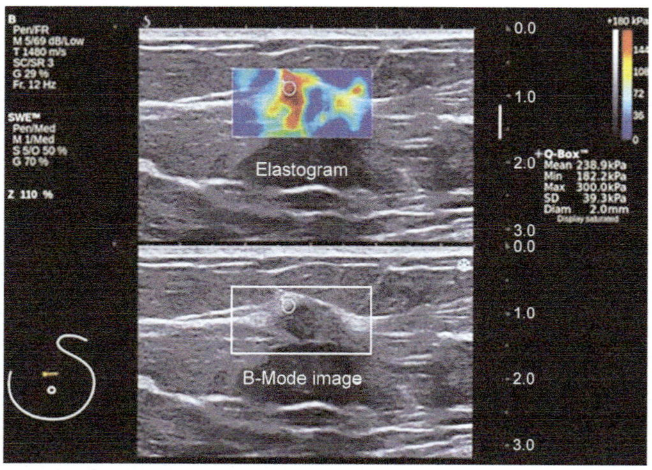

Fig. 23: Shear wave elastography. B-mode ultrasound image shows a subtle, 7 mm size, irregular solid mass. The real-time elastography image shows peritumoral stiffness (red areas) with high mean elasticity value of 238.9 kPa in the operator marked region of interest (ROI). Ultrasound-guided core biopsy confirmed invasive ductal carcinoma.

Table 8: Measurement parameters in shear wave elastography (SWE).

Parameter	*Meaning*	*Effect of region of interest (ROI) size*
E_{mean}	Sum of all elasticity values of each pixel within the ROI divided by the number of pixels	Decreases with an increase in ROI size
E_{max}	Maximum elasticity value (elasticity value of the stiffest pixels)	Not affected
E_{SD}	Average difference in elasticity value within the ROI to E_{mean}	Increases with size of ROI

3D SWE can demonstrate the stiffest part of the tumor much easily than a 2D SWE.[27,28]

Other promising applications of elastography as an adjunct to gray scale US include prediction of breast cancer prognosis and prediction of response to neoadjuvant therapy.

Recent advances in breast US (including automated breast volume US) will be discussed in a separate chapter.

BREAST MAGNETIC RESONANCE IMAGING

Since the early development of breast MRI, numerous technical developments, variations, and innovations have been described. This section describes the indications, techniques, ACR BI-RADS lexicon for MRI breast.

Indications of Breast Magnetic Resonance Imaging

The indications of breast MRI are listed in **Table 9**. Broadly, they can be divided into three categories: (1) screening, (2) diagnostic, and (3) as a problem solving tool. While there are conflicting reports regarding the utility of breast MRI in each of these scenarios; few of them have been unanimously proven to be of use.[29-33]

Technique

Coils and Patient Positioning

For breast MRI, the patient is placed in the prone position with the breasts in the "cups" of the coil, with judicious padding to minimize patient motion and transmitted vibration. Immobilization should be achieved by gently fixating the breast in the section-encoding direction (CC direction for transverse protocols).

Prone patient positioning minimizes the effects of respiratory motion on images and helps to move the breasts away from the chest wall and the resulting artifacts from cardiac and respiratory movement. Patient comfort is vital, as the breast MRI examination can last 30 minutes or longer, and any patient discomfort is likely to manifest as movement during or between scans.

MRI Field Strength

The current recommendations require that breast MRI be performed at 1.5 tesla (T) or higher. The higher field strength enables the acquisition of high-resolution imaging with adequate signal-to-noise ratio (SNR) and enables the use of fat suppression. Imaging at 3.0 T provides an opportunity for even greater improvement in SNR, increased image resolution, and faster imaging.

Imaging Protocols

Dynamic contrast-enhanced MRI is the key sequence of a breast MRI. It relies on the principle of neoangiogenesis in

Table 9: Indications for breast magnetic resonance imaging.[29-33]

Clinical scenario	*Suitable candidate/present status*
Screening	High-risk women (lifetime cancer risk 20% or higher); as a supplemental imaging technique to mammography • Several genetic mutations (e.g., BRCA1, BRCA2, PALPB2, TP53, PTEN, CHECK2, CDH1, ATM, and STK11) • Women who received chest radiation treatment before the age of 30 years Contralateral breast screening in known cancers
Preoperative staging in known breast cancer	• Young age at diagnosis • Interval cancer • Dense breasts • Hormone receptor-negative cancers • Breast conservation surgery (BCS) without radiation therapy contemplated • Invasive lobular carcinoma
Known cancers on treatment	• Presurgical treatment before BCS, and after neoadjuvant chemotherapy • Tumor response assessment on chemotherapy
Problem solving tool	• Discrepancy in mammography, US and clinical examination findings • Mammographic asymmetric density

a cancer; the new vessels being "leaky" capillaries. Hence, the cancers tend to show a very early enhancement.

Multiparametric breast MRI: The most widely used multiparametric MRI consists of the following sequences: T1-weighted spin-echo (T1W-SE), T2-weighted turbo spin-echo (T2W-TSE), diffusion-weighted imaging (DWI), and postcontrast sequences. T2W imaging can depict nonenhancing structures that correlate to mammographic or palpable findings, including simple or complex cysts, and dilated retroareolar ducts. T2W imaging can also help characterize certain benign lesions such as simple cysts, myxoid fibroadenoma or lymph nodes as these have very high signal intensity on T2W scans, whereas most cancers are dark. The contrast sequences can be acquired as an ultrafast dynamic contrast-enhanced series (for the first 1 minute); or the routine dynamic contrast-enhanced sequences. It is to be kept in mind that while imaging for the detection of post-neoadjuvant chemotherapy (NACT) residual disease; a delayed phase is more useful. To the contrary, the early dynamic imaging is useful for assessing tumor chemotherapy response.[29] Ultrafast dynamic contrast-enhanced MRI follows the same principle as the routine dynamic scans. The malignant lesions tend to show more early contrast wash-in, whereas benign lesions show enhancement at a later phase (>15 seconds).[29]

Implementation of the routine dynamic enhanced imaging requires careful monitoring by the radiologist. Precontrast T1W imaging should be checked carefully to ensure adequate breast coverage and lack of severe artifacts. A 0.1 mmol/kg gadolinium diethylenetriamine penta-acetic acid (Gd-DTPA) should be injected via an intravenous catheter placed in an antecubital vein before the patient is positioned in the coil. The patient must not be moved in and out of the magnet for the injection, to prevent motion and unnecessary time loss in the early postcontrast phase. The contrast agent is injected with a power injector at a rate of 3 mL/s, followed by a 20 mL saline flush. The first postcontrast acquisition is started after the volume of contrast material has been injected (i.e., during the application of the saline flush). Hand injections can also be used. T1-weighted scans are obtained at every 1 minute for at least 5–7 minutes after contrast injection. It is important to use the same T1 sequence and scan technique which was used for precontrast scan.

Bilateral imaging helps to avoid diagnostic errors (e.g., in patients with nonmass-like enhancement or enhancing foci). To categorize these areas or foci, it is very helpful to be able to assess symmetry by comparing with the contralateral breast.

Abbreviated breast MRI: This refers to a short MRI protocol consisting of only one pre- and one postcontrast T1W sequence. After its introduction in 2014;[34] it has been extensively evaluated worldwide for its accuracy in cancer detection. The results are promising, claiming a diagnostic accuracy similar to a full protocol.[35]

Plane of Imaging

Sagittal or axial planes of acquisition are preferred, as these planes allow for better depiction of the ductal organization of the breast glandular tissue than the coronal plane. Sagittal imaging provides the opportunity for much higher in-plane resolution because of the small imaging FOV obtainable. However, simultaneous bilateral sagittal imaging requires longer imaging time, and can lead to inadvertent exclusion of breast tissue in the axillary region. Axial imaging is therefore often used for bilateral breast MRI.

Fat Suppression

The ACR guidelines encourage the use of fat suppression techniques because, after contrast injection, enhancing lesions may become isointense to adjacent fatty tissue. Active fat suppression means that the signal from fatty tissue is specifically eliminated by additional radiofrequency pulses or by choosing selective water excitation. Both types add to the acquisition time and require a very homogeneous magnetic field across the entire FOV, which is difficult to achieve with bilateral imaging.

Subtraction does not require extra acquisition time and is not influenced by magnetic field inhomogeneities, which is why it is the preferred type of fat suppression for dynamic bilateral imaging. The main disadvantage of subtraction is that it may suffer from patient motion: Subtraction errors occur if the precontrast mask and the postcontrast image are not entirely congruent due to even subtle patient motion.

Kinetic Analysis

Kinetic data can be evaluated by visually assessing the lesion enhancement pattern, by placing an ROI to obtain kinetic curves, and by using a CAD system. The ROIs should be placed with wide window settings into the area that exhibits strongest enhancement on the first postcontrast image. Softwares which demonstrate color-coded areas of high enhancement with respect to predetermined threshold have now been developed and should be used if available, to place the ROI accurately. The ROI should include not >3–4 pixels, and care should be taken to ensure that the ROI is within the lesion throughout the entire dynamic series. If there is unrecognized patient movement during dynamic scans, the lesion moves out of the prescribed ROI after the first postcontrast image leading to false washout pattern. To quantify enhancement, the increase in signal intensity relative to baseline precontrast signal intensity is measured and is plotted over time.

Normal Magnetic Resonance Imaging Appearances

Normal glandular tissue has intermediate signal intensity on T1W and T2W sequences, whereas fat is of high signal. The fibrous trabeculae are seen as fine low signal intensity structures traversing the subcutaneous fat. Low axillary and intramammary lymph nodes can be recognized through their characteristic bean shape and central fatty hilum. The skin is of intermediate signal and uniformly thin except in the areolar region where it may be and few millimeters in thickness. After intravenous gadolinium, the nipple, blood vessels and lymph nodes normally enhance. Normal glandular parenchyma can also enhance gradually, especially in the second half of the menstrual cycle, reflecting hormonal-induced glandular proliferation. This enhancement, referred to as background enhancement, is often diffuse, patchy and progressive. Rarely, it may be intense or focal and difficult to interpret. Hence, if possible, breast MRI should be performed after menstruation in second week of the cycle.

Interpretation of Breast Magnetic Resonance Imaging

For differential diagnosis of enhancing lesions in breast MRI, morphologic information (type of enhancement, mass shape and margins, distribution of nonmass-like enhancement, internal architecture), kinetic information (initial enhancement increase and delayed phase enhancement), and information related to lesion signal intensity on T2W and T1W precontrast nonfat-suppressed images are analyzed systematically.

When interpreting breast MRI studies, the first step is to categorize any abnormal enhancement according to the 5th edition of ACR BI-RADS-MRI lexicon, published as a part of the American College of Radiology's Breast Imaging Reporting and Data System Atlas: a mass, an area of nonmass-like enhancement or a focus.

Focus

In the 4th edition of ACR BI-RADS Atlas, lesions smaller than 5 mm were termed as "foci". In the 5th edition, the size criteria are no more valid; rather the differentiation between mass/foci is largely based on morphology. A focus is a small isolated enhancing dot, too small for applying morphologic descriptors.[5,6]

Mass

A mass is a 3D space occupying lesion within the breast. Usually, it has a visible correlate on precontrast T1- or T2-weighted images. Masses are described in terms of shape, margin, and internal enhancement characteristics **(Table 10)**.

- *Shape*: A mass can be round, oval, or irregular **(Figs. 24A to C)**. "Lobulated" shape has been included in the "oval" category in the 5th edition. Irregular masses have an uneven shape that cannot be characterized as round or oval.
- *Margin*: Margins can be described as circumscribed (earlier designated "smooth") or noncircumscribed (includes irregular and spiculated) **(Figs. 25A to C)**. Spiculated margins frequently are a feature of malignant breast lesions and radial scars.
- *Internal enhancement characteristics*: Enhancement patterns of masses **(Figs. 26A to C)** have been divided into the following four types:
  1. Homogeneous enhancement is uniform and confluent enhancement throughout the mass.
  2. Heterogeneous enhancement is nonuniform enhancement that shows variations within the mass.

Table 10: ACR BI-RADS mass descriptors in magnetic resonance imaging.

Characteristic	*Term*	*Description*
Shape	Round	Spherical
	Oval	Elliptical
	Irregular	Uneven shape
Margin	Circumscribed	Smooth
	Noncircumscribed • Irregular • Spiculated	 Sharp lines projecting from the mass
Internal enhancement	Homogeneous	Uniform enhancement
	Heterogeneous	Nonuniform enhancement
	Rim enhancing	Enhancement concentrated at the periphery
	Internal nonenhancing septations	Dark septations within an enhanced lesion

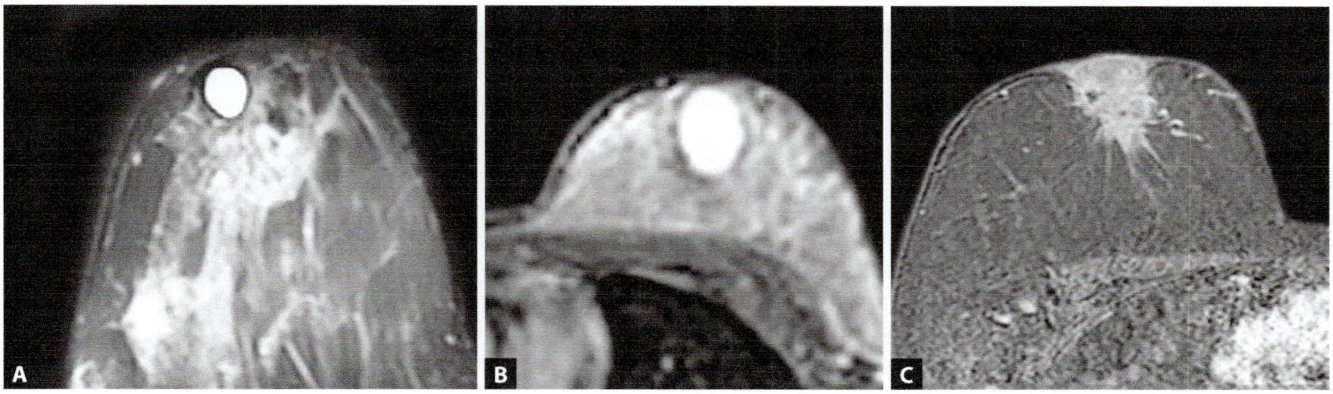

Figs. 24A to C: ACR BI-RADS descriptors for mass shape on magnetic resonance imaging (MRI). (A) Round; (B) Oval; (C) Irregular.

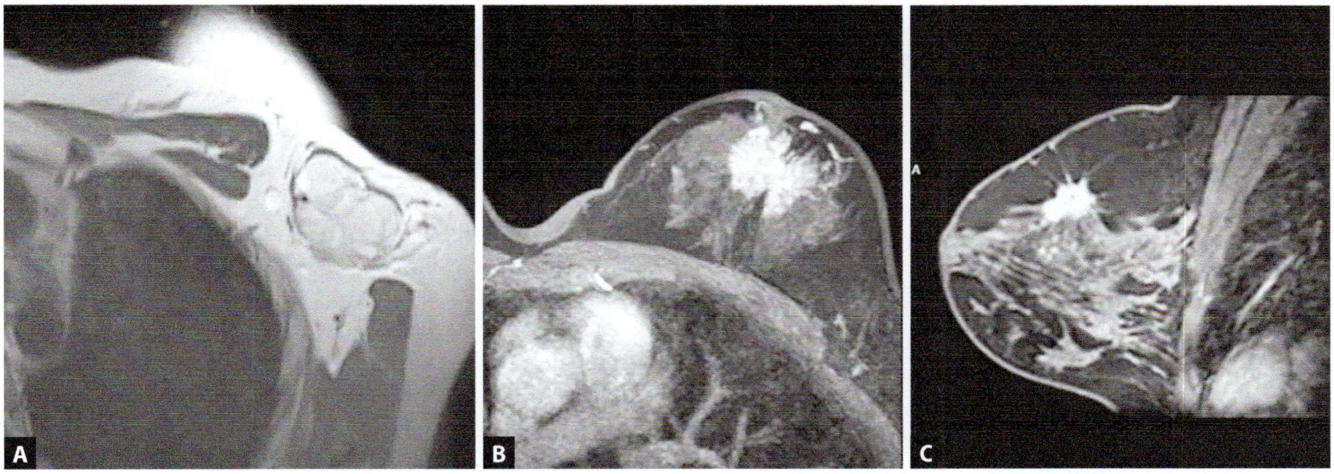

Figs. 25A to C: ACR BI-RADS descriptors for mass margin on magnetic resonance imaging (MRI): (A) Circumscribed; (B) Irregular; (C) Spiculated.

3. Rim enhancement is enhancement mainly concentrated at the periphery of the mass. This type of enhancement is most frequently a feature of high-grade invasive ductal cancer, fat necrosis, and cysts with inflammation.
4. Dark internal nonenhancing septations within an enhanced lesion are typical of fibroadenomas, especially when the lesion has smooth or lobulated borders.

Two types (enhancing internal septations and central enhancement) have been omitted in the 5th edition.

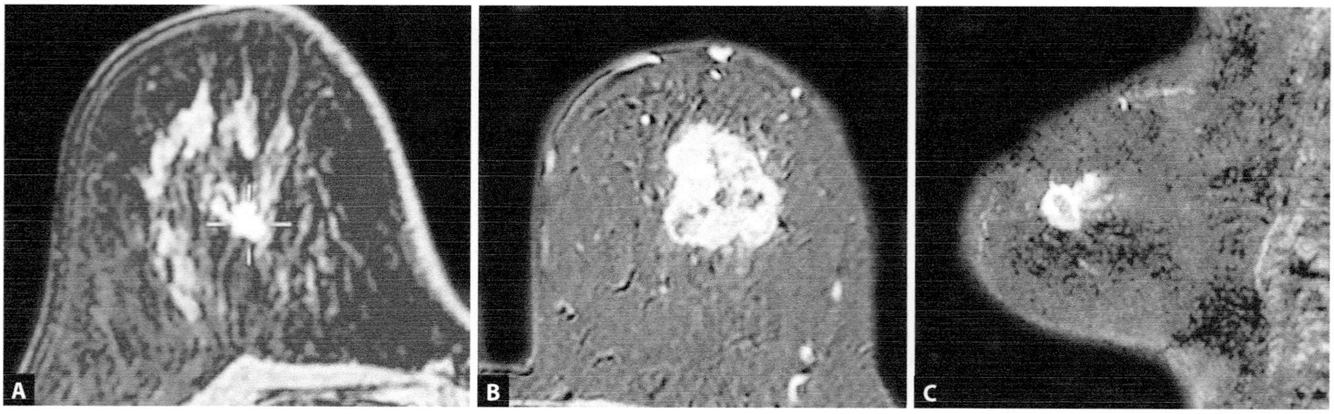

Figs. 26A to C: ACR BI-RADS descriptors for mass internal enhancement on magnetic resonance imaging (MRI): (A) Homogeneous; (B) Heterogeneous; (C) Rim enhancement.

Nonmass-like Enhancement

Nonmass-like enhancement means that enhancement occurs in an area of the fibroglandular tissue that otherwise appears normal on precontrast images. There is no space-occupying effect **(Fig. 27)**. The enhancing area usually has no correlate on fat-suppressed or nonfat-suppressed T2-weighted images. The distinction between mass and nonmass-like enhancement is important for further differential diagnosis. In a mass, the differential diagnostic consideration is either invasive breast cancer or a benign solid tumor (e.g., fibroadenoma). In nonmass-like enhancement, the main differential diagnosis is between intraductal or diffuse (e.g., lobular) cancer and mastopathic changes (focal adenosis), hormonal stimulation, or inflammatory changes. Features of nonmass-like enhancement[36] such as internal enhancement pattern, symmetry, and the distribution are assessed **(Table 11)**.

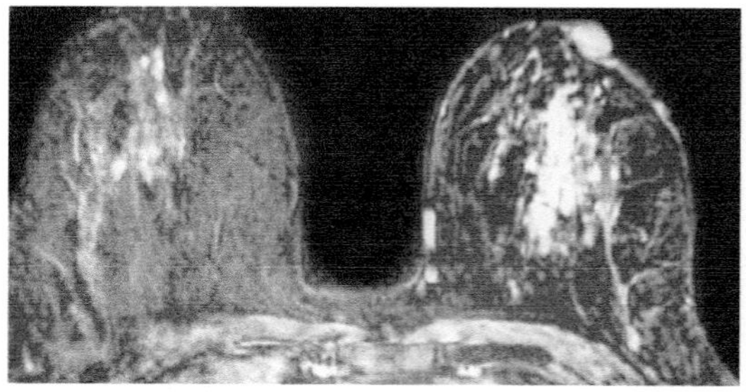

Fig. 27: Nonmass-like enhancement. Enhancement occurs in an area of the fibroglandular tissue that otherwise appears normal on precontrast images and there is no space-occupying effect.

*Distribution **(Figs. 28A to C)**:*

- A focal area is enhancement occupying <25% of the volume of a breast quadrant that has fat or normal glandular tissue between abnormally enhanced components. This type of enhancement usually manifests as clumped, irregular contrast enhancement.
- Linear enhancement is a sheet of enhancement that does not conform to the shape of a ductal system.
- Segmental enhancement is conical and probably represents one or more ductal systems. Segmental distribution of enhancement may be associated with in situ ductal cancer or invasive ductal cancer, atypical ductal hyperplasia, papillary neoplasms, or sclerosing adenosis.
- Regional enhancement is geographic enhancement involving one or more segments of the breast. A specific ductal or segmental configuration cannot be discerned.
- Multiple regions of enhancement are distributed in several areas of the breast.
- Diffuse enhancement is uniform enhancement of the entire parenchyma of the breast, usually associated with benign processes or normal fibroglandular tissue.

In the 5th edition, "ductal" enhancement has been omitted.

Internal enhancement pattern: The internal enhancement patterns are homogeneous, heterogeneous, clumped, and clustered ring. In the clustered ring pattern, the normal fat glandular tissue interface is lost. This finding is usually associated with inflammatory breast cancer or lymphatic involvement.

Symmetry is helpful in further characterization of nonmass-like enhancement. Bilateral symmetric nonmass-like enhancement in any distribution is more often caused by benign changes than by malignant lesions.

A new enhancement pattern "clustered ring" has been added in the 5th edition. Stippled/punctate calcification has been omitted.

Associated Findings

Associated findings have been expanded in the 5th edition; and divided into six categories.

1. Intramammary lymph node
2. Skin lesions

Table 11: ACR BI-RADS descriptors of nonmass-like enhancement in magnetic resonance imaging.

Characteristic	*Descriptor*	*Illustration*
Distribution	Focal	
	Linear	Enhancement in a line that may not conform to a duct
	Segmental	Triangular area of enhancement, apex pointing to nipple, suggesting a duct and its branches
	Regional	Enhancement in a large volume of tissue not conforming to a ductal distribution
	Multiple	Enhancement in at least two large volumes of tissues not conforming to a ductal distribution, multiple geographic areas, patchy areas of enhancement
	Diffuse	Enhancement distributed uniformly throughout the breast
Internal enhancement pattern	Homogeneous	Confluent uniform enhancement
	Heterogeneous	Nonuniform enhancement in a random pattern
	Clumped	Punctuate dot-like, enhancing foci
	Clustered ring	Enhancement with finger-like projections extending toward nipple (earlier included in reticular/dendritic pattern)

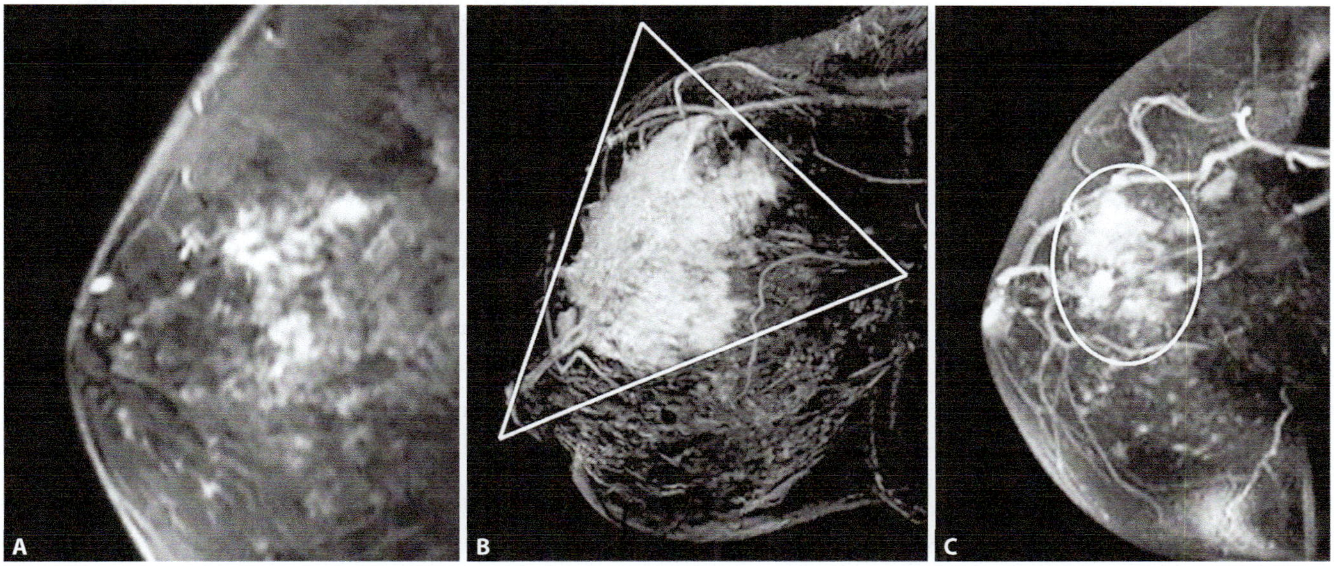

Figs. 28A to C: ACR BI-RADS descriptors of distribution of nonmass-like enhancement in magnetic resonance imaging (MRI). (A) Linear; (B) Segmental; (C) Regional.

3. Nonenhancing findings (include cyst, seroma, nonenhancing mass, foreign body/surgical clip, architectural distortion, etc.)
4. Associated findings (nipple retraction, nipple invasion, skin retraction, skin thickening, skin invasion, axillary adenopathy, chest wall/pectoralis muscle invasion, etc.)
5. Fat-containing lesions
6. Implants (a detailed evaluation of implants is newly added in the 5th edition).

Kinetic Curve Assessment

The analysis of enhancement kinetics is achieved by measuring the signal intensity in a small area of a lesion and tracking its course over the dynamic series to yield the kinetic curve (also referred to as time-signal intensity curve).

The most suspicious curve pattern derived from the fastest-enhancing part of a lesion is chosen to describe the enhancement curve. *Early phase enhancement*, i.e., enhancement within the first 2 minutes after contrast injection or until the curve starts to change, indicates the velocity and degree with which enhancement occurs and may be slow, medium, or fast.

Delayed phase enhancement refers to signal intensity changes that occur immediately after the early signal intensity increase, as early as 3 minutes after injection. Immediately after the early initial increase, the signal intensity may decline again, yielding a so-called washout curve (**type 3**) (**Fig. 29**); (1) exhibit a sharp bend and plateau (**type 2**); or (2) continue to rise after the early phase, yielding persistent enhancement until the delayed postcontrast phase (**type 1**). The main difference is that in types 2 (plateau) and type 3 (washout) curves, peak enhancement is reached early, usually within the first 2 minutes. This is the time course observed in most invasive breast cancers. Lesions with rapid early enhancement followed by a delayed phase plateau or washout have a positive predictive value of 77% for malignancy.[37] In persistent kinetics, the enhancement continues until the delayed postcontrast phase. This is the time course observed in most benign changes.

While enhancement kinetics is useful for the differential diagnosis of morphologically equivocal masses, it may be misleading and should, therefore, not be used for classification of nonmass-like enhancement. The reason is that in nonmass-like enhancement, the differential diagnosis includes DCIS and lobular cancers—two disease states known to exhibit inconsistent angiogenic activity.

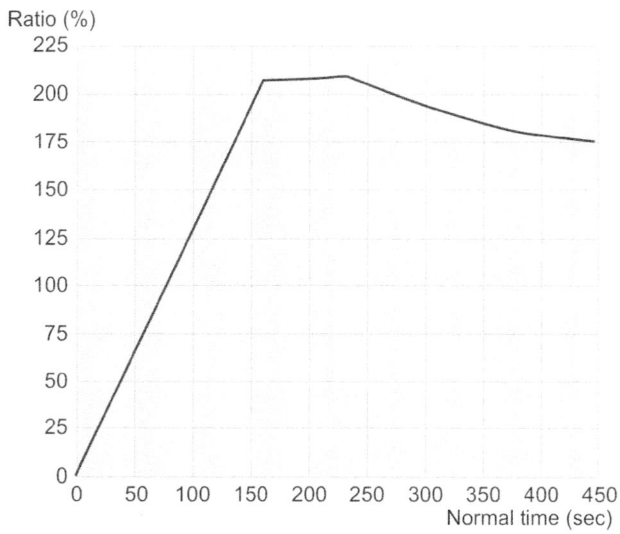

Fig. 29: Kinetic analysis of enhancing mass lesions on dynamic contrast-enhanced magnetic resonance imaging (DCE-MRI) showing type 3 curve. Immediately after the early initial increase, the signal intensity declines rapidly yielding a type 3 or washout curve.

Diffusion-weighted Imaging

Invasive breast cancers demonstrate restricted diffusion (lower apparent diffusion coefficient) relative to normal breast tissue or benign breast lesions.[38] This restricted diffusion of water in invasive cancers renders these lesions bright on diffusion-weighted images **(Figs. 30A and B)** and can potentially help identify malignant lesions when dynamic contrast-enhanced imaging is equivocal. Benign lesions with high intrinsic T2 signal intensity can also appear bright on DWI because of the phenomenon of "T2 shine-through". An apparent diffusion coefficient (ADC) pixel map should be generated from the component diffusion-weighted images produced from two or more DWI sets as hypointensity on these images confirms the restriction of diffusion. Thus, use of ADC quantification rather than DWI inspection alone is recommended for breast lesion characterization. The use of optimized ADC cutoff improves breast lesion characterization without decreasing sensitivity[39] with a potential reduction in the number of negative biopsies.

The changes in MRI section in BI-RADS 5th edition are highlighted in **Table 12**.

Sensitivity and Specificity of Magnetic Resonance Imaging

Detection of invasive breast carcinoma is extremely reliable on MRI as the sensitivity approaches 100%.[36] The sensitivity of breast MRI is not impaired by the density of the fibroglandular tissue or by scar tissue (e.g., after lumpectomy), radiation therapy, or prosthetic breast implants. It can, therefore, detect cancers which

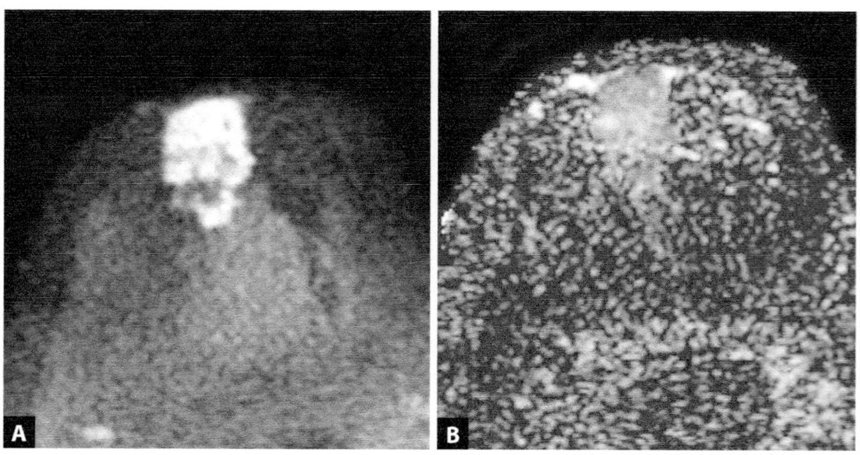

Figs. 30A and B: Diffusion-weighted magnetic resonance (MR) imaging. (A) Diffusion-weighted image; and (B) Apparent diffusion coefficient (ADC) pixel map in a malignant lesion showing marked restriction of diffusion.

Table 12: Changes in 5th edition ACR BI-RADS MRI section.[5]

Section	*Changes in 5th edition*
Amount of fibroglandular tissue	Newly added section (divided in four categories)
Background parenchymal enhancement	Newly added section (two categories with several subcategories included)
Focus	Definition changed (vide supra)
Mass descriptors: shape	Omitted "lobulated"
Mass descriptors: internal enhancement	Omitted two categories: enhancing internal septations and central enhancement
Nonmass-like enhancement: distribution	Omission of ductal distribution
Nonmass-like enhancement: internal enhancement patterns	Omission of stippled/punctate pattern Addition of "clustered ring" pattern
Associated findings	Expanded and divided in six categories (vide supra)

are occult on mammography and US. Normal breast MRI excludes the presence of gross focus of invasive cancer with high reliability. However, breast MRI has lower specificity and this is one of its biggest limitations. The detection of cancer relies on contrast enhancement but this can also be seen in many benign conditions like fibroadenoma, papilloma, fibrocystic disease, and lymph nodes. This results in significant false-positive examinations and hence unnecessary biopsies. False-negative breast MRI examinations can also occur but these are rare. Nonenhancing invasive breast cancers are exceedingly rare. More often, the reason for failure to diagnose invasive cancer with breast MRI is early and strong enhancement in the surrounding normal fibroglandular tissue that may mask the enhancing cancer. Invasive lobular carcinoma, well-differentiated invasive ductal carcinoma and few DCIS may be missed on breast MRI. A recent meta-analysis of 44 studies has estimated the sensitivity and specificity of MRI for the diagnosis of breast cancer as 90% and 72% respectively.[37] Because of the potential issue of a false-negative examination, a negative MRI examination should not deter biopsy of a suspicious lesion (BI-RADS 4 or 5) on mammography or US. Breast MRI is best used as an adjunct to conventional imaging, complementing but never replacing basic mammography and US.

Challenges in MRI interpretation have been shown in **Box 4**.

Box 4: Challenges in MRI interpretation.

False-positive
- Fibrocystic change
- Hormone-related enhancement
- Focal fibrosis, scar, fat necrosis
- Intraductal papilloma
- Fibroadenomas
- Intramammary lymph node

False-negative
- Strong background enhancement
- Nonenhancing ductal carcinoma in situ (DCIS)
- Nonenhancing invasive lobular carcinoma
- Recent radiotherapy

NUCLEAR MEDICINE IN BREAST IMAGING

Nuclear medicine techniques require intravenous administration of a radiotracer [technetium-99m-methoxyisobutyl isonitrile (MIBI)] and a camera that detects radiotracer activity. 99mTc-sestamibi preferentially accumulates in malignant tissue and this differential uptake is imaged. Its uptake and retention in the lesion depends on the regional blood flow, angiogenesis, and metabolic activity. The use of traditional gamma camera and radiotracer to image the breast is termed scintimammography,[40,41] where patients lie prone with breast dependent and imaging is performed in the lateral and anteroposterior positions. Malignant lesions are seen as focal increased uptake.

Breast-specific Gamma Imaging

Breast-specific gamma imaging (BSGI)[42] addresses the limited tumor visibility (minimum size, 15–20 mm) of large FOV sestamibi imaging. It provides optimal spatial resolution and sensitivity and is targeted at 95% detection rate of lesions 5 mm in diameter. For BSGI, the breast is positioned and compressed in a manner similar to a mammogram examination after intravenous injection of 20 mCi of technetium sestamibi. Routine CC and MLO views are obtained, with additional images as necessary resulting in an approximate 45-minute total examination time. If a focal area of uptake is seen, especially if there was no concern on mammogram, a directed US can be performed to determine if there is a suspicious finding that warrants biopsy.

Positron Emission Tomography

The ^{18}F-fluorodeoxyglucose (^{18}F-FDG) positron emission tomography (PET) has emerged as another imaging tool for many malignancies, including breast cancer. Rapidly dividing neoplastic cells have higher glucose metabolism compared with nonmalignant cells and hence, show preferential uptake of ^{18}F-FDG. The ^{18}F-FDG-PET, however, has poor anatomic resolution like other nuclear medicine techniques. Introduction of the hybrid FDG-PET/CT scanner, in which the FDG-PET scanner is equipped with a high-resolution multidetector CT for simultaneous acquisition of the FDG-PET and CT data, has greatly enhanced the spatial resolution of this technique. The FDG-PET/CT has proved to be useful in:

- Detection of breast cancers in mammographically dense breast, those with implants and those presenting with occult primary when other imaging modalities are indeterminate. A positive FDG-PET scan of the breast is highly suspicious for cancer with a high positive predictive value of 96%.
- *Locoregional staging of breast cancer*: Whole body FDG-PET can correctly estimate the true local and distant extent of the disease. PET can detect metastases to axillary lymph nodes as well as nodes at unsuspected areas such as internal mammary or supraclavicular lymph nodes owing to its large FOV.
- *Detection of unsuspected distant metastases*: 99mTc-methylene diphosphonate (MDP) bone scan has better sensitivity for sclerotic bone metastases and PET is more sensitive for lytic bone metastases. PET is unsatisfactory for detection of brain and small pulmonary metastases.
- Detection of recurrences in soft issues.
- *Early prediction of tumor response in patients with locally advanced breast cancer undergoing NACT.* Decreased uptake with chemotherapy suggests that pathologic remission may be achieved. Persistent high uptake with treatment predicts poor response.[43]
- Differentiation of scar tissue from cancer recurrence.

Limitations

Diagnostic accuracy of FDG-PET is dependent on tumor size and histology. The sensitivity of FDG-PET is 92% for lesions larger than 2 cm but is only 53% for primary lesions <5 mm.[44] PET also has poor sensitivity for detection of DICS and slow growing cancers such as invasive lobular carcinoma. PET is not suitable for screening even for high-risk patients, as negative study has limited value.

Positron Emission Mammography

Positron emission mammography (PEM) is a high spatial resolution (2 mm), dedicated breast PET device that can provide functional and anatomical information.[45] Dual moving head detectors are mounted opposite each other on compression paddles attached to a portable compact scanner to obtain tomographic images of the breast in the CC and MLO positions. It is primarily used for patients unable to undergo MRI.

CONCLUSION

The BI-RADS is a standardized system of reporting breast pathology on mammogram, ultrasonography (USG) and MRI and the standardized lexicon should be followed to ensure consistency between reports. The reporting structure should be such that there is clear communication to the clinician regarding diagnosis and management recommendations.

REFERENCES

1. Tabár L, Vitak B, Chen TH, Yen AM, Cohen A, Tot T, et al. Swedish two-county trial: impact of mammographic screening on breast cancer mortality during 3 decades. Radiology. 2011;260(3):658-63.
2. Mushlin AI, Kouides RW, Shapiro DE. Estimating the accuracy of screening mammography: a meta-analysis. Am J Prev Med. 1998;14:143-53.
3. Boyd NF, Guo H, Martin LJ, Sun L, Stone J, Fishell E, et al. Mammographic density and the risk and detection of breast cancer. N Engl J Med. 2007;356:227-36.
4. D'Orsi C, Sickles EA, Mendelson EB, Morris EA. ACR BI-RADS Atlas: Breast Imaging Reporting and Data System, 5th edition. Reston, VA: American College of Radiology; 2013.
5. Rao AA, Feneis J, Lalonde C, Ojeda-Fournier H. A pictorial review of changes in the BI-RADS fifth edition. Radiographics. 2016;36:623-39.
6. Spak DA, Plaxco JS, Santiago L, Dryden MJ, Dogan BE. BI-RADS® fifth edition: a summary of changes. Diagn Interv Imaging. 2017;98:179-90.
7. Rominger M, Wisgickl C, Timmesfeld N. Breast microcalcifications as type descriptors to stratify risk of malignancy: a systematic review and meta-analysis of 10,665 cases with special focus on round/punctate microcalcifications. Rofo. 2012;184(12):1144-52.
8. Price ER, Joe BN, Sickles EA. The developing asymmetry: revisiting a perceptual and diagnostic challenge. Radiology. 2015;274(3):642-51.
9. D'Orsi CJ, Newell MS. Digital mammography: clinical implementation and clinical trials. Semin Roentgenol. 2007;42(4):236-42.
10. Hendrick RE, Pisano ED, Averbukh A, Moran C, Berns EA, Yaffe MJ, et al. Comparison of acquisition parameters and breast dose in digital mammography and screen-film mammography in the American College of Radiology Imaging Network Digital Mammographic Imaging Screening Trial. AJR Am J Roentgenol. 2010;194(2):362-9.
11. Noble M, Bruening W, Uhl S, Schoelles K. Computer-aided detection mammography for breast cancer screening:

systematic review and meta-analysis. Arch Gynecol Obstet. 2009;279(6):881-90.
12. Poplack SA, Tosteson TD, Kogel CA, Nagy HM. Digital breast tomosynthesis: initial experience in 98 women with abnormal digital screening mammography. AJR Am J Roentgenol. 2007;189:616-23.
13. Gur D, Abrams GS, Chough DM, Ganott MA, Hakim CM, Perrin RL, et al. Digital breast tomosynthesis: observer performance study. AJR Am J Roentgenol. 2009;193:586-91.
14. Evans A, Trimboli RM, Athanasiou A, Balleyguier C, Baltzer PA, Bick U, et al. Breast ultrasound: recommendations for information to women and referring physicians by the European Society of Breast Imaging. Insights Imaging. 2018;9(4):449-61
15. Berg WA, Blume JD, Cormack JB, Mendelson EB, Lehrer D, Böhm-Vélez M, et al. Combined screening with ultrasound and mammography vs mammography alone in women at elevated risk of breast cancer. JAMA. 2008;299:2151-63.
16. Colin C, Foray N, Di Leo G, Sardanelli F. Radiation induced breast cancer risk in BRCA mutation carriers from low-dose radiological exposures: a systematic review. Radioprotection. 2017;52(4):231-40.
17. Stavros AT, Thickman D, Rapp CL, Dennis MA, Parker SH, Sisney GA. Solid breast nodules: use of sonography to distinguish between benign and malignant lesions. Radiology. 1995;196(1):123-34.
18. Graf O, Helbich TH, Fuchsjaeger MH, Hopf G, Morgun M, Graf C, et al. Follow-up of palpable circumscribed noncalcified solid breast masses at mammography and US: can biopsy be averted? Radiology. 2004;233(3):850-6.
19. Raza S, Goldkamp AL, Chikarmane SA, Birdwell RL. US of breast masses categorized as BI-RADS 3, 4, and 5: pictorial review of factors influencing clinical management. Radiographics. 2010;30(5):1199-213.
20. Sorelli PG, Cosgrove DO, Svensson WE, Zaman N, Satchithananda K, Barrett NK, et al. Can contrast-enhanced sonography distinguish benign from malignant breast masses. J Clin Ultrasound. 2010;38:177-81.
21. Jia WR, Chai WM, Tang L, Wang Y, Fei XC, Han BS, et al. Three-dimensional contrast-enhanced ultrasound score and dynamic contrast-enhanced magnetic resonance imaging score in evaluating breast tumor angiogenesis: correlation with biological factors. Eur J Radiol. 2014;83:1098-105.
22. Sidhu SP, Cantisani V, Dietrich CF, Gilja OH, Saftoiu A, Bartels E, et al. The EFSUMB guidelines and recommendations for the clinical practice of contrast-enhanced ultrasound (CEUS) in non-hepatic applications: update 2017 (Long Version). Ultraschall Med. 2018;39:e2-44.
23. Youk JH, Son EJ, Gweon HM, Kim H, Park YJ, Kim JA. Comparison of strain and shear wave elastography for the differentiation of benign from malignant breast lesions, combined with B-mode ultrasonography: qualitative and quantitative assessments. Ultrasound Med Biol. 2014;40:2336-44.
24. Chang JM, Moon WK, Cho N, Yi A, Koo HR, Han W, et al. Clinical application of shear wave elastography (SWE) in the diagnosis of benign and malignant breast diseases. Breast Cancer Res Treat. 2011;129:89-97.
25. Au FW, Ghai S, Moshonov H, Kahn H, Brennan C, Dua H, et al. Diagnostic performance of quantitative shear wave elastography in the evaluation of solid breast masses: determination of the most discriminatory parameter. AJR Am J Roentgenol. 2014;203:W328-36.
26. Berg WA, Cosgrove DO, Dore CJ, Schafer FK, Svensson WE, Hooley RJ, et al. Shear-wave elastography improves the specificity of breast US: the BE1 multinational study of 939 masses. Radiology. 2012;262:435-49.
27. Youk JH, Gweon HM, Son EJ, Chung J, Kim JA, Kim EK. Three-dimensional shear-wave elastography for differentiating benign and malignant breast lesions: comparison with two-dimensional shear wave elastography. Eur Radiol. 2013;23:1519-27.
28. Lee SH, Chang JM, Kim WH, Bae MS, Cho N, Yi A, et al. Differentiation of benign from malignant solid breast masses: comparison of two-dimensional and three-dimensional shear-wave elastography. Eur Radiol. 2013;23:1015-26.
29. Mann RM, Cho N, Moy L. Breast MRI: state of the art. Radiology. 2019;292:520-36.
30. National Comprehensive Cancer Network. (2018). Breast cancer screening and diagnosis. [online] Available from: https://www.nccn.org/professionals/physician_gls/pdf/breast-screening. pdf [Last accessed March, 2018].
31. National Institute for Health and Care Excellence. (2018). Early and locally advanced breast cancer: diagnosis and management. NICE guideline (NG101). [online] Available from: https://www.nice.org.uk/guidance/ng101 [Last accessed March, 2018].
32. Houssami N, Abraham LA, Kerlikowske K, Buist DS, Irwig L, Lee J, et al. Risk factors for second screen-detected or interval breast cancers in women with a personal history of breast cancer participating in mammography screening. Cancer Epidemiol Biomarkers Prev. 2013;22(5):946-61.
33. Lee JM, Abraham L, Lam DL, Buist DS, Kerlikowske K, Miglioretti DL, et al. Cumulative risk distribution for interval invasive second breast cancers after negative surveillance mammography. J Clin Oncol. 2018;36(20):2070-7.
34. Kuhl CK, Schrading S, Strobel K, Schild HH, Hilgers RD, Bieling HB. Abbreviated breast magnetic resonance imaging (MRI): first postcontrast subtracted images and maximum-intensity projection: a novel approach to breast cancer screening with MRI. J Clin Oncol. 2014;32(22):2304-10.
35. Leithner D, Moy L, Morris EA, Marino MA, Helbich TH, Pinker K. Abbreviated MRI of the breast: does it provide value? J Magn Reson Imaging. 2019;49:e85-100.
36. Saslow D, Boetes C, Burke W, Harms S, Leach MO, Lehman CD, et al. American Cancer Society guidelines for breast screening with MRI as an adjunct to mammography. CA Cancer J Clin. 2007;57(2):75-89.
37. Peters NH, Borel Rinkes IH, Zuithoff NP, Mali WP, Moons KG, Peeters PH. Meta-analysis of MR imaging in the diagnosis of breast lesions. Radiology. 2008;246:116-24.
38. Kuroki Y, Nasu K, Kuroki S, Murakami K, Hayashi T, Sekiguchi R, et al. Diffusion-weighted imaging of breast cancer with the sensitivity encoding technique: analysis of the apparent diffusion coefficient value. Magn Reson Med Sci. 2004;3(2):79-85.

39. Partridge SC, DeMartini WB, Kurland BF, Eby PR, White SW, Lehman CD. Quantitative diffusion-weighted imaging as an adjunct to conventional breast MRI for improved positive predictive value. AJR Am J Roentgenol. 2009; 193(6):1716-22.
40. Liberman M, Sampalis F, Mulder DS, Sampalis JS. Breast cancer diagnosis by scintimammography: a meta-analysis and review of the literature. Breast Cancer Res Treat. 2003;80(1):115-26.
41. Khalkhali I, Villanueva-Meyer J, Edell SL, Connolly JL, Schnitt SJ, Baum JK, et al. Diagnostic accuracy of 99mTc-sestamibi breast imaging: multicenter trial results. J Nucl Med. 2000;41(12):1973-9.
42. Brem RF, Floerke AC, Rapelyea JA, Teal C, Kelly T, Mathur V. Breast-specific gamma imaging as an adjunct imaging modality for the diagnosis of breast cancer. Radiology. 2008;247(3):651-7.
43. Smith IC, Welch AE, Hutcheon AW, Miller ID, Payne S, Chilcott F, et al. Positron emission tomography using [(18)F]-fluorodeoxy-D-glucose to predict the pathologic response of breast cancer to primary chemotherapy. J Clin Oncol. 2000;18:1676-88.
44. Kumar R, Das CJ. Hybrid PET-dynamic CECT in the management of breast cancer. Eur J Nucl Med Mol Imaging. 2009;36(3):413-5.
45. Berg WA, Madsen KS, Schilling K, Tartar M, Pisano ED, Larsen LH, et al. Breast cancer: comparative effectiveness of positron emission mammography and MR imaging in presurgical planning for the ipsilateral breast. Radiology. 2011;258(1):59-72.

CHAPTER

26

Benign and Malignant Lesions of the Breast

Smriti Hari, Smita Manchanda, Ekta Dhamija

INTRODUCTION

The primary role of breast imaging is to detect and characterize abnormalities that could represent malignancy. A large number of benign conditions of the breast are diagnosed and managed clinically. Imaging of benign conditions is required to detect underlying suspicious abnormalities, if any, and to evaluate patients of symptomatic breast diseases with equivocal clinical findings. Mammography is the primary breast imaging modality; ultrasound and magnetic resonance imaging (MRI) have an important complimentary role. Imaging findings are generally suggestive but not specific for most breast lesions.

PROLIFERATIVE BENIGN LESIONS OF THE BREAST

Benign proliferative breast disease is a pathological term used to describe breast conditions wherein there is more glandular and/or fibrotic tissue than expected for the patient's age and parity. It involves the lobules or ducts or both. The tissue is also morphologically abnormal. These conditions include fibrocystic disease, adenosis, fibroadenoma, cyst, ductal hyperplasia, and papilloma. These may coexist.

Fibrocystic Disease

This is the most common benign diagnosis in symptomatic women. It is a nonspecific term, which includes variations in the breast that histologically range from normal physiological changes to premalignant proliferative conditions. The breast is an end organ for cyclic hormonal changes during normal menstruation. The breast parenchyma is hyperemic and edematous in luteal phase of the menstruation. The response of the breast parenchyma to these hormonal changes varies considerably, from minimal to severe, time to time, and woman to woman. This heterogeneous response of breast leads to variable symptoms such as cyclical pain and lumpiness with clinical findings of nonspecific nodularity and tenderness. In addition, there is a long-term age-related actual involution resulting in replacement of glandular tissue with fat. The range of breast changes is often included under the broad heading of aberrations in normal development and involution (ANDI) of the breast.

Imaging findings are also variable. These include increased mammographic density or heterogeneous echotexture of the breast. Diffuse imaging findings do not correlate with histological changes and there is overlap in the normal and pathological conditions. Hence, imaging diagnosis of fibrocystic disease is discouraged.[1] Indication of imaging in symptomatic patient is to detect the underlying focal lesion, if any. If detected, further characterization and management such as biopsy or follow-up should be recommended.

Adenosis

Adenosis represents enlargement of the lobule secondary to a benign proliferation of the blunt ending intralobular ductules (acini). This proliferation is primarily an elongation and multiplication of the acini accompanied by overgrowth of epithelial and connective tissue elements in the lobule. If connective tissue proliferation is a predominant finding, then the term "sclerosing adenosis" is used. Adenosis is a relatively common benign condition of the breast, which is included under benign proliferative conditions.

Mammographically, adenosis rarely forms a visible mass. On occasion, it may be the cause of isolated cluster of uniform microcalcifications. These are extremely small deposits that precipitate in the acini of the lobule and their cystic dilated ends. These calcifications may be diffuse and scattered bilaterally. Adenosis may also cause nonspecific patchy or homogeneous areas of increased density. Adenosis is not visible by ultrasound.

Fibroadenoma

Fibroadenoma is the most common benign tumor of the breast in women of childbearing age. Fibroadenoma develops from overgrowth of the stromal connective tissue within the lobule. This idiopathic proliferation of collagen expands the lobule while simultaneously surrounding and compressing the acini and terminal ducts. Histologically, the proportion of stromal elements found in a fibroadenoma may vary, producing very cellular adenomas or preponderantly fibrotic lesions.

Clinical breast examination (CBE) reveals a firm, mobile, nontender mass. Fibroadenoma may be single or multiple, unilateral, or bilateral, vary in size from few millimeters to a very large size, though most are <3 cm in diameter. Fibroadenomas in women older than 35 years or those which are rapidly growing are excised. Fibroadenomas are hormone-dependent lesions. They regress with age and necrosis within the tumor results in coarse calcification. Fibroadenomas are not premalignant lesions. As there is epithelium within fibroadenoma, cancer can develop just as it can in normal ductal epithelium. Hence, ill-defined margins, microcalcifications, and increase in size on follow-up should raise concern.

On mammography, fibroadenoma is seen as a well-defined, round or oval mass with smooth margins **(Figs. 1A and B)**. Fibroadenomas may have somewhat flattened contours which if present help to distinguish them from cysts. Because, fibroadenomas follow the structure of the lobule, their margins are often lobulated. Occasionally, they have microlobulated margins. In the presence of microlobulations, however, cancer should be suspected. Fibroadenoma may partly or completely be surrounded by a radiolucent halo. Many fibroadenomas calcify as they undergo myxoid degeneration with age. There may be heavy, central, amorphous calcification or coarse, sharp, intermittent popcorn calcification. In postmenopausal age, there may be complete resolution of the soft tissue component of the fibroadenoma resulting in no residual soft tissue density on mammogram, but calcification remains unchanged.

On ultrasound, fibroadenomas are typically solid, round, or oval, well-circumscribed, homogeneously hypoechoic masses that are wider than taller. Like any round or oval masses, fibroadenomas may exhibit lateral wall refractive shadowing, the side lobe artifact. Posterior acoustic enhancement is frequently seen. Fibroadenomas can, however, produce varying sonographic and elastography appearances including ill-defined margins and posterior acoustic shadowing in more fibrotic adenomas.[2,3]

Magnetic resonance imaging is not recommended for a mammographically well-defined mass that is suspected to be a fibroadenoma. If MRI is performed, predominantly fibrous fibroadenomas are hypointense on all sequences and show no enhancement. Fibroadenomas, which are cellular and contain adenomatous or myxoid tissue, show an intermediate- to high-signal intensity on T2-weighted images and most have circumscribed margins with low-intensity internal septae. The enhancement is significant and homogeneous, usually delayed (type 1). Visualization of nonenhancing septae is diagnostic of fibroadenoma.[4]

A fibroadenoma with a diameter of >6 cm is defined as a giant fibroadenoma. It may fill a large part of the breast. It is a benign lesion and most commonly seen in adolescent females. Phyllode tumor is a close differential diagnosis; however, it is generally seen in later decades of life. Lactating fibroadenoma occurs in young females and is associated with pregnancy or lactation. The lactating fibroadenoma may attain enormous size. Juvenile fibroadenoma is another variant which may be seen in teenage females. It often grows rapidly and becomes very large.

Cysts

Breast cysts develop when lumina of ducts or acini become dilated and are lined by atrophic epithelium. Simple cysts are common lesions and vary in size from microscopic to large palpable masses. These are frequently bilateral and multiple but all may not be identified clinically or by imaging. Cysts are common in perimenopausal age but

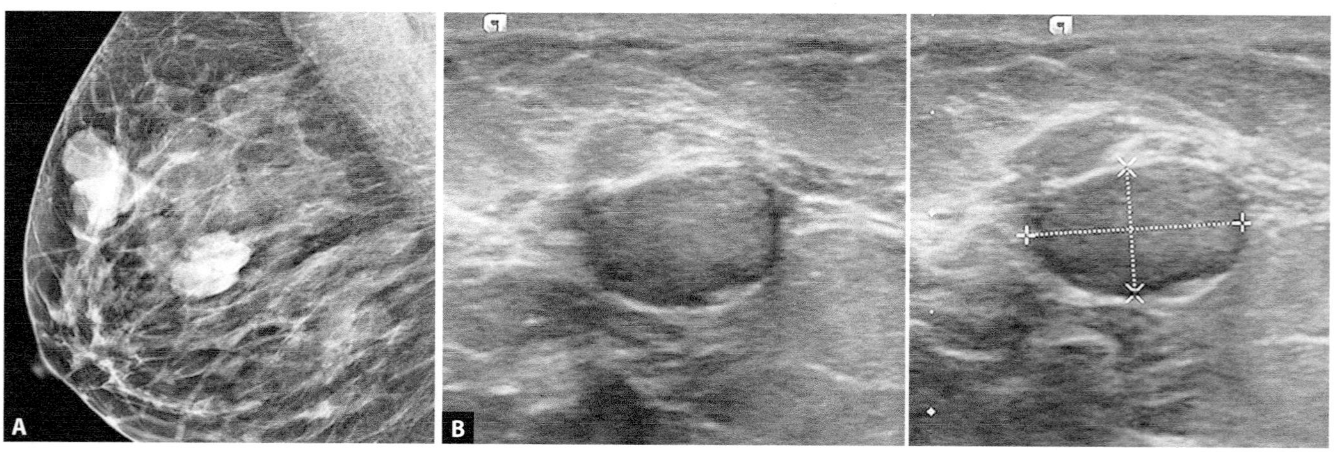

Figs. 1A and B: Fibroadenoma: (A) Mammogram shows two well-defined circumscribed masses with lobulations in upper outer quadrant of right breast. No internal calcification or surrounding architectural distortion is noted; (B) Corroborative ultrasound shows these lesions to have circumscribed margins and homogeneously hypoechoic echopattern.

may be seen in women of all ages. Cysts are benign lesions. Cysts may remain stable for many years or spontaneously resolve.

On mammography, a cyst is typically seen as well-defined, round or oval mass. The cyst may be of variable size, solitary or may occur in clumps. A tense cyst is round, but a lax cyst may vary in shape depending upon the degree of compression applied. Calcification is infrequent and it may be seen as a thin peripheral rim or flecks of calcium near the periphery. Rarely, microcysts may contain milk of calcium fluid which on erect lateral mammography layers on the cyst floor forming so-called "tea-cup" calcification. Cysts cannot be accurately diagnosed by mammography, because they cannot be distinguished from other circumscribed masses, unless they display characteristic pattern of calcification. However, bilateral multiple benign morphology masses on mammography most commonly represent cysts.[1] Ultrasound has an important role in the diagnosis of breast cysts. Typical simple breast cyst is sharply marginated, anechoic with posterior acoustic enhancement **(Fig. 2)**. It may have angular margins, few thin septations, or echogenic debris in the dependent part. These features do not necessarily make it suspicious for malignancy and can be ignored.[4] Posterior enhancement may not be seen if the cyst is small or close to the chest wall. Sometimes, multiple cysts may be seen forming a cluster. Ultrasound diagnosis of simple breast cyst is important as it obviates the need of any fine needle aspiration cytology (FNAC), treatment, or follow-up. Cysts with debris, wall thickening, and septations are referred to a complicated cysts. Chances of malignancy in a complicated cyst are <0.5% and hence, most complicated cysts are appropriately assigned BIRADS 3 (Breast Imaging Reporting and Data System 3) category.[5] Intracystic tumors are rare. If present, these are commonly intracystic papillomas; intracystic cancer is extremely rare. Indications for aspiration of complicated cysts include suspicion of cyst being an abscess, significant enlargement on follow-up, solid mass in the cyst, or suspicious mammographic findings. Symptomatic cysts may also require ultrasound-guided aspiration; however, half of these recur over 2 years.

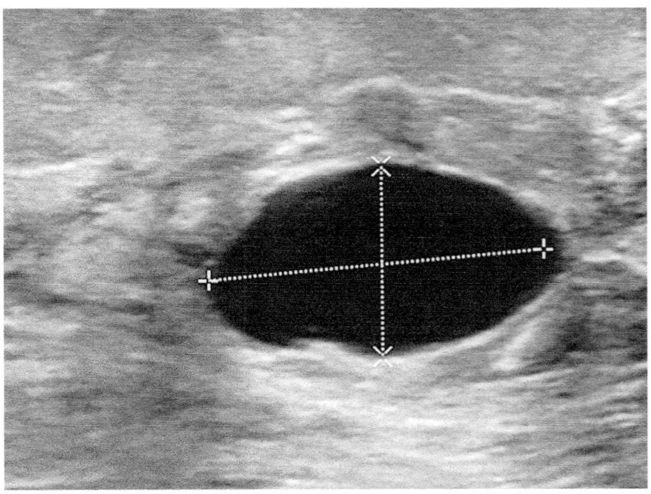

Fig. 2: Breast cyst. Ultrasound shows circumscribed anechoic lesion with smooth walls and posterior acoustic enhancement consistent with simple cyst. No internal septations or solid mural nodule is seen.

On MRI, most cysts are hypointense on T1-weighted images and brightly hyperintense on T2-weighted images. The presence of proteinaceous contents or blood products can modify the signal intensity pattern.

Intraductal Papilloma

Papilloma results from proliferation of the ductal epithelium. They project into the lumen of the duct and connected by a fibrovascular stalk to the epithelial lining. The duct around them can dilate forming a cystic structure giving the appearance of an intracystic papilloma. Benign papilloma is the most common cause of unilateral nipple discharge.[6] Most are located within few centimeters from the nipple in the major subareolar ducts and are usually single.

On mammography, most papillomas are not seen. Larger papillomas are seen as round or oval mass with benign morphology **(Fig. 3A)**. Sometimes, they grow over along length of the duct filling, but not enlarging it. Occasionally, mulberry-like calcification may be seen in the subareolar region. Ultrasound is the preferred modality for the evaluation of nipple discharge. On ultrasound, a typical finding of papilloma is a dilated duct with solid round or oval intraluminal mass **(Fig. 3B)**. Ductography shows dilated duct with intraluminal filling defect or complete obstruction of a duct with a meniscus **(Fig. 3C)**. On MRI, large papillomas behave similar to fibroadenomas.[7] Multiple papillomas arise more distally and are associated with increased risk of cancer.[8]

Duct Ectasia

Duct ectasia primarily affects the major ducts in the subareolar region. There is nonspecific dilatation of one or more ducts. It is generally associated with periductal inflammation. The distended ducts are filled with secretions and cellular debris.

On mammography, dilated ducts may or may not be appreciated. Ectatic ducts with thickened walls or periductal fibrosis are more visible. Intraluminal debris may calcify and produce calcifications called secretory deposits, resembling broken sticks. Ultrasound shows one or more dilated ducts without intraluminal mass. Depending on the composition of the contents, the duct may be anechoic, show debris or may be hyperechoic. Ductography is usually unnecessary and it shows a dilated duct with attenuated peripheral branches.

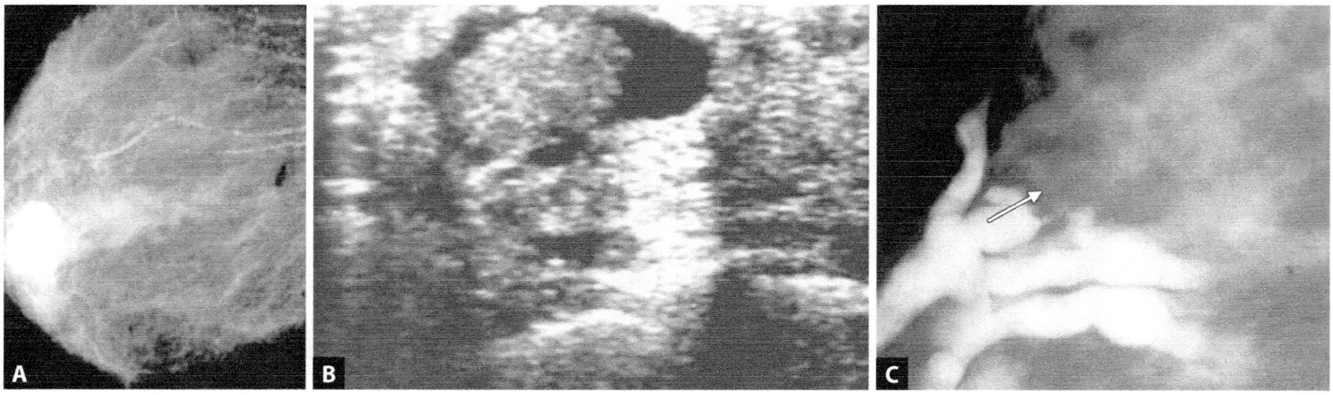

Figs. 3A to C: Duct papilloma: (A) Mammogram shows a small well-defined mass in subareloar location along with dilated duct; (B) Ultrasound shows a papilloma within a dilated duct; (C) Ductogram shows an abrupt cut-off of a duct with meniscus formation (arrow).

Ductal Epithelial Hyperplasia

Ducts are lined with a single layer of epithelial cells. In ductal hyperplasia, there is the benign multilayered cellular proliferation of the epithelium. If atypical cells are found in these, it is called atypical ductal hyperplasia (ADH). It is a high-risk condition as some of these progress into ductal carcinoma in situ (DCIS). Ductal hyperplasia is incidentally diagnosed on biopsy and does not have specific clinical or imaging features. Sometimes, suspicious masses or calcifications may be seen on mammography.

MISCELLANEOUS BENIGN BREAST CONDITIONS

Lipoma

As fat is frequently the preponderant tissue in the breast, it is difficult to differentiate a true lipoma from normal fat. Most lipomas are superficial and form a palpable mass. These are freely movable and generally soft. On mammography, they are lucent, have thin capsule and mass effect with displacement of surrounding structures **(Fig. 4)**. They are hypoechoic on ultrasound, just like the normal breast fat.

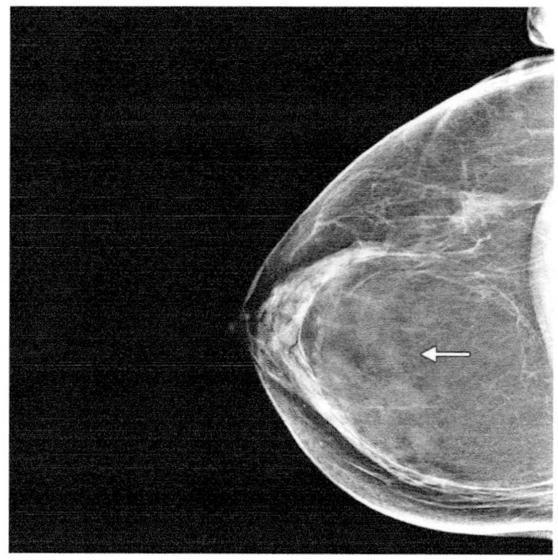

Fig. 4: Lipoma. Mammogram shows a well-defined fat density mass with a capsule (arrow).

Fat Necrosis

Fat necrosis is an inflammatory process of breast related to prior trauma or surgery. Patients are mostly asymptomatic and history of definite trauma is not always present. Some patients have a palpable painful mass with skin thickening or retraction. Occasionally, necrosed fat may form a gelatinous oil cyst with fibrous wall. Fat necrosis is an important lesion because it comes in the differential diagnosis of carcinoma and abscess on mammography.

On mammography, there is a wide spectrum of appearances. Most lesions are superficial in location. Surgical bed is also a common site. Fat necrosis may appear as a spiculated or irregular mass. Calcification is common in fat necrosis and may produce several patterns. Oil cyst shows a round smooth lucent mass, sometimes with calcified thin rim with egg shell appearance **(Figs. 5A and B)**. Cluster of microcalcifications or coarse calcification may also be seen. Post-traumatic oil cysts show varying echogenicity on ultrasound. MRI features of fat necrosis are variable and cannot be distinguished from malignancy. If a fat density is demonstrated within the center of the lesion on nonfat suppressed unenhanced T1-weighted images, fat necrosis can be confirmed.

Galactocele

Galactocele is a cyst filled with inspissated milk. It occurs during pregnancy or lactation and may persist long after cessation of lactation. It may be unilateral or bilateral or may present with multiple palpable masses.

Mammographic features vary with the fat content of the cyst. It may be a well-defined dense lesion like a cyst or a radiolucent mass surrounded by dense lactating breast parenchyma. The usual site is the retroareolar central breast area. Ultrasound shows features of a simple or complicated cyst or a solid mass with posterior enhancement **(Figs. 6A and B)**.

Radial Scar

Radial scar, also known as sclerosing duct hyperplasia, is a lesion of unknown etiology, possibly related to chronic inflammatory process or obliterative changes in blood vessels. There is no palpable mass and no history of trauma. Most are found incidentally on histopathology and some are detected on mammography. Radial scars cannot be accurately diagnosed on core biopsy and require an excisional biopsy. Radial scar is not a premalignant condition but it may rarely contain ADH and DCIS.

Mammographically, it is a spiculated lesion that cannot be differentiated from a cancer **(Figs. 7A and B)**. Central dense mass may or may not be seen. If central mass is absent, it appears like a spiculated architectural distortion only, which is well seen in one view but difficult to appreciate in the other.[9] Microcalcifications are rare. With the advent of digital breast tomosynthesis (DBT), the incidence of detection of radial scars have increased as it demonstrates architectural distortion better than standard two-dimensional (2D) digital mammography.[10] However, its association or upgradation to malignancy is less when seen only on DBT.[11] Ultrasound appearance is also similar to cancer and it shows an irregular, ill-defined, hypoechoic mass. On MRI, an irregular mass with variable contrast enhancement is seen.

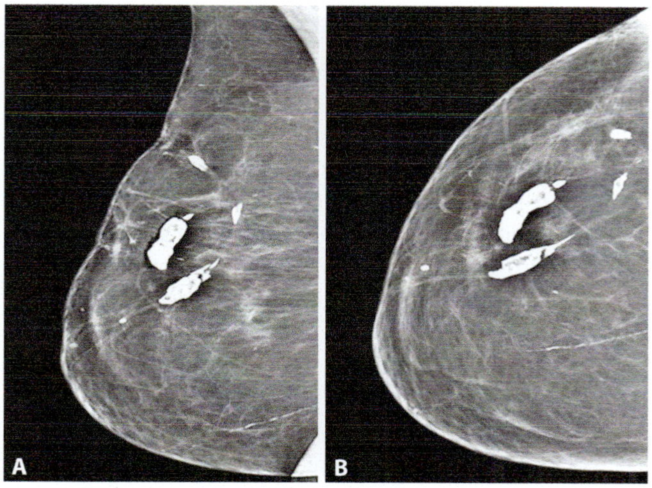

Figs. 5A and B: Fat necrosis. Mammogram shows multiple round and oval-calcified nodules suggestive of oil cyst formation at the operative site.

Hamartoma

Hamartoma or fibroadenolipoma is an uncommon lesion, which results from fibrous and adenomatous proliferation.

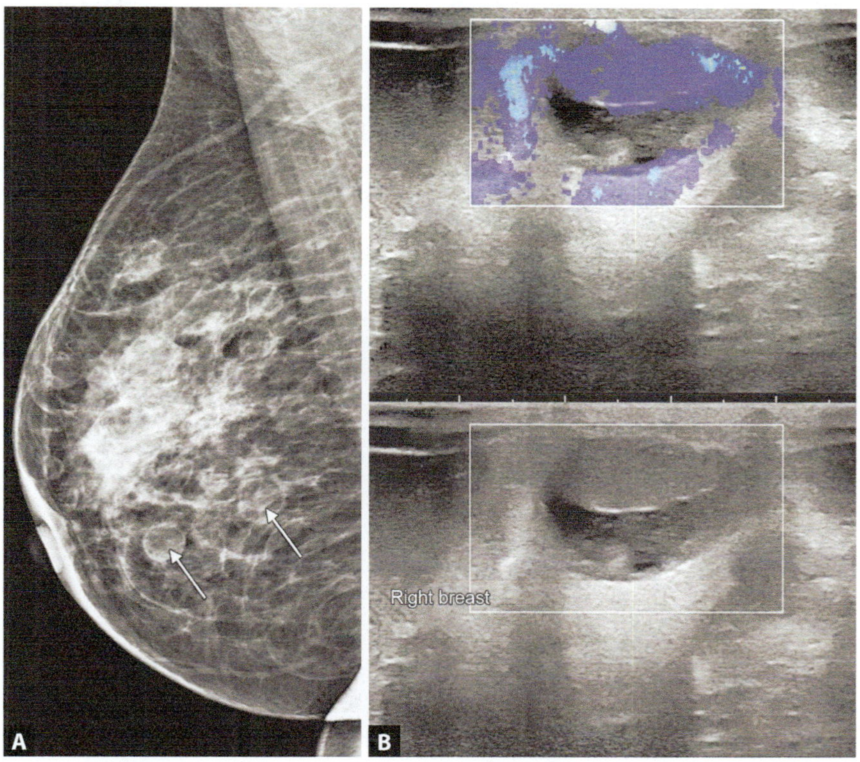

Figs. 6A and B: Galactocele: (A) Mammogram shows architectural distortion in upper quadrant with presence of multiple well-defined low-density circumscribed lesion; (B) Corroborative ultrasound shows cysts with debris in vicinity of a prominent duct. The apparent hypodense material in the cyst shows no vascularity and low elasticity on elastography.

The mammographic appearance is characteristic and is seen as sharply defined mass containing admixture of both fatty- and soft-tissue density. Ultrasound appearance is also similar and shows hypoechoic and hyperechoic areas within a well-defined mass.

Desmoid Tumor

Desmoid tumor, also known as fibromatosis, is a locally invasive, benign spindle cell tumor. It usually occurs in abdominal wall but may rarely be seen in the breast. It tends to develop deep in the breast, along the pectoralis fascia. Most patients have history of trauma or surgery. On mammography, it is seen as round or irregular mass with ill-defined or spiculated margins.[4]

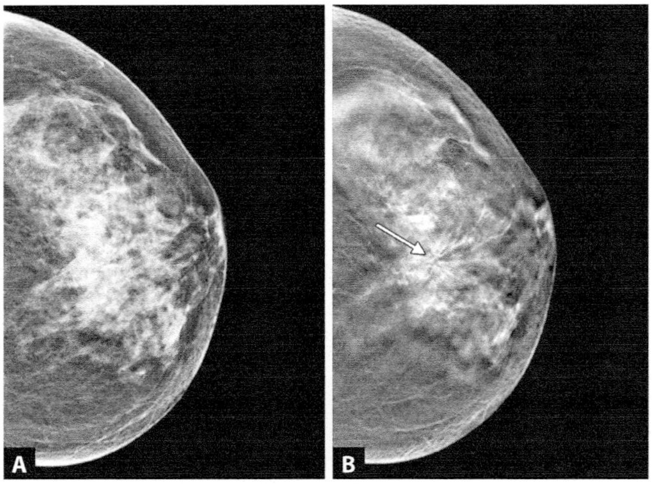

Figs. 7A and B: Radial Scar. Digital breast tomosynthesis shows area of architectural distortion in central inner quadrant (arrow in B) which was not appreciable on 2D mammogram (A).

Diabetic Mastopathy

It is a rare fibrous tumor that is found in young women with type 1 diabetes. It probably represents an autoimmune inflammatory process. They present with a hard palpable breast mass. Usual mammographic appearance is that of an asymmetric density. Ultrasound shows an ill-defined hypoechoic mass with posterior shadowing.[12]

Superficial Thrombophlebitis (Mondor's Disease)

It is a thrombophlebitis of superficial veins of the breast. It is clinically diagnosed and characterized by thickened and painful cord like veins. History of trauma, surgery, or breast biopsy may be present in some patients. It is a self-limiting process. It is difficult to demonstrate on mammography. The thrombosed vein may be seen as an elongated and beaded cord-like opacity on mammography **(Fig. 8A)**. A thrombosed subcutaneous vein can also be demonstrated on ultrasound **(Fig. 8B)**.

Breast Infections

Breast infections may be in the form of acute mastitis associated with lactation or a breast abscess. Acute mastitis may progress to form an abscess. Patient presents with painful, localized, or diffuse enlargement of the breast, with erythematous and edematous overlying skin. Breast infections are usually diagnosed and managed clinically.

Mammography is not required in acute mastitis. Breast abscess is painful and mammography is also difficult to perform. If performed, abscess formation is easily missed through the dense, edematous breast. In others, it is usually seen as a well- or ill-defined mass. Overlying skin thickening is often present. Ultrasound is preferred in evaluation of painful and tender breast as it does not require

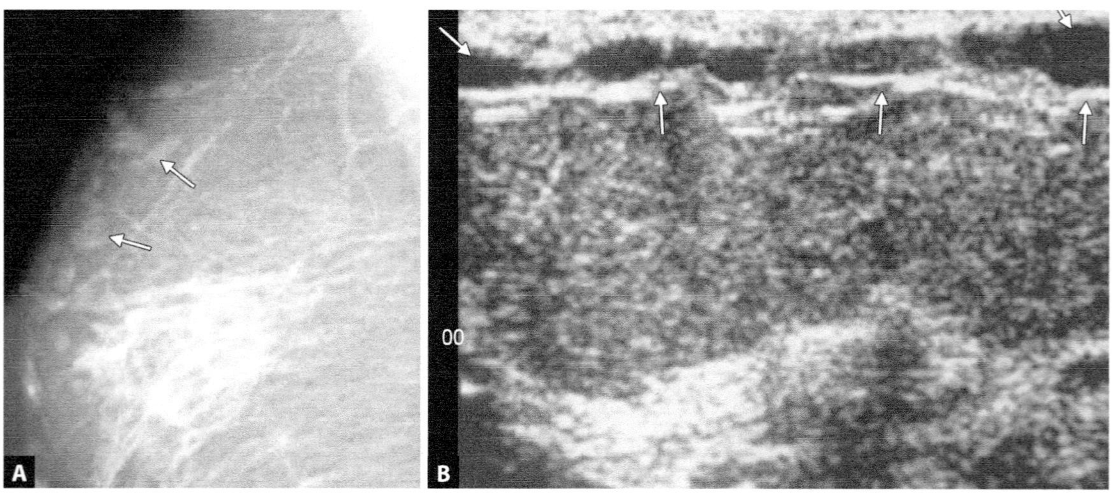

Figs. 8A and B: Mondor's disease: (A) Mammogram shows superficial tortuous linear opacities (arrows) representing a thrombosed vein; (B) Thrombosed subcutaneous vein (arrows) can be seen on ultrasound also.

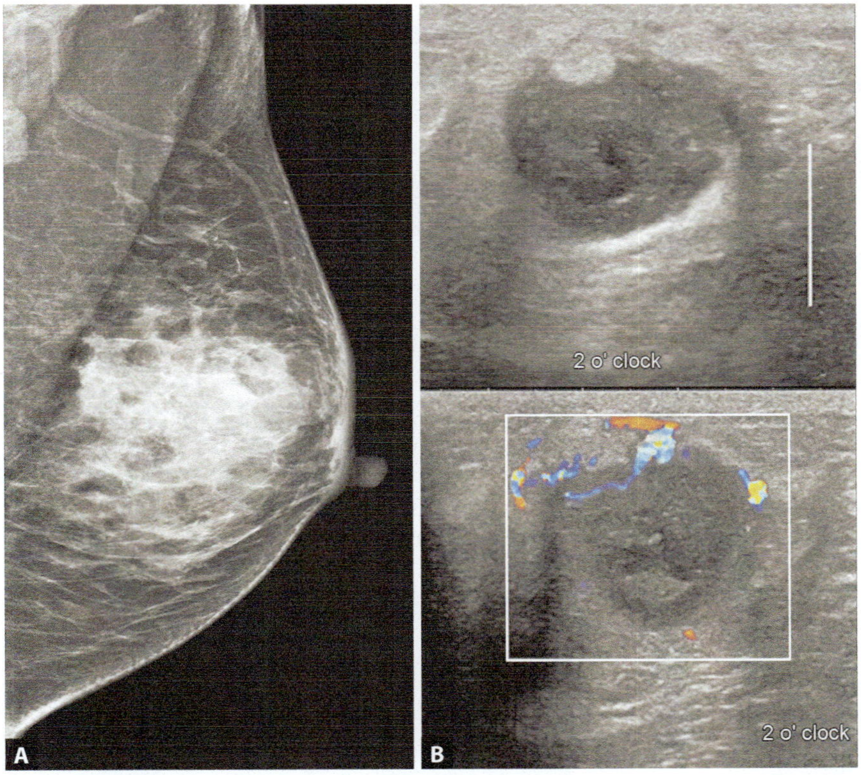

Figs. 9A and B: Breast abscess: (A) Left breast MLO view demonstrating irregular mass with obscured margins in central quadrant with overlying skin thickening in periareolar location; (B) Correlative ultrasound shows irregular complex solid cystic mass with surrounding inflammatory changes and vascularity in the periphery only. (MLO: mediolateral oblique)

breast compression. It is useful to localize the abscess, to exclude underlying inflammatory breast cancer (IBC), and for diagnostic or therapeutic aspiration.[13] On ultrasound, an abscess is seen as a complex irregular mass with solid/cystic components **(Figs. 9A and B)**. Gross subcutaneous edema is usually associated, which is seen as multiple thin, fluid-filled clefts beneath the skin. MRI is not required for evaluation of breast infections. If performed, it shows intense enhancement and secondary changes such as skin thickening, retraction, or architectural distortion. The enhancement tends to be delayed and diffuse but it cannot be differentiated from inflammatory carcinoma.

Granulomatous Mastitis

Granulomatous mastitis is a chronic inflammatory condition of breast for which underlying cause is uncertain. In developed countries, autoimmune etiology has been postulated whereas infection is thought to be the etiology in developing countries. Patients usually present with vague lumps. Clinical evaluation may mimic cancer. Mammography shows nonspecific features such as asymmetric increased density or an ill-defined mass with architectural distortion/trabecular thickening. Ultrasound may show an irregular mass, abscess, fluid-filled tracking channels, edema, or sinus tracts **(Figs. 10A and B)**.[14] Diagnosis is established on biopsy only.

Since tuberculosis is endemic in our country, it is thought to be the most common cause of any unresolving breast infection/mastitis. It has variable mammographic appearances. There are three types of lesions seen on mammography.[15] Nodular form is seen as a dense mass with irregular or spiculated margin, with or without calcification. It is the most common mammographic feature of breast tuberculosis and may mimic carcinoma.[16] Diffuse involvement produces multiple caseating confluent foci of tuberculosis. These also result in skin thickening, ulceration, and sinus formation. Mammography shows dense breast, or skin thickening with or without lymphadenopathy. These findings may mimic inflammatory carcinoma. Sclerosing form of breast tuberculosis is a slow-growing process with excessive fibrosis rather than caseation. Entire breast is hard with nipple retraction. Mammography is not contributory as it shows uniformly increased density of one breast. Ultrasound features of breast tuberculosis are nonspecific and these include a hypoechoic mass or abscess, skin thickening, sinuses, and duct ectasia. Computed tomography (CT) is useful in demonstrating the underlying chest wall involvement.

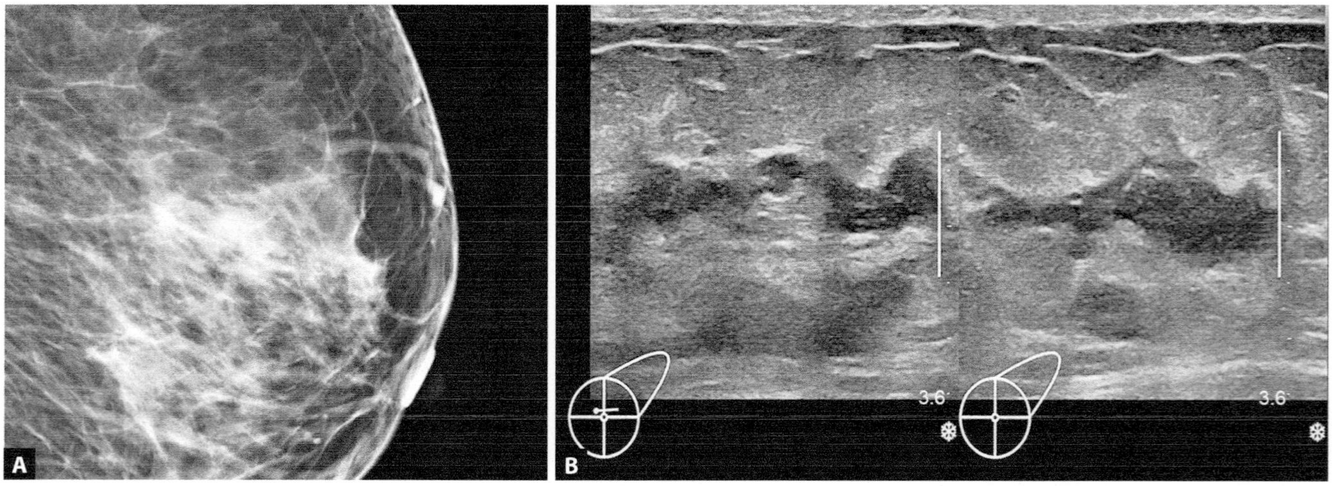

Figs. 10A and B: Granulomatous mastitis: (A) Mammogram shows an area of architectural distortion and trabecular thickening in central quadrant of left breast which is seen as fluid-tracking channels on ultrasound (B).

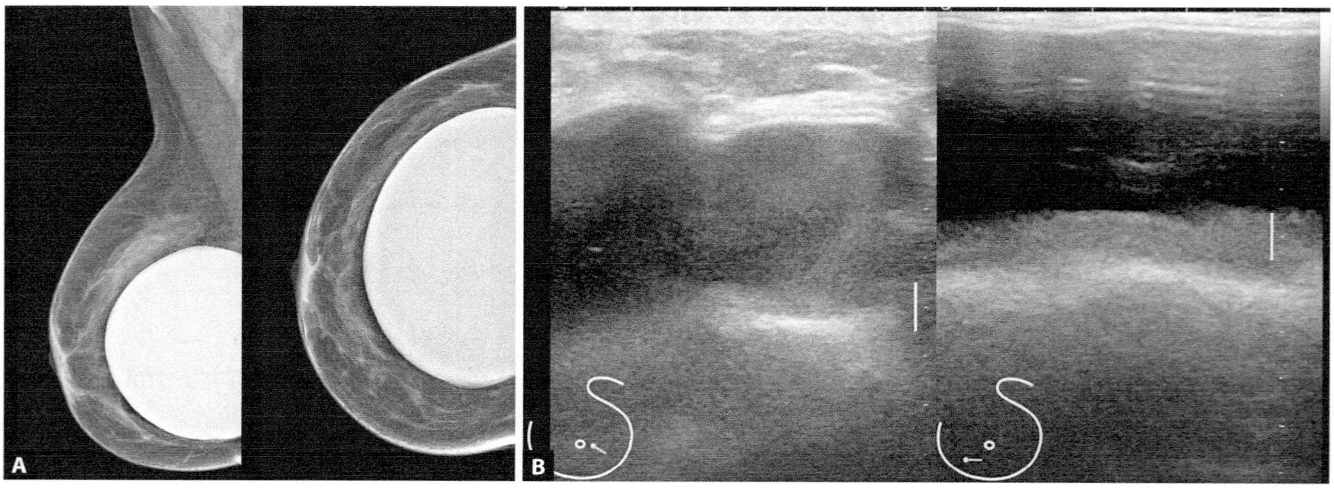

Figs. 11A and B: Breast implant: (A) Mammogram shows the implant as a large, semiovoid well-defined opacity; (B) Implant shows anechoic fluid content on ultrasound.

Breast Implants

Implants are used for cosmetic augmentation of the breast or for breast reconstruction after mastectomy. These are silicone rubber bags filled with silicone gel or saline. These are usually placed behind the breast tissue and anterior to pectoralis muscle. A fibrous capsule normally forms around the implant because of foreign body reaction. Implants appear semiovoid and opaque on mammography and these are anechoic on ultrasound **(Figs. 11A and B)**. During mammography, only the breast tissue anterior to implant can be pulled forward and compressed. Hence, complete visualization of breast parenchyma is not possible on mammography and this interferes with cancer detection. Ultrasound and MRI are useful for evaluation of implants. MRI is the modality of choice. Plain MRI is sufficient. Water- and fat-suppressed (silicone only) T2-weighted magnetic resonance (MR) sequences are particularly useful. Silicone is hypointense on T1-weighted images and hyperintense on T2-weighted images.

Common complications of implants are capsular contractions causing pain and deformity of the breast and implant rupture. Rupture may occur spontaneously due to capsular contracture or during the closed capsulotomy, a procedure in which a surgeon manually compress the capsule to break it and relieve the pain. Rupture can be intracapsular in which the extravasated gel remain inside fibrous capsule or it may be extracapsular leading to spread of the gel in breast parenchyma. The sequelae of noncontained silicone include granuloma formation, fibrosis, and migration. Migration of silicone into the axilla can involve the brachial plexus, resulting in neuropathy.

On ultrasound, intracapsular rupture is seen as folded membranes representing collapsed envelope in step-ladder pattern within the anechoic gel. On MRI, collapsed envelope is seen as low-intensity membranes floating in hyperintense gel on T2-weighted sequences.[17] With extracapsular rupture, ultrasound shows multiple hyperechoic foci in the breast. Extravasated gel in the parenchyma is very echogenic and produces shadowing.[18] On MRI, the extravasated gel appears as foci of low-signal intensity on T1-weighted sequences and high-signal intensity on T2-weighted sequences.[19]

MALIGNANT LESIONS OF THE BREAST

Breast cancer is the most common cancer in female population worldwide with over 2 million new cases detected in 2018 itself.[20] According to GLOBACON 2012, it constitutes approximately 25.1% of all cancers and is more common in developed countries but has more mortality in developing nations.[21] In India, breast cancer is number one cancer among females with age adjusted rate of 25.8 per 100,000 women and mortality of 12.7 per 100,000 women.[22]

Risk Factors for Breast Cancer

Female gender and increasing age are the most important risk factors for development of breast cancer. Other risk factors include early menarche, late menopause, nulliparity or late first pregnancy, and decreased breast feeding. All of these factors increase the overall duration of endogenous estrogen exposure, a hormone known to play a major role in the development of breast cancer. Exogenous estrogen exposure in hormonal replacement therapy (HRT) also increases the risk of breast cancer. Family history of breast cancer in a first-degree relative is also a risk factor, especially if they had breast cancer at an early age. The familial inheritance of the risk may be associated with or without genetic mutations. Women with Li-Fraumeni and Cowden syndromes have a high risk. History of benign breast disease, especially atypical hyperplasia also increases the risk of breast cancer. Mammographic breast density has also been identified as a risk factor. Women with >75% glandular density on mammogram are at fourfold greater risk for breast cancer development.[23]

BRCA1 and *BRCA2* genes mutations are major risk factors and these account for 5–10% of all breast cancers. The chances of breast cancer in the carriers of these mutations are variable in different races and range from 45 to 85%.[24] They also have an increase a risk for ovarian cancer, especially with *BRCA1* mutation. Breast cancer arising in these women is frequently aggressive and triple negative; negative for estrogen receptor (ER), progesterone receptor (PR), and human epidermal growth factor receptor (HER2). Management options in BRCA mutation carriers include close surveillance, chemoprevention, and prophylactic bilateral mastectomy with or without salpingo-oophorectomy.

Diagnosis of the Breast Cancer

Breast cancer may be detected in preclinical stage on screening mammography. Others are detected by self-breast examination (SBE) or CBE. Symptomatic breast cancers present with a palpable mass, focal tenderness, nipple discharge, skin retraction or ulceration, or sometimes as a metastatic disease with occult primary site. Mammography is the primary modality for detection of breast cancer; tomosynthesis, ultrasound, and MRI complement mammography in detection of breast cancer. Approach to the breast imaging and role of various imaging modalities in detection of breast cancer has been covered in the preceding chapter. However, there are no characteristic features of breast cancer on imaging. It is interesting to note that mammographic interpretation has a category of definitely benign lesions (BIRADS 2) but there is no category of definitely malignant lesions. Mammography only detects lesions which are either suspicious (BIRADS 4) or highly suspicious (BIRADS 5) for malignancy. Hence, all such lesions need to be subjected to biopsy for the definitive diagnosis of breast cancer. Image-guided breast biopsy is an important tool for the diagnosis of breast cancer, and it is described in detail in the following chapter. Pathological analysis routinely consists of assessment of invasion, histopathological characterization, and immunohistochemical analysis for ER, PR, and HER2 receptor status.[25] Classification of breast cancer into luminal and basal type, based on genetic expressions and molecular biology may also be performed.

BREAST CANCER SCREENING

Cancer screening is aimed at detection of a cancer when it is small, asymptomatic, and early stage. Chances of cure are highest with such cancers. Primary purpose of any screening program that targets healthy population is to reduce deaths from the disease and not just its early diagnosis. Mammography screening achieves this goal.

Mammography Screening

Mammography screening is the most widely used cancer screening modality in the world. It has been studied extensively and no other imaging modality has been subjected to as large scale and extensive research as mammography. There is level 1 evidence to suggest that mammography screening reduces the breast cancer mortality significantly in the screened population and it is cost effective. This evidence has primarily come from eight large randomized screening trials [randomized controlled trials (RCTs)] started in 1970s and early 80s in which half of women were invited to screening and the other half were not. These trials along with early benefits from these are given in **Table 1**.[26] Many of these trials are continuously analyzed. Health Insurance Plan (HIP) of

Table 1: Randomized controlled trials (RCTs) of mammography screening.

RCT	*Years of start*	*Number of women*	*Age group (years)*	*Mammography interval (months)*	*Early mortality reduction*
HIP, New York, USA	1963	62,000	40–64	12	29%
Two county, Sweden	1978	162,981	40–74	24	37%
Malmo, Sweden	1976	42,000	45–69	18	18%
Stockholm, Sweden	1981	59,176	40–64	24	20%
Gothenburg, Sweden	1982	52,000	39–59	18	14%
Edinburg, UK	1978	45,130	45–64	12	16%
NBSS 1, Canada	1980	50,430	40–49	12	Nil
NBSS 2, Canada	1980	39,476	50–59	12	30%

(HIP: Health Insurance Plan; NBSS: National Breast Screening Studies)

New York was the first trial and it also included CBE along with mammography. Twin county trial consisted of two simultaneous trials conducted at Swedish counties of Ostergotland and Kopparberg. It is the largest screening trial for which longest follow-up is available. National Breast Screening Studies (NBSS) of Canada performed two separate screenings for women of age groups 40–49 and 50–75 years, respectively. These were similar to HIP. The data and long-term follow-up of these trials have been analyzed and debated several times to determine the exact quantum of benefits from mammography screening. Overall, mammography screening effectively reduces the overall breast cancer mortality by 28–45%.[27] Most recent meta-analysis for US Preventive Services Task Force (USPSTF) also confirmed that mammography screening significantly reduces breast cancer mortality in women aged 39–69 years.[28] A three decade follow-up of the twin county trial has shown that cost-effectiveness and number of deaths prevented by screening improve over time.[29] Analysis of community screening programs, outside the RCTs, in developed countries of Europe, America, and Australia have also shown that the implementation of screening mammography reduces breast cancer deaths by as high as 35–50%.[28-31] Reviews and data analysis from the RCTs have been performed several times and using variable methods.[32] Some concluded that there is no benefit with screening mammography.[33] However, such reviews are few and their analysis is considered flawed by most experts.[34] Early detection is beneficial for diagnosis and treatment of any cancer and breast cancer is certainly not an exception to this logic.[35]

There are some variations in the recommendations for mammography screening. American College of Radiology and American Cancer Society recommend mammography every year from 40 to 74 years of age. However, USPSTF recommends 2 yearly mammography in the 50–75 years age group.[36] In some European countries, mammography is offered every 2 years from 50 to 70 years or 74 years.[37-39] After the age of 75 years, mammography is not cost-effective in term of number of lives saved as there are other competing causes of death.

Mammography screening must be organized and optimized for it to be successful. Mammography is the most regulated and legislated imaging modality in Europe and America. Licensing and accreditation of the facilities, regular QA programs, tests and training programs of radiographers and radiologists, reporting standards are regularly monitored, and audit of the outcome performed.

Screening mammography is a high-cost venture. At least 414 women must be screened for 7 years to prevent one breast cancer death.[27] It has several other drawbacks as well, which frequently generates controversies. Most important among these are false-positive mammograms and overdiagnosis. After a regular screening round, some women are recalled at the facility for additional imaging and/or biopsy. Although majority of them will not have a cancer, it causes anxiety in all of them and also increases the cost of screening. About half of women screened for 10 years have at least one recall and may be a biopsy. Screening mammography has also led to many fold increase in the DCIS detection rates.[40] This leads to biopsy and surgery, including mastectomies, in women with mammographic lesions. This may be unnecessary in some women since all DCIS do not grow into invasive carcinoma and cancer would have never been diagnosed in their lifetime, had screening not been done. Overdiagnosis and overtreatment of such indolent breast cancers is considered a major disadvantage of mammographic screening and often criticized. However, since there is no way to predict which DCIS will progress into invasive ductal carcinoma (IDC), this limitation of mammographic screening should be accepted for overall benefits. Screening mammography also does not detect all breast cancers. Some aggressive cancers may get diagnosed in between two sequential rounds of the screening. These are called interval cancers and their incidence may range from 10 to 43% in different age groups.[41]

True benefits from screening mammography have also been debated. In recent years, improved breast cancer treatment with better chemo/hormonal therapy and targeted therapy have improved the survival and it is difficult to determine the absolute contribution of screening mammography in reducing overall breast cancer mortality.[42] It is estimated that mammography has contributed by two-thirds and adjuvant treatment by one-third in present day breast cancer mortality reduction in developed countries.[30]

Magnetic Resonance Imaging Screening

Familial breast cancers account for 10–15% of all breast cancers and about half of these patients are *BRCA1* and *BRCA2* mutations carriers. Cancer occurs in these women at younger age and hence, screening must be started much earlier. Mammographic breast density is high in young women and as expected, the performance of mammography is poor in detection of breast cancer in these women. MRI does not depend on breast density and it is the most sensitive tool for breast cancer detection in these women.[43,44] Breast MRI is recommended for screening of high-risk women, if risk quantification is >25%.[44,45] Generally, annual breast MRI and mammograms are performed with 6-month gap between these two tests, resulting in imaging surveillance at every 6th month. Screening should be started at younger age of 25–30 years. Higher sensitivity of breast MRI comes with high false-positive rates. This leads to higher number of benign breast biopsies, when compared with mammographic screening.

Ultrasound Screening

Ultrasound, as a sole modality, has never been used for breast cancer screening. However, it is routinely used to evaluate mammographically dense breasts. It can show mammographically occult breast cancers in asymptomatic women with negative mammograms. However, the detection rate is <1%.[46,47] A blinded screening trial [ACRIN (American College of Radiology Imaging Network) 6666] comparing ultrasound and mammography for cancer detection in high-risk women found mammographic detection rate of 7.6 cancers per 1,000 women screened. It increased to 11.8 cancers with combined mammography and ultrasound use.[48] Additional cancers detected on ultrasound were invasive and node negative and hence, these women actually benefited from ultrasound screening. However, ultrasound is not likely to be used for population screening because of its inability to visualize microcalcifications, operator dependency, time consuming nature, and high false-positive rates, mostly from complicated cysts.

Breast Cancer Screening in Developing Countries

Population-based screening mammography is expensive and resource intensive. Hence, it is not an immediate option in countries with limited resources. SBE and CBE are widely encouraged for early diagnosis, or more precisely, to decrease the proportion of advanced breast cancers at presentation. However, the only RCT on SBE for breast cancer screening has shown no benefits.[49] Breast Health Global Initiative (BHGI), a nonprofit organization working in this area, has recommended the use of traditional "triple test" assessment comprising CBE, imaging (diagnostic mammography or ultrasound), and FNAC or biopsy for early diagnosis of breast cancer in low-resource countries.[50]

IMAGING FEATURES OF BREAST CANCER

Breast cancer is a group of malignant breast lesions. All breast cancers are believed to arise from the terminal duct lobular unit (TDLU). It is the distal most part of the ductal branching system which opens into the lobule of the gland and is the site of most active cellular proliferation. Breast cancers are classified into various pathological subtypes according to the World Health Organization (WHO) system. These cannot be determined on imaging. There are no imaging features which are specific to any pathological subtype of the breast cancer. Actually, imaging features are not even specific for cancer. However, some imaging characteristics are somewhat more commonly associated with particular type of cancer than others.

Preinvasive Breast Lesions

Preinvasive breast lesions include DCIS and lobular carcinoma in situ (LCIS). DCIS is the precursor of invasive breast cancer. On the other hand, most LCIS do not become invasive and this entity is hence, regarded as a high-risk condition rather than a true cancer.

Ductal Carcinoma In Situ

Ductal carcinoma in situ lies along a spectrum of preinvasive lesions of the breast tissue, with histologic progression from ADH to DCIS and then to the IDC. The pathological classification of DCIS is based on the nuclear grade of the tumor cells (low, intermediate, or high), the architectural pattern of tumor growth (solid, papillary, micropapillary, or cribriform), and the presence or absence of comedo necrosis.

Ductal carcinoma in situ is usually small but can grow to large size and become symptomatic. Presentations of DCIS include mammographically detected mass or calcification, palpable mass, Paget's disease, or an incidental finding on breast biopsy. DCIS is a precursor of IDC; however,

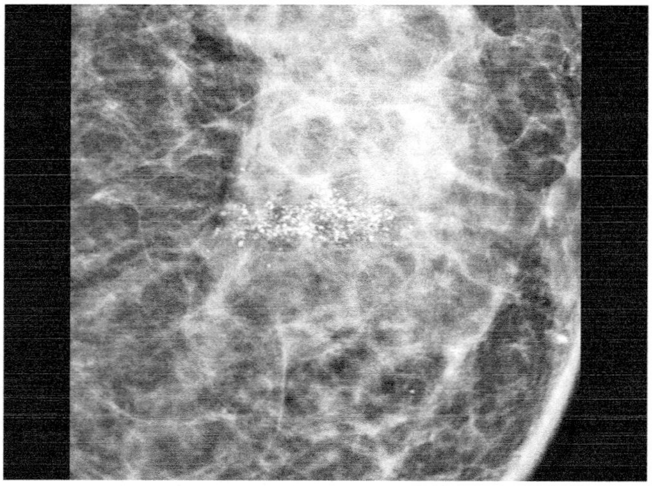

Fig. 12: DCIS. Mammogram shows pleomorphic, linear branching microcalcifications in the ductal orientation. (DCIS: ductal carcinoma in situ)

only some of DCIS develop into invasive cancer, while other remains indolent forever. True incidence of IDC in patients with DCIS is unknown. On mammography, DCIS is characterized by microcalcifications, usually of linear branching type **(Fig. 12)**. Less commonly, DCIS can produce a mass with ill-defined or lobulated borders, with or without calcification. Ultrasound is unsuitable to detect microcalcifications. Associated soft tissue component and architectural distortion may be appreciated as a hypoechoic mass on ultrasound. It may be suspected if there is an area of altered echotexture with parenchymal echogenicity, ductal changes, or few nonspecific cysts on ultrasound. Atypical ductal and parenchymal changes in comparison to normal rest of the breast parenchyma should be evaluated carefully to rule out possibility of DCIS. Calcifications are not seen on MRI; however, overall sensitivity of MRI is higher than mammography in detection of DCIS.[51] Both can detect DCIS not detected by the other modality. On MRI, about half of DCIS are seen as enhancing masses. Others show nonmass-like enhancement or no enhancement.[52] All three patterns of enhancement curves can be seen with DCIS. DCIS is treated with mastectomy or breast conservation treatment [lumpectomy followed by radiotherapy (RT)]. Since, it is not an invasive cancer, axillary dissection is not required.

Lobular Carcinoma In Situ

Atypical lobular hyperplasia (ALH) and LCIS are not true cancers but are high-risk or premalignant conditions. These are asymptomatic and incidentally detected on breast biopsy. Pathologically, these represent spectrum of atypical proliferation of loosely cohesive cells in the TDLU. LCIS is often multifocal and bilateral. It does not cause any clinical or imaging abnormalities. About one-third of the women with LCIS ultimately develop invasive lobular carcinoma (ILC) in the same or contralateral breast.[1] Management options include close surveillance or prophylactic mastectomy.

Invasive Breast Cancer

Invasive or infiltrating ductal carcinoma (IDC) is the most common histologic subtype of breast cancer. It is designated not otherwise specified (NOS) as it is not categorized into specific types such as medullary, lobular, mucinous, etc. In SEER data of National Cancer Institute, IDC (NOS) constituted 83.9% of all invasive breast cancers.[53] Others include invasive lobular (7.4%), medullary (3.1%), mucinous (2.3%), and Paget's disease (1%). Other subtypes accounted for <1% each. Depending on the nuclear pleomorphism and mitotic activity, all breast cancers are also graded histologically into grade 1 (well differentiated), grade 2 (moderately differentiated), and grade 3 (poorly differentiated). This tumor grading has prognostic significance.

Invasive Ductal Carcinoma

Invasive ductal carcinoma (NOS) is undifferentiated and has no specific histologic pattern. Desmoplastic reaction is common in IDC which accounts for its most common presentation of hard mass on palpation and spiculated mass on mammography **(Figs. 13A to C)**. It may also be seen as malignant calcifications, architectural distortion, or any combination of these. Ultrasound and MRI show a mass having one or more malignant features described in Chapter 25 **(Figs. 13A to C)**. Irregular mass with rim enhancement or heterogeneous internal enhancement is the most common MR appearance of IDC.

Invasive Lobular Carcinoma

Invasive lobular carcinoma is the second most common invasive breast cancer and a large number of these are multicentric or bilateral. Histologically, these show diffuse tumor foci invading the stroma. They spread in the form of a single file (line) of noncohesive malignant cells through intervening normal parenchyma, instead of a well-formed mass. They do not evoke desmoplastic response. Because of these features, ILC are difficult to detect on clinical examination, mammography, and even on MRI. Clinical presentation may be of an ill-defined mass, nonspecific induration, or tenderness. Other patients may present with symptoms from distant metastases. Mammographically, asymmetric breast density is the most common finding. Other mammographic findings include spiculated or ill-defined mass, or a normal mammogram.[1] Calcifications are distinctly rare. Ultrasound is useful to detect underlying mass in an asymmetric density seen on mammography **(Figs. 14A and B)**. MRI does not detect all ILC; however, it is more accurate than mammography for detection of ILC.[54]

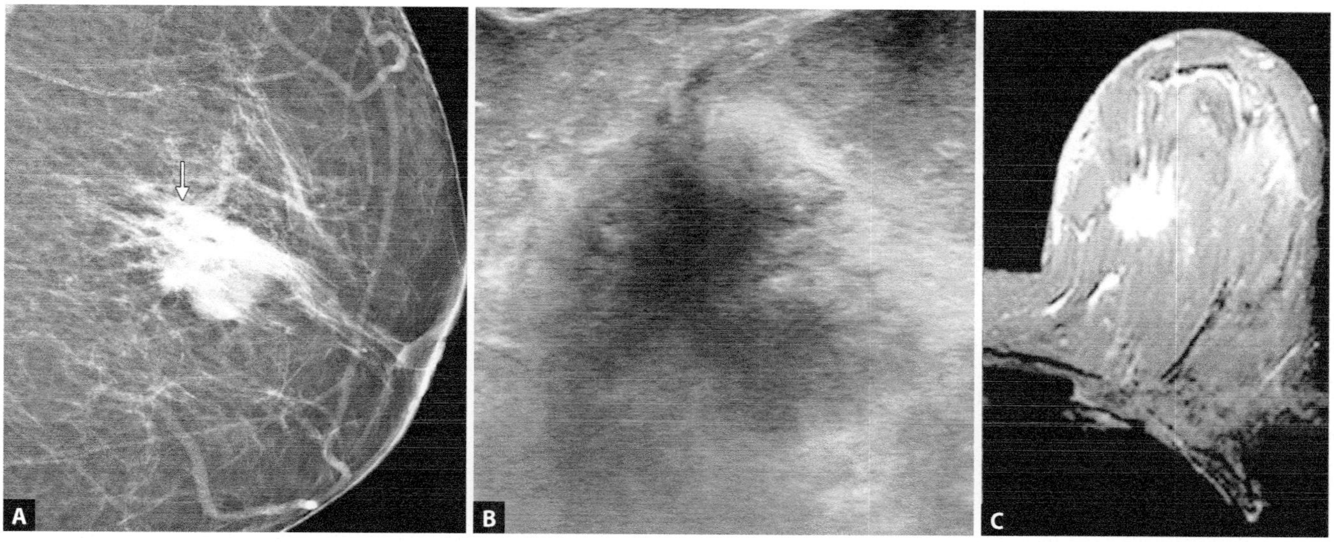

Figs. 13A to C: IDC: (A) Mammogram shows a high-density, irregular, spiculated mass (arrow); (B) Ultrasound shows a hypoechoic, irregular, spiculated mass with distal acoustic shadowing; (C) Contrast-enhanced T1-weighted MRI scan of another woman shows a spiculated, intensely enhancing mass. (IDC: invasive ductal carcinoma; MRI: magnetic resonance imaging)

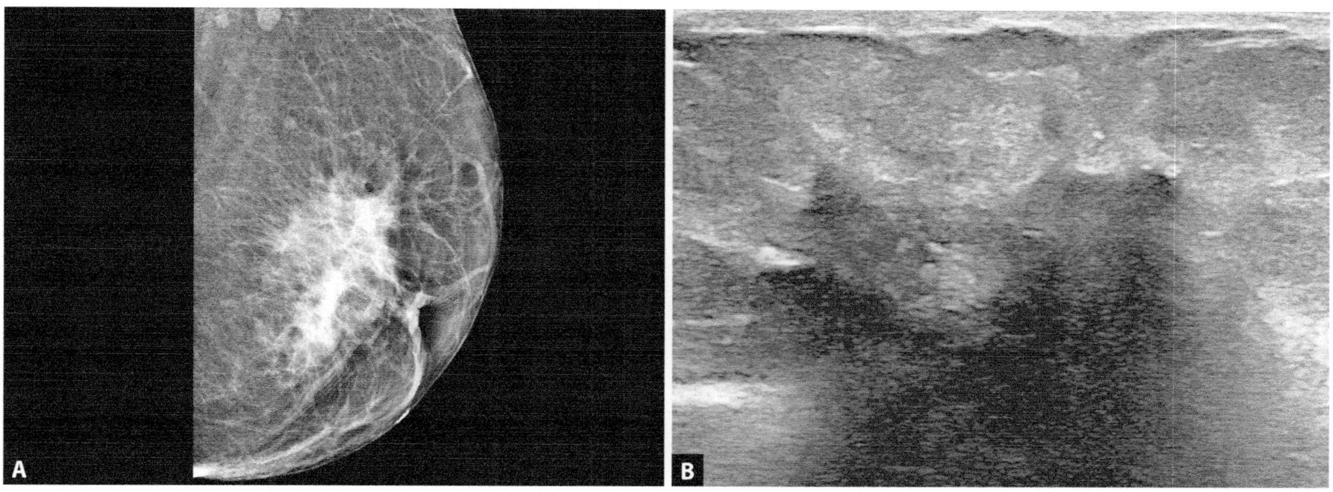

Figs. 14A and B: Invasive lobular carcinoma: (A) Left MLO view shows architectural distortion causing nipple retraction in the breast; (B) Ultrasound shows ill-defined hypoechoic mass with radiating spiculated margins. (MLO: mediolateral oblique)

On MRI, ILC are most commonly seen as enhancing mass with variable contrast enhancement patterns. Others may be seen as diffuse area of enhancement that is difficult to differentiate from normal parenchyma.[55] MRI detects additional foci of cancer in >50% of patients diagnosed with ILC.[56]

Medullary Carcinoma

Medullary carcinoma is usually seen in younger age. It is a rapidly growing tumor and often large in size when detected.[1] Histologically, they are high-grade tumors with abundant infiltration by inflammatory cells. Desmoplastic process is uncommon. The prognosis is poor as most have early lymphovascular invasion, lymph node, and distant metastases. On mammography, a well-defined or ill-defined mass, without spiculations or calcification is seen **(Fig. 15)**. On ultrasound, they are hypoechoic, well-circumscribed, or lobulated. Distal acoustic enhancement may be seen. These ultrasound features often simulate benign masses.

Mucinous Carcinoma

Mucinous (or colloid) carcinoma is a well-differentiated, slow growing tumor. It is generally seen in older women and has a better prognosis. It is characterized by abundant mucin production. Usual mammographic finding is of a low-density mass with ill-defined or microlobulated margins **(Figs. 16A and B)**. Calcification or desmoplastic reaction is uncommon. Ultrasound shows a well-defined, iso- or hypoechoic mass with microlobulated margins and posterior acoustic enhancement insome.[57] Rarely, it is seen as a complex cystic-solid mass on ultrasound. MR features are similar to mammography; however, the contrast enhancement pattern is frequently of benign type. Unlike most other breast cancers, mucinous cancer can demonstrate high-signal intensity on T2-weighted images.

Tubular Carcinoma

Tubular carcinoma is a rare well-differentiated invasive carcinoma which demonstrates poorly formed ductal structures. About one-third of these are multicentric and bilateral. They are slow growing and have better prognosis. On mammography, a small spiculated or ill-defined mass is usually seen.[1] Uncommonly, calcifications may be seen. There are no specific MR features.

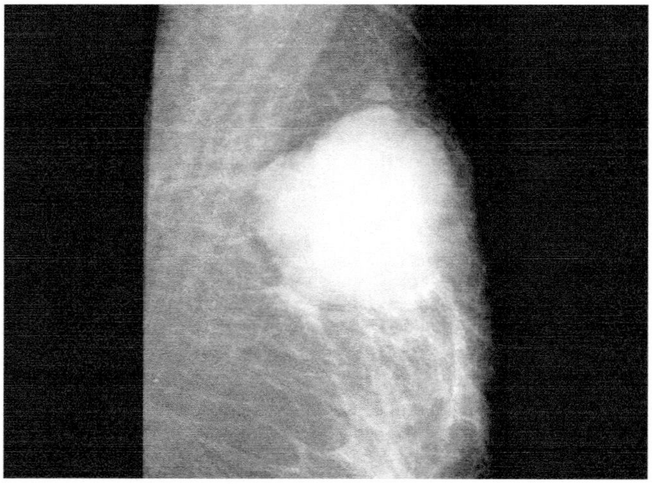

Fig. 15: Medullary carcinoma. Mammogram shows a round mass with lobulated, partially indistinct margin.

Papillary Carcinoma

Papillary carcinoma is seen with advanced age. There is villous epithelial proliferation that eventually fills the ductal lumen. Papillary carcinoma can develop as an intracystic lesion, although it is likely that the cyst represents a secondarily dilated duct.[1] These are slow growing and do not have desmoplastic reaction. On mammography, papillary carcinomas are seen as well-circumscribed masses because of their cystic nature. This is the only breast cancer which is commonly cystic on ultrasound; usual sonographic appearance is a complex solid-cystic mass or intracystic tumor with multiple fronds projecting into the lumen of the cyst **(Fig. 17)**.

Triple Negative Breast Cancer

Triple negative breast cancer (TNBC) is the term used for invasive breast cancers of any histologic type, which are negative for ER, PR, and HER2 receptors on immunohistochemistry. These are now separately classified because of their distinct clinical, radiological, and prognostic features. TNBC are characterized by occurrence at younger age, aggressive behavior, early metastases, and are refractory to treatment. TNBC are also difficult to diagnose on mammography. These are usually seen as well-defined or ill-defined masses. Spiculations and calcifications are rare. Hence, these may be difficult to differentiate from benign masses.[58] On ultrasound also, these have benign features of circumscribed masses with frequent posterior acoustic enhancement. MRI is most useful for their diagnosis. These are seen as mass- or

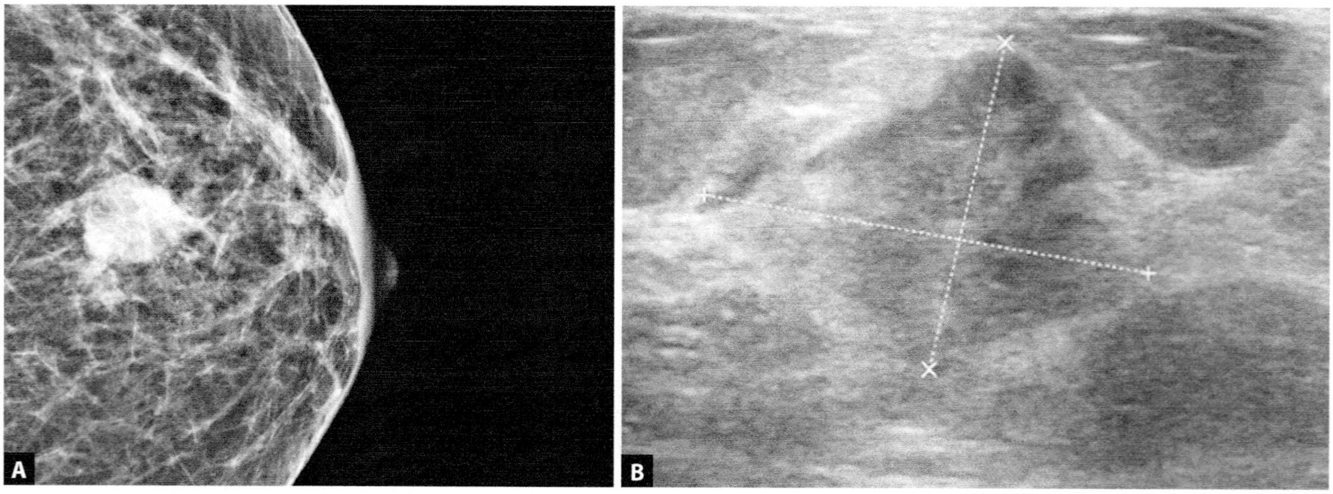

Figs. 16A and B: Mucinous carcinoma: (A) Mammogram shows an irregular high-density mass in central quadrant with partially obscured margins; (B) Ultrasound shows irregular, isoechoic mass with focal angular margins.

nonmass-like lesions with intense type 3 enhancement curve. These are frequently multicentric and are well-demonstrated on MRI.[59]

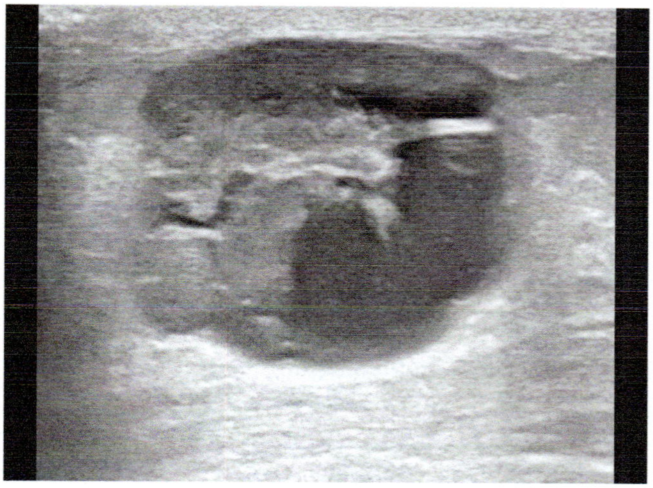

Fig. 17: Intracystic papillary carcinoma: ultrasound shows a complex cyst with irregular solid component projecting intraluminally from the lateral wall.

STAGING AND TREATMENT OF BREAST CANCER

Breast cancer is staged according to the TNM (Tumor size, Lymph Nodes affected, Metastases) staging system of AJCC (American Joint Committee on Cancer). An overview of the staging system is given in **Table 2**. After the diagnosis of breast cancer, clinical staging is performed based on both clinical as well as imaging findings. The clinical stage is denoted as cTNM. For metastatic workup, chest X-ray, ultrasound of the abdomen, and bone scan is sufficient in stage I and II tumors. CT or positron-emission tomography (PET) is recommended for stage III cancers. Surgery is the primary treatment of breast cancer in resectable patients and this includes breast conservation therapy (BCT) or mastectomy. After surgery, a final or pathological stage is assigned and it is denoted as pTNM. Final stage of the disease and other risk factors are considered to decide for adjuvant (postoperative) treatment with RT, chemotherapy, and hormone therapy.[60]

Table 2: Overview of staging of breast cancer.

Tis	*Carcinoma in situ*		*T-stage*		
T1	<2 cm			T1a: Up to 5 mm T1b: Up to 1 cm T1c: Up to 2 cm	
T2	2–5 cm				
T3	>5 cm				
T4	Chest wall/skin involvement			T4a: Chest wall invasion T4b: Skin invasion T4c: Both chest wall and skin invasion T4d: Inflammatory breast cancer	
			N-stage		
N0	No lymphadenopathy				
N1	Mobile level I, II axillary LN				
N2	Fixed level I, II axillary LN or internal mammary LN			N2a: Fixed or matted level I/II axillary LN N2b: Internal mammary LN without axillary LN	
N3	Level III axillary, internal mammary, supraclavicular LN			N3a: Level III axillary LN N3b: Both axillary and internal mammary LN N3c: Supraclavicular LN	
			M-stage		
M0	No distant metastases				
M1	Distant metastases				
			Stage groups		
	N0	N1	N2	N3	M1
T1	IA	IIA	IIIA	IIIC	IV
T2	IIA	IIB	IIIA	IIIC	IV
T3	IIB	IIIA	IIIA	IIIC	IV
T4	IIIB	IIIB	IIIB	IIIC	IV

(LN: lymph node)

Preoperative Breast Imaging

Surgery, either mastectomy or breast conservation surgery (BCS), is the mainstay of breast cancer treatment. Preoperative mammography, sometimes complimented with MRI, is important in patient selection for breast conservation. If mastectomy is planned, the role of mammography is limited to evaluation of the contralateral breast.

Main purpose of mammographic evaluation prior to BCS is to assess the extent and size of the tumor and to exclude multiple cancers. Breast cancers that are >5 cm are generally not treated with BCT. Mammography detects additional cancer in about 10% patients. Multifocal (located in same quadrant or within 4 cm) tumor can be considered for BCT **(Fig. 18)**. However, the extent of surgical resection will be wide and may not achieve the desired cosmesis. Also, women with multiple cancers have propensity to develop more cancers after the surgery resulting in treatment failure.[61] Multicentric (located in different quadrant) cancer is an absolute contraindication for BCT. Presence of suspicious calcification in and around the tumor should be carefully assessed. Clustered calcifications away from the tumor may indicate skip tumor areas. Invasive carcinoma frequently has associated component of DCIS which might extend along the ducts over a large area away from the tumor. This is known as extensive intraductal component (EIC). It is a frequent cause of positive margins in the surgically resected specimen.[62] Presence of linear branching calcifications extending from the primary tumor is a strong indicator of presence of EIC. Indeed, tumor may be more extensive than suspected on mammography. Many DCIS, especially the noncomedo type, are not always calcified and hence, not appreciated on mammography.[63,64] Contralateral breast must also be carefully evaluated on mammography to detect additional cancer, if any.

Preoperative mammographic evaluation is unsatisfactory in women with dense glandular breasts. Breast MRI is superior to mammography for preoperative evaluation of both breasts.[65] Routine preoperative MRI in women already diagnosed with breast cancer detects mammographically occult ipsilateral multicentric cancer in 20% women and contralateral synchronous cancer in 3–5% women **(Fig. 19)**.[66,67] Extent of surgical resection may be increased if multifocal cancer is detected. Similarly, BCS is converted into mastectomy if multicentric cancer is detected on MRI. Women in whom contralateral breast cancer is detected by MRI are also benefited as both cancers can be treated at the same time. Overall, preoperative breast MRI changes surgical management in 13% women; however, it may be due to false-positive MRI finding in half of these.[67] False-positive MRI, which results in unnecessarily more extensive breast surgery or mastectomy, is an important area of concern.[60] MRI is also useful for assessment of pectoralis muscle in patients with deep-seated tumors, as this cannot be evaluated on mammography.[68] Abnormal enhancement of the muscle is a specific indicator of muscle invasion; loss of fat plane is unreliable to diagnose muscle invasion. Breast MRI is the most preferred modality for preoperative breast evaluation, but not yet considered mandatory. Mammography remains the basic requirement of preoperative evaluation of the breasts before BCT.

Breast Conservation Therapy

Breast conservation therapy consists of wide local excision of the tumor with negative margins (BCS), followed by RT of the breast. It retains the affected breast and hence, has a

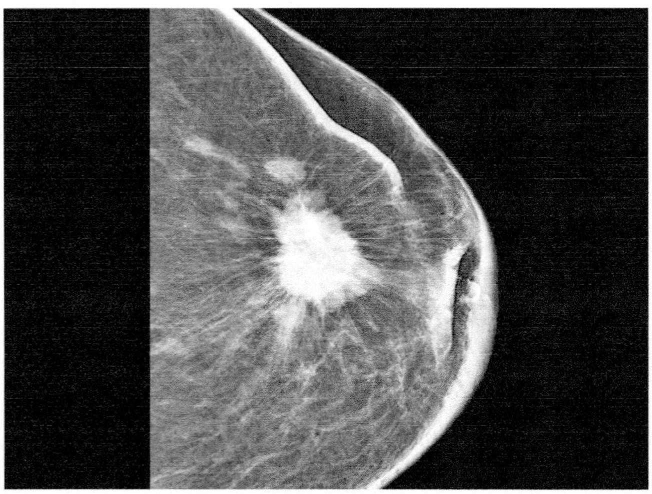

Fig. 18: Multifocal breast cancer. Mammogram shows multiple small ill-defined masses adjacent to an already diagnosed spiculated index tumor.

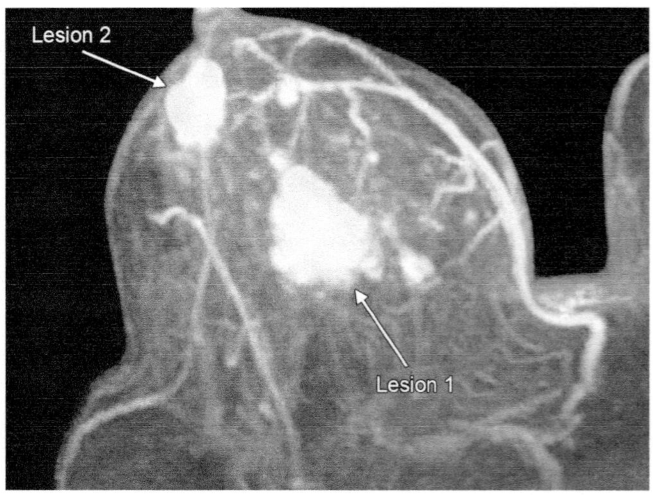

Fig. 19: Multicentric breast cancer. MIP image of a contrast-enhanced MRI shows a subareolar cancer in addition to an already diagnosed index tumor (MIP: maximum-intensity projection; MRI: magnetic resonance imaging)

cosmetic, and psychological advantage over mastectomy. BCT has low recurrence rates and its overall survival rates are comparable with those of mastectomy.[69,70] BCT is the preferred treatment modality for breast cancer in carefully selected patients. It is generally offered for the tumors up to 5 cm in size (T2). Ratio of tumor size and breast size is also considered. Patients with small breasts and large tumor size may be unsuitable, although some use neoadjuvant chemotherapy (NACT) for reduction of tumor size and to make it suitable for BCT. Large or multicentric tumors, pregnancy, and collagen vascular diseases are contraindications for BCT. Finally, patient's preference is also taken into account while selecting BCT or mastectomy.

Mastectomy

Mastectomy is the traditional surgery for breast cancer. It is performed in patients with contraindications for BCS or in those who opt for it. Total mastectomy removes skin, nipple-areola, and fascia anterior to pectoralis major along with the entire breast parenchyma. When combined with simultaneous axillary dissection, it is termed as modified radical mastectomy (MRM). Reconstruction of the breast for cosmetic purpose is also possible after skin sparing mastectomy. It is done in same sitting using myocutaneous flaps with intact vascular pedicle, such as transverse rectus abdominis muscle (TRAM) flap or latissimus dorsi (LD) flap to create a breast mound. Silicone or saline implants are also used for breast reconstruction.

Management of Axilla

Axillary lymph node involvement is the most important prognostic indicator for breast cancer survival. Axillary lymph node dissection is a standard part of surgery, whether BCS or mastectomy, in patients with invasive breast cancer. It is performed in same sitting. It is both therapeutic as well as a staging procedure used to determine pathological N-stage. Axillary lymph nodes are divided into three groups: level, II, and III which are located lateral, posterior, and medial to pectoralis minor muscle, respectively. Level III axillary nodes are also called as infraclavicular nodes. Axillary lymph node dissection, however, is a morbid procedure. It causes disruption of major lymphatic channels and fibrosis, which may be further complicated by axillary irradiation. This leads to various problems such as lymphedema of the arm, sensory loss, and restricted shoulder movements. This may be reported by up to one-third of the patients after axillary dissection and it is difficult to treat.

Sentinel lymph node mapping and biopsy is a technique, which helps to avoid axillary dissection in some of the patients who do not have axillary lymph nodes on clinical examination. In this, a radiotracer (^{99m}Tc labeled sulfur colloid) along with a blue dye is injected in or around the tumor. The lymphatics draining the tumor take up this dye with the radiotracer and course toward axilla. Intraoperatively, the first lymph node (sentinel node) draining the tumor is identified using a hand-held gamma camera sensor. This lymph node is removed and analyzed with frozen sections. If it is free of tumor, it is presumed that axillary nodes are also uninvolved and axillary dissection is avoided. If the sentinel node is involved, axillary dissection is performed to pathologically stage the axilla. False-negative rates of sentinel lymph node biopsy are low and its ability to correctly stage the axilla is comparable with direct axillary dissection.[71]

However, sentinel lymph node biopsy is a time-consuming and expensive procedure. The sentinel lymph node may not be localized in some patients and axillary dissection has to be performed. Allergic reactions to dye may also occur. Preoperative ultrasound evaluation of the axilla in patients selected for sentinel lymph node biopsy is fast gaining acceptance. It helps to avoid sentinel lymph node biopsy in some patients. A detailed description of ultrasound and ultrasound-guided FNAC of axillary lymph nodes is given in Chapter 27.

Perioperative Breast Imaging

If the tumor is nonpalpable, preoperative mammography or ultrasound-guided Hookwire localization is required before the BCS. These procedures are described in detail in Chapter 27. Although uncommonly utilized, intraoperative ultrasound is useful to assess gross tumor margins more accurately. Use of intraoperative ultrasound results in better margins of resection and lowers the chances of residual tumor.[72] Immediate postoperative mammograms may sometimes be requested but these are difficult to perform and interpret. The breast is tender and adequate compression cannot be given to the recently operated breast. The postoperative hematoma and edema also makes the mammographic interpretation difficult and residual mass, if any, cannot be reliably excluded on mammogram. Diagnosis of residual breast cancer after surgery and the decision to re-excise is primarily based on detection of positive tumor margins on postoperative histopathology and not on imaging. However, postoperative MRI after positive margins is desirable, if it was not performed preoperatively. It can identify gross residual tumor or unsuspected multifocal cancer and aid in planning of the extent of re-excision or to consider mastectomy.[73]

Adjuvant Treatment

Adjuvant (postoperative) treatment is given to treat microscopic disease. RT is used for local adjuvant treatment and is aimed at eradicating microscopic residual disease if any, so that chances of local recurrence are reduced. Systemic adjuvant treatment consists of chemotherapy or hormonal therapy, or more commonly, both. It is aimed at eradicating circulating micrometastases, if any, so that chances of distant metastatic recurrence are reduced.[74]

Radiotherapy is given to all patients after BCS. Generally, a total of 45–50 Gy of whole breast RT is given, which may be followed by 10–16 Gy of boost RT to the tumor bed. After mastectomy, RT is given to patients with adverse factors only, such as those with large tumors, close margins, lymphovascular invasion, and axillary lymph node involvement.[57]

Chemotherapy and hormonal therapy is the mainstay of systemic adjuvant treatment of breast cancer. All tumors of >1 cm require adjuvant chemotherapy. Standard anthracycline-based chemotherapy includes combination of 5 fluorouracil (5 FU) and cyclophosphamide along with doxorubicin or epirubicin [5-fluorouracil, adriamycin, cyclophosphamide (FAC)]. Newer regimes also incorporate taxanes.[57] Hormonal therapy with tamoxifen, an estrogen analog, is given for 5 years to all patients with ER-positive breast cancers. It significantly improves the disease-free survival and overall survival in these patients.[74] HER2 overexpression by the breast cancer is associated with high risk of early recurrence and resistance to standard chemotherapy and hormonal therapy. Trastuzumab (Herceptin) is a monoclonal antibody against HER2 protein. It improves survival in HER2 positive patients when given for 1 year, along with or after adjuvant chemotherapy.[60]

ADVANCED BREAST CANCER

Locally Advanced Breast Cancer

This term is used for breast cancers which are inoperable at presentation but without distant metastases **(Fig. 20)**. It includes all T4 tumors (invasion of chest wall, skin, or both), those with fixed axillary lymph nodes, and IBC. Some breast surgeons also include large (>5 cm) but operable tumors in locally advanced breast cancer (LABC). The pretreatment workup includes core biopsy for the diagnosis and receptors status, as well as metastatic workup to exclude distant metastases. These patients are treated with NACT with the intention of downstaging the tumor and making it operable.

Inflammatory Breast Cancer

Inflammatory breast cancer is an aggressive form of invasive duct carcinoma and accounts for 2.5% of all breast cancers.[75] Histopathologically, there is diffuse infiltration and obstruction of dermal lymphatics. It is characterized by younger age, rapid progression, early metastases, and high mortality. Patients present with enlarged painful breast with diffuse erythema, edema, sloughing, and ulceration of the skin over the breast. Clinical presentation mimics acute mastitis and the tumor though sizable, is difficult to palpate.

The diagnosis is usually clinical. Mammography is difficult to perform in a painful breast. Usual mammographic finding is of a dense edematous breast with skin and trabecular thickening **(Figs. 21A and B)**. Hence, primary tumor is uncommonly identified on mammography. Ultrasound is useful and it locates the primary tumor in more than half of patients.[73] It is seen as irregular or lobulated mass on ultrasound, usually large in size. Multicentric and diffusely infiltrating IBC is not localized on ultrasound. MRI and PET-CT are most accurate for evaluation of primary tumor as well as distant metastases.[76] MRI detects primary tumor in nearly all patients with IBC. The primary tumor is most often seen as single or multiple confluent masses with type three enhancement curve and skin involvement in majority of lesions.[77]

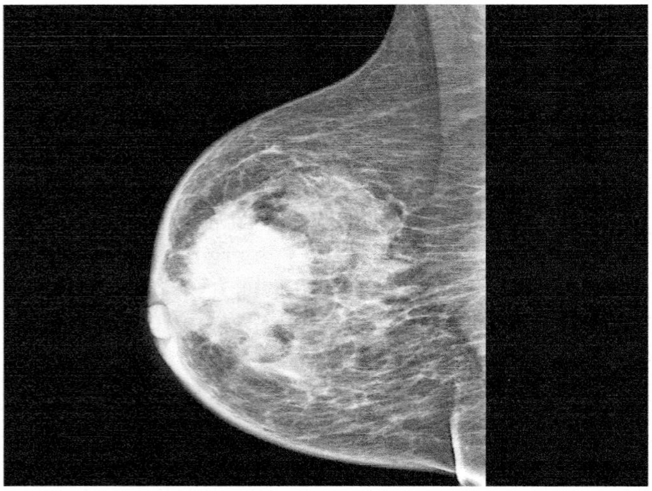

Fig. 20: Locally advanced breast cancer. Mammogram shows a large, infiltrating, spiculated mass with thickening of overlying skin.

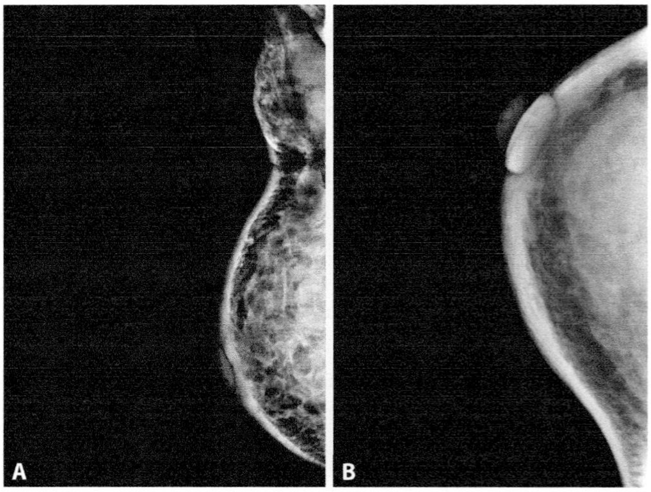

Figs. 21A and B: Inflammatory breast cancer. Mammogram shows diffuse increase in breast density along with thickening of trabeculi and skin. No definite mass is seen.

Neoadjuvant Chemotherapy

Locally advanced breast cancer is the most common indication for NACT. Patients with large but operable tumors who desire for BCT instead of mastectomy are also offered NACT. Traditional anthracycline-based chemotherapy is used. Majority of tumors respond well to chemotherapy and become operable. Mastectomy or BCT is offered after successful NACT, depending on the residual tumor size. About 15–25% patients achieve pathological complete response with NACT.[78]

Response to NACT is assessed with clinical examination and imaging. Mammography, ultrasound, MRI, and PET have been used for response assessment. Prediction of response after initial one or two cycles is important. Good responders can be continued with NACT, while it can be stopped in nonresponders. For this purpose, combination of mammography and ultrasound is more useful than clinical assessment alone.[78] PET-CT is also useful but MRI is most accurate.[79] Response to NACT is depicted by decrease in size and degree of contrast enhancement on MRI and decrease in standard uptake value (SUV) on PET.[80,81] Diffusion-weighted MRI evaluation is also useful to predict the response to NACT. Low-pretreatment apparent diffusion coefficient (ADC) values and high post one cycle ADC values predict good response.[82,83] After completion of NACT, residual tumor size is an important consideration for surgical planning. Both MRI and PET are highly sensitive to identify patients with pathological complete response, however, with moderate specificity.[84] Hence, all patients need to be operated, even if complete resolution of tumor is seen on post-NACT scans. It is prudent to insert a metallic marker clip in these tumors before starting NACT. If the tumor disappears on mammography, the marker clip is used to perform preoperative hook wire localization and surgery.[85]

Metastatic Breast Cancer

Metastatic breast cancer (MBC) is stage IV breast cancer that has spread beyond the breast, regional lymph nodes, and chest wall. Common sites of breast cancer metastases are liver, bone, lung, distant lymph nodes, and brain; however, any organ in the body can be involved. ER/PR positive cancers tend to spread to bones while receptor-negative cancers are more likely to involve the liver. Lobular carcinoma has propensity for serosal deposits involving pleura and peritoneum. Most women with MBC have already diagnosed breast cancer but small proportion of women present with symptoms of metastatic disease and breast cancer is subsequently diagnosed during workup for the occult primary cancer. Symptoms of MBC are nonspecific and include cough or dyspnea, bone pain, lymphadenopathy, or fatigue. Radionuclide bone scan, ultrasound, CT scan, and PET-CT are usually employed for diagnosis and response assessment of breast cancer metastases.

Bone is the most common site of distant metastases from breast cancer.[86] These preferentially involve spine and pelvis but any bone can be involved. Radionuclide bone scan is the primary imaging modality for detection of bone metastases.[87] It is sensitive, however, specificity is moderate. False-positive bone scan results are mainly from degenerative and inflammatory lesions. X-ray or CT-evaluation is required if metastases cannot be differentiated reliably from these on bone scan. On radiographs, bone metastases of breast cancer may be osteolytic, sclerotic, or mixed **(Fig. 22)**. PET is equally sensitive as bone scan but more specific. MRI is the most accurate modality for diagnosis of bone metastases from breast cancer.[88] However, it is not used as a routine investigation. PET-CT and MRI are also useful to monitor treatment response of the bone metastases. Liver metastases are hypovascular and hence, are identified on venous phase of the CT **(Fig. 23)**. Some liver metastases may be small and diffuse giving rise to the appearance of pseudocirrhosis.[89] Ascites and shrinkage of liver outline may also be present with these. Focal fatty infiltration is common in patients on chemotherapy or hormonal therapy. This may also be misinterpreted as metastases on CT. Lack of mass effect and preserved liver architecture is helpful to differentiate these from metastases. MRI is required in equivocal cases. Lung metastases from breast cancer are usually seen as single or multiple nodules. Breast cancer is a common cause of unusual manifestation of lung metastases such as lymphangitis carcinomatosis, airspace consolidation, and endobronchial metastases.[90] Breast cancer is the most common cause of ovarian metastases and its clinicoradiological features are usually similar to that of primary ovarian cancer. Breast cancer

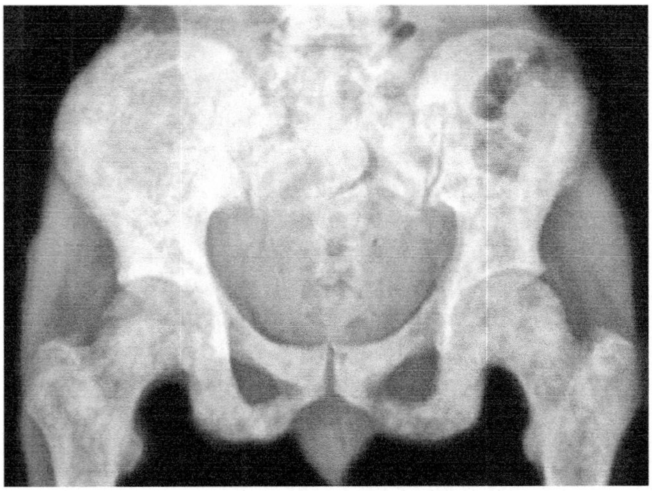

Fig. 22: Bone metastases. Pelvic radiograph shows multiple diffuse lytic and sclerotic metastases in all pelvic bones and both proximal femoral bones.

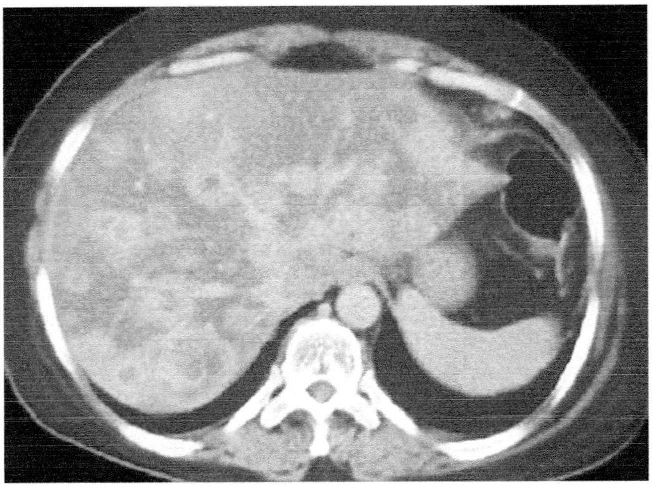

Fig. 23: Liver metastases. Multiple liver metastases are seen. In spite of being hypovascular, they appear hyperdense in the background of fatty infiltration of the liver.

metastases to small bowel produce long segment strictures and those to stomach may produce antral narrowing similar to linitis plastica.

Clinical and imaging diagnosis of metastases is usually unequivocal in majority. In others, biopsy may be required. If not already known, ER, PR, and HER2 status must be determined on biopsy, either from the breast lesion or the metastatic site.

Treatment of MBC is aimed at palliation and prolonging survival. Patients with less extensive metastases, fewer symptoms, and late development of metastases perform better. Chemotherapy is the mainstay of treatment in all MBC. Patients with ER/PR positive MBC are initially treated with hormonal therapy. HER2 positive patients benefit from trastuzumab. Other treatment options include bisphosphonates (pamidronate or zoledronic acid) to patients with bone metastases and RT to brain metastases and painful bone metastases.[60]

Occult Primary Breast Cancer

Mammography is standard part of workup in women presenting with metastatic adenocarcinoma anywhere from an occult primary site. Women presenting with axillary lymphadenopathy only are also evaluated with mammography. If clinical examination and mammography are negative but axillary lymph node biopsy is suspicious of primary breast carcinoma, MRI is recommended. MRI identifies mammographically occult breast cancer in majority of these patients.[91] If primary is not identified, the patients are treated with mastectomy or RT.

POST-TREATMENT BREAST IMAGING AND FOLLOW-UP

Patients treated with BCT need regular bilateral mammographic follow-up. It is primarily required to detect recurrence of cancer in treated or contralateral breast. A baseline mammogram of the treated breast should be obtained at 3–6 months after completion of the RT. This mammogram is compared with future serial mammograms. Patients treated with mastectomy are also followed with annual screening mammograms of the contralateral breast, as they are at high risk for development of second breast cancer. Breast cancer survivors have threefold increased risk of developing contralateral breast cancer. They are also at some risk for endometrial cancer, lung cancer, angiosarcoma, and acute leukemia.[58]

Several postsurgery and RT changes are apparent on follow-up mammogram after the BCT. A *fibrous scar* develops at the operative site, which is seen as an ill-defined density with adjacent architectural distortion **(Figs. 24A and B)**. Metallic surgical clips, intended to mark the tumor bed for boost radiation, may also be seen at the operative site. Sometimes, the fibrous scar has spiculated appearance and appears suspicious **(Figs. 25A and B)**. However, it does not have high-central density as in the case of a true mass. Exact site of the lumpectomy site must be known and review of preoperative mammograms is useful to determine this. Careful evaluation of scar in both craniocaudal (CC) and mediolateral oblique (MLO) views is also helpful. Unlike solid mass, the scar is a 2D structure formed by approximation and fibrosis of the lumpectomy cavity. Hence, size and density of the scar varies considerably in two views. *Seroma* is a fluid collection that is frequently seen at the operative site. It is usually seen as a round or oval mass which may persist for up to 2 years **(Figs. 26A to C)**.[92] It can be reliably characterized on ultrasound. Debris or septations are commonly seen in seroma and this should not lead to ultrasound-guided aspiration.

Radiation changes are seen in the form of diffuse thickening of trabeculi and skin, along with an overall increase in breast density. The changes are similar to breast edema due to any other cause. The severity of these changes varies in different patients; however, these remain stable or decrease on follow-up mammograms. Some distortion of the breast outline is also apparent after BCT and the degree of this depends on the extent of the excision. In addition to above changes, there may be development of benign calcifications in post-treatment mammograms. The causes include fat necrosis, sutural calcifications, and radiation-induced dystrophic calcifications.

Local recurrence at operative site occurs rarely and is seen in 2–7% of women followed for 10 years.[57] Younger age at diagnosis, high grade, and ER/PR negative breast tumors are more prone for local recurrence. Mammography is the primary modality of follow-up and detection of recurrences. However, its accuracy is lowered because of distortion of breast parenchyma by the post-treatment changes. Majority of local recurrences are detected by

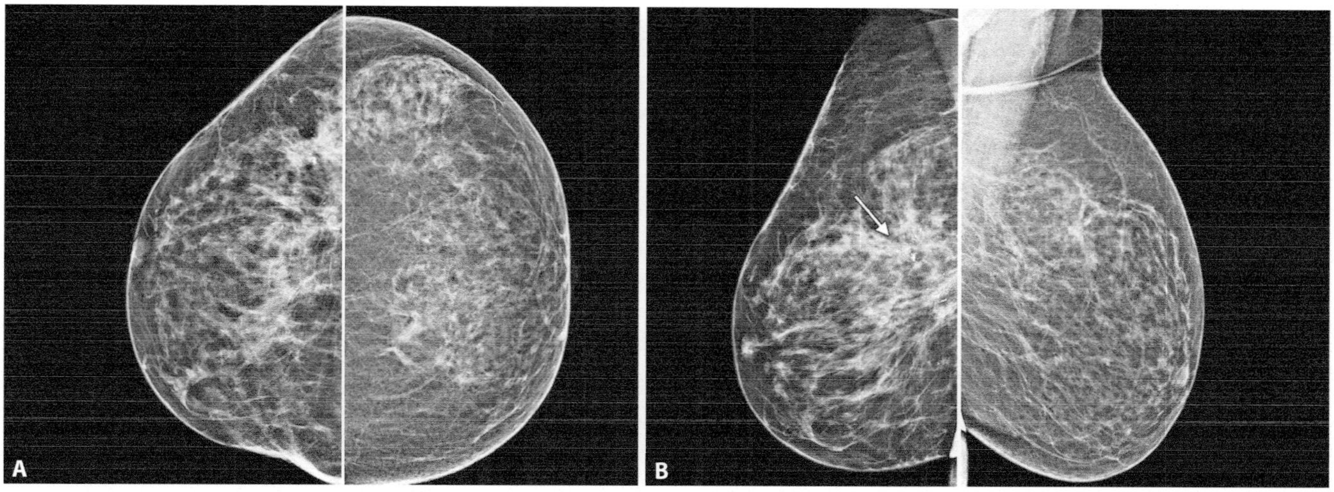

Figs. 24A and B: Post-treatment bilateral mammogram: Right breast shows fibrous scar at the operative site (arrow) with foci of dystrophic calcifications. There is diffuse trabecular thickening and increased density of the left breast, secondary to radiotherapy, as compared to the left breast.

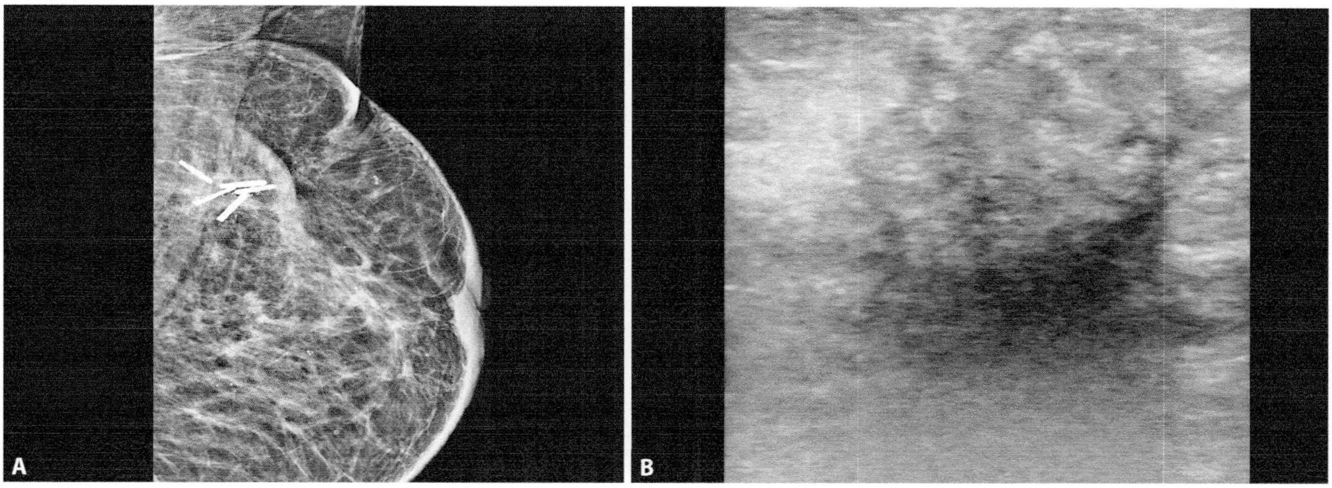

Figs. 25A and B: Postoperative scar. Mammogram shows architectural distortion and ultrasound shows spiculated scar at the operative site. This is an expected finding and does not suggest recurrence.

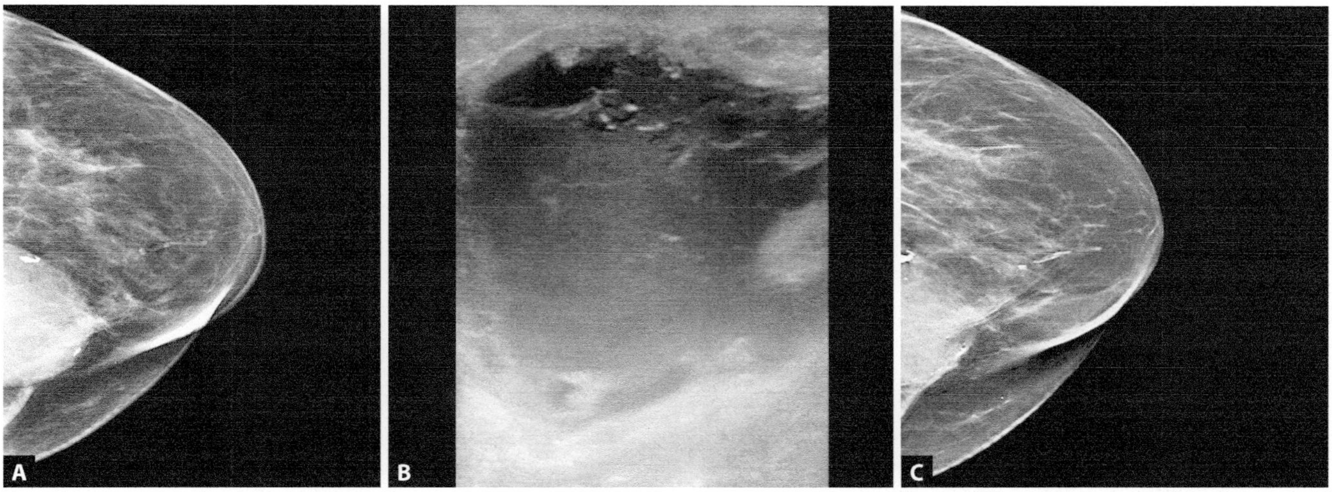

Figs. 26A to C: Seroma: (A) Mammogram shows a circumscribed equal density mass in inner quadrant with peripheral coarse calcification and overlying skin retraction along the surgical site; (B) Ultrasound shows it as a cyst with internal debris. Follow-up mammogram; (C) After 1 year shows reduction in size of the seroma with no upfront intervention.

mammography or by patients themselves on self-breast examination, while few are diagnosed on CBE.[93] The recurrences are most often seen as increased density and/or size of the scar, new mass, or suspicious calcifications on mammography. Their morphology is usually similar to that of the primary breast cancers in these patients and hence, review of the preoperative mammogram is useful for the detection of a recurrence.[94] MRI and percutaneous biopsy should be promptly obtained in case of suspicion of recurrence on mammogram.[95]

MISCELLANEOUS MALIGNANT LESIONS OF THE BREAST

Paget's Disease

In this condition, a centrally located ductal carcinoma grows along the ducts into the nipple with eczematous changes at the summit of the nipple (pagetoid changes). Nipple changes range from mild itching to extensive scaling, erosions, and ulceration in the nipple. Erosion extends to the areola and may cover a larger area of the skin. Fifty percent patients have a palpable mass. This disease is usually unilateral.

On mammography and ultrasound, underlying malignant mass or calcification is seen in most patients **(Figs. 27A and B)**. Nipple and areolar thickening is also present.[96] Malignant type of calcifications may be seen extending from deeper carcinoma to the nipple. MRI is recommended if mammogram is equivocal or normal.

Phyllodes Tumor

Phyllodes tumor (or phylloid tumor) is a stromal tumor composed of the epithelial elements of connective tissue stroma, similar to fibroadenoma. Its malignant potential is variable from completely benign lesion to fully malignant sarcoma. Most are benign. Clinically, they present as round multinodular palpable tumors like fibroadenomas. On mammography and ultrasound, they are well-defined and indistinguishable from fibroadenomas **(Figs. 28A and B)**. Occasionally, cystic component may be seen on ultrasound.[2] Phyllodes tumors are treated with wide local excision. Approximately 20% of these recur, if margins of excision are inadequate.[57] As malignant phyllodes tumor is a sarcoma, axillary lymphadenopathy is less common and lung metastases are more common.

Sarcoma

Sarcomas are rare tumors of breast. These include phyllodes tumor, angiosarcoma, fibrosarcoma, liposarcoma, malignant fibrous histiocytoma, and osteosarcoma. Their imaging features are nonspecific. Angiosarcoma is an aggressive, rapidly growing vascular tumor of young age. Presentation is similar to IBC. MRI shows a strongly enhancing, ill-defined, infiltrative mass with skin invasion. It metastasizes early and is rapidly fatal.

Metastases to Breast

Metastases to breast from other sites are rare. Usual primary sites of cancer are melanoma, lung, stomach, cervix, and ovary. Clinically, there are multiple palpable masses. In one-third of these patients, this may be the first manifestation of an occult primary cancer.[57] Another form of metastasis to breast is cross-lymphatic spread from the contralateral advanced breast cancer causing localized thickening of the skin.

On mammography, metastases to breast are usually multiple and bilateral **(Figs. 29A and B)**. These are seen as well-defined or ill-defined masses. Spiculations and calcifications are not commonly seen.

Although rare, *lymphoma* can secondarily involve the breasts. Large axillary lymph nodes are usually associated. Mammographically, single or multiple ill-defined masses

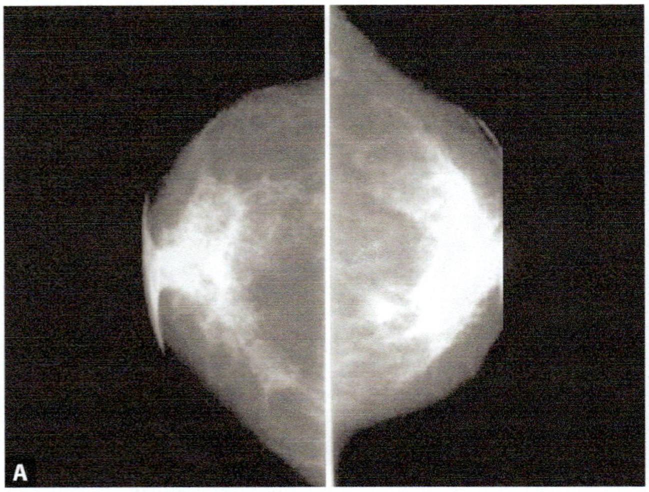

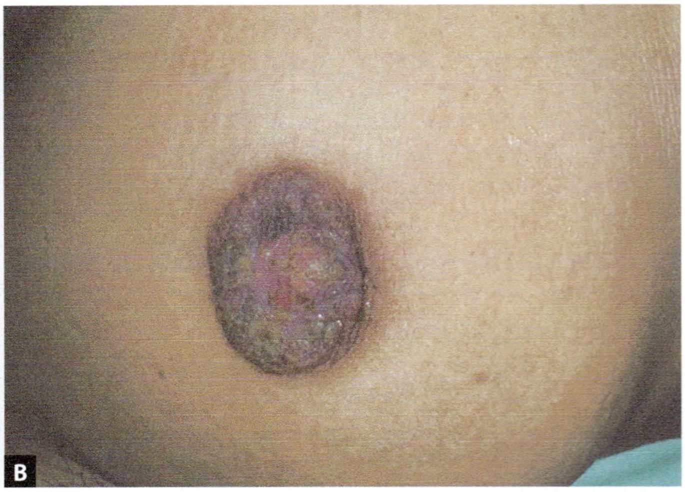

Figs. 27A and B: Paget's disease. Mammography shows nipple and areolar thickening in right breast with a subareolar mass. The NAC thickening corroborates with clinical picture of the patient. (NAC: nipple-areolar complex)

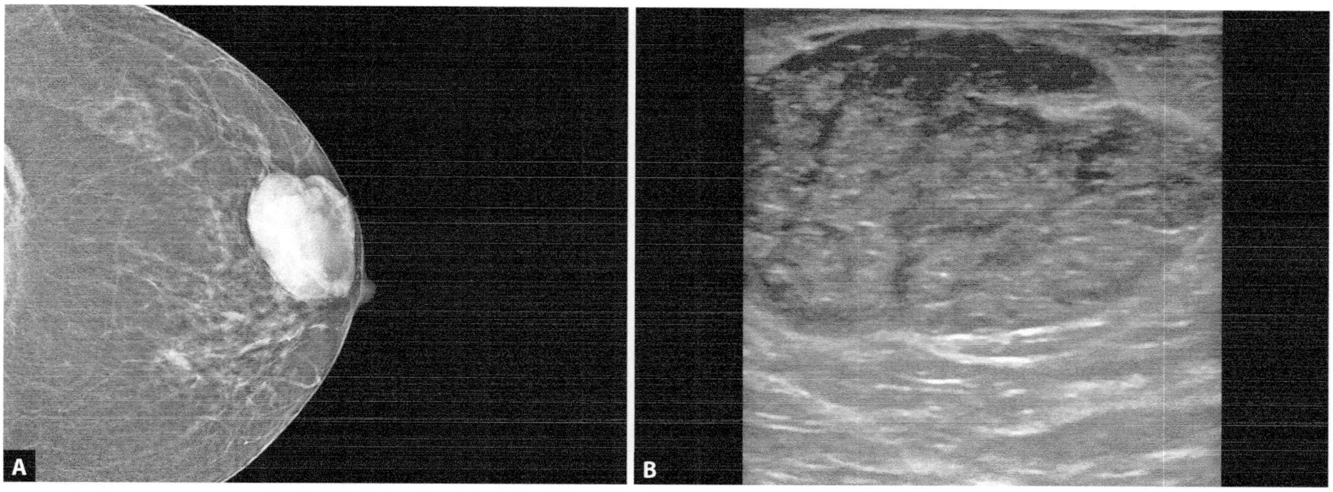

Figs. 28A and B: Phyllodes tumor: (A) Mammogram shows a dense breast with an irregular large mass in the anterior third of the breast; (B) Ultrasound shows a large hypoechoic mass with fluid clefts within.

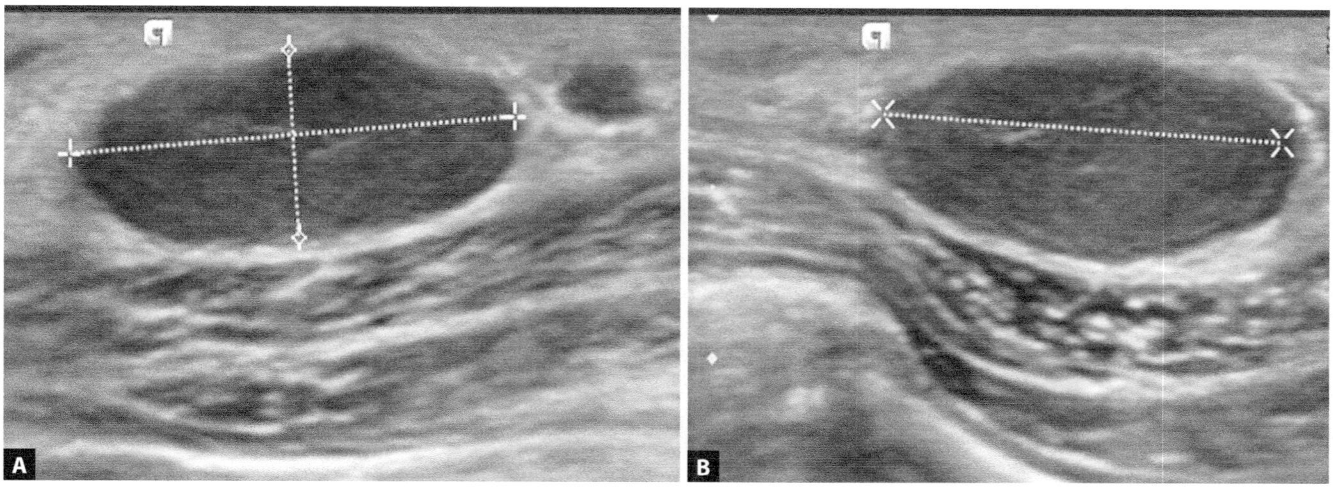

Figs. 29A and B: Metastases. Mammogram shows multiple variable-sized metastatic masses in the breast from Ewing's sarcoma (FNAC proven mets). (FNAC: fine needle aspiration cytology)

are seen. Spiculations and calcification are not seen. Lymphomatous lesion may also be seen as increased asymmetric density in the breast. Ultrasound shows single or multiple nonspecific solid masses.[97]

Male Breast Cancer

Male breast cancer accounts for about 1% of all breast cancers. Breast cancer in male patients occurs at an older age group than in female patients. Risk factors include Klinefelter's syndrome, BRCA mutation carriers, undescended testis, chronic liver disease, and alcoholism.[57] Gynecomastia is not a risk factor. Clinically, there is a painless hard mass. Nipple discharge or ulceration is seen in 25% cases. Mammographic features of male breast cancer are similar to those in females **(Figs. 30A and B)**.[98] Pathology and treatment of male breast cancer is also same. Due to small size of the breast, BCT is not performed.

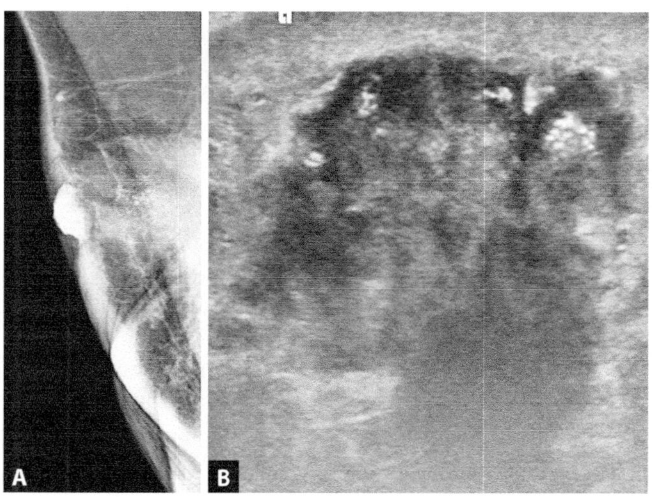

Figs. 30A and B: Male breast cancer: (A) Mammogram shows irregular retroareolar mass with pleomorphic calcification within; (B) Ultrasound confirms presence of an irregular hypoechoic mass with angular margins and internal microcalcifications.

REFERENCES

1. Kopans DB. Histologic, pathologic and imaging correlation. In: Kopans DB (Ed). Breast Imaging, 3rd edition. Philadelphia: Lippincott, Williams and Wilkins; 2007. pp. 783-888.
2. Goel NB, Knight TE, Pandey S, Riddick-Young M, de Paredes ES, Trivedi A. Fibrous lesions of the breast: imaging-pathologic correlation. Radiographics. 2005;25:1547-59.
3. Elseedawy M, Whelehan P, Vinnicombe S, Thomson K, Evans A. Factors influencing the stiffness of fibroadenomas at shear wave elastography. Clin Radiol. 2016;71(1):92-5.
4. Liberman L, Morris E, Lee MJ, Kaplan JB, LaTrenta LR, Menell JH, et al. Breast lesions detected on MR imaging: Features positive predictive value. AJR. 2002;179:171-8.
5. Venta LA, Kim JP, Pelloski CE, Morrow M. Management of complex breast cysts. AJR. 1999;173:1331-6.
6. Berg WA, Sechtin AG, Marques H, Zhang Z. Cystic breast masses and ACRIN 6666 experience. Radiol Clin N Am. 2010;48:931-87.
7. Lau S, Kuchenmeister I, Stachs A, Gerber B, Krause A, Reimer T. Pathologic nipple discharge: Surgery is imperative in post menopausal women. Ann Surg Oncol. 2005;12:546-51.
8. Orel SG, Dougherty CS, Reynolds C, Czerniecki BJ, Siegelman ES, Schnall MD. MR imaging in patients with nipple discharge: Initial experience. Radiology. 2000;216:248-54.
9. Neal L, Tortorelli CL, Nasser A. Clinicians guide to imaging and pathologic findings in benign breast disease. Mayo Clin Proc. 2010;85:274-9.
10. Phantana-Angkool A, Forster MR, Warren YE, Livasy CA, Sobel AH, Beasley LM, et al. Rate of radial scars by core biopsy and upgrading to malignancy or high-risk lesions before and after introduction of digital breast tomosynthesis. Breast Cancer Res Treat. 2019;173(1):23-9.
11. Alshafeiy TI, Nguyen JV, Rochman CM, Nicholson BT, Patrie JT, Harvey JA. Outcome of architectural distortion detected only at breast tomosynthesis versus 2D mammography. Radiology. 2018;288(1):38-46.
12. Wong KT, Tse GM, YangWT. Ultrasound and MR imaging of diabetic mastopathy. Clin Radiol. 2002;57:730-5.
13. Hook GW, Ikeda DM. Treatment of breast abscess with US guided percutaneous needle drainage without indwelling catheter placement. Radiology. 1999;213:579-82.
14. Memis A, Bilgen I, Ustun EE, Ozdemir N, Erhan Y, Kapkac M. Granulomatous mastitis: Imaging features with histopatholgical correlation. Clin Radiol. 2001;57:1001-6.
15. Sabate JM, Clotet M, Gomez A, Heras PD. Radiologic evaluation of uncommon and reactive breast disorders. Radiographics. 2005;24:411-24.
16. Sakr AA, Fawzy RK, Fadaly G, Baky MA. Mammographic and sonographic features of tuberculous mastitis. Eur J Radiol. 2004;51:54-60.
17. Herborn CU, Marincek B, Erfmann D, Meuli-Simmen C, Wedler V, Bode-Lesniewska B, et al. Breast augmentation and reconstructive surgery: MR imaging of implant rupture and malignancy. Eur Radiol. 2002;12:2198-206.
18. Debruhl ND, Gorczyca DP, Ahn CY, Shaw WW, Bassett P. Silicone breast implants: US evaluation. Radiology. 1993;189:95-8.
19. Caskey CI, Berg WA, Hamper UM, Sheth S, Chang BW, Anderson ND. Imaging spectrum of extracapsular silicone: Correlation of US, MR imaging, mammographic and histopathologic findings. Radiographics. 1999;19:S39-51.
20. Breast cancer statistics. (2018). World Cancer Research Fund. [online] Available from https://www.wcrf.org/dietandcancer/cancer-trends/breast-cancer-statistic [Last accessed March 2020].
21. Ghoncheh M, Pournamdar Z, Salehiniya H. Incidence and mortality and epidemiology of breast cancer in the world. Asian Pac J Cancer Prev. 2016;17(S3):43-6.
22. Malvia S, Bagadi SA, Dubey US, Saxena S. Epidemiology of breast cancer in Indian women. Asia Pac J Clin Oncol. 2017;13(4):289-95.
23. Boyd NF, Guo H, Martin LJ, Sun L, Stone J, Fishell E, et al. Mammographic density and the risk and detection of breast cancer. N Engl J Med. 2007;356:227.
24. Brose MS, Rebbeck TR, Catzone KA, Stopfer JE, Nathanson KL, Weber BL. Cancer risk estimates for BRCA1 mutation carriers identified in a risk evaluation program. J Natl Cancer Inst. 2002;94:1365.
25. Perou CM, Sorlie T, Eisen MB, van de Rijn M, Jeffrey SS, Rees CA, et al. Molecular portraits of human breast tumours. Nature. 2000;406:747-52.
26. Kopans DB. Screening mammography. In: Kopans DB (Ed). Breast Imaging, 3rd edition. Philadelphia, PA: Lippincott, Williams and Wilkins; 2007. pp. 121-90.
27. Tabar I, Vitak B, Chen HH, Yen MF, Duffy SW, Smith RA. Beyond randomized controlled trials: Organized mammographic screening substantially reduces breast cancer mortality. Cancer. 2001;91:1724-31.
28. Nelson HD, Tyne K, Naik A, Bougatsos C, Chan BK, Humphrey L. Screening for breast cancer: An update for the US Preventive Services Task Force. Ann Intern Med. 2009;151:727-42.
29. Tabar L, Vitak B, Chen THH, Yen AM, Cohen A, Tot T, et al. Swedish two county trial: Impact of mammographic screening on breast cancer mortality during 3 decades. Radiology. 2010;260:658-63.
30. Paci E, Duffy SW, Giorgi D, Crocetti E, Vezossi V, Bianchi S, et al. Quantification of the effect of mammographic screening on fatal breast cancers: The Florence programme 1990-96. Br J Cancer. 2002;87:65-9.
31. Elmore JG, Armstrong K, Lehman CD, Fletcher SW. Screening for breast cancer. JAMA. 2005;293:1245-56.
32. Elmore JG, Barton MB, Moceri VM, Polk S, Arena PJ, Fletcher SW. Ten year risk of false positive screening mammograms and clinical breast examinations. N Engl J Med. 1998;338:1089.
33. Schopper D, de Wolf C. How effective are breast cancer screening programs by mammography? Review of current evidence. Eur J Cancer. 2009;45:1916-23.
34. Gotzsche PC, Olsen O. Is screening for breast cancer with mammography justifiable? Lancet. 2000;355:129-34.
35. Bock K, Borisch B, Cawson J, Damtjernhaug B, de Wolf C, Dean P, et al. Effect of population based screening on breast cancer mortality. Lancet. 2011;378:1775-6.
36. US Preventive Services Task Force. Screening for breast cancer: US preventive services task force recommendation statement. Ann Intern Med. 2009;151:716-26.

37. ACOG. Breast cancer risk assessment and screening in average-risk women. [online] Available from https://www.acog.org/Clinical-Guidance-and-Publications/Practice-Bulletins/Committee-on-Practice-Bulletins-Gynecology/Breast-Cancer-Risk-Assessment-and-Screening-in-Average-Risk-Women?IsMobileSet=false [Last accessed March 2020].
38. Seely JM, Alhassan T. Screening for breast cancer in 2018—what should we be doing today? Curr Oncol. 2018; 25(Suppl 1):S115-24.
39. Breast Cancer Screening Guidelines for Women. [online] Available from https://www.cdc.gov/cancer/breast/pdf/breastcancerscreeningguidelines.pdf [Last accessed March 2020].
40. Ernster VL, Ballard BR, Barlow WE, Zheng Y, Weaver DL, Cutter G, et al. Detection of ductal carcinoma in situ in women undergoing screening mammography. J Natl Cancer Inst. 2002;94:1546-54.
41. Bordas P, Jonsson H, Nystom L, Lenner P. Interval cancer incidence and episode sensitivity in Norrbotten mammography screening programme. Sweden J Med Screen. 2009;16:39.
42. Kalager M, Zelen M, Langmark F, Zheng Y, Weaver DL, Cutter G, et al. Effect of screening mammography on breast cancer mortality in Norway. N Engl J Med. 2010;163:1203-10.
43. Warner E, Plewes DB, Hill KA, Causer PA, Zubovits JT, Jong RA, et al. Surveillance of BRCA1and BRCA2 mutation carriers with magnetic resonance imaging, ultrasound, mammography and clinical breast examination. JAMA. 2004;292:1317-25.
44. Gilbert FJ, Warren RM, Kwan-Lin G, Thompson DJ, Eeles RA, Evans DG, et al. Cancers in BRCA1 and BRCA2 carriers and in women with high risk for breast cancer: MR imaging and mammographic features. Radiology. 2009;254:358-68.
45. Saslow D, Boetes C, Burke W, Harms S, Leach MO, Lehman CD, et al. American Cancer Society guidelines for breast screening with MRI as an adjunct to mammography. CA Cancer J Clin. 2007;57:75-89.
46. Corsetti V, Houssami N, Ferrari A, Ghirardi M, Bellarosa S, Angelini O, et al. Breast screening with ultrasound in women with mammography negative dense breasts: Evidence on incremental cancer detection, false positives and associated cost. Eur J Cancer. 2004;4:539-44.
47. Nothaker M, Duda V, Hahn M, Warm M, Degenhardt F, Madjar H, et al. Early detection of breast cancer: Benefits and risks of supplemental breast ultrasound in asymptomatic women with mammographically dense breasts. A systematic review. BMC Cancer. 2009;9:335.
48. Berg WA, Blume JD, Cormac JB, Mendelson EB, Lehrer D, Böhm-Vélez M, et al. Combined screening with ultrasound and mammography vs mammography only in women at elevated risk of breast cancer. JAMA. 2008;299:2151-63.
49. Thomas DB, Gao DL, Ray RM, Wang WW, Allison CJ, Chen FL, et al. Randomized trial of breast self examination in Shanghai: Final results. J Natl Cancer Inst. 2002;94:1445-57.
50. Anderson BO, Shyyan R, Eniu A, Smith RA, Yip CH, Bese NS, et al. Breast cancer in limited resources countries: An overview of the Breast Health Global Initiative 2005 guidelines. Breast J. 2006;12:S3-15.
51. Kuhl CK, Shrading S, Bieling HB, Wardelmann E, Leutner CC, Koenig R, et al. MRI for diagnosis of pure ductal carcinoma *in situ*: A prospective observational study. Lancet. 2007;370:485-92.
52. Morris EA. Breast cancer imaging with MRI. RCNA. 2002;40:443-86.
53. Stalsberg H, Thomas DB. Age distribution of histologic types of breast cancer. Int J Cancer. 1993;54:1-7.
54. Weinstein SP, Orel SG, Heller R, Reynolds C, Czerniecki B, Solin LJ, et al. MR imaging of the breast in patients with invasive lobular carcinoma. AJR. 2001;176:399-406.
55. Yeh ED, Slanetz PJ, Edmister WB, Talele A, Monticciolo D, Kopans DB. Invasive lobular carcinoma: Spectrum of enhancement and morphology on magnetic resonance imaging. Breast J. 2003;9:13-8.
56. Liberman L, Morris EA, Dershaw DD, Abramson AF, Tan LK. MR imaging of ipsilateral breast in women with percutaneously proved breast cancer. AJR. 2003;180:901-10.
57. Lam WW, Chu WC, Tse GM, Ma TK. Sonographic appearance of mucinous carcinoma of the breast. AJR. 2004;182:1069-74.
58. Yang WT, Dryden M, Broglio K, Gilcrease M, Dawood S, Dempsey PJ, et al. Mammographic features of triple negative primary breast cancers in young premenopausal women. Breast Cancer Res Treat. 2008;111:405-10.
59. Dogan BE, Gonzalez-Angulo AM, Gilcreae M, Dryden MJ, Yang WT. Multimodality imaging of triple negative breast tumours with mammography, ultrasound and MRI. AJR. 2010;194:1160-6.
60. Burstein HJ, Harris JR, Morrow M. Malignant tumours of the breast. In: DeVita VT, Lawrence TS, Rosenberg SA (Eds). Cancer: Principles and Practice of Oncology, 9th edition. Philadelphia: Wolter Kluwer, Lippincott, Williams and Wilkins; 2011. pp. 1401-46.
61. Kutz JM, Jacquemier J, Amalric R, Brandone H, Ayme Y, Hans D, et al. Breast conserving therapy for macroscopically multiple cancers. Ann Surg. 1991;212:38-44.
62. Kurniawan ED, Wong MH, Windle I, Rose A, Mou A, Buchanan M, et al. Predictors of surgical margin status in breast conserving surgery within a breast screening program. Ann Surg Oncol. 2008;15(9):2542-9.
63. Holland R, Hendricks J, Verbee K, Mravunac M, Schuurmans Stekhoven JH. Extent, distribution and mammographic/histologic correlations of breast ductal carcinoma *in situ*. Lancet.1990;335:519-22.
64. Umetsu T, Yuen S, Kasami M, Uchida Y. Comparison of magnetic resonance imaging, multidetector row computed tomography, ultrasonography and mammography for tumour extension of breast cancer. Breast Cancer Res Treat. 2008;112:461-74.
65. Berg WA, Gutlerrez L, NessAlver MS, Carter WB, Bhargavan M, Lewis RS, et al. Diagnostic accuracy of mammography, clinical examination, US, and MR imaging in preoperative assessment of breast cancer. Radiology. 2004;233:830-49.
66. Lehman CD, Gatsonis C, Kuhl CK, Hendrick RE, Pisano ED, Hanna L, et al. MRI evaluation of contralateral breast in women with recently diagnosed breast cancer. N Engl J Med. 2007;356:1295-303.
67. Plana MN, Carreira C, Muriel A, Chiva M, Abraira V, Emparanza JI, et al. Magnetic resonance imaging in preoperative assessment of patients with primary breast cancer: Systematic review of diagnostic accuracy and meta-analysis. Eur Radiol. 2012;22:26-38.

68. Morris EA, Schwartz LH, Drotman MB, Kim SJ, Tan LK, Liberman L, et al. Evaluation of pectoralis major muscle in patients with posterior breast tumours on breast MR images: Early experience. Radiology. 2000;214:67-72.
69. Veronesi U, Cascinelli N, Mariani L, Greco M, Saccozzi R, Luini A, et al. Twenty year follow up of a randomized study comparing breast conserving surgery with radical mastectomy for early breast cancer. N Engl J Med. 2002;347:1227-32.
70. Fisher B, Anderson S, Bryant J, Margolese RG, Deutsch M, Fisher ER, et al. Twenty year follow up of a randomized trial comparing total mastectomy, lumpectomy, and lumpectomy plus irradiation for the treatment of invasive breast cancer. N Engl J Med. 2002;347:1233-7.
71. Mansel RE, Fellowfield L, Kissin M, Goyal A, Newcombe RG, Dixon JM, et al. Randomized multicenter trial of sentinel node biopsy versus standard axillary treatment in operable breast cancer: The ALMANC trial. J Natl Cancer Inst. 2006;98:599.
72. Moore MM, Whitney LA, Cerilli I, Imbrie JZ, Bunch M, Simpson VB, et al. Intraoperative ultrasound is associated with clear lumpectomy margins for palpable infiltrating ductal breast cancer. Ann Surg. 2001;233:761-8.
73. Lee JM, Orel SG, Czerniecki BJ, Solin LJ, Schnall MD. MRI before re-excision surgery in patients with breast cancer. AJR. 2004;182:473-80.
74. Early Breast Cancer Trialist Group. Effects of chemotherapy and hormonal therapy for early breast cancer on recurrence and 15-year survival: An overview of the randomized trials. Lancet. 2005;365:1687.
75. Le-Petraus H, Uppendahl L, Stafford J. Sonographic features of inflammatory breast cancer. Semin Roentgenol. 2011;46:275-9.
76. Le-Petross H, Cristofanilli M, Carkaci S, Krishnamurthy S, Jackson EF, Harrell RK, et al. MRI features of inflammatory breast cancer. AJR. 2011;197:W769-6.
77. Robertson FM, Bondy M, Yang W, Yamauchi H, Wiggins S, Kamrudin S, et al. Inflammatory breast cancer: The disease, the biology, the treatment. CA Cancer J Clin. 2010;60:351-75.
78. Peintinger F, Kuerer HM, Anderson K, Boughey JC, Meric-Bernstam F, Singletary SE, et al. Combination of mammography and sonography is useful in predicting tumor response in breast cancer patients after neoadjuvant chemotherapy. Ann Surg Oncol. 2006;13:1443-9.
79. Choi JH, Lim HI, Lee SK, Kim WW, Kim SM, Cho E, et al. The role of PET CT to evaluate the response to neoadjuvant chemotherapy in advanced breast cancer: Comparison with ultrasonography and magnetic resonance imaging. J Surg Oncol. 2009;4:1-6.
80. Yeh E, Slanetz P, Kopans DB, Rafferty E, Georgian-Smith D, Moy L, et al. Prospective comparison of mammography, sonography and MRI in patients undergoing neoadjuvant chemotherapy for palpable breast cancer. AJR. 2006;184:868-77.
81. Wang Y, Zhang C, Liu J, Huang G. Is ^{18}F-FDG PET accurate to predict neoadjuvant therapy response in breast cancer? A meta-analysis. Breast Cancer Res Treat. 2012;131:357-69.
82. Park SH, Moon WK, Cho N, Song IC, Chang JM, Park IA, et al. Diffusion weighted MRI imaging: Pretreatment prediction of response to neoadjuvant chemotherapy in patients with breast cancer. Radiology. 2010;257:56-63.
83. Fangberget A, Nilsen LB, Hole KH, Holmen MM, Engebraaten O, Naume B, et al. Neoadjuvant chemotherapy in breast cancer response evaluation and prediction of response to treatment using dynamic contrast enhanced and diffusion weighted MRI imaging. Eur Radiol. 2011;21:1188-99.
84. Park SH, Moon WK, Cho N, Chang JM, Im SA, Park IA, et al. Comparison of diffusion weighted MR imaging and FDG PET/CT to predict pathological complete response to neoadjuvant chemotherapy in patients with breast cancer. Eur Radiol. 2012;22:18-25.
85. Nadeem R, Chagla LS, Harris O, Desmond S, Thind R, Flavin A, et al. Tumour localization with a metal coil before administration of neoadjuvant chemotherapy. Breast. 2005;14:403-7.
86. Hamaoka T, Madewell JE, Podoloff DA, Hortobagyi GN, Ueno NT. Bone imaging in metastatic breast cancer. J Clin Oncol. 2004;22:2942-53.
87. Costelloe CM, Rohren EM, Madewell JE, Hamaoka T, Theriault RL, Yu TK, et al. Imaging bone metastases in breast cancer: Techniques and recommendations for diagnosis. Lancet Oncol. 2009;10:606-14.
88. Liu T, Cheng T, Xu W, Yan WL, Liu J, Yang HL. A meta-analysis of ^{18}FDG-PET, MRI and bone scintigraphy for diagnosis of bone metastases in patients with breast cancer. Skeletal Radiol. 2011;40:523-32.
89. Brookes M, MacVicar D, Husband J. Metastatic carcinoma of the breast: The appearances of metastatic spread to abdomen and pelvis as demonstrated by CT. Br J Radiol. 2007;80:284-92.
90. Jung JM, Kim HH, Park SH, Song SW, Chung MH, Kim HS, et al. Thoracic manifestations of breast cancer and its therapy. Radiographics. 2004;24:1269-85.
91. Olson JA Jr, Morris EA, Van Zee KA, Linehan DC, Borgen PI. Magnetic resonance imaging facilitates breast conservation for occult breast cancer. Ann Surg Oncol. 2000;7:411-5.
92. Brenner RJ, Pfaff JM. Mammographic features after conservation therapy for malignant breast disease: Serial findings standardized by regression analysis. AJR. 1996;167:171-8.
93. Montgomery DA, Krupa K, Cooke TG. Follow-up in breast cancer: Does routine clinical examination improve outcome? A systematic review of literature. Br J Cancer. 2007;97:1632-41.
94. Gunhan-Bilgen I, Oktay A. Mammographic features of local recurrence after conserving surgery and radiation therapy: Comparison with that of the primary tumour. Acta Radiologica. 2007;48:390-7.
95. Dao TH, Rahmount A, Campana F, Laurent M, Asselain B, Fourquet A. Tumour recurrence versus fibrosis in the irradiated breast: Differentiation with dynamic gadolinium contrast enhanced MR imaging. Radiology. 1993;187:751-5.
96. Gunhan-Bilgen I, Oktay A. Paget's disease of breast. Clinical, mammographic, sonographic and pathologic findings in 52 cases. Eur J Radiol. 2006;60:256-63.
97. Yang WT, Lane DL, Le-Petross HT, Abruzzo LV, Macapinlac HA. Breast lymphoma: Imaging findings in 32 tumours. Radiology. 2007;245:692-702.
98. Dershaw DD, Borgen PI, Deutch BM, Liberman L. Mammographic findings in men with breast cancer. AJR. 1993;160:267-70.

CHAPTER

27

Breast Interventions

Surabhi Vyas, Smriti Hari, Smita Manchanda

INTRODUCTION

Breast interventions primarily comprise of biopsy of suspicious breast lesions to obtain accurate pathological diagnosis. Breast biopsy is the mainstay of definitive and timely diagnosis of breast cancer and its treatment. Preoperative wire localization has both diagnostic and therapeutic applications. Ablative procedures for breast cancer treatment are still considered investigational.

BREAST BIOPSY

Mammography and other breast imaging modalities can detect nonpalpable breast abnormalities which may represent breast cancer and hence imaging-guided procedure for their sampling is mandatory for timely diagnosis of the breast cancer. The techniques and instrumentation of these procedures have evolved over years with improvement in accuracy of the diagnosis. Although palpable lesions can be sampled without image guidance, the sampling accuracy improves when the procedure is conducted under image guidance. For non-palpable lesions, imaging guidance is mandatory.[1] Special skills beyond those acquired in general radiology are required for radiologist who performs these procedures. As several of these techniques involve special equipment, assistance of an experienced technologist is desirable. The radiologist must have the basic knowledge of diagnostic breast imaging, limitations of imaging, cancer risks and treatment options for breast cancer so as to select appropriate lesion and the biopsy technique. This knowledge is also required for meaningful discussion with the patient, referring clinician and the pathologist. After the biopsy, follow-up of patient to diagnose and treat any complications is mandatory. Pathology results of the biopsy must also be correlated with baseline imaging findings to ensure that these are concordant with imaging.

BREAST BIOPSY TECHNIQUES

Surgical Biopsy

Surgical excision biopsy is the most accurate technique for the diagnosis of breast cancer as it completely removes the abnormality and hence there is no chance of sampling error. For nonpalpable lesions, this is performed after preoperative hookwire localization, so as to guide the surgeon to the exact location of the lesion. Surgical excision biopsy is the gold standard of breast cancer diagnosis and it is still routinely performed at few centers. However, the procedure is invasive and disfiguring. This disadvantage is especially important considering the fact that majority of breast biopsy results are benign and resultant scar and disfigurement of breast may be unacceptable to these patients. Even in patients with malignant diagnosis, this leads to two surgical procedures, one diagnostic and then another for treatment, leading to increased patient anxiety and cost of the treatment.

Percutaneous needle biopsy expedites the breast cancer diagnosis and is cost-effective. With modern biopsy techniques and instrumentations, the diagnostic accuracy is also nearly comparable to that of surgical excision biopsy. Percutaneous biopsy can be a fine needle aspiration cytology (FNAC) or core biopsy.

Fine Needle Aspiration Cytology

Fine needle aspiration cytology is a simple, less expensive and less traumatic technique. Generally, a 20-gauge (20G) to 22G needle is used to make multiple excursions in the lesion and fluid-containing dislodged cells is aspirated to make smears for cytological diagnosis. Results of FNAC are immediately available. However, FNAC has several limitations. It requires the availability of an experienced breast cytologist who can establish the adequacy of aspirated sample on site and also interpret it accurately. It has high insufficiency and false-negative rates. A negative FNAC cannot reliably exclude the presence of breast cancer. FNAC is especially unsuitable for nonpalpable breast lesions as up to 34% of FNAC samples may be insufficient for diagnosis.[2] Insufficiency rate is much higher for calcifications than for masses. FNAC gives cytological diagnosis only, i.e., it cannot differentiate in situ from invasive cancer. Modern treatment protocols often require immunohistochemical analysis for hormonal receptor status and this is difficult to obtain on FNAC. Benign FNAC results are often nonspecific and definitive diagnosis of a benign condition is rarely made. This affects the radiologic-pathologic correlation and may be a limitation in deciding further management. Diagnosis of papillary lesions is inaccurate on FNAC and it cannot differentiate fibroadenoma from phyllodes tumor.[3] FNAC results are frequently interpreted as atypical or suspicious only, which leads to a second more invasive biopsy. This leads to increased cost and delay in the diagnosis of breast cancer.[4] Although extremely rare, false-positive results on FNAC leading to an unnecessary surgery are also known. Because of these disadvantages, breast FNAC is less commonly employed at present and most breast care centers do not rely on breast FNAC to make the management decisions.

Core Needle Biopsy

Several of the disadvantages of FNAC have been addressed by percutaneous core needle biopsy (CNB) of the breast and this has become the standard of care for biopsy of breast lesions; whether palpable or not. Accuracy of CNB is better than FNAC and it allows cellular and architectural evaluation. With this, specific diagnosis of benign and malignant conditions can be made. The cores are also suitable for immunohistochemical and genetic analysis. However, CNB of breast is more traumatic, more expensive and requires higher skills to perform when compared with FNAC. Results of CNB are not immediately available and take few days at least.

Breast CNB is commonly performed using spring-loaded automated core biopsy needles, commonly known as biopsy guns. Earlier smaller gauge (16G or 18G) biopsy needles were used, but these suffered from lower sample sufficiency rates. Introduction of 14G core needles significantly improved the accuracy of breast CNB[5] **(Figs. 1A and B)**. False-negative rates of 14G CNB range from 0 to 9%.[6] Long throw (2 cm), 14G caliber is the standard size of biopsy guns used for breast CNB and smaller gauge biopsy guns which are routinely used in other body parts are not recommended for breast CNB. Typically, a minimum of 4–5 cores are obtained during a breast CNB.

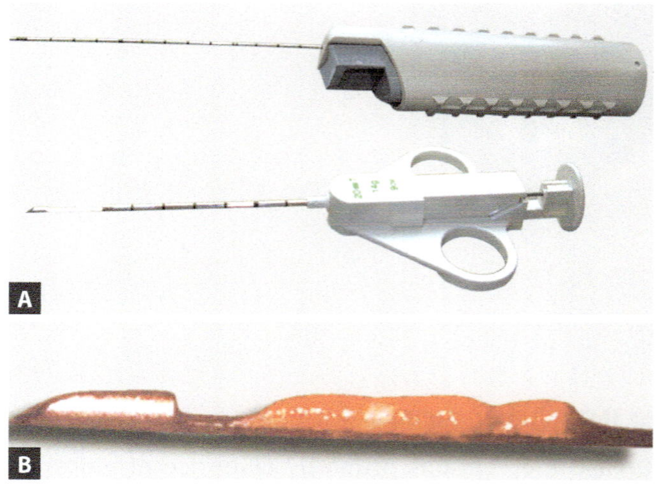

Figs. 1A and B: Core needle biopsy of breast: (A) 14G biopsy guns; (B) Open sample notch of the biopsy gun showing harvested tissue specimen.

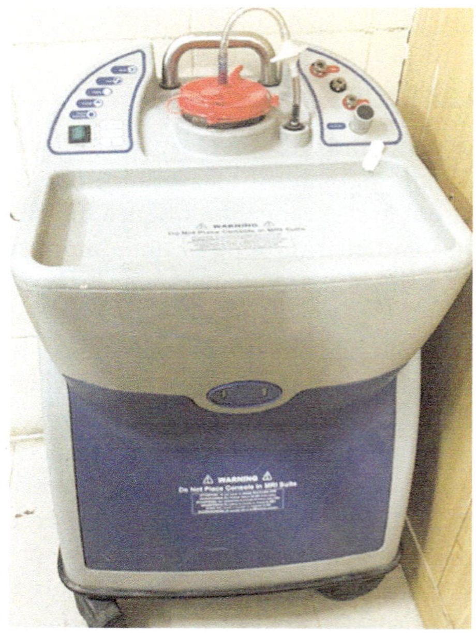

Fig. 2: Vacuum-assisted biopsy (VAB) device. Suros unit for vacuum-assisted breast biopsy.

Vacuum-assisted Biopsy

Directional vacuum-assisted biopsy (VAB) of breast is a modified and improved technique of large core breast biopsy. It was introduced in late 1990s.[7] It can be used under ultrasound, stereotactic or magnetic resonance (MR) guidance. The VAB device consists of a main unit housing the vacuum generator and the operating console and disposable biopsy probe (needle) attached to it **(Fig. 2)**. The probe consists of an outer cannula with a sample notch and an inner cutting cannula. When activated, a vacuum is applied which sucks and holds the tissue at the sample notch. Next, the inner cannula advances with high speed rotation to cut and enclose the tissue core within. Without removing the probe from the breast, the cut sample is then transported outside to the sample chamber using activation of another vacuum. Vacuum is also used to aspirate the oozed blood preventing hematoma formation. Saline irrigation or instillation of local anesthetic at the biopsy site through the probe is also possible during the procedure. All the steps of VAB are automated and contiguous multiple cores of tissue can be harvested without removing the probe from the breast. Some of the currently available

VAB devices include Mammotome® (previously Johnson and Johnson; now Devicor, Cincinnati, USA), Eviva® and Atec® (previously Suros; now Hologic, Bedford, USA) and Encore® (previously Senorx; now Bard, Tempe, USA). Thick caliber (11G–7G) probes are typically used in VAB.

Advantages of Vacuum-assisted Biopsy

Major advantage of the VAB is that it allows fast acquisition of multiple, large and contiguous tissue cores with single needle insertion into the breast. When compared with CNB using biopsy guns, a 10-fold greater tissue volume is obtained per core.[8] The probe can be rotated 360° within the lesion facilitating removal of tissue around the probe. Small lesions can be completely removed thereby eliminating the chances of sampling errors. Unlike biopsy guns, very accurate needle placement is not mandatory for VAB. The sample notch can be directed to the lesion and it can pull the lesion into the notch. This feature is particularly valuable when a small cluster of calcification is targeted. In VAB, the probe is placed close to or within the lesion before actually taking the biopsy and hence chance of cutting needle sliding by the side of the lesion, rather than penetrating it, is also eliminated. After the first few cores obtained during CNB, subsequent cores tend to contain tissue as well as clots. This does not happen in VAB as the oozing blood is continuously removed and all the harvested cores are of good quality.

Larger tissue removal with VAB increases the accuracy of breast biopsy. False-negative rates of VAB range from 0.6 to 5.2%.[6] The results of VAB are almost as good as surgical biopsy and negative predictive value as high as 99.9% can be achieved with VAB.[9,10] VAB is also more accurate than CNB in terms of frequency of histological underestimation, false negatives, and need for rebiopsy.[11,12]

Marker Clip Placement with Vacuum-assisted Biopsy

Vacuum-assisted biopsy probes also allow placement of radiopaque marker clips at the biopsy site before the removal of the probe from the breast **(Figs. 3A and B)**. If the small lesion is completely removed during the biopsy and histopathology result is positive for cancer, this clip can be used to direct preoperative hookwire placement to guide breast conservation surgery. If the result is benign, the small marker clip is left as such in the breast. Some marker clips have both metal and a gel which expands into the tissue. This type of clip can be visualized both on mammography and ultrasound for hookwire localization. Placement of marker clip is also important for breast mass of any size that is being considered for neoadjuvant chemotherapy.[13,14] After chemotherapy, some breast cancers may completely disappear on imaging and in this situation, tumor site can be identified with marker clip only and the surgery can be performed after performing hookwire localization of the marker clip.

Disadvantages of Vacuum-assisted Biopsy

Vacuum-assisted biopsy is more expensive than CNB using biopsy guns. The main unit with operating console as well as disposable biopsy probes is expensive. VAB probes are up to 10 times more expensive than the biopsy guns. One of the approaches toward better cost-effectiveness is that it could be selectively used as an alternative to open surgical biopsy for patients with nondiagnostic initial biopsy.[15] This approach is currently followed at author's institute. VAB also lacks the convenience of CNB. The probe is heavier and an experienced assistant is required during the procedure. However, advantages of VAB far outweigh

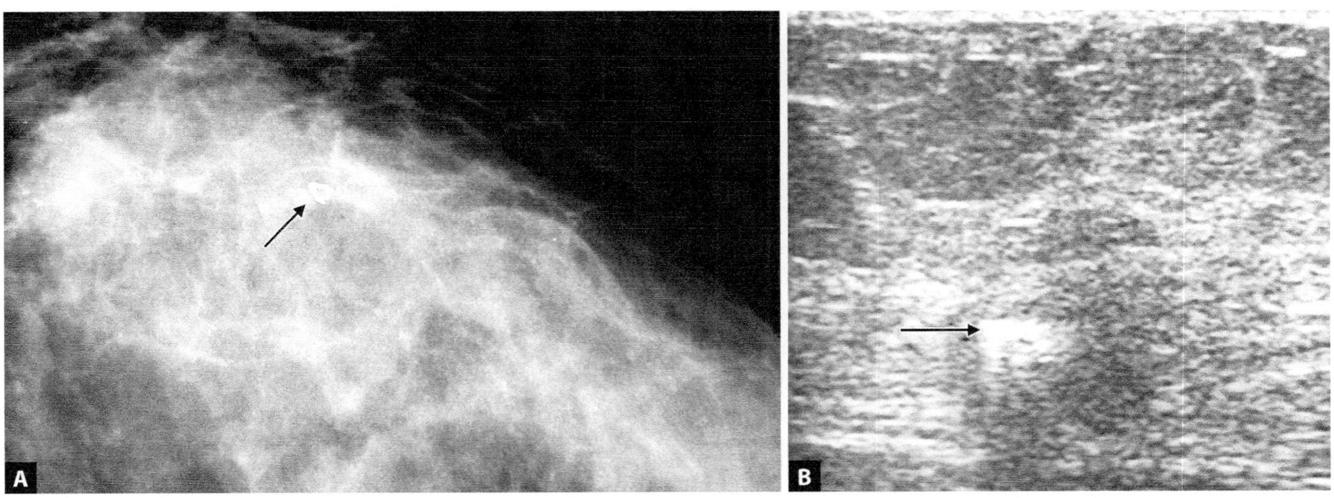

Figs. 3A and B: Marker clips: (A) Metallic marker clip Mammomark® deployed at the biopsy site (arrow) after VAB is seen on postbiopsy mammogram; (B) Gel-coated marker clip (arrow) can also be visualized on ultrasound.

the disadvantages and it has become the standard of breast biopsy in most breast care centers.

Complete Lesion Removal with Vacuum-assisted Biopsy

It is important to note that VAB instrument is intended for tissue sampling only and not for therapeutic removal of the lesion. Even if complete imaging evidence of the malignant lesion is removed with VAB, cancer is still found on surgery in majority of the patients.[16,17] Surgery for breast cancer requires en bloc removal of the tumor with adequate margins of normal parenchyma around it and not just the gross tumor removal. However, this is not an issue with the benign lesions. Although uncommonly performed, VAB has been used as a minimally invasive technique to remove small benign breast masses with high patient satisfaction rates.[18,19] VAB leaves a very small, 3–4 mm, scar on the breast and results in excellent cosmetic outcome when compared with surgical removal of a benign mass.

Lesion Selection for Breast Biopsy

Breast biopsy is indicated in all lesions classified as BI-RADS 4 (suspicious) or BI-RADS 5 (highly suspicious). BI-RADS 3 lesions have <2% chance of malignancy and these are best managed with imaging follow-up without significant delay in diagnosis or treatment of breast cancer. However, sometimes biopsy needs to be performed in BI-RADS 3 lesions as well. Such situations include inability to follow-up, anxious patient who refuses for follow-up, planned pregnancy, and presence of another breast lesion which is already diagnosed as breast cancer.

Selection of Guiding Modality

Image-guided breast biopsy can be performed under ultrasound, mammographic (stereotactic) or MR guidance. Ultrasound is the most commonly used modality, if the breast lesion is unequivocally demonstrated on ultrasound. No special ultrasound equipment is required and the modality as well as expertise is widely available. The procedure is real time and fast. The lying position is also comfortable to the patient. Ultrasound-guided procedures also allow greater flexibility of the approach and the puncture site. The needle can be inserted oblique or near parallel to the chest wall. Lesions located close to the chest wall, in the axillary tail or in the subareolar location may be difficult to position under stereotactic biopsy but these can be readily targeted with ultrasound guidance.

Microcalcifications only or masses which are seen on mammography only are indications for stereotactic breast biopsy. Personal preference and experience with biopsy techniques also govern the selection of guiding modality. At some centers, stereotactic biopsy is the preferred modality for all types of lesions, including masses that can be seen on ultrasound. MR-guided biopsy is cumbersome, expensive and time consuming. However, with increasing use of breast magnetic resonance imaging (MRI) and its higher sensitivity, MR-guided biopsy is required for lesions which are visible on MRI only. It is worthwhile to perform a careful "second look" targeted breast ultrasound in an attempt to localize the MRI-detected lesion. Many of the MR positive breast lesions can be demonstrated like this and ultrasound-guided biopsy can be performed.[20,21]

Suspicious areas of focal asymmetry or architectural distortion are generally not subjected to percutaneous biopsy. Excision biopsy is preferred in these situations. A suspicious dilated duct is also excised surgically unless there is an associated mass or calcification which can be used as a target for image-guided percutaneous biopsy.

Prebiopsy Assessment

Imaging on basis of which the breast biopsy has been recommended must be carefully evaluated. It should be ensured that a clearly visible abnormality is present which can be targeted accurately. Appropriate biopsy technique and guiding modality is then selected. If the imaging is inadequate or presence of the lesion is doubtful, additional imaging must be done before scheduling the biopsy. A brief history should be obtained from the patient and at the same time biopsy procedure, its risks and postbiopsy instructions may also be conveyed to the patient. History of allergy to Betadine or lignocaine, if any, should also be asked. No claims about outcome of the biopsy or future management should be made. The patient should be aware that a rebiopsy or excision may be required if the biopsy specimen is considered inadequate for definite pathological opinion. Informed consent must be obtained before the biopsy. Preprocedural coagulation profile is not required, unless patient has a bleeding tendency or is taking anticoagulants. Patients on aspirin or nonsteroidal anti-inflammatory drugs (NSAIDs) should stop it 3–5 days before the biopsy. Prophylactic antibiotics are not routinely required; however, these can be considered based on individual clinical judgment in patients with diabetes, rheumatic heart disease, artificial heart valves or joint replacement.

Ultrasound-guided Breast Biopsy

Wide availability, low cost, and ease of convenience to both the radiologist and the patient makes ultrasound the preferred modality for breast biopsy. Linear, 7.5 MHz (or more) transducer should be used. CNB must be performed with 14G long throw (2 cm or more) biopsy guns, even for a small subcentimeter lesion. Preprocedure test fire of the biopsy gun should be avoided. Correct patient positioning is important for ultrasound-guided breast biopsy. Ipsilateral arm of the patient should be raised above the head. Supine patient position is good for medial quadrant lesions. For lateral quadrant lesions, ipsilateral anterior supine oblique position should be made, preferably with a pillow under the patient's shoulder. This helps to spread and thin out the breast parenchyma over the lesion. Ultrasound unit should be aligned in such a way that a right-handed radiologist can conveniently scan with left hand and hold the needle in right hand, without twisting his or her body to see the image on the monitor.

Technique

After preliminary scanning, skin puncture site should be carefully chosen. Free hand technique with needle visualization in longitudinal plane of the scan field is used for ultrasound-guided breast biopsy. Instead of choosing shortest skin to lesion distance, puncture site should be at least 1 cm or more away from the edge of the transducer. This increases the distance which the needle has to travel in the breast, but it makes the needle path parallel to chest wall, thereby reducing the chances of injury or penetration of the chest wall. The needle remains parallel to the transducer improving the needle visibility **(Fig. 4)**.

The skin should be cleaned with Betadine and the draped with sterile sheets. Transducer surface is also cleaned or covered with sterile cover, as per the local practice. Local anesthesia should be given using 5–10 cc of 1% lignocaine and 22G or 23G needle. Local anesthetic should be injected under ultrasound guidance, first close to the lesion, then along the needle tract and finally, in the subcutaneous tissue at the puncture site. Raising a skin wheal with local anesthetic at the puncture site greatly reduces the pain during biopsy. A small skin incision is given at the puncture site using number 11 scalpel blade. Needle is then carefully inserted and turned horizontally. Some resistance may be felt initially as the needle penetrates through the fascia and ligaments attached to the skin, the needle advancement should be carefully controlled so as to avoid sudden give-in and deep penetration. In hard breast, counter pressure from opposite direction may be required to facilitate needle penetration. The needle should always be kept parallel to the chest wall and in the plane of the long axis of the transducer, i.e., the scan plane. Otherwise, the needle tip may not be seen. To achieve this transducer-needle alignment, sometimes the transducer needs to be rotated or repositioned during advancement of the needle. The needle tip should just pierce the lesion, if it is large enough, and has been stabilized with the transducer pressure **(Fig. 5A)**. Patient should be warned that a "thud" sound will be heard and she should not get scared or make sudden jerky moves. If an assistant is helping in taking the samples, phrases like "fire now" should be avoided as it may upset or scare the patient. The gun is then fired under real-time guidance. Before removing the needle, scanning in longitudinal and transverse planes should be done so as to ensure that the sample notch part of the gun is truly within the lesion **(Figs. 5B and C)**. It does not matter if the needle tip has crossed beyond the lesion. The needle is withdrawn; sample is retrieved and transferred to the sample bottle containing 10% formalin. The needle should not be dipped in formalin; instead, a scalpel blade should be used to remove the tissue from the sample notch. In this way multiple, at least four to five samples are collected and sample bottle is labeled. After the biopsy, light compression is applied at the biopsy site for about 10 minutes.

Technique of ultrasound-guided VAB is similar to that of ultrasound-guided CNB using biopsy gun **(Fig. 6A)**. The skin incision should be little wider so as to accommodate the large caliber VAB probes. The probe (needle) of VAB is not fired inside the lesion. Instead of hitting the lesion from the side, the probe tip is positioned below the lesion, in such a way that the sample notch remains just beneath the lesion **(Fig. 6B)**. This helps to obtain contiguous core of the lesion, beginning from the deeper part of the lesion and then probe gradually moves superficially through the lesion for each subsequent core. The probe of the VAB is thick and not removed from the breast until the end of the biopsy procedure. If it is placed in the superficial part, most part of the lesion will be obscured beneath the acoustic shadowing of the probe after obtaining initial cores. If a small lesion is completely removed during VAB, a marker clip must be deployed at the biopsy site through the probe before taking it out from the breast.

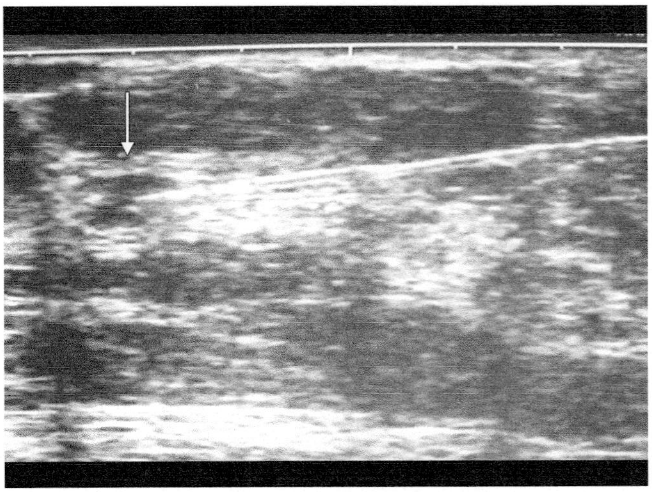

Fig. 4: Ultrasound-guided core needle biopsy (CNB). Horizontal needle approach improves the needle visualization, especially for targeting of small mass (arrow).

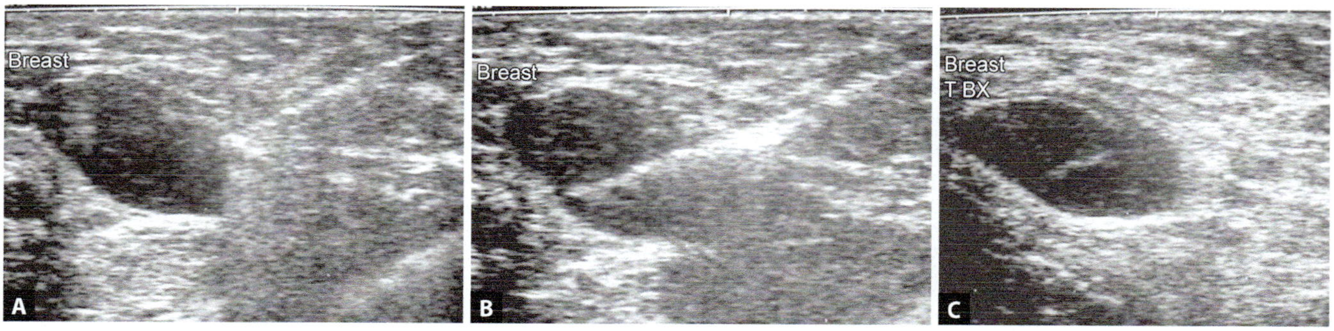

Figs. 5A to C: Ultrasound-guided core needle biopsy (CNB): (A) The tip of the biopsy needle is positioned at the periphery of the mass; (B) The mass and the needle are stabilized and the needle is fired. Area of sample notch is seen within the center of the mass indicating accurate positioning and sampling; (C) After withdrawal of the needle, small echogenic area of hemorrhage is seen within the mass at the site of biopsy.

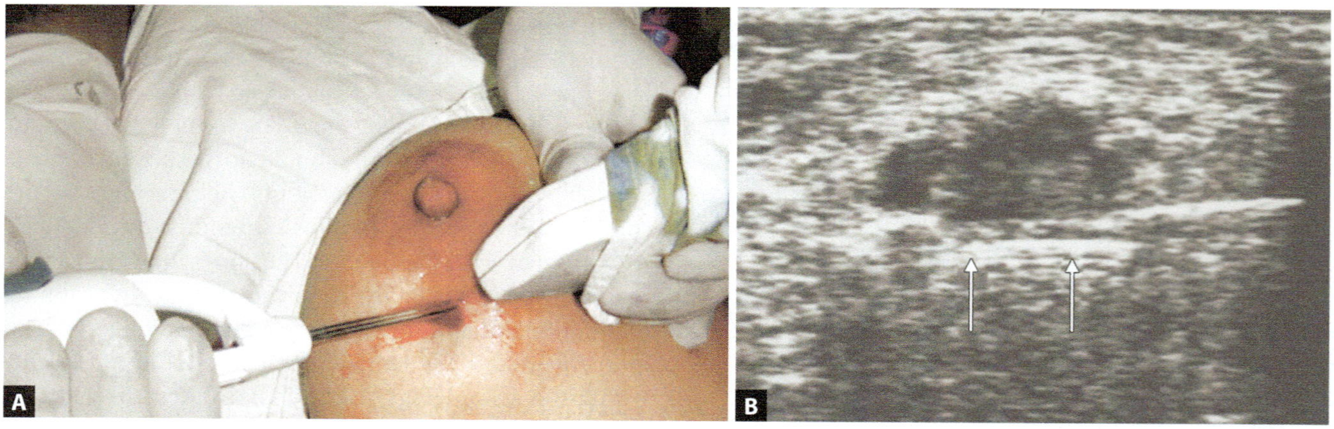

Figs. 6A and B: Ultrasound-guided vacuum-assisted biopsy (VAB): (A) Biopsy procedure is being performed with Mammotome® probe and transducer aligned in the same plane; (B) The open sample notch (arrows) is positioned just beneath the mass.

Stereotactic Breast Biopsy

The principle of stereotactic biopsy is based on the trigonometric determination of depth of the target lesion in the breast. The breast is positioned and compressed in the stereotactic unit and pair of mammographic spot exposures (stereo images) is obtained with +15° and –15° tube angulations. Relative position of the target will change in both views because of the parallax shift due to different tube angulations. Lesion situated close to the detector moves less and lesion situated away from the detector moves more in these two images. This movement is compared with the movements of a marker with known depth (reference marker at the base) to determine the depth (z-coordinate) of the target lesion in the breast. Actual process involves complex trigonometric calculations, which are fortunately performed by the system computer. The x- and y-coordinates are same in both views.

Equipment

Stereotactic biopsy equipment are of two types: (1) dedicated prone table and (2) add-on erect stereotactic device. Both of these were film-based in past but now digital systems are used as they make the procedure simpler and faster. In dedicated prone table unit, the patient lies prone on the table and the breast hangs down through an opening in the table **(Figs. 7A and B)**. The patient is comfortable and breast remains stable during the procedure which is performed below the table. As the patient does not see the procedure, her anxiety is reduced. There is also more working space for the radiologist. The lesion can be approached from any side (360°) around the breast. Dedicated prone table stereotactic biopsy units are more expensive, require large space and cannot be used for diagnostic mammography. Hence, these are cost-effective only if stereotactic biopsy is being routinely performed in the department. As thickness of the table will always remain between the chest wall and the breast, lesions situated too close to the chest wall may be difficult to access.

Add-on stereotactic biopsy device is actually an accessory device which can be attached to a standard diagnostic mammography unit to perform stereotactic biopsy **(Figs. 8A and B)**. It is cheaper and cost-effective. However, the biopsy can be performed in erect (sitting) patient position only. It is inconvenient to both the patient

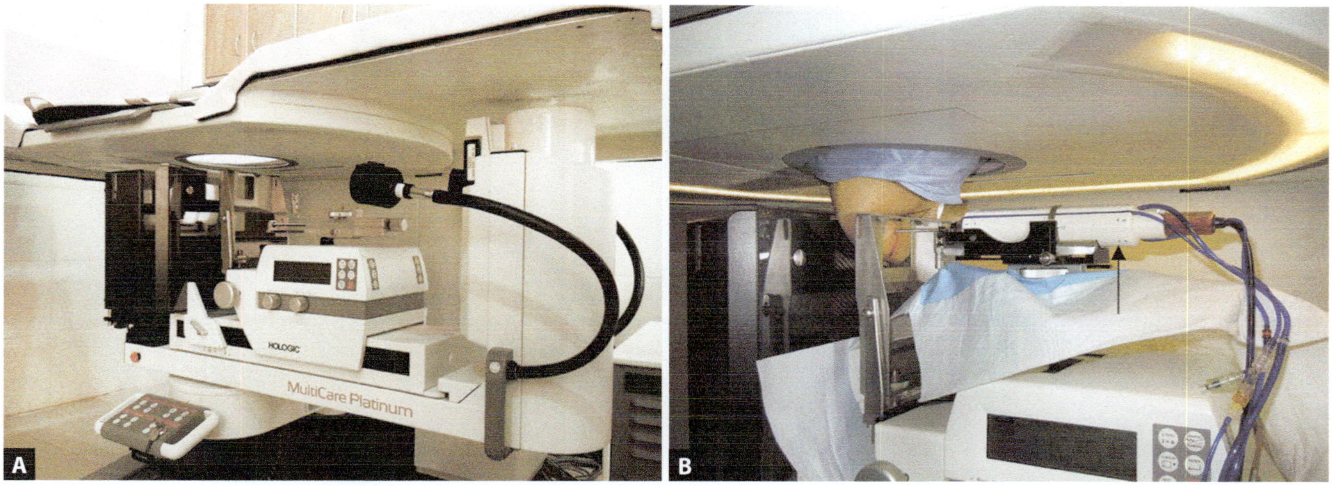

Figs. 7A and B: Dedicated prone table stereotactic biopsy: (A) Equipment (Mutlicare®, Hologic); (B) Stereotactic biopsy being performed using Atec® VAB device.

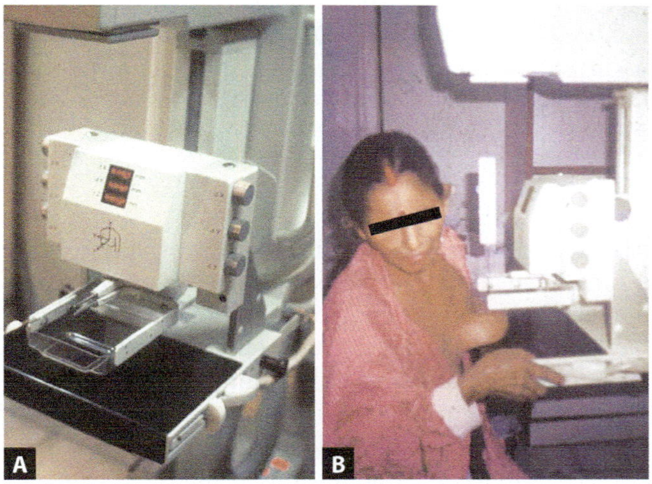

Figs. 8A and B: Add-on erect stereotactic biopsy equipment: (A) Biopsy unit (Opdima®, Siemens); (B) Stereotactic biopsy is being performed with biopsy gun in a sitting position.

and the radiologist as working space is limited. The needle must be inserted from cranial aspect only, even if the lesion is located in caudal part of the breast. The chances of breast movement resulting in unnoticed shifting of the target lesion during biopsy are more likely. The patient closely watches the approach and insertion of the biopsy needle in her breast and hence there are high chances of fainting and vasovagal reactions.

Technique

The technique of stereotactic biopsy is same for both types of units. The breast is positioned and compressed with a compression plate having an open window. An initial spot image is obtained without tube angulation to ensure that the lesion is seen in the center of the window. Once this is confirmed, a pair of stereo images is obtained without releasing the breast compression **(Fig. 9A)**. At the user interface of the computer, total needle length and distance from tip of the needle to the center of the sample notch is entered. Needle length must be measured in fired status of the needle. Single or multiple targets are then marked with mouse clicks in both images and transmitted to the device. Care must be taken to mark same part of the lesion in both images. The x-, y- and z-coordinates are calculated and displayed by the unit. The needle holder position is then moved and adjusted to appropriate position.

Presence of adequate breast tissues (thickness), both proximal and deep to the lesion, in compressed position of the breast is essential in stereotactic breast biopsy. The core biopsy sample is obtained from the sample notch and not from the tip of the needle. If the lesion is too close to the skin, the gun will have to be fired while the sample notch is partially outside the breast. This is not recommended. Similarly, if the lesion is too close to the table (bucky), the needle tip will puncture the skin and hit the table. These situations are called insufficient stroke margins and biopsy cannot be done. Some stereotactic units detect these errors automatically and warn the operator, while in others, safety of the stroke margin has to be calculated and determined by the radiologist. Changing breast position or rolling the breast before compression is sometimes useful in such situations. Prone table biopsy units are better in these situations as they allow greater flexibility in choosing the direction of needle entry.

Site preparation and biopsy procedure is same as that for ultrasound-guided breast biopsy. Needle is inserted through the needle holder in its selected final position. A prefire pair of stereo images is obtained with needle fully inserted **(Fig. 9B)**. In both of these images, the needle tip should be seen just before and at the same distance from the target. After that, the gun is fired and another set of postfire stereo images is obtained **(Fig. 9C)**. The needle tip should have symmetrically crossed the lesion in both

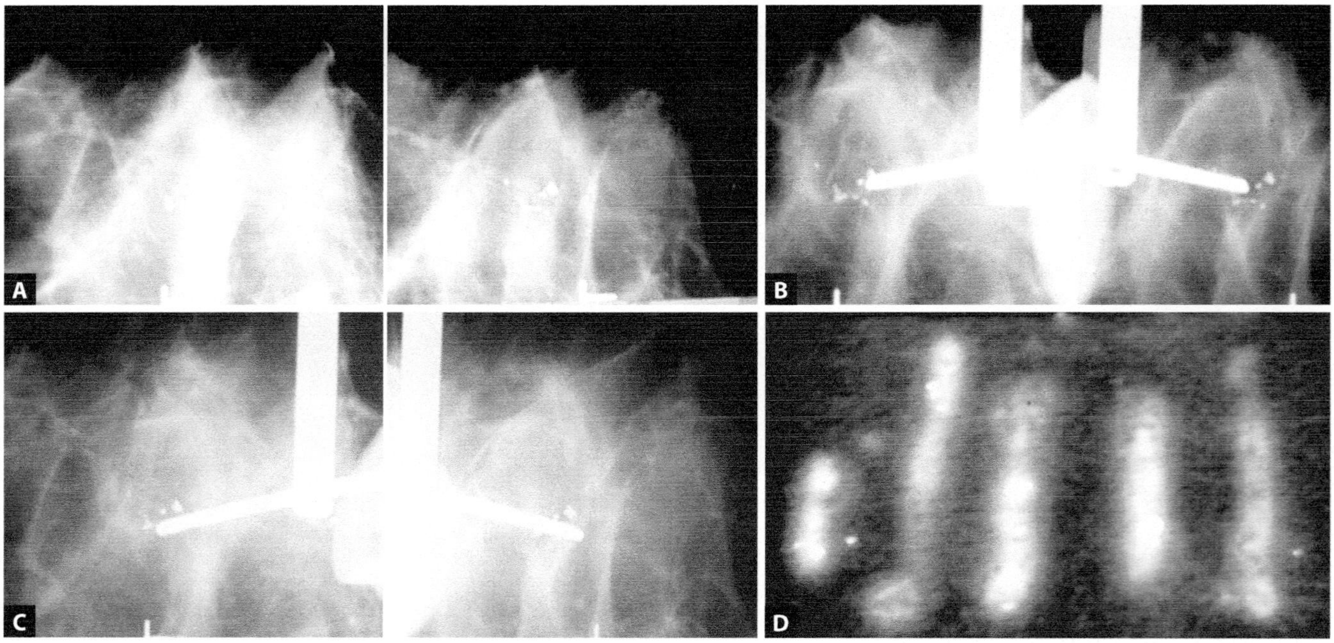

Figs. 9A to D: Stereotactic biopsy: (A) Pair of stereo images obtained at +10° and –10°. Targets are marked in both images on the lesion, i.e., cluster of calcifications in this case; (B) Prefire pair of images show needle tip close to the lesion in both images; (C) Postfire images show that needle has traversed the lesion; (D) Specimen radiography of the samples shows presence of calcifications in multiple cores, confirming accurate targeting and sampling.

of these images. The biopsy gun is then removed and sample retrieved. Subsequently, each target is selected, transmitted and fresh needle insertions are made to obtain multiple cores. It is not necessary to obtain pre- and postfire images for each subsequent core if these images are satisfactory during first sample. However, if the lesion has moved or if there is asymmetry of needle tip—lesion relationship in pre- or postfire images, a fresh pair of stereo images without needle should be obtained and biopsy continued with fresh target setting. When biopsy is being performed with vacuum-assisted probe, the probe is rotated in the same position to obtain multiple cores from all directions around the probe. At the end, the needle is withdrawn from the breast and compression is released.

Tomosynthesis-guided Core Biopsy

Digital breast tomosynthesis is a technique which improves detection and characterization of a breast lesion, by reconstructing the data into thin sections. It is especially helpful in dense breasts where the margin of a lesion may be obscured by overlapping fibroglandular parenchyma.[22] Tomosynthesis-guided core biopsy is a recent advance that allows histopathological diagnosis without resorting to more invasive surgical intervention.

Benefits

Tomoguided biopsy allows easier sampling of focal asymmetry, architectural distortion, calcifications and noncalcified masses by automatically providing a depth estimation without having to calculate the z-coordinate. It allows a sitting/upright biopsy and thus do away with the discomfort associated with prone biopsy. Posteriorly located lesions are also easily sampled compared to prone biopsy. However as some patients may experience vasovagal reaction, prone tomoguided setups are also now available. Studies have shown it to be a faster technique compared to the stereotactic biopsy as there is no intervening step of stereo-pair images.[23]

Technique

The steps of acquiring a tomoguided biopsy are similar to a stereotactic biopsy with few exceptions. After assessing the lesion on prior imaging and clinical examination, the approach for biopsy is planned as either craniocaudal/caudocranial or mediolateral/lateromedial, depending on the location of lesion and its nearest skin distance. After appropriate positioning, tomosynthesis data is acquired instead of the scout and stereo pairs. The suspicious area can then be targeted based on which tomo slice shows the lesion to best advantage. The depth calculation is not required. Further steps of biopsy, check view, clip placement and specimen radiography are similar to the stereotactic biopsy.

Disadvantages: Visualization of subtle and faint calcifications may sometimes be limited on tomosynthesis and may require two-dimensional (2D) imaging and 2D stereotactic biopsy.

Specimen Radiography

If the target lesion has calcifications, specimen radiography of the harvested cores is essential to document retrieval of calcifications in the specimen **(Fig. 9D)**. This is recommended both after ultrasound-guided and stereotactic core biopsy. The cores may be placed on a wet slide or film so that they do not stick to it and specimen radiography is performed on standard mammography unit using lowest exposure factors. Demonstration of calcifications in cores eliminates the risk of sampling error and improves the chances of specific diagnosis. If the calcifications are not demonstrated, pathological diagnosis can still be made; however, the accuracy of the diagnosis is lower than when calcifications are demonstrated.[24,25] Specimen mammography of cores is not required when the target is a mass lesion without calcification.

Postbiopsy Care

After ultrasound-guided or stereotactic core biopsy of the breast, a continuous light pressure is maintained over the biopsy site (and not at the skin puncture site) at least for 10 minutes to achieve good hemostasis. Sometimes, a longer compression is needed. After that the skin is cleaned with alcohol and the incision is closed using sterile adhesive tape. Procedure and instructions must be written in postbiopsy notes and explained to the patient. The patient should be advised to keep the biopsy site dry and watch for obvious bleeding or sudden breast enlargement; the latter would indicate internal bleed and hematoma formation. Although this is rare, the patient can apply light pressure herself and contact the radiologist immediately should this happen. A telephone number of the radiologist should be provided to her for this purpose. Patient should be asked to avoid strenuous ipsilateral arm movements, such as lifting heavy weights, pushing something exercise or cooking activities. The tape on the wound can be removed after 48 hours.

Mild pain and some heaviness of the breast may be experienced by the patient immediately after the biopsy. Ice fomentation using ice cubes in a plastic bag is useful to relieve postbiopsy pain and also to reduce chances of bleeding. Routine analgesics are not required and should be avoided as far as possible. Patients should also be told that small bruising or discoloration of the skin due to ecchymosed blood can occur and this clears subsequently. Local skin inflammation or small serous ooze from incision site may rarely be seen which is also self-limiting. The wound should be kept clean and dry and no ointment, etc., should be applied. Prolonged bloody or purulent discharge from the wound however, should be evaluated clinically as well radiologically to determine if any treatment is required.

COMPLICATIONS OF BREAST BIOPSY

Percutaneous core biopsy breast is a safe procedure and complications are rare. Vasovagal reaction, hematoma formation, and infection are main complications. Excessive bleeding or pain during biopsy necessitating termination of the procedure is extremely rare. Minor complication rate is 1.4%.[9] Significant hematoma formation or infection, defined as those requiring medical or surgical treatment, occurs only in 0.1% cases. Small hematoma formation at the biopsy site is an expected finding and it can be seen on ultrasound for a week in majority of patients.[26] Complication rates of biopsy with biopsy gun and VAB are similar.[27]

Vasovagal reaction is a potential but unpredictable risk of breast biopsy. It is caused by anxiety, fear, and pain. It is characterized by complaints of lightheadedness or fainting and signs of sweating, skin flushing and bradycardia. Distracting light conversation with patient during the biopsy procedure is helpful to avoid it. The patient should not be left alone during the biopsy. If vasovagal reaction occurs, she should be immediately placed in a supine position with feet raised and pulse and blood pressure monitored. This is usually adequate and active treatment with atropine is not generally required. Strict aseptic precautions during the biopsy are essential to minimize the chances of infection. A good compression after the biopsy and patient compliance of the postbiopsy instructions are important to reduce the chances of major hematoma formation.

Although complications of breast biopsy are uncommon, psychological impact of breast biopsy is important. The patient is worried and disturbed ever since she is told that there is a suspicious lesion in her breast that could be a cancer. Anxiety about the biopsy procedure itself is an additional cause of fear. These factors must also be considered while interacting with the patient.

Percutaneous breast biopsy does not cause seeding of tumor cells along the biopsy tract so as to cause spread or recurrence of the tumor in the breast or skin.[28] Although displaced tumor cells can be rarely found along the needle tract on histological examination of excised specimen, these cells probably do not sustain long enough to produce tumor seeding.[29,30] Needle tract cell displacement is more common with automated gun biopsies than with VAB, as unlike with biopsy guns, only single-time needle insertion is required with VAB.

Percutaneous breast biopsy generally does not produce any long-term changes, scarring or architectural distortion on follow-up mammograms. In <2% cases, a tiny round opacity may develop, which is seen in only one view of the mammogram.[31]

Magnetic Resonance Imaging-guided Breast Biopsy

Magnetic resonance imaging of breast is generally used as a problem-solving modality. It is also being used for high-risk screening and preoperative staging of breast cancer. Contrast-enhanced breast MRI is the most sensitive modality for breast cancer detection, which means that some breast lesions are seen only on MRI and not on conventional imaging. These are the lesions which require biopsy using MR guidance.

Magnetic resonance imaging-guided breast biopsy is performed with special breast coils and needle guide known as aiming device. It allows access on lateral aspect of breast only and hence, medially located lesions require deep needle insertion. Two types of localization devices are available. Most commonly used is a grid type device, a plate with multiple holes. The patient is positioned prone with breast in the coil. Mild compression is given with grid plate itself and contrast-enhanced MRI is performed. A fiducial (marker), usually a vitamin E capsule, is also placed in one of the holes. The lesion is localized in axial and sagittal planes. Its location and distance with respect to fiducial is determined. The needle holder is fixed in the grid hole which is in line with the lesion. Depth is determined by counting the sagittal slices between needle holder and the lesion. A coaxial needle is first introduced up to the lesion, through which biopsy is taken using MR compatible biopsy gun or VAB probe.[32] The other type of aiming device has a bar and column, which can be moved in horizontal and vertical directions respectively, instead of a grid. The lesion and fiducial are localized and bar and columns moved to align the needle holder with the lesion for performance of biopsy.

Magnetic resonance imaging-guided breast biopsy is difficult, time-consuming and expensive. It requires special hardware in the form of a special imaging coil with window for biopsy and localization device and MR compatible needles, usually made of titanium of nickel alloys. The biopsy must be done with contrast-enhanced MRI, which means that the procedure must be completed within 30–40 minutes when the lesion is enhancing and hence visible. The patient needs to be moved in and out of the gantry several times during the biopsy, making it cumbersome and time-consuming. As the lesion is seen only because of contrast enhancement in vivo, specimen imaging cannot be done.

Histopathological Correlation

Core biopsy is a reliable method of diagnosis of breast abnormalities. When malignancy is found, definitive surgery is undertaken. However, some cancers can be missed on core biopsy. False-negative rates of core breast biopsy can be as high as 9% for gun biopsy and 5% for VAB.[6] Core biopsy is a sampling procedure and sampling error cannot be eliminated altogether. However, steps should be taken to achieve best possible accuracy of the procedure. Accurate target setting and relationship of the needle with the lesion should be verified on imaging during breast biopsy. Whenever applicable, specimen radiography must be done to verify presence of calcifications in the harvested samples. After biopsy, the results of the biopsy should always be correlated with imaging findings. A rebiopsy is essential if the sample is considered inadequate for definitive pathological diagnosis. Rebiopsy, preferably a surgical excision biopsy, should also be performed when there is imaging-histologic discordance or if a high-risk lesion like atypical ductal hyperplasia (ADH) is reported on core biopsy. Imaging-histologic discordance is a situation when imaging findings are not consistent with the pathology report. Benign core biopsy diagnosis for a spiculated mass lesion or pleomorphic microcalcifications is not expected. Imaging-histologic discordance occurs in 3–7% of core biopsies and malignancy is found in about one-fourth of these cases on surgical excision.[33,34] Even if benign diagnosis of core biopsy is acceptable, such as for BI-RADS 4 lesions, it should be closely followed up with 6 monthly mammograms to rule out any sampling error.[35,36] Any suspicious development on follow-up mammogram is an indication for rebiopsy.

Histological underestimation is another limitation of core biopsy. When core biopsy result are correlated with final histopathology of the surgical specimen, a lesion diagnosed as atypical ductal hyperplasia or ductal carcinoma in situ (DCIS) on core biopsy may turn out to be DCIS or invasive carcinoma respectively. Biopsy may turn out to be DCIS or DCIS on core biopsy may turn out to be an invasive cancer. Histological underestimation occurs when core biopsy samples do not represent the pathologically most aggressive part of the lesion and this can occur in up to 40% of gun biopsies and 16% of VABs.[37] Hence, high-risk lesions like ADH should be subjected to rebiopsy with excision.

Close audit of the biopsy results at an individual center should be regularly performed to maintain the standard and accuracy of breast biopsy. Overall, malignant results are expected in 20–40% of all breast biopsies performed. This is known as positivity rate or positive predictive value (PPV) of the breast biopsy. If higher PPV is encountered, it indicates low index of suspicion on breast imaging. This means that some lesions which could have been cancers are not being recommended for biopsy and therefore, missed. On the other hand, if the PPV is low, the index of suspicion is very high and some lesions best suited for follow-up only are being referred for unnecessary biopsies.

PREOPERATIVE HOOKWIRE LOCALIZATION

Needle-hookwire localization followed by surgical excision was the standard procedure for obtaining pathological diagnosis of nonpalpable but suspicious breast lesions seen on the mammograms. With development of accurate percutaneous core biopsy techniques, hookwire localization is now rarely performed for initial diagnosis. At present, it is mainly used as a preoperative localization procedure for therapeutic excision (breast conservation surgery) of already diagnosed but nonpalpable breast cancer. Hookwire localization prior to breast conservation surgery helps to precisely resect the cancer with clear margins. Indications of hookwire localization for diagnostic surgical excision biopsy include nonavailability of stereotactic biopsy facility or rebiopsy after inconclusive or discordant percutaneous core breast biopsy. It is also recommended for biopsy of vaguely defined breast abnormalities lesions; such as suspicious focal asymmetry or architectural distortion without associated mass. Needle localization for excision biopsy helps to achieve accurate lesion retrieval with minimal removal of breast parenchyma.

Early preoperative localization procedures were performed using various types of dyes, such as methylene blue or Evans blue, mixed with iodinated contrast. The dye was injected in the lesion through a needle introduced under mammographic guidance. The dye could be seen on postlocalization films and also intraoperatively. However, spread of the dye and amount of tissue stained was unpredictable, leading to missed lesions or excision of much larger breast tissue than actually required. Charcoal powder was also used instead of aqueous dyes, so as to restrict the spread over large area, but this was also not very accurate.

Accuracy and reliability of preoperative needle localization greatly improved after the development of various needle-hookwire combinations. Kopans needle-hookwire assembly is most widely used. It consists of a 20G needle and a thin flexible wire which can be introduced through it. The distal end of the wire is folded back forming a sharp angle and overbent so that it has a spring action **(Fig. 10)**. The needle is introduced under mammographic guidance. After correct needle placement, the hookwire is introduced and needle withdrawn over it. This exposes the hook of the wire which then anchors itself in the lesion. Then it can only be removed surgically. A modification of this hookwire has a thick stiffened segment just proximal to the hook. This rigid segment of wire is useful to the surgeon as it allows manual palpation of the target lesion intraoperatively. Some versions of hookwire have double-folded hook forming a barb, which prevent their displacement with in or out of the breast. Another type of needle-hookwire assembly has a retractable curved J-tip instead of the angled hook. In this design, after positioning of the needle, the wire is advanced. The end of the wire which comes out of the needle forms a J-shaped curve and gets anchored. If final hookwire position is unsatisfactory, the curved part of the wire can be retracted back into the needle and repositioning can be performed. The needle stays in the breast after deployment and it provides a stiff guide to the surgeon.

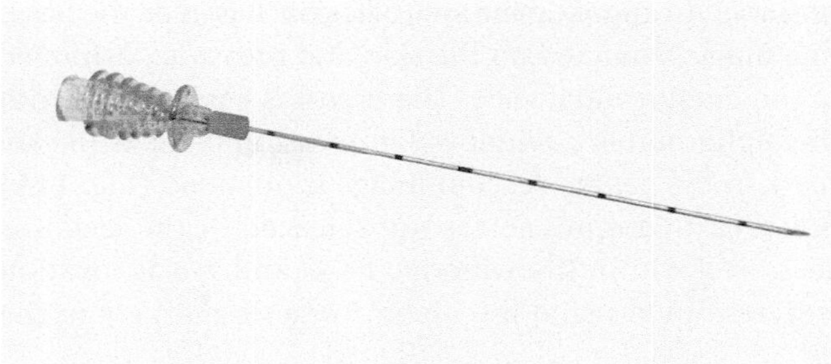

Fig. 10: Kopans needle-hookwire assembly. It consists of a 20G needle and a hookwire.

Equipment

Needle localization is usually performed under mammographic guidance. However, it may also be performed under ultrasound guidance if the lesion is clearly defined on ultrasound. MR compatible needle-hookwire assemblies are also available to localize the lesions seen only on MRI. Needle localization can be performed on all standard mammography machines. Only requirement is a special compression plate for needle localization. There are two types of compression plates. Alpha-numeric plate is the most widely used. It has a rectangular open window under which the lesion is positioned. There are radiopaque alpha-numeric centimeter markers on the margins of the window. The fenestrated compression plate has rows of multiple small round holes, like a sieve, instead of a single open window. These are also marked. The needle is introduced through the hole overlying the lesion. This type of compression is not preferred by many, as lesion frequently gets positioned under the solid part of the plate, rather than under the hole. Both digital and film-based mammography machines are suitable for needle localization. However, digital systems are preferred as images at each step are immediately available and procedure is therefore much faster.

Technique

Films on the basis of which needle localization has been recommended are reviewed and appropriate guiding modality and approach is selected. The procedure is scheduled just before the surgery. Informed consent inclusive of needle localization and excision is usually obtained by the surgeon. Mammographic needle localization is performed with the patient in a sitting position. An approximate area of lesion, based on the baseline films, is marked on the skin and breast is positioned in the craniocaudal view. The breast is compressed with the alpha-numeric window compression plate, with skin mark in the center. A scout image is obtained **(Fig. 11A)** but breast compression is not released. If the lesion is seen well within the window, its x- and y-axis location is determined using the alpha-numeric markers in the image. The point is marked on the skin at the crossing of same coordinates, as visible on the compression plate. Availability of movable cross-hair shadow marker in the light beam of mammography unit is greatly useful to mark the exact point on the skin.

After the skin entry point is marked, skin is prepared and local anesthetic is injected. If the target lesion is a mass or architectural distortion, care should be taken

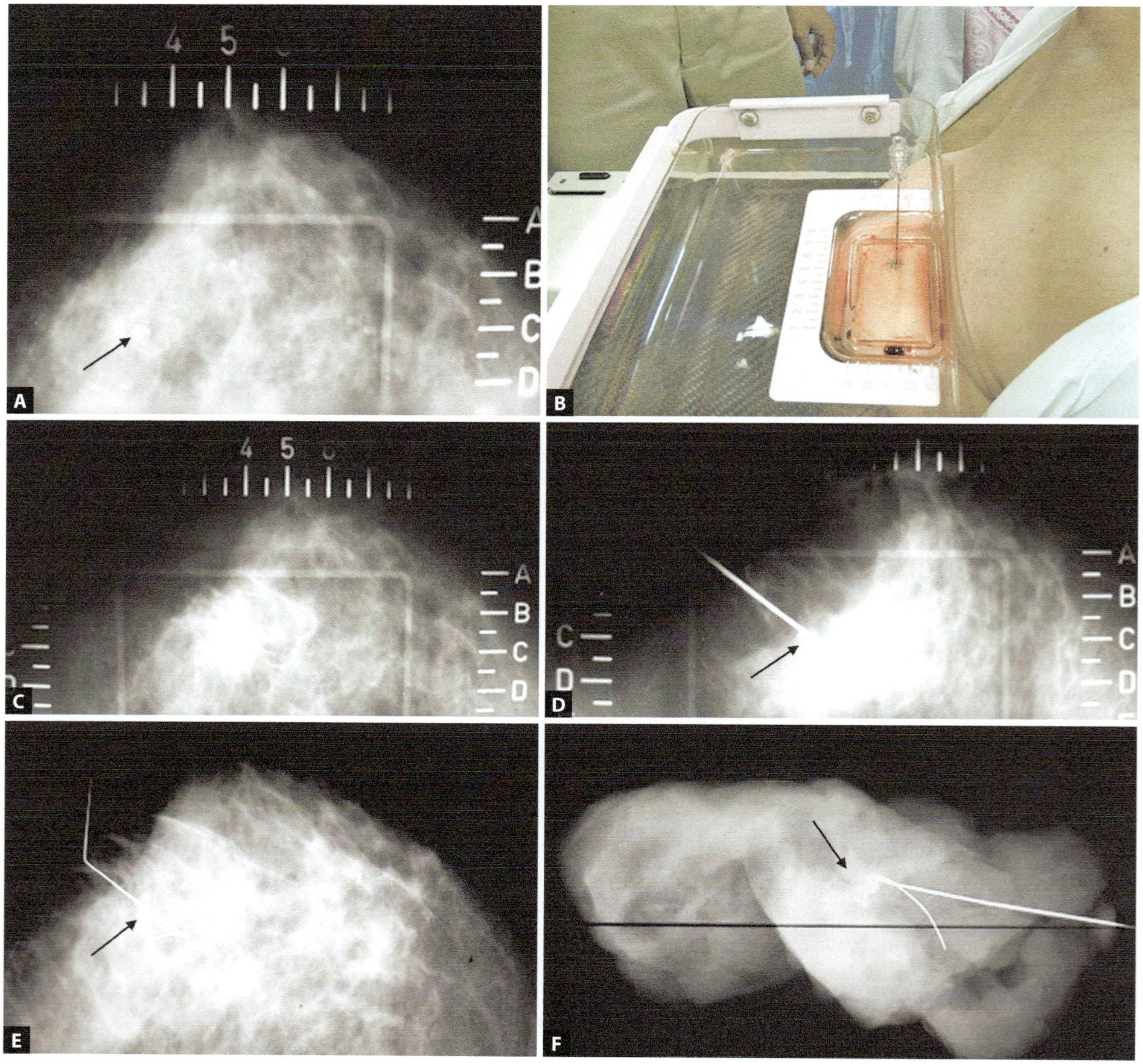

Figs. 11A to F: Preoperative hookwire localization: (A) Craniocaudal scout view shows cluster of calcification (arrow) in the center of the window of the compression plate. Its coordinates are determined in this film and skin entry point is marked; (B) Needle is inserted vertically. Note that the needle entry point is in the center of the shadow of the hub; thereby ensuring correct needle alignment in the direction of X-ray beam; (C) Another film is obtained. Needle is seen end on with its hub overlapping the lesion in this view; (D) Mediolateral view obtained thereafter shows that the needle tip has just crossed the lesion (arrow). Then the hookwire is inserted and the needle is withdrawn; (E) Posthookwire localization mammogram shows hookwire anchored correctly within the lesion (arrow); (F) Specimen radiograph of the excised tissue confirms accurate removal of the lesion (arrow).

not to inject too much local anesthetic as it can obscure lesion. The localization needle without hookwire is then inserted vertically into the breast. To improve the accuracy of needle hitting the target, the light beam of the mammography unit is turned on during insertion. It should be ensured that the shadow of the needle hub on the breast surrounds the needle entry point **(Fig. 11B)**. This maintains the needle in the direction of the X-ray beam and the needle remains perfectly perpendicular to the lesion. The needle is inserted to maximum depth and another image is obtained. With perfect positioning, the needle is seen enface in the form of a dot superimposed on the lesion **(Fig. 11C)**. Needle positioning is inaccurate if some length of the shaft is seen or if the needle is >5 mm away from the target. If this occurs, the needle should be withdrawn and reinserted. After satisfactory positioning, the compression released gradually. While the compression is being released, the breast bounces back and this may cause needle tip to come out from the lesion. To prevent this, the needle should be firmly supported and mild pressure is maintained to keep the needle tip deep in the breast during compression release. If the needle is not held, the needle hub may get entangled at the border of the compression plate window and come out with it. The breast is then repositioned in orthogonal (mediolateral) view using same compression plate. Then the exposure is made and the image obtained **(Fig. 11D)**. The needle should be seen crossing the lesion with tip about 1 cm beyond the lesion in this image. If this is not the case, then needle should be withdrawn accordingly while the breast is still compressed. Exact length to be withdrawn can be determined with the help of centimeter markings seen in the image. Presence of centimeter marks on the needle is useful in this depth adjustment.

After needle tip adjustment, the hookwire is inserted into the needle with the hook closed. The wire is inserted till a black mark on the wire reaches the hub. The tip of the hook is just at the needle tip at this position. A slight resistance to further advancement of wire is also be felt. The outside wire is then firmly held in position and needle withdrawn over it, releasing the hook in the breast. Wire should not be pushed during the withdrawal of the needle, as the hook may move further beyond the lesion, especially in fatty breasts.

After hookwire deployment, a mediolateral film is obtained for the surgeon **(Fig. 11E)**, craniocaudal view is not necessary. Procedure is considered successful if the hookwire is in the lesion or within 1 cm of it. If the wire is further away, procedure should be repeated with additional hookwire placement. The wire entry site is lightly covered with a gauze piece taking care that the wire is free to move in and out of the breast with changes in breast shape in supine and erect position of the patient. The wire should not be plastered to the breast at the skin entry site; otherwise the hook end of the wire inside the breast may get dislodged as the patient moves. The patient is then sent to the operation theater (OT) along with postlocalization film, with lesion marked on it, and a written note about the procedure and final hookwire-lesion relationship.

Other Localization Techniques

Hookwire localization is the most commonly performed and standard localization technique for nonplapable breast cancers. It requires a coordinated effort by breast intervention radiologist and breast surgeon, so that both are performed on the same day; however, there is a possibility of displacement or migration of the wire during patient transport from radiology to the operating theater.[38] The protruding wire has a bearing on route of dissection and may prove bothersome to the patient. There are recent advances in the localization techniques namely radioactive seed localization, magnetic seed for localization (Magseed) and infrared light/microimpulse radar reflector (SAVI scout).

1. *Radioactive seeds*: It was the first alternative to the wire localization systems and uses radioactive Iodine-125 seeds contained in a titanium shell. The placement of the seed can be performed under mammography or ultrasound guidance using 18G needle or by a preloaded assembly. The seed is localized at the time of surgery by a gamma probe, and confirmation is obtained by obtaining a specimen radiograph which shows the metallic seed within the resected specimen. Studies have shown it to be an effective alternate to wire localization with improved efficiency and convenience for the patient, intervention radiologist and the operating surgeon. The seed can be placed up to 5 days prior to the surgery. Disadvantages include exposure to radioactive material and the associated precautions required by the nuclear regulatory authorities, proper retrieval and safe disposal of the seed once it is used for localization.
2. *SAVI scout*: It is the first nonradioactive, nonwire localization method approved for use in humans. The localizer includes a reflector with antennae and is inserted in the breast lesion by a preloaded 16G introducer assembly. The reflector can be inserted as early as 30 days prior to surgery and remains inactive till it is activated by an extrinsic handpiece at the time of surgery.[39] It then reflects the RADAR signal and the location of the localizer can be deduced, which helps in guiding the surgery. The disadvantage of the system is that the reflector can be disabled by the electrocautery used during surgery. Also the antenna may be damaged during surgical dissection, causing failure of localization.
3. *Magseed*: Magseed is a paramagnetic seed made of steel and iron oxide of size 1 × 5 mm that may be used

to localize a nonpalpable breast lesion up to 30 days prior to surgery under ultrasound or mammography guidance. It is also available in a preloaded 18G needle. Its location is detected with a probe that generates magnetic field and thus detects the magnetic influx generated by the seed. A potential disadvantage is the interference created in its localization by other ferromagnetic instruments and equipment including electrocautery used in surgery, thereby necessitating use of special nonferromagnetic instruments. Moreover, the seed has to be placed after any MRI procedure.[38]

Specimen Radiography

The surgeon dissects the breast using hookwire in situ. The approach is usually along the wire. Rarely, a separate incision is made guided by the palpation of the thickened part of the wire and lesion approached. The breast tissue around the hook and the thickened wire segment is resected and sent to the mammography room for specimen radiography. The specimen radiography is done on mammography unit with minimal exposure factors **(Fig. 11F)**. Mild compression may be required, if the specimen is large. The specimen mammogram should confirm that the target lesion, along with good margins, has been removed within the resected specimen. The specimen mammogram must be correlated carefully with baseline mammogram for this purpose. This is especially important if the lesion has calcifications; all foci of suspicious calcifications should be within the specimen. Successful lesion removal should be communicated to the surgeon, who is waiting in the OT, so that the breast can be closed and sutured. If the lesion is incompletely seen or seen extending up to the margins, this should also be communicated in details, so that additional resection at the appropriate site is attempted.[40]

Complications

Preoperative hookwire localization is a well-established safe procedure. Complications are rare. These mainly include vasovagal reaction, bleeding, and pain. Unusual complications include hooking of pectoralis muscle and pneumothorax due to entry of the needle into the chest.

Migration of the hookwire after successful placement is an uncommon but serious problem. Risk factors for this include entirely fatty breast, excessive arm movements after the wire placement, and delay in surgery. Hookwire migration can also occur intraoperatively. Surgeon may hold and pull the wire during dissection and wire may come out. The wire may also get cut during dissection. The deeper segment of the wire then gets retracted and lost in the breast. If the surgeon is not familiar with this procedure, he should be cautioned about these complications.

Special Techniques of Localization

Placement of two or more hookwires in the same breast may be required for multiple lesions or to mark the extent of a large lesion (hookwire bracketing) before breast conservation surgery.[41] Stereotactic guidance is generally not preferred for needle localization procedures but this may be required for lesions seen in one view only. Needle localization can be accurately and quickly performed under ultrasound guidance and this modality should be preferred if the lesion is visible on ultrasound. Another advantage of ultrasound-guided needle localization is that it can be performed with anterior approach. Most surgeons prefer anterior approach for dissection. As with mammographic needle localization, postlocalization mammogram and specimen radiography should also be performed after ultrasound-guided localization. MRI-guided hookwire localization is also possible with MR compatible needle-hookwire devices. It is required for the lesions seen on MRI only.

Hematoma-guided localization has also been found useful for breast conservation surgery of nonpalpable breast cancers.[42,43] After a core biopsy, a small hematoma is always formed at the biopsy site. If the biopsy result is malignant and surgery is planned within 4–5 weeks, the small hematoma can be identified with intraoperative ultrasound. This can be used as a guide for dissection, without the need for any preoperative localization procedure. Radioguided occult lesion localization (ROLL) is another technique in which a radioisotope-containing colloid (also used for sentinel lymph node mapping) is injected into the tumor. Tumor is then localized intraoperatively using handheld gamma probe.[44]

Ultrasound-guided Intraoperative Excision

The use of intraoperative ultrasound is a relatively newer use of sonography in breast surgery. Palpable lesions are easy to identify and localize during surgery; however, nonpalpable, deep set, or smaller lesions may require use of ultrasound to objectively guide excision. Ultrasound-guided intraoperative excision helps in achieving tumor-free resection margins with sparing of surrounding healthy parenchyma and thus obtaining an optimum resection volume. It has been found that there is a difference in the adequacy of resection margins by ultrasound and wire localization with the former achieving 89% negative resection margins compared to around 50% in later.[45]

Various studies have shown that the use of ultrasound allows nearly 100% detection of nonpalpable lesions; however, smaller lesions of <5 mm may be missed, especially in obese patients.[46] In patients planned to undergo breast conservation surgery, ultrasound reduces the margin positivity rates and also reduces the reduction of breast volume thus achieving optimum cosmetic outcome.[47] There is also a consequent reduction in the re-excision rates.[48]

Technique

There are three basic techniques employed for ultrasound in intraoperative settings. The *first* involves a continuous use of ultrasound during resection to measure the distance of the resected margin from the ultrasound visualized mass. However, this technique offers some challenges due to fluid and air insinuating in the tissue planes during surgery which may preclude the proper visualization of the mass. Also, when the probe is inserted into the surgical bed, there is compression or displacement of the surrounding structures. The *second* technique involves marking the tumor margins on the skin prior to the resection in the OT. However, in this technique there may be mismatch of the surface markings and the actual tumor location, especially when there is mobilization of the breast during surgery. Moreover, depth measured prior to the surgery may not stay true after the mass is partially resected. The *third* technique involves a use of ultrasound-guided markers in the form of ultrasound contrast agents, visible dye, needle or wires to localize the mass with ultrasound so as to guide the surgeon during the procedure. All techniques include the ex vivo sonography of the resected specimen to ensure optimum margin to tumor distance.

MISCELLANEOUS BREAST INTERVENTIONS

Ductography

Ductography (or galactography) was a commonly performed procedure for evaluation of patients with nipple discharge, as ductal anatomy is not well seen on mammogram. With the advent of high-resolution ultrasound and contrast-enhanced MRI of the breast, ductal evaluation is now possible with reasonable accuracy with these modalities and hence ductography is rarely performed at present.

Indications of ductography include spontaneous solitary duct discharge that is serosanguineous, or bloody. Causes of such duct discharge are papilloma, fibrocystic disease, duct ectasia, and carcinoma.[49] Bilateral nipple discharge or discharge elicited by squeezing only is physiological not requiring ductography.

Ductography should be performed during active discharge. A 27G or 30G ductography cannula is used which is connected to a syringe containing 3–5 mL of nonionic contrast. All air from the cannula, tube and syringe must be removed. The duct is identified with a gentle squeeze and cannulated with gentle probing. The contrast is slowly injected till the patient feels some fullness. Usually, <1 cc of contrast is required. The cannula is then securely taped on the breast and mediolateral and craniocaudal mammographic views are obtained. Additional contrast can be injected if ductal opacification is incomplete.

Ductography demonstrates ductal anatomy of the drainage territory of the cannulated duct **(Fig. 12A)**. The size of the ductal territory is highly variable; this may be a small segment of the breast or it may cover a large area of the breast. Normal ducts show uniform and orderly branching of the ducts with smooth tapering from nipple to periphery. Single or multiple filling defects in the duct are most commonly produced by papillomas **(Fig. 12B)**, sometime by fibrocystic disease, blood clots, air bubbles or rarely by carcinoma. Abrupt cutoff may be produced by papilloma or a carcinoma. Ductal dilatation with abrupt tapering of distal ducts is a characteristic feature of duct ectasia **(Fig. 12C)**. Beaded appearance of the duct with multiple opacified cysts is seen in fibrocystic disease.[50]

Cyst Aspiration

Percutaneous cyst aspiration may be required for analysis of the contents of complex breast cysts. These usually represent inflammatory pathology, and extremely rarely, malignancy. Breast cyst aspiration may also be performed for symptomatic relief of large simple breast cysts. Breast

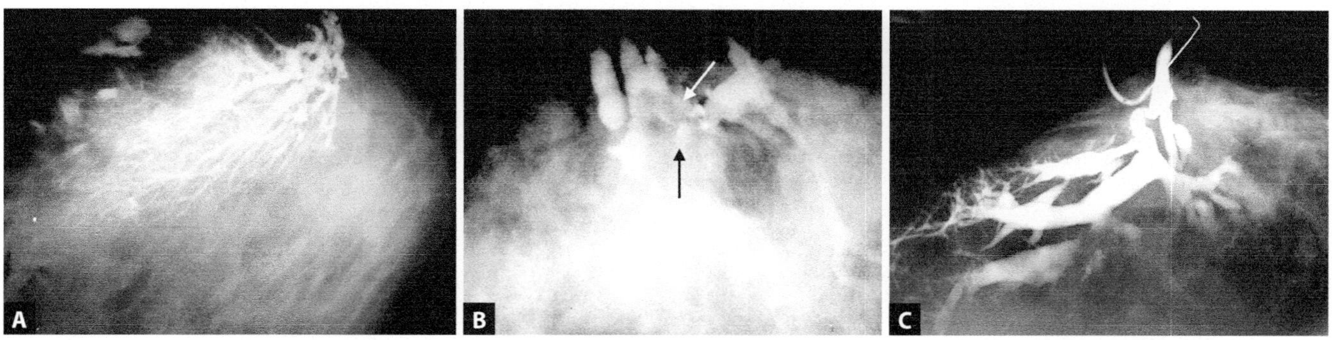

Figs. 12A to C: Ductogram: (A) Normal ductogram shows uniform branching pattern of the nondilated ducts opacified in segment of the breast; (B) Subareolar papilloma is seen as a filling defect (arrows) within a mildly dilated duct; (C) Duct ectasia is seen as moderately dilated ducts with pruning of side branches.

cyst aspiration is best performed under ultrasound guidance using 18G needle **(Fig. 13)**. Complete evacuation of the cyst should be attempted. If the fluid is clear or serous, cytological evaluation is not required.[51] If the fluid is bloody or purulent, it should be sent for cytological examination. Residual solid lesion after cyst aspiration is an indication for biopsy.

Ultrasound-guided Axillary Lymph Node FNAC

All patients with breast cancer require axillary lymph node dissection for sampling and pathological staging of the nodes, irrespective of their clinical nodal status.

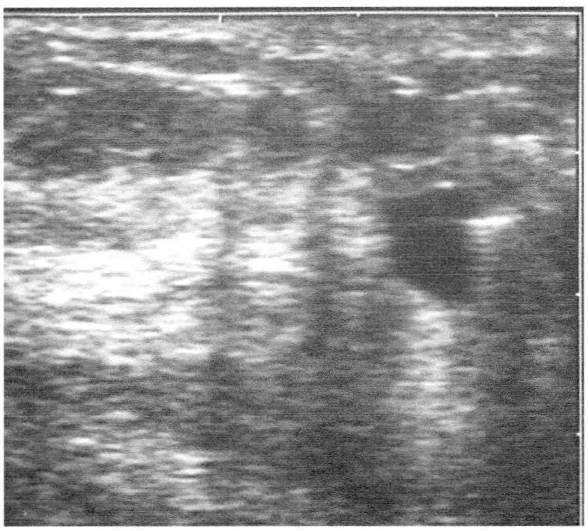

Fig. 13: Ultrasound-guided cyst aspiration. Needle tip is seen within the cyst with accompanied reverberations characteristically seen during cyst aspiration.

However, this procedure is morbid and many of the patients develop shoulder stiffness and lymphedema of the arm subsequently. Sentinel lymph node staging helps to avoid axillary lymph dissection in some of the patients who do not have axillary lymphadenopathy on clinical examination. In this procedure, a dye and radionuclide (99mTc-labeled sulfur colloid) is injected around the tumor. The first node draining the tumor area is localized with scintigraphy probe and excised. If this node is not pathologically involved, distal axillary lymph nodes are considered to be disease free and axillary dissection is avoided. However, the technique of sentinel lymph node staging is cumbersome, time-consuming and expensive.

Ultrasound of axilla in clinically node-negative patients, with ultrasound-guided FNAC of abnormal lymph nodes so detected, is fast gaining acceptance. Patients with confirmed axillary lymph node involvement can then be spared of sentinel lymph node staging and directly taken for axillary lymph node dissection. On ultrasound, size criteria or Doppler evaluation are not useful for identification of abnormal axillary lymph nodes. Lymph nodes of any size with focal or diffuse cortical thickening (>3 mm) or presence of hypoechoic deposits are considered suspicious[52] **(Figs. 14A and B)**. Absence of fatty hilum is also a reliable feature.[53] Abnormal lymph nodes are subjected to ultrasound-guided FNAC. Core biopsy is also done at some centers but FNAC is generally sufficient, as aim is to confirm the presence of malignancy and histological analysis is not essential. Overall, ultrasound-guided FNAC of axillary lymph nodes has high sensitivity and specificity of 80% and 98% respectively for axillary lymph node staging.[54]

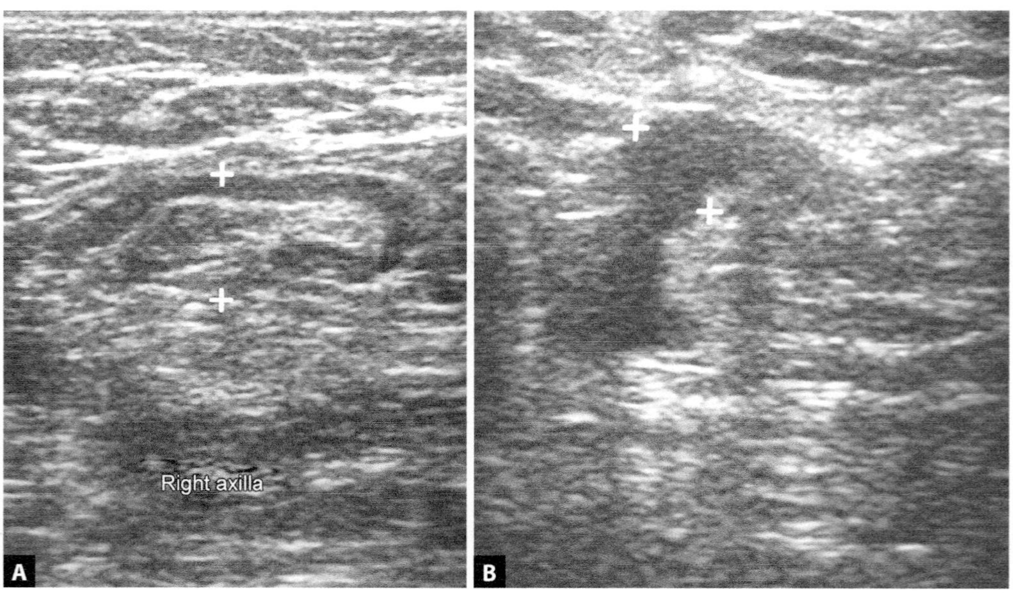

Figs. 14A and B: Ultrasound of axillary lymph nodes: (A) Central echogenic fatty hilum constitutes the most prominent part of a normal axillary lymph node. Peripheral cortex is seen as a thin hypoechoic rim of uniform thickness around the hilum; (B) A metastatic axillary lymph node showing irregular cortical thickening with normal fatty hilum.

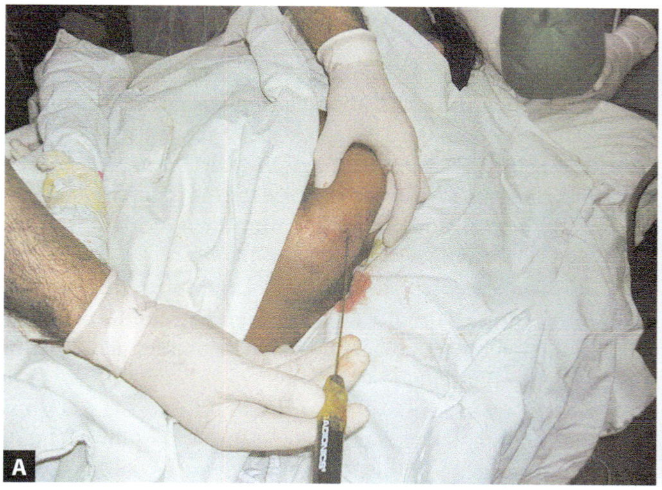

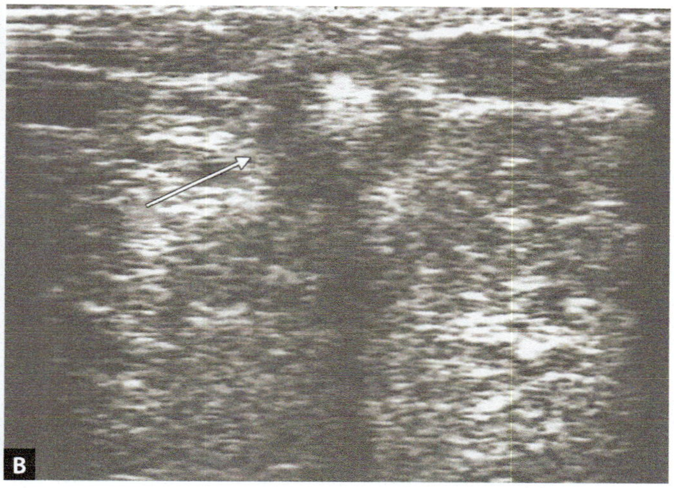

Figs. 15A and B: Breast cancer radiofrequency ablation (RFA): (A) RFA probe is percutaneously inserted into the breast mass using same technique as that for biopsy; (B) An echogenic area forms within the tumor (arrow) as energy is deposited during RFA procedure.

ABLATIVE PROCEDURES FOR BREAST CANCER

There are various image-guided ablative procedures increasingly used in both benign and malignant diseases. There is increasing data regarding potential of using radiofrequency ablation (RFA), cryoablation, high-intensity focused ultrasound (HIFU), laser ablation and electroporation in breast cancers and focal benign diseases like fibroadenoma. These methods are less invasive and give better cosmetic results due to small incision, if any, with reduced time and expenditure of hospitalization. Their role is proving useful especially in small early stage cancers and in poor surgical risk patients. Several studies have reported good pathological tumor ablation in most patients in both benign and malignant breast pathologies.[55,56] RFA seems the most promising modality as complete ablation of tumor and adjacent margin of breast parenchyma can be achieved with it[57-59] **(Figs. 15A and B)**.

Radiofrequency ablation: Similar to tumors throughout body, RFA has been used for breast cancers as well. It involves insertion of a needle electrode in the center of the tumor through which alternating current passes which cause heating and tumor necrosis. Ultrasound is the preferred modality for guidance as RFA may cause artifacts with MRI. Skin burns and injury to the underlying pectoralis muscle may complicate the procedure, especially when the tumor is abutting or invading these structures. Instillation of saline may be performed in such cases to increase the distance between skin/pectoralis and the tumor.

Cryoablation: Cryoablation is the only ablative method available which involves freezing for achieving tumor death instead of heating. It involves insertion of the cryoprobe through the skin under ultrasound/MRI or computed tomography (CT) guidance after a small skin incision. The procedure involves two phases of freezing and intervening thawing and formation of ice ball. The tumor cells are destroyed by means of intracellular ice formation, osmotic dehydration and ischemia followed by an enhanced immunological response by means of release of cytokines and stimulation of cytotoxic lymphocytes. Advantage of the technique is the added anesthetic effect due to freezing; however, the risk of skin injury remains.

Laser ablation: Laser ablation uses a laser light energy delivered to the target tissue by a thin optical wire introduced into the tumor under either ultrasonography (USG), CT or MRI guidance. Skin burn and pneumothorax are potential complications.

Microwave ablation: It uses electromagnetic waves which causes heating of the water molecules, and localized tissue destruction in breast cancer. An advantage of microwave ablation is that the tissue with lower water content like fat and glandular parenchyma of the breast remains unaffected. Complications include skin flap necrosis and skin blistering.

REFERENCES

1. Liberman L, Ernberg LA, Heerdt A, Zakowski MF, Morris EA, LaTrenta LR, et al. Palpable breast masses: is there a role of percutaneous imaging-guided core biopsy? AJR Am J Roentgenol. 2000;175:774-87.
2. Pisano ED, Fajardo LL, Tsimikas J, Sneige N, Frable WJ, Gatsonis CA, et al. Rate of insufficient samples from fine-needle aspiration for nonpalpable breast lesions in an multicenter clinical trial: the Radiologic Diagnostic Oncology Group 5 study. The RDOG5 investigators. Cancer. 1998;82:679-88.
3. Tse MG, Tan PH. Diagnosing breast lesions by fine needle aspiration cytology or core biopsy: which is better? Breast Cancer Res Treat. 2010;123:1-8.

4. Hukinen K, Kiwisaari L, Heikkelis PS, Von Simitten K, Leidenius M. Unsuccessful preoperative fine needle aspiration cytology or core biopsy, lead to increased cost of the diagnostic work-up in breast cancer. Acta Oncol. 2008;47:1037-45.
5. Parker SH, Jobe WE, Dennis MA, Stavros AT, Johnson KK, Yakes WF, et al. US-guided automated large-core breast biopsy. Radiology. 1993;187:507-11.
6. O'Flynn EA, Wilson AR, Michell MJ. Image-guided breast biopsy: state-of-the-art. Clin Radiol. 2010;65:259-70.
7. Burbank F, Parker SH, Fogarty TJ. Stereotactic breast biopsy: improved tissue harvesting with mammotome. Am Surg. 1996;62:738-44.
8. Berg WA, Krebs TL, Campassi C, Magder LS, Sun CC. Evaluation of 14- and 11-gauge directional vacuum-assisted biopsy probes and 14-gauge biopsy guns in a breast parenchymal model. Radiology. 1997;205:203-8.
9. Kettritz U, Rotter K, Schreer I, Murauer M, Schulz-Wendtland R, Peter D, et al. Stereotactic vacuum-assisted breast biopsy in 2,874 patients: a multicenter study. Cancer. 2004;100:245-51.
10. Jackman RJ, Marzoni FA Jr, Rosenberg J. False-negative diagnosis at stereotactic vacuum-assisted needle breast biopsy: long-term follow-up of 1,280 lesions and review of literature. AJR Am J Roentgenol. 2009;192:341-51.
11. Shah VI, Raju U, Chitale D, Deshpande V, Gregory N, Strand V. False-negative core needle biopsies of the breast: an analysis of clinical, radiologic, and pathologic findings in 27 consecutive cases of missed breast cancer. Cancer. 2003;97:1824-31.
12. Cho N, Moon WK, Cha JH, Kim SM, Kim SJ, Lee SH, et al. Sonographically guided core biopsy of the breast: comparison of 14-gauge automated gun and 11-gauge directional vacuum-assisted biopsy methods. Korean J Radiol. 2005;6:102-9.
13. Nadeem R, Chagla LS, Harris O, Desmond S, Thind R, Flavin A, et al. Tumour localisation with a metal coil before administration of neo-adjuvant chemotherapy. Breast. 2005;14:403-7.
14. Oh JL, Nguyen G, Whitman GJ, Hunt KK, Yu TK, Woodward WA, et al. Placement of radiopaque clips for tumor localization in patients undergoing neoadjuvant chemotherapy and breast conservation therapy. Cancer. 2007;110:2420-7.
15. Carpentier E, Maruani A, Michenet P, Bonneau C, Degand P, Lebas P. Can US-guided vacuum-assisted biopsies be an alternative to diagnostic surgery in cases of non-diagnostic core needle biopsy? J Radiol. 2005;86:475-80.
16. Liberman L, Dershaw DD, Rosen PP, Morris EA, Abramson AF, Borgen PI. Percutaneous removal of malignant mammographic lesions at stereotactic vacuum-assisted biopsy. Radiology. 1998;206:711-5.
17. March DE, Coughlin BF, Barham RB, Goulart RA, Klein SV, Bur ME. Breast masses: removal of all US evidence during biopsy by using a handheld vacuum-assisted device—initial experience. Radiology. 2003;227:549-55.
18. Fine RE, Whitworth PW, Kim JA, Harness JK, Boyd BA, Burak WE Jr. Low-risk palpable breast masses removal using a vacuum-assisted hand-held device. Am J Surg. 2003;186:362-7.
19. Thurley P, Evans A, Hamilton L, James J, Wilson R. Patient satisfaction and efficacy of vacuum-assisted excision biopsy of fibroadenomas. Clin Radiol. 2009;64:381-5.
20. LaTrenta LR, Menell JH, Morris EA, Abramson AF, Dershaw DD, Liberman L. Breast lesions detected with MR imaging: utility and histopathologic importance of identification with US. Radiology. 2003;227:856-61.
21. Meissnitzer M, Dershaw DD, Lee CH, Morris EA. Targeted ultrasound of the breast in women with abnormal MRI findings for whom biopsy has been recommended. AJR Am J Roentgenol. 2009;193:1025-9.
22. Hari S, Surabhi V, Chandrashekhara SH. Digital mammography. In: Gupta AK, Garg A, Sandhu S (Eds). Diagnostic Radiology: Recent Advances and Applied Physics in Imaging, 3rd edition. New Delhi, India: Jaypee Brothers Medical Publishers (P) Ltd.; 2019. pp. 279-86.
23. Shin K, Teichgraeber D, Martaindale S, Whitman GJ. Tomosynthesis-guided core biopsy of the breast: why and how to use it. J Clin Imaging Sci. 2018;8:28.
24. Liberman L, Smolkin JH, Dershaw D, Morris EA, Abramson AF, Rosen PP. Calcification retrieval at stereotactic 11-gauge directional vacuum-assisted breast biopsy. Radiology. 1998;208:251-60.
25. Margolin FR, Kaufman L, Jacobs RP, Denny SR, Schrumpf JD. Stereotactic core biopsy of malignant calcifications: diagnostic yield of cores with and without microcalcifications on specimen radiographs. Radiology. 2004;233:251-4.
26. Huber S, Wagner M, Medl M, Czembirek H. Benign breast lesions minimally invasive vacuum-assisted biopsy with 11-gauge needles: patient acceptance and effect on follow-up imaging. Radiology. 2003;226:783-90.
27. Philpotts LE, Hooley RJ, Lee CH. Comparison of automated versus vacuum-assisted biopsy methods for sonographically guided core biopsy of the breast. AJR Am J Roentgenol. 2003;180:347-51.
28. Parker SH, Burbank F, Jackman RJ, Aucreman CJ, Cardenosa G, Cink TM, et al. Percutaneous large-core breast biopsy: a multi-institutional study. Radiology. 1994;193:359-64.
29. Diaz LK, Wiley EL, Venta LA. Are malignant cells displaced by large-gauge needle core biopsy of the breast? AJR Am J Roentgenol. 1999;173:1303-13.
30. Hoorntje LE, Schipper ME, Kaya A, Verkooijen HM, Klinkenbijl JG, Borel Rinkes IH. Tumour cell displacement after 14G breast biopsy. Eur J Surg Oncol. 2004;30:520-5.
31. Lamm RL, Jackman RJ. Mammographic abnormalities caused by percutaneous stereotactic biopsy of histologically benign lesions evident on follow-up mammograms. AJR Am J Roentgenol. 2000;174:753-6.
32. Heywang-Köbrunner SH, Sinnatamby R, Lebeau A, Lebrecht A, Britton PD, Schreer I, et al. Interdisciplinary consensus on the uses and technique of MR-guided vacuum-assisted breast biopsy (VAB): results of a European consensus meeting. Eur J Radiol. 2009;72:289-94.
33. Liberman L, Drotman M, Morris EA, LaTrenta LR, Abramson AF, Zakowski MF, et al. Imaging-histologic discordance at percutaneous breast biopsy. Cancer. 2000;89:2538-46.

34. Ciatto S, Houssami N, Ambrogetti D, Bianchi S, Bonardi R, Brancato B, et al. Accuracy and underestimation of malignancy of breast core needle biopsy: the Florence experience of over 4,000 consecutive biopsies. Breast Cancer Res Treat. 2007;101:291-7.
35. Jackman RJ, Nowels KW, Roderiguez-Soto J, Marzoni FA Jr, Finkelstein SI, Shepard MJ. Stereotactic, automated, large-core needle biopsy of nonpalpable breast lesions: false-negative and histologic underestimation rates after long-term follow-up. Radiology. 1999;210:799-805.
36. Youk JH, Kim EK, Kim MJ, Oh KK. Sonographically guided 14-gauge core needle biopsy of breast masses: a review of 2,420 cases with long-term follow-up. AJR Am J Roentgenol. 2008;190:202-7.
37. Hoorntie LE, Peeters PH, Mali WP, Rinkes IH. Vacuum-assisted breast biopsy: a critical review. Eur J Cancer. 2003;39:1676-83.
38. Jeffries DO, Dossett LA, Jorns JM. Localization for breast surgery: the next generation. Arch Pathol Lab Med. 2017;141(10):1324-9.
39. Mango V, Ha R, Gomberawalla A, Wynn R, Feldman S. Evaluation of the SAVI scout surgical guidance system for localization and excision of nonpalpable breast lesions: a feasibility study. AJR Am J Roentgenol. 2016;207:W69-72.
40. Schaefer FK, Eden I, Schaefer PJ, Peter D, Jonat W, Heller M, et al. Factors associated with one step surgery in case of non-palpable breast cancer. Eur J Radiol. 2007;64(3):426-31.
41. Kirstein LJ, Rafferty E, Specht MC, Moore RH, Taghian AG, Hughes KS, et al. Outcome of multiple wire localization for larger breast cancers: when can mastectomy be avoided? J Am Coll Surg. 2008;207:342-6.
42. Thompson M, Tillman RH, Margulies A, Thostenson J, Bryant-Smith G, Fincher R, et al. Hematoma-directed ultrasound guided (HUG) breast lumpectomy. Ann Surg Oncol. 2007;14:148-56.
43. Arentz C, Baxter K, Boneti C, Henry-Tillman R, Westbrook K, Korourian S, et al. Ten-year experience with hematoma-directed ultrasound-guided breast lumpectomy. Ann Surg Oncol. 2010;17:378-83.
44. Nadeem R, Chagla LS, Harris O, Desmond S, Thind R, Titterrell C, et al. Occult breast lesions: a comparison between radioguided occult lesion localisation (ROLL) vs. wire-guided lumpectomy (WGL). Breast. 2005;14:283-9.
45. Rahusen FD, Bremers AJ, Fabry HF, van Amerongen AH, Boom RP, Meijer S. Ultrasound-guided lumpectomy of nonpalpable breast cancer versus wire-guided resection: a randomized clinical trial. Ann Surg Oncol. 2002;9:994-8.
46. Ngô C, Pollet AG, Laperrelle J, Ackerman G, Gomme S, Thibault F, et al. Intraoperative ultrasound localization of nonpalpable breast cancers. Ann Surg Oncol. 2007;14:2485-9.
47. Fisher CS, Mushawah FA, Cyr AE, Gao F, Margenthaler JA. Ultrasound-guided lumpectomy for palpable breast cancers. Ann Surg Oncol. 2011;18:3198-203.
48. Davis KM, Hsu CH, Bouton ME, Wilhelmson KL, Komenaka IK. Intraoperative ultrasound can decrease the re-excision lumpectomy rate in patients with palpable breast cancers. Am Surg. 2011;77:720-5.
49. Tabar L, Dean PB, Pentek Z. Galactography: the diagnostic procedure of choice for nipple discharge. Radiology. 1983;149:31-8.
50. Bassett LW, Kim CH. Ductography. In: Dershaw DD (Ed). Imaging-Guided Interventional Breast Techniques. New York: Springer-Verlag; 2003. pp. 1-30.
51. Ciatto S, Cariaggi P, Bularisis P. The value of routine cytologic examination of breast cyst fluid. Acta Cytol. 1987;31:301-4.
52. Choi YJ, Ko EY, Han BK, Shin JH, Kang SS, Hahn SY. High-resolution ultrasonographic features of axillary lymph node metastasis in patients with breast cancer. Breast. 2009;18:119-22.
53. Cho N, Moon WK, Han W, Park IA, Cho J, Noh DY. Preoperative sonographic classification of axillary lymph nodes in patients with breast cancer: node-to-node correlation with surgical histology and sentinel node biopsy results. AJR Am J Roentgenol. 2009;193:1731-7.
54. Houssami N, Ciatto S, Turner RM, Cody HS 3rd, Macaskill P. Preoperative ultrasound-guided needle biopsy of axillary nodes in invasive breast cancer: meta-analysis of its accuracy and utility in staging the axilla. Ann Surg. 2011;254:243-51.
55. Manenti G, Bolacchi F, Perretta T, Cossu E, Pistolese CA, Buonomo OC, et al. Small breast cancers: in vivo percutaneous US-guided radiofrequency ablation with dedicated cool-tip radiofrequency system. Radiology. 2009;251:339-46.
56. Zhao Z, Wu F. Minimally invasive thermal ablation of early-stage breast cancer: a systematic review. Eur J Surg Oncol. 2010;36:1149-55.
57. Grotenhuis BA, Vrijland WW, Klem TM. Radiofrequency ablation for early-stage breast cancer: treatment outcomes, and practical considerations. Eur J Surg Oncol. 2013;39(12):1317-24.
58. Mauri G, Sconfienza LM, Pescatori LC, Fedeli MP, Ali M, Di Leo G, et al. Technical success, technique efficacy and complications of minimally-invasive imaging-guided percutaneous ablation procedures of breast cancer: a systematic review and meta-analysis. Eur Radiol. 2017;27(8):3199-210.
59. Zhang W, Zhan-Qiang J, Baikpour M, Li JM, Zhang H, Liang T, et al. Clinical application of ultrasound-guided percutaneous microwave ablation for benign breast lesions: a prospective study. BMC Cancer. 2019;19:345.

CHAPTER

28

Advances in Breast Imaging

Tulika Singh, Veenu Singla, Uma Debi

INTRODUCTION

Among the cancers affecting women in the modern era, breast cancer has been at the forefront. In fact, it accounts for a major chunk of cancer-related mortality among women. Breast imaging plays an important role in screening as well as in diagnosis of breast cancer. In the last decade, many technological advancements have happened in the field of breast imaging. In this chapter, we have reviewed them with their clinical applications.

DIGITAL BREAST TOMOSYNTHESIS

Screen-film mammography (SFM) is being used for diagnostic and screening mammography for >30 years. For the last 10–15 years, it has been replaced by full-field digital mammography (DM) at most of the places.[1] It shows slightly higher sensitivity than SFM, but low density in women with dense breasts remain the limitation of conventional mammography.[2,3] The sensitivity of mammography ranges from about 30 to 48% in women with dense breasts, thus increasing the risk of interval cancer.[4,5] It is attributed mainly to overlapping of tissues which can obscure the breast cancer with similar attenuation as the breast tissue resulting in false-negative cases. In addition, overlapping of normal breast tissue can produce a pseudolesion, i.e., summation artifact resulting into false-positive cases. Digital breast tomosynthesis (DBT) is an emerging modality which can resolve this limitation to some extent. It acquires a series of low-dose projection images and then thin sections are reconstructed from the volumetric data on the workstation.[6] This has shown better sensitivity in various studies.[7,8]

Digital Breast Tomosynthesis Technology

Digital breast tomosynthesis is a mammography-based technology which uses X-rays but forms the image slices of the tissue volume. It has got US Food and Drug Administration (FDA) approval in 2012. These slices can be seen as thin as 1 mm in sharp focus with the tissue above and below out of focus.[9] Acquisition is similar to two-dimensional (2D) mammography and involves compression of the breasts between the compression paddle and the detector. A series of low-dose images is obtained by an X-ray tube head rotating in the arc across the breast from 15 to 50°, each from a different angle **(Fig. 1)**.[10] The time of acquisition varies between 5 and 25 seconds depending on the vendors. The total radiation exposure depends on breast density and thickness, but overall DBT radiation exposure is equivalent to that of SFM or DM. It usually acquires standard mammographic views which are craniocaudal (CC), mediolateral oblique (MLO), and mediolateral. Images can also be acquired with spot compression and implant displacement views. However, magnification view cannot be done with DBT.

The overall number of reconstructed images obtained depends on the thickness of the compressed breast. Images can be reviewed on the special workstation for tomosynthesis which allows the radiologist to scroll through the images. We can also adjust the slice thickness according to the lesion. DBT images are usually acquired in a combination mode which is FDA approved.[11] In a combination mode, DBT and 2D full-field DM are obtained in single breast compression. It acquires DBT first followed by 2D mammography; then 2D and 3D database can be coregistered and the radiologist can shuffle between 2D and 3D database. A synthesized 2D image reconstruction

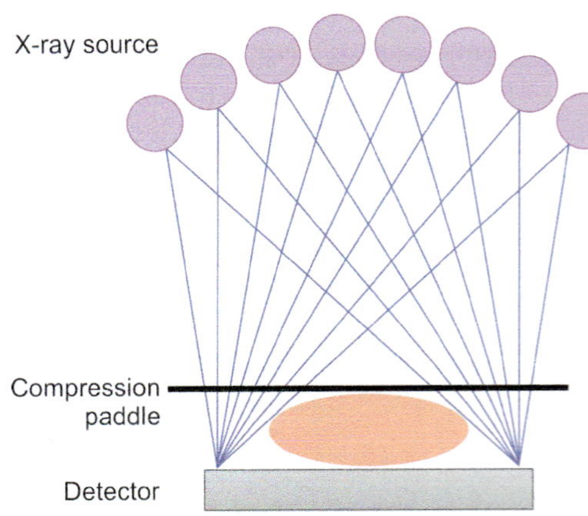

Fig. 1: Pictorial diagram of digital breast tomosynthesis image acquisition showing the X-ray tube movement in an arc, executing multiple sequential low-dose exposures of the compressed breast tissue with a sweep.

algorithm has been recently developed (C-View Hologic) to create a reconstructed 2D image from the volume of the DBT database.[12] It can reduce the patient radiation dose by acquiring only DBT and create a synthesized 2D view without acquiring any additional 2D view. Its performance is comparable to a conventional 2D mammogram in many studies.[13] DBT has demonstrated improved visibility of small invasive breast cancer which is subtle or occult on conventional mammography leading to interval cancer.[14] Mammographic visualization varies for different types of breast cancer. In invasive lobular carcinoma, the tumor growth is nonmass-like and sometimes it is difficult to detect on 2D and is better seen with DBT.[15] Several studies have concluded that DBT can also replace the need of additional compression view which is routinely done in diagnostic mammography. It also reduces the need of second-look ultrasound for better characterization of the lesion. Use of DBT can reduce the number of BI-RADS 3 (Breast Imaging Reporting and Data System 3) in a diagnostic setting by better characterization of breast lesions and changing these lesions into BIRADS 2 or 4.[16]

Digital Breast Tomosynthesis in a Screening Setting

Many studies done on screening with DBT show a decreased recall rate with increased cancer detection. These studies have been done by performing both conventional 2D mammography and DBT which resulted in increase in radiation dose as compared to mammography alone, but it was below the permissible limit.[7] The need of additional 2D mammography along with DBT screening is due to its better visualization of microcalcification which is an important sign of ductal carcinoma in situ (DCIS), for the comparison of previous mammography.

Use of Digital Breast Tomosynthesis in Diagnostic Workup

In clinical practice, DBT is generally used for the assessment of noncalcified lesions. Evaluation of calcification on DBT is limited; it may depict only a limited number of calcification with poor characterization.

Architectural distortion: Architectural distortion is a subtle finding better seen on DBT which is difficult to visualize on conventional imaging. It is a common manifestation of cancer. Architectural distortion on DBT shows a higher percentage of invasive lobular carcinoma (20%).[14] DBT also gives better visualization of radial scar; which are seen as a radiating lines converging to a point **(Figs. 2A and B)**. DBT is especially helpful in detection of suspected distortion at the fat–glandular interface and apex of the breast where summation shadows are frequent.

Focal asymmetry: Focal asymmetry is called when a small abnormal area of the fibroglandular density is seen in a similar shape in both views of a mammogram. The recent BI-RADS lexicon uses the term "asymmetry" when the finding is seen only in one view and is unilateral. DBT can be used to differentiate true asymmetry from the superimposed fibroglandular tissue or it can reclassify into a mass **(Figs. 3A and B)**. It has shown higher sensitivity (93%) in better characterization of focal asymmetry than the spot compression imaging (50%).[17]

Masses: Masses are described in terms of shape, margin, and density. These features are better visualized on DBT and a radiologist can give a better and accurate degree of suspicion of masses **(Figs. 4A and B)**. Use of an irregular shape descriptor is reduced with DBT, and the shape of masses is usually recategorized as round or

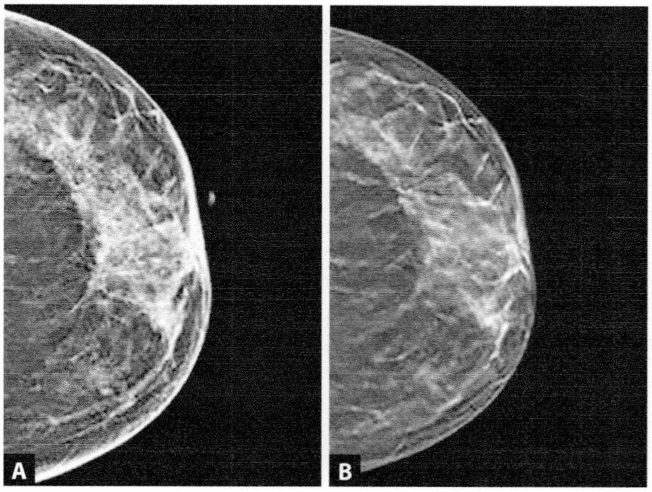

Figs. 2A and B: Better visualization of architectural distortion on digital breast tomosynthesis (DBT) (B) as compared to a 2D craniocaudal view (A). DBT image shows a multiple line radiating from a point in the lateral breast which is a suspicious finding. On stereotactic biopsy, it came out to be radial scar without atypia.

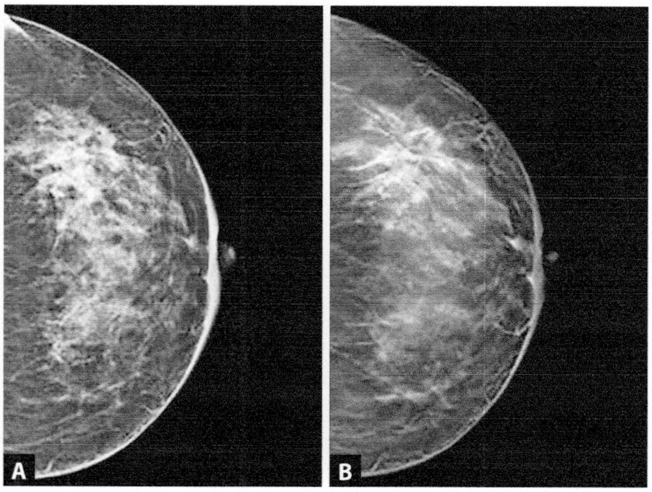

Figs. 3A and B: Better evaluation of focal asymmetry. 2D craniocaudal view (A) showing a focal asymmetry which on digital breast tomosynthesis image (B) shows well-defined mass with spiculated margins. Biopsy showed invasive ductal carcinoma.

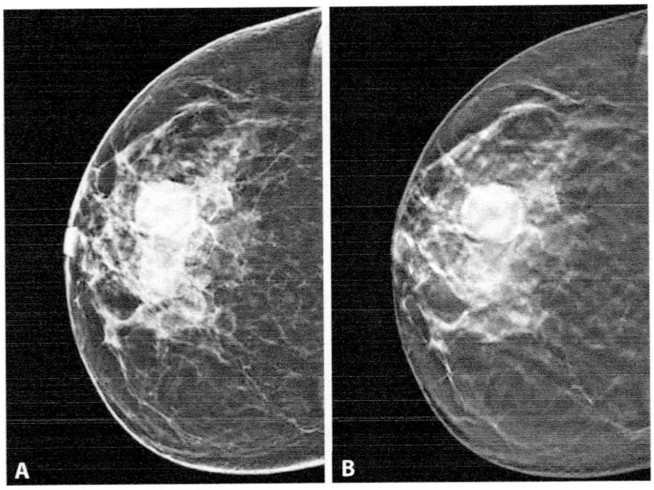

Figs. 4A and B: Improved visualization of mass shape and margins. (A) Right craniocaudal 2D image shows equal-density mass with obscured margins in the central breast; (B) Digital breast tomosynthesis image shows well-defined, round, equal-density mass with well-circumscribed margins. Biopsy showed fibroadenoma.

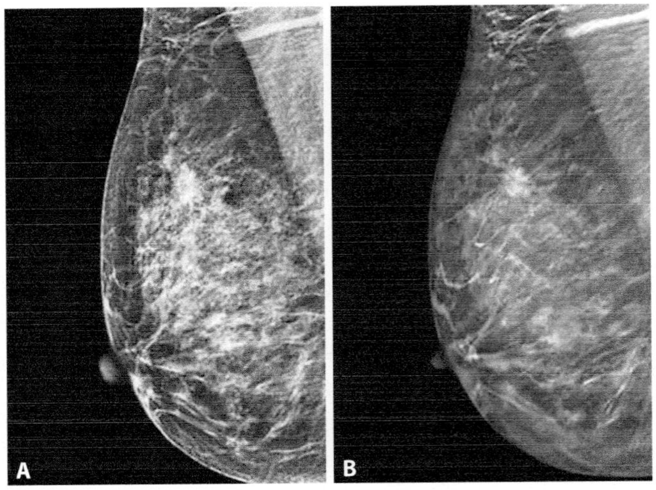

Figs. 5A and B: Improved visualization of mass margins. (A) Right mediolateral oblique 2D image shows high-density mass with indistinct margins in the upper breast; (B) Digital breast tomosynthesis image shows irregular mass with spiculated margins. Biopsy demonstrated invasive ductal carcinoma.

oval, specially in benign masses.[18] Margins of malignant masses are also better seen on DBT with improved details **(Figs. 5A and B)**. DBT is also useful in differentiation of spiculated and indistinct margins, which is difficult with 2D mammography. Associated architectural distortion is also better seen on DBT. Overall improved details result in an increase in degree of suspicion of malignant masses. Although the shape and margin of masses are better seen with DBT, the density of the mass is better appreciated on 2D mammography. Masses which are of high density on 2D mammography usually show lower density on 1-mm thin sections of DBT.

The overall need of spot compression decreases with DBT. It gives more patient satisfaction and is time-saving without any loss of diagnostic details for noncalcified lesions. Visualization of microcalcification is variable on DBT[19] and it needs dedicated magnification views for characterization which is currently recommended for microcalcification. However, if we adjust the slab thickness, we can evaluate the distribution of calcification better.

The drawbacks of DBT include radiation dose, cost, and workflow. The radiation dose is twice that of conventional DM, if we combine 2D mammography and DBT. Although it is less than the permitted limit, for screening population it may be of little concern. With the development of synthesized reconstructed 2D images which are made from a DBT volume dataset, we can eliminate the 2D mammography and reduce the radiation dose. The other limitation of DBT is the longer interpretation time for mammography plus DBT images as DBT can have 200 or more images. But it is compensated by decreasing the recall rate and additional views.[16] The cost of the DBT system is also higher than the cost of the 2D mammography system and with DBT there is additional expense of large storage space for large file size of DBT.

CONTRAST-ENHANCED MAMMOGRAPHY

Contrast-enhanced mammography (CEM) is an emerging imaging modality which combines intravenous (IV) contrast administration and DM. It utilizes the principle of dual-energy X-ray, also called contrast-enhanced dual-energy mammography (CEDM). CEM got FDA approval in 2011 as an adjunct to mammography. With the advanced full-field DM units, it can perform low-energy tomosynthesis in the same compression. Breast cancer is diagnosed on CEM by density, morphology, and neovascularity associated with malignancy.[20,21]

Contrast-enhanced Mammography Acquisition and Image Analysis

Contrast-enhanced mammography is done by using a standard DM system which is upgraded with a copper filter and special software to perform dual-energy scan.

For CEM, a nonionic iodinated contrast agent is first injected intravenously at 1.5 mL/kg at a rate of 3 mL/s. After 2 minutes of contrast injection, standard two-view mammography is performed. MLO and CC views using dual energy technique. In dual energy, low-energy imaging is done at kilovoltage which is below the K-edge of iodine (33.2 keV). In this image, no iodine is visualized and it appears similar to conventional digital 2D mammography with the same diagnostic performance.[22,23] High-energy

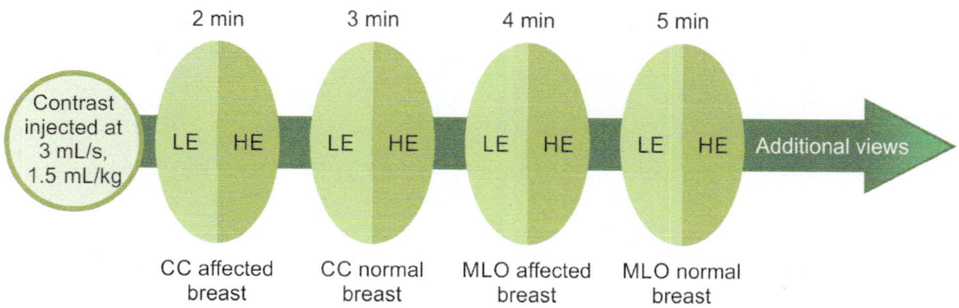

Fig. 6: Standard protocol of performing contrast-enhanced mammography. Low-energy (LE) images followed by high-energy (HE) images are taken for each view (CC: craniocaudal; MLO: mediolateral oblique).

imaging is acquired at above the K-edge of iodine, and it shows contrast agent uptake with other diagnostic information. The total duration of examination is around 5–6 minutes. Dual-energy images can be acquired up to 10 minutes after the contrast injection, if any extra view is required **(Fig. 6)**. These dual-energy images are subsequently postprocessed and the reconstructed image is formed which shows highlighted areas of contrast enhancement with suppression of background breast tissue densities. Both recombined and low-energy images are used for diagnostic evaluation. Additional spot compression and magnification views can be done after CEM, if needed. These can be done without the dual-energy technique.[24] Any abnormality found on a recombined image should be correlated with a low-energy image; if no correlate is identified on the low-energy image, additional ultrasound or magnetic resonance imaging (MRI) should be performed.

At present, there is no CEM-specific BI-RADS lexicon for image interpretation. Currently, mammography BI-RADS descriptors are used for low-energy images and MRI BI-RADS descriptors are used for evaluation of recombined images.[25,26]

Contrast-enhanced Mammography in Screening

The utility of CEM for breast cancer screening is being studied, but only limited data is available. Mammography is the first and best imaging modality for breast cancer screening, although its sensitivity is low in women with dense breast.[27] In these women, ultrasound is commonly used for additional screening. Women with a high risk of breast cancer were screened with supplemental MRI.[28] Doing MRI for these women is a challenge as MRI is expensive with long examination time and its lack of availability to all patients. Few studies have been done to evaluate the performance of CEM as an alternative to MRI in these patients. A study by Jochelson et al., which included 307 high-risk women for comparison of CEM and MRI, found that CEM and MRI are comparable with specificity of 94.1% and 94.7%, respectively.[29] These studies are preliminary, and more studies are needed to validate.

Diagnostic Performance of Contrast-enhanced Mammography

Breast Mass

CEM can be used for diagnostic workup of a palpable lump or a lesion found on imaging is diagnostic mammography. A retrospective study by Lalji et al., evaluated patients with breast lump in screening recall with mammography and CEM and found sensitivity of 97% and specificity of 70%.[22]

There are few studies that have compared the CEM with mammography and ultrasound in the setting of newly diagnosed cancer. CEM does not provide additional information in characterization of masses except the enhancement. However, it helps in identifying any additional lesion in breast **(Figs. 7A and B)**.[30]

Architectural Distortion

Architectural distortion is difficult to distinguish in mammography. It can be due to a benign or malignant cause and biopsy is the standard care as its chances of being malignant are as high as 50–70%.[31] In a study done with MRI, absence of enhancement with architectural distortion is more reliable on benign etiology.[32] Both CEM and MRI help differentiate the benign from the malignant cause of architectural distortion. Patel et al., conducted CEM in patients with architectural distortion and subsequent biopsy was performed in these patients, and 97% of patients who showed enhancement on CEM had malignancy.[33] CEM has high sensitivity and negative predictive values (NPV). It is useful to evaluate subtle architectural distortions detected on screening mammography which are not reproducible. If these do not show enhancement on CEM, then biopsy can be avoided.

Microcalcification

The most common cause of recall in screening mammography is microcalcification. Risk assessment of microcalcification is done by BI-RADS descriptors. Morphology of microcalcification can be well evaluated with the low-energy images in CEM and the recombined

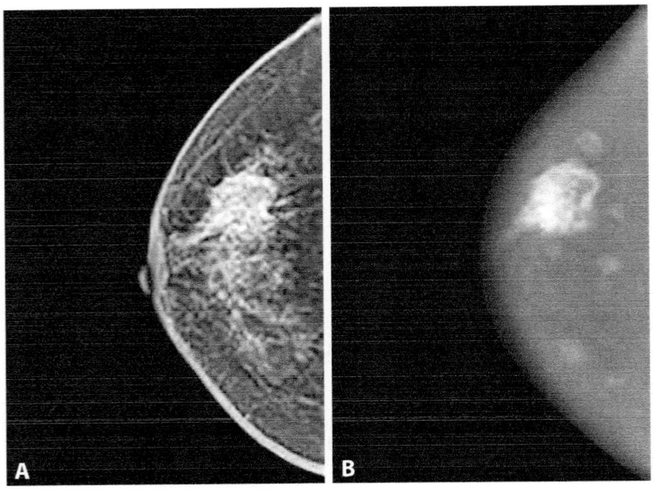

Figs. 7A and B: (A) Conventional craniocaudal view of right breast showing heterogeneously dense breast tissue suspicious of breast mass; (B) Contrast-enhanced subtracted image: Intensely enhancing right upper outer quadrant mass with multiple additional enhancing small masses in the same and other quadrants—s/o multicentric carcinoma right breast.
Source: Dr Rashmi Sudhir. Senior Consultant Radiologist, Indo American Cancer Hospital and Research Centre.

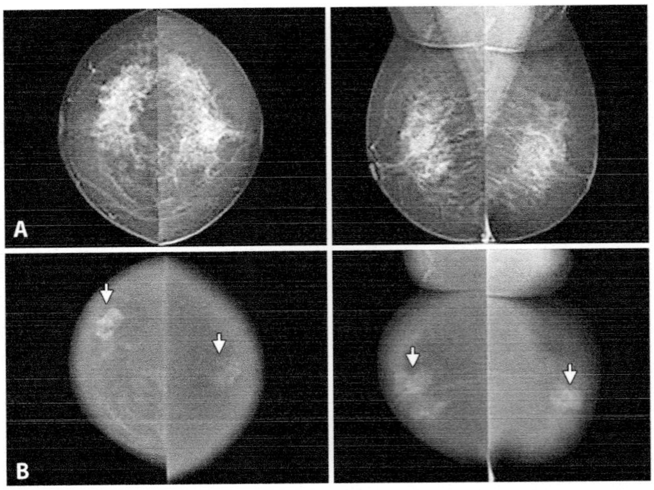

Figs. 8A and B: (A) Conventional mammogram shows heterogeneous dense breast tissue [American College of Radiology (ACR) category C] with asymmetric density and architectural distortion in retroareolar and upper outer quadrant of right breast. No definite mass lesion is seen in the left breast; (B) Contrast-enhanced subtracted mammogram shows enhancing mass lesions in bilateral breast (arrows).
Source: Dr Rashmi Sudhir. Senior Consultant Radiologist, Indo American Cancer Hospital and Research Centre.

images can show any associated enhancement. Many studies have been done to evaluate the role of CEM in a setting of microcalcification but they have shown mixed results. The overall results from these studies suggest that the presence of enhancement can suggest malignancy, but lack of enhancement cannot rule out malignancy. Suspicious calcification has to be biopsied. So, the role of CEM in the microcalcification is debatable and more studies are needed to evaluate this application.

Contrast-enhanced Mammography as an Alternative to Magnetic Resonance Imaging

With its comparable performance to show tumor enhancement, CEM can be used as an alternative to MRI evaluate the disease extent for the local staging. It can show a satellite lesion in ipsilateral or contralateral breast **(Figs. 8A and B)**. Many studies showed comparable performance and sensitivity for evaluating the disease extent in newly diagnosed breast cancer with satisfactory size correlation.[34,35] It can also be used as an alternative to MRI to evaluate the response assessment after neoadjuvant chemotherapy which is current practice for evaluating response. Multiple studies have been done to evaluate comparison of these two modalities in response assessment. Iotti et al., evaluated CEM and MRI before, during, and after neoadjuvant chemotherapy in patients of breast cancer.[36] CEM shows pathological complete response to treatment better than MRI.

Contrast-enhanced mammography may be used as an alternative to MRI to evaluate the disease extent and the chemotherapy response. It is especially useful in those places where MRI is not easily available. It is easy to upgrade the standard mammography machine with CEM and it costs less than MRI.

AUTOMATED BREAST VOLUME SCAN

Automated breast volume scan (ABVS) has recently developed for breast imaging and got FDA approval in 2012. These scanners are mainly developed to overcome few limitations of doing conventional handheld ultrasound for adjunct screening for women with dense breast on mammography. Although handheld ultrasound is the gold standard for breast ultrasound, the major limitation is that it is user dependent. In ABVS, continuous acquisition of B-mode pictures is done from which data is extrapolated and subsequent three-dimensional (3D) reconstruction of breast volume is done. Another advantage is that this data can be shared and analyzed separately by a specialist.[37]

Automated breast volume scan devices utilize wide linear-array transducers and making 3D imaging of whole breast volume possible.

A literature review comparing handheld ultrasound vis-a-vis ABVS has shown that although both these techniques allow detection of early breast cancer which are not detected on mammography, they tend to increase the false-positive recall rates. Screening programs utilizing mammography have mainly been successful due to their ability to detect breast cancer at an early stage albeit their sensitivity falls to as low as 61% in women with dense breasts, thus leading to an increase in the number of interval cancers in women with dense breasts. Small cancers are notorious in that they are silhouetted by normal glandular tissue reducing their rate of detection. Prospective trials in recent times have highlighted the ability of handheld ultrasound in the detection of early stage invasive breast cancer in apparently normal women with dense breasts which are not picked up on mammography.[38]

Optimum visualization using the ABVS system requires acquisition of minimum two, on an average three, consecutive B-mode ultrasound volumes per breast using high-frequency linear array transducers. The transducer utilizes a mechanical arm that automatically acquires in excess of 300 sections with the minimum thickness of 0.5 mm/volume. The technician is thus given the luxury of imaging the area of the breast between the midsternal line and the midaxillary line as a consequence of obtaining overlapping volumes.

Anteroposterior acquisition involves placement of nipple at the center of the ABVS image. Although lateral acquisition has some similarities with the anteroposterior acquisition, it involves placing the transducer in such a way that the lateral boundary of the transducer is kept in line with the midaxillary line so that the lateral part of breast sections can be imaged.

Water-based media need to be applied to the whole breast in order to prevent the air contact artifact. The patient should be instructed to breathe superficially and not to talk during ABVS acquisitions.

Automated breast volume scan acquisitions require a good workstation which can reconstruct the transverse images obtained to coronal and sagittal ones. These are subsequently displayed and interpreted using a multiplanar hanging protocol under appropriate conditions. Reporting of ABVS examinations generally requires 3–5 minutes for a normal case. The diagnostic accuracy and interpretation of ABVS are similar to those of handheld ultrasound.

Supplemental ABVS screening shows increased detection of small early stage invasive cancer specially in dense breast as compared to mammography alone. Detection of DCIS with ABVS is difficult, and this is the main cause for false-negative results in screening with ABVS. False-positive results on ABVS are mainly due to artifacts by Cooper's ligament and presence of a large number of benign lesions in healthy women.

The diagnostic performance of ABVS is comparable with handheld ultrasound. The commonly seen benign lesions on ABVS are cysts and fibroadenomas **(Fig. 9)**. It also beautifully depicts the intraductal papillary lesion **(Fig. 10)**. The other benign lesion is a complex sclerosing lesion which may raise suspicion of malignancy as it shows a retraction pattern on coronal ABVS images making it difficult to differentiate from malignancy.

The characteristics of a malignant lesion are the same as in handheld ultrasound. But a specific descriptor of the malignant mass on ABVS is the retraction phenomenon **(Fig. 11)**, commonly seen in breast cancer as stellate pattern around the mass likely a result of desmoplastic reaction in the surrounding tissue.[39] It is more common in low-profile indolent cancer and is usually not seen with fast-growing cancer like high-grade triple negative cancer.[40] ABVS is a novel technique that allows the whole breast ultrasound to be done by a technician in a standard way. The radiologist can read the images on the workstation and they are reproducible. It is useful as a supplemental screening tool for breast cancer in women with dense breast, and its diagnostic performance is comparable with

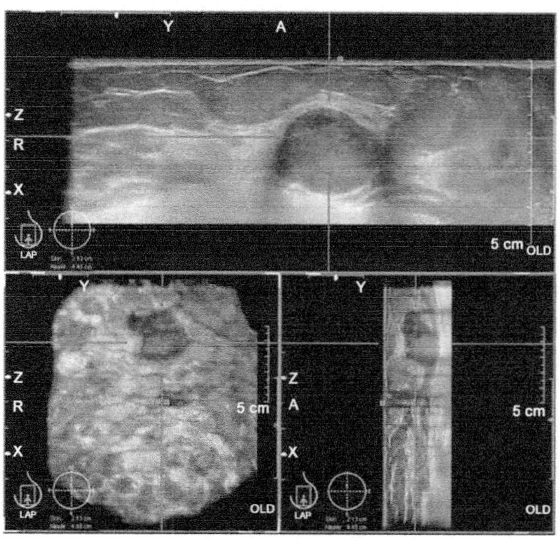

Fig. 9: Well-circumscribed iso- to hypoechoic mass with smooth margin at 12 o'clock position of left breast showing posterior acoustic enhancement by automated breast volume scan in three orthogonal planes. Biopsy showed fibroadenoma.

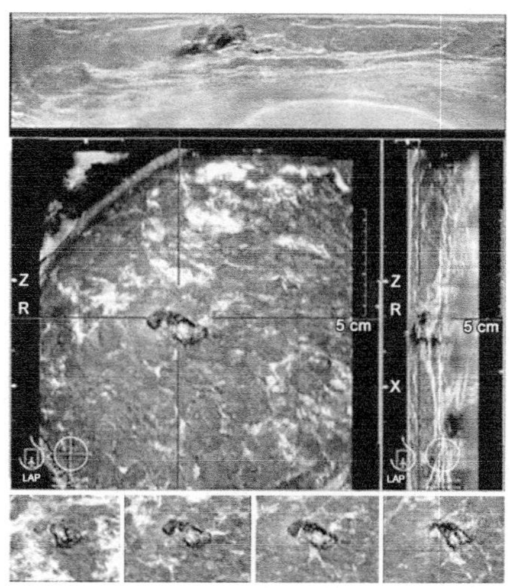

Fig. 10: Automated breast volume scan (ABVS) image showing a dilated duct at 10 o'clock position in the periareolar region reaching up to the nipple with an intraluminal polypoidal lesion. The course of the duct is better visualized in the coronal plane images of ABVS. (Biopsy showed intraductal papilloma).

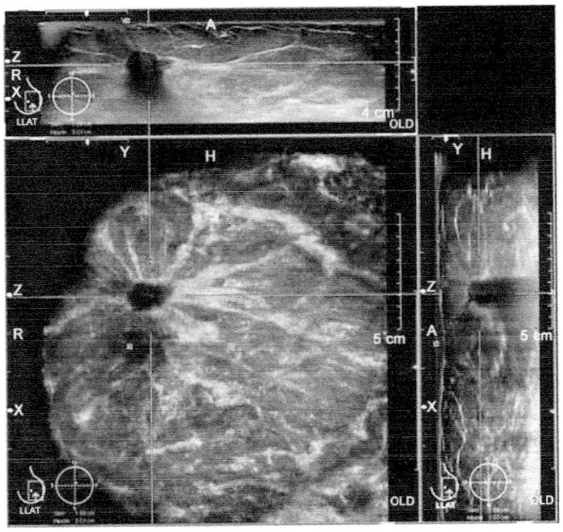

Fig. 11: Retraction phenomenon seen as converging bands of hyper- and hypoechogenicity in the coronal plane images of automated breast volume scan in a case of infiltrating ductal carcinoma.

conventional handheld ultrasound. There is a learning curve for the technologist as well as the radiologist for both acquisition and interpretation of ABVS images.

BREAST ELASTOGRAPHY

Elastography derives the information about the stiffness of the lesion under evaluation. It is a known fact that the malignant breast masses are harder than the adjoining normal breast parenchyma or any benign lesions, due to their desmoplastic reaction. The evaluation of breast masses to differentiate a benign lesion from a malignant one is one of the initial applications of the ultrasound elastography.[41] The evaluation of the stiffness has the same principle of that of conventional clinical examination just like palpation of any breast lump. Early works done in this area in 1997 showed that cancer generally appeared stiffer (darker) than a benign lesion and surrounding normal breast tissue on elastography.[42]

After that, many studies supported that when elastography is used as an adjunct to gray-scale ultrasonography, it can help a radiologist to give a more appropriate category of BI-RADS classification. Recently, elasticity of the breast masses was included as an associated feature in the 5th edition of BI-RADS ultrasound lexicon. Two most commonly used elastography techniques in breast are strain elastography and shear-wave elastography. This classification of elastography is based on the type of excitation for a region of interest (ROI) and measurement of induced disturbance. When this disturbance is measured as displacement in the field of view, it is called strain elastography. When it is measured as the velocity of an induced shear wave, it is called shear-wave elastography.[43,44]

Strain Elastography

Strain elastography utilizes different parameters to differentiate benign and malignant breast masses. The commonly used parameter is elasticity score (Tsukuba score).[45] It is a proposed scoring system for the lesions on color maps which is based upon the elastographic properties of the tissue (For details refer to Ultrasound Elastography chapter in Recent Advances and Applied Physics book).

When the elastography score cutoff point was taken between 3 and 4 for the malignant masses, it showed 86.5% sensitivity, 89.8% specificity, and 88.3% accuracy in the initial study.[45] This gives information about the strain at a given location in tissues, although the mechanical properties of the surrounding influence it. Another disadvantage is that it is not quantitative.[46] Therefore, other semiquantitative methods have been developed; one of them is the distance ratio in which the size of the lesion measured on elastogram is divided by the lesion size on gray-scale ultrasonography. It is noted that malignant masses almost invariably appeared larger on elastography due to stromal response to breast cancer. Distance ratio cutoffs >1 as malignant and <1 as benign show sensitivity and specificity (100% and 95%) in differentiating malignant from benign breast masses.[47] Other methods of semiquantitative assessment are the strain ratio of the nodule to the adjoining normal breast tissue for the differentiation of the benign verses malignant masses **(Fig. 12)**.[48]

Shear-wave Elastography

Shear-wave elastography gives information linked to the local elastic properties of the tissue, with a quantitative approach to elasticity values.[49] The interpretation and measurement of elasticity is done in terms of Young's modulus (in kilopascals, kPa). It is evaluated either as a single value in a small ROI or can be taken for each point in box (FOV) displayed as a color map **(Fig. 13)**.[50] On a color map, the scale ranges from 0 kPa (dark blue-soft) to 180 kPa (red-hard) for breast masses.[51] It is reported that mean elasticity values are significantly higher in malignant masses (153.3 ± 58.1 kPa) than in benign masses (46.1 ± 42.9 kPa).

With these methods, elastography can help in upgrading a mass of low suspicion, BI-RADS 3 which would be sent for biopsy otherwise or in downstaging a mass which is classified as BI-RADS 4A, when used as an adjunct to gray-scale ultrasound.[52]

Recently, elastography is also being used for the assessment of neoadjuvant chemotherapy response. Breast cancers stiff on strain elastography were less likely to have a pathological complete response after neoadjuvant chemotherapy than cancers which were soft on elastography **(Figs. 14A to C)**.[53]

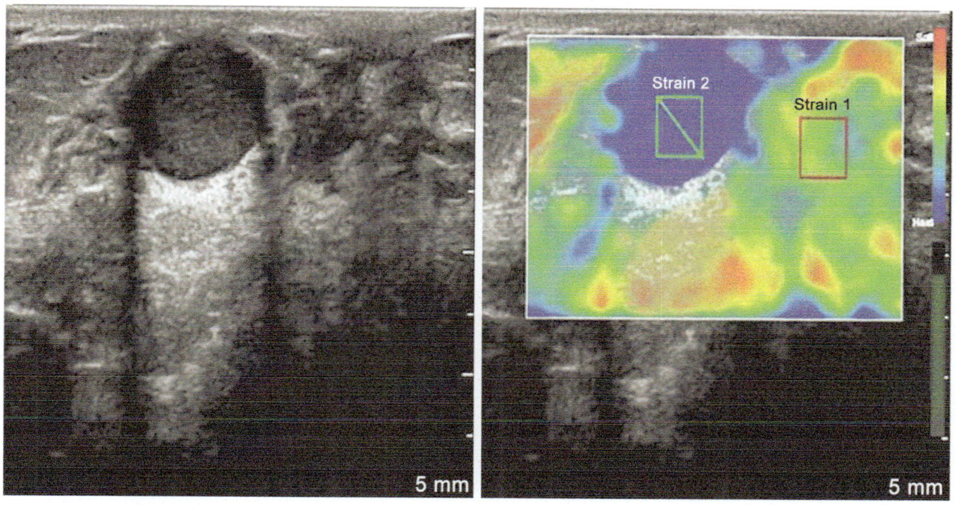

Fig. 12: Strain elastography image showing blue color in the lesion as well as in the surrounding parenchyma suggestive of malignancy. It is also showing a strain ratio of 4.5 between the lesion and the normal breast parenchyma which is highly suggestive of malignancy. Biopsy showed infiltrating ductal carcinoma.

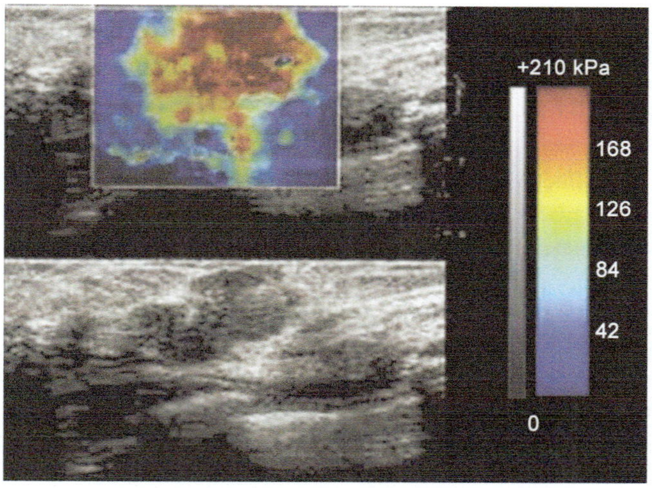

Fig. 13: On shear-wave elastography, image breast mass is showing red color suggestive of hard mass, with mean elasticity 210 kPa suggestive of malignancy. Biopsy showed invasive ductal carcinoma.

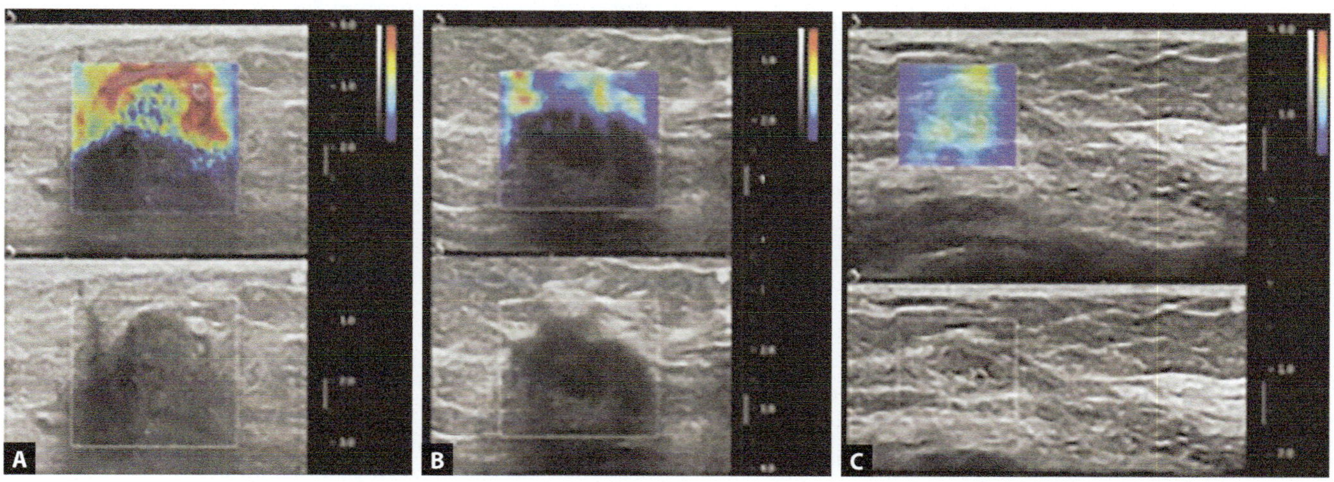

Figs. 14A to C: Change in mean elasticity after two cycles of neoadjuvant chemotherapy in a responder patient. (A and B) Elasticity measurements prechemotherapy and after two cycles, respectively. On completion of chemotherapy (C) the mass is faintly visible with marked reduction in elasticity.

Few studies show correlation between histological types of breast cancer with elastography features, but it is still an area of research and needs more studies for validation.

There are few limitations for the elastography of the breast masses. It is difficult to characterize complex masses with mixed solid and cystic components. Some benign masses such as hyalinized fibroadenoma and fat necrosis with fibrosis can also be stiff and some mucinous carcinoma can be soft. Posterior breast masses are difficult to assess with strain elastography.[54]

CONTRAST-ENHANCED ULTRASOUND

The role of contrast-enhanced ultrasound (CEUS) has been studied in the imaging of focal hepatic tumor, renal tumor, and gallbladder masses. Angiogenesis is the basic physiologic change which is growth of new microvessels, and it is essential for tumor growth and its prognostication. Color Doppler is commonly used for evaluation of vascularity on ultrasound in soft-tissue masses, but its role in detecting low flow and small vessels is limited. This limitation can be overcome by adding microbubble contrast agents along with specialized software. It enhances the signal of blood flow with suppression of intrinsic tissue signals making it as effective as MRI for the evaluation of soft-tissue masses.[55] CEUS was first utilized for the evaluation of the breast masses in the early 1990s. Early studies were focused on the enhancement pattern for the differential diagnosis of the breast lesions. Over the last decade, CEUS with quantitative and qualitative analysis studies has been developed for the breast masses for differentiating benign and malignant lesions.

Ultrasound Contrast Agent and Basic Principles

Ultrasound contrast agents are gas-filled microbubbles with phospholipid covering. The size of the microbubbles is <7 m to pass through capillaries. There are two generations of an ultrasound contrast agent depending on the type of gas in microbubbles. The first generation has air covered by a galactose shell. These agents undergo early destruction. The second-generation agents contain sulfur hexafluoride gas with a phospholipid shell on outside. These agents stay longer and can be used for continuous imaging. It is injected intravenously and it acts like a blood-pool contrast agent and improves the detection of blood flow. It causes an acoustic impedance difference causing ultrasound signal backscattering and vascular enhancement on the ultrasound images. It increases echoes from blood 500–1,000 times. Previous CEUS studies used Doppler flow signals to visualize the microbubbles but they were associated with many artifacts. Now with contrast-specific nonlinear harmonic imaging, pulse sequences are used to actually separate nonlinear microbubble signals at the second harmonic and suppress the linear tissue signals from the surrounding stationary tissues.[56] Ultrasound contrast agents are excreted via breathing and through liver. No renal excretion makes it valuable in patients with kidney disease.[55]

Contrast-enhanced Ultrasound Acquisition and Evaluation

For contrast-enhanced imaging, 2–4 mL of an ultrasound contrast agent is injected in a peripheral vein in a bolus followed by 5–10 mL of saline flush. Continuous imaging is done just after the injection for 2–3 minutes and video clips are stored. Acquired clips can be analyzed on a qualitative or quantitative basis. Qualitative analysis of breast masses includes the following features:

- Lesion enhancement as compared to the surrounding parenchyma. There can be hyperenhancement, isoenhancement, or hypoenhancement.
- *Internal homogeneity*: It can be homogeneous enhancement or heterogeneous enhancement.
- *Enhancement direction*: It can be centripetal or centrifugal.
- *Perfusion defect*: It can be present or absent.
- Presence or absence of radially penetrating vessels.[57]

Benign masses usually show slow wash-in with homogeneous and centrifugal enhancement with clear margins and the size will be equal to or less than the size on the 2D gray-scale images **(Figs. 15A to C)**. No perfusion defect will be seen. Malignant masses will show hyperenhancement with centripetal perfusion, irregular shape, and perfusion defects **(Figs. 16 and 17)**. The size will appear larger than the size on a 2D gray-scale image. Penetrating vessels can be seen **(Fig. 18)**. This is because malignant masses show abnormally

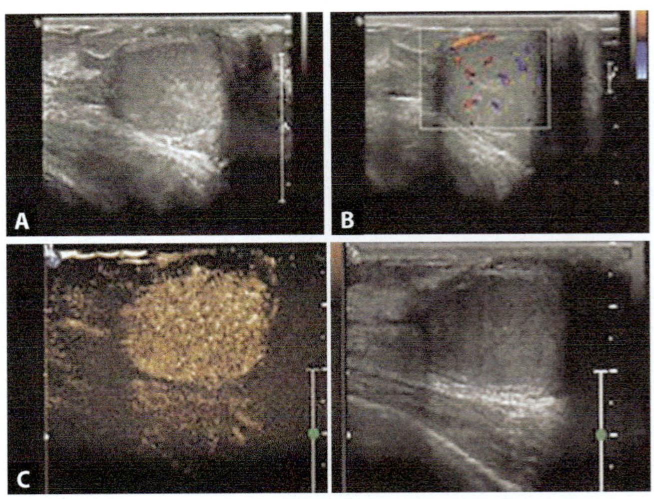

Figs. 15A to C: (A) Gray-scale ultrasound shows oval circumscribed isoechoic mass in parallel orientation; (B) Color Doppler shows significant internal vascularity; (C) Contrast-enhanced ultrasound shows well-defined hyperenhancing mass with uniform postcontrast appearance with a regular shape and no enlargement of diameter. Biopsy showed fibroadenoma.

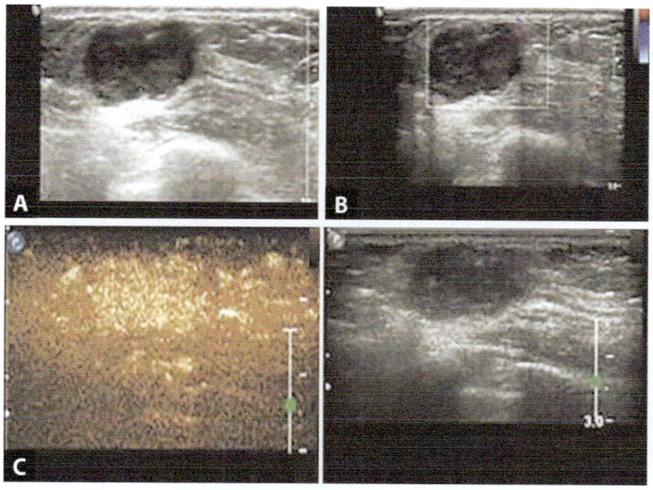

Figs. 16A to C: (A) Gray-scale ultrasound shows hypoechoic mass with a microlobulated outline in parallel orientation; (B) Color Doppler shows mild internal vascularity; (C) Contrast-enhanced ultrasound shows poorly defined hyperenhancing mass with irregular margins. Biopsy demonstrated invasive ductal carcinoma.

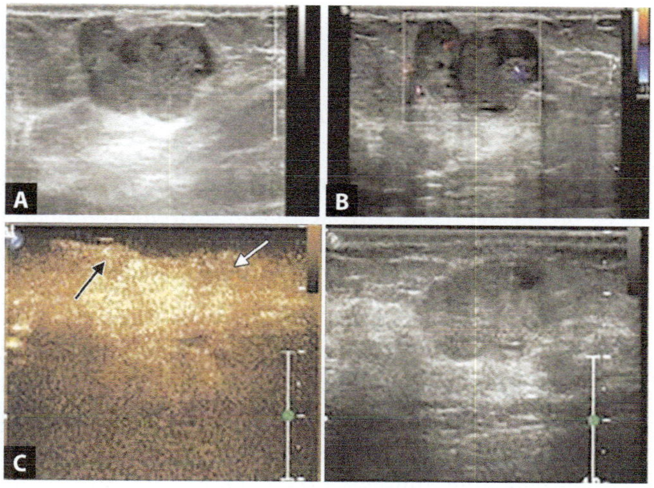

Figs. 17A to C: (A) Gray-scale ultrasound shows heterogeneously hypoechoic mass with a microlobulated outline in parallel orientation; (B) Color Doppler shows internal vascularity and surrounding vessel; (C) Contrast-enhanced ultrasound shows poorly defined heterogeneously hyperenhancing mass areas of perfusion defect within (white arrow) and surrounding vessel (black arrow). Biopsy showed intraductal carcinoma.

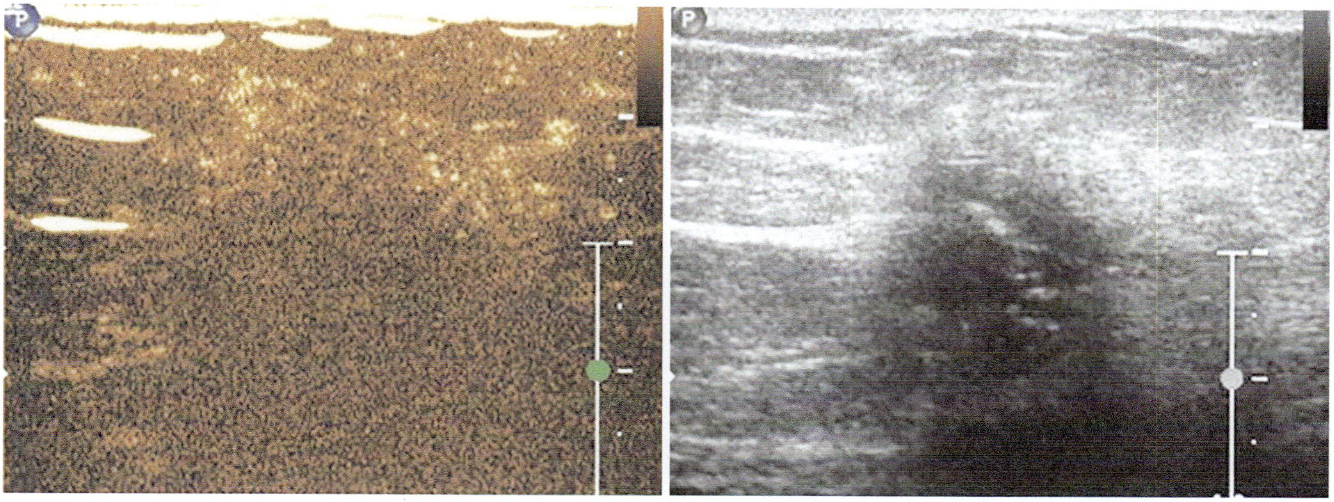

Fig. 18: Contrast-enhanced ultrasound shows poorly defined heterogeneously enhancing mass (predominantly peripheral) with enlargement of transverse diameter and surrounding vessel. Biopsy showed invasive ductal carcinoma.

arranged clusters of cells with increased desmoplastic stroma. There is increased vascularity in tumors with abnormally arranged vessels. As the tumor size increases, blood vessel formation increases in periphery which is more tortuous and dilated. Rapid growth of tumors leads to difference in demand and supply of oxygen causing hypoxia and necrosis. These are the factors responsible for irregular heterogeneous enhancement of contrast radially penetrating vessels and central perfusion defect seen on CEUS.

Quantitative analysis: It is derived from the time–intensity curve and the following parameters can be analyzed:

- *Peak intensity (PEAK)*: It is the maximum intensity value of the time-intensity curve, calculated by the formula

$$\frac{\text{Postcontrast intensity} - \text{Precontrast intensity}}{\text{Precontrast intensity}} \times 100\%$$

- *Time to peak (TTP)*: It is the time taken between the point when the contrast medium reaches first in the lesion and the time of maximum intensity of contrast enhancement.
- *Mean transit time (MTT)*: It is the total duration of contrast enhancement.[57]

For *qualitative analysis*, malignant masses show significantly higher and faster enhancement than the benign masses and their TTP is usually shorter. They also show larger wash-in area under the curve (AUC) and shorter MTT.[58]

Lymphosonography is another area in which CEUS has a promising role in breast imaging. Identification and localization of the first line of lymph nodes in the tumor pathway that is called the sentinel node are important for staging. Conventionally, lymphography is done with the dermal injection of lymphatic dye and visualizing tracking the lymphatic channels directly into surgical bed[59] and it also performed with the radiotracer dye and the node with gamma probe.[60]

Lymphosonography is also done with the same method of periareolar dermal injection and visualization of the nodes after 5 minutes of ultrasound contrast injection. Initial studies of lymphosonography have shown the sentinel node in breast cancer patients.[61]

Use of CEUS combined with gray-scale ultrasound for breast imaging is a promising technique with significant clinical application. More research is being done to develop newer techniques in this field for better visualization and quantifying breast masses vascularity.

THERMAL IMAGING

Thermography, or thermal imaging, is a noninvasive and radiation-free modality of breast imaging. This was extensively evaluated in the 1970s and 1980s and was approved by US FDA as an adjunct tool for diagnosis of breast cancer.

A special type of camera is used to measure the temperature of the skin on the breast's surface based on infrared radiation which the human body normally emits. It gives a pictorial representation. The physiological principle behind this imaging modality is that as the cancer cells grow and multiply very fast as compared to normal tissue, the blood flow and metabolism are higher in that area. So, the skin temperature in that area also becomes higher than the surrounding skin which can be detected in thermal imaging.

The infrared cameras used in thermal imaging are ultrasensitive. Sophisticated computers are used to detect the small temperature variations. The data is then analyzed to produce high-resolution images of the skin temperature.

Thermal imaging has been in use for many decades, but till now no concrete evidence exists to prove that it can be used as a good screening tool for early detection of breast cancer. The US FDA has given a safety communication that thermal imaging is not to be used as a substitute for mammography.

ARTIFICIAL INTELLIGENCE IN BREAST IMAGING

Various attempts have been made previously in order to augment human perception, such as computer-aided detection (CAD) used in breast imaging. Artificial intelligence (AI) has become an umbrella term and includes various training techniques, such as machine learning (ML), artificial neural networks (ANNs), and deep learning (DL).[62]

Artificial intelligence has been used in various other fields such as military, communications, finance, corporate, and entertainment sectors. Recently, there is a growing focus on health care, especially radiology. The techniques used in AI are well suited for radiology because images themselves, whose pixel values can be quantitated, are primary source data that can inform and train some AI algorithms.

Recent breast imaging studies have focused on ways to improve multimodality detection and diagnosis, workflow, and clinical decision-making. Beginning in the 1990s, articles about CAD appeared in the radiology literature as aids to radiologists in marking calcifications and masses on mammograms, findings that might have gone undetected or misclassified.[62] Many false-positives reduced the benefit-to-harm ratio before sensitivity and specificity thresholds were calibrated better to attain the desired location on a receiver operating characteristic curve (ROC).

A 2011 study undertaken to determine whether an ANN could predict breast cancer from analysis of patient age and mammographic and ultrasound BI-RADS features of masses in 800 patients with biopsy established breast cancer yielded disease prediction of 90.5%, thus validating the process.[62] AI research based on voxel analysis in 3D CT and MRI is not as far as is image analysis based on pixel quantification.

Reading mammograms in a screening setting is one of the most difficult tasks in radiology. A system that supports radiologists with the decision to refer a woman for further examination appears to be more effective than a classical CAD system. AI systems are now available for mammography analysis with accuracy that is on par with that of average but dedicated, breast radiologists on heterogeneous datasets of mammograms. Deep learning will contribute significantly to increase the application areas of MRI and make it an economically viable breast cancer screening method. AI will open more ways to detect breast cancer earlier and reduce mortality, decrease the variance in performance between radiologists, and improve the screening program as a whole by supporting less-experienced radiologists with their decisions. High-quantity and quality data are needed to train such algorithms. Various algorithmic errors are possible in AI and still there is no solid evidence supporting it. AI should not be relied on solely for a clinician's decisions that may affect survival.

CONCLUSION

Breast imaging has an important place in the field of radiology. Mammography is the first and best method of breast cancer screening. DBT has been developed to overcome few limitations of conventional mammography with an improved cancer detection rate. CEM has a promising role as it has comparable results as MRI in detecting enhancing masses in breast. ABVS has shown significant benefit over conventional mammography in women with dense breast. Other emerging ultrasound techniques such as breast elastography and contrast-enhanced breast ultrasound are expected to continue to expand their role in breast imaging.

REFERENCES

1. Lee CI, Lehman CD. Digital breast tomosynthesis and the challenges of implementing an emerging breast cancer screening technology into clinical practice. J Am Coll Radiol. 2013;10(12):913-7.
2. Pisano ED, Gatsonis C, Hendrick E, Yaffe M, Baum JK, Acharyya S, et al. Diagnostic performance of digital versus film mammography for breast-cancer screening. N Engl J Med. 2005;353(17):1773-83.
3. Bick U, Diekmann F. Digital mammography: what do we and what don't we know? Eur Radiol. 2007;17(8):1931-42.
4. Mandelson MT, Oestreicher N, Porter PL, White D, Finder CA, Taplin SH, et al. Breast density as a predictor of mammographic detection: comparison of interval- and screen-detected cancers. J Natl Cancer Inst. 2000;92(13):1081-7.
5. Kolb TM, Lichy J, Newhouse JH. Comparison of the performance of screening mammography, physical examination, and breast US and evaluation of factors that influence them: an analysis of 27,825 patient evaluations. Radiology. 2002;225(1):165-75.
6. Lei J, Yang P, Zhang L, Wang Y, Yang K. Diagnostic accuracy of digital breast tomosynthesis versus digital mammography for benign and malignant lesions in breasts: a meta-analysis. Eur Radiol. 2014;24(3):595-602.
7. Skaane P, Bandos AI, Gullien R, Eben EB, Ekseth U, Haakenaasen U, et al. Comparison of digital mammography alone and digital mammography plus tomosynthesis in a population-based screening program. Radiology. 2013;267(1):47-56.
8. Skaane P, Bandos AI, Gullien R, Eben EB, Ekseth U, Haakenaasen U, et al. Prospective trial comparing full-field digital mammography (FFDM) versus combined FFDM and tomosynthesis in a population-based screening programme using independent double reading with arbitration. Eur Radiol. 2013;23(8):2061-71.
9. Caumo F, Bernardi D, Ciatto S, Macaskill P, Pellegrini M, Brunelli S, et al. Incremental effect from integrating 3D-mammography (tomosynthesis) with 2D-mammography: increased breast cancer detection evident for screening centres in a population-based trial. Breast. 2014;23(1):76-80.
10. Andersson I, Ikeda DM, Zackrisson S, Ruschin M, Svahn T, Timberg P, et al. Breast tomosynthesis and digital mammography: a comparison of breast cancer visibility and BIRADS classification in a population of cancers with subtle mammographic findings. Eur Radiol. 2008;18(12):2817-25.
11. Gur D, Zuley ML, Anello MI, et al. Dose reduction in digital breast tomosynthesis (DBT) screening using synthetically reconstructed projection images: an observer performance study. Acad Radiol. 2012;19(2):166-71.
12. Zuley ML, Guo B, Catullo VJ, Chough DM, Kelly AE, Lu AH, et al. Comparison of two-dimensional synthesized mammograms versus original digital mammograms alone and in combination with tomosynthesis images. Radiology. 2014;271(3):664-71.
13. Skaane P, Bandos AI, Eben EB, Jebsen IN, Krager M, Haakenaasen U, et al. Two-view digital breast tomosynthesis screening with synthetically reconstructed projection images: comparison with digital breast tomosynthesis with full-field digital mammographic images. Radiology. 2014;271(3):655-63.
14. Dang PA, Humphrey KL, Freer PE, Halpern EF, Saksena MA, Rafferty EA. Comparison of lesion detection and characterization in invasive cancers using breast tomosynthesis versus conventional mammography [abstr]. In: Radiological Society of North America Scientific Assembly and Annual Meeting Program. Oak Brook, Ill: Radiological Society of North America, 2013;156.
15. Hilleren DJ, Andersson IT, Lindholm K, Linnell FS. Invasive lobular carcinoma: mammographic findings in a 10-year experience. Radiology. 1991;178(1):149-54.
16. Raghu M, Hooley RJ, Philpotts LE, et al. Digital breast tomosynthesis in diagnostic mammography: can tomo affect the final assessment categories? [abstr]. In: Radiological Society of North America Scientific Assembly and Annual Meeting Program. Oak Brook, Ill: Radiological Society of North America, 2013;156.
17. Nicholson BT, Raymond S, Rochman CM, Peppard HR, Harvey JA. Comparison of tomosynthesis in the diagnostic setting to 2D mammography for the evaluation of focal asymmetry recalled from screening. Presented at the annual meeting of the American Roentgen Ray Society, San Diego, California, May 4-9, 2014.
18. Zuley ML, Bandos AI, Ganott MA, Sumkin JH, Kelly AE, Catullo VJ, et al. Digital breast tomosynthesis versus supplemental diagnostic mammographic views for evaluation of noncalcified breast lesions. Radiology. 2013;266(1):89-95.
19. Destounis SV, Arieno AL, Morgan RC. Preliminary clinical experience with digital breast tomosynthesis in the visualization of breast microcalcifications. J Clin Imaging Sci. 2013;3:65.
20. Dromain C, Thibault F, Muller S, Rimareix F, Delaloge S, Tardivon A, et al. Dual-energy contrast-enhanced digital mammography: initial clinical results. Eur Radiol. 2011;21(3):565-74.

21. Lewin JM, Isaacs PK, Vance V, Larke FJ. Dual-energy contrast-enhanced digital subtraction mammography: feasibility. Radiology. 2003;229(1):261-8.
22. Lalji UC, Jeukens CR, Houben I, Nelemans PJ, van Engen RE, van Wylick E, et al. Evaluation of low-energy contrast-enhanced spectral mammography images by comparing them to full-field digital mammography using EUREF image quality criteria. Eur Radiol. 2015;25(10):2813-20.
23. Francescone MA, Jochelson MS, Dershaw DD, Sung JS, Hughes MC, Zheng J, et al. Low energy mammogram obtained in contrast-enhanced digital mammography (CEDM) is comparable to routine full-field digital mammography (FFDM). Eur J Radiol. 2014;83(8):1350-5.
24. Dromain C, Balleyguier C, Adler G, Garbay JR, Delaloge S. Contrast-enhanced digital mammography. Eur J Radiol. 2009;69(1):34-42.
25. Knogler T, Homolka P, Hoernig M, Leithner R, Langs G, Waitzbauer M, et al. Application of BI-RADS descriptors in contrast-enhanced dual-energy mammography: comparison with MRI. Breast Care (Basel). 2017;12(4):212-6.
26. Kamal RM, Helal MH, Mansour SM, Haggag MA, Nada OM, Farahat IG, et al. Can we apply the MRI BI-RADS lexicon morphology descriptors on contrast-enhanced spectral mammography? Br J Radiol. 2016;89(1064):20160157.
27. Patel BK, Davis J, Ferraro C, Kosiorek H, Hasselbach K, Ocal T, et al. Value Added of Preoperative Contrast-Enhanced Digital Mammography in Patients With Invasive Lobular Carcinoma of the Breast. Clin Breast Cancer. 2018;18(6):e1339-45.
28. Mainiero MB, Moy L, Baron P, Didwania AD, diFlorio-Alexander RM, Green ED, et al. (2017). ACR Appropriateness Criteria: Breast Cancer Screening. American College of Radiology. [online] Available from https://acsearch.acr.org/docs/70910/Narrative/. [Last accessed March 2019].
29. Jochelson MS, Pinker K, Dershaw DD, Hughes M, Gibbons GF, Rahbar K, et al. Comparison of screening CEDM and MRI for women at increased risk for breast cancer: A pilot study. Eur J Radiol. 2017;97:37-43.
30. Patel BK, Garza SA, Eversman S, Lopez-Alvarez Y, Kosiorek H, Pockaj BA. Assessing tumor extent on contrast-enhanced spectral mammography versus full-field digital mammography and ultrasound. Clin Imaging. 2017;46:78-84.
31. Luczyńska E, Heinze S, Adamczyk A, Ryś J, Mituś JW, Hendrick E. Comparison of the mammography, contrast-enhanced spectral mammography and ultrasonography in a group of 116 patients. Anticancer Res. 2016;36(8):4359-66.
32. Si L, Zhai R, Liu X, Yang K, Wang L, Jiang T. MRI in the differential diagnosis of primary architectural distortion detected by mammography. Diagn Interv Radiol. 2016;22(2):141-50.
33. Patel BK, Naylor ME, Kosiorek HE, Lopez-Alvarez YM, Miller AM, Pizzitola VJ, et al. Clinical utility of contrast-enhanced spectral mammography as an adjunct for tomosynthesis-detected architectural distortion. Clin Imaging. 2017;46:44-52.
34. Fallenberg EM, Dromain C, Diekmann F, Engelken F, Krohn M, Singh JM, et al. Contrast-enhanced spectral mammography versus MRI: Initial results in the detection of breast cancer and assessment of tumour size. Eur Radiol. 2014;24(1):256-64.
35. Lee-Felker SA, Tekchandani L, Thomas M, Gupta E, Andrews-Tang D, Roth A, et al. Newly diagnosed breast cancer: Comparison of contrast-enhanced spectral mammography and breast MR imaging in the evaluation of extent of disease. Radiology. 2017;285(2):389-400.
36. Iotti V, Ravaioli S, Vacondio R, Coriani C, Caffarri S, Sghedoni R, et al. Contrast-enhanced spectral mammography in neoadjuvant chemotherapy monitoring: a comparison with breast magnetic resonance imaging. Breast Cancer Res. 2017;19(1):106.
37. Wojcinski S, Farrokh A, Hille U, Wiskirchen J, Gyapong S, Soliman AA, et al. The automated breast volume scanner (ABVS): initial experiences in lesion detection compared with conventional handheld B-mode ultrasound: a pilot study of 50 cases. Int J Womens Health. 2011;3:337-46.
38. Van Zelst JCM, Mann RM. Automated three-dimensional breast us for screening: technique, artifacts, and lesion characterization. Radiographics. 2018;38(3):663-83.
39. Chen L, Chen Y, Diao XH, Fang L, Pang Y, Cheng AQ, et al. Comparative study of automated breast 3-D ultrasound and handheld B-mode ultrasound for differentiation of benign and malignant breast masses. Ultrasound Med Biol. 2013;39(10):1735-42.
40. Zheng FY, Lu Q, Huang BJ, Xia HS, Yan LX, Wang X, et al. Imaging features of automated breast volume scanner: correlation with molecular subtypes of breast cancer. Eur J Radiol. 2017;86:267-75.
41. Cespedes I, Ophir J, Ponnekanti H, Maklad N. Elastography: elasticity imaging using ultrasound with application to muscle and breast in vivo. Ultrasonic imaging. 1993;15(2):73-88.
42. Garra BS, Cespedes EI, Ophir J, Spratt SR, Zuurbier RA, Magnant CM, et al. Elastography of breast lesions: initial clinical results. Radiology. 1997;202(1):79-86.
43. Barr RG, Sonographic breast elastography. J Ultrasound Med. 2012;31(5):773-83.
44. Barr RG. Elastography in clinical practice. Radiol Clin North Am. 2014;52(6):1145-62.
45. Itoh A, Ueno E, Tohno E, Kamma H, Takahashi H, Shiina T, et al. Breast Disease: Clinical Application of US Elastography for Diagnosis. Radiology. 2006;239(2):341-50.
46. Burnside ES, Hall TJ, Sommer AM, Hesley GK, Sisney GA, Svensson WE, et al. Differentiating benign from malignant solid breast masses with US strain imaging. Radiology. 2007;245(2):401-10.
47. Barr RG. Real-time ultrasound elasticity of the breast: initial clinical results. Ultrasound Q. 2010;26(2):61-6.
48. Zhi H, Xiao Y, Yang HY, Wen Y, Ou B, Luo B-M, et al. Semi-quantitating stiffness of breast solid lesions in ultrasonic elastography. Acad Radiol. 2008;15(11):1347-53.
49. Tanter M, Bercoff J, Athanasiou A, Deffieux T, Gennisson JL, Montaldo G, et al. Quantitative assessment of breast lesion viscoelasticity: initial clinical results using supersonic shear imaging. Ultrasound Med Biol. 2008;34(9):1373-86.
50. Cosgrove D, Piscaglia F, Bamber J, Bojunga J, Correas JM, Gilja O, et al. EFSUMB guidelines and recommendations on the clinical use of ultrasound elastography. Part 2: Clinical applications. Ultraschall Med. 2013;34(3):238-53.

51. Lee SH, Chang JM, Cho N, Koo HR, Yi A, Kim SJ, et al. Practice guideline for the performance of breast ultrasound elastography. Ultrasonography. 2014;33(1):3-10.
52. Shiina T, Nightingale KR, Palmeri ML, Hall TJ, Bamber JC, Barr RG, et al. WFUMB guidelines and recommendations for clinical use of ultrasound elastography: Part 1: basic principles and terminology. Ultrasound Med Biol. 2015;41(5):1126-47.
53. Hayashi M, Yamamoto Y, Ibusuki M, Fujiwara S, Yamamoto S, Tomita S, et al. Evaluation of tumor stiffness by elastography is predictive for pathologic complete response to neoadjuvant chemotherapy in patients with breast cancer. Ann Surg Oncol. 2012;19(9):3042-9.
54. Faruk T, Islam MK, Arefin S, Haq MZ. The Journey of elastography: background, current status and future possibilities in breast cancer diagnosis. Clin Breast Cancer. 2015;15(5):313-24.
55. Cosgrove D. Ultrasound contrast agents: An overview. Eur J Radiol. 2006;60(3):324-30.
56. Wan C, Du J, Fang H, Li F, Wang L. Evaluation of breast lesions by contrast enhanced ultrasound: qualitative and quantitative analysis. Eur J Radiol. 2012;81(4):e444-50.
57. Vraka I, Panourgias E, Sifakis E, Andreas K, Galanis P, Dellaportas D, et al. A correlation between contrast-enhanced ultrasound characteristics (qualitative and quantitative) and pathological prognostic factors in breast cancer. In Vivo. 2018;32(4):945-54.
58. Ji CL, Li XL, He YP, Li DD, Gu XG, Xu HX. Quantitative parameters of contrast-enhanced ultrasound in breast invasive ductal carcinoma: The correlation with pathological prognostic factors. Clin Hemorheol Microcirc. 2017;66(4):333-45.
59. Goldberg BB, Merton DA, Liu JB, Forsberg F, Zhang K, Thakur M, et al. Contrast-enhanced ultrasound imaging of sentinel lymph nodes after peritumoral administration of Sonazoid in a melanoma tumor animal model. J Ultrasound Med. 2011;30(4):441-53.
60. Rautiainen S, Sudah M, Joukainen S, Sironen R, Vanninen R, Sutela A. Contrast-enhanced ultrasound-guided axillary lymph node core biopsy: diagnostic accuracy in preoperative staging of invasive breast cancer. Eur J Radiol. 2015;84(11):2130-6.
61. Omoto K, Matsunaga H, Take N, Hozumi Y, Takehara M, Omoto Y, et al. Sentinel node detection method using contrast-enhanced ultrasonography with sonazoid in breast cancer: preliminary clinical study. Ultrasound Med Biol. 2009;35(8):1249-56.
62. Mendelson EB. Artificial intelligence in breast imaging: potentials and limitations. Am J Roentgenol. 2019;212(2):293-9.

CHAPTER

29

Male Breast Imaging

Veenu Singla, Tulika Singh, Nidhi Prabhakar

INTRODUCTION

The male breast is structurally identical to that of the female breast at birth. However, the testosterone surge during puberty causes atrophy and involution of the ductal units, making it nonfunctional and rudimentary. The male breast is susceptible to similar pathologies as that of the female breast. The incidence of breast-related complaints in males is on the rise, though the pathologies affecting the male breast are predominantly benign. The incidence of breast cancer in males is approximately 1%. More than half of men over 44 years show palpable stroma.[1]

IMAGING METHODS

Imaging of the male breast has been a challenge as there are no set protocols for its evaluation and because of the lesser breast volume, breast malignancies tend to involve the chest wall much earlier. The use of mammography and ultrasound for radiological evaluation of the male breast varies among different radiologists. Mammography is a reliable imaging investigation to differentiate between gynecomastia and breast cancer as it allows accurate assessment of relationship of mass with nipple, and eccentric location of mass favors malignancy. In daily practice, all masses which are suspicious clinically in patients >25 years of age should undergo mammography as the first imaging investigation. Bilateral mammograms should always be obtained as they allow comparison, and as risk factors predisposing to carcinoma on one breast are also applicable to the other breast. Despite the lesser breast volume in males, mammography is easy to acquire and standard craniocaudal (CC) and mediolateral oblique (MLO) views should be routinely done. Magnification and spot compression views should be done as per case-based requirement. Ultrasonography is performed if mammography findings are questionable or not typical of gynecomastia. Ultrasonography is easy to perform because of the small breast size and can also guide tissue sampling. Magnetic resonance imaging (MRI) is technically difficult to perform in males and is recommended when lesion identification is difficult because of associated gynecomastia, for evaluating chest wall or skin invasion, and for demonstrating primary breast mass in cases of axillary metastasis when both ultrasound and mammography are negative.

ANATOMY

Knowing the anatomy of male breast is crucial to identify and differentiate various benign and malignant processes on imaging. The male breast extends from the 2nd to 6th anterior ribs craniocaudally, and from the sternum in the midline to the midaxillary line mediolaterally. It comprises skin, subcutaneous tissue, fibroglandular stroma and involuted ducts. However, the fatty component of the breast predominates in the male breast, unlike fibroglandular stromal predominance in females. The suspensory ligaments of Cooper are not seen in male breasts. As the lobular development is dependent on estrogen and progesterone, pathologies that involve the lobular units viz., fibroadenoma, phyllodes tumor, lobular carcinoma in situ, and invasive lobular carcinoma are rare, with the gamut of diseases affecting the ductal and stromal units predominating in males.[2] The male breast receives its blood supply from the branches of the axillary artery, internal mammary artery and intercostal arteries, with the venous drainage into the intercostal veins. Lymphatics of the breast drain into the axillary, internal mammary, and the supraclavicular nodes.[3]

NORMAL IMAGING APPEARANCE

On mammography, due to the predominant fatty component, male breast appears homogeneously radiolucent, with minimal retroareolar ductal tissue and a prominent pectoralis muscle **(Fig. 1)**. On ultrasonography, the nipple appears as an echogenic nodule with posterior acoustic shadowing. The skin is hyperechoic. The subcutaneous tissue is hypoechoic with echogenic fibrous septa **(Fig. 2)**. The rudimentary fibroglandular tissue appears hypoechoic.[3]

Though gynecomastia and breast cancer are considered mainly in a male patient with a palpable breast mass, masses arising from skin and subcutaneous tissue like lipomas and epidermal inclusion cysts are also common.

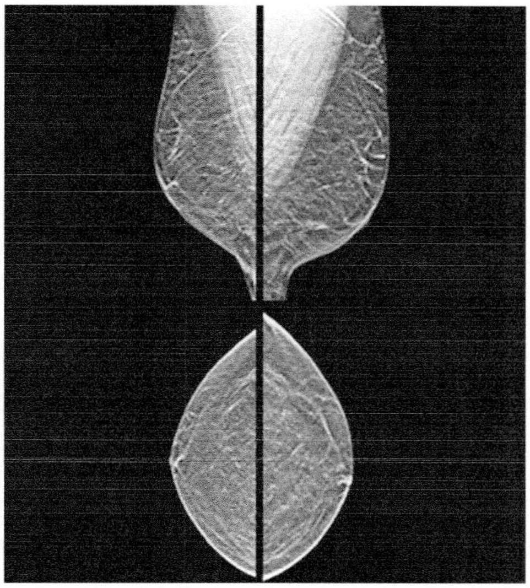

Fig. 1: Mammographic appearance of a normal male breast showing predominantly fatty tissue and minimal fibroglandular component.

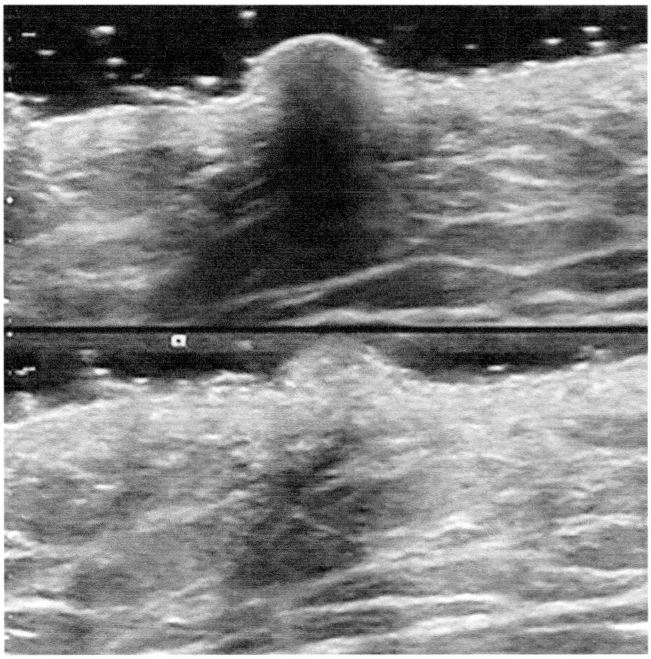

Fig. 2: Ultrasonographic appearance of the normal male breast. The nipple appears as a small heteroechoic nodule with mild posterior attenuation. The small volume of glandular tissue appears hypoechoic. The overlying skin is hyperechoic, and the subcutaneous tissue is hypoechoic with hyperechoic streaks that represent fibrous striae.

Gynecomastia

It is the most common breast abnormality in males and is due to benign proliferation of the stromal and ductal elements. Gynecomastia presents with clinical manifestations and imaging signs which may be unilateral or bilateral. Gynecomastia can be physiological during infancy, puberty and senescence, when there is increased estrogen and reduced testosterone. It can also be seen with the use of drugs (such as marijuana, steroids, leuprolide, thiazides, etc.), in patients with cirrhosis, syndromic hypogonadism, hyperthyroidism, chronic kidney disease and neoplasms such as germ cell tumors, Sertoli and Leydig cell tumors, adrenocortical tumors, and pituitary tumors.[2]

Men commonly present with a palpable, tender lump, or burning sensation. Clinically, gynecomastia is seen as a concentric subareolar mass contrary to other pathologies, which show eccentric growth in relation to the nipple-areola complex. This should also be differentiated from pseudogynecomastia, which occurs due to fat proliferation with no significant proliferation of the stroma.

On mammography, three characteristic patterns of gynecomastia are seen, namely—(1) nodular, (2) dendritic and (3) diffuse glandular.[2,4] The *nodular pattern* is seen as a *fan-shaped* density which radiates from the nipple. It is usually more prominent in the upper outer quadrant. This correlates with the pathological class of early phase of gynecomastia known as "florid gynecomastia", where there is hyperplastic ductal epithelium, with loose stroma and edema surrounding it. Clinically, it correlates with the phase of a painful lump. On mammography, a fan-shaped or triangular density is seen behind the nipple. On ultrasonography, it is seen as a focal hypoechoic nodular discoid structure or triangular hypoechoic area in the retroareolar location, with long axis parallel to the skin. It is reversible if the precipitant stimulus is removed. The *dendritic pattern* of gynecomastia is seen as a *flame-shaped* soft tissue density in the retroareolar location. This form correlates with the pathological class of long-standing, quiescent, or "fibrous gynecomastia", which shows dense fibrotic stroma. On mammography, it is seen as a dendritic density in the subareolar location with finger-like projections extending into deeper fatty tissue. On ultrasonography, irregular subareolar hypoechoic is seen with linear projections extending into surrounding adipose tissue. As fibrosis has set in, the process becomes irreversible from this phase **(Figs. 3A and B)**.[5] The *diffuse glandular pattern* resembles that of a heterogeneously dense breast seen in females and is seen in patients on high-dose estrogen therapy.[2] On mammography, there is generalized increase in breast density; and on ultrasonography, there is increase in volume and echogenicity of breast tissue resembling sonologically dense female breast. Gynecomastia may be confused with malignancy, although malignancies rarely involve the subareolar location. However, careful history with special attention to patient's medical history, and clinical examination can help in differentiating gynecomastia from malignancy.

As breast malignancy is uncommon in younger males, nearly all men <30 years of age having breast symptoms have

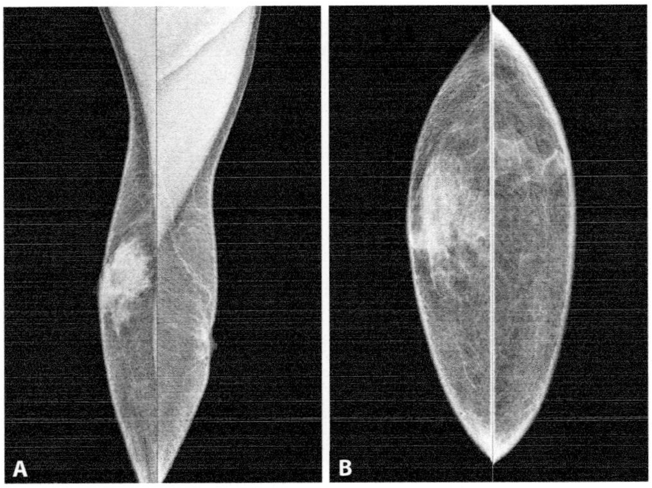

Figs. 3A and B: Mammography of a male patient showing dendritic subareolar density interdigitating into underlying fatty tissue. Features suggestive of gynecomastia—dendritic type.

gynecomastia. Imaging features that favor gynecomastia over malignancy are central/subareolar location of mass, lack of spiculations and absence of secondary signs of malignancy like skin changes. Occasionally, it becomes difficult to differentiate gynecomastia from malignancy on imaging,[6] and biopsy is required for confirmation of the diagnosis.[2]

Gynecomastia is self-regressing and may resolve when the precipitating factors are eliminated. However, in later stages, when the disease is refractory to medical management, reduction mammoplasty can be undertaken.

BENIGN NEOPLASMS OF THE MALE BREAST

Angiolipoma

It is a common fatty tumor in rest of the body; however, its occurrence in the breast is rare. On mammography, it appears as a mixed density mass having fatty as well as soft tissue components. On ultrasonography, it is seen as a homogeneously hyperechoic mass. The patient is usually kept on imaging follow-up. The tumor is rarely treated by excision.

Schwannoma

They are extremely rare neoplasms in the male breast; however, when associated with neurofibromatosis type 2, they have increased malignant potential. They present as soft, smooth, and often painless mass. On mammography, they are seen as nonspecific, round or oval, well-defined masses. On ultrasonography, they are seen as well-demarcated, solid hypoechoic masses with variable degrees of posterior acoustic enhancement. Occasionally, these tumors may show central cystic regions.

Intraductal Papilloma

It is characterized by proliferation of the ductal epithelium, supported by a core of fibrovascular stroma and myoepithelial cells. Men usually present with a palpable lump in the subareolar location or with discharge from the nipple. Ultrasonography has shown increased sensitivity in the detection of these lesions, which are seen as an intraluminal masses within a dilated duct. On color Doppler, the fibrovascular stalk shows internal vascularity. When the duct is not dilated at the time of the ultrasound examination, the intraluminal mass may be become inconspicuous and may lead to false-negative results.[2] Surgical excision is the preferred diagnostic as well as therapeutic modality as core biopsy may underestimate the lesion histologically.[2]

Lipomas

They are the second most common benign lesion of the male breast after gynecomastia; and are characterized by benign proliferation of mature adipocytes. They present as nonpainful, soft palpable masses. On mammography, they are seen as a well-defined, encapsulated lesion showing fat density; and on ultrasonography as mildly echogenic, avascular masses. However, they may also appear isoechoic or hypoechoic to the surrounding fat. They do not warrant surgery unless they are cosmetically disturbing.

Benign Spindle Cell Neoplasms

These are rare mesenchymal lesions, which include myofibroblastoma, spindle cell lipoma, leiomyoma, solitary fibrous tumor, and fibrous histiocytoma. The imaging features are nonspecific, and often, histopathology is needed for validation of diagnosis. Mammography and ultrasonography may show well-defined masses with coarse calcifications. Myofibroblastomas have been reported to occur in cases of previous malignancies of pancreas, kidney, and prostate.

BENIGN NON-NEOPLASTIC LESIONS OF MALE BREAST

Pseudogynecomastia

This is a bilateral or less commonly unilateral condition, which is seen commonly in obese adolescent males, overweight persons, or in neurofibromatosis. It occurs due to excessive fat deposition. On clinical examination, it is non-nodular, diffuse, and symmetrical. On mammography, there is excessive fatty tissue in the breast without any fibroglandular tissue. On ultrasonography, homogeneously hypoechoic lobules of adipose tissue are seen to be separated from one another by thin hyperechoic bands representing fibrous tissue.

Intramammary Lymph Nodes

They are common lesions, usually seen in the upper outer quadrant, however, can be located anywhere within the breast. On mammography, they appear oval with radiodense peripheral cortex and radiolucent central fatty hilum. On ultrasonography, normal lymph nodes appear homogeneous with a cortical thickness of <2–3 mm, with hyperechoic fatty hilum and echogenic cortex. Lymph nodes which measure >10 mm in short axis diameter, rounded nodes, irregular nodes, or nodes with cortical thickening >3 mm are taken as abnormal.

Epidermal Inclusion Cyst

They are benign intradermal lesions, which occur secondary to obstruction of hair follicles and contain lamellated keratin within a wall of epidermis. They are the third most common benign lesion in male breast. On imaging, they are indistinguishable from sebaceous cysts, which occur due to obstruction of hair follicles. On mammography, both are seen as a well-defined high density, superficial lesion, which is continuous with the skin. On ultrasonography, they are seen as oval, well-demarcated, hypoechoic, subcutaneous lesions adjacent to the skin surface with no internal vascularity **(Figs. 4A and B)**. However, infected cysts may show peripheral hyperemia. Due to the lamellated keratin, they may give onion skin appearance on sonography, with alternate hypoechoic and hyperechoic concentric rings. Such lesions are seldom sampled for diagnosis as their rupture may lead to inflammatory response and subsequent formation of breast abscess, hence these are considered "no biopsy" lesions and diagnosis should be clinched on imaging.

Duct Ectasia

Duct ectasia is rare in men. It may present with signs of chronic inflammation and nipple discharge. Imaging reveals dilated subareolar ducts with inspissated secretions. These secretions may occasionally calcify. As benign duct dilatation is present centrally; if located peripherally, malignancy needs to be ruled out.

Diabetic Mastopathy

It is a rare fibroinflammatory disease seen in patients with a long-standing history of type 1 diabetes mellitus. On mammography, it may appear as a discrete, nonspecific mass, or focal asymmetry. On ultrasonography, appearance may be as solitary or multiple hypoechoic masses which show minimal or no internal vascularity, and may show posterior acoustic attenuation. Imaging appearance may be similar to that of malignancy; hence biopsy is often required for diagnosis. On histopathology, it shows sclerosis of the stroma with dense infiltration by lymphocytes. Diagnosed cases do not necessitate surgery as these lesions have no increased malignant potential.

Post-traumatic Hematoma/Fat Necrosis

It is usually seen following breast trauma or surgery, however, may follow a trivial trauma in patients with coagulopathy or patients on anticoagulant medications. In acute phases, hematoma as well as fat necrosis may appear as an atypical mass, which shows associated thickening of skin and accentuation of the trabeculae. On mammography, hematomas are radiopaque, circumscribed or irregular, having appearance that may be similar to that of an abscess or malignancy. With time, hematomas progress to discrete masses showing fluid-fluid levels due to conversion of acute blood into serum; and fat necrosis may evolve to masses showing fat-fluid levels due to necrosis/liquefaction of fat. Acute hematomas are hyperechoic on sonography. However, on ultrasonography, both hematoma and fat necrosis may appear similar as well-defined masses showing fluid-debris level and internal septations with no internal vascularity.

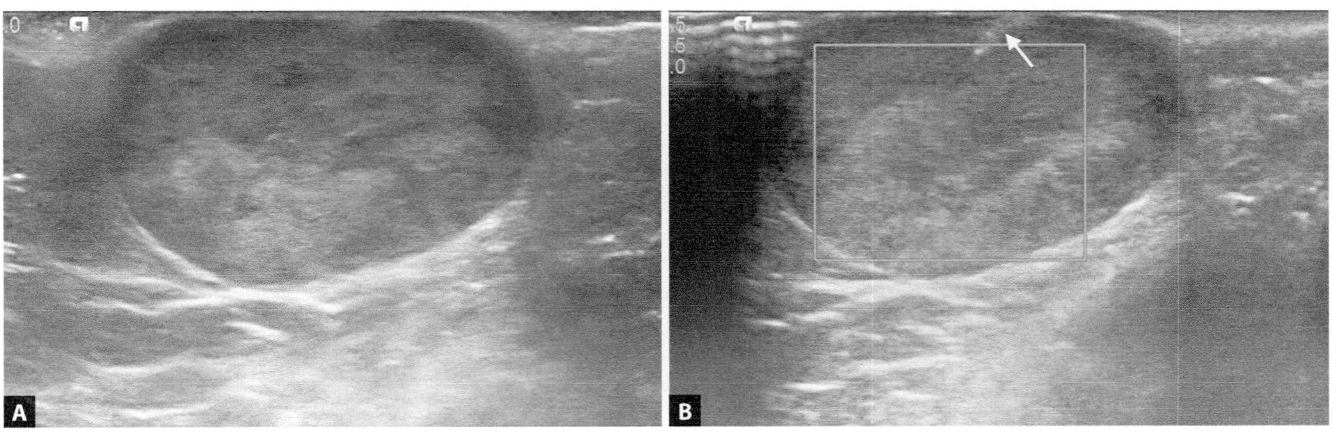

Figs. 4A and B: Epidermal inclusion cyst. Ultrasonography of the breast showing presence of a superficial, well-defined heteroechoic lesion lying parallel to the chest wall and showing positive "claw sign" with the surrounding subcutaneous tissue and an echogenic tract (arrow) reaching up to the skin surface. Color Doppler shows no vascularity within the lesion.

Ultrasound examination in the decubitus views is crucial to look for the mobility of debris and exclude underlying soft tissue. Internal vascularity suggests an underlying neoplastic etiology. Chronic hematomas and fat necrosis may appear as persistent masses, architectural distortion, and dystrophic calcifications on imaging **(Fig. 5)**.

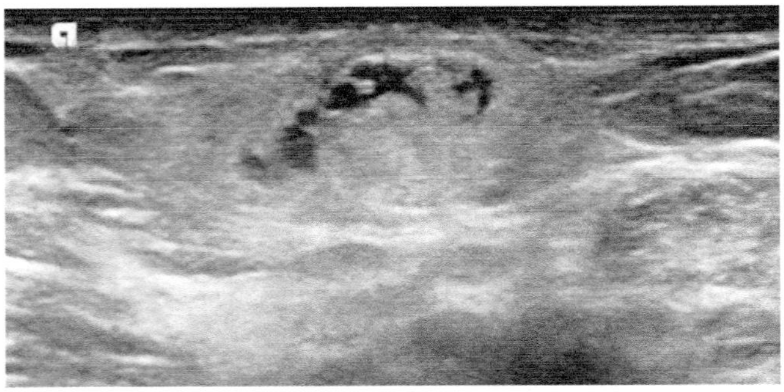

Fig. 5: Ultrasonography of breast in a male with history of chest trauma showing a superficial, ill-defined, predominantly echogenic lesion with few hypoechoic areas within which show internal debris. Features suggestive of traumatic fat necrosis.

Mastitis

It is a diffuse inflammation of the breast which may present with or without abscess formation within ectatic ducts. It is usually caused by staphylococci or less commonly streptococci. These bacteria enter the nipple due to trauma or nipple piercing. On mammography, they appear as diffuse enlargement of the breast with thickened trabeculae **(Figs. 6 and 7)**. In the presence of an abscess, ill-defined masses are seen which may or may not show calcifications. They may be confused with gynecomastia; however, presence of skin thickening helps in differentiating between them. Treatment is by percutaneous drainage and antibiotics with or without excision of ectatic ducts.

Subareolar Abscess

It is due to a localized infection, which occurs secondary to ductal ectasia, chronic ductal obstruction, and inflammation. Men present with nipple swelling, discharge and pain. On mammography, they are seen as an ill-defined mass with trabecular thickening.

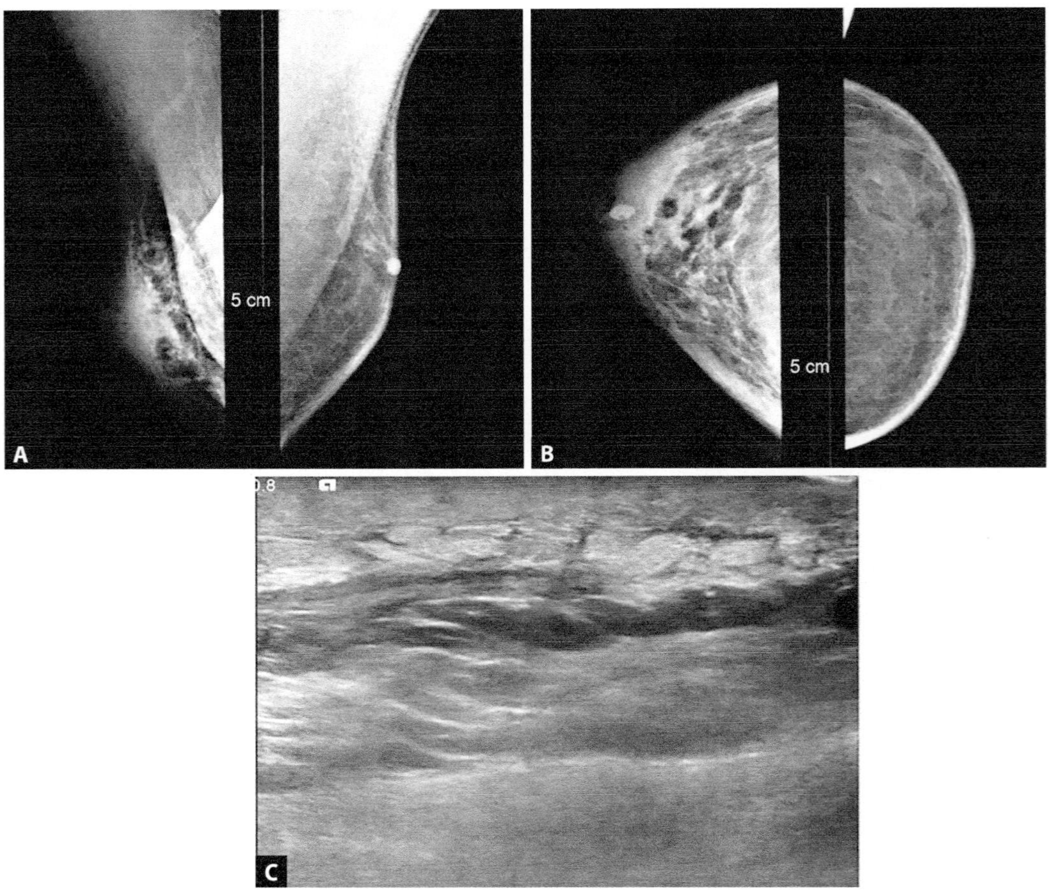

Figs. 6A to C: (A and B) Mammogram of a male with painful swelling in right breast showing diffuse skin thickening and coarsened trabeculae, suggesting an inflammatory pathology; (C) Ultrasonography of breast in the same patient showing diffuse thickened echogenic subcutaneous tissue with thin streaks of fluid tracking between the fibrous septae. Features suggestive of diffuse edema.

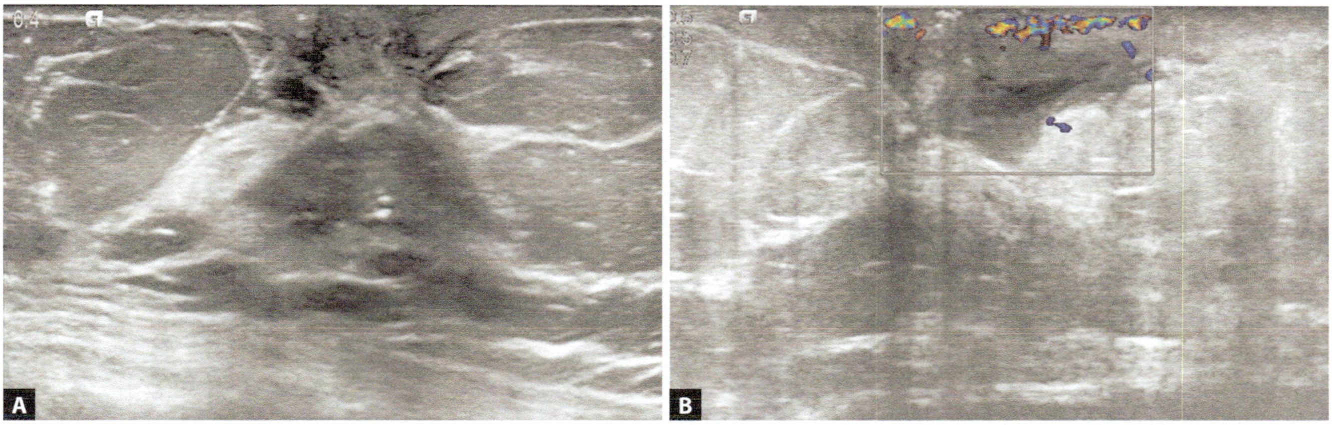

Figs. 7A and B: Ultrasonography of breast in a male presenting with painful lump showing presence of focal heteroechoic area in the subareolar location with increased peripheral vascularity. Features suggestive of mastitis.

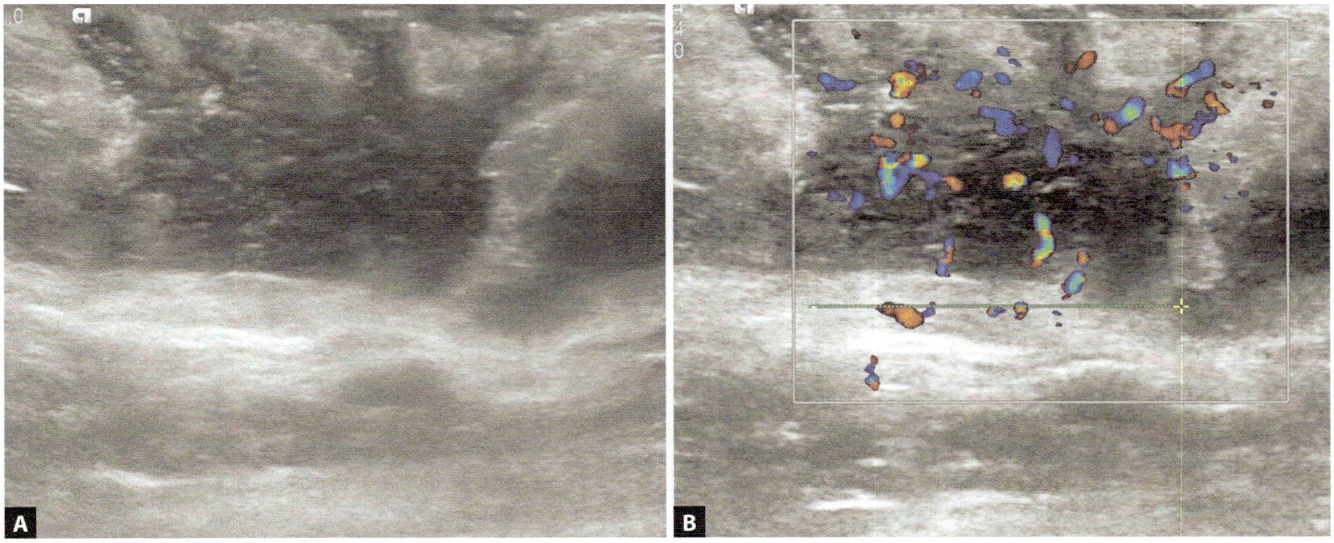

Figs. 8A and B: Ultrasonography of breast in a male presenting with painful breast lump showing presence of a heteroechoic lesion in the subcutaneous tissue showing shaggy walls and dense internal echoes within. Color Doppler showing hypervascularity. Features suggestive of evolving breast abscess.

On ultrasonography, they are seen as an ill-circumscribed mass showing complex fluid within and showing peripheral hyperemia and no internal vascularity **(Figs. 8A and B)**. Treatment is by surgical excision of the abscess and the regional ducts to avoid recurrence of the disease.

Tuberculosis of the Breast

Primary tuberculosis of the male breast is rare, as its incidence increases in females during pregnancy and lactation due to increased vascularity as well as dilated ducts. HIV infection is also a major risk factor. Commonly it presents with lump with surrounding inflammatory signs with or without axillary lymphadenopathy. They can be of three types, namely—(1) nodular tuberculosis (characterized by a malignant looking mass with or without sinus formation), (2) diffuse or disseminated mastitis (characterized by multiple foci which may lead to the formation of draining sinuses) and (3) sclerosing type (characterized by hard, painless lump with nipple retraction due to extensive fibrosis).

Pseudoangiomatous Stromal Hyperplasia

Pseudoangiomatous stromal hyperplasia (PASH) is a benign proliferation of the stroma which is commonly seen incidentally on biopsy specimens, which were done for other indications. However, it may also present with a palpable lump. On mammography and ultrasonography, it may show well defined or partially defined margins. Symptomatic or fast growing lesions can be treated by wide local excision taking 1–2 cm surgical margins, as they carry high rates of recurrence.[1]

Hamartomas

They are uncommon lesions containing fibroglandular and fatty elements of the breast. These lesions rarely can harbor foci of ductal carcinoma within them.

On mammography, these lesions are well defined with stromal as well as fat density areas within. On ultrasonography, they have varied appearances and can appear hyperechoic, heteroechoic, or isoechoic well-defined lesions.

Augmented Male Breasts

Hormonal therapy is used as a nonsurgical option in transsexual patients for breast augmentation. This is done by the administration of exogenous estrogen and suppression of androgen secretion. This results in dense breasts similar to that of female breasts. In addition, injected high viscous fluids (like petroleum jelly, paraffin, automobile transmission fluid, etc.) may show extensive calcifications, which in some cases may cause extensive surrounding inflammation leading to a condition called sclerosing lipogranulomatosis. Sclerosing lipogranulomatosis may require treatment by radical debridement and even mastectomy.

Venous Malformation

It is the most common vascular malformation of the male breast, which is characterized by slow flow and absence of arteriovenous shunting. It usually presents as unilateral painless, gradual breast enlargement. On mammography, they are seen as multiple serpiginous densities. On ultrasonography, they show multiple tubular, anechoic cystic spaces showing internal color flow, which differentiate them from a lymphatic malformation. They may show associated features such as phleboliths or thrombosis.

Secondary Syphilis

It can be transmitted during vaginal delivery in cases of congenital syphilis or sexually transmitted in cases of acquired syphilis. Secondary syphilis manifests several months after the primary chancre and shows periareolar mucous excrescences, nipple retraction, and skin thickening. On mammography, they are seen as diffuse skin thickening and diffuse asymmetry of fibroglandular pattern. Similar mammographic appearances can be seen in cases of Paget's disease of the breast, subareolar abscesses, and inflammatory carcinomas.

Nodular Fasciitis

It is a benign, reactive fibroblastic proliferation, usually affecting forearms and rarely affecting the breast presenting as a firm mass. On mammography, they are seen as ill-defined irregular densities. On ultrasonography, they are seen as solid hypoechoic masses which may mimic malignancy, and hence biopsy is often needed for confirmation of diagnosis.

MALE BREAST CANCER

Male breast cancer constitutes <1% of all breast cancers. Hence, the screening for male breast cancer is not justified, and imaging of the male breast is usually for diagnostic purposes. It is associated with multiple risk factors such as advanced age, Klinefelter's syndrome, mutations of *BRCA1* or *BRCA2*, history of breast cancer in a first-degree male or female relative, hyperestrogenic states, cryptorchidism, testicular injury, liver dysfunction, and prior irradiation to the chest. There is two- to four times increased risk of breast cancer in patients with a positive family history. These cancers are more commonly unilateral, with the incidence of bilateral cancers being <1% of all male breast cancers. The mean age of diagnosis of male breast cancers is about 5–10 years later than that of female breast cancers; with more than half the men (>50%) presenting with axillary nodal metastasis at presentation. Majority of the cancers are infiltrating ductal carcinoma of "not otherwise specified" subtype (up to 80%) or ductal carcinoma in situ (DCIS); with the rarer subtypes being infiltrating mammary carcinoma and invasive papillary carcinoma.[7] However, papillary carcinomas are seen to be more commoner in men than in women.[8]

Men usually present with a palpable painless breast lump which may be associated with skin thickening, nipple retraction, nipple discharge or axillary lymphadenopathy. The mass can be immobile and fixed to the skin or the subcutaneous tissue. These lesions most commonly occur at the subareolar location, eccentric to the nipple or less commonly in the peripheral breast. The predominance in subareolar location can be explained by the fact that in females breast tissue is mainly present in upper outer quadrant, while in males, breast tissue is confined mainly to subareolar location. Nipple discharge may be the only presenting symptom in carcinoma in situ.[9] Mammography remains the initial imaging modality, and a supplementary ultrasonographic examination is done whenever necessary. On mammography, bilateral CC and MLO views should be acquired. These lesions can have a wide spectrum of mammographic appearances, ranging from having well-defined, ill-defined, to spiculated margins; and round, oval to irregular shapes **(Figs. 9 and 10)**. In contrary to the female breast cancers, calcifications are fewer, more coarser and scattered and seldom rod-shaped. In other words, the benign patterns of calcifications in female breast lesions need not necessarily be benign in male breast lesions, i.e., calcifications which are accepted as benign in female breast (e.g., punctate), may indicate malignancy in male breast . On ultrasonography, these lesions may appear as taller than wider hypoechoic masses with angulated or microlobulated or spiculated margins with or without calcifications. Lesions may also show variable degrees of posterior acoustic attenuation or enhancement or both. Rarely these lesions can also

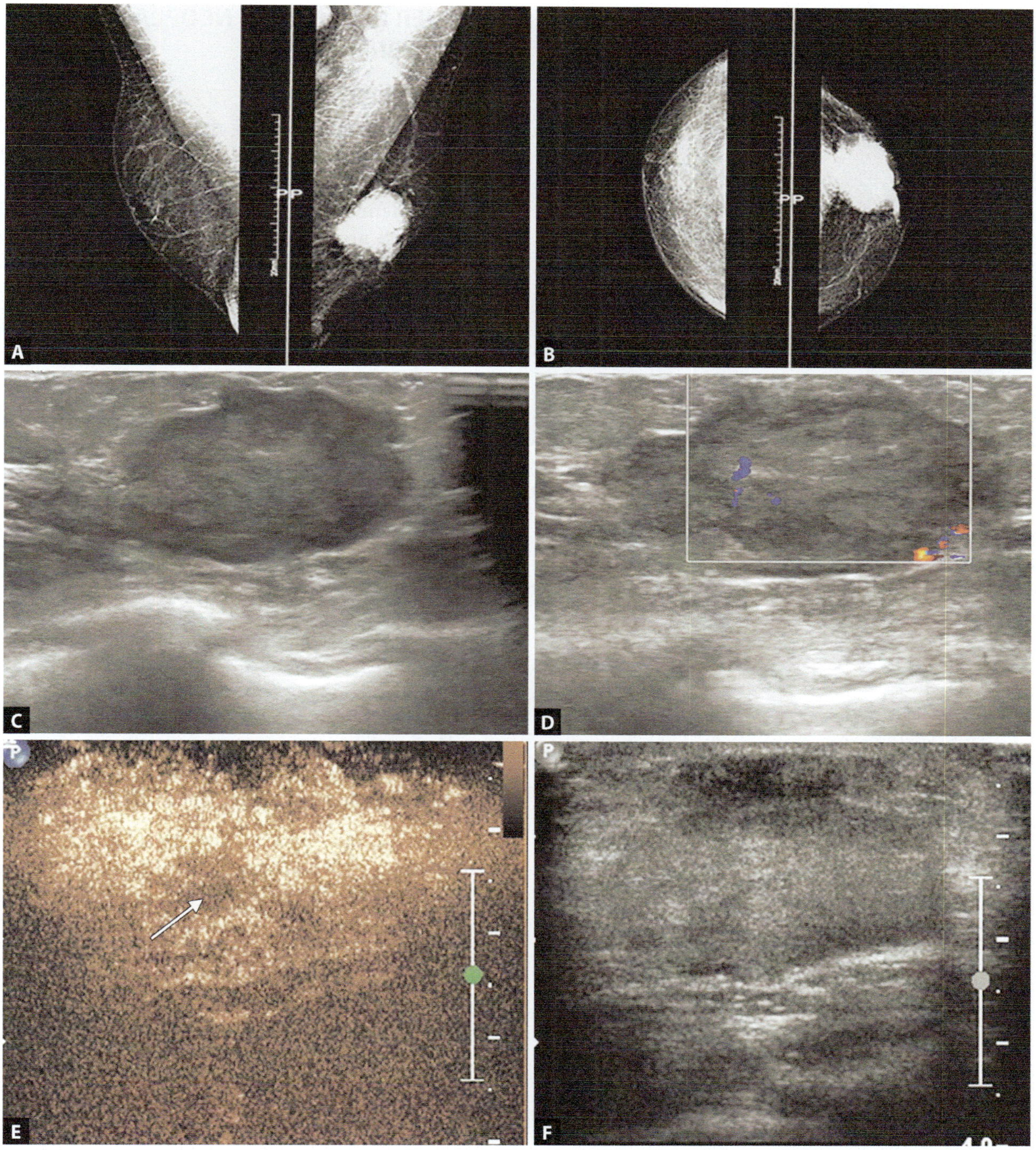

Figs. 9A to F: (A and B) Mediolateral oblique and craniocaudal views of mammogram of a male presenting with painless breast lump showing presence of an oval, high-density lesion with microlobulated margins in the outer central aspect of left breast showing surrounding architectural distortion and associated axillary lymphadenopathy. Note the eccentric location of the lesion; (C and D) Ultrasonography of breast shows presence of an oval heteroechoic mass with lobulated margins with mild architectural distortion. Color Doppler shows peripheral as well as internal vascularity; (E and F) Contrast-enhanced ultrasound showed florid enhancement with central perfusion defect (arrow). Biopsy from the lesion revealed infiltrating ductal carcinoma.

appear as complex cystic masses as in cases of papillary carcinomas. On color Doppler, they may show variable degrees of internal vascularity.[10] Ultrasonography provides added advantage of assessment of chest wall or nipple invasion and axillary nodal assessment. Any suspicious lesion on any of the modalities should be sampled for diagnosis.

Imaging of cancer in men with concomitant gynecomastia is challenging and has similar pitfalls of imaging a female breast cancer with background breast dysplasia. The increase in mammographic density in gynecomastia can mask the presence of an underlying malignancy. Also, a mass appearing benign on imaging can turn out to be malignant on histology and vice versa.

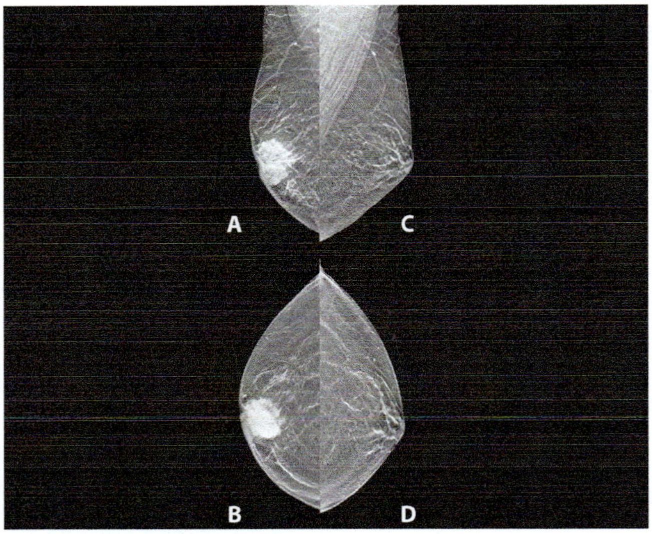

Figs. 10A to D: Mammogram of another male patient. (A and B) Mediolateral oblique (MLO) and craniocaudal (CC) views of right breast showing an irregular high-density mass with spiculated margins present in retroareolar location. There is associated skin thickening and nipple retraction. This mass was proven to be breast carcinoma on biopsy; (C and D) MLO and CC views of left breast of the same patient showing normal mammogram.

Table 1: Differentiating features of male breast carcinoma from gynecomastia.

Sr. No.	*Gynecomastia*	*Carcinoma*
1.	Age: infancy, puberty, senescence	Age > 60 years
2.	Soft	Hard
3.	Mobile	Immobile
4.	Tender in acute phase	Painless
5.	Subareolar (central) in location	Eccentric in location
6.	Unilateral or bilateral	Usually unilateral
7.	No skin thickening or nipple retraction	Skin thickening or nipple retraction may be present

The differentiating features of male breast carcinoma from gynecomastia are summarized in **Table 1**.

Although no standard guidelines are available for the screening of high-risk patients for cancer, it is recommended that screening should be done in patients with a strong family history of breast cancer, genetic predispositions for breast cancers, and men with previous history of breast cancer. Screening should be done in the form of:

- Self-examination of the breast every month
- 6 monthly clinical examination, after the age of 35
- Baseline mammography, at 40 years of age and annually thereafter if the breast density is increased on baseline imaging [National Comprehensive Cancer Network (NCCN) clinical practice guidelines in oncology].[11]

OTHER MALIGNANT NEOPLASMS OF THE MALE BREAST

Primary Lymphoma

Primary lymphoma affecting the breast is extremely rare and shares a similar frequency of occurrence as that of the female breast. Majority of the patients show lesions as a part of disseminated disease. Mammographic findings of the disease are nonspecific and show a wide spectrum of features, of which the most typical pattern is the presence of a well-defined lesion with a thin radiolucent halo. On ultrasonography, the lesions commonly appear hypoechoic and parallel to the chest wall; however, findings are nonspecific. These masses are usually hypervascular **(Figs. 11A and B)**. Axillary lymphadenopathy may be seen as a part of disseminated disease.

Dermatofibrosarcoma

Dermatofibrosarcoma, also known as spindle cell tumor of the breast, is characterized by a locally aggressive slow-growing mass. Its occurrence is more common in males in the second to fifth decades as compared to females. These lesions appear as ill-defined high-density masses on mammography, and on ultrasonography, they are seen as lobulated echogenic or mixed density masses. Complete surgical resection is indicated as it has high recurrence rates.[12]

Multiple Myeloma

Multiple myeloma involving the breast is very rare, and involvement may be as a part of disseminated disease, or in the form of a solitary plasmacytoma of the breast. Also, the most common cause of a new breast mass in cases of multiple myeloma is carcinoma breast. Myeloma lesions of the breast are well-defined, solid masses that may appear hypoechoic or anechoic on ultrasonography due to good transmission of echoes.

Glomus Tumors

Glomus tumors arise from the specialized neurovascular organ known as the glomus body. Breast is an unusual site of presentation, and very few case reports are available in the literature. These lesions tend to present as chronic breast pain with pinpoint severe tenderness, increasing in cold temperatures. On imaging, they are seen as tender, well-defined, superficially situated hypervascular masses. They are treated by surgical excision. They show high recurrence rates after surgery.

Inflammatory Myofibroblastic Tumor

Inflammatory myofibroblastic tumor, very rarely, involves the breast and has intermediate malignant potential. They present with a nonspecific lump adherent to the skin. Imaging features are nonspecific.

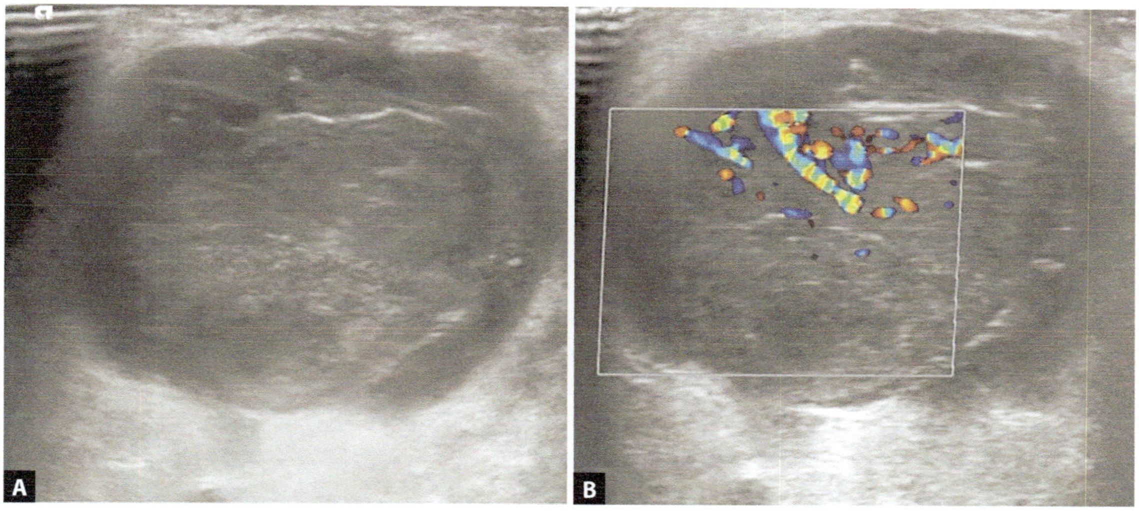

Figs. 11A and B: Ultrasonography of breast in an elderly male with generalized lymphadenopathy and painless breast lump, showing a well-defined, lobulated, heteroechoic lesion showing florid internal vascularity. Tissue sampling showed it to be a lymphomatous deposit.

Metastasis

Metastasis to the breast is very rare, and the most common extramammary cancers metastasizing to the breast are from melanoma, carcinomas of the gastrointestinal tract, lung, thyroid, urogenital tract, and prostate. They present as well-defined solid masses, which may show necrosis and dystrophic calcification. On ultrasonography, they are seen as well-defined homogeneously hypoechoic masses with no significant changes in the surrounding tissues.

CONCLUSION

- Though the male breast is rudimentary anatomically and nonfunctional physiologically, a wide spectrum of diseases occurs in the male breast.
- The most common abnormality of male breast is gynecomastia, which is the proliferation of ducts and stroma and classically presents as a soft mobile mass in subareolar location. It is tender and reversible in the acute florid phase but not in the chronic fibrotic phase.
- The dictum is that any gynecomastia must be subareolar, and any mass which is not subareolar does not fit into gynecomastia.
- As in women, there is no lobular proliferation in men; hence tumors of lobular origin like fibroadenoma, phyllode tumors, invasive lobular carcinomas are extremely rare.
- Myofibroblastoma is the only breast mass that occurs more frequently in men than in women.
- Male breast cancer has similar imaging appearance as that in women. It may appear as a taller than wider, spiculated mass, eccentric to the nipple, in contrast to gynecomastia which is central (subareolar). Invasive ductal cancer is the most common subtype. Calcifications are less frequently seen with male breast cancer, but when seen are coarser, and on imaging look like benign calcifications of the female breast.
- For male breast, the rule of thumb is that if imaging appearance is not fitting into normal or benign findings, biopsy should be performed.

REFERENCES

1. Iuanow E, Kettler M, Slanetz PJ. Spectrum of disease in the male breast. Am J Roentgenol. 2011;196:W247-59.
2. Nguyen C, Kettler MD, Swirsky ME, Miller VI, Scott C, Krause R, et al. Male breast disease: pictorial review with radiologic-pathologic correlation. Radiographics. 2013;33:763-79.
3. Draghi F, Tarantino CC, Madonia L, Ferrozzi G. Ultrasonography of the male breast. J Ultrasound. 2011;14:122-9.
4. Popli MB, Popli V, Bahl P, Solanki Y. Pictorial essay: mammography of the male breast. Indian J Radiol Imaging. 2009;19:278-81.
5. Günhan-Bilgen I, Bozkaya H, Ustün EE, Memiş A. Male breast disease: clinical, mammographic, and ultrasonographic features. Eur J Radiol. 2002;43:246-55.
6. Appelbaum AH, Evans GF, Levy KR, Amirkhan RH, Schumpert TD. Mammographic appearances of male breast disease. Radiographics. 1999;19:559-68.
7. Mathew J, Perkins GH, Stephens T, Middleton LP, Yang WT. Primary breast cancer in men: clinical, imaging, and pathologic findings in 57 patients. Am J Roentgenol. 2008;191:1631-9.
8. Yitta S, Singer CI, Toth HB, Mercado CL. Image presentation. Sonographic appearances of benign and malignant male breast disease with mammographic and pathologic correlation. J Ultrasound Med. 2010;29:931-47.
9. Muñoz Carrasco R, Álvarez Benito M, Rivin del Campo E. Value of mammography and breast ultrasound in male patients with nipple discharge. Eur J Radiol. 2013;82:478-84.
10. Yuan WH, Li AF, Chou YH, Hsu HC, Chen YY. Clinical and ultrasonographic features of male breast tumors: a retrospective analysis. PLoS One. 2018;13(3):e0194651.
11. Block WD, Muradali D. Breast cancer in men. Can Med Assoc J. 2013;185:1247.
12. Chen L, Chantra PK, Larsen LH, Barton P, Rohitopakarn M, Zhu EQ, et al. Imaging characteristics of malignant lesions of the male breast. Radiographics. 2006;26:993-1006.

Index

Page numbers followed by *b* refer to box, *f* refer to figure, *fc* refer to flowchart, and *t* refer to table

B

C

D

E

F

I

O

P

T

U

V

W

Z